TEXTBOOK OF
DIAGNOSTIC
SONOGRAPHY

SEVENTH EDITION   VOLUME ONE

TEXTBOOK OF
DIAGNOSTIC SONOGRAPHY

Sandra L. Hagen-Ansert,
MS, RDMS, RDCS, FASE, FSDMS

Cardiology Department
Supervisor, Echo Lab
Scripps Clinic—Torrey Pines, California

with 3,463 illustrations

ELSEVIER
MOSBY

3251 Riverport Lane
St. Louis, Missouri 63043

TEXTBOOK OF DIAGNOSTIC SONOGRAPHY   ISBN: 978-0-323-07301-1
Copyright © 2012 by Mosby, Inc., an affiliate of Elsevier Inc.

Notices

Knowledge and best practice in this field are constantly changing. As new research and experience broaden our understanding, changes in research methods, professional practices, or medical treatment may become necessary.

Practitioners and researchers must always rely on their own experience and knowledge in evaluating and using any information, methods, compounds, or experiments described herein. In using such information or methods they should be mindful of their own safety and the safety of others, including parties for whom they have a professional responsibility.

With respect to any drug or pharmaceutical products identified, readers are advised to check the most current information provided (i) on procedures featured or (ii) by the manufacturer of each product to be administered, to verify the recommended dose or formula, the method and duration of administration, and contraindications. It is the responsibility of practitioners, relying on their own experience and knowledge of their patients, to make diagnoses, to determine dosages and the best treatment for each individual patient, and to take all appropriate safety precautions.

To the fullest extent of the law, neither the Publisher nor the authors, contributors, or editors, assume any liability for any injury and/or damage to persons or property as a matter of products liability, negligence or otherwise, or from any use or operation of any methods, products, instructions, or ideas contained in the material herein.

Previous editions copyrighted 2006, 2001, 1995, 1989, 1983, 1978

Publisher: Andrew Allen
Executive Editor: Jeanne Olson
Developmental Editor: Linda Woodard
Publishing Services Manager: Julie Eddy
Project Manager: Richard Barber
Design Direction: Paula Catalano

Printed in the United States

Last digit is the print number: 9 8 7 6 5 4 3 2 1

To my daughters,
Becca, Aly, *and* **Kati,**
who are changing the world one day at a time

Joan Baker, MSR., RDMS, RDCS
President, Sound Ergonomics
Kenmore, Washington

Carolyn Coffin, MPH, RDMS, RDCS, RVT
CEO, Sound Ergonomics
Kenmore, Washington

Marveen Craig, RDMS
Diagnostic Ultrasound Consultant
Tucson, Arizona

M. Robert De Jong, RDMS, RDCS, RVT
Radiology Technical Manager, Ultrasound
The Russell H. Morgan Department of Radiology and Radiological Science
The Johns Hopkins Hospital
Baltimore, Maryland

Terry J. DuBose, MS, RDMS
Associate Professor and Director
Diagnostic Medical Sonography Program
University of Arkansas for Medical Sciences
Little Rock, Arkansas

Pamela Foy, M.S., RDMS
Clinical Instructor, Department OB/ GYN
The Ohio State University Medical Center
Columbus, Ohio

Candace Goldstein, BS, RDMS
Sonographer Educator
Scripps Clinic Carmel Valley
San Diego, California

Charlotte G. Henningsen, MS, RT (R), RDMS, RVT
Chair and Professor
Diagnostic Medical Sonography Department
Florida Hospital College of Health Sciences
Orlando, Florida

Mira L. Katz, PhD, MPH
Associate Professor
Division of Health Behavior and Health Promotion
School of Public Health
The Ohio State University
Columbus, Ohio

Fredrick Kremkau, PhD
Professor & Director
Center for Medical Ultrasound
Wake Forest University School of Medicine
Winston-Salem, North Carolina

Salvatore LaRusso, MEd, RDMS, RT (R)
Technical Director
Penn State Hershey/ Hershey Medical Center
Department of Radiology
Hershey, Pennsylvania

Daniel A. Merton, BS, RDMS
Technical Coordinator of Research
The Jefferson Ultrasound Research and Educational Institute
Thomas Jefferson University
Philadelphia, Pennsylvania

Carol Mitchell, PhD, RDMS, RDCS, RVT, RT(R)
Quality Assurance Coordinator, UW AIRP
Program Director, University of Wisconsin School of Diagnostic Medical Ultrasound
University of Wisconsin Hospitals & Clinics
Madison, Wisconsin

Cindy A. Owen, RT, RDMS, RVT
Global Luminary and Research Manager
Radiology & Vascular Ultrasound
GE Healthcare
Memphis, Tennessee

Mitzi Roberts, BS, RDMS, RVT
Chair, Assistant Professor
Diagnostic Medical Sonography Program
Baptist College of Health Science
Memphis, Tennessee

Jean Lea Spitz, MPH, RDMS
Maternal Fetal Medicine Foundation
Nuchal Translucency Quality Review Program
Oklahoma City, Oklahoma

Susan Raatz Stephenson, MEd, BSRT-U, RDMS, RT(R)(C)
International Foundation for Sonography Education & Research
AIUM communities.org
Sandy, Utah

Diana M. Strickland, BS, RDMS, RDCS
Clinical Assistant Professor and Co-Director
Ultrasound Program
Department of Obstetrics and Gynecology
Brody School of Medicine
East Carolina University
Greenville, North Carolina

Shpetim Telegrafi, M.D.
Assistant Professor
Director, Diagnostic Ultrasound
NYU School of Medicine, Department of Urology
New York City, New York

Barbara Trampe, RN, RDMS
Chief Sonographer
Meriter/University of Wisconsin Perinatal Ultrasound
Madison, Wisconsin

Barbara J. Vander Werff, RDMS, RDCS, RVT
Chief Sonographer
University of Wisconsin-Madison
  Hospitals and Clinics
Madison, Wisconsin

Kerry Weinberg, MS, RDMS, RDCS
Director
Diagnostic Medical Sonography
  Program
New York University
New York, New York

Ann Willis, MS, RDMS, RVT
Clinical Coordinator, Diagnostic
  Medical Sonography Program
Baptist College of Health Sciences
Memphis, Tennessee

Dennis Wisher, BS, RDMS, RVT
Director of Education and Product
  Management
Medison America, Inc.
Cypress, California

Jan Blend, MS, RT(R), RDMS, ARDMS
Program Coordinator, Diagnostic Medical Sonography
El Centro College
Dallas, Texas

Katherine K. Borok, BS, RDMS, RDCS
Clinical Coordinator
American Institute of Ultrasound in Medicine
Laurel, Maryland

Joie Burns, MS, RT(R)(S), RDMS, RVT
Associate Professor, Program Director, Diagnostic Medical Sonography
Boise State University
Boise, Idaho

Saretta C. Craft, MS, RDCS, RVT
Program Director, Diagnostic Sonography
St. Catharine College
St. Catharine, Kentucky

Laura L. Currie, BS, RT(R), RDMS, RVT
Clinical Coordinator
Cape Fear Community College
Wilmington, North Carolina

Marianna C. Desmond, BS, RT(R), RDMS
Clinical Coordinator, Diagnostic Medical Sonography Program
Triton College
River Grove, Illinois

Jann Dolk, MA, RT(R), RDMS
Adjunct Faculty, Diagnostic Medical Sonography Program
Palm Beach State College
Palm Beach Gardens, Florida

Ken Galbraith, MS, RT(R), RDMS, RVT
State University of New York
Syracuse, New York

Karen M. Having, MS Ed, RT, RDMS
Associate Professor, School of Allied Health
Southern Illinois University-Carbondale
Carbondale, Illinois

Bridgette Lunsford, BS, RDMS, RVT
Adjunct Faculty, George Washington University
Washington, D.C.

Kasey L. Moore, ARRT, RDMS, RT(R) (M) (RDMS)
Sonography Instructor
Danville Area Community College
Danville, Illinois

Susan M. Perry, BS, ARDMS
Program Director, Diagnostic Medical Sonography
Owens Community College
Toledo, Ohio

Kellee Ann Stacks, BS, RTR, RDMS, RVT
Program Director, Medical Sonography
Cape Fear Community College
Wilmington, North Carolina

INTRODUCING THE SEVENTH EDITION

The seventh edition of *Textbook of Diagnostic Sonography* continues the tradition of excellence that began when the first edition published in 1978. Like other medical imaging fields, diagnostic sonography has seen dramatic changes and innovations since its first experimental days. Phenomenal strides in transducer design, instrumentation, color-flow Doppler, tissue harmonics, contrast agents, and 3D imaging continue to improve image resolution and the diagnostic value of sonography. The seventh edition has kept abreast of advancements in the field by having each chapter reviewed by numerous sonographers currently working in different areas of medical sonography throughout the country. Their critiques and suggestions have helped ensure that this edition includes the most complete and up-to-date information needed to meet the requirements of the modern student of sonography.

Distinctive Approach

This textbook can serve as an in-depth resource both for students of sonography and for practitioners in any number of clinical settings, including hospitals, clinics, and private practices. Care has been taken to cultivate readers' understanding of the patient's total clinical picture even as they study sonographic examination protocol and technique. To this end, each chapter covers the following:

- Normal anatomy (including cross-sectional anatomy)
- Normal physiology
- Laboratory data and values
- Pathology
- Sonographic evaluation of an organ
- Sonographic findings
- Pitfalls in sonography
- Clinical findings
- Differential considerations

The full-color art program is of great value to the student of anatomy and pathology for sonography. Detailed line drawings illustrate the anatomic information a sonographer must know to successfully perform specific sonographic examinations. Color photographs of gross pathology help the reader visualize some of the pathology presented, and color Doppler illustrations are included where relevant.

To make important information easy to find, key points are pulled out into numerous boxes; tables throughout the chapters summarize the pathology under discussion and break the information down into Clinical Findings, Sonographic Findings, and Differential Considerations.

Sonographic findings for particular pathologic conditions are always preceded in the text by the following special heading:

◀ **Sonographic Findings.** This icon makes it very easy for students and practicing sonographers to locate this clinical information quickly.

Study and review are also essential to gaining a solid grasp of the concepts and information presented in this textbook. Learning objectives, chapter outlines, comprehensive glossaries of key terms, full references for cited material, and a list of common medical abbreviations printed on the back inside cover all help students learn the material in an organized and thorough manner.

Scope and Organization of Topics

The *Textbook of Diagnostic Sonography* is divided into eight parts:

Part I introduces the reader to the foundations of sonography and patient care and includes the following:
- Basic principles of ultrasound physics and medical sonography
- Terminology frequently encountered by the sonographer
- Overview of physical findings, physiology, and laboratory data
- Patient care for the sonographer
- Ergonomics and musculoskeletal issues for practitioners
- Basics of other imaging modalities
- Image artifacts

Part II presents the abdomen in depth. The following topics are discussed:
- Anatomic relationships and physiology
- Abdominal scanning techniques and protocols
- Abdominal applications of ultrasound contrast agents
- Ultrasound-guided interventional techniques
- Emergent abdominal ultrasound procedures
- Separate chapters for the vascular system, the liver, gallbladder and biliary system, pancreas, gastrointestinal tract, urinary system, spleen, retroperitoneum, and peritoneal cavity and abdominal wall

Part III focuses on the superficial structures in the body including the breast, thyroid and parathyroid glands, scrotum, and musculoskeletal system.

Part IV explores sonographic examination of the neonate and pediatric patient.

Part V focuses on the thoracic cavity and includes:
- Anatomic and physiologic relationships within the thoracic cavity
- Echocardiographic evaluation and techniques
- Fetal echocardiography

Part VI comprises four chapters on extracranial and intracranial cerebrovascular imaging and peripheral arterial and venous sonographic evaluation.

Part VII is devoted to gynecology and includes the following topics:
- Normal anatomy and physiology of the female pelvis
- Sonographic and Doppler evaluation of the female pelvis
- Separate chapters on the pathologic conditions of the uterus, ovaries, and adnexa
- Updated chapter on the role of sonography in evaluating female infertility

Part VIII takes a thorough look at obstetric sonography. The following topics are discussed:
- The role of sonography in obstetrics
- Clinical ethics for obstetric sonography
- Normal first trimester and first-trimester complications
- Sonography of the second and third trimesters
- Obstetric measurements and gestational age
- Fetal growth assessment
- Prenatal diagnosis of congenital anomalies, with a separate chapter on 3D and 4D evaluation of fetal anomalies
- Chapters devoted to the placenta, umbilical cord, and amniotic fluid, as well as to the fetal face and neck, neural axis, thorax, anterior abdominal wall, abdomen, urogenital system, and skeleton

New to This Edition

Ten new contributors joined the seventh edition to update and expand existing content, bringing with them a fresh perspective and an impressive knowledge base. They also helped contribute the more than 1000 images new to this edition, including color Doppler, 3D, and contrast-enhanced images. More than 30 new line drawings complement the new chapters found in the seventh edition.

Essentials of Patient Care for the Sonographer (Chapter 3) covers all aspects of patient care the sonographer may encounter, including taking and understanding vital signs, handling patients on strict bed rest, patients with tubes and oxygen, patient transfer techniques, infection control, isolation techniques, emergency medical situations, assisting patients with special needs, and patient rights.

Ergonomics and Musculoskeletal Issues in Sonography (Chapter 4) outlines the importance of proper technique and positioning throughout the sonographic examination as a way to avoid long-term disability problems that may be acquired with repetitive scanning.

Understanding Other Imaging Modalities (Chapter 5) is a comparative overview of the multiple imaging modalities frequently encountered by the sonographer: computerized tomography, magnetic resonance, positron emission tomography (PET), nuclear medicine, and radiography.

Artifacts in Scanning (Chapter 6) is an outstanding review of all the artifacts commonly encountered by sonographers. There are numerous examples of the various artifacts and detailed explanations of how these artifacts are produced and how to avoid them.

3D and 4D Evaluation of Fetal Anomalies (Chapter 54) has a three-fold focus: (1) to introduce the sonographer to the technical concepts of 3D ultrasound; (2) to acquaint the sonographer with the 3D tools currently available; and (3) to provide clinical examples of the integration of 3D ultrasound into conventional sonographic examinations. Although a chapter with this title appeared in the last edition, this chapter has been entirely rewritten and includes all new illustrations.

Student Resources

Workbook. Available for separate purchase, *Workbook for Textbook of Diagnostic Sonography* has also been completely updated and expanded. This resource gives the learner ample opportunity to practice and apply the information presented in the textbook.

- Each workbook chapter covers all the material presented in the textbook.
- Each chapter includes exercises on image identification, anatomy identification, key term definitions, and sonographic technique.
- A set of 30 case studies using images from the textbook invites students to test their skills at identifying key anatomy and pathology and describing and interpreting sonographic findings.
- Students can also test their knowledge with the hundreds of multiple choice questions found in the four exams covering different content areas: General Sonography, Pediatric, Cardiovascular Anatomy, and Obstetrics and Gynecology.

Evolve. On the *Evolve* site, students will find a printable list of the key terms and definitions for each chapter; a printable selected bibliography for each chapter, and Weblinks.

Instructor Resources

Resources for instructors are also provided on the *Evolve* site to assist in the preparation of classroom lectures and activities.

- PowerPoint lectures for each chapter that include illustrations
- Test bank of 1500 multiple-choice questions in Examview and Word
- Electronic image collection that includes all the images from the textbook both in PowerPoint and in jpeg format

Evolve Online Course Management. *Evolve* is an interactive learning environment designed to work in coordination with *Textbook of Diagnostic Sonography.* Instructors may use *Evolve* to include an Internet-based course component that reinforces and expands upon the concepts delivered in class. *Evolve* may be used to:

- Publish the class syllabus, outlines, and lecture notes
- Set up virtual office hours and email communication
- Share important dates and information on the online class calendar
- Encourage student participation with chat rooms and discussion boards
- Post exams and manage grade books

For more information, visit http://www.evolve.elsevier.com/HagenAnsert/diagnostic/ or contact an Elsevier sales representative.

ACKNOWLEDGMENTS

I would like to express my gratitude and appreciation to a number of individuals who have served as mentors and guides throughout my years in sonography. Of course it all began with Dr. George Leopold at UCSD Medical Center. His quest for knowledge and his perseverance for excellence have been the mainstay of my career in sonography. I would also like to recognize Drs. Dolores Pretorius, Nancy Budorick, Wanda Miller-Hance, and David Sahn for their encouragement throughout the years at the UCSD Medical Center in both Radiology and Pediatric Cardiology.

I would also like to acknowledge Dr. Barry Goldberg for the opportunity he gave me to develop countless numbers of educational programs in sonography in an independent fashion and for his encouragement to pursue advancement. I would also like to thank Dr. Daniel Yellon for his early-hour anatomy dissection and instruction; Dr. Carson Schneck, for his excellent instruction in gross anatomy and sections of "Geraldine;" and Dr. Jacob Zutuchni, for his enthusiasm for the field of cardiology.

I am grateful to Dr. Harry Rakowski for his continued support in teaching fellows and students while I was at the Toronto Hospital. Dr. William Zwiebel encouraged me to continue writing and teaching while I was at the University of Wisconsin Medical Center, and I appreciate his knowledge, which found its way into the liver physiology section of this textbook.

My good fortune in learning about and understanding the *total patient* must be attributed to a very dedicated cardiologist, James Glenn, with whom I had the pleasure of working while I was at MUSC in Charleston, South Carolina. It was through his compassion and knowledge that I grew to appreciate the total patient beyond the transducer, and for this I am grateful.

For their continual support, feedback, and challenges, I would like to thank and recognize all the students I have taught in the various diagnostic medical sonography programs: Episcopal Hospital, Thomas Jefferson University Medical Center, University of Wisconsin-Madison Medical Center, UCSD Medical Center, and Baptist College of Health Science. These students continually work toward the development of quality sonography techniques and protocols and have given back to the sonography community tenfold.

The continual push towards excellence has been encouraged on a daily basis by our Scripps Clinic Cardiologists and David Rubenson, Medical Director of the Echo Lab at Scripps Clinic.

The sonographers at Scripps Clinic have been invaluable in their excellent image acquisition. Special thanks to Ewa Pikulski, Megan Marks and Kristen Billick for their echocardiographic images. The general sonographers at Scripps Clinic have been invaluable in providing the excellent images for the Obstetrics and Gynecology chapters.

I would like to thank the very supportive and capable staff at Elsevier who have guided me though yet another edition of this textbook. Jeanne Olson and her excellent staff are to be commended on their perseverance to make this an outstanding textbook. Linda Woodard was a constant reminder to me to stay on task and was there to offer assistance when needed. Jennifer Moorhead has been the mainstay of this project from the beginning and has done an excellent job with the manuscript. She is to be commended on her eye for detail.

I would like to thank my family, Art, Becca, Aly, and Kati, for their patience and understanding, as I thought this edition would never come to an end.

I think that you will find the 7th Edition of the *Textbook of Diagnostic Sonography* reflects the contribution of so many individuals with attention to detail and a dedication to excellence. I hope you will find this educational experience in sonography as rewarding as I have.

Sandra L. Hagen-Ansert
MS, RDMS, RDCS, FSDMS, FASE

CONTENTS

PART VIII   Obstetrics

Foundations of Sonography

Foundations of Sonography

Sandra L. Hagen-Ansert

The words *diagnostic medical ultrasound, ultrasound,* and *ultrasonography* have all been used to describe the instrumentation utilized in ultrasound. S*onography* is the term used to describe a specialized imaging technique used to visualize soft tissue structures of the body. The term *echocardiography*, or simply *echo*, refers to an ultrasound examination of the cardiac structures. A sonographer is an allied health professional who has received specialized education in ultrasound and has successfully completed the national boards given by the American Registry of Diagnostic Medical Sonography. Sonologists are physicians who have received specialized training in ultrasound and have successfully completed the national boards given by their respective specialty.

The field of diagnostic ultrasound has grown to become a well-respected and important part of diagnostic imaging, providing pertinent clinical information to the physician and to the patient. The applications of diagnostic ultrasound are extensive. They include but are not limited to the following:

1. Abdominal, renal, and retroperitoneal ultrasound
2. Interventional and therapeutic guided ultrasound
3. Thoracic ultrasound
4. Ultrasound of superficial structures (breast, thyroid, scrotum)
5. Cardiovascular and endoluminal ultrasound
6. Obstetric and gynecologic ultrasound
7. Intraoperative ultrasound
8. Neonatal and pediatric ultrasound
9. Musculoskeletal ultrasound
10. Ophthalmologic ultrasound

Extensive research has verified the safety of ultrasound as a diagnostic procedure. No harmful effects of ultrasound have been demonstrated at power levels used for diagnostic studies when performed by qualified and nationally certified sonographers under the direction of a qualified and board certified physician, using appropriate equipment and techniques.

Diagnostic ultrasound has come to be such a valuable diagnostic imaging technique for so many different body structures for many reasons, but two are especially significant. First is the lack of ionizing radiation for ultrasound as compared with the other imaging modalities of magnetic resonance imaging (MRI), computed tomography (CT), or nuclear medicine. The second reason is the portability of the ultrasound equipment. The ultrasound system can easily be moved into the intensive care unit (ICU), surgical suite, or small doctor's office, or packed into small planes for distant clinical sites. Ultrasound is unique in other ways as well. It allows an image to be presented in a real-time format, which makes it possible to image rapidly moving cardiac structures or a moving fetus. The flexible multiplanar imaging capability allows the sonographer to "follow" the path of a tortuous vessel or a moving cardiac structure or fetus to capture the necessary images. Moreover, Doppler techniques allow the qualitative and quantitative evaluation of blood flow within a vessel. Finally, the cost analysis of an ultrasound system is superior when compared with the other imaging systems.

Today nearly every hospital and medical clinic has some form of ultrasound instrumentation to provide the clinician with an inside look at the soft tissue structures within the body. Ultrasound manufacturers continue their research to improve image acquisition, develop efficient transducer functionality and design, and create software to improve computer assessment of the acquired information. Two-dimensional information can be re-created in a three- or four-dimensional format to provide a surface rendering of the area in question. Color flow Doppler, harmonics, tissue characterization, and spectral analysis have greatly expanded the utility of ultrasound imaging.

To obtain even more information from the ultrasound image, various medical centers and manufacturers have been working toward the development of effective contrast agents that may be ingested or administered intravenously into the bloodstream to facilitate the detection and diagnosis of specific pathologies. Early attempts at producing a contrast effect with ultrasound imaging involved administration of aerated saline or carbon dioxide. Research today is focused on the development of gas microspheres, which are injected into the patient to provide visual contrast during the ultrasound study. Specific applications of ultrasound contrast are found in Chapter 18.

The purpose of this chapter is to introduce the sonographer to the basics of sonography as a career and as a diagnostic imaging technique. And because you can't know where you are going until you know where you have been, this introductory chapter also provides a discussion of the history of the development of medical ultrasound.

THE ROLE OF THE SONOGRAPHER

A role is a specific behavior that an individual demonstrates to others. A function involves the tasks or duties that one is obligated to perform in carrying out a role. With these definitions in mind, we can say that a sonographer is someone who performs ultrasound studies and gathers diagnostic data under the direct or indirect supervision of a physician. Sonographers are known as "image makers" who have the ability to create images of soft tissue structures and organs inside the body, such as the liver, pancreas, biliary system, kidneys, heart, vascular system, uterus, and fetus. In addition, sonogra-

phers can record hemodynamic information with velocity measurements through the use of Doppler spectral analysis to determine if a vessel or cardiac valve is patent (open) or restricted.

Sonographers work directly with physicians and patients as a team member in a medical facility. They also interact with nurses and other medical staff as part of the health care team. The sonographer must be able to review the patient's records to assess clinical history and clinical symptoms; to interpret laboratory values; and to understand other diagnostic examinations. The sonographer is required to understand and operate complex ultrasound instrumentation using the basic principles of ultrasound physics.

To produce the highest quality sonographic image for interpretation, the sonographer must possess an in-depth understanding of anatomy and pathophysiology and be able to evaluate a patient's problem. Sonographers use their knowledge and skills to provide physicians with information such as evaluation of a trauma victim's injury or detection of fetal anomalies, or to measure fetal growth and progress, or even to evaluate the patient for cardiac abnormalities or injury. In addition to technical expertise and knowledge of anatomy and pathophysiology, several other qualities contribute to the sonographer's success (Box 1-1).

What makes the sonographer distinct from the other health care professionals?

- The sonographer talks directly with patients to identify which of their symptoms relate directly to the ultrasound examination.

BOX 1-1 | Qualities of a Sonographer

The sonographer must possess the following qualities and talents:

Intellectual curiosity to keep abreast of developments in the field

Perseverance to obtain high-quality images and the ability to differentiate an artifact from structural anatomy

Ability to conceptualize two-dimensional images into a three-dimensional format

Quick and analytical mind to continually analyze image quality while keeping the clinical situation in mind

Technical aptitude to produce diagnostic-quality images

Good physical health because continuous scanning may cause strain on back, shoulder, or arm

Independence and initiative to analyze the patient, the history, and the clinical findings and tailor the examination to answer the clinical question

Emotional stability to deal with patients in times of crisis; this means the ability to understand the patient's concerns without losing objectivity

Communication skills for interactions with peers, clinicians, and patients; this includes the ability to clearly communicate ultrasound findings to physicians and the ability *not* to disclose or speculate on findings to the patient during the examination

Dedication because a willingness to go beyond the "call of duty" is often required of the sonographer

- The sonographer explains the procedure to the patient and performs the examination using the protocol established by the department.
- The sonographer analyzes each image and correlates the information with patient information.
- The sonographer uses independent judgment in recognizing the need to make adjustments on the sonogram to answer the clinical question.
- The sonographer reviews the previous sonogram and provides an oral or written summary of the technical findings to the physician for the medical diagnosis.
- The sonographer alerts the physician if dramatic or new changes are found on the sonographic examination.

Advantages and Disadvantages of a Sonography Career

Sonographers with specialized education in ultrasound have demonstrated their ability to produce high-quality sonographic images, thereby earning the respect of other allied health professionals and clinicians. Every day, sonographers are faced with varied human interactions and opportunities to solve problems. These experiences give sonographers an outlet for their creativity by requiring them to come up with innovative ways to meet the challenges of performing quality ultrasound examinations on difficult patients. New applications in ultrasound and improvements in instrumentation create a continual challenge for the sonographer. Flexible schedules and variety in examinations and equipment, not to mention patient personalities, make each day interesting and unique. Certified sonographers find that employment opportunities are abundant, schedule flexibility is high, and salaries are attractive.

On the other hand, some sonographers find their position to be stressful and demanding, with the constant changes in medical care and decreased staffing causing increased workloads. Hours of continual scanning may lead to tendinitis, arm and shoulder pain, and back strain. (Chapter 4 focuses on ergonomics and musculoskeletal issues in sonography.) Also, sonographers may become frustrated when dealing with terminally ill patients, which can lead to fatigue and depression.

Employment. The field of sonography is growing faster than all other imaging modalities and is at the top of all medical imaging pay scales. The demand for certified sonographers exceeds the supply nationwide. Sonographers may find employment in the traditional setting of a hospital or medical clinic. Staffing positions within the hospital or medical setting may include the following: Director of Imaging, Technical Director, Supervisor, Chief Sonographer, Sonographer Educator, Clinical Staff Sonographer, Research Sonographer, or Clinical Instructor. Clinical research opportunities may be found in the major medical centers throughout the country. Sonographers with advanced degrees (i.e., BS, MS, or PhD) may serve as faculty in Diagnostic Medical Sonography programs as Program Director, department head, or Dean of Allied Health. Many sonographers have entered the commercial world as application specialists and directors of education, continuing education, marketing, product design/engineering, sales, service, or quality control. Other sonographers have become independent business partners in medicine by offering mobile ultrasound services to smaller community hospitals.

Resource Organizations. Specific organizations are devoted to developing standards and guidelines for ultrasound:

- AIUM: American Institute of Ultrasound in Medicine: www.aium.org. This organization represents all facets of ultrasound to include physicians, sonographers, biomedical engineers, scientists, and commercial researchers.
- ASE: American Society of Echocardiography: www.asecho.org. This very active organization represents physicians, sonographers, and scientists involved with cardiovascular applications of sonography.
- SDMS: Society of Diagnostic Medical Sonography: www.sdms.org. This is the principal organization for more than 25,000 sonographers. The website contains information regarding the SDMS position statement on the code of ethics for the profession of diagnostic medical ultrasound; the nondiagnostic use of ultrasound; the scope of practice for the diagnostic ultrasound professional; and diagnostic ultrasound clinical practice standards.
- SVU: Society for Vascular Ultrasound: www.svunet.org. This is the principal organization representing physicians, sonographers, and scientists in vascular sonography.

The National Certification Examination for Ultrasound is provided by the following:

- ARDMS: American Registry for Diagnostic Medical Sonography: www.ardms.org.

The national review boards for educational programs in sonography are provided by two groups:

- JRC-DMS: Joint Review Committee on Education in Diagnostic Medical Sonography (includes general ultrasound, echocardiology, and vascular technology): www.jrcdms.org
- JRC-CVT: Joint Review Committee on Education in Cardiovascular Technology (includes noninvasive cardiology, invasive cardiology, and vascular technology): www.jrccvt.org

Several journals are devoted to ultrasound; however, these journals are connected to their respective national organizations:

- JDMS (SDMS) Journal of Diagnostic Medical Sonography
- JUM (AIUM) Journal of Ultrasound in Medicine
- JASE (ASE) Journal of the American Society of Echocardiography
- JVU (SVT) Journal for Vascular Ultrasound

HISTORICAL OVERVIEW OF SOUND THEORY AND MEDICAL ULTRASOUND

A complete history of sound theory and of the development of medical ultrasound is beyond the scope of this book. The following is a brief overview, designed to give readers a sense of the long history and exciting developments in this area of study. For a more detailed outline of historical data, the reader is referred to Dr. Joseph Woo's excellent online article entitled "A Short History of the Development of Ultrasound in Obstetrics and Gynecology" and other resources listed in the Selected Bibliography at the end of this chapter.

The story of acoustics begins with the Greek philosopher **Pythagoras** (6th Century BC), whose experiments on the properties of vibrating strings led to the invention of the sonometer, an instrument used to study musical sounds. Several hundred years later, in 1500 AD, **Leonardo da Vinci** (1452–1519) discovered that sound traveled in waves and discovered that the **angle of reflection** is equal to the **angle of incidence**. **Galileo Galilei** (1564–1642) is said to have started modern studies of acoustics by elevating the study of vibrations to scientific standards. In 1638, he demonstrated that the frequency of sound waves determined the pitch. **Sir Isaac Newton** (1643–1727) studied the speed of sound in air and provided the first analytical determination of the speed of sound. **Robert Boyle** (1627–1691), an Irish natural philosopher, chemist, physicist, and inventor, demonstrated the physical characteristics of air, showing that it is necessary in combustion, respiration, and sound transmission. **Lazzaro Spallanzani** (1729–1799), an Italian biologist and physiologist, essentially discovered echolocation. Spallanzani is famous for extensive experiments on bat navigation, from which he concluded that bats use sound and their ears for navigation in total darkness. **Augustin Fresnel** (1788–1827) was a French physicist who contributed significantly to the establishment of the theory of wave optics, forming the theory of wave diffraction named after him. **Sir Francis Galton** (1822–1911) was an English Victorian scholar, explorer, and inventor. One of his numerous inventions was the Galton whistle used for testing differential hearing ability. This is an ultrasonic whistle, which is also known as a dog whistle or a silent whistle. **Christian Johann Doppler** (1803–1853) was an Austrian mathematician and physicist. He is most famous for what is now called the Doppler effect, which is the apparent change in frequency and wavelength of a wave as perceived by an observer moving relative to the wave's source. In 1880, **Paul-Jacques Curie** (1856–1941) and his brother **Pierre Curie** (1859–1906) discovered **piezoelectricity,** whereby physical pressure applied to a crystal resulted in the creation of an electric potential. **John William Strutt (Lord Rayleigh)** (1842–1919) wrote *The Theory of Sound.* The first volume, on the mechanics of a vibrating medium which produces sound, was published in 1877; the second volume on acoustic wave propagation was published the following year. **Paul Langevin** (1872–1946) was a French physicist and is noted for his work on paramagnetism and diamagnetism. He devised the modern interpretation of this phenomenon in terms of spins of electrons within atoms. His most famous work was on the use of ultrasound using Pierre and Jacques Curie's piezoelectric effect. During World War I, he began working on the use of these sounds to detect submarines through echo location.

SONAR is an acronym for *sound navigation and ranging.* Sonar is a technique that uses sound propagation, usually underwater, to navigate, communicate with, or detect other vessels. Sonar may be used as a means of acoustic location and measurement of the echo characteristics of "targets" in the water. The term *sonar* is also used for the equipment used to generate and receive the sound. The acoustic frequencies used in sonar systems vary from very low (infrasonic) to extremely high (ultrasonic). World War II brought sonar equipment to the forefront of military defense, and medical ultrasound was influenced by the advances in sonar instrumentation. In the 1940s, **Dr. Karl Dussik** (1908–1968) made one of the earliest applications of ultrasound to medical diagnosis when he used two transducers positioned on opposite sides of the head to measure ultrasound transmission profiles. He discovered that tumors and other intracranial lesions could be detected by this technique. **Dr. William Fry,** an electrical engineer whose primary research was in the field of ultrasound, is credited with being the first to introduce the use of computers in diagnostic ultrasound. Around this same time, he and **Dr. Russell Meyers** performed craniotomies and used ultrasound to destroy parts of the basal ganglia in patients with Parkinsonism.

Between 1948 and 1950, three investigators, Drs. **Douglass Howry,** a radiologist, **John Wild,** a clinician interested in tissue characterization, and **George Ludwig,** who was interested in reflections from gallstones, each demonstrated independently that when ultrasound waves generated by a piezoelectric crystal transducer are transmitted into the body, ultrasound waves of different acoustic impedances are returned to the transducer.

One of the pioneers in the clinical investigation and development of ultrasound was **Dr. Joseph Holmes** (1902–1982). A nephrologist by training, Dr. Holmes' initial interest in ultrasound involved its ability to detect bubbles in hemodialysis tubings. Holmes began work in ultrasound at the University of Colorado Medical Center in 1950, in collaboration with a group headed by **Douglass Howry.** In 1951, supported by Joseph H. Holmes, Douglass Howry, along with **William Roderic Bliss** and **Gerald J. Posakony,** both engineers, produced the "immersion tank ultrasound system," the first two-dimensional B-mode (or PPI, plan position indicator mode) linear compound scanner. Two-dimensional (2D) cross-sectional images were published in 1952 and 1953, which demonstrated that interpretable 2D images of internal organ structures and pathologies could be obtained with ultrasound. The Pan Scanner, put together by the Holmes, Howry, Posakony, and **Richard Cushman** team in 1957, was a landmark invention in the history of B-mode ultrasonography. With the Pan Scanner, the patient sat on a modified dental chair strapped against a plastic window of a semicircular pan filled with saline solution, while the transducer rotated through the solution in a semicircular arc (Figure 1-1).

In 1954, echocardiographic ultrasound applications were developed in Sweden by Drs. **Hellmuth Hertz** and **Inge Edler,** who first described the M-mode (motion) display.

An early obstetric contact compound scanner was built by **Tom Brown** and **Dr. Ian Donald** (1910–1987) in Scotland in 1957. Dr. Donald went on to discover many fascinating image patterns in the obstetric patient; his work is still referred to today. Meanwhile, in the early 1960s in Philadelphia, **Dr. J Stauffer Lehman** designed a real-time obstetric ultrasound system (Figure 1-2).

In 1959 the Ultrasonic Institute (UI) was formed at the National Acoustic Laboratory in Sydney, Australia. **George Kossoff** and his team, including **Dr. William Garrett** and **David Robinson,** developed diagnostic B-scanners with the use of a water bath to improve resolution of the image (Figures 1-3 and 1-4). This group

was also responsible for introducing gray-scale imaging in 1972. Kossoff and his colleagues were pioneers in the development of large-aperture, multitransducer technology in which the transducers are automatically programmed to operate independently or as a whole to

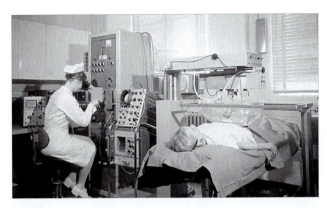

FIGURE 1-2 Dr. Lehman used a water path system to scan his obstetric patients.

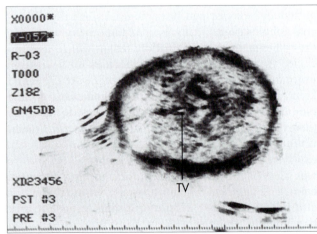

FIGURE 1-3 The Octoson used eight transducers mounted in a 180-degree semicircle and completely covered with water. The patient would lie on top of the covered waterbed, and the transducers would automatically scan the patient.

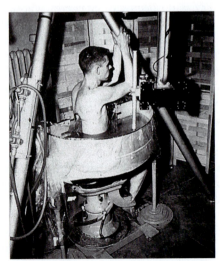

FIGURE 1-1 One of the early ultrasound scanning systems used a B-52 gun turret tank with the transducer carriage moved in a 360-degree path around the patient.

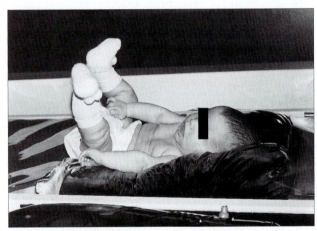

FIGURE 1-4 Real-time image of the neonatal head. *TV,* Third ventricle.

provide high-quality images without operator intervention, as was required with the contact static scanner that had been developed in 1962 at the University of Colorado.

The advent of real-time scanners changed the face of ultrasound scanning. The first real-time scanner (initially known as a fast B-scanner) was developed by **Walter Krause** and **Richard Soldner.** It was manufactured as the Vidoscan by Siemens Medical Systems of Germany in 1965. The Vidoscan used three rotating transducers housed in front of a parabolic mirror in a water coupling system and produced 15 images per second. The image was made up of 120 lines, and basic gray-scaling was present. The use of fixed-focus large-face transducers produced a narrow beam to ensure good resolution and a good image. Fetal life and motions could be demonstrated clearly. In 1973 **James Griffith** and **Walter Henry** at the National Institutes of Health produced a mechanical oscillating real-time scanning device that could produce clear 30-degree sector real-time images with good resolution. The phased-array scanning mechanism was first described by **Jan Somer** at the University of Limberg in the Netherlands and was in use from 1968, several years before the appearance of linear-array systems.

Medical applications of ultrasonic Doppler techniques were first implemented by **Shigeo Satomura** and **Yasuhara Nimura** at the Institute of Scientific and Industrial Research in Osaka, Japan, in 1955 for the study of cardiac valvular motion and pulsations of peripheral blood vessels. The Satomura team pioneered transcutaneous Doppler flow measurements in 1959. In 1966, **Kato** and **T. Izumi** pioneered the directional flow-meter using the local oscillation method whereby flow directions were detected and displayed. This was a breakthrough in Doppler instrumentation because reverse flow in blood vessels could now be documented. In the United States, **Robert Rushmer** and his team did groundbreaking work in Doppler instrumentation, starting in 1958. They pioneered transcutaneous continuous-wave flow measurements and spectral analysis in 1963. **Donald Baker,** a member of Rushmer's team, introduced a pulsed-Doppler system in 1970. In 1974 Baker, along with **John Reid** and **Frank Barber** and others, developed the first duplex pulsed-Doppler scanner, which allowed 2D scale imaging to be used to guide placement of the ultrasound beam for Doppler signal acquisition. In 1985 a work entitled "Real-Time Two-Dimensional Blood Flow Imaging Using an Autocorrelation Technique" by **Chihiro Kasai, Koroku Namekawa,** and **Ryozo Omoto** was published in English translation. The autocorrelation technique described in this publication could be applied to estimating blood velocity and turbulence in color flow imaging. The autocorrelation technique is a method for estimating the dominating frequency in a complex signal, as well as its variance. The algorithm is both computationally faster and significantly more accurate compared with the Fourier transform, since the reso-lution is not limited by the number of samples used. This provided the rapid means of frequency estimation to be performed in real-time that is still used today.

In 1987 The Center for Emerging Cardiovascular Technologies at **Duke University** started a project to develop a real-time volumetric scanner for cardiac imaging. In 1991 they produced a matrix array scanner that could image cardiac structures in real-time and in 3D. By the second half of the 1990s, many other centers throughout the world were working on laboratory and clinical research into 3D ultrasound. Today 3D ultrasound has developed into a clinically effective diagnostic imaging technique.

INTRODUCTION TO BASIC ULTRASOUND PRINCIPLES

To produce high-quality images that are free of artifacts, the sonographer must have a firm understanding of the basic principles of ultrasound. This section reviews basic principles of acoustics, measurement units, instrumentation, real-time sonography, 3D ultrasound, harmonic imaging, and optimization of gray-scale and Doppler ultrasound to reinforce the sonographer's understanding of scanning techniques.

Acoustics

Acoustics is the branch of physics that deals with sound and sound waves. It is the study of generating, propagating, and receiving sound waves. Within the field of acoustics, *ultrasound* is defined as sound frequencies that are beyond (ultra-) the range of normal human hearing, which is between 20 **hertz (Hz)** and 20 **kilohertz (kHz).** Thus, ultrasound refers to sound frequencies greater than 20 kilohertz. Sound is the result of mechanical energy that produces alternating **compression** and **rarefaction** of the conducting medium as it travels as a wave (Figure 1-5). (A **wave** is a propagation of energy that moves back and forth or vibrates at a steady rate.) Diagnostic ultrasound uses short sound pulses at frequencies of 1 to 20 million **cycles**/sec (**megahertz [MHz]**) that are transmitted into the body to examine soft tissue anatomic structures (Table 1-1). In medical ultrasound, the piezoelectric vibrating source within the transducer is a ceramic element that vibrates in response to an electrical signal. The vibrating motion of the ceramic element in the transducer causes the particles in the surrounding tissue to vibrate. In this way the ultrasound transducer converts electrical energy into mechanical energy as patients are examined. As the sound beam is directed into the body at various angles to the organs, reflection, absorption, and scatter cause the returning signal to be weaker than the initial impulse. Over a short period of time, multiple anatomic images are acquired in a real-time format.

The **velocity** of propagation is constant for a given tissue and is not affected by the frequency or wavelength

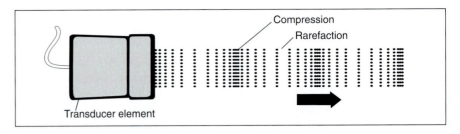

FIGURE 1-5 As the transducer element vibrates, waves undergo compression and expansion, or rarefaction, by which the molecules are pulled apart.

TABLE 1-1	Applications of Sound Frequency Ranges	
Frequency Range	**Manner of Production**	**Application**
Infrasound 0–25 Hz	Electromagnetic vibrators	Vibration analysis of structures
Audible 20 Hz–20 kHz	Electromagnetic vibrators, musical instruments	Communications, signaling
Ultrasound 20–100 kHz	Air whistles, electric devices	Biology, sonar
100 kHz–1 MHz	Electric devices	Flaw detection, biology
1–20 MHz	Electric devices	Diagnostic ultrasound

Hz, Hertz; *kHz*, kilohertz; *MHz*, megahertz.

of the pulse. In soft tissues, the assumed average propagation velocity is 1540 m/sec (Table 1-2). It is the stiffness and the density of a medium that determine how fast sound waves will travel through the structure. The more closely packed the molecules, the faster is the speed of sound.

The velocity of sound differs greatly among air, bone, and soft tissue, although the velocity of sound varies by only a little from one soft tissue to another. Sound waves travel slowly through gas (air), at intermediate speed through liquids, and quickly through solids (metal). Air-filled structures, such as the lungs and stomach, or gas-filled structures, such as the bowel, impede the sound transmission, while sound is attenuated through most bony structures. Small differences among fat, blood, and organ tissues that are seen on an ultrasound image may be better delineated with higher-frequency transducers that improve resolution.

Measurement of Sound. The **decibel (dB)** unit is used to measure the intensity (strength), amplitude, and power of an ultrasound wave. Decibels allow the sonographer to compare the intensity or **amplitude** of two signals. **Power** refers to the rate at which energy is transmitted. Power is the rate of energy flow over the entire beam of sound and is often measured in watts (W) or milliwatts (mW). **Intensity** is defined as power per unit area. It is the rate of energy flow across a defined area of the beam and can be measured in watts per square meter (W/m^2) or milliwatts per square centimeter. Power and intensity are directly related: If you double the power, the intensity also doubles.

TABLE 1-2	Characteristic Acoustic Impedance and Velocity of Ultrasound	
Material	**Acoustic Impedance** $(g/cm/sec \times 10)$	**Velocity**
Air	0.0001	331
Fat	1.38	1450
Water	1.50	1430
Blood	1.61	1570
Kidney	1.62	1560
Liver	1.65	1550
Muscle	1.70	1580
Skull	7.80	4080

Frequency. Sound is characterized according to its frequency (Figure 1-6). Frequency may be explained by the following analogy: If a stick were moved into and out of a pond at a steady rate, the entire surface of the water would be covered with waves radiating from the stick. If the number of vibrations made in each second were counted, the frequency of vibration could be determined. In ultrasound, **frequency** describes the number of oscillations per second performed by the particles of the medium in which the wave is propagating:

1 oscillation/sec = 1 cycle/sec = 1 **hertz** (1 **Hz**)

1000 oscillations/sec = 1 kilocycle/sec = 1 **kilohertz** (1 **kHz**)

1,000,000 oscillations/sec = 1 megacycle/sec

= 1 **megahertz** (1 **MHz**)

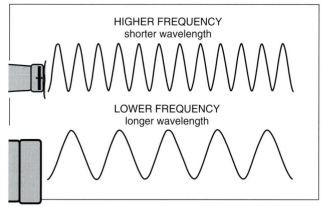

FIGURE 1-6 Wavelength is inversely related to frequency. The higher the frequency, the shorter is the wavelength and the less is the depth of penetration. The longer wavelength has a lower frequency and a greater depth of penetration.

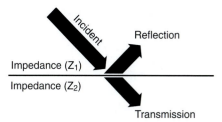

FIGURE 1-7 Reflection occurs when a sound wave strikes an interface between two objects with different acoustic impedances, causing some of the energy to be transmitted across the interface and some of it to be reflected.

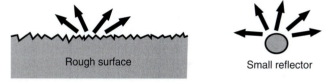

FIGURE 1-8 If the difference between two materials is small, most of the energy in a sound wave will be transmitted across an interface between them, and the reflected echo will be weak. If the difference is large, little energy will be transmitted; most will be reflected.

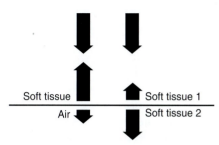

FIGURE 1-9 Nonspecular reflectors reflect, or scatter, the sound wave in many directions.

TABLE 1-3	Units Commonly Used in Ultrasound	
Quantity	**Unit**	**Abbreviation**
Amplifier gain	Decibels	dB
Area	Meters squared	m^2
Attenuation	Decibels	dB
Attenuation coefficient	Decibels per centimeter	dB/cm
Frequency	Hertz (cycles per second)	Hz
Intensity	Watts per square meter	W/m^2
Length	Meter	m
Period	Microseconds	μsec
Power	Watts	W
Pressure amplitude	Pascals	Pa
Relative power	Decibels	dB
Speed	Meters per second	m/sec
Time	Seconds	sec
Volume	Meters cubed	m^3

The sonographer should be familiar with the units of measurement commonly used in the profession (Table 1-3).

Propagation of Sound Through Tissue. Once sound pulses are transmitted into a body, they can be reflected, scattered, refracted, or absorbed. Reflection occurs whenever the pulse encounters an **interface** between tissues with different acoustic impedances (Figure 1-7). **Acoustic impedance** is the measure of a material's **resistance** to the propagation of sound. The strength of the reflection depends on the difference in acoustic impedance between the tissues, as well as the size of the interface, its surface characteristics, and its orientation with respect to the transmitted sound pulse. The greater the acoustic mismatch, the greater is the backscatter or reflection (Figure 1-8). Large, smooth interfaces are called specular reflectors. If specular reflectors are aligned

perpendicular to the direction of the transmitted pulse, they reflect sound directly back to the active crystal elements in the transducer and produce a strong signal. Specular reflectors that are not oriented perpendicular to the sound produce a weaker signal.

Scattering refers to the redirection of sound in multiple directions. This produces a weak signal and occurs when the pulse encounters a small acoustic interface or a large interface that is rough (Figure 1-9).

Refraction is a change in the direction of sound that occurs when sound encounters an interface between two tissues that transmit sound at different speeds. Because the sound frequency remains constant, the **wavelength** changes to accommodate differences in the speed of sound in the two tissues. The result of this change in wavelength is a redirection of the sound pulse as it passes through the interface.

Absorption describes the loss of sound energy secondary to its conversion to thermal energy. This is greater in soft tissues than in fluid and greater in bone than in soft tissues. Absorption is a major cause of acoustic shadowing.

Instrumentation

Piezoelectric Crystals. When a ceramic **crystal** is electronically stimulated, it deforms and vibrates to produce the sound pulses used in diagnostic sonography (Figure 1-10). **Pulse duration** is the time that a piezoelectric element vibrates after electrical stimulation. Each pulse consists of a band of frequencies referred to as *bandwidth*. The center frequency produced by a transducer is the resonant frequency of the crystal element and depends on the thickness of the crystal. The echoes that return to the transducer distort the crystal elements and generate an electric pulse that is processed into an image. The higher-amplitude echoes produce a greater crystal deformation and generate a larger electronic voltage, which is displayed as a brighter pixel. These 2D images are known as B-mode, or brightness mode, images.

Image Resolution. **Resolution** is the ability of an imaging process to distinguish adjacent structures in an object and is an important measure of image quality. The resolution of the ultrasound image is determined by the size and configuration of the transmitted sound pulse. Resolution is always considered in three dimensions: axial, lateral, and azimuthal. **Axial resolution** (Figure 1-11) refers to the ability to resolve objects within the imaging plane that are located at different depths along the direction of the sound pulse. This depends on the direction of the sound pulse, which, in turn, depends on the wavelength. Because wavelength is inversely proportional to frequency, the higher-frequency probes produce shorter pulses and better axial resolution, but with less penetration. These probes are best for superficial structures such as thyroid, breast, and scrotum. **Lateral resolution** (Figure 1-12) refers to the ability to resolve objects within the imaging plane that are located side by side at the same depth from the transducer. Lateral resolution can be varied by adjusting the **focal zone** of the

transducer, which is the point at which the beam is the narrowest. Azimuthal (elevation) resolution refers to the ability to resolve objects that are the same distance from the transducer but are located perpendicular to the plane of imaging. Azimuthal resolution is also related to the thickness of the tomographic slice (Figure 1-13). **Slice thickness** is usually determined by the shape of the crystal elements or the characteristics of fixed acoustic lenses.

Attenuation. **Attenuation** is the sum of acoustic energy losses resulting from absorption, scattering, and reflection. It refers to the reduction in intensity and amplitude of a sound wave as it travels through a medium as some of the energy is absorbed, reflected, or scattered (Figure 1-14). Thus, as the sound beam travels through the body, the beam becomes progressively weaker. In human soft tissue, sound is attenuated at the rate of 0.5 dB/cm per

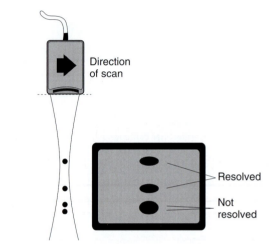

FIGURE 1-11 Axial resolution refers to the minimum distance between two structures positioned along the axis of the beam where both structures can be visualized as separate objects.

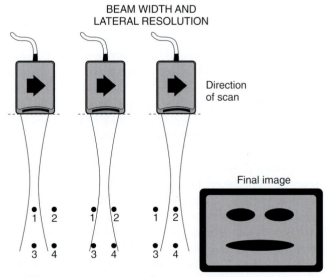

FIGURE 1-12 Beam width determines lateral resolution. If two reflectors are closer together than the diameter or width of the transducer, they will not be resolved.

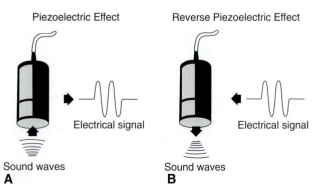

FIGURE 1-10 Piezoelectric effect. **A,** In certain crystals, when a sound wave is applied perpendicular to its surface, an electric charge is created. **B,** If the element is exposed to an electric shock, it will begin to vibrate and transmit a sound wave.

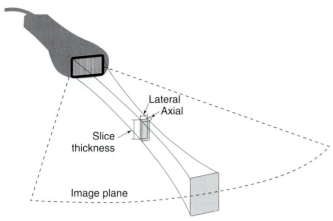

FIGURE 1-13 Slice thickness refers to the thickness of the section in the patient that contributes to the echo signals on any one image.

ATTENUATION

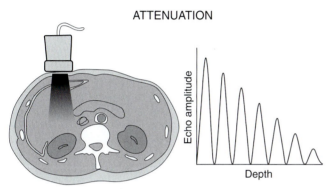

FIGURE 1-14 As the sound travels through the abdomen, it becomes attenuated, as some of it is reflected, scattered, and absorbed.

million hertz. If air or bone is coupled with soft tissue, more energy will be attenuated. Attenuation through a solid calcium interface, such as a gallstone, will produce a shadow with sharp borders on the ultrasound image.

With the exception of air-tissue and bone interfaces, the differences in acoustic impedance in biologic tissues are so slight that only a small component of the ultrasound beam is reflected at each interface. The lung and bowel have a detrimental effect on the ultrasound beam, causing poor transmission of sound. Therefore, anatomy beyond these two areas cannot be imaged because of air interference. Bone conducts sound at a much faster speed than soft tissue. (Normal transmission of sound through soft tissue travels at 1540 m/sec.) Much of the sound beam is absorbed or scattered as it travels through the body, undergoing progressive attenuation. The sound is reflected according to the acoustic impedance, which is related to tissue density. Most of the sound is passed into tissues deeper in the body and is reflected at other interfaces. Because acoustic impedance is the product of the velocity of sound in a medium and the density of that medium, acoustic impedance increases if the density or propagation speed increases.

Real-Time Ultrasound

Real-time compound imaging allows the sound to be steered at multiple angles, as well as perpendicular to the body, to produce the best image. These signals are then "averaged" from the multiple angles, and accentuation of the high-level reflectors is produced over the weaker reflectors and noise. This vastly improves the signal-to-noise ratio and tissue contrast.

Harmonic Imaging

Sound waves contain many component frequencies. Harmonics are those components whose frequencies are integral multiples of the lowest frequency (the "fundamental" or "first harmonic"). Harmonic imaging involves transmitting at frequency f and receiving at frequency $2f$, the second harmonic. Because of the finite bandwidth constraints of transducers, the transducer insonates at half of its nominal frequency (e.g., 3 MHz for a 6 MHz transducer) in harmonic mode and then receives at its nominal frequency (6 MHz in this example). The harmonic beams generated during pulse propagation are narrower and have lower side-lobe artifacts than the fundamental beam. The strength of the harmonics generated depends on the amplitude of the incoming beam. Therefore, the image-degrading portions of the fundamental beam (i.e., scattered echoes, reverberations, and slice-thickness side lobes) are much weaker than the on-axis portions of the beam and generate weaker harmonics.

Harmonic formation increases with depth, with few harmonics being generated within the near field of the body wall. Therefore, filtering out the fundamental frequency and creating an image from the echoes of the second harmonic should result in an image that is relatively free of the noise formed during the passage of sound through the distorting layers of the body wall.

Transducer Selection

A **transducer** is a device that converts energy from one form to another. Figure 1-15 illustrates the single-element transducer design. Most of the transducers used today are not a single element but rather a combination of elements that form an array. The transducer array scan head contains multiple small piezoelectric elements, each with its own electrical circuitry. These elements are very small in diameter, which greatly reduces beam divergence. A reduction in beam divergence leads to beam steering and focusing. The focus of the array transducers occurs on reception and on transmission (Figure 1-16). The focusing is done dynamically during reception. Shortly after pulse transmission, the received focus is set close to the transducer. As time elapses and the echoes from the distant targets return, the focal distance is gradually lengthened. Some instruments have multiple

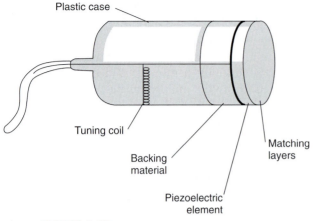

FIGURE 1-15 Single-element transducer design.

METHODS OF FOCUSING

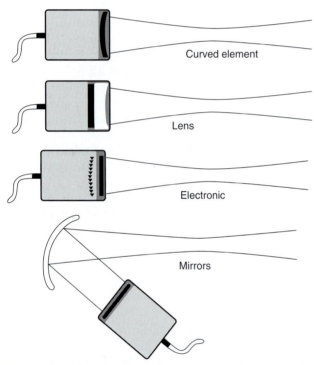

FIGURE 1-16 Focusing effectively narrows the ultrasound beam. Multiple methods may be used to achieve this effect.

ELECTRONICALLY SCANNED ARRAYS

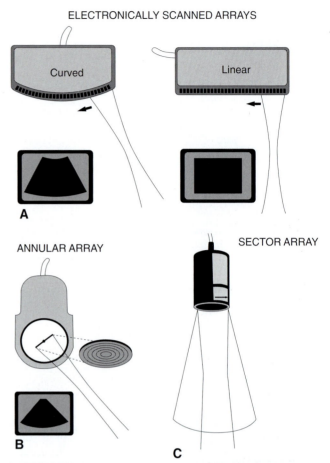

FIGURE 1-17 Comparison of transducer models. **A,** Electronically scanned arrays may be curved or linear. **B,** Annular array has a larger diameter with multiple rings of focus. **C,** Sector array with multiple small elements within the transducer face.

transmit focal zones to allow better control of the resolution of the beam at certain depths of field in the image.

The type of transducer selected for a particular examination (Figure 1-17) depends on several factors: the type of examination, the size of the patient, and the amount of fatty or muscular tissue present. High-frequency linear array probes are generally used for smaller structures (carotid artery, thyroid, scrotum, or breast). The abdomen is usually scanned with a curved linear array and/or a sector array; the frequency will depend on the size of the patient. An echocardiographic examination is performed with a phased-array transducer to allow the smaller probe to scan in between the ribs. The transesophageal studies are obtained with the transesophageal probe to image detailed anatomy of the cardiac structures. Obstetric and gynecologic scans are usually performed with a linear or curved array transducer. The transvaginal probe is used to scan intercavity areas.

Multielement Transducer. These transducers contain groups of small crystal elements arranged in a sequential fashion. The transmitted sound pulses are created by the summation of multiple pulses from many different elements. The timing and sequence of activation are altered to steer the transmitted pulses in different directions while focusing at multiple levels.

Phased-Array Transducer. With this transducer, every element in the array participates in the formation of each transmitted pulse. The sound beams are steered at varying angles from one side of the transducer to the other to produce a sector format. The transducer is smaller and is better able to scan in between ribs (especially useful in echocardiography). The transducer permits a large, deep field of view. The limitations of this transducer are a reduced near field focus and a small superficial field of view (Figure 1-18).

Linear-Array Transducer. The linear-array transducer activates a limited group of adjacent elements to generate each pulse. The pulses travel in the same direction (parallel) and are oriented perpendicular to the transducer surface, resulting in a rectangular image. The pulses may also be steered to produce a trapezoidal image (Figure 1-19). This transducer provides high resolution in the near field. The transducer is quite large and cumbersome for accessing all areas and is used more often in obstetric ultrasound.

Curved-Array Transducer. The curved-array transducer uses the linear-array transducer with the surface of the transducer re-formed into a curved convex shape to produce a moderately sized sector-shaped image with a convex apex. This allows for a wider far field of view,

with slightly reduced resolution. This type of probe can be formatted into many different applications with varying frequencies for use in the abdomen for smaller endoluminal scanning.

Intraluminal Transducer. These transducers are very small and can be placed into different body lumens that are close to the organ of interest. Much higher frequencies are used with high resolution. Elimination of the body adipose tissue greatly enhances image quality. The drawback of a high-frequency transducer is a limited depth of field. These transducers have been labeled as transvaginal and endorectal when used to image the female organs and rectum, respectively (Figure 1-20). Cardiologists have used the transesophageal probe to produce exquisite views of the cardiac valvular apparatus. Interventional physicians have used the intra-arterial probes that fit onto the end of a catheter.

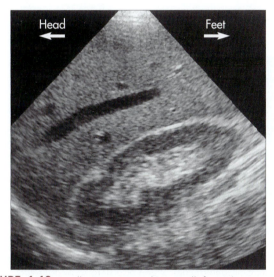

FIGURE 1-18 Small sector array has small footprint to get in between ribs, but visualization of the near field is limited.

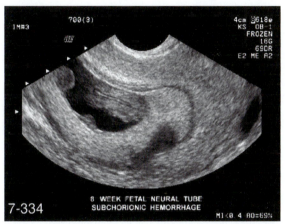

FIGURE 1-20 Transvaginal probe may provide 90- to 120-degree sector field of view to image this 8-week gestation with a subchorionic hemorrhage.

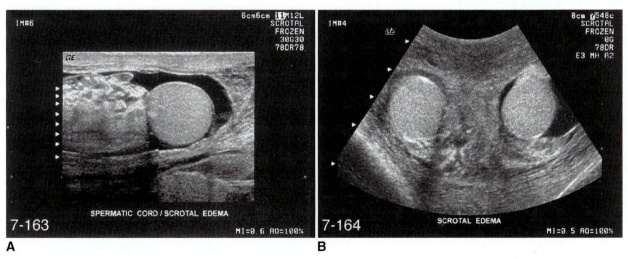

A   **B**

FIGURE 1-19 Comparison of linear array **(A)** versus curved array **(B)** images of the scrotal sac. The linear array produces a "rectangular" image display, whereas the curved array shows a wide "pie" curve display.

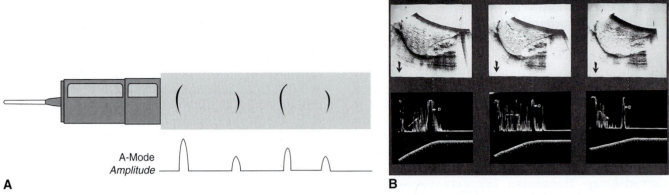

FIGURE 1-21 A, Amplitude is shown along the vertical axis, and time is shown along the horizontal axis. **B,** Earlier instrumentation used the A-mode display to help determine proper settings for the two-dimensional image. The bottom images show the A-mode and time gain compensation scale below.

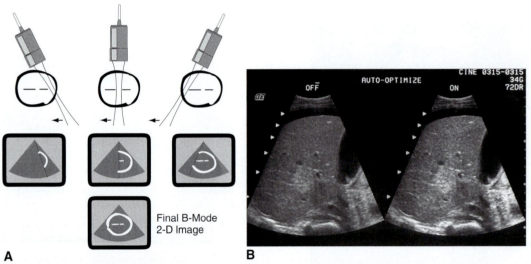

Final B-Mode
2-D Image

FIGURE 1-22 A, Acquisition of multiple image planes over a period of time is made to produce a B-mode image. **B,** B-mode image of the liver with a hemangioma in the center of the right lobe. The auto-optimize control is used in the right-hand display to show improved focus.

Pulse-Echo Display Modes

A-Mode (Amplitude Modulation). A-mode, or amplitude modulation, produces a one-dimensional image that displays the amplitude strength of the returning echo signals along the vertical axis and the time (distance) along the horizontal axis. The amplitude display represents the time or distance it takes the beam to strike an interface and return the signal to the transducer. The greater the reflection at the interface, the taller the amplitude spike will appear (Figure 1-21).

B-Mode (Brightness Modulation). The B-mode, or brightness modulation, method displays the intensity (amplitude) of an echo by varying the brightness of a dot to correspond to echo strength. **Gray scale** is an imaging technique that assigns to each level of amplitude a particular shade of gray to visualize the different echo amplitudes. The B-mode is the basis for all real-time imaging in ultrasound (Figure 1-22). In B-mode imaging,

the ultrasound beam is sent in various directions into the region of interest to be scanned. Each beam interrogates the reflectors along a different line. The echo data picked up along the beam line are displayed in a B-mode format. The B-mode display "tracks" the ultrasound beam line as it scans the region, "sketching out the 2D image" of the body. As many as 200 beam lines may be used to construct each image.

M-Mode (Motion Mode). The M-mode, or motion mode, displays time along the horizontal axis and depth along the vertical axis to depict movement, especially in cardiac structures (Figure 1-23).

Real-time. Real-time imaging provides a dynamic presentation of multiple image frames per second over selected areas of the body. The **frame rate** is dependent on the frequency and depth of the transducer and depth selection. Typical frame rates are 30 frames per second or less. The principal barrier to higher scanning speeds is the speed of sound in tissue, dictating the time required

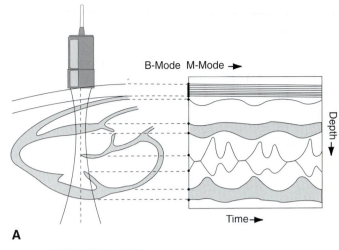

A

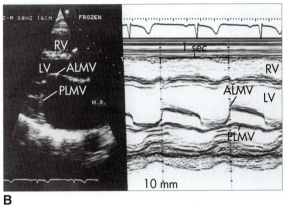

B

FIGURE 1-23 **A,** M-mode imaging. From the B-mode image, one line of site may be selected to record a motion image of a moving structure over time and distance. **B,** The M-mode is recorded through the stenotic mitral valve to show decreased opening and closing of the valve leaflet over time. On the M-mode, the vertical scale represents depth, and the space between the markers represents time. The distance between these two markers is 1 second. *ALMV,* Anterior leaflet mitral valve; *LV,* left ventricle; *PLMV,* posterior leaflet mitral valve; *RV,* right ventricle.

to acquire echo data for each beam line. The **temporal resolution** refers to the ability of the system to accurately depict motion.

Three-Dimensional Ultrasound

Conventional ultrasound offers a 2D visualization of anatomic structures with the flexibility of visualizing images from different orientations or "windows" in real-time. The sonographer acquires these 2D images in at least two different scanning planes and then forms a 3D image in his or her head. Recent developments in technology allow ultrasound images to be acquired on their *x, y,* and *z* axes, manually realigned, and then reconstructed into a 3D format. This technique has been useful in reconstructing the fetal face, ankle, and extremities in the second- and third-trimester fetus (Figure 1-24). Clinical investigations are currently under way to discover additional applications of 3D imaging.

Three-dimensional ultrasound (3DU) has continued to develop, with improvements in resolution and accuracy. Data for the 3DU are acquired as a stack of parallel cross-sectional images with the use of a conventional ultrasound system or as a volume with the use of an electronic array probe. These images can be reconstructed in a variety of formats to produce the desired

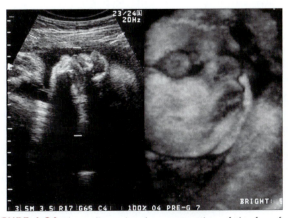

FIGURE 1-24 Three-dimensional reconstruction of the face from the two-dimensional fetal profile image in a third-trimester fetus.

image. More information on this technique will be found in Chapter 54.

System Controls for Image Optimization

Pulse-Echo Instrumentation. The critical component of the pulse-echo instrument is the B-mode (2D) imager. The beam former includes the electronic transmitter and the receiver. The transmitter supplies electrical signals to

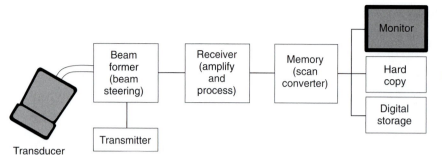

FIGURE 1-25 Components of an ultrasound system.

the transducer for producing the sound beam. The transducer may be connected to the transmitter and receiver through a beam-former system. Echoes picked up by the transducer are applied to the receiver. At this point, the echoes are amplified and processed into a suitable format for display. An image memory (scan converter) retains data for viewing or storage on digital media (Figure 1-25).

Power Output. The power output determines the strength of the pulse that is transmitted into the body. The returning echoes are stronger when the transmitted pulse is stronger, and thus the image is "brighter." The power output is displayed as a decibel (dB) or as a percent of maximum.

Gain. Once the sound wave strikes the body, sound attenuation occurs with each layer the beam transverses, causing an interface in the deep tissues to produce a weaker reflection and less distortion of the crystal than a similar interface in the near tissues. To compensate for this attenuation of sound in the deeper tissues, the sound is "electronically amplified" after the sound returns to the transducer. The receiver **gain** allows the sonographer to amplify or boost the echo signals. It may be compared with the volume control on a radio—as one increases the volume, the sound becomes louder. The acoustic exposure to the patient is not changed when the receiver gain is increased. If the gain is set too high, artifactual echo noise will be displayed throughout the image.

Recall the discussion of how the signal is absorbed, reflected, and attenuated as the beam traverses the body. The depth of the interface is determined by the amount of time it takes for the transmitted sound pulse to return to the transducer. The **time gain compensation (TGC)** control, sometimes referred to as *DGC (depth gain compensation)*, allows the sonographer to amplify the receiver gain gradually at specific depths (Figure 1-26). Thus, the echoes well seen in the near field may be reduced in amplitude, while the echoes in the far field may be amplified with the TGC controls. The TGC control will be continually adjusted during the sonographic examination to highlight or display various signals within the body.

Focal Zone. The focal zone control allows the transducer to focus the transmitted sound at different depths (Figure 1-27). It is usually indicated on the side of the image as single or multiple arrowheads and may be

TIME GAIN COMPENSATION (TGC)

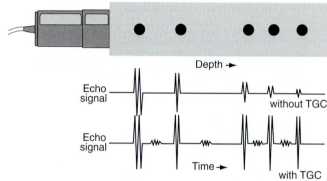

FIGURE 1-26 The time gain compensation (TGC) allows the sonographer to amplify the receiver gain gradually at specific depths to adjust for attenuation.

FOCAL ZONE CHARACTERISTICS

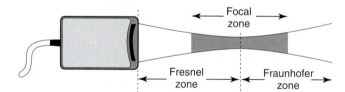

FIGURE 1-27 The near field (**Fresnel zone**) is the area closest to the transducer. The far field (**Fraunhofer zone**) is farthest from the transducer.

adjusted in depth to focus on specific areas of interest. As multilevel focusing is utilized, a decrease in the frame rate will occur.

Field of View. This control allows the sonographer to adjust the depth and width of the image. The larger or deeper field of view will directly cause the frame rate to decrease. Depth is displayed as centimeters on the side of the image. Width adjusts the horizontal axis of the image and may be used to reduce side-lobe artifacts.

Reject. The reject control eliminates both electronic noise and low-level echoes from the display.

Dynamic Range. The **dynamic range** of a device is the range of input signal levels that produce noticeable changes in the output of the device. The dynamic range capabilities vary among different ultrasound machines. The sonographer usually notes the low dynamic range as one of high contrast (echocardiography and peripheral vascular), whereas the high dynamic range shows more shades of gray and lower contrast (abdominal and obstetric).

Doppler Ultrasound

Two basic modes of transducer operation are used in medical diagnostic applications: continuous wave and pulsed wave. Real-time instrumentation uses only the pulse-echo amplitude of the returning echo to generate gray-scale information. Doppler instrumentation uses both continuous and pulse-wave operations.

Doppler Effect. The Doppler effect is the apparent change in frequency of sound or light waves emitted by a source as it moves away from or toward an observer (Figure 1-28). Sound that reflects off a moving object undergoes a change in frequency. Objects moving toward the transducer reflect sound at a higher frequency than that of the incident pulse, and objects moving away reflect sound at a lower frequency. The difference between the transmitted and the received frequency is called the Doppler **frequency shift.** This Doppler effect is applied when the motion of laminar or turbulent flow is detected within a vascular structure. When the source moves toward the listener, the perceived frequency is higher than the emitted frequency, thus creating a higher-pitched sound. If the sound moves away from the listener, the perceived frequency is lower than the transmitted frequency, and the sound will have a lower pitch.

In the medical application of the Doppler principle, the frequency of the reflected sound wave is the same as the frequency transmitted only if the reflector is stationary. If the red blood cell (RBC) moves along the line of the ultrasound beam (parallel to flow), the Doppler shift is directly proportional to the velocity of the RBC. If

the RBC moves away from the transducer in the plane of the beam, the fall in frequency is directly proportional to the velocity and direction of RBC movement (Figure 1-29). The frequency of the echo will be higher than the transmitted frequency if the reflector is moving toward the transducer, and lower if the reflector is moving away. **Doppler Shift.** The difference between the receiving echo frequency and the frequency of the transmitted beam is called the **Doppler shift.** This change in the frequency of a reflected wave is caused by relative motion between the reflector and the transducer's beam. Generally the Doppler shift is only a small fraction of the transmitted ultrasound frequency.

The Doppler shift frequency is proportional to the velocity of the moving reflector or blood cell. The frequency at which a transducer transmits ultrasound influences the frequency of the Doppler shift. The higher the original, or transmitted, frequency, the greater is the shift in frequency for a given reflector velocity. The returning frequency increases if the RBC is moving toward the transducer and decreases if the blood cell is moving away from the transducer. The Doppler effect produces a shift that is the reflected frequency minus the transmitted frequency. When interrogating the same blood vessel with transducers of different frequencies, the higher-frequency transducer will generate a larger Doppler shift frequency.

The angle that the reflector path makes with the ultrasound beam is called the **Doppler angle.** As the Doppler angle increases from 0 to 90 degrees, the detected Doppler frequency shift decreases. At 90 degrees, the Doppler shift is zero, regardless of flow velocity. The frequency of the Doppler shift is proportional to the cosine of the Doppler angle. The beam should be parallel to flow to obtain the maximum velocity. The closer the Doppler angle is to zero, the more accurate is the flow velocity (Figure 1-30). If the angle of the beam to the reflector exceeds 60 degrees, velocities will no longer be accurate.

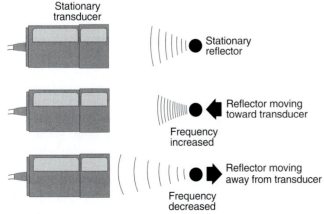

FIGURE 1-28 The Doppler effect refers to a change in frequency of a sound wave when the source or the listener is moving relative to the other.

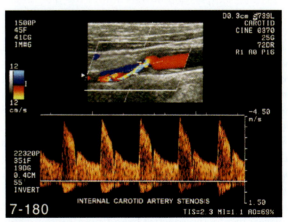

FIGURE 1-29 Color Doppler with spectral wave shows stenosis of the internal carotid artery and increased velocity through the area of stenosis.

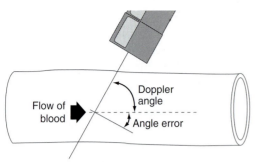

FIGURE 1-30 The closer the Doppler angle is to zero, the more accurate is the flow velocity. Thus the more parallel the transducer is to flow, the more accurate is the velocity.

Laminar flow

Turbulent flow

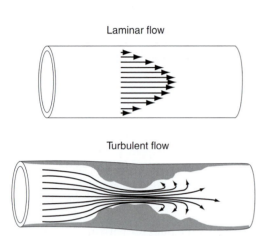

FIGURE 1-31 Laminar flow is smooth and has uniform velocity, whereas turbulent flow has multiple flow velocity characteristics.

Spectral Analysis. Blood flow through a vessel may be laminar or turbulent (Figure 1-31). **Laminar** flow is the normal pattern of vessel flow, which occurs at different velocities, as flow in the center of the vessel is faster than it is at the edges. When the range of velocities increases significantly, the flow pattern becomes turbulent. The audio of the Doppler signal enables the sonographer to distinguish laminar flow from turbulent flow patterns. The process of **spectral analysis** allows the instrumentation to break down the complex multifrequency Doppler signal into individual frequency components.

The spectral display shows the distribution of Doppler frequencies versus time (Figure 1-32). This is displayed as velocity on the vertical axis and time on the horizontal axis. Flow toward the transducer is displayed above the baseline, and flow away from the transducer is displayed below the baseline.

When the area of the vessel that is examined contains red blood cells moving at similar velocities, they will be represented on the spectral display by a narrow band. This area under the band is called the "window." As flow becomes more turbulent or disturbed, the velocity increases, producing **spectral broadening** on the display. A very stenotic (high-flow velocity) lesion would cause the window to become completely filled in.

VELOCITIES ON
SPECTRAL WAVEFORM

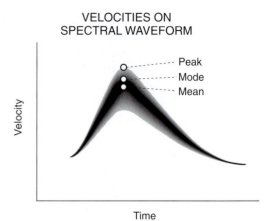

FIGURE 1-32 The spectral display shows the distribution of Doppler frequencies versus time.

Continuous Wave Doppler. Continuous wave (CW) Doppler uses two piezoelectric elements: one for sending and one for receiving. The sound is transmitted continuously rather than in short pulses. Continuous wave is used to record the higher velocity flow patterns, usually above 2 m/sec, and is especially useful in cardiology (Figure 1-33). Unlike pulsed wave Doppler, continuous wave cannot pinpoint exactly where along the beam axis flow is occurring, as it samples all of the flow along its path. In the example of a five-chamber view of the heart, a sample volume placed in the left ventricular outflow tract will sample all the flow along that "line" to include the flows in the outflow tract and in the ascending aorta.

Pulsed Wave Doppler. Pulsed wave (PW) Doppler is used for lower velocity flow and has one crystal that pulses to transmit the signal while also listening or receiving the returning signal. The pulsed wave Doppler uses brief bursts of sound like those used in echo imaging. These bursts are usually of a longer duration and produce well-defined frequencies. The sonographer may set the **gate** or Doppler window to a specific area of interest in the vascular structure so interrogated. This means that a specific area of interest may be examined at the point the gate or sample volume is placed. For example, in a five-chamber view of the heart, the sample volume may be placed directly in the outflow tract, and recordings only from that particular area "within the gate or window" will be measured.

With pulsed Doppler, for accurate detection of Doppler frequencies to occur, the Doppler signal must be sampled at least twice for each cycle in the wave. This phenomenon is known as the **Nyquist sampling limit**. When the Nyquist limit is exceeded, an artifact called aliasing occurs. **Aliasing** presents on the spectral display as an apparent reversal of flow direction and a "wrapping around" of the Doppler spectral waveform. The highest velocity, therefore, may not be accurately demonstrated when aliasing occurs; this usually happens when the flows are greater than 2 m/sec. One can avoid aliasing by

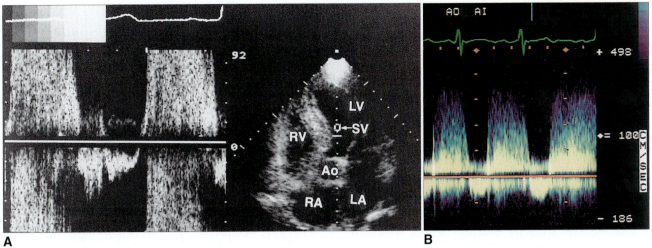

FIGURE 1-33 A, The sample volume *(SV)* is placed in the left ventricular outflow tract. Aortic insufficiency exceeds the Nyquist limit of the pulsed wave Doppler. Flow is seen above and below the baseline. When the continuous wave transducer is used **(B),** the velocity measures 3.5 m/sec. *Ao,* Aorta; *LA,* left atrium; *LV,* left ventricle; *RA,* right atrium; *RV,* right ventricle.

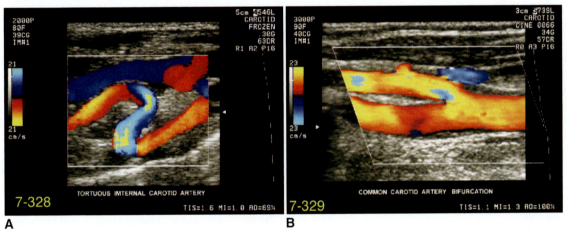

FIGURE 1-34 Color Doppler has been helpful to outline the direction and velocity of flow. The color box **(A)** shows which color assignment has been made for the image. The color toward the transducer is blue. **B,** This image shows that the color bar has assigned red to flow toward the transducer.

changing the Doppler signal from pulsed wave to continuous wave to record the higher velocities accurately.

Color Doppler. Color Doppler is sensitive to Doppler signals throughout an adjustable portion of the area of interest. A real-time image is displayed with both gray scale and **color flow** in the vascular structures. Color Doppler is able to analyze the phase information, frequency, and amplitude of returning echoes.

Velocities are quantified by allocating a pixel to flow toward the transducer and flow away from the transducer. Each velocity frequency change is allocated a color. Color maps may be adjusted to obtain different color assignments for the velocity levels; signals from moving red blood cells are assigned a color (red or blue) based on the direction of the phase shift (i.e., the direction of blood flow toward or away from the transducer) (Figure 1-34). Flow velocity is indicated by color brightness: The higher the velocity, the brighter is the color.

Aliasing also occurs in color flow imaging when Doppler frequencies exceed the Nyquist limit, just as in spectral Doppler. This appears as a wrap-around of the displayed color. The velocity scale (PRF) may be adjusted to avoid aliasing. Color arising from sources other than moving blood is referred to as flash artifact or ghosting.

Power Doppler. Power Doppler estimates the power or strength of the Doppler signal rather than the mean frequency shift. Although the Doppler detection sequence used in power Doppler is the same as that used in frequency-based color Doppler, once the Doppler shift has been detected, the frequency components are ignored in lieu of the total energy of the Doppler signal. The color and hue relate to the moving blood volume rather than to the direction or the velocity of flow.

This principle provides power Doppler several advantages over color Doppler imaging. In power Doppler, low-level noise is assigned as a homogeneous color

PULSING CHARACTERISTICS

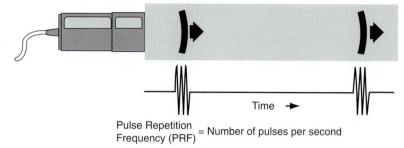

FIGURE 1-35 The pulse repetition frequency (PRF) may be adjusted in Doppler applications to record the lower or higher velocity signals.

background, even when the gain is increased. With color Doppler, the higher gains produce noise in the signal that obscures the image. The Doppler angle is not affected in power Doppler; with color Doppler the angle is critical in determining the exact flow velocity.

The downside of power Doppler is that it provides no information about the direction or velocity of blood flow, and it is susceptible to flash artifact (zones of intense color that results from motion of soft tissues and motion of the transducer).

Doppler Optimization

Transducer Frequency. The Doppler frequency shift is proportional to the transmitted frequency. Therefore, higher-frequency transducers cause a higher Doppler frequency shift that is easier to detect. Higher-frequency probes also result in stronger reflections from red blood cells. Remember that the higher-frequency probes are not sensitive to deeper structures; therefore multiple probes may be necessary, depending upon the type of ultrasound examination.

Gain. Doppler gain is the receiver end amplification of the Doppler signal. This can be applied to either the waveform itself or to the color Doppler image. The Doppler gain is usually increased to the maximum limit where "noise" scatter is seen in the background.

The gain is then slowly decreased until that noise disappears. The Doppler gain is independent of the gray scale gain.

Power. Power refers to the strength of the transmitted ultrasound pulse. The stronger pulse will produce stronger reflections that are more easily detected. Power will affect both gray-scale and Doppler images. Increasing the power may be helpful in the deeper structures, but increasing power increases patient exposure and may cause increased artifacts. For these reasons, power controls generally are not modified as frequently by the sonographer as the other controls.

Pulse Repetition Frequency (PRF). The **pulse repetition frequency** (PRF) refers to the number of sound pulses transmitted per second. A high PRF results in a high Doppler scale (to record higher velocities, i.e., aortic stenosis), whereas a lower PRF results in a lower Doppler scale (to record lower velocities, i.e., venous return or low-flow states). The PRF is adjusted for the higher flows to eliminate aliasing (Figure 1-35).

Wall Filter. The wall filter allows the sonographer to eliminate artifactual or unwanted signals arising from pulsating vessel walls or moving soft tissues. This filter allows frequency shifts above a certain level to be displayed while lower-frequency shifts are not displayed.

Introduction to Physical Findings, Physiology, and Laboratory Data

Sandra L. Hagen-Ansert

OBJECTIVES

On completion of this chapter, you should be able to:
- Explain how to interview a patient, obtain a health history, and perform a physical assessment
- Recognize the clinical signs and symptoms of diseases discussed in this chapter
- Recall the anatomy and physiology discussed in this chapter
- Be familiar with common laboratory tests and what their results may indicate

OUTLINE

The sonographer soon discovers that a good patient history and pertinent clinical information are very important in planning the approach to each sonographic examination. Slight changes in the laboratory data (i.e., white blood cell differential, serum enzymes, or fluctuations in liver function tests) may enable the sonographer to tailor the examination to provide the best information possible to answer the clinical question. Specific questions related to the current health status of the patient will direct the sonographer to examine the critical area of interest with particular attention as part of the routine protocol. Knowledge of the patient's previous surgical procedures will also help tailor the examination—the sonographer will not spend time looking for the gallbladder or ovaries that have been removed.

THE HEALTH ASSESSMENT

Obtaining a health history and performing a physical assessment are essential steps to analyzing the patient's medical problem. Although the health assessment is done by the health care practitioner before the patient's arrival in the ultrasound department, an understanding of the health assessment helps the sonographer better understand patient symptoms and laboratory values. Any health assessment involves collecting two types of data: objective and subjective. Objective data are obtained through observation and are verifiable. For example, a red swollen leg in a patient experiencing leg pain constitutes data that can be seen and verified by someone other than the patient. Subjective data are derived from the patient alone and include such statements as, "I have back pain," or "My stomach hurts."

The Interview Process

The purpose of the health history is to gather subjective data about the patient and while exploring previous and current problems. This information is gathered during a patient interview that typically occurs in a limited amount of time just before the ultrasound examination.

Be sure to introduce yourself to the patient, and explain that the purpose of the assessment is to identify the problem and provide information for the ultrasound examination. First, ask the patient about his or her general health, and then specifically about body systems and structures, with questions tailored to the ordered examination. Remember that your interviewing techniques will improve and become smoother with practice.

Successful patient interviews include the following considerations:

- Reassure the patient that everything will be kept confidential.
- Be sure the patient understands English and can hear well.
- Use language that the patient can understand, and avoid a lot of medical terms. If the patient does not understand, repeat the question in a different format using different words or examples. For example, instead of asking, "Did you have gastrointestinal difficulty after eating?" ask, "What foods make you sick to your stomach?"
- Always address the patient respectfully by a formal name, such as Mr. Delado or Ms. Peligrino.
- Listen attentively and make notes of pertinent information on the ultrasound data sheet.
- Remember that the patient may be worried that a problem will be found. Explain the procedure that will occur after the examination is complete (i.e., the images will be shown to the clinician, and the patient may contact his or her referring physician to find out the results).
- Briefly explain what you are planning to do, why you are doing it, how long it will take, and what equipment you will use.

Professional Demeanor. Remember to maintain professionalism throughout the interview process and examination. Remain neutral by avoiding sarcasm and keeping jokes in good taste. Do not let your personal opinions interfere with your assessment, and do not share your own medical problems with the patient. Do not offer advice. Know enough to answer questions the patient may have about the ultrasound examination, but leave the diagnostic interpretation to the physician. Be careful if the patient asks how everything looks. If you respond,

"It looks fine," meaning the technique was good, the patient will likely think you mean the examination is normal when it may not be.

Two Ways to Ask Questions. Questions may be characterized as open-ended or closed. Open-ended questions require the patient to express feelings, opinions, and ideas. They may also help the clinician to gather further information. Such a question as, "How would you describe the problems you have had with your abdomen?" is an example of an open-ended question.

Closed questions elicit short responses that may help you to zoom in on a specific point. These questions would include, "Do you ever get short of breath?" or "Do you have nausea and vomiting after fatty meals?"

Important Interview Questions. The sonographer usually does not have a great deal of time to obtain extensive histories; thus it is important to ask the right questions.

Biographical Data. The patient's name, address, phone number, birth date, marital status, religion, and nationality likely have been obtained already. Be sure to always check the patient's name and birth date on the report with the patient you are interviewing to make sure it is the correct patient. The primary care or referring physician is important to include for contact information.

Chief Complaint. Try to pinpoint why the patient is here for the ultrasound examination. Ask what his/her symptoms are and what prompted him/her to seek medical attention.

Medical History. Ask the patient about past and current medical problems and hospitalizations that may be pertinent to the examination.

Questions Specific to Body Structures and Systems. The structures and systems that are most frequently encountered by the sonographer are presented below.

Neck. Do you have swelling, soreness, lack of movement, or abnormal protrusions in your neck? How long have you had the problem? Have you done anything specific to aggravate the condition?

Respiratory System. Do you have shortness of breath on exertion or while lying in bed? Do you have a productive cough? Do you have night sweats? Have you been treated for a respiratory condition before? Have you ever had a chest x-ray?

Cardiovascular System. Do you have chest pain, palpitations, irregular heartbeat, fast heartbeat, shortness of breath, or a persistent cough? Have you ever had an electrocardiogram or echocardiogram or nuclear exercise study before? Do you have high blood pressure, peripheral vascular disease, swelling of the ankles and hands, varicose veins, cold extremities, or intermittent pain in your legs? Does heart disease run in your immediate family?

Breasts. Do you perform monthly breast self-examinations? Have you noticed a lump, a change in breast contour, breast pain, or discharge from your nipples? Have you ever had breast cancer? If not, has anyone else in your family had it? Have you ever had a mammogram?

Gastrointestinal Tract. Have you ever had nausea, vomiting, loss of appetite, heartburn, abdominal pain, frequent belching, or passing of gas? Have you lost or gained weight recently? How frequent are your bowel movements, and what color, odor, and consistency are your stools? Have you noticed a change in your regular pattern? Have you had hemorrhoids, rectal bleeding, hernias, gallbladder disease, or a liver disease, such as hepatitis?

Urinary System. Do you have urinary problems, such as burning during urination, **incontinence**, urgency, retention, reduced urinary flow, or dribbling? Do you get up during the night to urinate? What color is your urine? Have you ever noticed blood in it? Have you ever had kidney stones?

Female Reproductive System. Do you have regular periods? Do you have clots or pain with them? What age did you stop menstruating? Have you ever been pregnant? How many live births? How many miscarriages? Have you ever had a vaginal infection or a sexually transmitted disease? When did you last have a gynecologic examination and Pap test?

Male Reproductive System. Do you perform monthly testicular self-examinations? Have you ever noticed penile pain, discharge, lesions, or testicular lumps? Have you had a vasectomy? Have you ever had a sexually transmitted disease?

Musculoskeletal System. Do you have difficulty walking, sitting, or standing? Are you steady on your feet, or do you lose your balance easily? Do you have arthritis, gout, a back injury, muscle weakness, or paralysis?

Endocrine System. Have you been unusually tired lately? Do you feel hungry or thirsty more than usual? Have you lost weight for unexplained reasons? How well can you tolerate heat and cold? Have you noticed changes in your hair texture or color? Have you been losing hair? Do you take hormonal medications?

Performing the Physical Assessment

The physical assessment is another important part of the health assessment. Most likely this assessment will be performed by the primary physician or nurse practitioner. The information is presented here so that the sonographer gains a better understanding of the process the patient has been through before arriving for the ultrasound examination. Performing a physical assessment usually includes the following:

Height and Weight. These measurements are important for evaluating nutritional status, calculating medication dosages, and assessing fluid loss or gain.

Body Temperature. Body temperature is measured in degrees Fahrenheit (F) or degrees Celsius (C). Normal body temperature ranges from 96.7°F to 100.5°F (35.9°C to 38°C), depending on the route used for measurement.

Pulse. The patient's pulse reflects the amount of blood ejected with each heartbeat. To assess the pulse, palpate, with the pads of your index and middle fingers, one of the patient's arterial pulse points (usually at the wrist, on the radial side of the forearm), and note the rate, rhythm, and amplitude (strength) of the pulse. Press lightly over the area of the artery until you feel pulsations. If the rhythm is regular, count the beats for 10 seconds and multiply by 6 to obtain the number of beats per minute. A normal pulse for an adult is between 60 and 100 beats/min.

Although the radial pulse is the most easily accessible pulse site (on the wrist, same side as the thumb), the femoral or carotid pulse may be more appropriate in cardiovascular emergencies because these sites are larger and closer to the heart and more accurately reflect the heart's activity.

Respirations. Along with counting respirations, note the depth and rhythm of each breath. To determine the respiratory rate, count the number of respirations for 15 seconds and multiply by 4. A rate of 16 to 20 breaths/min is normal for an adult.

Blood Pressure. Systolic and diastolic blood pressure readings are helpful in evaluating cardiac output, fluid and circulatory status, and arterial resistance. The systolic reading reflects the maximum pressure exerted on the arterial wall at the peak of the left ventricular contraction. Normal systolic pressure ranges from 100 to 120 mmHg.

The diastolic reading reflects the minimum pressure exerted on the arterial wall during left ventricular relaxation. This reading is usually more notable because it evaluates the arterial pressure when the heart is at rest. Normal diastolic pressure ranges from 60 to 80 mmHg.

The **sphygmomanometer**, a device used to measure blood pressure, consists of an inflatable cuff, a pressure manometer, and a bulb with a valve. To record a blood pressure, the cuff is centered over an artery just above the elbow, inflated, and deflated slowly. As it deflates, listen with a stethoscope for Korotkoff sounds, which indicate the systolic and diastolic pressures. Blood pressures can be measured from most extremity pulse points, but the brachial artery is commonly used because of accessibility.

Auscultation. Auscultation is usually the last step in physical assessment. It involves listening for various breath, heart, and bowel sounds with a stethoscope. Hold the diaphragm (flat surface) firmly against the patient's skin—firmly enough to leave a slight ring afterward. Hold the bell lightly against the skin, enough to form a seal. Do not try to auscultate over the gown or bed linens because they can interfere with sounds. Be sure to warm the stethoscope in your hand.

FURTHER EXPLORATION OF SYMPTOMS

A clear understanding of the patient's symptoms is essential for guiding the specific examination. If symptoms are acute and severe, you may need to pay particular attention to a specific area. If symptoms seem mild to moderate, you may be able to take a more complete history. Most likely, the primary or referring physician has performed a detailed physical examination to define the specific patient symptoms.

The following five areas should be assessed:

1. *Provocative or palliative.* Your questions should be directed to finding out what causes the symptom and what makes it better or worse.
   - What were you doing when you first noticed it?
   - What seems to trigger it? Stress? Position? Activity?
   - What relieves the symptom? Diet? Position? Medication? Activity?
   - What makes the symptom worse?
2. *Quality or quantity.* Try to find out how the symptom feels, looks, or sounds.
   - How would you describe the symptom?
   - How often are you experiencing the symptom now?
3. *Region or radiation.* It is important to pinpoint the location of the patient's symptom. Ask the patient to use *one finger to point to the area of discomfort.*
   - Where does the symptom occur?
   - If pain is present, does it travel down (radiate from) your back or arms, up your neck, to your shoulder, etc.
4. *Severity.* The acuity of the symptom will have an impact on the timeliness of further assessments. The patient may be asked to rate the symptom on a scale of 1 to 10, with 10 being the most severe.
   - How bad is the symptom at its worst? Does it force you to lie down, sit down, or slow down?
   - Does the symptom seem to be getting better, getting worse, or staying the same?
5. *Timing.* Determine when the symptom began and how it began, whether gradually or suddenly. If it is intermittent, find out how often it occurs.

GASTROINTESTINAL SYSTEM

The gastrointestinal (GI) system consists of two major divisions: the GI tract and the accessory organs. The GI tract is a hollow tube that begins at the mouth and ends at the anus. About 25 feet long, the GI tract includes the pharynx, esophagus, stomach, small intestine, and large intestine. Accessory GI organs include the liver, pancreas, gallbladder, and bile ducts. The abdominal aorta and the gastric and splenic veins also aid the GI system.

Major functions of the gastrointestinal system include ingestion and digestion of food and elimination of waste products. Gastrointestinal complaints can be especially difficult to assess and evaluate because the abdomen has so many organs and structures that may influence pain and tenderness.

Normal Findings for the GI System

Visual Inspection
- Skin is free from vascular lesions, jaundice, surgical scars, and rashes.
- Faint venous patterns (except in thin patients) are apparent.
- Abdomen is symmetrical, with a flat, round, or scaphoid contour.
- Umbilicus is positioned midway between the xiphoid process and the symphysis pubis, with a flat or concave hemisphere.
- No variations in the color of the patient's skin are detectable.
- No bulges are apparent.
- The abdomen moves with respiration.

Auscultation
- High-pitched, gurgling bowel sounds are heard every 5 to 15 seconds through the diaphragm of the stethoscope in all four quadrants of the abdomen.
- A venous hum is heard over the inferior vena cava.
- No bruits, murmurs, friction rubs, or other venous hums are apparent.

Percussion
- **Tympany** is the predominant sound over hollow organs, including the stomach, intestines, bladder, abdominal aorta, and gallbladder.
- Dullness can be heard over solid masses, including the liver, spleen, pancreas, kidneys, uterus, and a full bladder.

Palpation
- No tenderness or masses are detectable.
- Abdominal musculature is free from tenderness and rigidity.
- No guarding, rebound tenderness, distention, or ascites is detectable.
- The liver is impalpable, except in children.
- The spleen is impalpable.
- The kidneys are impalpable, except in thin patients or those with a flaccid abdominal wall.

Inspecting the Abdomen

When visually inspecting the abdomen as part of the physical assessment, mentally divide the abdomen into four quadrants. Keep in mind these three terms: *epigastric* (above the umbilicus and between the costal margins), *umbilical* (around the navel), and *suprapubic* (above the symphysis pubis).

- Observe the abdomen for symmetry, checking for bumps, bulges, or masses.
- Note the patient's abdominal shape and contour.
- Assess the umbilicus; it should be midline and inverted. Pregnancy, ascites, or an underlying mass can cause the umbilicus to protrude.
- The skin of the abdomen should be smooth and uniform in color.
- Note any dilated veins.
- Note any surgical scars.
- Note the abdominal movements and pulsations. Visible rippling waves may indicate bowel obstruction. In thin patients, aortic pulsations may be seen.

Guidelines for GI Assessment

Temperature. Fever may be a sign of infection or inflammation.

Pulse. Tachycardia may occur with shock, pain, fever, sepsis, fluid overload, or anxiety. A weak, rapid, and irregular pulse may point to hemodynamic instability, such as that caused by excessive blood loss. Diminished or absent distal pulses may signal vessel occlusion from embolization associated with prolonged bleeding.

Respirations. Altered respiratory rate and depth can result from hypoxia, pain, electrolyte imbalance, or anxiety. Respiratory rate also increases with shock. Increased respiratory rate with shallow respirations may signal fever and sepsis. Absent or shallow abdominal movement on respiration may point to peritoneal irritation.

Blood Pressure. Decreased blood pressure may signal compromised hemodynamic status, perhaps from shock caused by GI bleed. Sustained severe **hypotension** results in diminished renal blood flow, which may lead to acute renal failure. Moderately increased systolic or diastolic pressure may occur with anxiety or abdominal pain. **Hypertension** can result from vascular damage caused by renal disease or renal artery stenosis. A blood pressure drop of greater than 30 mmHg when the patient sits up may indicate fluid volume depletion.

Common Signs and Symptoms of GI Diseases and Disorders

The most significant signs and symptoms related to gastrointestinal diseases and disorders are abdominal pain, diarrhea, bloody stools, nausea, and vomiting (Table 2-1).

Abdominal Pain. Abdominal pain usually results from a GI disorder, but it can be caused by a reproductive, genitourinary, musculoskeletal, or vascular disorder; use of certain drugs; or exposure to toxins.

- Constant, steady abdominal pain suggests organ perforation, ischemia, inflammation, or blood in the peritoneal cavity.
- Intermittent and cramping abdominal pain suggests the patient may have obstruction. Ask if the pain radiates to other areas. Ask if eating relieves the pain.
- Abdominal pain arises from the abdominopelvic viscera, the parietal peritoneum, or the capsule of the liver, kidney, or spleen, and may be acute or chronic, diffuse or localized.
- Visceral pain develops slowly into a deep, dull, aching pain that is poorly localized in the epigastric, periumbilical, or hypogastric region.
- Mechanisms that produce abdominal pain, including stretching or tension of the gut wall, traction on the peritoneum or mesentery, vigorous intestinal contraction, inflammation, or ischemia, may cause sensory nerve irritation.

Diarrhea. Diarrhea is usually a chief sign of intestinal disorder. Diarrhea is an increase in the volume, frequency, and liquidity of stools compared with the patient's normal bowel habits. It varies in severity and may be acute or chronic.

- Acute diarrhea may result from acute infection, stress, fecal impaction, or use of certain drugs.
- Chronic diarrhea may result from chronic infection, obstructive and inflammatory bowel disease, malabsorption syndrome, an endocrine disorder, or GI surgery.
- The fluid and electrolyte imbalance may precipitate life-threatening arrhythmias or hypovolemic shock.

Hematochezia. Hematochezia is the passage of bloody stools and may be a sign of GI bleeding below the ligament of Treitz. It may also result from a coagulation disorder, exposure to toxins, or a diagnostic test. It may lead to hypovolemia.

Nausea and Vomiting. Nausea is a sensation of profound revulsion to food or of impending vomiting. Vomiting is the forceful expulsion of gastric contents through the mouth that is often preceded by nausea.

- Nausea and vomiting may occur with fluid and electrolyte imbalance, infection, metabolic, endocrine, labyrinthine, and cardiac disorders, use of certain drugs, surgery, and radiation.
- Nausea and vomiting may also arise from severe pain, anxiety, alcohol intoxication, overeating, or ingestion of distasteful food or liquids.

GENITOURINARY AND URINARY SYSTEMS

It is important to recognize that a disorder of the genitourinary system can affect other body systems. For example, ovarian dysfunction can alter endocrine balance,

TABLE 2-1	Signs and Probable Indications of Gastrointestinal Diseases and Disorders	
Signs or Symptoms		**Probable Indication**
Abdominal Pain		
• Localized abdominal pain, described as steady, gnawing, burning, aching, or hunger-like, high in the midepigastrium slightly off center, usually on the right		Duodenal ulcer
• Pain begins 2 to 4 hours after a meal.		
• Ingestion of food or antacids brings relief.		
• Changes in bowel habits		
• Heartburn or retrosternal burning		
• Pain and tenderness in the right or left lower quadrant, may be sharp and severe on standing or stooping		Ovarian cyst
• Abdominal distention		
• Mild nausea and vomiting		
• Occasional menstrual irregularities		
• Slight fever		
• Referred, severe upper abdominal pain, tenderness, and rigidity that diminish with inspiration		Pneumonia
• Fever, shaking, chills, aches, and pains		
• Blood-tinged or rusty sputum		
• Dry, hacking cough		
• Dyspnea		
Diarrhea		
• Diarrhea occurs within several hours of ingesting milk or milk products.		Lactose intolerance
• Abdominal pain, cramping, and bloating		
• Flatus		
• Recurrent bloody diarrhea with pus or mucus		Ulcerative colitis
• Hyperactive bowel sounds		
• Cramping lower abdominal pain		
• Occasional nausea and vomiting		
Hematochezia		
• Moderate to severe rectal bleeding		Coagulation disorders
• Epistaxis (nosebleed)		
• Purpura (skin rash resulting from bleeding into the skin from small blood vessels)		
• Bright-red rectal bleeding with or without pain		Colon cancer
• Diarrhea or ribbon-shaped stools		
• Stools may be grossly bloody		
• Weakness and fatigue		
• Abdominal aching and dull cramps		
• Chronic bleeding with defecation		Hemorrhoids
• Painful defecation		
Nausea and Vomiting		
• May follow or accompany abdominal pain		Appendicitis
• Pain progresses rapidly to severe, stabbing pain in the right lower quadrant (McBurney sign).		
• Abdominal rigidity and tenderness		
• Constipation or diarrhea		
• Tachycardia		
• Nausea and vomiting of undigested food		Gastroenteritis
• Diarrhea		
• Abdominal cramping		
• Hyperactive bowel sounds		
• Fever		
• Headache with severe, constant, throbbing pain		Migraine headache
• Fatigue		
• Photophobia		
• Light flashes		
• Increased noise sensitivity		

or kidney dysfunction can affect the production of certain hormones that regulate red blood cell production.

The primary functions of the urinary system are the formation of urine and the maintenance of homeostasis. These functions are performed by the kidneys. Kidney dysfunction can cause trouble with concentration, memory loss, or disorientation. Progressive chronic kidney failure can also cause lethargy, confusion, disorientation, stupor, convulsions, and coma. Observation of the patient's vital signs may give indication of hypertension, which may be related to renal dysfunction if the hypertension is uncontrolled.

Anatomy and Physiology of the Urinary System

The urinary system consists of the kidneys, ureters, bladder, and urethra.

Kidneys. The kidneys are highly vascular organs that function to produce urine and maintain homeostasis in the body. The two bean-shaped organs of the kidneys are located in the retroperitoneal cavity along either side of the vertebral column. The peritoneal fat layer protects the kidneys. The right kidney lies slightly lower than the left because it is displaced by the liver. Each kidney contains about 1 million nephrons. Urine gathers in the collecting tubules and ducts and eventually drains into the ureters, then the bladder, and through the urethra (via urination).

Ureters. The ureters are 25 to 30 cm long. The narrowest part of the ureter is at the ureteropelvic junction. The other two constricted areas occur as the ureter leaves the renal pelvis and at the point it enters into the bladder wall. The ureters carry urine from the kidneys to the bladder by peristaltic contractions that occur one to five times per minute.

Bladder. The bladder is the vessel where urine collects. Bladder capacity ranges from 500 to 1000 ml in healthy adults. Children and older adults have less bladder capacity. When the bladder is empty, it lies behind the symphysis pubis; when it is full, it becomes displaced under the peritoneal cavity and serves as an excellent "window" for the sonographer to view the pelvic structures.

Urethra. The urethra is a small duct that carries urine from the bladder to the outside of the body. It is only 2.5 to 5 cm long and opens anterior to the vaginal opening. In the male, the urethra measures about 15 cm as it travels through the penis.

Common Signs and Symptoms Related to Urinary Dysfunction

The most common symptom of urinary dysfunction for both women and men is urinary incontinence. For women, a common symptom is dysuria, which often means a urinary tract infection. For men, common signs of urinary dysfunction include urethral discharge and

TABLE 2-2	Signs and Probable Indications of Urinary Dysfunction in Women	
Signs or Symptoms	**Probable Indication**
Dysuria	
• Urinary frequency • Nocturia • Straining to void • Hematuria • Perineal or low-back pain • Fatigue • Low-grade fever	Cystitis
• Dysuria throughout voiding • Bladder distention • Diminished urinary stream • Urinary frequency and urgency • Sensation of bloating or fullness in the lower abdomen or groin	Urinary system obstruction
• Urinary urgency • Hematuria • Cloudy urine • Bladder spasms • Feeling of warmth or burning during urination	Urinary tract infection
Urinary Incontinence	
• Urge or overflow incontinence • Hematuria • Dysuria • Nocturia • Urinary frequency • Suprapubic pain from bladder spasms • Palpable mass on bimanual examination	Bladder cancer
• Overflow incontinence • Painless bladder distention • Episodic diarrhea or constipation • Orthostatic hypotension • Syncope • Dysphagia	Diabetic neuropathy
• Urinary urgency and frequency • Visual problems • Sensory impairment • Constipation • Muscle weakness	Multiple sclerosis

urinary hesitancy. Tables 2-2 and 2-3 summarize the most common symptoms and probable causes of urinary dysfunction for women and men, respectively.

Dysuria. Dysuria is painful or difficult urination and is commonly accompanied by urinary frequency, urgency, or hesitancy. This symptom usually reflects a common female disorder of a lower urinary tract infection (UTI).

Pertinent questions for the patient would include how long the patient has noticed the symptoms, whether anything precipitates them, if anything aggravates or alleviates them, and where exactly the discomfort is felt. You might also ask if the patient has undergone a recent

TABLE 2-3	Signs and Probable Indications of Urinary Dysfunction in Men	
Signs or Symptoms		**Probable Indication**
Scrotal Swelling		
• Swollen scrotum that is soft or unusually firm • Bowel sounds may be heard in the scrotum		Hernia
• Gradual scrotal swelling • Scrotum may be soft and cystic or firm and tense • Painless • Round, nontender scrotal mass on palpation • Glowing when transilluminated		Hydrocele
• Scrotal swelling with sudden and severe pain • Unilateral elevation of the affected testicle • Nausea and vomiting		Testicular torsion
Urethral Discharge		
• Purulent or milky urethral discharge • Sudden fever and chills • Lower back pain • Myalgia (muscle pain) • Perineal fullness • Arthralgia • Urinary frequency and urgency • Cloudy urine • Dysuria • Tense, boggy, very tender, and warm prostate palpated on digital rectal examination		Prostatitis
• Opaque, gray, yellowish, or blood-tinged discharge that is painless • Dysuria • Eventual anuria		Urethral neoplasm
• Scant or profuse urethral discharge that is thin and clear, mucoid, or thick and purulent • Urinary hesitancy, frequency, and urgency • Dysuria • Itching and burning around the meatus		Urethritis
Urinary Hesitancy		
• Reduced caliber and force of urinary stream • Perineal pain • Feeling of incomplete voiding • Inability to stop the urine stream • Urinary frequency • Urinary incontinence • Bladder distention		Benign prostatic hyperplasia
• Urinary frequency and dribbling • Nocturia • Dysuria • Bladder distention • Perineal pain • Constipation • Hard, nodular prostate palpated on digital rectal examination		Prostate cancer
• Dysuria • Urinary frequency and urgency • Hematuria • Cloudy urine • Bladder spasms • Costovertebral angle tenderness • Suprapubic, low back, pelvic, or flank pain • Urethral discharge		Urinary tract infection

invasive procedure such as a cystoscopy or urethral dilatation.

Urinary Incontinence. Urinary incontinence is the uncontrollable passage of urine. Incontinence results from a bladder abnormality or a neurologic disorder. A common urologic sign may involve large volumes of urine or dribbling. This condition would be important for the sonographer if a full bladder were required. It may be difficult for the patient to hold large enough volumes of fluid to fill the bladder for proper visualization.

Male Urethral Discharge. Male urethral discharge is discharge from the urinary meatus that may be purulent, mucoid, or thin; sanguineous or clear. It usually develops suddenly. The patient may have other signs of fever, chills, or perineal fullness. Previous history of prostate problems, sexually transmitted disease, or urinary tract infections may be associated with this condition.

Male Urinary Hesitancy. Male urinary hesitancy is a condition that usually arises gradually with a decrease in urinary stream. When the bladder becomes distended, the discomfort increases. Often prostate problems, previous urinary tract infection or obstruction, or neuromuscular disorders are associated with this condition.

PHYSIOLOGY AND LABORATORY DATA

The Circulatory System

Fundamental to an understanding of human physiology is knowledge of the circulatory system. Circulation of the blood throughout the body serves as a vital connection to the cells, tissues, and organs to maintain a relatively constant environment for cell activity.

Functions of the Blood. The blood is responsible for a variety of functions, including transportation of oxygen and nutrients, defense against infection, and maintenance of pH. Blood is thicker than water and therefore flows more slowly than water. The specific gravity of blood may be calculated by comparing the weight of blood versus water; with water being 1.00, blood is in the range of 1.045 to 1.065.

Acidic versus Alkaline. The hydrogen ion and the hydroxyl ion are found within water. When a solution contains more hydrogen than hydroxyl ions, it is called an **acidic** solution. Likewise, when it contains more hydroxyl ions than hydrogen ions, it is referred to as an **alkaline** solution. This concentration of hydrogen ions in a solution is called the pH, with the scale ranging up to 14.0.

In water, an equal concentration of both ions exists; water is thus a neutral solution, or 7.0 on the pH scale. Human blood has a pH of 7.34 to 7.44, being slightly alkaline. A blood pH below 6.8 is a condition called *acidosis;* blood pH above 7.8 is known as *alkalosis.* Both conditions can lead to serious illness and eventual death unless proper balance is restored. To help in this process, blood plasma is supplied with chemical compounds called *buffers.* These buffers can act as weak acids or bases to combine with excess hydrogen or hydroxyl ions to neutralize the pH. Plasma is the basic supporting fluid and transporting vehicle of the blood. It constitutes 55% of the total blood volume.

The volume of blood in the body depends on the body surface area; however, the total volume may be estimated as approximately 9% of total body weight. Therefore, blood volume is approximately 5 quarts in a normal-sized man.

The red blood cells (**erythrocytes**), the white blood cells (**leukocytes**), and the platelets (**thrombocytes**) make up the remainder of the blood. The percent of the total blood volume containing these three elements is called the **hematocrit.** Normally, the hematocrit is described as 45, or 45% of the total blood volume (with plasma accounting for the remaining 55%).

Red Blood Cells. Red blood cells (RBCs) are disk-shaped, biconcave cells without a nucleus. They are formed in the bone marrow and are the most prevalent of the formed elements in the blood. Their primary role is to carry oxygen to the cells and tissues of the body. Oxygen is picked up by a protein in the red cell called *hemoglobin.* Hemoglobin releases oxygen in the capillaries of the tissues.

The production of red blood cells is called *erythropoiesis.* Their life span is approximately 120 days. Vitamin B_{12} is necessary for complete maturity of the red blood cells. The inner mucosal lining of the stomach secretes a substance called the intrinsic factor, which promotes absorption of vitamin B_{12} from ingested food. **Anemia** is an abnormal condition where the blood lacks either a normal number of red blood cells or normal concentration of hemoglobin. If too many red blood cells are produced, **polycythemia** results.

As old red blood cells are destroyed in the liver, part of the hemoglobin is converted to bilirubin, which is excreted by the liver in the form of **bile.** When excessive amounts of hemoglobin are broken down, or when biliary excretion is decreased by liver disease or biliary obstruction, the plasma bilirubin level rises. This rise in plasma bilirubin results in a yellow-skin condition known as jaundice.

White Blood Cells. White blood cells (WBCs) are the body's primary defense against infection. WBCs lack hemoglobin, are colorless, contain a nucleus, and are larger than RBCs. White cells are extremely active and move with an ameboid motion, often against the flow of blood. They can pass from the bloodstream into intracellular spaces to phagocytize foreign matter found between the cells. A condition called *leukopoiesis* is WBC formation stimulated by the presence of bacteria.

Granulocytes. Neutrophils, eosinophils, and basophils are the groups of leukocytes called granulocytes because of the presence of granules in their cytoplasm. Their function is to ingest and destroy bacteria with the formation of pus.

The basophils contain heparin and control clotting. The eosinophils increase in patients with allergic diseases.

Lymphocytes and Monocytes. The lymphocytes are WBCs formed in lymphatic tissue. They enter the blood by way of the lymphatic system and contain antibodies responsible for delayed hypersensitivity reactions. Monocytes are large white cells capable of phagocytosis and are quite mobile. Their numbers are few, and they are produced in the bone marrow.

The differential complete blood count (CBC) is a laboratory blood test that evaluates and states specific values for all these subgroups of white blood cells.

White cells have two main sources: (1) red bone marrow (granulocytes) and (2) lymphatic tissue (lymphocytes). When an increase in the white cells arises from a tumor of the bone marrow, it is called *myelogenous leukemia* and is noted as an increase in granulocytes. On the other hand, an increase in WBCs caused by overactive lymphoid tissue is called *lymphatic leukemia*, with an increase in lymphocytes. Splenomegaly and prominent lymph nodes may be imaged during an ultrasound examination.

In bacterial infections, the white cells increase in number (leukocytosis), with most of the increase noted in the neutrophils. A decrease in the total white cell count (leukopenia) is a result of a viral infection.

Thrombocytes. Thrombocytes, or blood platelets, are formed from giant cells in the bone marrow. They initiate a chain of events involved in blood clotting together with a plasma protein called fibrinogen. Thrombocytes are destroyed by the liver and have a life span of 8 days.

Blood Composition. Plasma makes up 55% of the total blood volume and consists of about 92% water. The remaining 8% comprises numerous substances suspended or dissolved in this water. Hemoglobin of the red cells accounts for two thirds of the blood proteins, with the remaining consisting of plasma proteins. These include serum albumin, globulin, fibrinogen, and prothrombin.

Serum album constitutes 53% of the total plasma proteins. It is produced in the liver and serves to regulate blood volume. Globulin can be separated into alpha, beta, and gamma globulin. The latter is involved in immune reactions in the body's defense against infection. Fibrinogen is concerned with coagulation of blood. Prothrombin is produced in the liver and participates in blood coagulation. Vitamin K is essential for prothrombin production.

The Liver and the Biliary System

Both the liver and the biliary system play a role in the digestive and circulatory systems. As food enters the small intestine, nutrients are absorbed by the walls of the intestine. These nutrients enter the blood through the walls of the portal system. The portal venous system is a special transporting system that serves to carry nutrient-rich blood from the intestines to the liver for metabolic and storage purposes. The hepatic artery supplies nutrient-rich blood to the liver through the porta hepatis, whereas the biliary system drains bile products from the liver and gallbladder through the porta hepatis.

The liver consists of rows of cubical cells that radiate from a central vein. On one side of these cells lie blood vessels that are slightly larger than capillaries and are called *sinusoids*. Blood from the portal vein and the hepatic artery is brought into the liver to be filtered by these sinusoids, which in turn empty into the central vein. The bile ducts lie on the other side of the sinusoids. The bile pigment—old, worn-out blood cells and materials derived from phagocytosis—is removed from the blood by special hepatic cells called *Kupffer cells* and is deposited into the bile ducts as bile.

The **Kupffer cells** are located in the sinusoids and are capable of ingesting bacteria and other foreign matter from the blood. These cells are part of the reticuloendothelial system of the liver and spleen.

The bilirubin arises from the hemoglobin of disintegrating red blood cells, which have been broken down by the Kupffer cells. After the bilirubin is formed, it combines with plasma albumin. The primary function of albumin is to maintain the osmotic pressure of the blood. When this serum albumin is lowered, conditions such as liver disease, malnutrition, and chronic nephritis should be considered.

The combination of bilirubin with plasma albumin is considered as unconjugated, or indirect, bilirubin. The parenchyma cells of the liver excrete this bile pigment into the bile canaliculi. It is during this process that the bilirubin-plasma albumin chemical bond is broken and becomes conjugated, or direct, bilirubin, which is excreted into the biliary passages. This conjugation process occurs only in the hepatic parenchymal cells. Excreted bilirubin forced back into the bloodstream in cases of biliary obstruction results in elevated serum bilirubin of the direct type. If an abnormal amount of indirect bilirubin is found, it was probably caused by an increase in red blood cell breakdown and hemoglobin conversion.

Direct bilirubin enters the small bowel by way of the common bile duct and is acted upon by bacteria to form urobilinogen (urine) or stercobilinogen (feces). A portion of the pigment is reabsorbed and is carried by the portal circulation to the liver, where it is reconverted into bilirubin. A small amount escapes into the general circulation and is excreted by the kidneys. The pooling of these bile pigments as a result of biliary obstruction or liver disease causes spillover into the tissues and general circulation, resulting in jaundice.

Jaundice. Jaundice is identified by its site of disruption of normal bilirubin metabolism: prehepatic, hepatic, or posthepatic. In prehepatic jaundice, no intrinsic disease is present in the liver or biliary tract. It is simply increased amounts of bilirubin being presented to the liver for excretion. No obstruction is present; therefore, bilirubin is not forced back into the bloodstream, and no significant increase in direct bilirubin is found. However, increased amounts of urobilinogen are present in the intestinal tract and subsequently in the feces and urine.

Hepatic jaundice is caused by intrinsic hepatic parenchymal injury or disease. This may be the result of infection with hepatitis, drugs, tumor growth, or injury from toxic agents. Lack of bilirubin transfer by the hepatic cells results in piling up of unconjugated bilirubin and increased amounts of conjugated bilirubin in the body's circulation. Clinically, the patient has an enlarged and tender liver (with or without splenomegaly). Also noted are decreased appetite, nausea, and vomiting. Laboratory data would show elevation of total serum bilirubin, positive urinary bilirubin, urinary urobilinogen as normal or elevated, and fecal urobilinogen as normal or decreased.

Posthepatic jaundice is a partial or complete blockage of the biliary tract by calculi, tumor, fibrosis, or extrinsic pressure that results in a conjugated bilirubin. Biliary calculi are classically manifested by colicky upper abdominal pain in the right upper quadrant that radiates to the shoulder. It may be accompanied by intermittent or increasing jaundice. On the other hand, tumor obstruction at the common bile duct tends to be painless, with increasing and unremitting jaundice. The total serum bilirubin is elevated, the urinary bilirubin is positive, the urinary urobilinogen is decreased or normal, and the fecal urobilinogen is decreased.

In addition to the transport of nutrients to the body, the liver provides energy for body tissues. This process is done through the use of carbohydrates and their storage and by the release of sugars. After the nutrient sugars are absorbed by the small intestine, the sugars are transported to the liver by way of the portal system (superior mesenteric vein). The hepatic cells convert most of the sugars into glycogen, during a process called glycogenesis, for storage.

If the levels of available glucose in the blood are lower than normal, the liver can break down the available glycogen back into glucose (glycogenolysis) to maintain a normal blood glucose level. The most important use of glucose is the oxidation of glucose by tissue cells. When glucose is oxidized by the tissues, carbon dioxide and water are formed, and energy is released. Most tissues use glucose for their supply of energy.

The Pancreas. The pancreas plays an important role in the regulation of these carbohydrates. The secretion of insulin and glucagons from the islets of Langerhans provides for cellular control by promoting oxidation of glucose by the tissue cells. Inside the cell, released energy is stored as adenosine triphosphate (ATP) in the mitochondria. Only small molecules can enter the mitochondrial membrane; this can occur only by breakdown of nutrient molecules to pyruvic acid and then to acetic acid. Once inside the mitochondria, the components

combine to form citric acid. This series of reactions is called the *Krebs cycle*. The result is the release of carbon dioxide and energy. The Krebs cycle is also involved in the metabolism of fat and proteins. This is the principal energy cycle in the body.

Fat. Fat enters the system in the form of fatty acids, glycerol, phospholipids, and cholesterol. A small amount is produced in the liver, but most is synthesized in adipose tissue. Fat deposits in the body provide a concentrated source of energy and furnish about 40% of the energy used. Absorbed fats are acted upon by special cells in the liver (lipolysis), and the resultant products are channeled into the Krebs cycle for the release of energy. The production of fats (lipogenesis) results from an excess of fatty acids and glycerol, which combine to form triglyceride.

Besides being a source of energy, stored fats act as a cushion for the internal organs. The phospholipids are used in the formation of plasma membranes. Fats are completely broken down to carbon dioxide and water with release of energy, and this process occurs predominantly in the liver. The end product of fatty acid oxidation is ketone or acetone bodies, which are secreted in the urine. In patients with uncontrolled diabetes, the sugar is not used properly and excessive fat metabolizes.

Cholesterol. Cholesterol is found in fats and is derived from a diet of animal foods, such as egg yolks and meats. Cholesterol may serve as the substance from which various hormones are synthesized. High cholesterol levels have an adverse effect on the cardiovascular system. An increase in cholesterol levels is seen in liver disease, whereas a decrease in serum cholesterol is found in acute infections, malnutrition, and anemias.

Amino Acids. Amino acids absorbed from the intestine are used in the production of proteins. They may be converted to fatty acids and glycogen, or they may be oxidized as an energy source. The transfer of the amino group to other substances is called transamination. Enzymes associated with this process are useful in the diagnosis of hepatic disease. These enzymes are found in the blood: aspartate aminotransferase (AST) (formerly serum glutamic-oxaloacetic transaminase [SGOT]); and alanine aminotransferase (ALT) (formerly serum glutamic-pyruvic transaminase [SGPT]). An increase in these enzymes is noted in the presence of hepatic cell necrosis caused by viral hepatitis and toxic hepatitis. However, a significant increase in chronic liver disease or in obstructive jaundice has not been observed.

Another important enzyme is alkaline phosphatase. This is normally found in the serum in an acid or alkaline state. (Acid phosphatase is used primarily in assessing prostate cancer.) Alkaline phosphatase is helpful in identifying disorders of the liver and biliary tract. An increase may be seen in patients with biliary obstruction.

Lactic dehydrogenase (LDH) is another enzyme found in the liver. This level may be increased in conditions such as liver disease, acute leukemia, malignant lymphoma, and carcinoma. LDH is also found in cardiac tissue, and an increase may indicate myocardial infarction.

Blood Clotting. Another important function of the liver is the production of various factors involved in blood clotting. Prothrombin is converted to thrombin in the clotting process. The prothrombin content in the blood is lower in liver diseases, drug therapy, and vitamin K deficiency.

Detoxification. An essential function of the liver is detoxification. The liver breaks down a variety of toxins by way of chemical reactions.

The Gallbladder. Bile is constantly being secreted by the liver cells. It collects in the bile canaliculi, which are tiny channels in the liver, and from there, flows into bile ducts. The bile canaliculi merge to form bile ductules, which eventually become the common bile duct. The common bile duct joins the pancreatic duct where it enters the duodenum at the ampulla of Vater. If no food is in the upper digestive tract, then most of the bile is diverted into the gallbladder. The gallbladder stores and concentrates the bile. After food is consumed, three events occur: (1) The bile enters the small bowel because of relaxation of the sphincter of Oddi; (2) the gallbladder contracts; and (3) liver secretions increase. This process is initiated by the enzyme cholecystokinin, which is released when fats and proteins reach the duodenum. Therefore, bile plays an important role in the intestinal breakdown and absorption of fat and is the vehicle of excretion of the end product of hemoglobin breakdown.

The amount of bile excreted daily ranges from 250 to 1000 ml. Bile is made up mostly of water, bile salts, and other organic substances in small amounts, including cholesterol. Bile salts are derived from metabolism of hemoglobin. In addition to digesting and absorbing fats, bile emulsifies fats into minute particles. This provides a pathway by which the pancreatic lipase can act upon the fats to further aid digestion. At the completion of their digestive function, bile salts are returned via the portal system to the liver for reuse. Gallstones may form as the result of excessive cholesterol and bile salt deposits.

Obstruction of a bile duct prevents flow of bile, and increases in liver secretions cause a backflow of bile in the liver, with spillover into the blood and tissue, resulting in jaundice. As a result of obstruction, excessive excretion of fat is noted in the feces because of lack of digestion and absorption in the intestine secondary to the absence of bile salts.

Laboratory Tests for Hepatic and Biliary Function

No single laboratory test can fully evaluate liver function in a healthy or diseased state. The most commonly used tests to evaluate hepatic and biliary function are pre-sented in Table 2-4. Normal laboratory values should be obtained from your respective laboratory.

The Pancreas

Endocrine Function. The pancreas functions both as an exocrine gland and as an endocrine gland. Endocrine function is carried out by small areas of specialized tissue called the *islets of Langerhans,* which are scattered throughout the gland. Two important hormones secreted are insulin and glucagon. Insulin is responsible for causing an increase in the rate of glucose metabolism.

Glucose does not readily pass through the cell pores without the help of some transport mechanism provided by insulin. In the absence of insulin, the rate of glucose transport is about one-fourth the normal value. Conversely, an excess of insulin multiplies the normal rate. Insulin is also responsible for regulation of blood glucose levels.

In the presence of insulin, glucose is transported to the tissue cells so fast that the blood glucose level may drop. Diabetes mellitus is a disease caused by inadequate secretion of insulin by the pancreas. This results in the cells' inability to use glucose and an increase in the blood sugar level (hyperglycemia).

Glucagon mobilizes glucose from the liver, which causes an increase in blood glucose concentration. When the blood glucose concentration falls, the pancreas secretes large quantities of glucagons to compensate.

Exocrine Function. The pancreas is the most active and versatile of the digestive organs. In the absence of other digestive secretions, its enzymes alone are capable of almost completing total digestion. Pancreatic juice consists of three basic groups of enzymes: carbohydrate, fat, and trypsin.

The carbohydrate enzyme is pancreatic amylase, which acts upon starch and glycogen and produces the sugar maltose. The fat enzyme is pancreatic lipase and is capable of breaking down fats to monoglycerides and fatty acids. Trypsin ultimately digests proteins and peptides partially digested in the stomach. The end products of trypsin digestion are amino acids and polypeptides.

The digestion of food is incomplete without the action of the pancreatic enzymes. Lack of these enzymes may be due to obstruction in the pancreatic duct or to diseases that impair the ability of the pancreas to produce these enzymes in proper amounts. If adequate digestion and absorption do not occur, amounts of carbohydrates increase, and protein is found in the feces.

Pancreatic juice also contains a high concentration of sodium bicarbonate, which is responsible for neutralization of gastric acid and a decrease in chloride concentration. The release of pancreatic juice is stimulated by secretin and pancreozymin (similar to cholecystokinin in the gallbladder). These hormones increase the volume of pancreatic secretion and increase the amount of bicarbonate in secretion. They also increase sodium levels but

TABLE 2-4	Laboratory Tests for Hepatic and Biliary Function
Laboratory Test	**Description and Possible Indications**
White blood count	White blood count (WBC) depicts the number of white cells in the blood. A high WBC may be a sign of infection.
Red blood count	Red blood cells (RBCs) are the most common type of blood cell. These are oxygen-rich cells that deliver oxygen to all parts of the body. Blood disease that impedes the production of RBCs includes many types of anemia (sickle cell, thalassemia, pernicious anemia). A surplus of RBCs is seen in polycythemia vera. Decreased RBCs may be associated with leukemia, Hodgkin's disease, or severe diarrhea.
Hemoglobin (Hgb)	Hemoglobin is the amount of oxygen-carrying protein contained within the red blood cells. A low count may suggest anemia. A high count may occur with pulmonary disease or excessive bone marrow production of blood cells.
Hct	This is the packed cell volume that is the proportion of blood occupied by RBCs.
Prothrombin time (PT)	This test is used to determine the clotting tendency of blood, in liver damage, to assess vitamin K status, and to measure the warfarin dosage.
Bilirubin	Bilirubin is derived from the breakdown of hemoglobin in red blood cells and is excreted by the liver in the bile. When destruction of red cells increases greatly, or when the liver is unable to excrete the normal amounts of bilirubin produced, the concentration in the serum rises. If it rises too high, jaundice may appear. The bilirubin test will spot the increase early before the onset of jaundice. Intrahepatic and extrahepatic obstruction may be determined by knowing the levels of direct and indirect bilirubin. This may be seen as an increase in conjugated or direct bilirubin. An increase in unconjugated or indirect bilirubin is indicative of an increase in red blood cell destruction or hemolysis.
Cholesterol	Cholesterol is found in the blood and in all cells. Hepatic disease may alter its metabolism. Total cholesterol is normal or decreased in hepatitis or cirrhosis, but increased in primary biliary cirrhosis and extrabiliary obstruction.
Glucose (blood)	Abnormal blood glucose levels may indicate problems with the liver's ability to metabolize glucose. Decreased glucose levels are associated with extensive liver disease, and elevated levels are associated with chronic renal failure, renal disease, and pancreatitis. The use of glucose by the body cells is intimately related to the blood level of insulin, the hormone secreted by the islets of Langerhans in the pancreas.
Alkaline phosphatase	This is found in the serum, and the value rises in disorders of the liver and biliary tract when excretion is impaired (i.e., obstruction). Alkaline phosphatase levels are elevated typically in obstructive jaundice, biliary cirrhosis, acute hepatitis, and granulomatous liver disease.
Aspartate aminotransferase (AST) (formerly SGOT)	This enzyme is increased in the presence of liver cell necrosis secondary to viral hepatitis, toxic hepatitis, and other acute forms. No significant increase is usually seen in chronic liver disease, such as cirrhosis or obstructive jaundice.
Alanine aminotransferase (ALT) (formerly SGPT)	This enzyme rises higher than AST in cases of hepatitis. It falls slowly and reaches normal levels in 2 to 3 months.
Lactic acid dehydrogenase	Lactic acid dehydrogenase (LDH) is present in nearly all metabolizing cells, with highest concentrations in tissues of kidneys, heart, skeletal muscle, brain, and liver, and in RBCs. Tissue damage causes this enzyme to be released into the bloodstream. Persistent, slightly increased LDH levels are associated with hepatitis, cirrhosis, and obstructive jaundice.
Prothrombin time	Prothrombin is converted to thrombin in the clotting process. This is made possible by the action of vitamin K that is absorbed in the intestine and stored in the liver.
Urinary bile and bilirubin	Spillover into the blood may occur in obstructive liver disease, or where an excess of red blood cell destruction occurs. Bile pigments are found in the urine with obstruction of the biliary tract. Bilirubin is found alone with excessive breakdown of red blood cells.
Urinary urobilinogen	This test may be used to differentiate between complete and incomplete obstruction of the biliary tract. Urobilinogen is a product of hemoglobin breakdown that may be found in hemolytic diseases, liver damage, and severe infections. In cases of complete obstructive jaundice, no excess of urobilinogen is usually seen in the urine.
Fecal urobilinogen	Considerable amounts of urobilinogen are found in the feces, but an increase or decrease in normal amounts may indicate hepatic digestive abnormalities. In complete obstruction of the biliary tree, values are decreased, whereas an increase in fecal urobilinogen may suggest an increase in hemolysis.

TABLE 2-5	Laboratory Tests for Pancreatic Function
Laboratory Test	**Description and Possible Indications**
Serum amylase	An increase in serum amylase levels may be a result of pancreatic disease, which causes the digestive enzymes to escape into the surrounding tissue and results in necrosis and severe pain with inflammation. **Example:** acute pancreatitis and obstruction, acute cholecystitis–high serum amylase
Serum lipase	In diseases such as acute pancreatitis and carcinoma of the pancreas, both amylase and lipase rise at the same rate, but lipase persists for a longer time.
Glucose tolerance test (GTT)	Large amounts of glucose are administered and blood sugar levels are monitored. The glucose should be metabolized in less than 3 hours, otherwise diabetes is suspected. If slow to return to normal, liver disease may also be involved.
Urinary amylase	Amylase in the serum is excreted in the urine and can be measured. Will remain higher in abnormal disease states than the serum amylase.
Ketone bodies	Ketone bodies are excreted in the urine as a result of faulty metabolism. Sugar is not used properly and excessive fat metabolizes. The fats produce ketone bodies and acetone, and when these levels rise, spillover into the urine occurs. This is usually a result of improperly controlled or uncontrolled diabetes.

TABLE 2-6	Laboratory Tests for Urinary Disease
Laboratory Test	**Description and Possible Indications**
Urine pH	• pH refers to the strength of the urine as a partly acidic or alkaline solution. • Abundance of hydrogen ions in a solution is called pH. When urine has more hydrogen ions than hydroxyl ions, it is acidic. It is alkaline when it has more hydroxyl ions. • Important in diagnosing and managing bacteriuria and renal calculi. Renal calculi are somewhat dependent on pH of urine. • Alkaline urine is associated with renal tubular acidosis, chronic renal failure, and other urinary tract disorders.
Specific gravity	• Measurement of kidney's ability to concentrate urine • The urine concentration factor is dependent on the quantity of dissolved waste products within it. • Excessive intake of fluids or decrease in perspiration may cause large output of urine and decrease in specific gravity (also low in renal failure, glomerular nephritis, and pyelonephritis). • Low fluid intake, excessive perspiration, or diarrhea will cause the output of urine to be low and the specific gravity to increase (may also be high in nephrosis).
Blood (hematuria)	• Appearance of blood cell casts in the urine • Can be associated with early renal disease
Protein (albuminuria)	• Found when glomerular damage is apparent—albumin and other plasma proteins may be filtered in excess—allows overflow to enter the urine, which lowers the blood serum albumin concentration • Found with benign and malignant neoplasms, nephritis, calculi, chronic infection, and pyelonephritis
Red cell casts	• Occur when red blood cells in lumen of nephron tubule become trapped and elongated gelled proteins • Indicate bleeding has occurred into the nephrons • Abundance of casts may indicate renal trauma, calculi, or pyelonephritis.
White cells and white cell casts	• Leukocytes may be present whenever there is inflammation, infection, or tissue necrosis originating from anywhere within the genitourinary tract.
Creatinine clearance	• Specific measurements of creatinine concentrations in urine and blood serum are considered an accurate index for determining the glomerular filtration rate (GFR). • A decreased urinary creatinine clearance indicates renal dysfunction because it prevents the normal excretion of creatinine.
Hematocrit	• Refers to the relative ratio of plasma to packed cell volume in the blood • Decrease in hematocrit will occur with acute hemorrhagic process secondary to disease or blunt trauma.
Hemoglobin	• Presence of hemoglobin in urine occurs whenever there is extensive damage or destruction of functioning erythrocytes. • Hemoglobinuria can cause acute renal failure.
Blood urea nitrogen (BUN)	• Concentration of urea nitrogen in blood—end product of cellular metabolism • Urea is formed in the liver and is carried to the kidneys through the blood to be excreted in the urine. • Impairment of renal function and increased protein catabolism will result in blood urea nitrogen (BUN) elevation in relation to the degree of renal impairment and the rate of urea nitrogen excreted by the kidneys.
Serum creatinine	• Renal dysfunction will result in elevation of serum creatinine. • More sensitive than BUN in determining renal impairment

decrease chloride and potassium. Incompletely digested proteins and peptides are found as increased amounts of total fecal nitrogen.

Laboratory Tests for Pancreatic Function

Tests most commonly used to evaluate pancreatic function are presented in Table 2-5.

The Kidneys

The renal arteries carry approximately 25% of the cardiac output to the kidneys. This ensures the maintenance of an increased level of blood pressure as it reaches the cortical portion of the kidneys via the interlobar and arcuate arteries. These arteries branch into smaller afferent arterioles, which leads to a complex network of capillaries, called the glomeruli. From this point, the capillaries branch into the efferent arterioles to the peritubular capillaries and course through the venules to the returning blood supply of the renal veins and inferior vena cava.

The vascular anatomy is critical in supplying vital nutrients for the important functional unit of the kidney, the *nephron*. At least 1 million nephrons are present in each normal adult kidney. Within the nephron complex, a diffusion process takes place to maintain continual homeostasis of blood plasma and other nutrient components for the body.

The two major parts of the nephron are the glomerulus and the renal tubules. These structures have a direct role in the production of urine by means of three processes: filtration, reabsorption, and secretion.

1. Glomerular filtration is the first step in urine formation. This filtration process takes place through the glomerular capsular membrane, which surrounds the glomerulus. Glomerular filtration is directly affected by the blood pressure of the glomerular arterial capillaries, which forces an essentially protein-free filtrate consisting mainly of blood plasma through the permeable glomerular capsular membrane, *Bowman's capsule*.
2. *Bowman's capsule* provides the basis for determining the filtration permeability factor and the glomerular filtration rate.
3. Most of the filtered volume is reabsorbed back into the renal tubules along with many vital components of the filtrate, such as glucose, sodium, potassium, chlorides, and other essential nutrients in extracellular fluid.
4. As the remaining filtrate continues through the renal tubules, more solutes are added by secretions from the tubular epithelial cells.
5. Some of these cells are excreted with the remaining constituents of urine.

Laboratory Tests for the Kidney

Urinary tract disorders are usually detected through analysis of urine (urinalysis). Urine samples may be collected randomly or over a prolonged period of time. Table 2-6 lists the most common laboratory tests for urinary disease.

Essentials of Patient Care for the Sonographer

Marveen Craig

On completion of this chapter, you should be able to:
- Define patient-focused care
- Discuss the basic patient care techniques covered in this chapter
- Describe patient transfer techniques
- Discuss infection control and isolation techniques
- Demonstrate the ability to respond to common medical emergencies
- Describe how to assist patients with special needs
- Define patient rights and HIPAA

OUTLINE

A Sonographer's Obligations
   Patient-Focused Care
Basic Patient Care
   Vital Signs
Patients on Strict Bed Rest
   Bedpans and Urinals
   Emesis Basins
Patients with Tubes and Tubing
   Intravenous Therapy
   Nasogastric Suction Tubes
   Catheters
   Oxygen Therapy
   Wounds, Drains, and Dressings
   Ostomies

Patient Transfer Techniques
   Body Mechanics
   Moving Patients Up in Bed
   Assisting Patients To and From the Scanning Table
   Wheelchair Transfers
   Stretcher Transfers
Infection Control
   Standard Precautions
   Additional Precautions
   Nosocomial Infections
Isolation Techniques
Emergency Medical Situations
   Choking
   Cardiopulmonary Resuscitation
   Basic Cardiac Life Support

Professional Attitudes
   Reestablishing Patient-Focused Care
Assisting Patients with Special Needs
   Crying Patients
   Pediatric Patients
   Adolescent Patients
   Elderly Patients
   Culturally Diverse Patients
Evaluating Patient Reactions to Illness
   Terminal Patients
Patient Rights
   The Patients' Bill of Rights
   Health Insurance Portability and Accountability Act (HIPAA)

As a sonographer in training, the majority of your studies will focus on anatomic and clinical knowledge as well as the technical skills necessary to produce diagnostic ultrasound images. But another important area of study includes the basic patient care you will be expected to provide in clinical practice. The goal of this chapter is to prepare you to provide that care confidently, proficiently, and safely to the patient entrusted to your care.

A SONOGRAPHER'S OBLIGATIONS

As a sonographer, you have four main obligations: to your patients; to your sonologist, department, or institution; to the profession; and to yourself. Compassion, patience, and the desire to help people are qualities that will help you meet your obligations to your patients. Meeting the obligations to your sonologist and institution requires the ability to produce high-quality diagnostic studies, to project self-confidence and maturity, and to practice good interpersonal skills. A profession in diagnostic medical sonography requires you to act professionally at all times, to pass your registry examinations, and thereafter to continue your education in order to keep abreast of the growth and changes in the field. To achieve all of these goals, you have an important obligation to maintain good physical and mental health by practicing proper nutrition, engaging in adequate exercise, and getting the rest and relaxation you need.

Patient-Focused Care

Florence Nightingale advocated focusing on the patient, rather than on the disease, as a way to recognize the many unique dimensions of the sick and wounded. By distinguishing patient care from medicine, Nightingale established the value of nurses and created the earliest patient advocates.

The most important facet of being a sonographer is seeing the patient as the primary focus of your efforts. Despite personal or philosophical concerns, you must be considerate of the patient's age, cultural traditions, personal values, and lifestyle. Good patient care goes beyond procedural skills. It includes communicating with patients and allowing them to express their individual problems, fears, and frustrations. It also requires you to cooperate with other departments and facilities and health care professionals in order to deliver the best and most complete patient care through a team effort.

Patient-focused care (PFC) represents a national movement to recapture the respect and goodwill of the American public. It is the beginning of a larger objective to ensure that every patient receives the best possible medical care. The patient-focused approach encourages sonographers to relate to patients as people with needs, who are to be respected and cared for in a mature and dignified manner.

BASIC PATIENT CARE

Vital Signs

Vital signs are the observable and measurable signs of life and include the following: pulse, respiratory rate, body temperature, and blood pressure. Vital signs are monitored as indicators of how a patient's body is functioning and to establish a baseline for further study. Changes in age and medical condition can alter the normal vital sign ranges. Box 3-1 provides a concise, age-related reference for normal vital signs. It is essential to take careful and accurate measurements of each of the vital signs, as well as to include observations about the patient's skin color and any comments patients make about how they feel or how they react while in your care.

Sonographers are not routinely required to assess vital signs unless performing specific ultrasound studies (e.g., cardiovascular, obstetrical) or in an emergency situation. When they do, the focus is on pulse, respiration and blood pressure. Practicing how to perform vital sign measurements on yourself or others will help you sharpen your skills before the need arises.

Pulse. When the heart actively pumps, blood is forced into large and small arteries during contractions of the left ventricle. The amount of force created when blood hits the arterial walls produces an advancing pressure wave that causes the arterial walls to expand. This expansion produces the feeling of a pulse that can be felt

---

BOX 3-1	Normal Vital Signs

Adult
Oral temperature: 96.8F to 99.5F
Normal pulse: 60–100
Normal respirations: 12–20
Normal blood pressure range: 100–139 diastolic; 60–89 systolic

Adolescent
Oral temperature: 97.5F–98.6F
Pulse: 55–90
Respirations: 12–20
Blood pressure: 121/70

School-Age Child
Oral temperature: 97.5F–98.6F
Pulse: 60–100
Respirations: 16–20
Blood pressure: 107/64

Preschool Child
Axillary temperature: 97.5F–98.6F
Pulse: 70–110
Respirations: 16–22
Blood pressure: 95/57

Toddler
Axillary temperature: 97.5F–98.6F
Pulse: 80–120
Respirations: 20–30
Blood pressure: 92/55

One-Year Old
Axillary temperature: 97.0F–99.0F
Pulse: 90–130
Respirations: 20–40
Blood pressure: 90/56

Newborn
Axillary temperature: 97.7F–99.5F
Pulse: 120–160
Respirations: 30–60
Blood pressure: 73/55 systolic

Data from *Mosby's expert physical exam handbook: rapid inpatient and outpatient assessments,* ed 3, St. Louis, 2009, Mosby.
Data from Silvestri LA: *Saunder's comprehensive review for the NCLEX-RN examination,* ed 4, Philadelphia, 2008, Saunders.

---

in the abdomen, wrists, neck, inside of the elbow, ankles, feet, scalp, behind the knee, and near the groin (peripheral pulses). The places where the pulse is measured are named after the artery that is palpated in that area. Any artery that passes over bone can be used to find the pulse, but the arteries that are most commonly used for recording the pulse are the radial and carotid arteries.

The **pulse** offers an easy and effective way to measure heart rate and is recorded as beats per minute (bpm). The beat of the pulse should be evaluated for rate, rhythm, and regularity as well as for strength and tension (Table 3-1). Normal adult pulse rates should be between 60 and 100 bpm and should have a regular rhythm (see Box 3-1). However, there are some normal variations. For example, rates in children, women, and

TABLE 3-1	Pulse Patterns	
Pulse Type	**Rhythm: Rate**	**Factors Involved**
Normal adult female	Steady: 60-100 bpm	
Normal adult male	Steady: 55–95 bpm	
Dysrhythmia	Irregular: uneven intervals between beats	Hypoxia Low potassium Occasional premature beats are normal
Tachycardia	Rapid: >100 bpm	Activity or exercise Acute pain Alcohol Anemia Anxiety Asthma medications Atropine Decongestants Extreme heat Fever Heart disease Hyperthyroidism Stimulants (caffeine, amphetamines, diet pills, cigarettes) Stress
Bradycardia	Steady: <60 bpm	Antidysrhythmics Beta-blockers Digitalis Heart disease Hypothyroidism Well-conditioned athletes

Data from Mosby's *PDQ for LPN,* ed 2, St. Louis, 2008, Mosby.
Data from Pagana KD, Pagana TJ: *Mosby's manual of diagnostic and laboratory tests,* ed 3, St. Louis, 2006, Mosby.
bpm: Beats per minute.

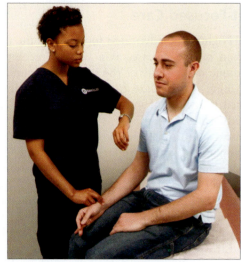

FIGURE 3-1 Taking a radial pulse. Never use the thumb to feel the patient's pulse.

- Changes in heart muscle
- Injury from a heart attack
- Healing process after heart surgery

Among the most common arrhythmias are **tachycardia** and **bradycardia** (see Table 3-1). Tachycardia is defined as a heart rate of more than 100 bpm. This finding may only be temporary, caused by exertion or nervousness, or it may be secondary to cardiac disease.

A heart rate of fewer than 60 bpm is bradycardia and may arise from disease in the heart's electrical conduction system. Examples include sinus node dysfunction and heart block. However, it is important to remember that irregular heart rhythms can also occur in "healthy" hearts as a normal physical response. In normal adults, the strength of the pulse should be full and strong, a factor that is influenced by arterial wall elasticity, blood volume, and the mechanical actions of the heart. If no abnormalities are detected, the pulse should be counted for 30 seconds and multiplied by 2. If irregularities *are* noted, the pulse should be counted for a full minute.

When taking a pulse, first explain the procedure to the patient and then have the patient bend his elbow with his arm at his side, palm side down. The radial artery can be located by placing the index, middle, and ring fingers on the anterior surface of the thumb side of the patient's hand (Figure 3-1). Gentle pressure should be applied to avoid obstructing blood flow. Never use your thumb to take the patient's pulse, as the strong pulse within your own thumb may be confused with that of the patient's. Using your finger, gently feel for the radial artery on the inner side of the wrist. When found, record the pulse rate and anything you notice about the pulse, such as its being weak, strong, or missing beats. If an irregularity is detected, determine if it occurs in a pattern or is random.

the elderly are slightly higher than they are for adult males, whereas rates in athletes in good condition are slightly lower.

An increased pulse volume sounds full and bounding, whereas a decreased volume sounds weak and thready. Any irregular heartbeat is termed an **arrhythmia** or *dysrhythmia.* The following conditions may cause arrhythmias:

- Strenuous exercise
- Strong emotions
- Fever
- Pain
- Coronary artery disease
- Electrolyte imbalances in the blood (such as sodium or potassium)

If the radial pulse is difficult to count, try the carotid artery. To find the carotid artery, place your fingers just below the angle of the patient's mandible (Figure 3-2).

Pulse Oximetry. Oximetry is a convenient, noninvasive method of monitoring blood oxygen levels. For a variety of reasons, this information is useful to determine whether the heart, lungs, and blood are working synchronously to deliver oxygen to various parts of the body. A low blood oxygen reading can be a sign of an illness or injury.

The test is performed by using an oximeter, a specially designed photoelectric device that measures the difference between levels of the red pigment hemoglobin, which carries oxygen in the blood. The most commonly used oximeters are called pulse oximeters because they

respond only to pulsations such as those of the pulsating capillaries in the area to be tested (Figure 3-3). One end of the device is attached like a clothespin to the end of the patient's index finger or ear lobe. The index finger is usually selected, but a smaller finger may be used if the index finger is too large to accommodate the clip. The other end of the oximeter is attached to a monitor so that the patient's oxygenation level can be seen at all times. The patient's hand should be positioned at heart level to eliminate venous pulsations and to promote accurate readings.

The amount of oxygen in the blood is given as a percentage. A normal reading for a person breathing room air is in the high 90s. A reading of 90% or less will trigger visual and audible alarms, requiring immediate action.

Pulse oximetry cannot offer a profile of blood gas analysis nor can it act as a substitute for taking a blood sample and examining its content. The oximeter acts purely as an indicator that something somewhere is interfering with the oxygenation of blood levels and that further investigation is required. The test may not be accurate in certain conditions such as when a patient has very low blood pressure or very poor heart function, or with conditions that can change blood color (e.g., exposure to carbon monoxide). A variety of factors may cause readings to be lower than expected:

- The patient's wearing of nail polish
- Improper positioning of the probe
- Excessive movement by the patient
- Hypothermia or cold injury to the extremities
- Anemia
- Chronic obstructive pulmonary disease (COPD)
- Carbon monoxide poisoning
- Shock associated with blood loss or poor perfusion

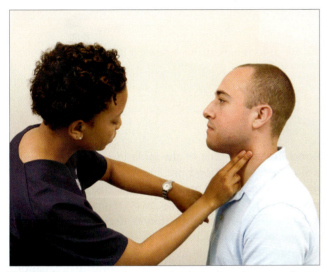

FIGURE 3-2 To locate the carotid pulse point, place your fingers just below the angle of the mandible.

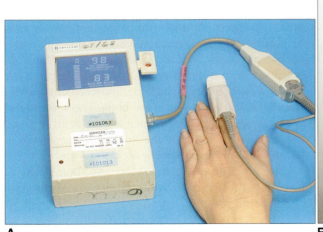
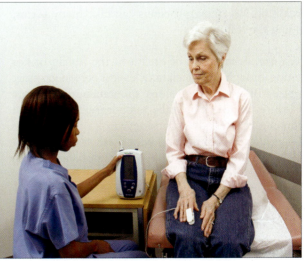

A   **B**

FIGURE 3-3 Pulse oximeters are used to detect problems with blood oxygen levels before clinical signs appear. **A,** Portable pulse oximeter with digit probe. **B,** The pulse oximeter sensor is attached to the patient's finger to measure the oxygen saturation levels in the blood.

BOX 3-2 | Evaluating Patient Respiration

Rate. The number of respirations per minute.
Rhythm. The regular rate of breathing and a symmetric movement of the chest.
Depth. The amount of air taken in with each respiration (e.g., normal, shallow, deep).
Character. The quality of respiration (quiet, labored, wheezing, coughing).

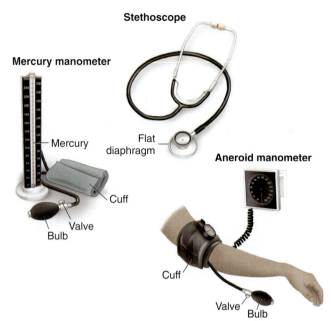

FIGURE 3-4 Instruments for measuring blood pressure. Mercury and aneroid types of manometers and accessories (stethoscope and cuff).

Respiration. Respiration, or breathing, is the process of inhaling and exhaling air. Its primary function is to obtain oxygen for use by the body's cells and to eliminate the cells' production of carbon dioxide.

Normal breathing is quiet, effortless, and has a regular rhythm. In an adult at rest, respiration occurs at a rate of 12 to 20 breaths per minute. However, the normal rates change depending on age and condition (see Table 3-1). Measuring respiration for less than a full minute may lead to inaccuracies.

When assessing a patient's respiratory rate, the rhythm, depth, and character of the respiration also should be noted (Box 3-2). Any injuries to the lungs, chest muscles, or diaphragm will affect breathing. Note whether the patient needs to sit up or stand up to breathe easily as opposed to lying down. Any difficulty in breathing (**dyspnea**) or changes in the patient's color (pallor or **cyanosis**) should be noted.

To count respirations, note the number of inhalations per minute. Counting respirations is often done while continuing to hold the patient's wrist—after the pulse has been counted—to prevent patients from being aware that you are monitoring their breathing. Aware patients sometimes force a change in their respirations.

In addition to counting the respiratory rate, it is important to note whether the patient has any difficulty in breathing. Breathing problems can take many forms, including the following:

- *Dyspnea.* A shortness of breath or the feeling of not getting enough air, which may leave a person gasping.
- *Apnea.* Breathing that stops spontaneously for any reason is **apnea**. It may be temporary, starting and stopping at intervals, or prolonged.
- *Wheezing.* Hard breathing with a whistling or high-pitched sound, resulting from constriction, or obstruction of the breathing tubes.
- *Hyperventilation.* Rapid breathing in excess of body requirements. Such breathing results in an excessive loss of carbon dioxide from the body.
- *Respiratory arrest.* A life-threatening stoppage of breathing that requires emergency medical assistance. It is caused either by an excessive loss of oxygen or by an increase of excessive carbon dioxide in the blood.

Blood Pressure. One of the most important vital signs is blood pressure. Blood pressure is the pressure exerted by circulating blood against the walls of the blood vessels. As the blood travels away from the heart, the pressure of the circulating blood *decreases*, spreading through arteries and capillaries, and back toward the heart through the veins.

Unless qualified, the term *blood pressure* generally refers to the brachial arterial pressure in the major blood vessel of the upper arm. The manual measurement of blood pressure is usually performed with a sphygmomanometer, blood pressure cuff, and stethoscope. The blood pressure cuff consists of an air pump, a pressure gauge, and a rubber cuff (Figure 3-4). The instrument measures the blood pressure in units called millimeters of mercury (mmHg). Electronic blood pressure monitors may also be used to measure heart rate or pulse.

Two numbers, systolic and diastolic, are recorded when measuring blood pressure. The higher number is the *systolic* pressure, which occurs when the ventricles contract to pump blood to the body. The lower number is the *diastolic* pressure, which occurs near the end of the cardiac cycle when the ventricles are filling with blood. Both numbers are important and are written as a fraction: the top number is the systolic number and the bottom number is the diastolic number. Both the systolic and diastolic pressures are recorded as mmHg, representing how high the mercury column is raised by the pressure of the blood. A normal, resting blood pressure in an adult is 115 mmHg systolic and 75 mmHg diastolic, and it would be written as 115/75 mmHg.

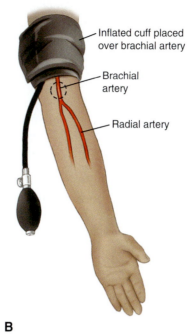

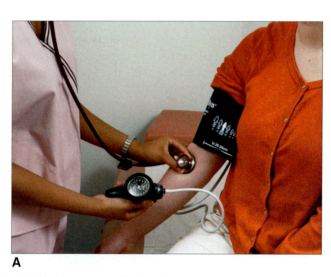

FIGURE 3-5 A, The blood pressure cuff should be snugly wrapped approximately 1 inch above the bend of the arm. **B,** The stethoscope should be placed over the brachial artery at the bend of the arm.

When manually taking a patient's blood pressure, you should explain the procedure, including the fact that it will take several minutes and that the patient will feel the cuff tighten and then deflate.

For the most accurate readings, wait 5 minutes before taking the blood pressure of a patient who is quiet and relaxed. Wait 15 to 30 minutes before taking the blood pressure of a patient who has been actively exercising. The proper protocol for obtaining a blood pressure includes the following steps (Figure 3-5):

- If the patient is sitting, be sure he has both feet on the floor.
- The brachial artery in the upper arm is the usual site for manually taking a blood pressure. Move any clothing out of the way to be able to put the blood pressure cuff on properly.
- Place the cuff above the elbow, making sure it is about an inch above the elbow.
- You should be able to put only one finger under a cuff that is tightened correctly.
- Position the patient's arm, placing it on a table, desk, or the bedside.
- Choose a stethoscope with a flat style diaphragm for taking blood pressures. Place the stethoscope earpieces into your ears; then feel for the brachial artery pulsation (usually found at the crease of the elbow) and place the diaphragm there.
- Squeezing the balloon, rapidly inflate the cuff to about 200 mmHg, or until no sound is heard. If you inflate too slowly, you will get a false reading.

- Loosen the valve slowly (no faster than 5 mmHg/second) to let some air out and listen for the first heart beat. Check the position of the pointer of the dial. This first sound is the systolic reading.
- Continue deflating the cuff slowly. Check the position of the pointer for the diastolic number. The last audible sound is the diastolic reading.
- Release the cuff and record both readings as a fraction (e.g., 110/70).

The sound produced by a normal heart is heard as a *lub-dub.* Every time you hear this sound, it means the heart is contracting once. When you hear the *lub* sound, the atrioventricular valves are closing. The *dub* sound represents the pulmonic and aortic valves.

Always use a blood pressure cuff that is correctly sized for the patient. Cuffs that are too small may yield readings 10 to 50 mmHg too high, falsely indicating hypertension.

On occasion, blood pressure may be measured in the main artery of the ankle. The ratio of the blood pressure measured at the ankle—to the brachial blood pressure—gives the ankle brachial pressure index (ABPI).

Hypertension. High blood pressure, or **hypertension**, directly increases the risk of coronary heart disease and stroke. When blood pressure is high, the arteries may have increased resistance against the flow of blood, causing the heart to pump harder.

According to the National Institutes of Health (NIH), high blood pressure for adults is defined as 140 mmHg or greater systolic pressure and 90 mmHg or greater diastolic pressure. In 2003, the NIH guidelines for hypertension were updated and a new blood pressure category, **prehypertension**, was added. The blood pressure readings associated with prehypertension are 120 mmHg to 139 mmHg systolic pressure and 80 mmHg to 89 mmHg diastolic pressure.

These numbers should be used only as guides, because a single elevated blood pressure measurement is not necessarily an indication of a problem. Multiple blood pressure measurements over several day or weeks are necessary before the diagnosis of hypertension is made and treatment initiated.

Isolated Systolic Hypertension. Isolated systolic **hypertension** exists when the systolic pressure is above 140 mmHg, with a diastolic pressure that is still below 90 mmHg. This condition primarily affects older people. It is characterized by an increased pulse pressure. **Pulse pressure** is the difference between the systolic and diastolic blood pressures. When the systolic pulse pressure measurement is elevated—without an elevation of the diastolic pressure—there is an increase in the pulse pressure. Hardening of the arteries contributes to the pulse pressures associated with isolated systolic high blood pressure.

Previously thought to be harmless, a high pulse pressure is now considered a precursor of health problems and potential end-organ damage. Patients with this type of hypertension have a 2 to 4 times greater risk for enlarged heart, heart attack, and stroke. At the opposite end of the spectrum is **hypotension**, or abnormally low blood pressure. Pressure that falls too far below <90/60 mmHg normal blood pressure is considered hypotension.

Blood pressure readings can be affected by a variety of factors, including cardiovascular disorders, neurologic conditions, kidney and urologic disorders, obesity, and some medications.

PATIENTS ON STRICT BED REST

Occasionally, patients on bed rest are brought to the ultrasound lab for diagnostic testing. For these patients, a full bladder can be very uncomfortable, making it difficult to remain still during scanning. Unless a full urinary bladder is needed for the study, always ask patients if they need to void before starting any lengthy procedures and be prepared with the proper equipment (a urinal, bedpan, or wheelchair, and bathroom facilities).

Bedpans and Urinals

There are two types of bedpans. Fracture pans have a flat lip in the front that makes them easy to slide under a patient who has problems lifting the pelvis for bedpan placement. The regular bedpan is somewhat larger and deeper, with a rounded lip designed to support the buttocks (Figure 3-6). Single-use disposable containers (including bedpans and urinals) are now available in many short-stay hospital departments. There are special disposal containers for these bedpans and urinals that accept both the container and contents to minimize handling.

Assisting with Patient Elimination. When assisting with patient elimination, assemble the supplies you will need, don protective gloves, and follow the procedure as outlined in Box 3-3. Be sure the patient is adequately covered for privacy. When helping female patients with a bedpan, the upper torso needs to be slightly elevated to prevent urine from running up the patient's back. You may need to help male patients use a urinal if they are unable to do so by themselves. Put on protective gloves and explain the procedure. Spread the patient's legs, lifting the sheet with one hand and sliding the penis into the urinal with the other. It may be necessary to hold the urinal in position until the patient is finished. Always

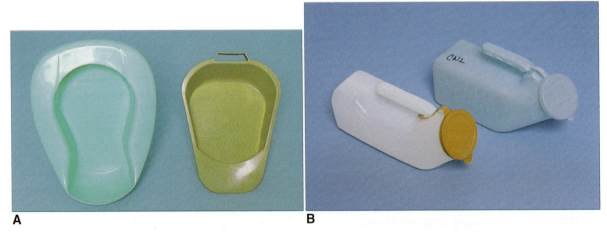

FIGURE 3-6 A, Regular bedpan (*left*) and fracture bedpan (*right*). **B,** Types of male urinals.

- Assemble the equipment: bedpan with cover; toilet tissue, disposable moist towelettes and a sheet.
- Wash your hands, and don disposable gloves.
- Explain the procedure and the purpose.
- Ask the patient to bend the knees and raise the hips.
- Assist the patient by lifting with one hand under the small of the back while you slide the bedpan under the patient's buttocks with your other hand.
- Ask the patient to call when finished. Elevate the side rails of the bed or stretcher, leaving the toilet tissue within reach.
- Provide the patient with privacy.
- When the patient is finished, provide a moist towelette for the patient's hands.
- Ask the patient to raise his or her hips, and then remove the bedpan.
- Cover the bedpan and place it aside until the patient is settled and secure.
- If blood is present in *either stool or urine*, record your observation.
- Dispose of the contents in the toilet (or specimen container if necessary). Remove and dispose of your gloves and repeat hand washing.

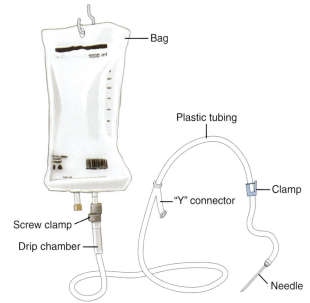

FIGURE 3-7 IV equipment. Plastic tubing leads from a solution-filled bag at one end and connects to a needle at the other end. Clamping the tubing controls the rate of flow.

check the chart before emptying bedpans or urinals to see if there is an order for a specimen collection or if urinary intake and output need to be measured. The nursing staff should indicate this and provide the correct container.

Emesis Basins

Vomiting often accompanies illness or injury. Emesis basins are kidney-shaped containers that are used to collect the vomit (emesis). (Emesis basins are also sometimes used to collect the run-off from medical procedures involving the application of liquid to the body.) If a patient is nauseated, place an emesis basin below his chin and against his neck to collect any vomit. After the patient finishes vomiting, offer him a glass of water to rinse his mouth and a tissue to dry his face.

It is important to observe the emesis with respect to its color, odor, and for the presence of undigested food. Emesis that is dark brown or reddish brown may be evidence of undigested blood and should be reported. Do not dispose of the emesis until you have been cleared to do so. Check the chart for any orders to collect the emesis for laboratory study. If the order exists, place the emesis in the proper specimen container and see that it is delivered to the lab. Once the emesis has been removed, the basin, which may be made of stainless steel or plastic, should be cleansed or properly discarded, if disposable.

PATIENTS WITH TUBES AND TUBING

The most common types of tubing that sonographers encounter when working with hospital patients are the following:

- IV infusion tubing
- Nasogastric suction tubing
- Urinary catheters
- Nasal catheters/cannulae used for oxygen administration

Sonographers are generally not responsible for starting any of the procedures that use such equipment, but they are required to know how to handle and care for patients who have such tubes in place.

Intravenous Therapy

The practice of giving liquid substances directly into a vein is called **intravenous (IV) therapy**. The intravenous route is the fastest way to way to deliver fluids and medications. IV therapy is often used to correct dehydration or electrolyte imbalances or to deliver medications or blood transfusions. Fluids can be administered intermittently or continuously, with the continuous method called an *IV drip*.

Figure 3-7 shows the chief components of a standard IV infusion set: a prefilled, sterile plastic bag (or glass container) of fluids. There is an attached drip chamber that makes it easy to see the rate of flow and allows the fluid to flow one drop at a time. A long sterile tube with a clamp leads from the drip chamber to the insertion site of the IV. The clamp regulates or stops the flow. The IV "line" is attached to a short catheter that is inserted into a peripheral vein. For adult patients, arm and hand veins are commonly used; for infants, the scalp veins are sometimes used.

Patients who are receiving IV fluids may come to the ultrasound department with either a standard IV set or possibly an electronic flow regulator in place. Once the patient is transferred to the scanning table, it is important to check the height of the IV fluid container. It should always be 18 to 20 centimeters above the level of the patient's vein. An IV container placed too high may cause too rapid a flow rate and fluid may infiltrate into the surrounding tissues. Conversely, if the container is placed too low, blood may flow back into the catheter or tubing and may clot, causing the fluid to stop flowing.

If the needle is accidentally dislodged, the IV fluid may enter the surrounding tissue rather than the vein. The patient may complain of discomfort, and you may observe swelling (edema) of the tissues around the injection site. Clamp off the flow and notify the nursing staff for instructions and to determine if you should continue the study.

Medication pumps (electronic flow regulators) are often used for patient-controlled pain medications, parenteral nutrition, and the continuous administration of medicine (Figure 3-8). These regulators will emit a warning sound when the solution supply is low, when flow is interrupted, or when the battery power of the pump is too weak. If an alarm sounds while you are scanning, avoid the temptation to work rapidly to complete the study and have the patient returned to ward. If this situation arises, call the nursing service immediately for instructions.

Nasogastric Suction Tubes

A nasogastric suction tube (NG tube) is a flexible tube made of rubber or plastic (Figure 3-9). An NG tube is passed through the nose and down through the nasopharynx and esophagus into the stomach to (1) remove the contents of the stomach, including air; (2) decompress the stomach; and (3) remove small solid objects or

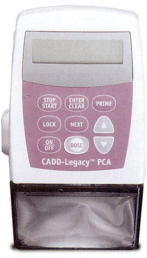

FIGURE 3-8 Patient-controlled analgesia pump. (Courtesy Smiths Medical, ASD, Inc.)

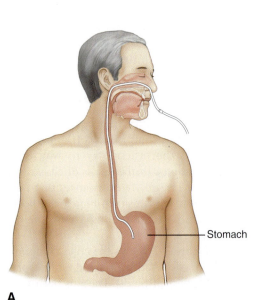

Stomach

A

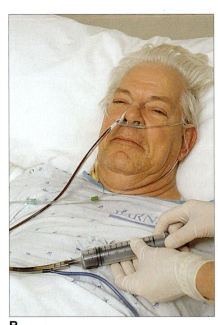

B

FIGURE 3-9 A, A nasogastric (NG) tube is inserted through one nostril and down through the esophagus until it reaches the stomach. **B,** A syringe can be used to suction the stomach contents.

fluid, such as poison, from the stomach. NG tubes can also be used to instill medications and put substances such as nutrients directly into the stomach when a patient cannot take food or drink by mouth.

If used for drainage, the NG tube is usually attached to a collector bag placed below the level of the patient's stomach, thus using gravity to empty the stomach contents. If used for continuous drainage, the drainage bag is placed below the level of the patient's stomach and suction drainage is employed. When patients connected to mechanical suction machines come to the ultrasound department, there are rules for working with them:

- Never pull on the tube when moving the patient.
- Check for leaks in both the NG tube and suction equipment. If found, report them immediately.
- Never raise or open the drainage bottle.
- Never disconnect the tubing.
- If the amount of material being suctioned rapidly increases, report it immediately.
- If the patient begins to gag or vomit while the tube is in place, report it immediately.

Catheters

Urinary catheters are used for removing fluids from the body. They are thin, sterile tubes that are inserted into the bladder as a way to manage urinary incontinence, urinary retention, to collect sterile fluid for laboratory diagnosis, and to fill the bladder prior to imaging studies (Figure 3-10, *A*).

Catheters come in a large variety of sizes, types, and materials (latex, silicone, and Teflon). The most commonly used catheter is the Foley catheter, a flexible latex tube that has openings in the tip and below the opening; the tubing inflates on demand like a small balloon. Once placed properly, the balloon is inflated with sterile water to effectively occlude the cervix of the bladder where the urethra begins and to prevent the catheter from sliding out of the bladder. Urine flows through the openings in the catheter tubing and into the tubing itself, instead of through the urethra and out of the urinary meatus. The urine drains into a collecting bag (Figure 3-10, *B*).

When catheterized patients are transferred from wheelchairs or stretchers to the scanning table, the collecting bag must be held below the level of the patient's bladder. This will prevent urine in the tube or bag from being siphoned back into the bladder, which would cause patient discomfort and give bacteria potential access to the bladder. Because it can be left in the bladder for a period of time, the Foley catheter is also called an indwelling catheter. A sterile urinary catheterization kit needs to be provided if the patient must be catheterized while in the ultrasound department. A doctor or medical assistant is normally called to insert the Foley catheter.

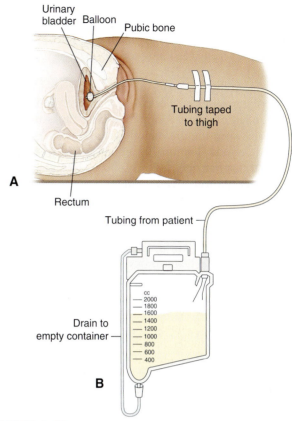

FIGURE 3-10 Catheterization equipment. **A,** A plastic/rubber urinary catheter is inserted through the urethra and into the bladder. **B,** Urine drains into a container.

Oxygen Therapy

Oxygen therapy is an essential treatment for many conditions. Its primary purpose is to decrease the work of breathing for patients experiencing respiratory difficulties. Oxygen should be treated as a drug whose dosage or concentration is ordered by a physician. There are important safety issues involving the use of oxygen. Although oxygen itself cannot burn, it will ignite and burn if it comes in contact with any combustible substance (even a spark). When large concentrations of oxygen are present, ignition could cause an explosion.

A variety of oxygen systems exist to provide either high-flow or low-flow oxygen delivery. The type of system selected depends on the concentration of oxygen needed and the age and the activity level of the patient. Oxygen systems consist of three main parts: (1) a container, (2) a breathing device (mask or cannula), and (3) a connecting tube.

Oxygen tanks have different parts:

- A pressure gauge to show how much oxygen is left in the tank
- A flow meter to control the rate of oxygen coming out of the tank

- A humidifier bottle, where water is mixed with the oxygen and the oxygen is warmed before delivery to prevent the membranes of the patient's nose, mouth, and throat from becoming too dry

Portable oxygen systems deliver compressed oxygen in either large tanks on a cart or in smaller cylinders that can be rolled on a small cart. The large tanks are used for patients who require high flow rates of oxygen over extended periods. The smaller cylinders are used during patient transportation or for short duration needs. Ambulatory patients who require continuous oxygen generally use an over-the-shoulder strap or a rolling stand to hold the cylinder.

For scanning labs equipped with in-room piping, both oxygen and suction are usually provided through wall outlets. Figure 3-11 illustrates the appearance of an oxygen flow meter. The dial on the side is used to adjust the flow rate, which is indicated by the level of the small ball shown near the center of the gauge.

Whether patients come to the ultrasound department with a tank or a cylinder, or will be using in-wall systems, there are special safety precautions to follow:

- Do not transport any oxygen tank unless it is secured to a tank/cylinder cart.
- Secure the tank in an upright position and away from any heat source because of the risks of combustion. This includes electrical equipment, such as heating pads and radios.
- No one should smoke where oxygen is being used.
- Any combustible material, such as alcohol, perfumes, and propane, must be kept away from oxygen tanks.
- Do not place a cylinder beside a patient when transporting the patient by stretcher.

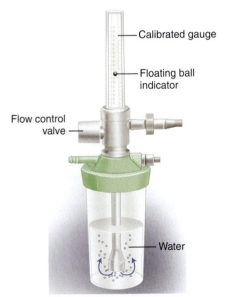

Calibrated gauge

Floating ball indicator

Flow control valve

Water

FIGURE 3-11 Schematic drawing of a typical wall-mounted oxygen flowmeter. Water levels must be kept high enough to bubble as oxygen flows through the flowmeter.

Nasal Cannulae and Nasal Catheters. Delivery of oxygen to the patient requires tubing connected to the oxygen source on one end and attached at the other end to a patient's mask, **nasal cannula**, or a tent. Nasal cannulae are usually used to deliver low-to-medium concentrations of oxygen in situations when precise accuracy is not required. The patient-end of the nasal cannula is placed into each of the patient's nostrils and held in place by an elastic band around the patient's head (Figure 3-12, A).

A **nasal catheter** (oropharyngeal catheter) is a piece of tubing that is longer than a cannula. It is inserted through the nostril and into the back of the patient's mouth. This method provides more effective oxygen delivery and is used when the patient must have additional oxygen at all times. The nasal catheter is fastened to the patient's forehead or cheek by a piece of adhesive tape to hold it steady, and it must be long enough with enough slack to allow the patient to move around comfortably.

Oxygen Masks. There are a variety of oxygen masks for delivering oxygen to patients with specific needs. The simple mask is used to provide short-term therapy; it delivers both oxygen and humidity. This type of oxygen mask is typically made of transparent material that conforms to the patient's face. It is held in place by an elastic strap that is fitted over nose, mouth, and chin (Figure 3-12, B). The reservoir mask is a low-flow device identified by the presence of a bag, which must remain constantly inflated by one third. There are several types: partial and non-rebreather masks. The partial re-breather mask delivers oxygen concentrations of 40% to 60%. Openings in the mask allow the patient to inhale room air if the oxygen source fails. The non-rebreather mask delivers the highest possible oxygen concentrations (60% to 90%) because the patient only breathes air from the bag. It is effective for short-term therapy (Figure 3-12, C).

Both masks cover the nose and mouth of the patient and are attached with an elastic band around the patient's head. These masks have an attached reservoir bag that is inflated approximately two-thirds full of oxygen before placing it on the patient. Sonographers should especially note the level of inflation on the non-rebreather mask, because if the bag completely deflates, the patient no longer has a source of air to breathe.

The Venturi mask is a high-flow mask designed to administer precisely controlled low oxygen concentrations, but with variable air flow to produce a constant oxygen concentration regardless of breathing rate. This is accomplished by a Venturi device and is identified by the presence of a hard plastic adapter with large "windows" on either side.

The following precautions should be observed whenever working with patients receiving oxygen therapy:

- Observe all fire regulations in effect at your institution.

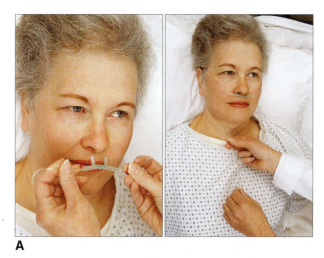

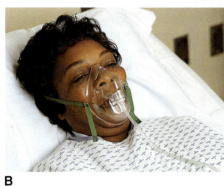

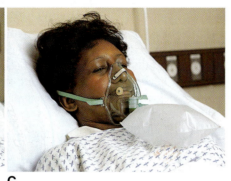

A

B   **C**

FIGURE 3-12 A, Nasal cannula. The two prongs of the cannula should be inserted a short distance into the patient's nostrils. An elastic headband behind the ears is used to keep the cannula in place. **B,** A simple oxygen face mask should cover the nose and mouth of the patient. **C,** Reservoir, or partial rebreathing, mask. This low-flow device is equipped with an inflatable bag.

- Check the flow meter to be sure oxygen is being delivered to the patient. The water level in the humidifying chamber should be high enough so that it bubbles as the oxygen goes through it.
- Be sure the tubing connected to the oxygen source is taped to the patient to help keep it from accidentally being pulled when moving the patient.
- Make sure the patient is not lying on the tubing or that it is not kinked, which can slow or stop the oxygen flow.
- In most hospitals, inhalation therapy or respiratory therapy departments are responsible for the patient's treatment. They should be called to make any needed adjustments after checking with the patient's physician or nurse.

Wounds, Drains, and Dressings

Some postsurgical patients sent for abdominal ultrasound studies may present with wound drains. A wound drain is created by inserting a wick inside of the wound to provide drainage. It is important not to pull or dislodge the drain whenever positioning, scanning or transferring the patient. For the wounds that are actively draining, a gauze pad can be taped over the area until the scan is completed.

If the wound is situated within the scanning field, sterile technique is required to scan over the open wound. After gloving, apply sterile gel to the wound area and cover it with thin plastic film. Next, more sterile gel should be applied over the film to create an airless contact between the transducer and the wound area.

Some wounds may be covered by a dressing to protect them from injury or infection. If it becomes necessary to remove the dressing to gain scanning access, you should always check with the nursing staff before removing or replacing any dressings. It is important to determine if wound precautions are in place, because if they are, the nursing staff is responsible for changing any dressings. If the dressings are considered nonsterile, the procedure for changing dressings is as follows:

- Wash hands and glove.
- Use sterile scanning gel to prevent wound infection.
- Remove the old dressing carefully to avoid dislodging any scabs or causing any pain.
- Remove the soiled dressing and dispose of it properly.

- Apply a clean dressing, using paper tape if possible.
- Report the presence of bleeding, drainage or foul odor.
- Report any patient complaints such as pain, itching or burning.

Ostomies

Ostomies are sometimes created for patients with certain health conditions or diseases. Patients with colostomies or ileostomies have undergone surgical resection of the colon in which the distal end of the remaining functioning bowel terminates in an artificial opening in the abdominal wall called a stoma. A stoma appears as a small hole surrounded by a ring of mucosal tissue (Figure 3-13). This opening may be temporary or permanent, depending on the patient's condition.

Ostomy patients must wear an external bag or pouch to collect liquefied fecal matter. The disposable ostomy bags are attached to the skin with a double-faced adhesive substance that seals the bag to the skin. The bags are equipped with a clamp or other closure device to keep the bag closed and secure between emptyings. Ostomy bags require frequent changing because of the constant flow of fecal material.

Another product designed for the ostomy patient's use is a stoma cap or cover to be placed on the stoma when the stoma is not actively draining. The cover or cap is attached to the skin in the same fashion as the ostomy bag. If your department schedules ostomy patients, keeping a small supply of the following items on hand is encouraged:

- New bags
- Plastic bags for disposal
- Closure clamps
- Water or bag-cleaning solution
- Washcloths and towels
- Toilet or bedpan
- Gloves
- Facial tissues
- Paper tape

Changing an ostomy bag requires clean rather than sterile technique. After gloving, remove and discard the old bag. Gently wipe the stoma and the peristomal skin with a facial tissue. Carefully wash and dry the peristomal skin, then apply a closure clamp if necessary. If desired, apply paper tape in a picture-frame fashion to the edges of the bag for additional security. The patient should be encouraged to stay quietly in position for about 5 minutes to improve adherence of the bag. Record the date and time of bag removal and replacement and the character of the drainage (color, amount, type, and consistency).

PATIENT TRANSFER TECHNIQUES

Patient safety is a prime component of patient care. Equally important is sonographer safety. Some of the most common injuries among members of the health care team are severe musculoskeletal strains. Sonographers can avoid many injuries with conscious use of body mechanics in their everyday activities, work activities, and especially when performing patient transfers. By protecting themselves from injury, they are also protecting their patients.

Body Mechanics

The term **body mechanics** refers to using the correct muscles to complete a task safely, efficiently, and without undue strain on any joints or muscles.

The basic principles of body mechanics require the following:

- Maintaining a stable center of gravity by keeping your center of gravity low, your back straight, and bending at the hips and knees.
- Maintaining a strong base of support by keeping your feet apart, placing one foot slightly ahead of the other with toes pointed in the direction of activity, then flexing your knees to absorb jolts and turning with your feet, instead of your hips.
- Maintaining a center of gravity by keeping your back straight and keeping any objects that are being lifted, close to your body.
- Maintaining proper body alignment through good posture: Tuck in your buttocks, pull your abdomen in and up, keep your back flat, your head up, and your chin in as you keep your weight forward and supported on the outside of your feet (Figure 3-14).

Sonographers benefit greatly from using body mechanics techniques when lifting and reaching. Their first consideration should be whether the object or patient is too heavy to lift alone. The potential for injury to themselves and their patients can be avoided by enlisting the help of another person.

Lifting should be done using the strong leg muscles—not the back—and lifting straight upward in one smooth motion (Figure 3-15). When reaching, it is important to stand directly in front of the object or patient and to

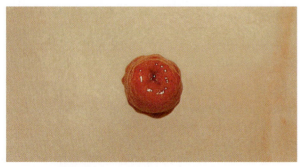

FIGURE 3-13 Typical colostomy stoma.

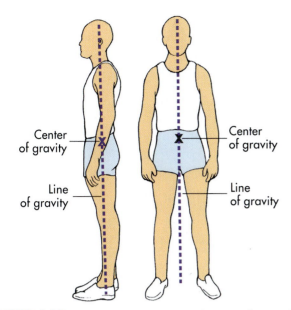

FIGURE 3-14 Correct body alignment when standing. Before lifting, feet should be placed shoulder width apart, with weight evenly distributed to provide a strong support base.

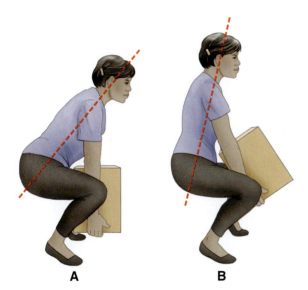

FIGURE 3-15 Proper body mechanics for lifting. **A,** Keep the back straight. When lifting, use the large muscles of the thigh instead of the smaller muscles of the back. **B,** Before the lift, tighten abdominal and pelvic muscles, tuck buttocks in, and keep head and chest up.

avoid any twisting or stretching motions. One of the most common causes of muscle strains or tears as well as skeletal injuries is stooping by bending at the waist.

The techniques of body mechanics are important if you will be walking patients or lifting or moving them via wheelchair or stretcher. In many hospitals, using wheeled transport is a strict policy when moving patients from one place to another. It is a safety precaution based on the possibility that ambulatory patients could become weak or faint while traveling from their room to the ultrasound department. For patients who can sit and stand comfortably, a wheelchair may be sufficient for transfer, but patients who cannot stand or walk alone should only be transferred by stretcher.

Active toddlers and infants are usually transported in their crib. The high sides provide better safety than side rails on a stretcher. An added advantage is that if the child must be unattended for any period of time, he or she will be safe. On rare occasions, patients whose condition makes it painful or difficult to move may come to the ultrasound department in a bed.

When preparing to transfer patients, always check with the nursing station to obtain the patient's chart and ask if there are any special instructions before or during transfer. The transfer equipment should be checked for safety and function. Sonographers assigned to transfer patients also are responsible for checking safety straps, buckles, brakes, and side rails (if a stretcher is used). If any extra equipment must accompany a patient (IV stands, urine bags, etc.), check with the nursing station before disconnecting any equipment or moving the patient. Once the patient is cleared for transfer, identify yourself to the patient and explain the reason for the transfer. Then ask the patient's name and check his ID bracelet to verify his identity.

Moving Patients Up in Bed

First assess the patient's size and condition. If the patient is alert and cooperative and you are confident that you do not need help, follow these steps:

- Explain to the patient that on the count of 3, you are going to shift him up in bed.
- Lower the side rails to the level of patient's shoulders.
- Move close to the side of the bed, keeping your back straight, knees bent, and one foot forward to provide a base of support.
- Ask the patient to bend his knees with his feet placed firmly on the bed.
- Place your hand and arms under the patient's hips, while keeping your back straight, knees bent, and feet apart.
- Count to 3 and pull the patient up to the head of the bed, while he pulls with his arms and pushes with his feet.

If the patient is very large or unable to assist you, it will be easier to slide the patient up in bed by using a draw sheet and the help of another person (Figure 3-16):

- Ask the patient to bend his knees, then slide a draw sheet under his hips and buttocks.
- Put the head of the bed down.
- Grasp the draw sheet, pointing one of your feet in the direction in which you are moving toward the patient.

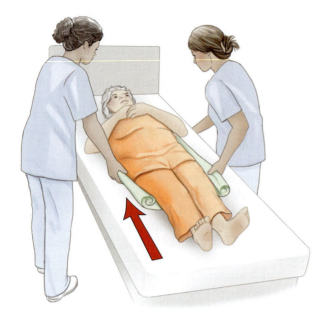

FIGURE 3-16 Using a lifting/turning sheet to move helpless patients. It is advisable to slide or pull rather than to lift. With the help of a colleague, this technique affords the safest way to move patients who are heavy or unable to help themselves.

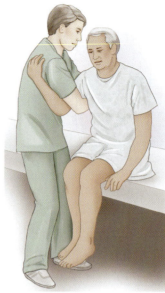

FIGURE 3-17 Assisting patients to and from a bed or scanning table. The sonographer should provide support under the arms of the patient and rotate or shift his or her weight as the person is brought closer to the sonographer.

- Lean in the direction of the move, using your legs and body weight.
- On the count of 3, both of you slide the draw sheet toward the head of the bed.
- Reposition the patient comfortably and raise bedside rails if the patient is to remain in bed.

Assisting Patients To and From the Scanning Table

- When dealing with an ambulatory patient, if necessary, simply provide the patient with a gown and a private area in which to change.
- While the patient is changing, place a step stool near the middle of the scanning table and arrange the pillows, linens, and any supplies you will be using.
- When the patient is ready, escort him to the table and help him up and into the proper position for scanning.
- Once the exam is completed, help the patient down from the table and back to the changing area (Figure 3-17).

Wheelchair Transfers

It is always important to have everything ready for patient transfers before you begin. If you are moving the patient from the bed to a wheelchair, you may require the patient's help, so clear communication is essential. If patients are unable to help, you will need two people to make the transfer.

When working alone, first position and lock the wheelchair close to the bed and facing the foot of the bed. Then, remove the armrest nearest the bed and swing away both leg rests (Figure 3-18):

- Adjust the bed to its lowest position to make it easy for the patient to step down to the floor.
- Sit the patient up by putting one arm under patient's neck, with your hand supporting his shoulder blade, and putting the other hand under the patient's knees.
- Swing the patient's legs over the edge of the bed, helping him to sit up.
- Place your arms around the torso of the patient for support. Put one arm of the patient over your shoulder or on your hip, while his other arm is extended with his hand flat on the bed to help support the position.
- Ask the patient to scoot to the edge of the bed until his feet are on the floor.
- Widen the distance of your feet with your right foot forward and left foot back, to easily shift of your weight as you lift the patient.
- Put your arms around the patient's chest and clasp your hands behind his back. If available, you may also use a transfer belt around the patient's waist to provide a firmer handhold.
- While your arms are still supporting the patient's torso, one arm of the patient should still be on your shoulder and his other arm should still be extended, palm flat on the bed.
- Position your right foot alongside the patient's left foot to provide stability and to keep the patient's foot

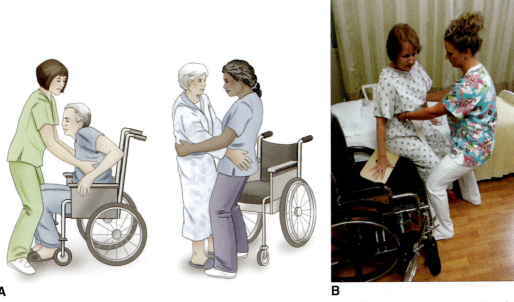

A   **B**

FIGURE 3-18 A, When moving patients to and from a wheelchair, bend at the knees and hips when lowering or raising the patient. Keep your shoulders level with the patient's shoulders and enlist the patient's help, if possible, by having the patient support his or her own weight when rising from or sitting down into the wheelchair. **B,** A friction-reducing device may be used to transfer a patient from the bed to the wheelchair.

and knee from buckling when he is lifted to a standing position.

- Slightly bend your knees and lean your body forward. Instruct the patient to get ready to push the arm that's extended on the bed, as you lift him up to a standing position.
- Count to 3, as you assist the patient to a standing position while he is pushing off the bed at the same time.
- Have the patient pivot toward the chair as you continue clasping your hands around the patient.
- Stand in front of the patient, keeping your knees bent and your feet about 12 inches apart.
- Make sure the backs of the patient's legs are against the chair seat. A helper can stabilize the wheelchair or the patient from behind. Always be sure the wheelchair is locked.
- As the patient bends toward you, bend your knees and lower the patient down and toward the back of the wheelchair.

Stretcher Transfers

Patient safety is the primary concern when moving patients from a bed to a stretcher. Remember not to lift at the expense of your own back. If you move the patient's legs first, you can decrease the stress on your back. If at all possible, enlist the aid of a second person to help in making the move.

- Put the head of the bed down and adjust the bed height.

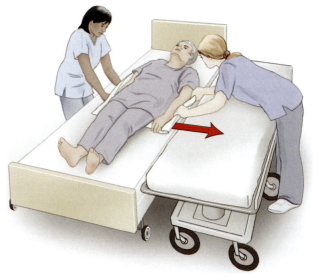

FIGURE 3-19 Transferring patients from bed to stretcher. Use of a "pulling sheet" is recommended whenever transferring patients who cannot help themselves.

- Put a plastic slide board (or plastic trash bag) between the sheet and the draw sheet, beneath one edge of the patient's torso.
- Move the patient's legs closer to the edge of the bed.
- Instruct the patient to cross his arms across his chest, and then explain the move to the patient.
- For a two-person transfer, grasp the draw sheet on both sides of the bed (Figure 3-19).
- Adjust the bed slightly higher than the stretcher and then position the stretcher, locking it in place.

- Move the patient's legs onto the stretcher and have the helper kneel on the bed while holding onto the draw sheet.
- On the count of 3, grasp the draw sheet and slide the patient onto the stretcher.
- Raise the stretcher side rails, and unlock the brakes.
- See that the patient is comfortable and modestly covered.

INFECTION CONTROL

In the early 1800s, people believed that fresh air and sunlight were all that was needed to kill germs, and those working in the medical profession were not much more enlightened. Physicians spent little time washing their hands; a patient's skin was seldom cleansed before surgery; instruments were simply rinsed off between operations; and sponges were routinely reused. That all changed when Joseph Lister decided to spray carbolic acid on wounds, dressings, and surgical instruments. This one simple act significantly reduced postsurgical deaths. Not until the early 1900s would nurses began using gloves—not to protect the patients but to protect their hands against the harsh chemicals used during surgery. It would take many years for the medical profession to realize that wearing gloves also protects patients and to begin routinely using them as barriers to infection.

Standard Precautions

In the 1980s, the outbreak of HIV/AIDS triggered the development of *universal precautions* to fight the ravaging disease. It would be another decade before the Centers for Disease Control (CDC) would establish *standard precautions* and *additional precautions* to expand the universal precautions' guidelines by including additional body fluids and sites to the earlier protocols. These precautions apply to *all* patients regardless of their diagnoses and even if they appear asymptomatic.

It is extremely important to observe standard precautions when performing ultrasound studies on outpatients as well as inpatients.

Standard precautions are the basic infection-control guidelines used to reduce the risks of infection spread through the following three transmission modes: airborne infection, droplet infection, and contact infection.

The most important weapon against the spread of infection is proper hand washing, followed by the use of barriers (gloves, gowns, and masks) and the proper handling and disposal of infectious waste materials. You should wash your hands whenever you come in contact with the following substances:

- Blood
- All body fluids: secretions, excretions, and contaminated items—even if blood is not visible. The only body fluid exception is perspiration.

BOX 3-4 | Infectious Materials

- Blood
- Semen
- Vaginal secretions
- Cerebrospinal fluid
- Synovial fluid
- Pleural fluid
- Pericardial fluid
- Amniotic fluid
- Saliva in dental procedures
- Any body fluid visibly contaminated with blood
- Mixtures of fluids where you cannot differentiate among body fluids
- Unfixed human tissue or organs (other than intact skin)
- Certain cell tissue or organ cultures and mediums

- Broken skin.
- Mucous membranes (inside the mouth, nose, and eyelids).
- Dried blood or dried bloody fluids.

Box 3-4 lists infectious materials you should be aware of. Included in the standard precautions are the following important protocols:

Hand Washing

- Wash your hands after touching blood, body fluids, or contaminated items—*whether or not gloves are worn*.
- Wash your hands after removing gloves, between patient contacts, and whenever indicated, to avoid transfer of microorganisms to other patients or the environment.
- It may be necessary to wash hands between tasks and procedures on the same patient, to prevent cross-contamination of different body sites.
- Use plain soap for routine hand washing and an antimicrobial agent or waterless agent for specific situations (e.g., to control outbreaks or for hyperendemic infections).

Gloves

- Wear clean, nonsterile gloves when touching blood, body fluids, secretions, excretions, and contaminated items.
- Put on clean gloves just before touching mucous membranes and nonintact skin.
- Change gloves between tasks and procedures on the same patient after contacting material that may contain a high concentration of microorganisms.
- Remove gloves promptly after use, before touching noncontaminated items and surfaces, and before going to another patient.
- Wash hands immediately to avoid transfer of microorganisms to other patients or environments.

Masks, Eye Protection, and Face Shields

- Wear a mask, eye protection, and face shields whenever performing procedures likely to generate splashes or sprays of blood, body fluids, secretions, and excretions.

Gown

- Wear a clean, nonsterile gown to protect skin and clothing from blood and body fluids during procedures or patient care activities likely to generate splashes or sprays of blood, body fluids, secretions, and excretions.
- Remove dirty gowns and gloves as soon as possible, and then wash your hands to avoid transfer of microorganisms to other patients or environments.

Patient Care Equipment

- Handle used patient-care equipment that is soiled with blood, body fluids, secretions, and excretions in a way that prevents skin and mucous membrane exposure, contamination of clothing, and transfer of microorganisms to other patients and environments.
- If disposable items are used, they must be disposed of properly and never used again. Ensure that reusable equipment is not used for another patient unless it has been properly cleaned and reprocessed.
- Thoroughly clean the transducer after every patient with the Steri-septic cleaner.

Linens

- Handle, transport, and process used linen soiled with blood, body fluids, secretions and excretions in a way that prevents skin and mucous membrane exposures and contamination of clothing and that avoids transfer of microorganisms to other patients and environments.
- A patient's used linens should not be shaken, but rolled up and placed into a laundry hamper or bag for cleaning. Always hold the used linens away from your clothes.

Environmental Control

- Keep the work environment as clean as possible, especially after any spills.
- Be sure your institution has adequate procedures for routine care, cleaning, and disinfection of environmental surfaces, beds, or side rails.
- Equipment (blood pressure cuffs, basins, bedpans, or wheelchairs) should be cleansed according to your institution's policies.

For your own safety, change your uniform or lab coat daily, and bathe or shower daily, paying special attention to hair and body areas not covered by clothing. By keeping your hair covered or pinned, you will reduce the chance of it coming in contact with the blood or body fluids of patients. This is especially true with longer hair that can brush against open wounds, if not properly

BOX 3-5	What Are Your Facility's Infection Procedures?

- To whom should you report?
- Who determines the source of exposure?
- How do *you* get care?
- Who performs follow-up?

secured. Wash your hair daily to remove germs and debris. It is important to know what your facility's infection procedures are (Box 3-5).

Additional Precautions

Recognizing that some patients require more than basic methods of infection control, the CDC developed extra guidelines known as additional precautions. These are divided into disease categories related to specific transmission patterns:

1. *Airborne transmission.* Germs capable of floating airborne for long periods of time are often very contagious and can travel long distances. Some of the diseases spread by airborne transmission include the following:
   - Tuberculosis
   - Measles
   - Chicken pox
   - Shingles

   If you are immune to diseases such as measles or chicken pox, you can work with infected patients without concern for becoming infected with the disease. However, you must still follow all infection control precautions ordered for that patient.

2. *Droplet transmission.* Germs that are too heavy to remain airborne can drop quickly. Diseases spread via droplet transmission include the following:
   - Mumps
   - Measles (rubella)
   - Whooping cough (pertussis)
   - Pneumonia
   - Meningitis (specific forms)
   - Strep throat

   Because droplets are too heavy to float, they usually don't travel more than 3 feet. They are most commonly spread by coughing, sneezing, and talking. Patients on droplet precautions may be placed in private rooms and wear surgical masks if they are around uninfected people for short time periods. You should wear a surgical mask when working within 3 feet of these patients.

3. *Contact transmission.* Germs spread directly or indirectly by touching the germ include the following diseases:
   - Methicillin-resistant *Staphylococcus aureus* (MRSA)

- *E. coli*
- Wound infections
- Flu
- Impetigo
- Pinkeye
- Scabies
- Hepatitis A

One of the most serious of these diseases is the MRSA infection. MRSA is a form of staph bacteria that live on the skin and nasal passages of a third of the world's population. These bacteria are resistant to certain broad-spectrum antibiotics. MRSA infections can be divided into two categories: (1) community-acquired infections and (2) hospital-acquired infections. The primary differences between them are that community-acquired forms typically produce skin infections, whereas the hospital-acquired forms can develop into more serious lung and blood stream infections. MRSA is primarily spread on the hands of health care workers and infected persons. Draining wounds and infected discharge are other methods of transmission.

It is not possible to eliminate MRSA in health care settings, because new patients, visitors, and employees will reintroduce the infection. The best defense against MRSA in hospital settings is hand washing and the proper use of barrier devices. Proper maintenance of restrooms, soap and towel dispensers, and proper room cleansing also are essential to preventing the spread of infection.

Risk factors for MRSA are greatest among health care workers and patients in hospital and assisted living settings. MRSA skin infections may resemble boils or spider bites with a painful, red, and swollen ring of skin surrounding the bite. Pus drainage may occur. If MRSA spreads to other body areas (e.g., lungs or into the bloodstream), more serious symptoms may develop, such as fatigue, fever, chills, and shortness of breath.

Whereas mild infections are often treated with oral antibiotics, more serious infections, which travel in the bloodstream, frequently require intravenous antibiotic therapy (e.g., Vancomycin, Septra, or Bactrim).

As mentioned earlier, there are two forms of infection contact: direct contact, which refers to touching the skin of an infected person, and indirect contact, which refers to touching an object that has been touched by an infected person. Examples of contact transmission include the following:
- Changing the clothes/gown of a patient infected with staph germs without wearing gloves
- Failing to change gloves between patients

Patients on contact precautions may be isolated from other patients. When caring for such patients, you may need to do the following:
- Glove before entering the patient's room.

- Change gloves during patient contact, especially after touching highly contaminated items.
- Remove gloves before leaving the patient's room and wash your hands immediately.
- Gown while in contact with the patient and remove the gown right before leaving the patient area.
- Discard disposable items and disinfect equipment used on patients with a contact infection.

Biohazardous waste—refuse that has been contaminated with germs, such as discarded dressings, used needles, contents of bedpans or urinals, and so on—should be bagged and labeled. In some cases, items may need to be double bagged. Used sharps must always be placed in puncture-proof containers.

4. *Blood-borne transmission.* Blood-borne diseases are those spread when the blood of an infected person comes in contact with the blood of another person. HIV/AIDS and hepatitis are two of the most common diseases spread by blood-borne transmission.

Nosocomial Infections

Hospital-acquired infections are known as **nosocomial infections**. Contracted as a result of medical treatment, they usually manifest within the first 48 hours of treatment. The most common of these are urinary tract infections (UTI), pneumonia, and surgical incision site infections. The patients at most risk are those whose general health is compromised: intensive care unit (ICU) and neonatal intensive care unit (NICU) patients and immunocompromised patients who are already fighting or at risk for infection. Transmission of nosocomial infections occurs through the following means:

- *Direct contact.* Person to person.
- *Indirect contact.* Touching an infected surface or a surface treated with improperly sterilized equipment.
- *Droplet infection.* Via sneezing and coughing.
- *Airborne transmission.* Via sneezing and coughing.
- Common vehicle transmission. Resulting from food, water, or medical devices.
- *Vector transmission.* As a result of contact or bites from an insect or animal.

The symptoms of nosocomial infection should be suspected when patients develop fever and other symptoms not associated with their primary complaint. Prevention of nosocomial infections relies on following stringent quality infection control procedures.

Preventive Measures. Do not underestimate the importance of personal protective equipment (PPE). Many health care workers who become ill are unsure of the proper order in which PPE should be donned and removed. The CDC recommends the following:

- Put on PPE before contact and generally before entering the patient's room.

- Once PPE is on, use it carefully to avoid contamination.
- Keep your hands away from your face.
- Work from clean to dirty areas.
- Limit the surfaces you touch.
- Change the PPE when torn or heavily contaminated.

Basic PPE Protocols. The proper way to don a gown is to select the appropriate size and type. With the opening at the back, secure the gown at the neck and waist. If the gown is too small to provide full coverage, wear two—the first with the opening in the front and the second placed over it with the opening in the back.

To don a mask, place it over the nose, mouth, and chin. Fit the flexible nose pieces over the bridge of your nose, and then secure it on the head with ties or elastic.

Gloves should be the last of the PPE to be applied. Extend your hands into the gloves and stretch the gloves to cover the wrist of an isolation gown. Tuck the cuffs of the gown securely in place under each glove. Adjust the gloves for comfort and dexterity (Figure 3-20).

Once the patient care tasks are completed, carefully remove the PPE and discard it properly. Immediately wash your hands. While removing gloves, gowns, or masks, the goal is to avoid contaminating yourself or the environment. The outside front of gloves and masks are considered contaminated, regardless of their appearance. The outside front and sleeves of a gown are considered contaminated. Where to remove PPE depends on the type of equipment as well as the patient category of isolation. If only gloves are worn, they may be discarded in the patient's room. When a gown and full PPE are used, they should be discarded at the door of the patient's room or in an anteroom and in a designated container.

To remove a gown, unfasten the ties and peel the gown away from your neck and shoulders. Turn the outside toward the inside, then fold or roll the gown into a bundle and discard it in a designated receptacle. To remove a mask, *do not t*ouch the front of it. First, untie the bottom, then the top ties. Lift the mask away from your face and discard in a designated receptacle. To remove gloves, grasp the outer edge near the wrist. Peel the glove away from the hand, turning the glove inside out. Hold it in the opposite glove, then slide an ungloved finger under the wrist of the remaining glove and peel it off from the inside, creating a "bag" for both used gloves. Discard properly and again perform hand washing after using and discarding the PPE.

Preparing a Sterile Field. Medical aseptic technique is designed to rid an area or object of pathogenic microorganisms. Aseptic technique is commonly used in procedures that involve puncturing the skin or when placing objects into normally sterile body cavities. These are the recommended principles to follow:

- All materials in a sterile field *must be sterile* and *all objects added* to a sterile field *must also be sterile.*

When placing hands into a sterile field, they must be covered with sterile gloves.
- Any sterile field that has been compromised by punctures, tears, or moisture is considered contaminated.
- Once a sterile package is opened, a 1-inch border around the edge is considered unsterile.
- If there are any questions or doubts about an object's sterility, the object should be considered unsterile.
- Movement around or in the sterile field must not compromise or contaminate the sterile field. Never reach across a sterile field and never turn your back on a sterile field. Bring all tables used in the procedure up to waist level to avoid bending over the field.
- Most procedures today use disposable equipment wrapped in paper or plastic.
- Always read the directions on the package in advance of the actual procedure.

Nondisposable equipment from central supply is usually double-wrapped in cloth and sealed with tape stating the expiration dates or with an indicator tape of a predetermined color, confirming sterilization. All such packs are wrapped in a standardized fashion and should be opened as outlined here (Figure 3-21):

- Place the pack on a clean surface within reach of the physician.
- Just before the procedure begins, break the seal and open the pack.
- Unfold the first corner *away* from you; then unfold the two sides.
- Pull the front fold down toward you and drop it without touching the inner surface. If there is an inner wrap, open it in the same manner.
- A sterile field has now been established. Any nondisposable items (wrapped separately) may now be added to the sterile field.
- Stand back from the table and grasp the object through the wrapping, using one hand. With the other hand, unseal the wrappings, allowing them to fall down over your wrist.
- Hold the edges of the wrapper with your free hand and drop the object onto the sterile field without dropping the wrapper.
- Add any disposable items (sponges, gloves, etc.) These will be supplied in "peel down" paper wraps. Separate the paper layers of the wraps. Invert the package and let the object fall onto the sterile field.
- If a liquid medium is to be added, read the label carefully and position the liquid toward your hand.
- Open the spout and squirt a few drops into a wastebasket or sink, to wash the container lip.
- Pour the required amount into the sterile receptacle on the tray.
- Items in the sterile field may be manipulated with sterile forceps. Replace the forceps with the tips in the

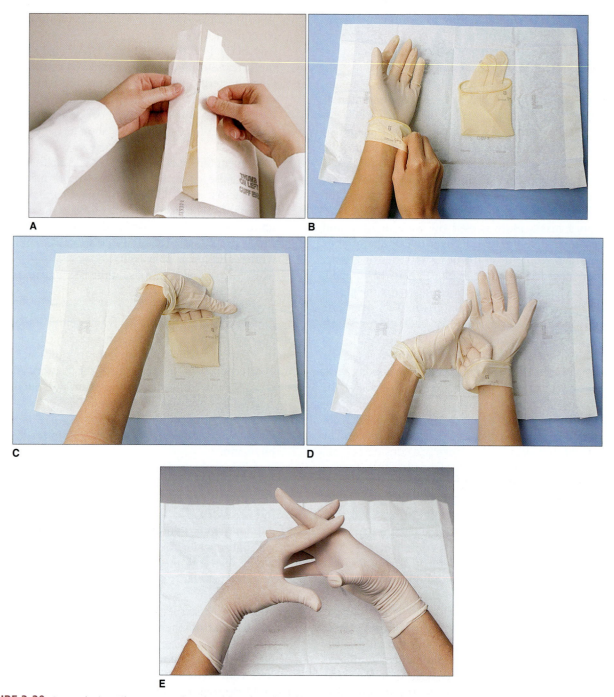

FIGURE 3-20 Open gloving. The sonographer should perform hand hygiene. Choosing the correct size glove is important. **A,** Remove outer glove package and lay it on a clean, flat surface just above waist level. Open package, keeping gloves on wrapper's inside surface. **B,** Glove the dominant hand first. With thumb and first two fingers of nondominant hand, grasp edge of cuff of glove for dominant hand. Touch only the glove's inside surface. Carefully pull the glove over the dominant hand, leaving cuff and being sure cuff does not roll up wrist. **C,** With gloved dominant hand, slip fingers underneath second glove's cuff. **D,** Carefully pull second glove over nondominant hand. Do not allow fingers and thumb of gloved dominant hand to touch any part of exposed nondominant hand. Keep thumb of dominant hand abducted back. **E,** After second glove is on, interlock hand. The cuffs usually fall down after application.

sterile field and the handles protruding toward you, to use again.
• If the procedure is delayed, do not open the pack. If it has already been opened, cover it at once with a sterile drape or discard it.

After the procedure is completed, don gloves and thoroughly clean all reusable items before returning the pack to central supply. Discard disposable items, placing needles in sharps containers and the remainder in a bio-hazard bag.

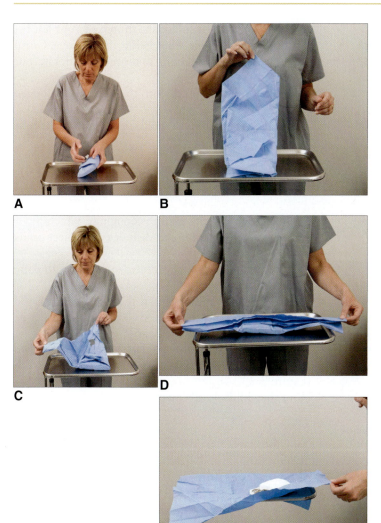

FIGURE 3-21 Preparing a sterile field. **A, B,** Open the first corner away from yourself. **C,** Open one side by grasping a corner tip. **D,** Open the second side in the same manner. **E,** Pull the remaining corner toward yourself. If there is an inner wrap, it should be opened in the same manner.

ISOLATION TECHNIQUES

Before the development of universal precautions, the diagnosis or even the suspicion of communicable disease resulted in patient isolation. Formerly, hospital isolation procedures were adopted that were either disease specific or category specific, which included seven different types of isolation. With the advent of standard precautions and additional precautions, the following isolation techniques evolved:

1. *Blood-borne isolation techniques.* In addition to standard precautions, patients who contaminate the environment or cannot be expected to assist in maintaining appropriate hygiene or environmental control should be placed in a private room.
2. *Airborne precautions.* When working with patients known to have or suspected of having serious illnesses that are transmitted by droplet nuclei, you should always wear respiratory protection, especially when entering the room of a patient suspected of having tuberculosis.

EMERGENCY MEDICAL SITUATIONS

Each year thousands of emergency medical situations end in death because the victim did not receive immediate and proper first aid. This section focuses on the two medical emergencies that sonographers are most likely to encounter during their work with patients. In addition, being proficient in performing emergency measures can make a critical difference in the lives of your family and all other people with whom you interact outside of your daily work activities.

Choking

Choking typically results from a blockage of the upper airway by food or other objects, preventing normal breathing. In some cases, victims can dislodge the object by coughing; however, if this is not possible, choking becomes a medical emergency requiring fast, appropriate action. When someone with a completely blocked airway begins to choke, no oxygen can enter the lungs. Brain cells, which are extremely sensitive to oxygen deprivation, will begin to die within 4 to 6 minutes. If first aid is not initiated quickly, brain death can occur in as little as 10 minutes.

The universal sign of choking is that of clutching the throat while having difficulty breathing. At times, the victim's attempts to inhale may produce a high-pitched sound. The symptoms can rapidly progress to cyanosis and loss of consciousness. Even partial air exchange (involving a partial obstruction) should be treated as a complete airway obstruction.

To assist a choking victim, you must be ready to perform the **Heimlich maneuver**. This emergency treatment involves the application of sudden, upward pressure on the upper abdomen (abdominal thrusts) to create an artificial "cough" and force foreign objects from the windpipe. There are separate techniques for adults and children over 1 year of age and for babies under the age of 1.

The Heimlich maneuver (abdominal thrusts) for adults and children over age 1: If the victim can breathe, speak, and cough, *do not* interfere. If the victim cannot breathe, cough, or speak, begin the Heimlich maneuver (Figure 3-22):

- Stand behind the victim.
- Make a fist and place it below the rib cage and above the navel of the victim.
- Grasp your fist with your other hand.
- Give 6 to 10 quick, sharp thrusts backward and upward.

- If the victim is obese, place the thumb of your left fist against the breastbone—not below the rib cage. Grasp the fist with your right hand and squeeze quickly, four times.
- Continue, uninterrupted, until the object is dislodged or help arrives.
- When the object is dislodged, seek medical help at once.

To clear the airway of a choking infant under the age of 1 year, follow these steps:

- *Do not* proceed if the infant is coughing forcefully or has a strong cry, as this can dislodge the object on its own.
- *Do not* grasp or pull the object out if the choking infant is conscious.
- *Do not* perform these steps if the child has stopped breathing for other reasons such as asthma, allergic reaction, or a blow to the head.
- Assume a seated position and lay the infant face down along your forearm, which is resting on your thigh (Figure 3-23, *A*).
- Hold the child's head lower than its body.

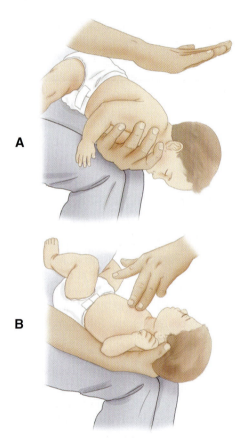

A

B

FIGURE 3-23 The Heimlich maneuver on infants. **A,** Back blows are administered between the shoulder blades to an infant supported on the arm and thigh. **B,** Chest thrusts are administered in the same position as for cardiac compressions, using two or three fingers.

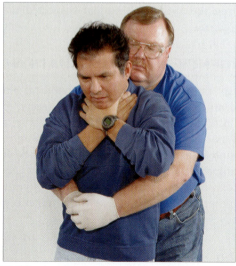

FIGURE 3-22 The Heimlich maneuver (abdominal thrusts) may be applied to choking patients either in the standing or in the supine position. The victim here is giving the universal sign of choking, with the hands crossed over the throat.

- Thump the infant gently but firmly five times on the middle of the back between the shoulder blades, using the heel of your hand. The combination of gravity and back blows should release the blocking object.
- If the objection doesn't dislodge by itself, turn the infant face up on your forearm with its head lower than its body (Figure 3-23, *B*).
- Using two fingers placed in the center of the breastbone between the nipples, give five quick chest compressions.
- Continue five back blows and five chest thrusts until the object is dislodged.
- If breathing doesn't resume or the child loses consciousness, call for emergency medical help.
- If the object is dislodged, seek medical help to prevent complications that can arise from the choking or from the first aid provided.

If the victim is unconscious and breathing, follow these steps:

- Place the child down on his back.
- Place the heel of one hand (fingers pointing in the direction of the child's head) against the middle of his abdomen, just above the navel and well below his sternum.
- Place the other hand on top of the first hand. Using both hands, administer five thrusts, pressing inward and upward. Each thrust should be a separate and distinct effort to dislodge the object.
- Maintain your heel hand contact with the abdomen between thrusts.
- If the object is visible, perform a finger sweep by grasping the child's tongue and jaw, lifting upward to pull the tongue away from the back of the child's throat and the lodged object.
- Using the index finger of your other hand, slide the finger inside the baby's cheek and use a sweeping, hooking action across the interior of the mouth, to the other cheek.
- If the object is within reach, you can dislodge it, grasp it, and remove it. *Do not* force the object deeper, which can happen easily in young children.

To clear the airway of an unconscious person:

- Lower the person on his or her back, onto the floor.
- Clear the airway.
- If there is a visible blockage at the back of the throat or high in the throat, reach a finger into the mouth and sweep out the cause of the blockage.
- Be careful not to push the food or object deeper into the airway.
- Begin cardiopulmonary resuscitation (CPR) as described next, if the object remains lodged and the person doesn't respond after you take these measures. The chest compressions used in CPR may dislodge

the object, so remember to recheck the mouth periodically.

Only perform finger sweeps on unconscious victims, as the action could cause a conscious person to gag or vomit. If the victim is obese or in advanced pregnancy, performing a chest thrust would be safer.

Cardiopulmonary Respiration

Cardiopulmonary respiration (CPR) can be defined as a combination of emergency life-saving techniques aimed at restarting lung and heart function in patients in cardiac arrest (breathing and heart beat have stopped). CPR is most successful when an irregular heartbeat is the cause of the cardiac arrest.

The heart is a muscle that can rapidly deteriorate when oxygenated blood stops flowing to the brain and other vital organs. The goal of CPR is to maintain circulation and breathing until emergency help arrives. It is important to note that if done improperly, CPR can result in serious injury. Therefore, it should not be performed unless a person has stopped breathing and does not demonstrate signs of circulation (normal breathing, coughing, or movement in response to rescue breathing).

CPR measures include chest compressions to pump blood out of the heart and into the body and rescue breathing. Time is the critical factor when initiating CPR, because death can occur within 8 to 10 minutes. Approximately 95% of sudden cardiac arrest victims will die without treatment, but given CPR assistance, the survival rate triples.

For 50 years, CPR consisted of the combination of artificial blood circulation with chest compressions and lung ventilation. However, in March 2010, the American Heart Association and the European Resuscitation Council reversed their previous positions and endorsed the effectiveness of chest compressions alone—without artificial respiration—for adult victims who collapse suddenly in cardiac arrest.

Providing basic life support requires an orderly progression of activities. The American Heart Association coined the phrase *Think ABC: Airway, Breathing and Circulation* as an easily remembered reminder of that progression.

Persons untrained in CPR should provide hands-only, uninterrupted chest compressions (two per second) until trained professionals arrive. They should not attempt rescue breathing. For the person with training come the options to alternate between 30 chest compressions and two rescue breaths or to perform only chest compressions.

The first step in administering CPR is to evaluate the situation and check the patient for consciousness by tapping or gently shaking the victim's shoulder and loudly asking, "Are you OK?" *Do not* shake victims if there is a possibility of a neck or spinal injury. If there

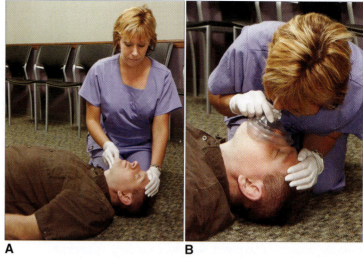

FIGURE 3-24 Methods of artificial ventilation. **A,** Backward head-tilt position. **B,** Mouth-to-mouth resuscitation technique.

is no response and you are alone, call out for help. If other people are present, send them for help.

Adult CPR

*   Roll the victim onto his back and pull him slowly toward you.
*   Open his airway by putting the palm of your hand on his forehead and gently tilting his head back (Figure 3-24, *A*).
*   With your other hand, gently lift his chin.
*   Check for normal breathing by looking listening and feeling, for no more than 10 seconds. Gasping is not normal breathing.
*   Initiate chest compressions by locating the sternal notch. Place the heel of your other hand on the notch, next to your fingers.
*   Remove your hand from the notch and put it on top of the other hand, keeping your fingers off the chest.
*   Position your shoulders over your hands and compress the breastbone 2 inches. Push hard and push fast.
*   Perform two compressions per second.
*   Do four cycles of compressions and breaths, rechecking the pulse after 1 minute.
*   If no pulse is found, continue CPR until help arrives.
*   If the victim has not responded after five cycles (about 2 minutes) and an automatic external defibrillator (AED) is available, apply it and follow the prompts.
*   Alternate one shock and resume CPR starting with chest compressions for 2 minutes before administering a second shock.

Child CPR

For children ages 1 through 8, the CPR procedure is essentially the same as that for an adult. The only differences are these:

*   If you are alone, perform five cycles of compressions and breaths for about 2 minutes before calling for help or using an AED.
*   Use only one hand to perform chest compressions.
*   Breathe more gently.
*   If there is no response after 2 minutes (five cycles) and an AED is available, use pediatric pads and follow the prompts. If no pediatric pads are available, use the adult pads.
*   Continue until the child moves or help arrives.

Infant CPR

Infant cardiac arrests occur primarily from lack of oxygen such as might result from drowning or choking. Perform first aid for choking if you know the infant has an airway obstruction. Perform CPR if you don't know why the infant isn't breathing:

*   Assess the situation by stroking the baby and watching for a response such as movement. *Do not* shake the child.
*   If there is no response and you are the only rescuer, do CPR for 2 minutes before calling for help.
*   If other persons are available, have one of them call for help immediately while you attend the infant.
*   Place the baby on his back on a firm flat surface such as a table, the floor, or the ground.
*   Open the airway by gently tipping the head back and lift the chin with your other hand.
*   Check for breathing for no more than 10 seconds, by putting your ear near the infant's mouth. Look for chest motion, listen for breath sounds and feel for breath on your cheek and ear.
*   If the chest still doesn't rise, check the infant's mouth to make sure no foreign material is inside. If you see

such an object, sweep it out with your finger. If the airway appears blocked, perform the same first aid indicated for a choking infant.
- Begin chest compressions to restore circulation.

Barrier Devices. As a result of the risk of exposure to infectious diseases, many CPR practitioners prefer to use barrier devices when providing artificial respiration. The barrier device is of no help to the victim; it is solely used to protect the practitioner. Such devices are designed to restrict the airflow in one direction and prevent direct contact between the mouths of the victim and the rescuer. There are two commonly used CPR barrier devices. One consists of a single sheet of thin plastic; the other is a larger pear-shaped plastic apparatus that will form a seal around the mouth (Figure 3-24, *B*).

After opening an airway and checking for any obstructions, the CPR barrier device should be positioned over the victim's mouth. Two quick rescue breaths are then directed into the CPR barrier. The device is removed, and a cycle of chest compressions should be performed. After approximately 30 chest compressions, the barrier device should be replaced and two more rescue breaths given. The cycle is repeated as outlined previously. As soon as the victim shows signs of recovery such as a cough or a gasp, the CPR barrier must be removed to give the victim adequate space to breathe. In some instances, vomiting will occur. Time should never be wasted trying to locate a barrier device because it will delay the onset of CPR. The lack of a barrier device should not prevent you from performing CPR in an emergency situation, as the threat of infectious diseases is relatively small.

Basic Cardiac Life Support

Automatic External Defibrillators. An automatic external defibrillator (AED) is a portable device used to diagnose cardiac rhythms and to detect the absence of them (Figure 3-25). In the latter case, it is used to administer an electrical shock to reestablish a normal cardiac rhythm. AEDs are very effective, even when used by individuals with only a limited amount of training, and many public places (schools, malls, gyms, airports, sports venues, and large office buildings) are beginning to have them available. The devices use audio and visual prompts to guide users through the process. Built-in computers assess the patient's heart rhythm, judge whether defibrillation is necessary, and administer the shock.

Before using an AED unit, check for signs of life. Never use an AED on a person who is breathing and has a pulse. If the victim's chest is not rising and there is no pulse, send someone for help and to bring back an AED unit, if one is available. Before using an AED unit, make sure the surroundings are safe. Tell people to step back, and then follow the prompts given by the AED machine:

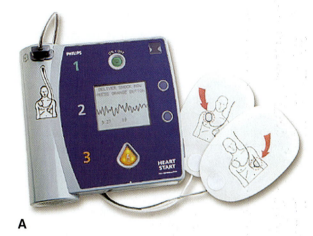

A

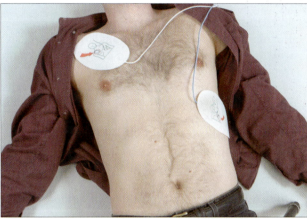

B

FIGURE 3-25 A, Automated external defibrillator (AED). **B,** Connect the adhesive pads to the AED cables, then apply the pads to the patient's chest at the upper-right sterna border and the lower-left ribs over the cardiac apex.

- Place one pad on the upper right side of the victim's chest and one on the lower left.
- The AED unit will diagnose the heart rhythm and indicate if a shock is needed.
- Only apply shock if there is no pulse and the unit instructs you to do so.
- Continue CPR until another shock command is issued.
- If only one shock was needed, simply follow the unit's commands until help arrives.

PROFESSIONAL ATTITUDES

Professionalism is composed of attitudes and behaviors. Often we behave in a manner to achieve optimal outcomes in our professional tasks and interactions. Whether it's attitudes or behaviors, how we interact with patients will have a significant effect on their reactions to us and their willingness to work together to improve their medical conditions.

The first step in caring for our patients is in how we communicate with them. Accurate communications is essential not only for the immediate situation but also for ongoing patient care. The way to establish rapport with our patients is by showing respect and by listening and responding to them as well as by giving instructions. Nonverbal communication is a process of communicating by sending and receiving wordless messages through body language, gesture, facial expression, eye contact, physical proximity, and touching. Patients will not entirely trust information given them when the body language and the verbal language of the speaker are not harmonious. The following suggestions are helpful in making sure that your patients fully understand you:

- Make eye contact with the patients to demonstrate that they have your full attention and to see that they are listening to you attentively.
- Sit rather than stand. Looking down on patients when communicating with them is intimidating. Sitting also will make the conversation seem less rushed and more respectful.
- Maintain a relaxed posture when speaking to patients. Do not cross your arms over your chest, as that gesture indicates negativity.
- Use a calm steady voice whenever communicating sensitive or important information. Patients will be more receptive to a lower, softer voice than a shrill one.
- Do not speak rapidly or use medical jargon because it will overwhelm your patients.
- Ask comprehensive questions that require a mixture of responses from the patient rather than just a yes or a no.
- If you explain a diagnosis or give instructions, be sure to ask if the patient understands. Many patients will say yes, but after additional conversation, you should be able to determine whether they *really* do understand.

Reestablishing Patient-Focused Care

A patient is someone in need. Patients come to us because they have health problems, and our job is to assist them. The move toward patient-focused care comes at a time when it is important to stem the tide against the long trend of turning health care into a business by treating patients as *clients* or *users* and by focusing primarily on *cost-cutting* and *maximizing productivity*. The term *patient* should be defended. It implies suffering over time. Patients should be treated with dignity and as individuals, and they should be empowered to make choices about their own care. This can only be done if they are not hurried along, if they are provided information in a form they can understand, and if their views are listened to. It is hoped that among all health professionals, the return to this kind of focus will rekindle the long-admired traits of caring, compassion, and respect and encourage a sharing of skills to enhance the patient's existence.

ASSISTING PATIENTS WITH SPECIAL NEEDS

Although much of your studies focus on the art and science of producing valuable diagnostic studies, another important dimension to being a sonographer is that of assessing not only your patients' illnesses or diseases but also any special needs that they may have. This section provides suggestions on how to deal with many types of patients, including the elderly, those with sensory challenges, and culturally diverse patients whose religious and ethnic backgrounds may run counter to our own.

Crying Patients

People respond to news in many different ways. Part of your job is to comfort patients. You may not have to *do* anything if your patient is crying. Sometimes, the best thing is just be with them, sending the message that at times it is alright to cry. Sharing a burden with someone else can make bad news tolerable. If you acknowledge the situation in a calm manner, you communicate to the patient that you are concerned about him or her and that although there may be nothing you can do to fix the situation, you would like to offer what help you can. If you don't know what to do, ask. Ask the patient what would be most helpful at that moment. You may have a great opportunity to heal, even if you cannot cure.

Pediatric Patients

Small children may have difficulty expressing themselves when in unfamiliar surroundings. Usually, however, they respond to a smile and a firm and gentle touch. The following tips may make it easier for you to effectively work with the pediatric patient:

- Ask the child's name and use that familiar name throughout the exam.
- Allow the child to take a favorite toy into the ultrasound lab to promote a sense of security.
- Reassure a small child by talking to him in a cheerful voice, even though he may not understand all that you say.
- Remain calm, cheerful, and unhurried to give the child the opportunity to respond to the strange surroundings and frightening machines in a medical setting.

Children over the age of 4 or 5 respond differently because they are able to share information and may be able to cooperate more fully. Practice the following suggestions when dealing with this age group:

- Children fear the loss of control. By giving them simple options such as getting onto the scanning table by themselves, or with your help, their feeling of control may be restored.

- Never tell a child, "This won't hurt very much." The only word the child will hear is *hurt*.
- Always explain what you are going to do and why you need to do it, in words that the child can understand.
- If the child asks questions, answer them simply. Do not force information on children, as it only makes them apprehensive.
- Keep directions simple and honest and assure the child that you will work as fast as you can.
- When dealing with a disruptive child or one who refuses to follow directions, set limits such as "You must lie still" or "You may not get down."

If you have been patient, and reasonable attempts are not working, ask for help. If hospital policies permit, immobilize the child gently but firmly, and complete the exam as quickly as possible.

Adolescent Patients

Working with adolescent patients can be challenging and will require creativity, flexibility, and openness. Young adolescents often try to act like adults, while hiding the fact that they are confused or frightened. In this age group, modesty and privacy are very important. You can earn the adolescent patient's trust by adopting a friendly and nonjudgmental approach and being sensitive to their concerns about privacy and confidentiality.

Elderly Patients

Patients should be treated according to their clinical needs rather than their age. However, we must also acknowledge that aging does have adverse effects on the systems of the body (Box 3-6) and allowances must be made for those who may have multiple health issues as well as patterns of disease and responses to treatment that differ from those of younger patients. Patients over age 85 represent the fastest growing segment of our population and are most vulnerable to adverse outcomes. It is important that you become competent and comfortable in dealing with an older patient, especially the frail elder with an unstable disability for whom even the smallest event may affect the ability to function on a daily basis.

Some elderly patients may be incontinent, immobile, unstable, confused, and even display dementia as a result of their diseases. Box 3-7 lists strategies for dealing with some of the more common physical limitations of older patients. Be aware that older patients often experience a rapid onset of illness coupled with an increase in complications and delayed recovery because they lack physiologic reserves. Diseases of the elderly tend to be chronic and progressive, evolving over a long period of time. Minor insults can produce major problems, and the more coexisting health issues an elderly patient has and the more medications he or she must take lead to higher risks and more rapid deterioration.

Culturally Diverse Patients

Culture has a profound effect on our attitudes and the way in which we communicate and perceive others. There are more than 100 ethnic groups and more than 500 American Indian groups in the United States, making it one of the most culturally diverse countries in the world. Studies have shown that patients from other cultures feel alienated by the language and communication

---

BOX 3-6 | The Effects of Aging on the Body

Sensory
The development of nearsightedness and cataracts increases sensitivity to light, glare, and the risk of falling.

Cardiovascular
As systolic blood pressure rises, elder patients are at increased risk of stroke, if untreated. As their cardiovascular reserves decline, they become more likely candidates for congestive heart failure or orthostatic hypotension.

Pulmonary
Older patients with pulmonary disease, rather than aging changes alone, will experience atrophy of the respiratory muscles and a decline in the elasticity of their lungs.

Genitourinary
Reduced bladder capacity and residual urine increase the incidences of nocturia and functional incontinence in the elder patient.

Gastrointestinal
Loss of teeth can lead to poor nutrition or malnutrition. Declining liver function increases the chance of drug toxicity with respect to drugs metabolized by the liver. Peristalsis declines and, with it, diet and fluid intake suffer.

Mulsculoskeletal
Muscle mass declines 30% with age, thereby decreasing muscle strength, bulk, and endurance. Bone density declines in both men and women may yield fractures. Degeneration of joints produces pain and increased falls.

Neurologic
Neurologic decline is more profound after age 75 and may manifest as slowed reaction times, accidents, and falls as well as a decline in the responsiveness of the autonomic nervous system.

Immune System
The skin's ability to serve as a protective barrier begins to decline. Cellular immune responses decline, increasing the risk of infection. Cough reflexes decline, increasing the risk of pneumonia and influenza and prolonged recovery times.

Homeostatic Responses
Postural hypotension predisposes to falls. Thirst mechanisms decline, producing dehydration.

BOX 3-7	Strategies for Dealing with Physical Limitations of the Elderly Patient

Vision and Hearing Problems

Provide good lighting. Ask patients if they wear corrective lenses or hearing aids.

Slowed Physical Pace

Aging produces a tendency to proceed at one's own pace. Most elderly patients respond poorly to a feeling of being pushed or hurried.

Mental Confusion

Older patients may not understand why they find themselves in unfamiliar surroundings. Medication, illness, senility, or injury may be the reason for mental confusion. However, Alzheimer's disease or organic brain syndrome may also play a role. Treating elder patients calmly, patiently, and with respect will help them maintain their sense of identity and increases their desire to be cooperative.

Patients who appear confused respond best to familiar situations. Use the patient's full name and ask questions about his past (e.g., where she was born, etc.). Such questions give them a sense of comfort because their distant memories may be much clearer than their short-term memory.

barriers of the dominant culture and by their strong allegiance to family and folk medicine. Any alienation they feel in their daily life is carried over into their perceptions and experiences with the health care system. Box 3-8 outlines some cultural differences you may encounter in a clinical setting.

Culturally appropriate care is that which respects individuality, creates mutual understanding, caters to spiritual needs, and maintains dignity. One universal principle germane to this topic is that health professionals may have to challenge their own assumptions and develop an understanding of the many cultures and subcultures with which they may deal on a daily basis. The starting point for improving any service is to understand the expectations of its users and to manage areas of conflict between personal and institutional values and individual patients' cultural requirements. The following suggestions are intended to help both you and your culturally diverse patients:

- Document any request to be treated by only male or female staff.
- Thoroughly explain the procedure that you need to conduct, including which body parts you will need to touch and the reason for examining them.
- Understand that there may be a cultural reluctance to discuss certain topics, particularly if you, or an interpreter, are not of the same gender as the patient.
- Use words—not gestures—to convey your meaning (see Box 3-8). Gestures acceptable in one culture may be offensive in others.

BOX 3-8	Cultural and Language Differences among Multicultural Patients

Gestures

- Gestures commonly used in the United States may have different meanings or be offensive to patients of different cultures. For example, using a finger or hand to indicate *come here* is a gesture used in some cultures to summon dogs. Pointing with one finger may also be considered rude. In Asian cultures, the entire hand is used to point to something.

Touch

- In American culture, patting a child's head is considered friendly or affectionate. However, many Asians consider touching someone's head inappropriate, as the head is believed to be a sacred part of the body.
- Physical contact while speaking may lead to discomfort because touching may be viewed as too intimate. Do not put your arm around the patient's shoulder or touch the person's face or hold his or her hand. Shaking hands upon meeting is acceptable, but only momentarily.
- In the Middle East, the left hand is reserved for bodily hygiene and should not be used to touch another part or to transfer objects.
- In Muslim cultures, touch between individuals of the opposite gender is generally considered inappropriate.

Eye Contact

- Americans interpret eye contact as attentiveness and honesty. In many cultures (Hispanic, Asian, Middle Eastern, and Native American), however, eye contact is considered disrespectful or rude, especially from children. Lack of eye contact does not mean that a person is not paying attention.
- Women, in particular, may avoid eye contact with men because it can be seen as a sign of sexual interest.

Babies

- Admiring babies and young children and commenting on how cute they are is avoided in Hmong and Vietnamese cultures for fear that these comments will be overheard by a spirit who will try to steal the baby or otherwise cause it some harm.

Personal Space

- The average acceptable personal distance varies from culture to culture. Americans tend to require more personal space than people in other cultures and will back away if they feel that their personal space has been invaded.
- In many Hispanic cultures, personal and physical spaces are not emphasized and an individual may stand less than a foot away from another when conversing. In these cultures, it is considered rude to step back.

Time

- Many Hispanic cultures have a relaxed attitude toward time. Tardiness or last-minute changes are perfectly acceptable, as things will get done "in good time."

Speaking

- Americans value courtesy when engaging in discussions. They will wait until there is an opportune time to state their views or ask questions.
- Taking turns when speaking is not always the rule in many foreign cultures. People will interrupt conversations, and often many people will speak simultaneously.

- Be aware of the personal wishes of patients regarding their condition. In some cultures, medical decisions are only made by the family.
- Respect the patient's privacy at all times. Some patients may prefer to converse or pray in private with family members while in your department.
- Respect the patient's dietary requirements, and be aware that some patients may be fasting for religious reasons at certain times.
- Respect the patient's dress requirements as decreed by the individual's faith.

Asking a patient's views about his illness or condition can be culturally and clinically valuable as it may reveal health beliefs and the names of diseases with which you are unfamiliar. The following list of questions may be useful when working with multicultural patients:

- What do you call your problem? Does it have a special name?
- What caused your problem?
- Why do you think it started when it did?
- How does your sickness affect you? How severe is it?
- What problems has your sickness caused you?
- What have you done to treat your sickness?
- What results do you hope to achieve?

As we interact with others of different cultures, there is no good substitute for receptiveness to interpersonal feedback, good observation skills, effective questions, and plain common sense.

EVALUATING PATIENT REACTIONS TO ILLNESS

When patients are ill, they are under stress and many emotional pressures. Fear of pain, prolonged illness, or death and feeling a loss of control are just a few. Being able to recognize the signs and symptoms of stress and identify how the patient is coping is essential to providing effective care. Some patient fears are so great that they will avoid seeking professional help.

Beside concerns about their bodies, patients have worries that their illness may separate them their loved ones, create financial problems, and isolate them from other people. The latter fear is particularly reinforced by not having questions answered by medical staff and being subjected to staff that talk too fast or fail to explain the reasons for tests or treatments.

Patients go through many emotional and psychological changes with regard to personal illness:

- *Denial or disbelief.* Patients may avoid, refuse, or *forget* needed care or appointments.
- *Acceptance.* During the acceptance phase, some patients may become dependent on the health care

team as they focus attention on their symptoms and illness.
- *Recovery.* Depending on how much a patient's lifestyle must change as a result of the illness, the patient will eventually begin to recover, rehabilitate, or convalesce.

The patient will go through a process of resolving perceived loss or impairment of normal function.

Fear is one of the greatest emotional responses to illness and may actually produce symptoms such as tachycardia, dry mouth, constipation/diarrhea, hypertension, increased perspiration, and a flight-or-flight reaction. Anxiety is another major reaction and can lead to fatigue, insomnia, urinary urgency, diarrhea or constipation, nausea, anorexia, and excessive perspiration. Ultimately, patients experience stress or tension. When the body is stressed by physical, psychological, or physiologic changes, it attempts to rid itself of the cause of the stress and the patient may develop ulcers, hair loss, or insomnia. Increasing feelings of helplessness may lead some patients to become overly dependent while searching for help and understanding. The overly dependent patient may also become fearful or angry.

Though as a sonographer you may not often be involved in the long-term care of your patients, you must understand that there are as many reactions to illness as there are patients. You also must learn that kindness, courtesy, and understanding will help your patients go through the illness with a minimum of stress and anxiety.

Terminal Patients

Despite the fact that we all realize our mortality, there is no easy way to discuss death. To strong and healthy patients, death is a frightening thought and many consciously put that reality out of mind. Terminally ill patients have many of the same basic needs as those of other patients: spiritual, psychological, cultural, economic, and physical. What makes these patients different is a sense of urgency to resolve the majority of their needs within a limited amount of time.

Accepting mortality and mourning loss are complicated processes. Not every patient will experience, in order, the oft-quoted five stages of dying—denial, anger, bargaining, depression, and acceptance—that were first introduced in Elisabeth Kübler-Ross's book *On Death and Dying* (1969). And for some, the stage of acceptance may never be reached. Patients traditionally view death from the perspective of their own cultural heritage, and many seek comfort and support in religious faith. Patients who do learn to accept their imminent deaths often feel the need to get their affairs in order as part of their preparation for dying, and they may want to use you as a sounding board for their plans. On the other hand, it is sometimes the case that the patient's family needs more emotional support than the patient does.

Caucasian Anglo-European culture expects a dying patient to show peaceful acceptance of his or her prognosis, and the bereaved are expected to show grief. Patients who belong to other ethnic groups may demonstrate a very different response, crying loudly and inflicting pain upon themselves. Death affects not only the individual patient but also family, friends, staff, and even other patients. For this reason, it is essential that all members of the health care team understand the process of dying and its possible effects on those left behind. Your partnership with your patients and their families will provide a unique insight into their values, spirituality, and relationship dynamics that will be especially helpful at the end of life.

PATIENT RIGHTS

The Patients' Bill of Rights

When patients seek health care, they expect that they have certain rights, including the rights to open and honest communication, respect for their person and their values, and sensitivity to any differences that may affect their care. In 2004, the American Hospital Association replaced an earlier Patients' Bill of Rights with a plain-language brochure called *The Patient Care Partnership: Understanding Expectations, Rights and Responsibilities*. This document is available is eight different languages (English, Arabic, Simplified Chinese, Traditional Chinese, Russian, Spanish, Tagalog, and Vietnamese).

The brochure outlines how patients have a right to do the following:

- Be treated with respect
- Make a treatment choice
- Refuse treatment
- Obtain their medical records
- Protect privacy of their medical records
- Have informed consent
- Make decisions about end-of-life care

Patients also must understand that that they have a responsibility to do the following:

- Maintain healthy habits
- Be respectful to providers
- Be honest with providers
- Comply with treatment plans
- Prepare for emergencies
- Read behind the headlines
- Make decisions responsibly

Unlike our nation's Bill of Rights, few of the patients' rights are clearly spelled out, except those relating to privacy and access to medical records. Compounding the problem, there are a number of rights that patients believe they have, but which are, in fact, not rights, like

access to health care and the right to *total* privacy of medical records. Patients also must understand the rights they do *not* have, so it will be easier for them to get the care and outcomes that they seek.

The Health Insurance Portability and Accountability Act (HIPAA)

The Health Insurance Portability and Accountability Act of 1996 (HIPAA) established new standards for the uses of health care information. HIPAA created three types of standards: privacy, security, and administrative simplification (e.g., transaction standards). Together, these regulations impact the day-to-day functioning of the nation's hospitals, medical providers, and medical community. They affect virtually every department of every entity that provides or pays for health care.

HIPAA has created national standards to protect individuals' medical records and other personal health information. It does the following:

- Gives patients more control over their health information
- Sets boundaries on the use and release of health records
- Establishes appropriate safeguards that health care providers and others must achieve to protect the privacy of health information
- Holds violators accountable with civil and criminal penalties that can be imposed if they violate patients' privacy rights
- Strikes a balance when public responsibility supports disclosure of some forms of data (i.e., in the case of protecting public health)

For patients, the HIPAA act means the following:

- Being able to make informed choices when seeking care and reimbursement for care, based on how personal health information may be used
- Being able to find out how their information may be used, and about certain disclosures of their information that have been made
- Generally, obtaining the right to examine and obtain a copy of their own health records and request corrections
- Empowering individuals to control certain uses and disclosures of their health information

For sonographers, the HIPAA act means the following:

- Putting patient information away after hours
- Taking files out of sight of any lingering staff and custodians
- Setting screensavers on computers for the shortest time possible
- Taking care that other patients do not overhear any conversations (including phone conversations)

- Removing patient identification from any scans that will be used for publication or presentation
- Keeping any patient charts filed with the names facing the wall to ensure that passersby or visitors to the ultrasound area cannot see the names or any information on the charts
- Honoring patient requests that students, other observers, medical personnel, and families leave the room during their sonography examination
- Explaining to patients the hospital or department policies regarding the rights of friends and family to view their ultrasound procedure
- Meeting the patient's expectation of a pleasant physical and emotional environment where comfort, safety, and respect as an individual are ensured.

The following links to the Patients' Bill of Rights and the Health Insurance Portability and Accountability Act (HIPAA) should be reviewed for any updates:

www.cc.nih.gov/participate/patientinfo/legal/bill_of_rights.shtml

www.hhs.gov/ocr/privacy/hipaa/understanding/consumers/index.html

Providing competent and excellent patient care in today's health care environment is challenging, both because today's patients are often better informed and more demanding and because many are newcomers to the United States who bring with them different cultural and religious views on how they should be treated. Patients expect reliable care, prompt responses to their requests, and assurances that they will be safe under a sonographer's care. They expect not only proficiency, but empathy.

The modern sonographer must meet a growing list of needs while competently and efficiently carrying out his or her sonographic duties. Most diagnostic medical sonography programs do a good job of educating and training students in the scientific and technical aspects of sonography. However, they must also focus equal attention on helping sonography students to develop a humanistic approach when dealing with their patients. They must also stress the critical importance of continuing education after graduation, to stay current with the rapid and exciting developments that are a hallmark of diagnostic medical sonography.

Ergonomics and Musculoskeletal Issues in Sonography

Carolyn Coffin and Joan P. Baker

HISTORY OF ERGONOMICS

Broadly defined, **ergonomics** is the science of designing a job to fit the individual worker. One of its primary goals is increasing productivity and decreasing injury by modifying products, tasks, and environments to better fit people.

The term *ergonomics* comes from the Greek words *ergon*, meaning *work*, and *nomos*, meaning *study of* or *natural laws*. The word first entered the modern lexicon when Wojciech Jastrzebowski used it in his 1857 philosophical tract titled *The Science of Work, Based on the Truths Taken from the Natural Science*. The association between work activities and musculoskeletal injuries has been documented for centuries. Bernardino Ramazinni (1633–1714) was the first physician to write about work-related injuries and illnesses in his 1700 publication *De Morbis Artificum (Diseases of Workers)*, which he researched by visiting the workplaces of his patients.

In the early 1900s, industry production was still largely dependent on human power and motion, rather than on machines, and ergonomic concepts were developing to improve worker productivity. Frederick Winslow Taylor pioneered the "scientific management" method, which sought to improve worker efficiency by discovering the optimum way to do any given task. Frank and Lillian Gilbreth expanded upon Taylor's methods in the early 1900s with their time and motion studies aimed at improving efficiency by eliminating unnecessary steps and motion.

The assembly line developed by Ford Motor Company between 1908 and 1915 was heavily influenced by the emerging field of ergonomics. In assembly line manufacturing, parts are added to a product in a sequential, well-planned manner to create a finished product much faster than with handcrafting-type methods. Although assembly line production improved productivity in the Ford Motor Company, it also reduced the need for workers to move throughout their workday and, thus, resulted in static work postures.

World War II brought about a greater interest in human-machine interaction, a natural result of the development of new and complex machines and weaponry. It was not only observed that the success of the machine depended on its operator but also that the design of the machine influenced how successful its operator was. It was important that equipment fit the size of the soldier and that controls were logical and easy to understand. After World War II, the equipment design focus expanded to include worker safety as well as productivity.

In the decades since the war, the field of ergonomics has continued to flourish and diversify with the advent of the Space Age and the Computer Age.

History of Work-Related Musculoskeletal Disorders (WRMSD) in Sonography

Awareness of pain and discomfort associated with the occupation of sonography surfaced around 1980 just before the widespread use of real-time scanners. The most common complaint was shoulder pain in the sonographer's scanning arm. The increasing number of complaints reached the attention of Marveen Craig, a well-known sonographer, educator, and author. Craig published an article in 1985 summarizing the results of a survey done of 100 sonographers who had between 5 and 20 years of scanning experience.[2] The survey respondents complained of stress and burnout, vision problems that improved when images switched from black on white to white on black, infections, and allergies. Electric shock was not uncommon, especially when doing bedside studies and when removing transducers from the articulated arm of static scanners. Muscle strain involving the wrist, base of the thumb, and shoulder was also reported. Sonographers complained of heavy transducers and cables, and carpal tunnel syndrome claimed its first victim. The term "sonographer's shoulder" came into use.

In the early 1980s, ultrasound systems underwent a complete redesign to real-time two-dimensional scanners, and although articulated arm scanners were used for many more years, real-time scanners were slowly introduced to most faculties.

As more real-time systems came into use, sonographer's shoulder appeared to diminish. However, this decline lasted only 10 years, and by 1995, the Society of Diagnostic Medical Sonography (SDMS) started receiving increasingly more and varied complaints. In 1997, an extensive 125-question survey was developed by the Health Care Benefit Trust of Vancouver Canada (HBT), in collaboration with the SDMS, the Canadian Society of Diagnostic Medical Sonography (CSDMS), and the British Columbia Ultrasound Society (BCUS). Through this survey, the incidence of work-related musculoskeletal disorder (WRMSD) was found to be 81% in the United States and 87% in Canada, for a combined average incidence in North America of 84%.[3,4]

In 2008, a follow-up survey was conducted, and the incidence increased from 81% to 90% in the United States. Several variables may account for this increase: aging workforce, increased awareness of WRMSD among sonographers, and increased willingness by sonographers to report injury.

History of OSHA's Involvement in Sonography

In 1970 Congress passed the federal **Occupational Safety and Health Act (OSHA)**. The purpose of OSHA is to ensure, as far as possible, that every working man and woman in the nation has safe and healthful working conditions. Employers may be subjected to civil, and sometimes, criminal penalties if they violate this act.[5]

The act is administered by the Occupational Safety and Health Agency of the U.S. Department of Labor, although individual states had the option to create their own agency to enforce the act. Approximately 50% of the states opted to be regulated by federal OSHA. The other states created their own agencies, which operate under a "state plan." For example, California has a state plan and created its own agency, Cal/OSHA, to enforce safety regulations within that state.[5]

Where industry-specific guidelines do not exist within OSHA, the general duty clause can be used. Lawyers representing injured sonographers seeking legal recourse refer to this clause. The criteria for applying the general duty clause are as follows:

- No acceptable standard for an industry
- Exposure to hazard that causes serious physical harm
- Hazard is recognized by the industry
- Feasible abatement method exists to correct the hazard

Section 5B to the general duty clause states that each employee shall comply with occupational safety and health standards and all rules, regulations, and orders issued pursuant to this act that are applicable to his or her own actions and conduct.[6]

It is under the provisions of paragraph 5A(1) that OSHA addresses ergonomic disorders. The language in paragraph 5B gives the impression that the employee holds significant responsibility for complying with health and safety standards; however, the employer bares most of the responsibility for compliance in the eyes of OSHA.[6]

Over the years, OSHA has used many different labels for occupational injury:

- Cumulative trauma disorder (CTD)
- Repetitive motion injury (RMI)
- Overuse syndrome
- Repetitive strain injury (RSI)
- Musculoskeletal strain injury (MSI)

The term **work-related musculoskeletal disorder** (**WRMSD**) is currently in use. WRMSD incidents are defined as injuries that result in (1) restricted work, (2) days away from work, (3) symptoms of musculoskeletal disorder (MSD) that remain for 7 or more days, and (4) MSD requiring medical treatment beyond first aid.

According to Liberty Mutual, which collects data on WRMSD and the associated costs, repetitive motion injuries cost U.S. industries 2.3 billion dollars. Ultrasound exam specialties such as echocardiography, high-risk OB and, to a lesser extent vascular sonography, involve repetitive motion.

Liberty Mutual also reports that 95% of chief executive officers support workplace safety. Benefits include improved employee health. Indirect costs such as morale, productivity, and hiring of replacement staff are significantly reduced, whereas direct costs such as wage replacement and medical expenses are avoided.[1]

Over the years, the Department of Labor received numerous requests from workers' unions to create a way for employees to deal with their WRMSDs. This resulted in the development of an Alliance Program, which enables organizations to work with OSHA to prevent workplace injuries by educating and leading employers and their employees in advancing workplace safety and health.

In May 2003, an International Ultrasound Industry Consensus Conference was hosted by the SDMS to develop injury risk-reducing standards to address the problem of work-related musculoskeletal disorders in sonography. Twenty-six organizations represented by 32 participants attended the conference with the goal of discussing how they might design new platforms and procedures that incorporate better ergonomics. The industry standards address the role of employees and employers, educators, medical facilities, and equipment manufacturers in reducing the impact of these injuries on the workforce and are intended to assist all stakeholders in making informed decisions.

Separately, but at the same time, administrators addressed the issues of workload, scheduling, and room size, while sonographers discussed best practices, education, and training. The need for accredited programs to include curriculum related to ergonomics and injury prevention, as well as certifying bodies testing knowledge of risk factors, was covered.

INJURY DATA IN SONOGRAPHY

Definitions

Work-related musculoskeletal disorders are injuries of muscles, tendons, and joints that are caused by or aggravated by workplace activities. These injuries are the main reason for long-term absence among health care workers,[8] accounting for up to 60% of all workplace illnesses. Survey data have shown that more than 80% of sonographers have some form of MSD that can be attributed to their work activities.

Surveys

Table 4-1 outlines the numerous surveys that have been conducted on the incidence of this injury in sonography. These surveys have produced other data relevant to the study of occupational injury in ultrasound, and their results support the presence of risk factors in the sonography profession. A number of other factors contribute to reported injury rates, including worker awareness; unwillingness to work in pain; busier patient schedules; job dissatisfaction; an aging workforce; and computerization of the workplace.

A positive relationship has been demonstrated between the severity of MSDs and the performance of repetitive work tasks or tasks that require forceful movements, with or without repetitive motion.[9] Increased use of technology has resulted in workers' being able to accomplish the same work tasks with fewer movements. Thus, the relationship between the user and the workstation equipment has become "frozen," and the worker is often forced into a static posture. This combination of repetitive motions and prolonged static postures results in musculoskeletal discomfort and eventually injury.

TABLE 4-1	Surveys of Work-Related Musculoskeletal Disorders				
Author	**Year**	**Number Surveyed**	**Number Responded**	**Incidence**	**Scope**
Vanderpool	1993	225	101	86%	Random ARDMS
BCUS	1994	232	211	91%	BC Canada
SDMS	1995	3,000	983	81%	Random ARDMS
CSDMS	1995	Unknown	427	87%	Canada
Smith	1997	220	113	80%	National cardiac
Wihlidal	1997	156	96	89%	Alberta Canada
Gregory	1998	Unknown	197	77.8%	Australia
Magnavita	1999	2670	2041	74%	Italy MD's
McCullough	2002	Unknown	295	82%	United States
Ransom	2002	Unknown	300	89%	United Kingdom
Sound Ergonomics	2008	5,800	3,244	90%	United States

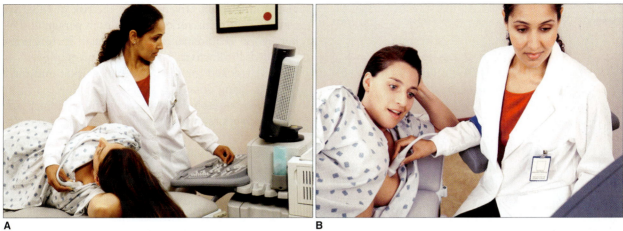

FIGURE 4-1 **A,** Bad ergonomics. Right-handed cardiac scanning is likely to cause injury to the sonographer because of the abduction of the arm over the patient's back, the hyperflexion of the right wrist, and the need to lean to the right and twist the neck to view the monitor. Moreover, it is the obese patient population that requires this type of test, making the level stretching and twisting even worse. **B,** Good ergonomics. It is difficult to reduce these risk factors, but one way is to turn the patient around to perform the study. (Courtesy Siemens Healthcare, Ultrasound USA Division.)

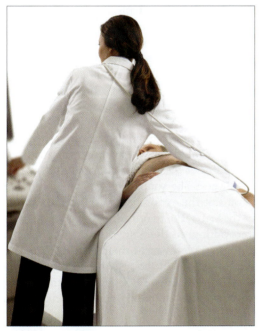

FIGURE 4-2 Asymmetric forces are exerted on the spine when more weight is put on one side of body. This means that the head must be turned further to view the monitor, resulting in a twisted neck. (Courtesy Philips Healthcare, Ultrasound, North America.)

Risk Factors

Risk factors include forceful exertions, awkward postures and prolonged static postures, repetitive motions, "pinch" grip, and exposure to environmental factors such as extreme heat, cold, humidity, or vibrations (Figure 4-1). The accumulated exposure to one or more of these risk factors over time leads to injury, because repeated exposure interferes with the ability of the body to recover. WRMSDs cause pain, inflammation, swelling, deterioration of tendons and ligaments, and spinal degeneration. Muscles and joints are further stressed once their support structures are weakened.

Mechanisms of Injury

Sustained awkward postures can cause imbalances between the muscles that move and the muscles that stabilize. Repeatedly rotating the head, neck, and trunk causes one set of muscles to become stronger and shorter and the opposing muscles to become weaker and elongated. Asymmetric forces are exerted on the spine causing misalignment (Figure 4-2). Nerve entrapment syndromes can result from increased muscle and tendon pressure on major nerves that run behind tightened muscles. Tasks that require the worker to continually lean forward or to bend the head down or laterally are examples of these types of postures. Prolonged static postures, whether sitting or standing, increase the load on soft tissues and the compressive forces on the spine. Additionally, the contraction of more than 50% of the body's muscles is required to maintain static postures.[10] Human physiology depends on movement, which promotes normal muscle contraction and relaxation. Muscle activity circulates blood to carry nutrients to and remove toxins from muscles. Awkward and static postures cause muscles to continuously be contracted; therefore, they cannot receive oxygen or get rid of toxins.[11]

Types of Injury

Tendonitis and tenosynovitis. Inflammation of the tendon and the sheath around the tendon. These often occur together.

de Quervain's disease. Specific type of tendonitis involving the thumb that can result from gripping the transducer.

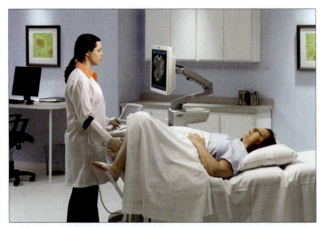

FIGURE 4-3 Epicondylitis can result from repeated twisting of the forearm, a motion performed when scanning transvaginally from the patient's side. Twisting of the forearm can be reduced or avoided by scanning from the foot of the table with the patient in leg supports (stirrups). (Courtesy Sound Ergonomics, LLC, Kenmore, Washington.)

Carpal tunnel. Entrapment of the median nerve as it runs through the carpal bones of the wrist. This results from repeated flexion and extension of the wrist and also from mechanical pressure against the wrist.

Cubital tunnel. Entrapment of the ulnar nerve as it runs through the elbow. This can result from repeated twisting of the forearm and mechanical pressure against the elbow when you rest it on the exam table while scanning.

Epicondylitis (lateral and medial). Inflammation of the periosteum in the area of the insertion of the biceps tendon into the distal humerus. This can result from repeated twisting of the forearm (Figure 4-3).

Thoracic outlet syndrome. Nerve entrapment can occur at different levels, resulting in a variety of symptoms.

Trigger finger. Inflammation and swelling of the tendon sheath in a finger entraps the tendon and restricts motion of the finger.

Bursitis (shoulder). Inflammation of the shoulder bursa from repeated motion.

Rotator cuff injury. Repeated motion results in fraying of the rotator cuff muscle tendons. This injury increases with age and is even more prevalent when work-related stresses are added. Repeated arm abduction contributes to this injury by restricting blood flow to the soft tissues of the shoulder.

Spinal degeneration. Intervetebral disc degeneration results from bending and twisting and improper seating

INDUSTRY AWARENESS AND CHANGES

The increase in MSDs in industry led to research into the causes and to legislation in the United States regulating the design of office furniture and duration of video terminal work. Appropriate ergonomic adaptations have been found to effectively reduce the risk of MSD symptoms. Adapting a workstation to each person and his or her work requirements ensures that it functions as intended. Productivity is increased if an employee's work area is arranged for the individual worker and the type of work being done.

Developing solutions to occupational injury among sonographers requires a combined effort on the part of equipment companies, employers, and sonographers. Because MSD is caused by multiple factors, injury prevention requires solutions from many sources as well. By taking a multidisciplinary approach, significant impacts can be made on the risk for work-related injury in the sonography profession.

Mitigating risk for injury involves a strategy for control. The first solutions to consider are engineering solutions, which involve a change in the physical features of a workplace. This is the preferred method for control because it can effectively eliminate the workplace hazard. However, these solutions also tend to be the most expensive initially.[7]

When engineering controls are not feasible or cost prohibitive, administrative controls can be implemented. These solutions are not as effective as engineering controls and include changes in workplace policies, changes in patient scheduling and sonographer rotations, and the implementation of rest breaks. Administrative controls lessen the duration and frequency of exposure to an injury risk.[7]

The least effective control is the use of personal protective equipment (PPE) or professional practices. This method addresses best practices and the use of arm support devices. The sonographer is still exposed to the risk factor, but the exposure is somewhat reduced.[7]

Over the years, the major ultrasound equipment manufacturers addressed the issue of occupational injury by redesigning the platform of their systems. This involved changing the aspects of the system's control panel, monitors, and transducers. As a result, many features of today's ultrasound systems are designed with ergonomics in mind.

Ergonomically Designed Ultrasound Systems

The well-designed ultrasound system should be easily mobile and have brakes. The control panel should be height adjustable and swivel. The monitor should also be height adjustable, independent of the control panel, and should turn and tilt. Controls should be easy to access without overreaching. Transducers should not be too wide, which causes stretching of the fingers, or too narrow, which causes a "pinch grip." Transducer cables should be thin, flexible, and lightweight, and the transducer cable should be supported during an exam. In addition, transducers should be easy to activate with readily accessible connecting ports and storage.

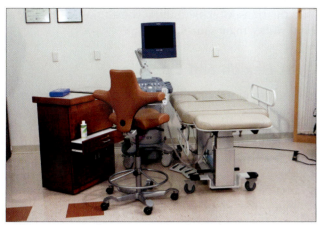

FIGURE 4-4 An ultrasound workstation with an ergonomically designed table and chair. (Courtesy Oakworks Medical, Inc., New Freedom, Pennsylvania.)

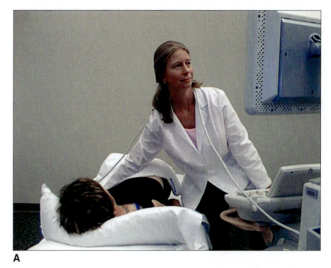

A

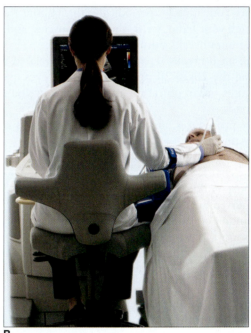

B

FIGURE 4-5 **A,** You must take responsibility for your postural alignment. **B,** Sit up straight with the top of the monitor level with your eyes and arms length away. Support your feet on the ring of the chair, and support your forearm on a cushion. (**A,** Courtesy Susan Rantz Stephenson. **B,** Courtesy Philips Healthcare, Ultrasound, North America.)

Other engineering controls involve the workstation, which includes the exam table and the chair and accessories (Figure 4-4). An electronically height adjustable exam table is an important component of an ergonomically designed workstation. It should be specialty specific by providing options that adapt it for use in certain procedures. Examples would be a drop section for apical cardiac views or stirrups for OB/GYN examinations. If the sonographer sits to scan, a height-adjustable chair with an appropriate height range is equally as important as the exam table. The sonographer also should be able to support his or her arms while scanning and have an exam room that is large enough to allow for a flexible setup. The room must have appropriate lighting to avoid glare on the monitor and reduce eyestrain.

Administrative Controls

Patient exams should be carefully scheduled to prevent repetition of the same type of exam back to back. It is important to perform a variety of exams, allowing different muscles to fire. The schedule should allow enough time between exams for muscle recovery. Exam gloves should have textured fingers to prevent the need to grip the transducer too tightly. Take short "mini" breaks during exams to relax muscles, especially in the shoulder and neck. If it is necessary to perform bedside exams, make sure that the ultrasound system can be moved easily and has a small footprint. Try to share bedside exams with other staff, and do these exams only when absolutely necessary, not because it is just more convenient. Bedside exams should be reserved for those patients whose condition prohibits transporting them.

Provide separate monitors so that the patient and the sonographer do not have to share the monitor mounted on the system. Provide ergonomically designed scanning rooms to reduce the risk of injury to the

sonographer, including appropriately adjustable ancillary equipment.

PPE/Professional Controls

You are the only person who can control your work postures and behaviors, some of which may be injury producing (Figure 4-5). You must take responsibility for your postural alignment and take the time to arrange the exam room equipment to suit you and the study you are performing. Best practices address how to prevent or reduce your exposure to known risk factors. Be aware of what causes pain and make changes in technique and postures immediately:

- Minimize sustained bending, twisting, reaching, lifting, and transducer pressure.
- Avoid awkward postures.
- Alternate sitting and standing throughout exams.
- Vary scanning techniques and transducer grips.
- Adjust all equipment to suit each user's size.
- Have accessories on hand before beginning the exam.
- Use appropriate measures to reduce arm abduction.
- Avoid forward and backward reach.
- Instruct the patient to move as close to you as possible.
- Adjust the height of the table and chair.
- Use support for your arms.
- Relax your muscles periodically throughout the day.
- Stretch your hand, wrist, shoulder muscles, and spine.
- Take mini breaks during the procedure.
- Take meal breaks separate from work-related tasks.
- Using the 20-20-20 rule, refocus your eyes every 20 minutes on an object about 20 feet from you for 20 seconds.
- Vary procedures, tasks, and skills as much as reasonably possible.
- Use correct body mechanics when moving patients, wheelchairs, beds, stretchers, and ultrasound systems.
- Report and document any persistent pain to your employer, and seek competent medical advice.
- Maintain a good level of physical fitness in order to perform the demanding work tasks required.
- Collaborate with employers on staffing solutions that allow sufficient time away from work.

WORK PRACTICE CHANGES

Gripping the Transducer

Use mild transducer pressure. Avoid the temptation to be "image-driven"—sacrificing your body for a "pretty picture" that does not affect the diagnosis. It is unnecessary to grip the transducer tightly. This might be no more than a bad habit and you may be unaware that you are doing it. This is also a difficult habit to break, as it is as natural as holding a pen.

Manufacturer improvements, such the lightweight flexible cables, can reduce the weight and torque that the transducer produces on the scanning hand. If they are available in your department, use lightweight transducers. Keeping the transducer handle free of excess gel will also reduce the amount of force needed to grip the transducer. It is also important to use gloves that fit properly. Gloves that are too large require more muscle force to grip than gloves that fit. Additionally, it takes 40% more effort to hold a transducer in a ergonomic pinch grip versus a power grip. Therefore, it is important to learn different ways to hold the transducer that allow you to use more of your hand rather than your fingers.

Wrist Flexion and Extension

It is important to keep the wrist in a neutral or "normal" position. Dorsiflexion of the wrist can lead to pressure and resultant injury in the carpal tunnel. This position requires the muscles of the forearm to fire continuously. When transporting the equipment, push from the legs not the arms and wrists, keeping your wrists in a neutral position. Avoid resting your wrist on the keyboard while scanning or typing. Be sure to support your forearm while scanning to reduce muscle fatigue of the forearm, neck, and shoulder.

Twisting Your Neck

This position produces increased pressure on the intervertebral discs and should be minimized as much as possible. Position the ultrasound system so that it is as close to the exam table as possible with the monitor facing you to reduce neck twisting. Do not share the monitor with the patient. An external monitor for patient viewing is strongly recommended. Also remember to keep your shoulders relaxed as much as possible, rolling them periodically during the scan to release your neck muscles.

Abduction of Your Scanning Arm

The main reason for shoulder pain associated with right-handed scanning is due to the abduction of the shoulder. Shoulder abduction must be reduced to 30 degrees or less (Figure 4-6). Lower the exam table or elevate the chair to achieve the correct posture. The sonographer must also position the patient by having him or her move to the edge of the exam table so that the patient's side is touching the sonographer's right hip to further reduce abduction and reach. One study showed that decreasing the angle of abduction from 75° to 30° and supporting the forearm on support cushions could achieve a reduction of up to 88% in muscle activity of the shoulder. Sonographers who are short in stature may have to stand to scan. It may also be helpful to sit for part of the scan and stand for other parts, as long as the equipment is readjusted to suit the two different positions. Support your scanning arm by placing support cushions or a rolled-up towel under your elbow.

Transducer Cable Management

Current transducers inherently create torque on the wrist forcing the muscles of the hand and forearm to fire constantly to counteract the drag. Cable braces can be used to hold and support the cable of ultrasound transducers. This takes the strain off the operator's hand and forearm

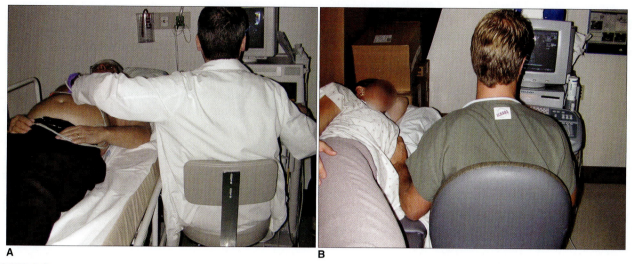

FIGURE 4-6 **A,** Bad ergonomic practice in left-handed cardiac scanning. **B,** Good ergonomics. In left-handed cardiac scanning, it is easy to adjust the height of the chair up and the table down to reduce the angle of abduction to 30 degrees or less. This often requires that you bring the patient to the edge of the table. (Courtesy Sound Ergonomics, LLC, Kenmore, Washington.)

created by the imbalance of the transducer and cable, significantly reducing torque on the wrist. Additionally, cable braces can alleviate the need to grip as tightly or the need to put the cable around your neck or between your hip and the table. This latter position creates issues of spinal alignment and weight imbalance.

Trunk Twisting

Trunk twisting is often necessary in small rooms where equipment cannot be optimally positioned to reduce twisting. Sonographers with poor scanning technique also exhibit this posture (Figure 4-7). If you stand to scan, have your weight evenly distributed over both feet so that your spine remains straight. If you are uncertain as to whether you have the habit of leaning on one leg, ask a colleague to watch you scan and observe your spine position. When seated, use your abdominal muscles to support your trunk, and sit upright with good postural alignment. This often takes some practice but can be more readily achieved by using a specially designed chair that puts you into a more natural position. These chairs have a saddle-type seat and are ideal for maintaining the natural lordosis of the spine. Another option is an air-filled cushion, which forces you to maintain a stable, more neutral, position by engaging your abdominal muscles to help you balance on the cushion.

Reaching

This occurs when you reach for the controls while scanning with the opposite hand. To reduce reach, the ultrasound system must be brought as close as possible to you. Frequently used controls should be in the middle of the control panel, so that regardless of the hand used to manipulate them, they can be adjusted without causing strain. If you sit to scan, you must be able to fit your legs under the control panel in order to position the system close enough. Be sure your feet are fully supported when sitting, either on the system, the floor, chair, or footstool. If this is not possible, it may be better to stand while scanning. Don't get into the habit of leaving your nonscanning arm in an extended position over the control panel, especially over the freeze frame control.

All these work practices also apply to your computer workstation and the PACs station. These environments are part of your workday and can be another source for injury. The heights of the computer monitor, work desk, and chair should all be adjustable. The keyboard should be positioned to minimize reach and maximize a neutral wrist posture.

Exercise

Sonographers should also learn and perform a regular maintenance exercise program designed to strengthen and stretch the shoulder, arms, hands, and trunk (Figure 4-8).

ECONOMICS OF ERGONOMICS

The cost of occupational injury to both the employer and the employee is phenomenal. The losses to the employer encompass not only the medical costs of an injury, but also the cost of replacement staff, workers' compensation, and loss of revenue. The loss of experienced professionals and a skilled, stable workforce also affect productivity. The cost to the worker includes not only monetary hardship, but also the possibility of permanent injury, chronic pain, and loss of profession.

Acute and chronic MSDs are the most prevalent workplace injury in all industries. The Bureau of Labor

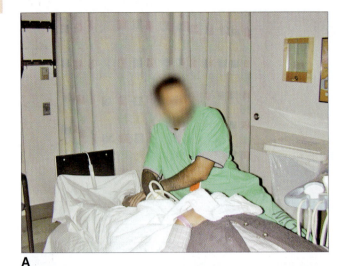

A

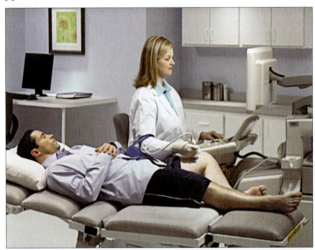

B

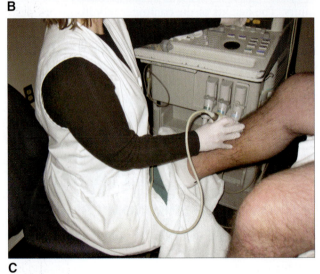

C

FIGURE 4-7 A, Ultrasound performed for evaluation of deep vein thrombosis (DVT) can be very injury producing if not performed correctly. **B,** When scanning the patient's left leg, turn the patient so that the left leg is closest to you. **C,** This is the most ergonomic way to perform a scan for the evaluation of DVT if you have a mobile patient. (**A, C,** Courtesy Sound Ergonomics, LLC, Kenmore, Washington. **B** Courtesy Siemens Healthcare Ultrasound, USA Division.)

Statistics states that more than 300,000 MSDs are reported annually. They account for 56% of the work-related illnesses reported to the Occupational Safety and Health Administration (OSHA) and are responsible for 640,000 lost workdays. MSDs are also the most costly of all occupational problems, accounting for the majority of workers' compensation costs. The costs related to occupational musculoskeletal disorders are both direct and indirect. MSDs cost $60 billion overall per year and to businesses, $5 billion to $20 billion per year in direct costs. These costs include workers' compensation and medical expenses, the latter of which are increasing 2.5 times faster than any other benefit cost:

- $1 of every $3 of workers' compensation costs are spent on occupational MSDs.
- Employers pay $15 billion to $20 billion per year in workers' compensation costs for lost workdays.
- The mean cost per cause of upper extremity WRMSD is $8070 versus a mean cost of $4075 per case for all types of work-related injury. With regard to incurred claim costs (which include indemnity and medical payments), the average for all claims is $10,105, but for carpal tunnel syndrome, it is $13,263.
- Indirect costs are three to five times higher, reaching approximately $150 billion per year. These include absenteeism, staff replacement and retraining, and loss of productivity or quality.
- The cost of hiring temporary replacement staff is between $130,000 and $166,000 per year. The estimated average cost to find and hire a new sonographer is $10,000
- If an ultrasound exam room is down because of the loss of worker time, the loss of chargeable income is equal to between $4500 per day, $22,500 per week, or $1,170,000 per year in lost revenue.

The cost of equipping a sonography examination room is minimal compared to addressing a workers' compensation injury. The quality of the patient's examination may also suffer if the sonographer is in pain while performing the examination. Quality diagnostic images take time to produce, and sonographers should not feel rushed to produce images because of scheduling conflicts or pain.

Accessory equipment that can mitigate injury risk includes the following:

- *A height-adjustable stool.* Cost: $750 reimbursement on two to three patient studies.
- *A set of support cushions.* Cost: $250 reimbursement on one patient study.
- *An ergonomic exam table.* Cost: $7,400 reimbursement from 2 days work.

It is very important that work-related injuries be reported immediately to occupational health or risk management departments. These injuries should be

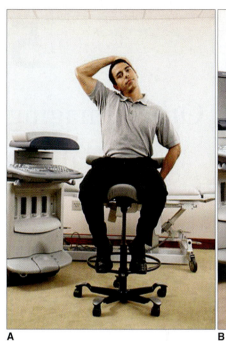
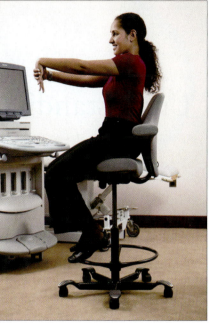

FIGURE 4-8 Simple stretches and exercises like these done throughout the day for a few minutes makes a significant difference to your health and well-being. (Courtesy Siemens Healthcare Ultrasound, USA Division.)

A   B

recorded on OSHA logs. Failure to do this may result in denial of claims.

REFERENCES

1. Ergoweb Inc., www.ergoweb.com/resources/reference/history.cfm.
2. Craig, M: Sonography: an occupational health hazard? J Diagnostic Medical Sonographers (JDMS) in May/June 1985.
3. Pike I, Russo A, Berkowitz J, et al: The prevalence of musculoskeletal disorders among diagnostic medical sonographers, JDMS 13(5):219-227, 1997.
4. Murphy C, Russo, A: *An update on ergonomic issues in sonography (Canada) healthcare benefit trust,* July 2000.
5. www.dol.gov/oasam/programs/history/mono-osha13introtoc.htm.
6. www.osha.gov/pls/oshaweb/owadisp.show_document?p_id=3359&p_table=OSHACT.
7. www.sdms.org/pdf/wrmsd2003.pdf Industry Standards for the Prevention of Work-Related Musculoskeletal Disorders in Sonography.
8. Bongers PM, deWinter CR, Kompier MAJ, Hildebrandt, VH: Psychosocial factors at work and musculoskeletal disease, *Scand J Work Environ Health* 19(5):297-312, 1993.
9. Barr AE, Safadi FF, Gorzelany I, et al: Repetitive, negligible force reaching in rates induces pathological overloading of upper extremity bones, *J Bone Miner Res* 18(11):2023-2032, 2003.
10. Valachi B, Valachi K: Mechanisms leading to musculoskeletal disorders in dentistry, *J Am Dent Assoc*, October (134):1344-1350, 2003.
11. Kroemer K, Grandjean E: *Fitting the task to the human,* ed. 5, Philadelphia, 2000, Taylor & Francis.

Understanding Other Imaging Modalities

Salvatore LaRusso

OBJECTIVES

On completion of this chapter, you should be able to:
- List the properties of x-rays and gamma rays
- Define radiographic contrast and density
- Discuss the use of contrast media in diagnostic imaging

- Compare and contrast how images are produced using computed tomography, nuclear medicine, positron emission tomography, and diagnostic ultrasound

OUTLINE

History and Use of X-Rays
Radiographic Density and Contrast
General Diagnostic Referrals to
  Ultrasound

Pleural Effusion
Ventriculoperitoneal Shunt
Voiding Cystourethrogram
Computed Tomography

Nuclear Medicine
Positron Emission Tomography

It is becoming increasingly important that sonographers understand how other imaging modalities work, especially computed tomography (CT) and positron emission tomography and computed tomography (PET/CT), which most frequently complement sonography. No longer does each of the various imaging modalities operate within a "silo," independent of each other. Instead, many diagnostic algorithms require two or more imaging modalities to be employed, and diagnosis requires that specific comparisons be made between them. In this way, ultrasound now interacts extensively with CT and other imaging methods to optimize the workup of a patient. Many patients referred to ultrasound for evaluation of a potential abnormality have already been imaged by another modality, which has detected an abnormality but was unable to characterize it or vice versa. Understanding what each modality has to offer is of prime importance in crafting the multimodality imaging workup for any particular problem.

It is also becoming more common for physicians to follow up an abnormality—even one that has been previously characterized—by using another imaging method like ultrasound. Ultrasound is often preferred over CT, which involves ionizing radiation, or magnetic resonance imaging (MRI), which is both time consuming and costly. To effectively meet the patient's needs, the sonographer must be able to tailor his or her exam appropriately so

as to exploit the unique strengths of ultrasound and to minimize its limitations. The sonographer must also understand how the ultrasound examination in each setting may be influenced or guided by findings from previous CT or other studies. To effectively evaluate patients who have had or will undergo additional imaging by other modalities, the sonographer must be able to understand the basics of each of the other imaging modalities within the radiology armamentarium.

What are the other modalities that interact most closely with ultrasound? The most common modalities include the CAT scan, PET/CT, and nuclear medicine. Minimally there will also be some crossover from general diagnostic radiology. This chapter reviews the most common indications for imaging with each modality that might lead to a second referral for sonographic examination or correlation imaging, or for sonographic evaluation in an attempt to further characterize a lesion detected by other means. We review the basic characteristics of abnormalities seen with other imaging technologies and explore how these correlate with ultrasound imaging. We also compare the appearance of various pathologies between sonography and the other imaging modalities.

The various imaging modalities ultimately depict and evaluate the same abnormalities, and they are generally equivalent in identifying the physical size and shape of pathologic lesions. However, each modality approaches the problem from a different standpoint, using differing physical properties of the normal tissue and pathologic lesions to derive image contrast and resolve important details. Ultrasound and MRI both have a safety advantage in that they do not use ionizing radiation. CT scanning and general diagnostic (x-ray) imaging, on the other hand, both image the body by use of ionizing radiation, often in significant doses. The radiation for both CT and x-ray is produced by an external source and tends to produce sharp images with high anatomic detail. Nuclear medicine also images the body by using a radiation source, but that modality utilizes radiation, which is internal, or within the patient's body, relying on the inherent biodistribution of radiotracers to construct the images, which generally lack anatomic detail.

HISTORY AND USE OF X-RAYS

Dr. Wilhelm Conrad Roentgen discovered x-rays on November 8, 1895. After weeks of meticulous research on the new "ray," his findings were published in a scientific paper on December 28, 1895. Ultimately Roentgen's discovery was rewarded with the first Nobel Prize presented for physics in 1901. Roentgen's x-rays are a type of electromagnetic radiation, which has both electrical and magnetic properties. It moves through space in waves that have wavelength and frequency, and it also demonstrates properties like those of a stream of solid particles, or photons. As with ultrasound, wavelength and frequency are inversely related. Higher energy x-rays have decreased wavelength and increased frequency.

You should be aware of the following characteristics of x-rays: they have no mass; they travel at the speed of light; they can penetrate matter and are sufficiently energetic as to cause chemical and biologic changes in living tissues. X-rays are invisible to the human eye and are electrically neutral. Currently, all medical x-rays are produced the same way. The production of x-rays requires a stream of high-energy electrons accelerated across a high voltage and then suddenly halted by impacting a positively charged metal barrier called an *anode*. The source of the stream of electrons is a negatively charged electrode called a *cathode*. The movement of electrons between the cathode to anode is possible because of the difference in charges, and the electrons are accelerated because of the high voltage generated between the cathode and the anode, generally thousands of volts (kilovolts).

X-rays must pass though tissue and interact with an image receptor to produce images. The receptor can be film or detectors (digital imaging). As with ultrasound, the resultant image is dependent on the interaction of the beam with various tissues of the body. Some of the beam is absorbed, scattered, and transmitted through the tissues. The characteristics of the x-ray beam are affected by the thickness of the tissue, the atomic number of the material through which the x-ray beam passes, and the electron-density of the tissue it passes through. The remainder of the beam that exits the body part being imaged will be composed of varying energy and will cause different responses from the detector, leading to different shades of gray in the final image.

RADIOGRAPHIC DENSITY AND CONTRAST

Tissues that absorb a greater number of the x-rays create whiter areas on the resultant image. These are displayed areas of higher density. This is because more of the beam was attenuated, and, therefore, less x-ray energy exited the body to interact with the detector or film. The blacker areas on the x-ray image indicate areas of lower density, or less absorption of the beam as it passed through the tissue. High and low density refers to the amount of energy that reached the film or the detector and its subsequent display on the image. Different tissue densities thus create the various shades of gray, which allows their discrimination on the final image. In a normal x-ray, bones absorb the beam the most and are displayed as white. Air absorbs the beam the least and is displayed as black.

Contrast is the difference between adjacent densities (structures) and is the feature of an image that affects the ability to visualize detail and detect lesions. Contrast allows the interpreter to distinguish differences in anatomic tissue. Radiographic contrast comprises two parts: **film/detector contrast** and **subject contrast**. Film/detector contrast is inherent in the film type and the processing techniques. Film contrast is not changeable by the operator. Subject contrast is affected by the absorption characteristics of the tissue being imaged and by the imaging parameters utilized by the radiologic technologist (kilovoltage and mAs). Subject contrast can be further defined as low and high subject contrast. If the image is composed of multiple tissues with similar absorption characteristics, it is difficult to differentiate anatomic structures. Imaging of the entire abdomen would fall into this category (Figure 5-1). Conversely, on an image of tissues with differing absorption characteristics, it is easier to differentiate adjacent structures. A chest x-ray is a good example of a high-contrast image (Figure 5-2).

When it becomes necessary to accurately image areas of low subject contrast, a contrast media can be used to alter the absorption characteristics of tissue. Contrast media can be ingested or injected into the body, depending on the organ to be imaged. Contrast media can either increase or decrease the absorption of x-rays. The atomic number of the contrast media influences the absorption rate. Iodine and barium are generally safe, have high atomic numbers, and thus absorb a high percentage of the x-rays. These are the "active ingredients" in almost all medical radiographic contrast media. Subsequently, the organs containing contrast will appear whiter on the final image (Figure 5-3). Iodine and barium are considered **positive contrast agents**. Conversely, air has a low

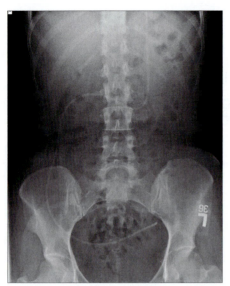

FIGURE 5-1 AP radiograph of the abdomen is characteristic of multiple tissue interfaces with similar absorption characteristics, which make it difficult to differentiate anatomic structures.

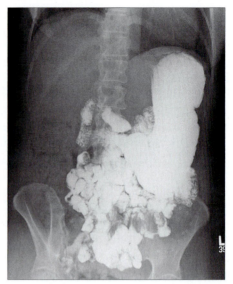

FIGURE 5-3 Barium is a positive contrast agent in radiographic imaging. It has filled the stomach and small bowel and appears as white on this image.

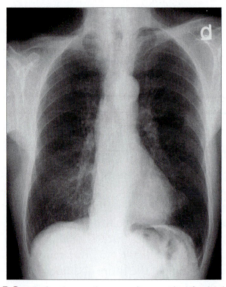

FIGURE 5-2 AP chest x-ray is a good example of a high-contrast image, with the black lungs in sharp contrast with the white of the thoracic cavity and spine.

atomic number and decreases the amount of x-ray absorption compared to the surrounding tissues. Air is a *negative* contrast agent. Air-filled structures appear to be darker than the surrounding tissues (Figure 5-4, *A* and *B*). To summarize, positive contrast agents add radiographic density to the adjacent tissues, whereas negative contrast agents produce less radiographic density.

GENERAL DIAGNOSTIC REFERRALS TO ULTRASOUND

Ultrasound receives minimal referrals as a direct consequence of findings from general diagnostic radiology. In

the adult population, ultrasound primarily evaluates pleural effusions detected on chest x-ray and also is used for evaluations of **ventriculoperitoneal (VP) shunts**, which can be seen radiographically. In the pediatric population, ultrasound referrals are commonly made for evaluation of ventriculoperitoneal shunts and to follow up positive voiding cystourethrogram (VCUG) studies without subjecting the patient to further radiation exposure.

Pleural Effusion

When the patient is referred for the evaluation of pleural effusion, the lung bases and diaphragm are the area of interest for the sonographer. In a normal chest x-ray, the lateral areas of the lung come to a point called the costophrenic angle (Figure 5-5, *A*). Pleural fluid will cause blunting of the costophrenic angles so that they will not come to a sharp point on the chest radiograph (Figure 5-5, *B*). As fluid increases, the base (inferior portion) of the lung will rise superiorly. The lung bases will not be symmetrical (Figure 5-5, *C*).

Ventriculoperitoneal Shunt

A **ventriculoperitoneal (VP) shunt** is a tube that is placed by a neurosurgeon to relieve intracranial pressure caused by increased cerebrospinal fluid (hydrocephalus). This typically occurs in the pediatric population, but the patency of the shunt is evaluated throughout a patient's lifetime. The shunt tubing connects from the ventricles of the brain to the abdominal cavity to allow fluid to drain from the ventricular system of the brain into the peritoneal cavity. One end of the shunt is located in the brain ventricle as the tube is tunneled through the

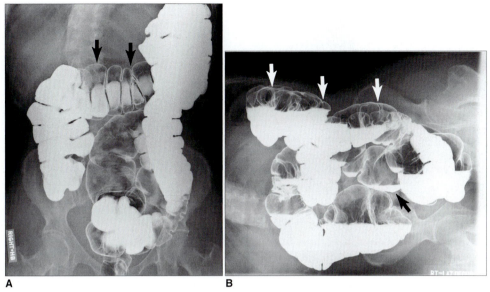

FIGURE 5-4 A, B, Air-filled structures (*arrows*) appear to be darker than the surrounding tissues on these radiographic images.

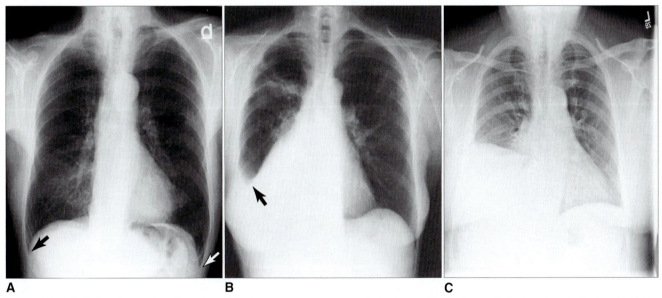

FIGURE 5-5 A, Pointed costophrenic angles of the lung as seen on a normal chest x-ray. **B,** Chest x-ray indicates pleural effusion. **C,** Notice the loss of the costophrenic angle from fluid in the pleural space pushing the lung superiorly in the chest cavity.

subcutaneous tissue through the neck and chest, and terminates in the abdominal cavity. In the event the patient's intracranial pressure increases, the clinical concern would be for a shunt malfunction, possibly because of the development of a "CSFoma" (a loculated cerebrospinal fluid collection). If the patient has signs and symptoms of increasing intracranial pressure, one of the potential causes is a blockage of the VP shunt within the abdomen.

Ultrasound may be used to evaluate for this possibility, by allowing visualization of a small CSFoma at the tip of the tubing. A plain film radiograph should be obtained before performing the ultrasound for accurate identification and targeted ultrasound imaging. The abdominal

x-ray is done to determine the position of the tube end (Figure 5-6, *A*). It is imperative to identify the tip before scanning the patient. The sonographer should review the radiographs to determine where to focus the ultrasound examination to search for a loculated anechoic fluid collection adjacent to the tip of the echogenic tubing. It is imperative to find the tip of the shunt and evaluate that area with sonography to ascertain if there is a loculated fluid collection at that location.

Figure 5-6, *B*, illustrates how tortuous a VP shunt can be. If the tube is functioning correctly, there will be fluid within the abdomen. The clinical concern is to determine whether the fluid is loculated—that is, limited in its mobility—or whether instead it is free to flow

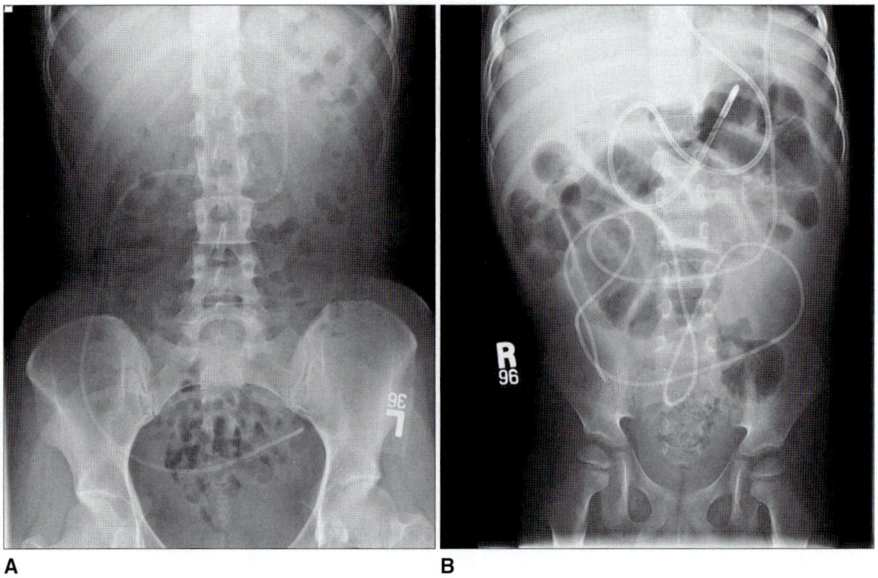

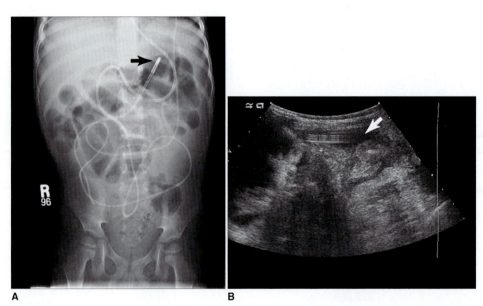

FIGURE 5-6 A, Abdominal radiograph demonstrating the position of the tube end of a VP shunt. **B,** This image illustrates just how tortuous a VP shunt can be.

FIGURE 5-7 A, The tip (*arrow*) of a VP shunt on a radiograph. **B,** The subsequent sonographic image demonstrates the tip of the shunt and a small amount of free fluid without a loculated fluid collection (*arrow*).

throughout the abdomen. One must visualize the tube tip accurately to make that determination (Figure 5-7). In the pediatric population, enough tubing is placed to allow for the child to grow without the end being pulled into a less desirable location. Figure 5-8, *A*, demonstrates a coiled VP shunt with the tip located medially in the pelvis. Sonographic interrogation (Figure 5-8, *B*) targeted to the area of the shunt indicates a small amount of free fluid present but no loculated fluid collection.

Voiding Cystourethrogram (VCUG)

Voiding cystourethrogram (VCUG) studies are primarily performed within the pediatric patient population. A child who has recurrent urinary tract infections is typically evaluated by an ultrasound of the kidneys and also a VCUG. The VCUG is performed by placing a small catheter into the bladder for the purpose of instilling a contrast agent. The sonographer should also evaluate the VCUG images to determine the degree of hydronephrosis or scarring that may be present during the ultrasound examination. The VCUG is used to determine whether the patient has reflux, which means that urine refluxes back up the ureter into the kidney. Reflux can be graded 1 through 5, and a higher number of reflux can indicate damage to the kidneys. Figure 5-9 shows reflux into both kidneys, with the right kidney being more prominent than the left. Both ureters are also identified. The contrast can be imaged as either black-on-white background format

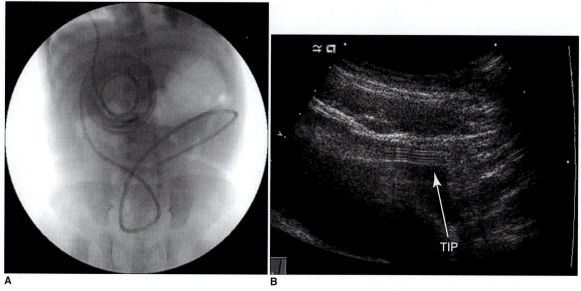

A   B

FIGURE 5-8 A, This radiograph of the abdomen demonstrates a coiled VP shunt with the tip located medially in the pelvis. **B,** Sonographic interrogation targeted to that area indicates a small amount of free fluid present, but no loculated fluid collection.

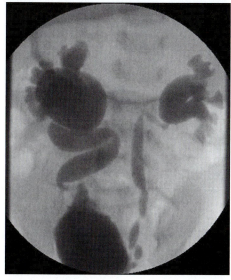

FIGURE 5-9 This radiographic image indicates reflux into both kidneys, with the right kidney been more prominent than the left.

or a white-on-black background format. This image uses a black-on-white background format. The subsequent ultrasound images demonstrate hydronephrosis on the right side, which is worse than the left side; this corresponds well with the VCUG image (Figure 5-10).

Computed Tomography (CT)

The first available CT scanner was invented by Sir Godfrey Hounsfield in the United Kingdom at the EMI Central research laboratories. Although his research began in 1967, Hounsfield did not publicly announce his discovery until 1972. His invention employed x-rays to spatially determine the location of an object within a box. Allen McLeod Cormack independently invented a similar process at the Tufts University of Massachusetts. Both Hounsfield and Cormack shared the Nobel Prize in physiology and medicine in 1979.

The typical appearance of a CT scanner is a square "doughnut" with a hole in the center called a **gantry**. Inside the gantry of the machine there is an x-ray-producing source (tube) opposite banana-shaped x-ray sensors. As x-rays are produced, they leave the anode in a fan-type fashion and are directed toward the sensors. Early in CT technology, the anode and sensors would make one full revolution and stop. The patient table would move at a predetermined rate, typically 1 mm to 10 mm. A whole body x-ray image would be produced that indicated the image slices, or tomographic cuts, the machine would ultimately render (Figure 5-11). The anode and detectors would then make a revolution in the direction opposite the previous revolution. This would create a slice through the patient's body and produce one tomographic "slice" image. This process would continue until the entire area of interest was imaged.

Because CT imaging uses x-rays, its physical basis is similar to general diagnostic x-ray imaging. As the x-rays pass through the body, they are absorbed and attenuated at different levels by the tissues, normal or otherwise. The detectors absorb the final x-rays in each tube position, generating a large amount of digital data, which is then sent through a computer system. The computer system subjects the data to a mathematical analysis known as "back projection" to create the two-dimensional image. At this juncture, the image consists merely of a two-dimensional array of numbers reflecting the densities of the materials and tissues through which the x-ray beam has passed. To produce a viewable image,

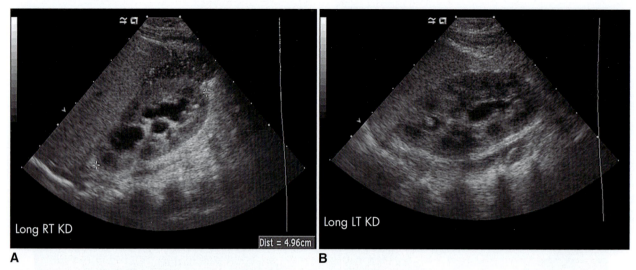

A **B**

FIGURE 5-10 The subsequent ultrasound images demonstrate hydronephrosis on the right side **(A)**, which is worse than the left side **(B)**.

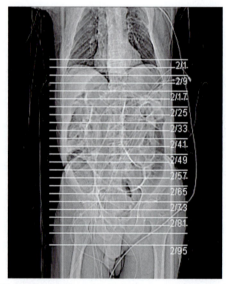

FIGURE 5-11 A whole body x-ray image is produced by the CT scan. The image indicates the image slices, or *tomographic cuts*, the machine would ultimately render.

BOX 5-1	**Hounsfield Units**
Air	−1000
Fat	−120
Water	0
Muscle	+40
Bone	+400 or more

a gray scale is applied, according to parameters set by the user (usually referred to as "window" and "level"). The final viewable image is then transferred either to film media or (currently) a PACS system. The computer allows the data stored to be displayed or photographed or used as input for additional further processing such as multiplanar reconstruction.

New scanners with much faster computer systems and newer software strategies can process not only individual cross sections but also continually changing cross sections. As the x-ray tube rotates continuously in one direction within the gantry, the object to be imaged smoothly slides through the x-ray opening. This process allows for rapid imaging of large areas of the body. The entire torso can generally be imaged in exquisite detail during the time of a single breath-hold. The common name for this newer method is *spiral* or *helical* CT scanning. The computer systems integrate the data of moving slices to generate three-dimensional (3D) volume imaging, which then can be reconstructed and be viewed in multiple different perspectives on the workstation monitors. Images can be configured in 3D as a "solid" object or displayed as traditional tomographic imaging slices in the transverse, coronal, sagittal or nonstandard, user-chosen planes.

The numeric scale for representing the different tissue characteristics by their x-ray density (or "electron density") is known as the **Hounsfield unit,** in honor of the inventor of CT, Sir Godfrey Hounsfield. The Hounsfield unit scale is a linear transformation of the attenuation coefficient using the radiodensity of pure, distilled water at a standard pressure and temperature. The attenuation of pure water is arbitrarily defined as zero Hounsfield units (Box 5-1). CT scanners are calibrated to this standard.

CT scan images have the same range of grays, blacks, and whites as ultrasound images. The same density configuration is seen in general x-ray and CT, wherein black is a less dense structure and white is a denser structure. Because air is less dense, x-rays with typical exposure will display air as black (Figure 5-12). Figure 5-13 is an

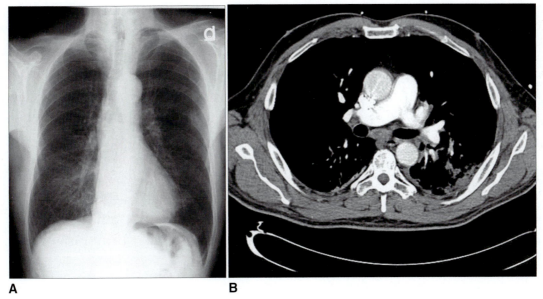

A   **B**

FIGURE 5-12 **A,** This AP chest x-ray demonstrates the lungs as *black*. **B,** This CT scan is a thoracic cross section through the lungs, which are black in nearly all viewing windows.

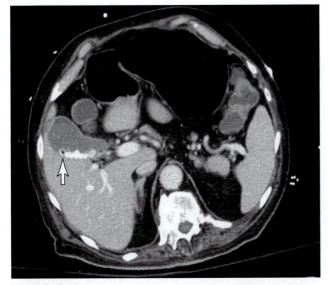

FIGURE 5-13 This CT scan demonstrates multiple gallstones layered along the floor of the gallbladder. The *arrow* indicates a gallstone that has a small focus of air density within it.

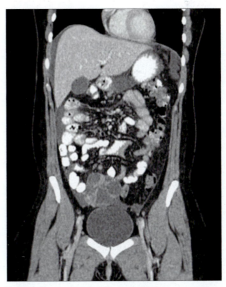

FIGURE 5-14 This sagittal CT image demonstrates all of the varying tissue characteristics. The bright white areas demonstrate contrast within the bowel and colon. The black areas demonstrate air. Fluid appears similar to muscle.

interesting example of the appearance of air on a CT scan. A series of gallstones lies along the floor of the gallbladder, but one gallstone has a small focus of air density within it.

All of the varying tissue characteristics can be demonstrated on a CT scan (Figure 5-14). The bright white areas demonstrate contrast within the bowel and colon. The black areas demonstrate air. Fluid appears similar to muscle. This cross-sectional CT scan demonstrates the subcutaneous fat as the same brightness as intraperitoneal fat. Like Figure 5-14, Figure 5-15 is in "abdominal window," in which the gray scale is optimized for viewing

structures within the abdomen. In this setting, the lungs appear black and featureless. To view the lungs with this same CT data, one would merely change to "lung window" viewing settings. It would not be necessary to rescan the patient.

Fluid on CT appears as gray, whereas fluid on ultrasound appears as black. Figures 5-16 and 5-17 illustrate two different cases of fluid. Figure 5-16 shows a loculated fluid collection outside the abdominal cavity, whereas Figure 5-17 shows free fluid in the abdomen (not loculated). In both cases, however, the fluid appears gray on the CT scan and black on the ultrasound image.

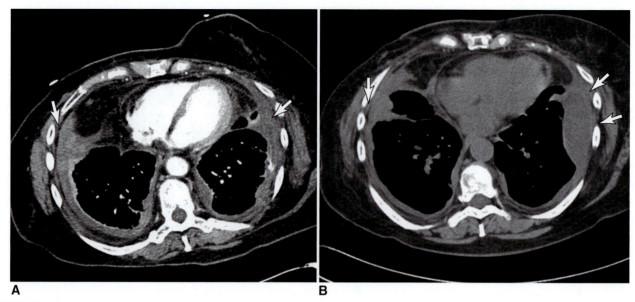

A   **B**

FIGURE 5-15 This patient has had intravenous contrast that highlights the heart and the pulmonary vasculature. The lungs are black because they contain air. There are bilateral pleural effusions (*arrows*) present. **B,** This CT image does not demonstrate contrast, and the blood within the heart has the same characteristic as the pleural fluid. Arrows indicate regions of fluid.

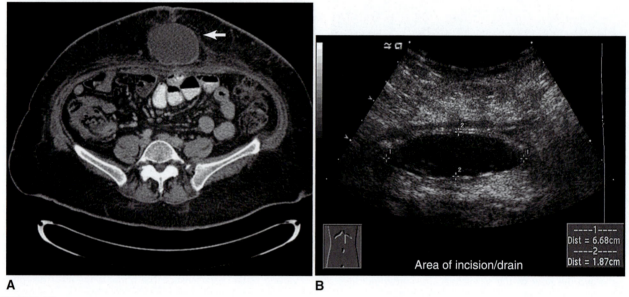

A   **B**

FIGURE 5-16 A, An anterior abdominal wall fluid collection *(arrow)* is visualized on this CT scan. **B,** The fluid collection appears as black on the corresponding sonographic image.

As in general diagnostic x-ray, contrast is used to change the appearance of tissues for improved imaging. Depending on the indications of the scan, one may elect to use oral contrast (Figure 5-18) or rectal contrast. For oral contrast, a dilute suspension of barium sulfate is most commonly used. The concentrated barium sulfate preps used for fluoroscopy (i.e., barium enemas) are too dense for CT imaging, as they cause "streak" artifacts on CT. Iodinated contrast agents may be used if barium is contraindicated. Other agents such as air or water may be used if the colon and bowel must be imaged.

Iodine-based IV contrast may also be used. In Figure 5-19, *A*, the heart appears gray, indicating the presence of fluid. After the intravenous injection of a contrast medium (Figure 5-19, *B*), the heart appears bright white, highlighting the presence of fluid in the heart. Similarly, in Figure 5-20, *A*, there is no evidence of vessel delineation in the CT image without IV contrast. Administering contrast enhances visualization of the anatomy, and the portal vein and liver vessels appear white (Figure 5-20, *B*). Figure 5-21 is a cross-sectional CT image through the abdomen and liver. Notice

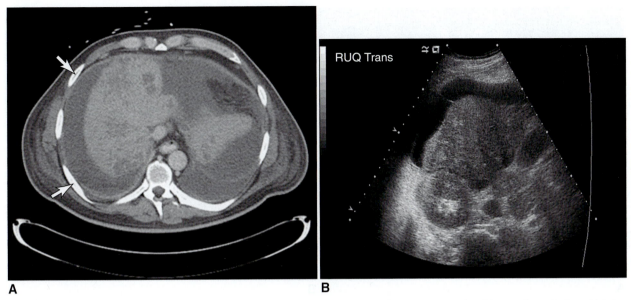

FIGURE 5-17 A, Ascites (*arrows*) within the abdominal cavity is shown as gray on this CT cross-sectional image through the midabdomen. **B,** The corresponding sonographic image demonstrates the fluid as black, as it separates the abdominal wall from the border of the liver.

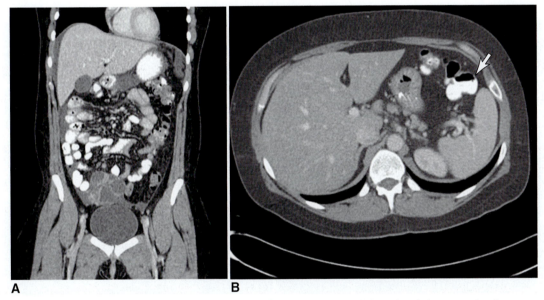

FIGURE 5-18 The bright white areas indicate oral contrast, which has coated the small bowel and the stomach adjacent to the liver. The *arrow* on the cross-sectional image **(B)** indicates a loop of small bowel, which has dependent contrast displayed as bright white and air anterior displayed as black within the same loop of bowel.

the difference in the appearance of each kidney. IV contrast is excreted through the urinary system and is present throughout the normal right kidney soon after injection. The left kidney, however, is obstructed, which prevents the contrast from being excreted through to the ureter. Hence, the left kidney appears "bright" on the image.

Case Studies. Several examples are provided here to illustrate how ultrasound confirms the findings of other imaging modalities, namely computed tomography (CT). In Figure 5-22, both cross-sectional and sagittal CT

images through the abdomen demonstrate a bilobed, low-density structure anterior/superior to the upper pole of the left kidney. The corresponding ultrasound image confirms the shape and location of the legion, showing a bilobed, hypoechoic mass superior/anterior to the kidney. Ultrasound was able to demonstrate that the mass was solid and confirm that the lesion was adrenal in nature and not part of the kidney.

In Figure 5-23, a cross-sectional CT image shows an ill-defined mass posterior to the lower pole of the left kidney. Angiomyolipoma was suspected. The

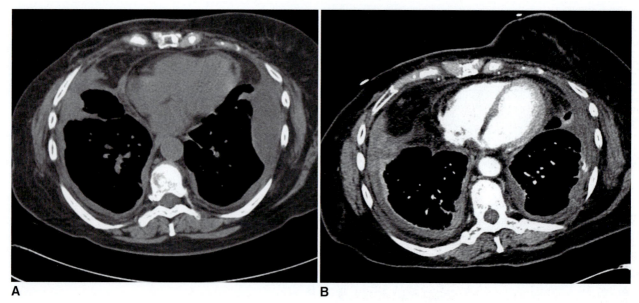

A   B

FIGURE 5-19 A, This cross-sectional CT image is made through the midchest. The heart is shown with a gray appearance, indicating fluid. **B,** The corresponding image displays the heart as bright white after injection of IV contrast.

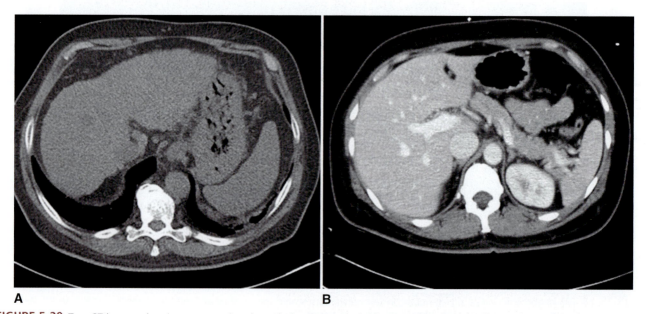

A   B

FIGURE 5-20 Two CT images showing cross section through the abdomen and liver. **A,** There is no evidence of vessel delineation. **B,** With the use of an intravenous contrast material, the portal vein and liver vessels appear white.

corresponding ultrasound images indicate a slightly hyperechoic mass compatible with angiomyolipoma. (Angiomyolipoma is characteristically hyperechoic on ultrasound.) Angiomyolipoma is a benign condition.

The CT scan in Figure 5-24 reveals a small bright mass in the anterior aspect of a cystic mass that has the same density approximately as bone, which suggested a calcification. Ultrasound examination revealed a calcification adherent to the anterior wall with shadowing compatible with a teratoma. Two CT images through the

patient's neck demonstrate a complex mass in the left thyroid gland (Figure 5-25, A and B). Subsequent ultrasound examination corroborates the CT findings, demonstrating a complex mass in the left thyroid gland (Figure 5-25, C).

In our final case, CT images through the gallbladder demonstrate a focal thickening in the gallbladder wall, which might suggest gallbladder carcinoma (Figure 5-26, A and B). Ultrasound, however, did not corroborate the CT findings. The corresponding ultrasound image of the

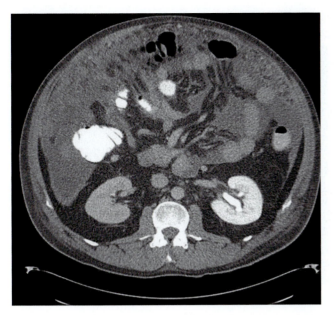

FIGURE 5-21 CT cross section through the abdomen and kidneys taken after administration of IV contrast. The left kidney is obstructed, which prevents the contrast from being excreted through to the ureter, hence the appearance of being bright on the image.

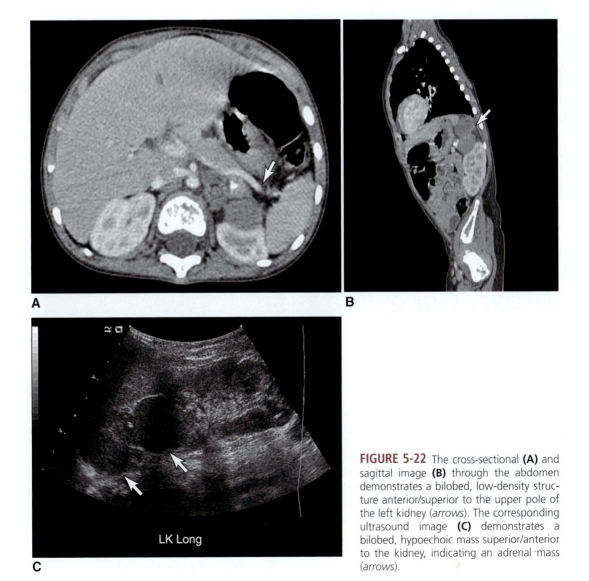

FIGURE 5-22 The cross-sectional **(A)** and sagittal image **(B)** through the abdomen demonstrates a bilobed, low-density structure anterior/superior to the upper pole of the left kidney (*arrows*). The corresponding ultrasound image **(C)** demonstrates a bilobed, hypoechoic mass superior/anterior to the kidney, indicating an adrenal mass (*arrows*).

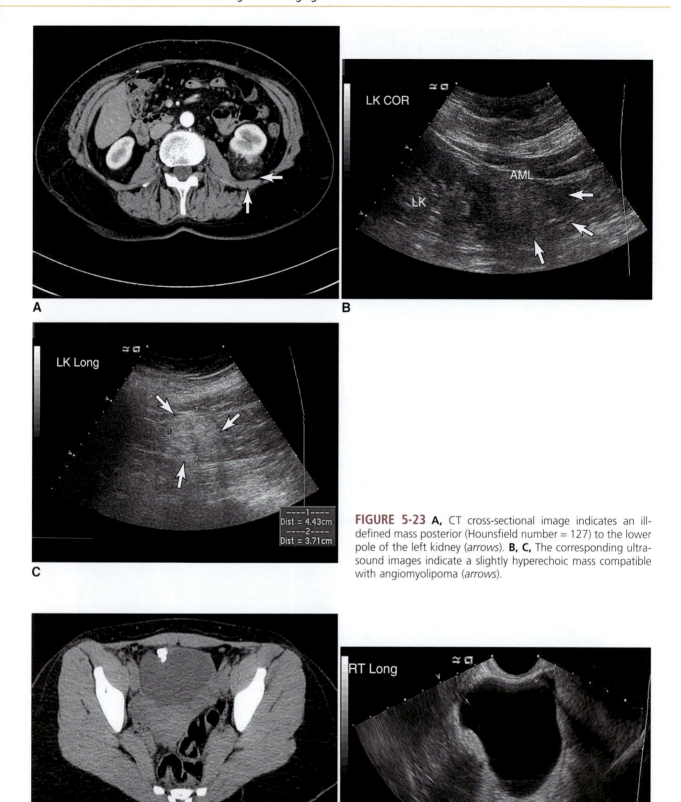

FIGURE 5-23 A, CT cross-sectional image indicates an ill-defined mass posterior (Hounsfield number = 127) to the lower pole of the left kidney (*arrows*). **B, C,** The corresponding ultrasound images indicate a slightly hyperechoic mass compatible with angiomyolipoma (*arrows*).

FIGURE 5-24 A, CT scan indicates a small bright mass in the anterior aspect of a cystic mass approximately the same density as bone. **B,** The corresponding ultrasound image indicates a calcification adherent to the anterior wall with shadowing.

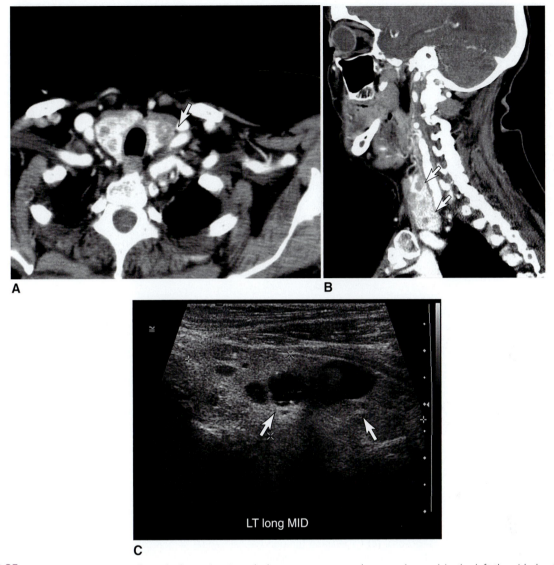

FIGURE 5-25 A, B, These CT images through the patient's neck demonstrate a complex mass (*arrows*) in the left thyroid gland. **C,** Subsequent ultrasound image corroborates the CT findings and demonstrates a complex mass in the left thyroid gland (*arrows*).

same area in the fundus of the gallbladder indicates a normal gallbladder (Figure 5-26, C).

Nuclear Medicine

Nuclear medicine is a descendent of the scientific discovery of x-rays made in 1895 and the discovery of artificial radioactivity in the mid-1930s. In 1946, a thyroid cancer patient's treatment with radioactive iodine led to the complete disappearance of the patient's cancer. In the 1950s, nuclear medicine was used to measure the functional thyroid and diagnose thyroid disease. After the 1970s, visualization of organs in addition to the thyroid became prevalent. The use of nuclear medicine for diagnosing heart disease, as well as the addition of digital computers, occurred in the 1980s.

Nuclear medicine images the human body by utilizing radiation. However, unlike CT and general x-ray, which produces radiation from an external source, nuclear medicine uses radiation from an internal source. Nuclear medicine employs **gamma rays**, which are physically similar to x-rays but are generated spontaneously from the decay of radioactive isotopes. Gamma rays that are used to image tissues are generally fairly short in wavelength, similar to the range of diagnostic x-rays generated artificially by kilovoltage x-ray tubes. Clinical nuclear medicine utilizes radioactive pharmaceuticals, in which the radioactive atom is bound chemically to a tracer molecule that is inhaled, taken orally, or administered intravenously (Figure 5-27). The terminology commonly used to describe these imaging agents may be "radionuclide," "radiopharmaceuticals," or "radiotracers."

When these radionuclide substances are administered, they are distributed according to the patient's physiology to certain tissues or sites (i.e., the "target' tissues") via the pharmaceutical, whereas some is distributed diffusely

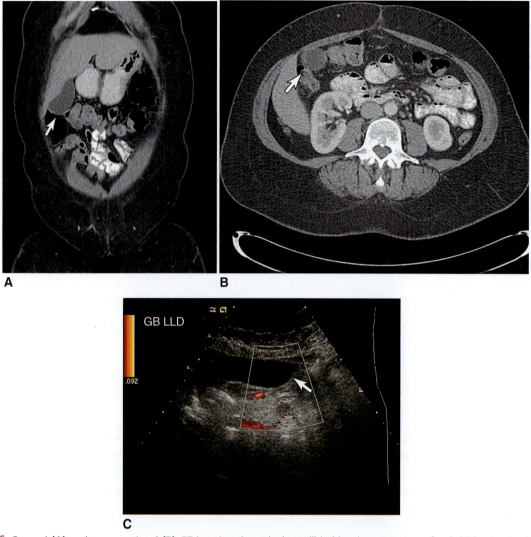

A   **B**

C

FIGURE 5-26 Coronal **(A)** and cross-sectional **(B)** CT imaging through the gallbladder demonstrates a focal thickening in the gallbladder wall (*arrows*). **C,** The corresponding ultrasound image of the same area in the fundus of the gallbladder demonstrates the gallbladder to be normal.

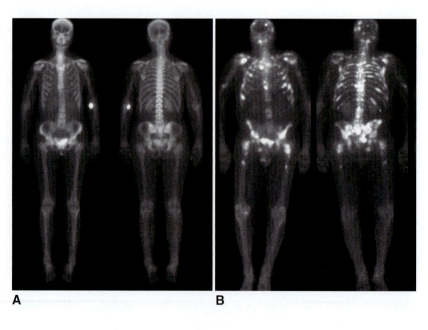

FIGURE 5-27 A, Normal bone scan. The bright dot on the arm is the injection site of the radionuclide. The radionuclide is a molecule that is highly absorbed by the bones, especially at sites of bony destruction and repair. **B,** Metastasis to the bones. All of the intensely bright spots are areas of increased uptake of the radionuclide by the tumors (increased cellular activity and bone turnover) within the skeleton.

A   **B**

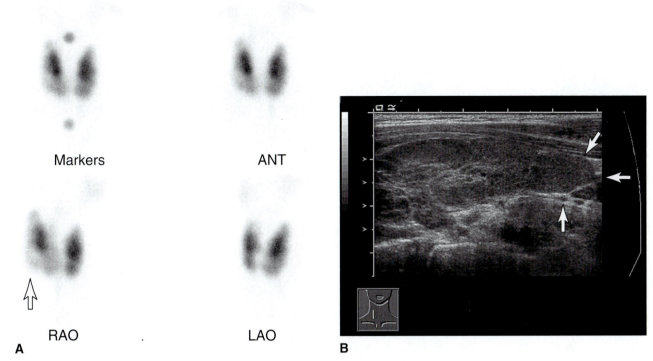

FIGURE 5-28 A, A "cold nodule" (*arrow*) in the inferior right lobe of the thyroid. **B,** Sonography demonstrates the area of interest as a solid lesion (*arrows*) in this sagittal image of the thyroid.

to all tissues (i.e., the "background"). After the radionuclides are distributed or attached to the specific organ(s) of interest, special sensing equipment is used to detect the radioactivity emitted by the tracer to yield an image. The basic technique is known as scintigraphy, and the radiation is detected by a device called a Gamma camera or "Anger camera," after its inventor, the late Dr. Hal Anger. Once obtained, the data are processed by computer to produce a two-dimensional image or a series of images of the particular organ being interrogated. This technique utilizes a computer to process data to construct three-dimensional images using nuclear medicine imaging while exposing the patient to a small dose of a short-lived radiation. The technique is helpful in assessing physiologic or functional activity such as blood flow kidney function, tumor growth, or infection. The most commonly imaged tissues and organs are the gallbladder, heart, liver, lungs, thyroid, and bones.

Nuclear medicine often is able to determine the cause of clinical problems caused by *physiologic* malfunction of the bone, organ, or tissue. This is different from other imaging modalities that detect and characterize pathology based on *structural* appearance. Nuclear medicine often evaluates tissue at the cellular level. The resultant images tend to lack anatomic detail and are often described as "cold spots" or "hot spots." In general, a cold spot has reduced uptake of the radionuclide, whereas a hot spot demonstrates increased uptake or hyper functioning tissue. The hot spots generally indicate more

cellular function or tracer accumulation than the surrounding tissue, whereas the cold areas demonstrate decreased cellular function or radiotracer affinity. The correlation with corresponding sonograms may not be straightforward. Decreased cellular function may indicate a solid lesion that is not functioning (Figure 5-28), or it may represent a cyst (which would not have any functioning tissue within it), or it may merely represent a type of living tissue that has no affinity for the particular tracer used.

The most common clinical question of the patient sent for ultrasound evaluation after nuclear medicine imaging involves thyroid (Figure 5-29) and parathyroid lesions, for which ultrasound may be used either for further characterization or to provide needle biopsy guidance.

Positron Emission Tomography (PET)

Another nuclear medicine imaging technique is positron emission tomography (PET). The scanner appears similar to the CT in which there is a table that moves the patient through a double gantry—one for CT and one for detection of emitted gamma rays (Figure 5-30).

The PET camera detectors surround the patient in a fixed ring, much like the x-ray detectors in a CT gantry. A computer digitally correlates the output to formulate a three-dimensional image by detecting pairs of emitted gamma rays resulting from decay of the isotope and subsequent annihilation of the emitted positron to

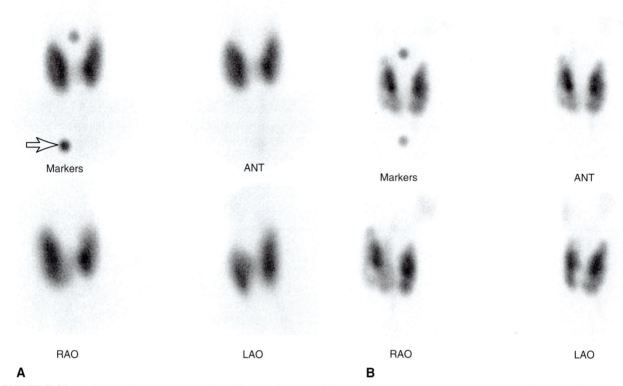

FIGURE 5-29 Nuclear medicine scans of a thyroid. **A,** Both thyroid lobes are symmetrical in the displayed "blacks." The dot (*arrow*) represents a marker that is placed by the nuclear medicine technologist and is not an abnormality. **B,** The mottled appearance of radionuclide uptake on this scan demonstrates a difference in tissue composition of the thyroid gland.

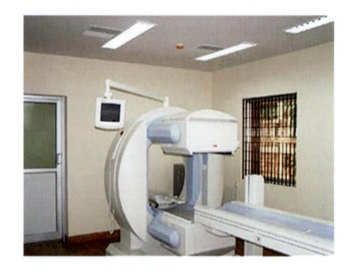

FIGURE 5-30 A positron emission tomography (PET) scanner.

produce a pair of gamma photons oriented at 180° from each other. A CT scanner is incorporated in the PET scanner, and the system generates a composite image that consists of a CT scan image with a colorized nuclear medicine image superimposed. This hybrid image provides detailed anatomic data blended with physiologic and function nuclear medicine data as well (Figure 5-31).

To perform PET, the patient is injected with pharmaceutical substances that are tagged with a radioactive atom that emits a "positron," the antimatter opposite of an electron. Such atoms are manufactured in a cyclotron device by neutron bombardment at high energies and include Carbon-11, Oxygen-15, Fluorine-18, and Nitrogen-13. These are all short lived radioactive isotopes, which decay with emission of a positron.

The positron travels a short distance in the patient's body before encountering an electron, which is its antiparticle, and undergoing annihilation, with complete conversion of its mass into energy in the form of two identical gamma photons with a characteristic energy and directed in 180° opposite directions. The PET detectors localize the origin of the paired gamma rays generated at the site where a positron emitted by the radioactive substance interacts with an electron of the patient's tissues, and a mathematical back-projection algorithm produces the PET image.

The CT portion is exactly as any other CT scanner. For most machines, the CT exam is performed first, and then the table returns and stays in position to acquire the gamma radiation component of the images. Both images are "co-registered," so they match up anatomically and then are fused together by a computer to generate composite images containing both anatomic and physiologic detail. The most commonly used tracer is the glucose analog, F-18-fluorodeoxy-glucose (FDG), which is accumulated in metabolically active tissues that utilize glucose to a greater extent than in "normal" tissue. PET images areas that are metabolically active, primarily cancers and inflammation (Figure 5-32). With the FDG tracer, the brain will always image as bright because it is highly metabolically active and relies exclusively on glucose. The heart is capable of utilizing glucose or free fatty acids for its metabolic needs and therefore may or may not accumulate FDG.

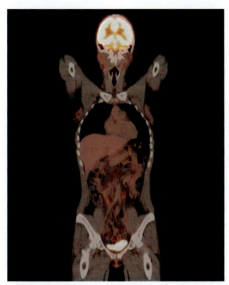

FIGURE 5-31 Normal PET scan. Notice the brightness of the brain, which is metabolically active. Also, the bladder is bright because the radionuclide is being excreted in the urine.

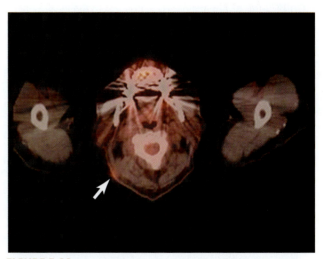

FIGURE 5-32 Inflammations are metabolically active. This PET scan reveals an incidental finding of a sebaceous cyst (arrow).

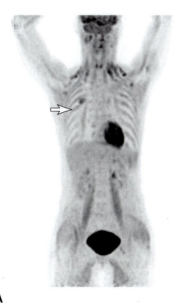

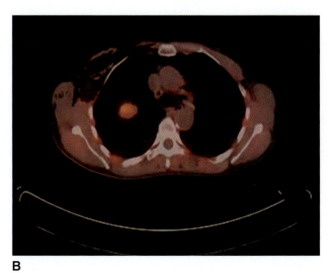

A   B

FIGURE 5-33 A, Conventional nuclear medicine identifies a lesion in the right lung (arrow). B, Adding the CT scan to the nuclear medicine image enables determination of where the lesion is located in the second plane (AP).

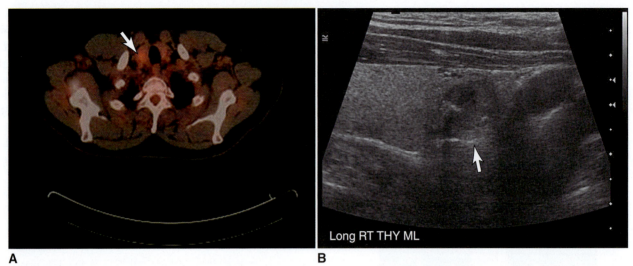

FIGURE 5-34 A, A metabolically active area in the lower pole of the thyroid gland (*arrow*). **B,** The subsequent ultrasound image confirms a solid lesion (*arrow*).

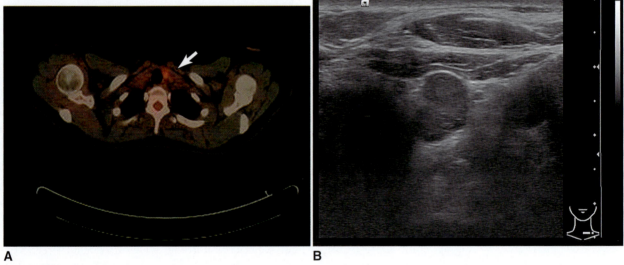

FIGURE 5-35 A, The PET image demonstrates a metabolically active area in the left neck in a patient who has had a total thyroidectomy (*arrow*). **B,** Subsequent ultrasound imaging demonstrates an abnormal focus of tissue.

Although conventional nuclear medicine can identify lesions (Figure 5-33, *A*), it cannot determine the depth or specific location of a lesion, which is something that CT can do. Figure 5-33, *B*, is a composite image showing where the lesion is located in the second plane.

Case Studies. The PET image in Figure 5-34, *A*, reveals a metabolically active area in the lower pole of the thyroid gland. Ultrasound examination confirmed a solid lesion

(Figure 5-34, *B*) that turned out to be malignant. Both benign and malignant lesions can be metabolically active.

This PET image demonstrates a metabolically active area in the left neck of a patient who had had a total thyroidectomy (Figure 5-35, *A*). The patient should not have any metabolically active areas after the thyroid is removed. Subsequent ultrasound imaging revealed a localized area of abnormal tissue (Figure 5-35, *B*).

Artifacts in Scanning*

Frederick W. Kremkau

In sonographic imaging, an artifact is the appearance of anything that does not properly present the structures or motion imaged. An artifact is caused by some problematic aspect of the imaging technique. Some artifacts are helpful. They should be used to advantage in the diagnostic imaging process. Others hinder proper interpretation and diagnosis. These artifacts must be avoided or handled properly when encountered.

Artifacts in sonography occur as apparent structures that are one of the following:

1. Not real
2. Missing
3. Misplaced
4. Of improper brightness, shape, or size

Some artifacts are produced by improper equipment operation or settings (e.g., incorrect gain and compensation settings). Others are inherent in the sonographic and Doppler methods and can occur even with proper equipment and technique.

The assumptions in the design of sonographic instruments are that sound travels in straight lines, that echoes originate from objects located on the beam axis, that the amplitudes of returning echoes are related directly to the echogenicity of the objects that produced them, and that the distance to echogenic objects is proportional to the roundtrip travel time (13 μs/cm of depth). If any of these assumptions is violated, an artifact occurs.

Several artifacts are encountered in Doppler ultrasound, yielding incorrect presentations of Doppler flow information, either in spectral or in color Doppler form. The most common of these is aliasing. Others include spectrum mirror image and those that occur in anatomic imaging.

PROPAGATION

Section Thickness

Axial and lateral (detail) resolutions are artifactual because a failure to resolve means a loss of detail, and two adjacent structures may be visualized as one. These artifacts occur because the ultrasound pulse has finite length and width in the scan plane. Increasing frequency improves both resolutions, whereas focusing improves

---

*This chapter is adapted from Forsberg F, Kremkau FW: Artifacts. Chapter 6 in Kremkau FW: *Sonography: principles and instruments*, ed 8, Philadelphia, 2011, Saunders.

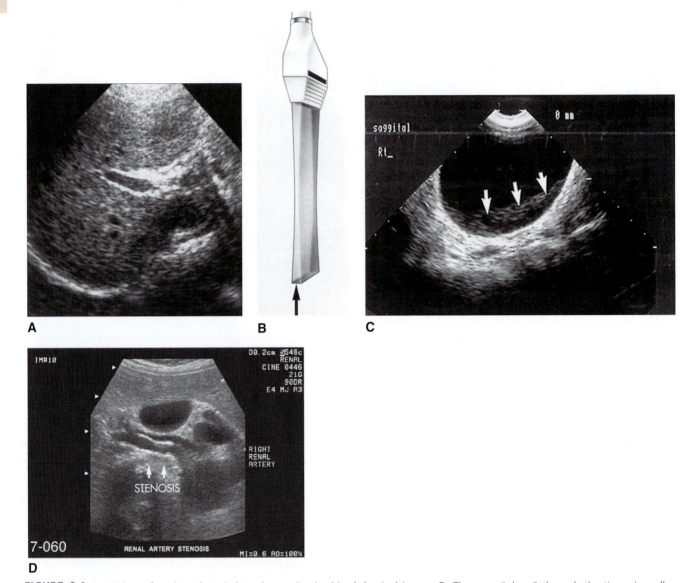

FIGURE 6-1 A, Without focusing, there is lateral smearing in this abdominal image. **B,** The scan "plane" through the tissue is really a three-dimensional volume. Two dimensions (axial and lateral) are in the scan plane, but there is a third dimension (called section thickness or slice thickness). The third dimension *(arrow)* is collapsed to zero thickness when the image is displayed in two-dimensional format. **C,** An ovarian cyst that should be echo-free has an echogenic region *(arrows)*. These off-axis echoes are a result of scan-plane section thickness. **D,** Section-thickness artifact appears as low-level echoes within hypoechoic structures.

lateral (Figure 6-1, *A*). The beam width perpendicular to the scan plane (the third dimension in Figure 6-1, *B*) results in **section-thickness** artifacts; for example, the appearance of false debris in what should be echo-free areas (Figure 6-1, *C* and *D*). These artifacts occur because the interrogating beam has finite thickness as it scans through the patient. Echoes are received that originate not only from the center of the beam but also from off-center. These echoes are all collapsed into a thin (zero-thickness) two-dimensional image that is composed of echoes that have come from a not-so-thin tissue volume scanned by the beam. Section-thickness artifact is also called slice-thickness or partial-volume artifact.

Speckle

Apparent image resolution can be deceiving. The detailed echo pattern often is not related directly to the scattering properties of tissue (called tissue texture) but rather is the result of the interference effects of the scattered sound from the distribution of scatterers in the tissue. There are many scatterers in the ultrasound pulse at any instant as it travels through tissue. Their echoes can combine constructively or destructively. The result varies as the beam is scanned through the tissue, producing the pattern of bright and dark spots. This phenomenon is called acoustic **speckle** (Figure 6-2).

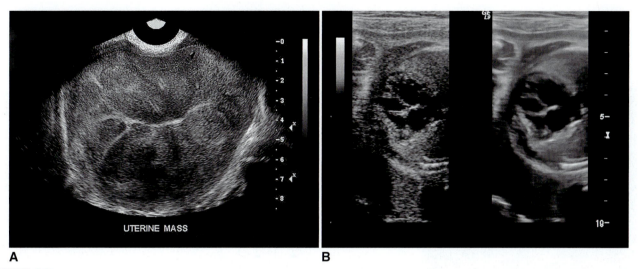

FIGURE 6-2 A, The typically grainy appearance of this ultrasound image is not primarily the result of detail resolution limitations but rather of speckle. Speckle is the interference pattern resulting from constructive and destructive interference of echoes returning simultaneously from many scatterers within the propagating ultrasound pulse at any instant. **B,** Approaches to speckle reduction (right image compared with the left) are being implemented in modern instruments.

Reverberation

Multiple reflection (reverberation) can occur between the transducer and a strong reflector (Figure 6-3, *A* and *B*). The multiple echoes may be sufficiently strong to be detected by the instrument and to cause confusion on the display (additional echoes that do not represent additional structures). The process by which they are produced is shown in Figure 6-3, *B*. This results in the display of additional reflectors that are not real (Figure 6-4, *A,B*). The multiple reflections are placed beneath the real reflector at separation intervals equal to the separation between the transducer and the real reflector. Each subsequent reflection is weaker than prior ones, but this diminution is counteracted at least partially by the attenuation compensation (TGC) function. Reverberations can originate between two anatomic reflecting surfaces also. When closely spaced, they appear in a form called comet tail (Figure 6-5, *A-I*). **Comet tail**, a particular form of reverberation, is a series of closely spaced, discrete echoes. Figure 6-6 shows an artifact that appears similar but is fundamentally different. Discrete echoes cannot be identified here because continuous emission of sound from the origin appears to be occurring. This continuous effect, termed **ring-down artifact**, is caused by a resonance phenomenon associated with the presence of a collection of gas bubbles. **Resonance** is the condition in which a driven mechanical vibration is of a frequency similar to a natural vibration frequency of the structure. The bubbles are stimulated into vibration by the incident ultrasound pulse. They then pulsate (expand and contract) for several cycles, acting as a source of ultrasound, producing a continuous stream of ultrasound that progresses distal to the bubble collection as the echo stream returns.

Mirror Image

The **mirror-image artifact**, also a form of reverberation, shows structures that exist on one side of a strong reflector as being present on the other side as well. Figure 6-7, *A-C*, explains how this happens and shows examples. Mirror-image artifacts are common around the diaphragm and pleura because of the total reflection from air-filled lung. They occasionally occur in other locations (Figure 6-7, *C*). Sometimes the mirrored structure is not in the unmirrored scan plane.

Refraction

Refraction of light enables lenses to focus and distorts the presentation of objects, as shown in Figure 6-8, *A* and *B*. Refraction can cause a reflector to be positioned improperly (laterally) on a sonographic display (Figure 6-9). This is likely to occur, for example, when the transducer is placed on the abdominal midline (Figure 6-10, *A-C*), producing doubling of single objects. Beneath are the rectus abdominis muscles, which are surrounded by fat. These tissues present refracting boundaries because of their different propagation speeds.

Grating Lobes

Side lobes are beams that propagate from a single transducer element in directions different from the primary beam. Grating lobes are additional beams emitted from an array transducer that are stronger than the side lobes of individual elements (Figure 6-11). Side and grating lobes are weaker than the primary beam and normally do not produce echoes that are imaged, particularly if they fall on a normally echogenic region of

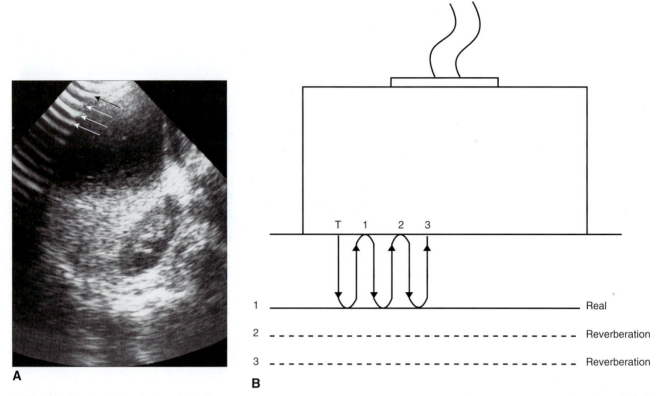

A

B

FIGURE 6-3 A, Reverberation artifact appearing as multiple presentations of a rib *(arrows).* **B,** The behavior in **A** is explained as follows: A pulse (T) is transmitted from the transducer. A strong echo is generated at the rib and is received *(1)* at the transducer, allowing correct imaging of the object. However, the echo is reflected partially at the transducer so that a second echo *(2)* is received, as well as a third (3) and possibly more. Because these echoes arrive later, they appear deeper on the display, where there are no reflectors. The lateral displacement of the reverberating sound path is for figure clarity. In fact, the sound travels down and back the same path repeatedly.

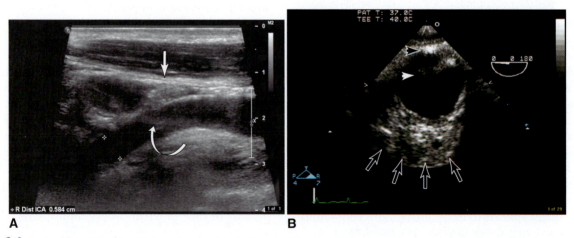

A   **B**

FIGURE 6-4 A, Reverberation *(curved arrow)* appearing in the carotid artery. This is a second echo from the proximal echogenic layer *(straight arrow)* **B,** Transesophageal scan of ascending aorta shows reverberation *(curved arrowhead)* as the second echo from the proximal margin *(straight arrow).* Enhancement *(arrows)* is also evident.

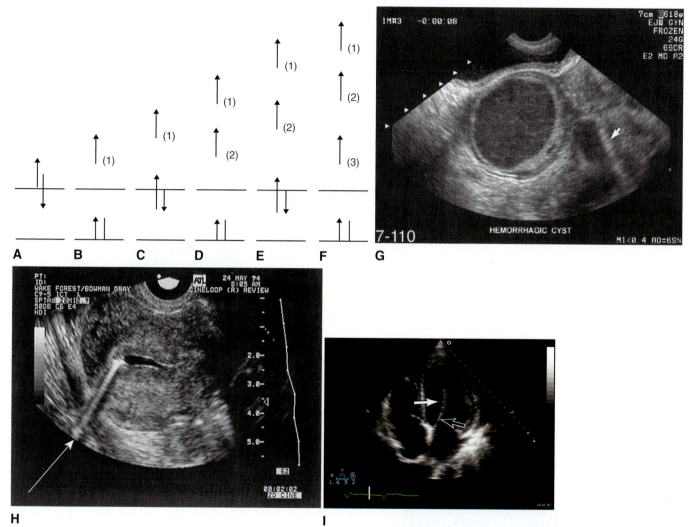

FIGURE 6-5 Generation of comet-tail artifact (closely spaced reverberations). Action progresses in time from left to right. **A,** An ultrasound pulse encounters the first reflector and is reflected partially and is transmitted partially. **B,** Reflection and transmission at the first reflector are complete. Reflection at the second reflector is occurring. **C,** Reflection at the second reflector is complete. Partial transmission and partial reflection are again occurring at the first reflector as the second echo passes through. **D,** The echoes from the first (1) and second (2) reflectors are traveling toward the transducer. A second reflection (repeat of **B**) is occurring at the second reflector. **E,** Partial transmission and reflection are again occurring at the first reflector. **F,** Three echoes are now returning—the echo from the first reflector (1), the echo from the second reflector (2), and the echo from the second reflector (3)—that originated from the back side of the first reflector (**C**) and reflected again from the second reflector (**D**). A fourth echo is being generated at the second reflector (**F**). **G,** Comet tail appears as a strong acoustic interface (arrow) from gas-filled bowel. **H,** Comet tail (arrow) from bubbles in an intrauterine saline injection. **I,** Apical four-chamber view of comet tail artifact (top left arrow) in the left ventricle. Artifact is connected to anterior mitral leaflet (lower right arrow).

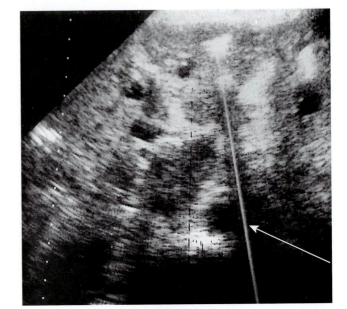

FIGURE 6-6 Ring-down artifact *(arrow)* from air in the bile duct.

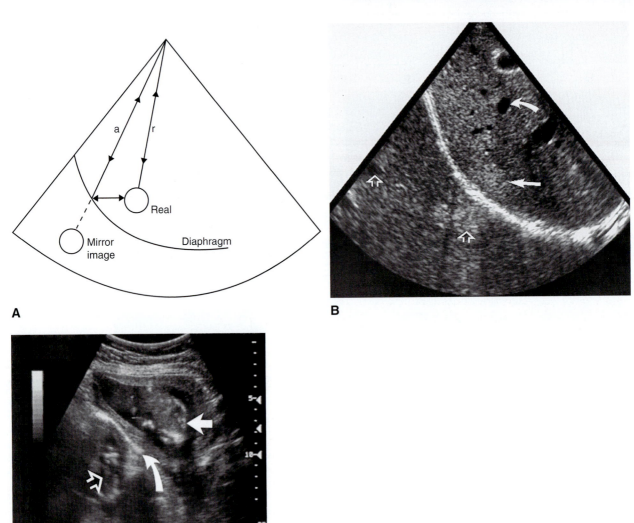

FIGURE 6-7 A, When pulses encounter a real hepatic structure directly (scan line *r*), the structure is imaged correctly. If the pulse first reflects off the diaphragm (scan line *a*) and the echo returns along the same path, the structure is displayed on the other side of the diaphragm. **B,** A hemangioma *(straight arrow)* and vessel *(curved arrow)* with their mirror images *(open arrows)*. **C,** A fetus *(straight arrow)* also appears as a mirror image *(open arrow)*. The mirror *(curved arrow)* is probably echogenic muscle.

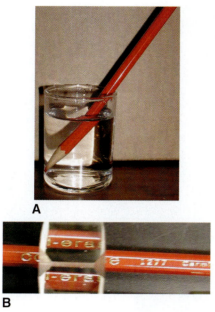

FIGURE 6-8 **A,** A pencil in water appears to be broken. **B,** A pencil beneath a prism appears to be split in two.

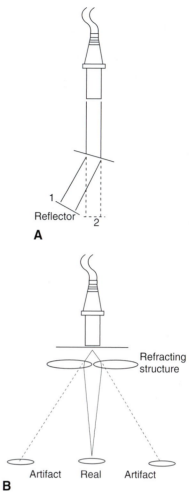

FIGURE 6-9 Refraction **(A)** results in improper positioning of a reflector on the display. The system places the reflector at position 2 (because that is the direction from which the echo was received) when in fact the reflector is actually at position 1. **B,** One real structure is imaged as two artifactual objects because of the refracting structure close to the transducer. If unrefracted pulses can propagate to the real structure, a triple presentation (one correct, two artifactual) will result.

the scan. However, if grating lobes encounter a strong reflector (e.g., bone or gas), their echoes may well be imaged, particularly if they fall within an **anechoic** region. If so, they appear in incorrect locations (Figure 6-12).

Speed Error

Propagation **speed error** occurs when the assumed value for propagation speed (1.54 mm/µs, leading to the 13 µs/cm roundtrip travel-time rule) is incorrect. If the propagation speed that exists over a path traveled is greater than 1.54 mm/µs, the calculated distance to the reflector is too small, and the display will place the reflector too close to the transducer (Figure 6-13). This occurs because the increased speed causes the echoes to arrive sooner. If the actual speed is less than 1.54 mm/µs, the reflector will be displayed too far from the transducer (Figure 6-14) because the echoes arrive later. Refraction and propagation speed error also can cause a structure to be displayed with incorrect shape.

Range Ambiguity

In sonographic imaging, it is assumed that for each pulse all echoes are received before the next pulse is emitted. If this were not the case, error could result (Figures 6-15 and 6-16). The maximum depth imaged correctly by an instrument is determined by its pulse repetition frequency (PRF). To avoid **range ambiguity**, PRF automatically is reduced in deeper imaging situations. This also causes a reduction in frame rate. Sometimes two artifacts combine

to present even more challenging cases. An example involving range ambiguity is shown in Figure 6-17.

ATTENUATION

Shadowing

Shadowing is the reduction in echo amplitude from reflectors that lie behind a strongly reflecting or attenuating structure. A strongly attenuating or reflecting structure weakens the sound distal to it, causing echoes from the distal region to be weak and thus to appear darker, like a shadow. Of course, the returning echoes also must pass through the attenuating structure, adding to the shadowing effect. Examples of shadowing structures include calcified plaque, bone, and stone (Figure 6-18).

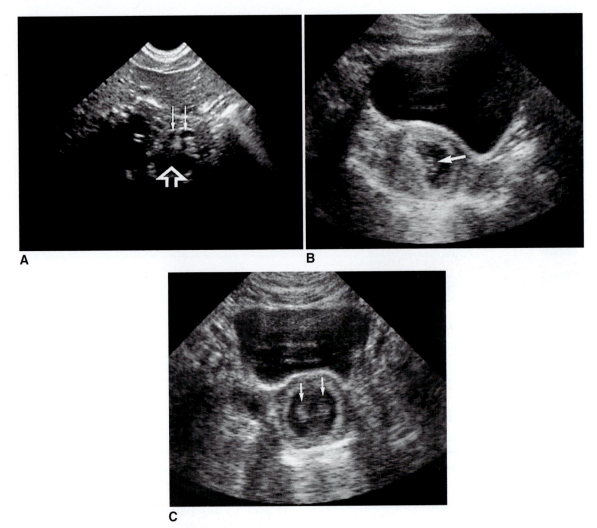

A

B

C

FIGURE 6-10 A, Refraction (probably through the rectus abdominis muscle) has widened the aorta *(open arrow)* and produced a double image of the celiac trunk *(arrows).* Refraction may cause a single gestation **(B)** to appear as a double gestation **(C).**

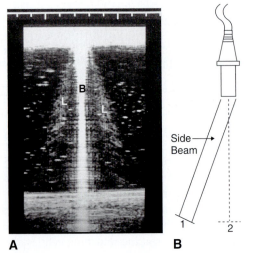

A   B

FIGURE 6-11 A, The primary beam *(B)* and grating lobes *(L)* from a linear array transducer. **B,** A side lobe or grating lobe can produce and receive a reflection from a "side view."

Shadowing also can occur beyond the edges of objects that are not necessarily strong attenuators (Figure 6-19). In this case, the cause may be the defocusing action of a refracting curved surface. Alternatively, it may be attributable to destructive interference caused by portions of an ultrasound pulse passing through tissues with different propagation speeds and subsequently getting out of phase. In either case, the intensity of the beam decreases beyond the edge of the structure, causing echoes to be weakened.

Enhancement

Enhancement is the strengthening of echoes from reflectors that lie behind a weakly attenuating structure (Figures 6-16; 6-18, *B*; and 6-20, *A-D*). Shadowing and enhancement result in reflectors being placed on the image with amplitudes that are too low and

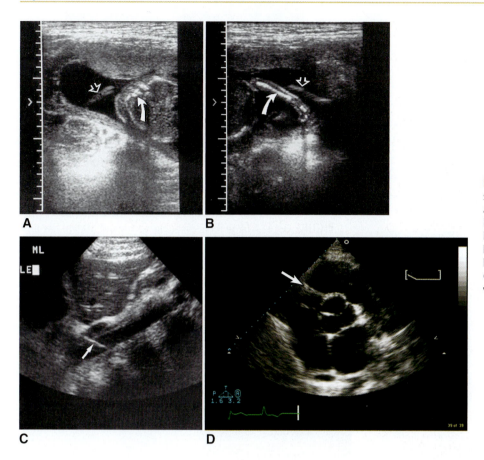

A **B**

C **D**

FIGURE 6-12 Grating lobes in obstetric scans can produce the appearance of amniotic sheets or bands. **A, B,** Grating lobe duplication *(open arrows)* of fetal bones *(curved arrows)* resembles amniotic bands or sheets. **C,** Artifactual grating lobe echoes *(arrow)* cross the aorta. **D,** Grating lobe *(arrow)* in the cardiac right ventricle.

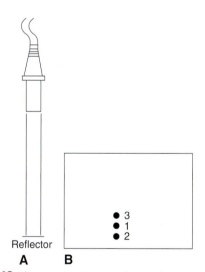

A **B**

FIGURE 6-13 The propagation speed over the traveled path **(A)** determines the reflector position on the display **(B)**. The reflector is actually in position *1*. If the actual propagation speed is less than that assumed, the reflector will appear in position *2*. If the actual speed is more than that assumed, the reflector will appear in position *3*.

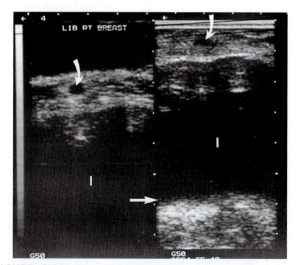

FIGURE 6-14 The low propagation speed in a silicone breast implant (I) causes the chest wall *(straight arrow)* to appear deeper than it should. Note that a cyst *(curved arrows)* is shown more clearly on the left image than on the right because a gel standoff pad has been placed between the transducer and the breast, moving the beam focus closer to the cyst.

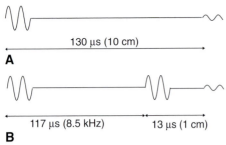

A

130 μs (10 cm)

B

117 μs (8.5 kHz)   13 μs (1 cm)

FIGURE 6-15 A, An echo (from a 10-cm depth) arrives 130 μs after pulse emission. **B,** If the pulse repetition period were 117 μs (corresponding to a pulse repetition frequency of 8.5 kHz), the echo in **A** would arrive 13 μs after the next pulse was emitted. The instrument would place this echo at a 1-cm depth rather than the correct value. This range location error is known as the range-ambiguity artifact.

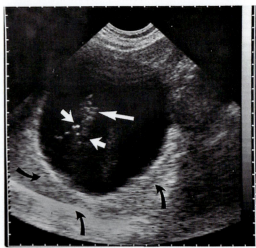

FIGURE 6-16 A large renal cyst (diameter about 10 cm) has artifactual range-ambiguity echoes within it *(white arrows)*. They are generated from structure(s) below the display. These deep echoes arrive after the next pulse is emitted. Because the time from the emission of the last pulse to echo arrival is short, the echoes are placed closer to the transducer than they should be. Echoes arrive from much deeper (later) than usual in this case because the sound passes through the long, low-attenuation paths in the cyst. These echoes may have come from bone or far body wall. Low attenuation in the cyst is indicated by the strong echoes (enhancement) below it *(curved black arrows)*.

FIGURE 6-17 A large pelvic cyst produces a large echo-free region in this scan. A structure is located at a depth of about 13 cm *(straight arrows)*. Located in the anechoic region at a depth of about 6 cm is a structure *(curved arrows)* shaped like that at 13 cm. How could this artifact appear closer than the actual structure, implying that these echoes arrived earlier than those from the correct location? It turns out that the artifact is actually a combination of two phenomena: reverberation and range ambiguity. The artifact seen is a reverberation from the deep structure and the transducer. But a reverberation should appear at twice the depth of the actual structure—that is, at about 26 cm. However, the arrival of the reverberation echoes occurs about 78 μs after the next pulse is emitted so that they are placed at a 6-cm depth. Single artifacts are difficult enough. Fortunately, combinations like this occur infrequently.

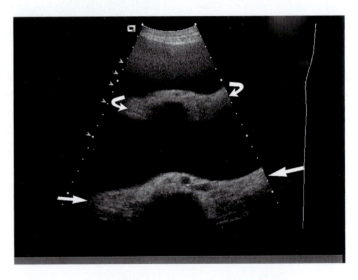

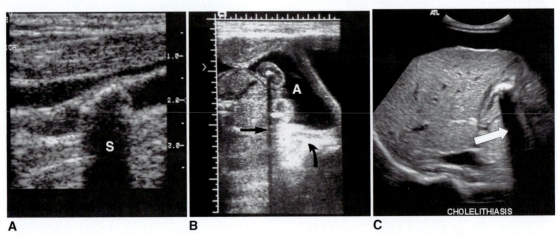

A   **B**   **C**

FIGURE 6-18 A, Shadowing from a high-attenuation calcified plaque in the common carotid artery. **B,** Shadowing *(straight arrow)* from a fetal limb bone and enhancement *(curved arrow)* caused by the low attenuation of amniotic fluid through which the ultrasound travels. **C,** Shadowing *(arrow)* from gallstones.

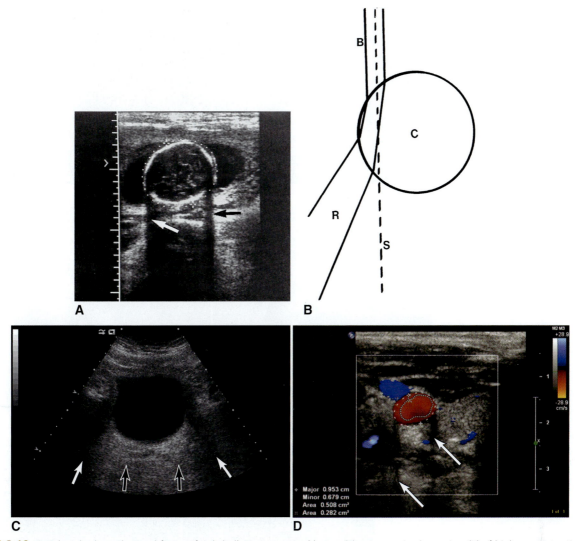

FIGURE 6-19 A, Edge shadows *(arrows)* from a fetal skull. **B,** As a sound beam *(B)* enters a circular region *(C)* of higher propagation speed, it is refracted, and refraction occurs again as it leaves. This causes spreading of the beam with decreased intensity. The echoes from region R are presented deep to the circular region in the neighborhood of the dashed line. Because of beam spreading, these echoes are weak and thus cast a shadow *(S)*. **C,** Enhancement *(black arrows)* and edge shadows *(white arrows)* from pediatric bladder. **D,** Transverse carotid scan showing edge shadows *(arrows)*.

too high, respectively. Brightening of echoes also can be caused by the increased intensity in the focal region of a beam because the beam is narrow there. This is called *focal enhancement* or *focal banding* (Figure 6-21, *A*). Banding can also be caused by incorrect gain and TGC settings (Figure 6-21, *B*). Shadowing and enhancement are often useful for determining the nature of masses and structures. Shadowing is reduced with spatial compounding because several approaches to each anatomic site are used, allowing the beam to "get under" the attenuating structure. This is useful with shadowing because it can uncover structures (especially pathologic ones) that were not imaged because they were located in the shadow. Noise, generated internally or from external influences, also can produce artifacts (Figure 6-22).

SPECTRAL DOPPLER

Aliasing

Aliasing is the most common artifact encountered in Doppler ultrasound. The word *alias* comes from Middle English *elles*, Latin *alius*, and Greek *allos*, which mean *other* or *otherwise*. Contemporary meanings for the word include (as an adverb) *otherwise called* or *otherwise known as* and (as a noun) *an assumed or additional name*. Aliasing in its technical use indicates improper representation of information that has been sampled insufficiently. An optical form of temporal aliasing occurs in motion pictures when wagon wheels appear to rotate at various speeds and in reverse direction. Similar behavior is observed when a fan is lighted with a strobe light. Depending on the flashing rate of the strobe light, the

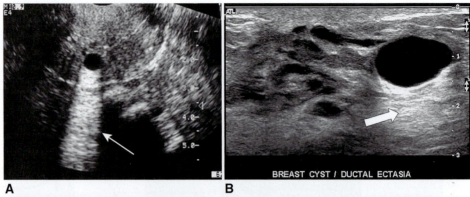

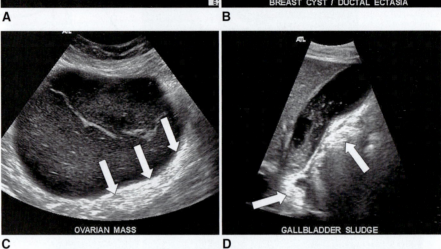

FIGURE 6-20 A, Enhancement *(arrow)* beyond a cervical cyst. **B** to **D,** Examples of enhancement *(arrows).*

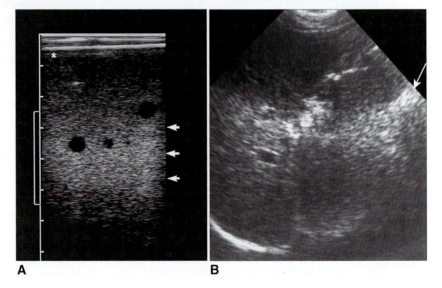

FIGURE 6-21 A, Focal banding *(arrows)* is the brightening of echoes around the focus, where intensity is increased by the narrowing of the beam. **B,** Banding *(arrow)* caused by incorrect TGC settings. The midfield gain is too high compared to near- and far-field.

fan may appear stationary or rotating clockwise or counterclockwise at various speeds.

Nyquist Limit

Pulsed wave Doppler instruments are sampling instruments. Each emitted pulse yields a sample of the desired Doppler shift. The upper limit to Doppler shift that can be detected properly by pulsed instruments is called the **Nyquist limit.** If the Doppler-shift frequency exceeds one half the pulse-repetition frequency (PRF) (which, for Doppler functions, is normally in the 5 to 30 kHz range),

temporal aliasing occurs. Improper Doppler shift information (improper direction and improper value) results. Higher PRFs (Table 6-1) permit higher Doppler shifts to be detected but also increase the chance of the range-ambiguity artifact occurring. Continuous-wave Doppler instruments do not experience aliasing. However, recall that neither do they provide depth localization. Figure 6-23 illustrates aliasing in the popliteal artery and in the heart of a normal subject. This figure also illustrates how aliasing can be reduced or eliminated (Box 6-1) by increasing PRF, increasing Doppler angle (which decreases the Doppler shift for a given flow), or by

TABLE 6-1	Aliasing and Range-Ambiguity Artifact Values	
Pulse Repetition Frequency (kHz)	**Doppler Shift Above Which Aliasing Occurs (kHz)**	**Range Beyond Which Ambiguity Occurs (cm)**
5.0	2.5	15
7.5	3.7	10
10.0	5.0	7
12.5	6.2	6
15.0	7.5	5
17.5	8.7	4
20.0	10.0	3
25.0	12.5	3
30.0	15.0	2

BOX 6-1	Methods of Reducing or Eliminating Aliasing

Shift the baseline.*
Increase the pulse repetition frequency.*
Increase the Doppler angle.
Use a lower operating frequency.
Use a continuous wave device.

*These are the most convenient and commonly used. Both are required in extreme cases.

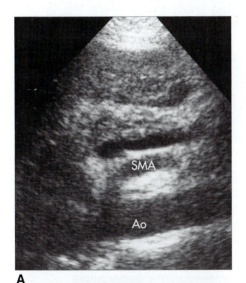

A

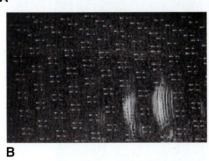

B

FIGURE 6-22 A, Noise is seen with "fill-in" of anechoic vascular structures. *Ao,* Aorta; *SMA,* superior mesenteric artery. **B,** Interference (repeating white specks) from nearby electronic equipment.

baseline shift. The latter is an electronic cut-and-paste technique that moves the misplaced aliasing peaks over to their proper location. The technique is successful as long as there are no legitimate Doppler shifts in the region of the aliasing. If there are legitimate Doppler shifts, they will be moved over to an inappropriate location along with the aliasing peaks. (This would happen if the baseline were shifted farther down in Figure 6-23, *E.*) Baseline shifting is not helpful if the desired informa-

tion (e.g., peak systolic Doppler shift) is buried in another portion of the spectral display, as in Figure 6-23, *H.* Other approaches to eliminating aliasing include changing to a lower-frequency Doppler transducer (Figure 6-23, *F* and *G*) or switching to continuous wave operation (Figure 6-23, *H* and *I*). The common and convenient solutions to aliasing are shifting the baseline, increasing PRF, or doing both in extreme cases.

In Figure 6-23, *A,* the vertical axis is calibrated in Doppler-shift frequency units so that we can see that aliasing occurs at Doppler shifts greater than 1.75 kHz. The aliased peaks add another 1.25 kHz of Doppler shift, so the correct peak systolic shift is 3 kHz. With the higher PRF in Figure 6-23, *C,* this result is confirmed. Thus, at the lower PRF, the peak shift can be determined and baseline shifting is not necessary (but *is* convenient). However, if the peaks were buried in other portions of the Doppler signal (as in Figure 6-23, *H*), baseline shifting would not help, but a higher PRF (most convenient method), a larger Doppler angle, or a lower operating frequency would. Aliasing occurs with the pulsed system because it is a sampling system; that is, a pulsed system acquires samples of the desired Doppler shift frequency from which it must be synthesized. If samples are taken often enough, the correct result is achieved. Figure 6-24 shows temporal sampling of a signal. Sufficient sampling yields the correct result. Insufficient sampling yields an incorrect result.

The Nyquist limit, or Nyquist frequency, describes the minimum number of samples required to avoid aliasing. At least two samples per cycle of the desired Doppler shift must be made for the image to be obtained correctly. For a complicated signal, such as a Doppler signal containing many frequencies, the sampling rate must be such that at least two samples occur for each cycle of the highest frequency present. To restate this rule, if the highest Doppler-shift frequency present in a signal exceeds one half the PRF, aliasing will occur (see Figure 6-24).

Lesser-used correction methods include increasing the Doppler angle (which reduces the Doppler shift), reducing the operating frequency, and switching to continuous wave operation. Continuous wave operation, because it is not pulsed, is not a sampling mode and is thus not subject to aliasing. However, it does not have range selectivity ability.

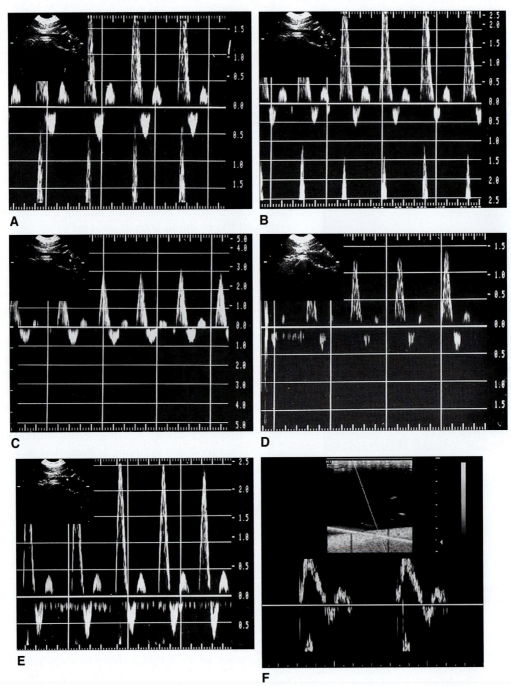

FIGURE 6-23 A, Aliasing in the popliteal artery. **B,** Pulse repetition frequency (PRF) is increased. **C,** The PRF is increased further. **D,** Doppler angle is increased with original PRF. **E,** Baseline is shifted down with original PRF. **F,** Aliasing is occurring with an operating frequency of 6 MHz.

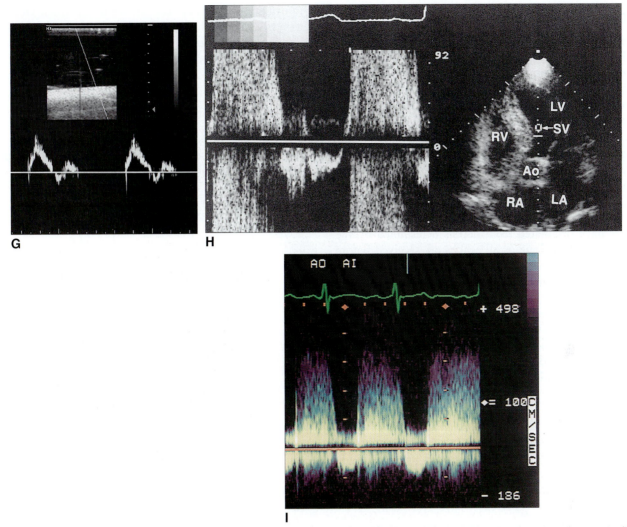

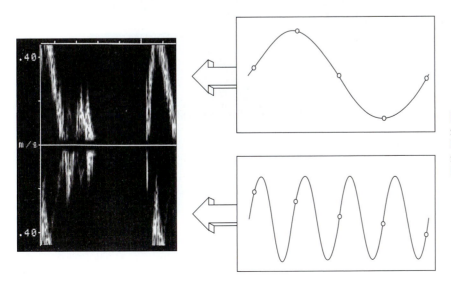

FIGURE 6-23, cont'd **G,** When operating frequency is reduced to 4 MHz, the Doppler shifts are reduced to less than the Nyquist limit, thereby eliminating the aliasing seen in **F. H,** The sample volume *(SV)* is placed in the left-ventricular outflow tract. There is aortic insufficiency that causes the Doppler shifts to exceed the Nyquist limit producing aliasing. *Ao,* aorta; *LA,* left atrium, *LV,* left ventricle; *RA,* right atrium; *RV,* right ventricle. **I,** Using continuous-wave (CW) ultrasound eliminates the aliasing because there is no sampling.

FIGURE 6-24 In this spectral display, the presentation above the baseline is correct (unaliased, five samples per cycle), whereas the systolic peaks appear incorrectly below the baseline (aliased, one sample per cycle).

Range Ambiguity

In attempting to solve the aliasing problem by increasing the PRF, one can encounter the range-ambiguity problem. As described previously under the propagation group, this problem occurs when a pulse is emitted before all the echoes from the previous pulse have been received. When this happens, early echoes from the last pulse are received simultaneously with late echoes from the previous pulse. The instrument is unable to determine whether an echo is an early one (superficial) from the last pulse or a late one (deep) from the previous pulse. To solve this difficulty, the instrument simply assumes that all echoes are derived from the last pulse and that these echoes have originated from depths determined by the 13 μs/cm rule. As long as all echoes are received before the next pulse is sent out, this is true. However, with high PRFs, this may not be the case. Doppler flow information therefore may come from locations other than the assumed one (the gate location). In effect, multiple gates or sample volumes are operating at different depths. Table 6-1 lists, for various PRFs, the ranges beyond which ambiguity occurs. Multiple sample volumes are shown on the display to indicate this condition.

Mirror Image

A mirror image of a Doppler spectrum can appear on the opposite side of the baseline when, indeed, flow is unidirectional and should appear only on one side of the baseline. This is an electronic duplication of the spectral information. The duplication can occur when Doppler gain is set too high, causing overloading in the amplifier and leakage, called **cross-talk**, of the signal from the proper-direction channel into the opposite-direction channel (Figure 6-25).

Noise

Doppler spectra have a speckle quality to them that is similar to that observed in sonography. Internally generated electronic noise appears if Doppler gain is set too high (Figure 6-26, *A*). Electromagnetic interference from nearby equipment can cloud the spectral display with lines or "snow" (Figure 6-26, *B* and *C*).

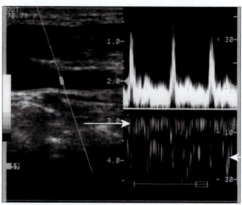

FIGURE 6-25 High gain produces a mirror image *(arrows)* of the carotid artery spectrum below the baseline.

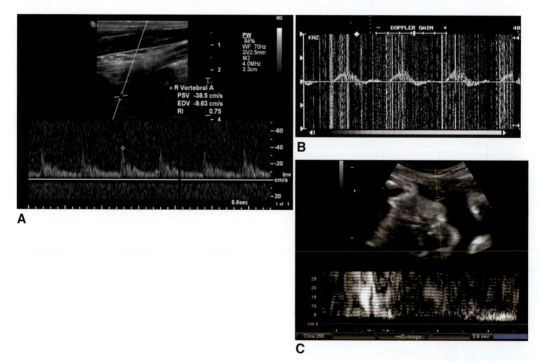

FIGURE 6-26 A, Doppler gain is set too high, causing noise to appear on the spectral display. **B,** Interference from nearby electrical equipment clouds the spectral display with electric noise (the vertical "snow" lines). **C,** Interference (wavy horizontal lines in the spectral display) from an external source.

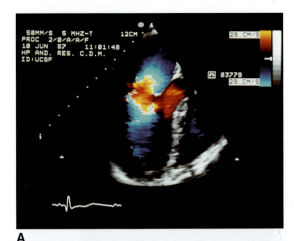

A

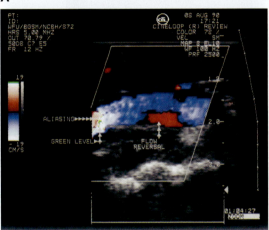

B

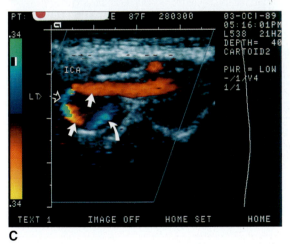

C

FIGURE 6-27 A, A transesophageal cardiac color Doppler image of the long axis in diastole. The blue colors in the left atrium *(upper)* and left ventricle *(lower)* represent blood traveling away from the transducer, but where the flow speeds exceed the Nyquist limit (29 cm/s), aliasing occurs and the yellow and orange colors have replaced the blue colors. **B,** Color Doppler presentation of common carotid artery flow, including flow reversal and aliasing. The two can be distinguished because the boundary between the different directions with flow reversal passes through the baseline *(black)*, whereas the aliasing boundary passes through the upper and lower extremes of the color bar *(white)*. In this particular color bar assignment, the maximum positive Doppler shifts are assigned the color green, so that a thin green region shows the exact boundary where aliasing occurs. The aliasing occurs in the distal portion of the vessel

COLOR DOPPLER

Artifacts observed with color Doppler imaging are two-dimensional color presentations of artifacts that are seen in gray-scale sonography and Doppler spectral displays. They are incorrect presentations of two-dimensional motion information, the most common of which is aliasing. However, others occur, including anatomic mirror image, Doppler angle effects, shadowing, and clutter.

Aliasing

Aliasing occurs when the Doppler shift exceeds the Nyquist limit (Figure 6-27). The result is incorrect flow direction on the color Doppler image (Figure 6-28).

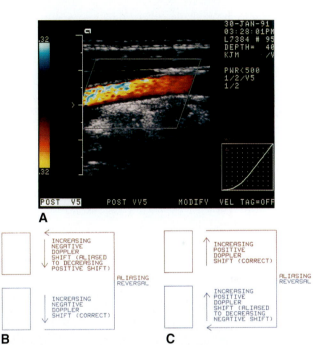

FIGURE 6-28 A, Positive *(blue)* Doppler shifts are shown in the arterial flow in this image. **B,** These are actually negative Doppler shifts that have exceeded the lower Nyquist limit (converted here to the equivalent flow speed: −0.32 m/s) and are wrapped around to the positive portion of the color bar **(C)**. Positive shifts that exceed the +0.32 m/s limit would alias to the negative side.

because it is curving down, reducing the Doppler angle between the flow and the scan lines. **C,** In a tortuous internal carotid artery, negative Doppler shifts are indicated in the red regions *(solid straight arrows)*. Two regions of positive Doppler shifts *(blue)* are seen *(open arrow* and *curved arrow)*. In the latter, legitimate flow toward the transducer is indicated. In the former, the flow away from the transducer has yielded high Doppler shifts (because of a small Doppler angle; i.e., flow is approximately parallel to scan lines), which produces a color shift to the opposite side of the map because of aliasing. The boundaries from and to normal negative Doppler shifts into and out of the aliased region are bright yellow and cyan from the ends of the color bars. The transition from unaliased negative Doppler shift into unaliased positive Doppler shift (near bottom) is black, representing the baseline of the color bar. The flow direction is counterclockwise.

Increasing the flow speed range (which is actually an increase in PRF) can solve the problem (Figure 6-29). However, too high a range can cause loss of flow information, particularly if the wall filter is set high (Figure 6-29, *D* and *E*). Baseline shifting can decrease or eliminate the effect of aliasing (Figure 6-29, *C*), as in spectral displays.

Mirror Image, Shadowing, Clutter, and Noise

In the mirror (or ghost) artifact (Figure 6-30), an image of a vessel and source of Doppler-shifted echoes can be duplicated on the opposite side of a strong reflector (e.g., pleura or diaphragm). This is a color Doppler extension

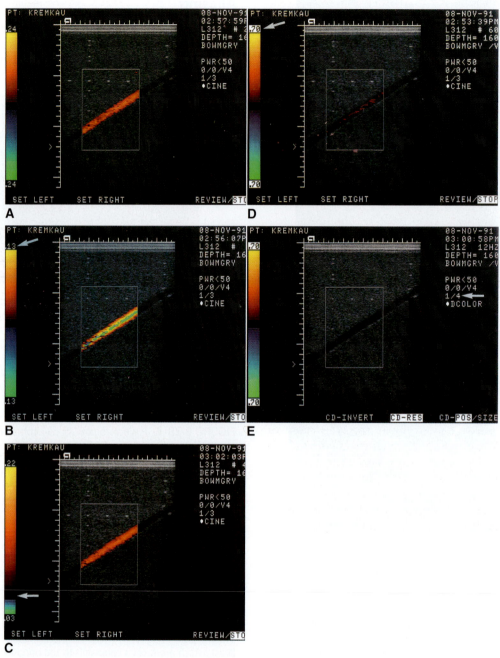

FIGURE 6-29 A, Flow is toward the upper right, producing positive Doppler shifts. **B,** The pulse repetition frequency and Nyquist limit (0.13, *arrow*) are too low, resulting in aliasing (negative Doppler shifts) at the center of the flow in the vessel. **C,** With the same pulse repetition frequency setting as in **B,** the aliasing has been corrected by shifting the baseline *(arrow)* down 10 cm/s below the center of the color bar. **D,** The Nyquist limit setting (0.70, *arrow*) is too high, causing the detected Doppler shifts to be well down the positive scale, producing a dark red appearance. **E,** With the Nyquist limit set as in **D,** an increase in the wall filter setting *(arrow)* eliminates what little color flow information there was in **D.**

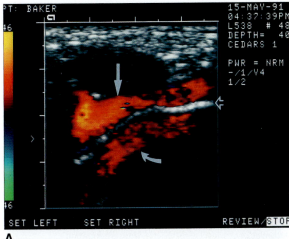

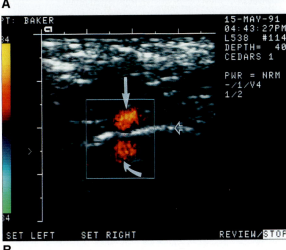

FIGURE 6-30 Color Doppler imaging of the subclavian artery *(straight arrow)* in longitudinal **(A)** and transverse **(B)** views. The pleura *(open arrow)* causes the mirror image *(curved arrow)*.

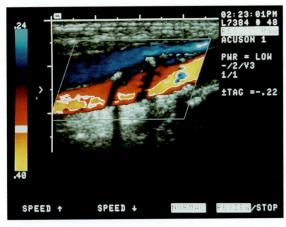

FIGURE 6-31 Shadowing from calcified plaque follows the gray-scale scan lines straight down while following the angled color scan lines parallel to the sides of the parallelogram.

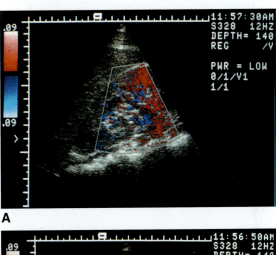

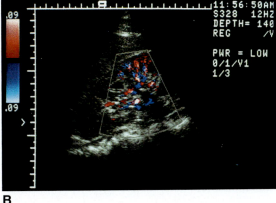

FIGURE 6-32 A, Clutter from tissue motion (caused by respiration) obscures underlying blood flow in the renal vasculature. **B,** An increased wall filter setting removes the clutter, revealing the underlying flow.

of gray-scale mirror. Shadowing is the weakening or elimination of Doppler-shifted echoes beyond a shadowing object, just as occurs with non–Doppler-shifted (gray-scale) echoes (Figure 6-31). Clutter results from tissue, heart wall or valve, or vessel wall motion (Figure 6-32). Such clutter is eliminated by wall filters. Doppler angle effects include zero Doppler shift when the Doppler angle is 90 degrees, as well as the change of color in a straight vessel viewed with a sector transducer. Noise in the color Doppler electronics can mimic flow, particularly in **hypoechoic** or anechoic regions (Figure 6-33). The "twinkling" artifact (Figure 6-34) has been observed at strongly reflecting scattering surfaces. It is thought to occur with complications in the phase detection process of Doppler detection when a finite number of strong scatterers is encountered.

This chapter has discussed several ultrasound imaging and flow artifacts, which are listed in Table 6-2, along with their causes. In some cases the names of the artifacts are identical to their causes. Shadowing and enhance-

ment are useful in interpretation and diagnosis. Other artifacts can cause confusion and error. Artifacts seen in two-dimensional imaging are evidenced in three-dimensional imaging also, sometimes in unusual ways. All of these artifacts can hinder proper interpretation

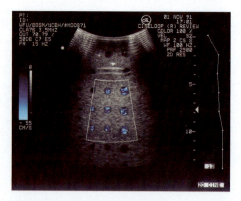

FIGURE 6-33 Color appears in echo-free (cystic) regions of a tissue-equivalent phantom. The color gain has been increased sufficiently to produce this effect. The instrument tends to write color information preferentially in areas where non–Doppler-shifted echoes are weak or absent.

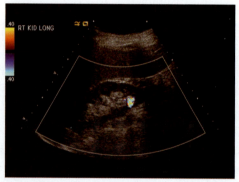

FIGURE 6-34 Twinkling artifact associated with a renal stone.

TABLE 6-2	Artifacts and Their Causes
Artifact	**Cause**
Axial resolution	Pulse length
Comet tail	Reverberation
Grating lobe	Grating lobe
Lateral resolution	Pulse width
Mirror image	Multiple reflection
Refraction	Refraction
Reverberation	Multiple reflection
Ring down	Resonance
Section thickness	Pulse width
Speckle	Interference
Speed error	Speed error
Range ambiguity	High pulse repetition frequency
Shadowing	High attenuation
Edge shadowing	Refraction or interference
Enhancement	Low attenuation
Focal enhancement	Focusing
Aliasing	Low pulse repetition frequency
Spectrum mirror	High Doppler gain

and diagnosis and so must be avoided or handled properly when encountered. A proper understanding of artifacts and how to deal with them when they are encountered enables sonographers and sonologists to use them to advantage while avoiding the pitfalls that they can cause.

Abdomen

Anatomic and Physiologic Relationships Within the Abdominal Cavity

Sandra L. Hagen-Ansert

To understand the complexity of the human body and how the parts work together to function as a whole truly is to gain an appreciation of anatomy and physiology. The science of body structure (anatomy) and the study of body function (physiology) are intricately related, for each structure of the human body system carries out a specific function. Anatomy and physiology can take many forms: Gross anatomy studies the body by dissection of tissues; histology studies parts of body tissues under the microscope; embryology studies development before birth; and pathology is the study of disease processes.

FROM ATOM TO ORGANISM

A review of the composition of the human body begins with an understanding that all materials consist of chemicals. The basic units of all matter are tiny invisible particles called *atoms*. An atom is the smallest compo-

nent of a chemical element that retains the characteristic properties of that element. Atoms can combine chemically to form larger particles called *molecules*. For example, two atoms of hydrogen combine with one atom of oxygen to produce a molecule of water.

The next level of complexity in the human body is a microscopic unit called a *cell*. Although they share common traits, cells can vary in size, shape, and specialized function. In the human body, atoms and molecules associate in specific ways to form cells, and trillions of different types of cells are found within the body. All cells have specialized tiny parts called *organelles*, which carry on specific activities. These organelles consist of aggregates of large molecules, including those of such substances as proteins, carbohydrates, lipids, and nucleic acids. One organelle, the *nucleus*, serves as the information and control center of the cell.

Cells that are organized into layers or masses that have common functions are known as *tissue*. The four primary types of tissue in the body are muscle, nervous, connective, and epithelial tissues.

Groups of different tissues combine to form *organs*—complex structures with specialized functions, such as the liver, pancreas, or uterus. One organ may have more than one type of tissue (i.e., the heart mainly consists of muscle tissue, but it is also covered by epithelial tissue and contains connective and nervous tissue).

A coordinated group of organs are arranged into organ or *body systems*. For example, the digestive system consists of the mouth, esophagus, stomach, intestines, liver, gallbladder, and pancreas. Body systems make up the total part or *organism* that is the human body.

Metabolism

All physical and chemical changes that occur within the body are referred to as **metabolism.** The metabolic process is essential to digestion, growth and repair of the body, and conversion of food energy into forms useful to the body. Other metabolic processes maintain the routine operations of the nerves, muscles, and other body parts.

Homeostasis

The anatomic structures and functions of all body parts are directed toward maintaining the life of the organism. To sustain life, an organism must have the proper quantity and quality of water, food, oxygen, heat, and pressure. Maintenance of life depends on the stability of these factors. **Homeostasis** is the ability to maintain a steady and stable internal environment. Stressful stimuli, or *stressors*, disrupt homeostasis.

Vital signs are medical measurements used to ascertain how the body is functioning. These measurements include body temperature and blood pressure and rates and types of pulse and breathing movements. A close relationship has been noted between these signs and the homeostasis of the body, as vital signs are the result of metabolic activities. Death is the absence of such signs.

BODY SYSTEMS

A body system consists of a group of tissues and organs that work together to perform specific functions. Each system contributes to the dynamic, organized, and carefully balanced state of the body. The sonographer should be familiar with at least the integumentary, skeletal, muscular, respiratory, and nervous systems of the body. The remaining systems—endocrine, digestive, circulatory, lymphatic, urinary, and reproductive—should be thoroughly understood by the sonographer. Table 7-1 lists the components and functions of human body systems.

ANATOMIC DIRECTIONS

The anatomic position assumes that the body is standing erect, the eyes are looking forward, and arms are at the

TABLE 7-1	Systems in the Human Body	
System	**Components**	**Functions**
Integumentary	Skin, hair, nails, sweat glands	Covers and protects tissues, regulates body temperature, supports sensory receptors
Skeletal	Bones, cartilage, joints, ligaments	Supports the body, provides framework, protects soft tissues, provides attachments for muscles, produces blood cells, stores inorganic salts, provides calcium storage
Muscular	Skeletal, cardiac, smooth muscle	Moves parts of skeleton, provides locomotion, pumps blood, aids movement of internal materials, produces body heat
Nervous	Nerves and sense organs, brain, and spinal cord	Receives stimuli from external and internal environment, conducts impulses, integrates activities of other systems
Endocrine	Pituitary, adrenal, thyroid, pancreas, parathyroid, ovaries, testes, pineal, and thymus gland	Regulates body chemistry and many body functions
Lymphatic	Lymph nodes	Returns tissue fluid to the blood, carries specific absorbed food molecules, defends the body against infection
Circulatory	Heart, blood vessels, blood, lymph and lymph structures	Moves the blood through the vessels and transports substances throughout the body
Respiratory	Lungs, bronchi, and air passageways	Exchanges gases between blood and external environment
Digestive	Mouth, tongue, teeth, salivary glands, pharynx, esophagus, stomach, liver, gallbladder, pancreas, small and large intestines	Receives, breaks down, and absorbs food and eliminates unabsorbed material from the body
Urinary	Kidney, bladder, ureters	Excretes waste from the blood, maintains water and electrolyte balance, and stores and transports urine
Reproductive	Testes, scrotum, spermatic cord, vas deferens, ejaculatory duct, penis, epididymis, prostate, uterus, ovaries, fallopian tubes, vagina, breast	Reproduction; provides for continuation of the species

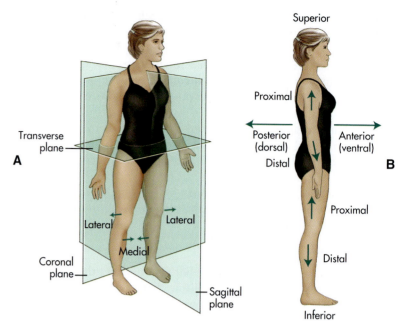

FIGURE 7-1 A, Anterior view of the body in the anatomic position. Note the directions and body planes. **B,** Lateral view of the body.

sides with the palms and toes directed forward. Refer to Figure 7-1 for the four anatomic directions of the body discussed here.

1. **Superior/inferior.** The top of the head is the most superior point of the body. The inferior point of the body is the bottom of the feet. All anatomic structures are designated relative to these two terms. The liver is considered to be superior to the bladder because the liver is closer to the head. The gallbladder is inferior to the diaphragm because it is closer to the feet. Other terms that are interchanged with *superior* are *cephalic* and *cranial* (toward the head). *Caudal* (toward the tail) is sometimes used instead of *inferior*.

2. **Anterior/posterior.** The front (belly) surface of the body is anterior, or *ventral*. The back surface of the body is posterior, or *dorsal*. This concept is very important to sonographers and to their understanding of sectional anatomy. If the patient is lying supine (face up), the aorta is anterior to the vertebral column. The right kidney is posterior to the head of the pancreas.

3. **Medial/lateral.** The body axis is an imaginary line from the center of the top of the head to the groin. *Medial* is described as the superior-inferior body axis as it goes right through the midline of the body. Structures are said to be medial if they are closer to the midline of the body than to another structure (e.g., the hepatic artery is medial to the common duct). The structure is *lateral* if it is toward the side of the body (e.g., the adnexae are lateral to the uterus).

4. **Proximal/distal.** When a structure is closer to the body midline or point of attachment to the trunk, it is described as *proximal* (e.g., the hepatic duct is

proximal to the common bile duct). *Distal* means farther from the midline or point of attachment to the trunk (e.g., the sphincter of Oddi is distal to the common bile duct).

5. **Superficial/deep.** Additionally, structures may be identified as being superficial or deep. Structures located close to the surface of the body are *superficial*. The rectus abdominis muscles are superficial to the transverse abdominis muscles. Structures located farther inward (away from the body surface) are *deep*.

Anatomic Terms

The ability of the sonographer to understand anatomy as it relates to cross-sectional, coronal, oblique, and sagittal projections is critical to performing a quality sonographic examination. Normal anatomy has many variations in size and position, and the sonographer must be able to demonstrate these findings on the sonogram. A thorough understanding of anatomy as it relates to anteroposterior relationships and variations in sectional anatomy is required (see Figure 7-1). The following list contains anatomic terms grouped loosely by category:

anatomic position—individual is standing erect, arms are by the sides with the palms facing forward, face and eyes are directed forward, and heels are together, with the feet pointed forward

median plane—vertical plane that bisects the body into right and left halves

supine—lying face up

prone—lying face down

anterior (ventral)—toward the front of the body or in front of another structure

posterior (dorsal) —toward the back of the body or in back of another structure
medial—nearer to or toward the midline
lateral—farther from the midline or to the side of the body
proximal—closer to the point of origin or closer to the body
distal—away from the point of origin or away from the body
internal—inside
external—outside
superior—above
inferior—below
cranial—toward the head
caudal—toward the feet

PLANES OR BODY SECTIONS

The sonographer observes the body in three different planes: transverse, sagittal, and coronal (see Figure 7-1).

1. **Transverse.** The transverse plane is horizontal to the body. This plane divides the body or any of its parts into upper and lower portions.
2. **Sagittal.** The sagittal plane is a lengthwise plane running from front to back. It divides the body or any of its parts into right and left sides, or two equal halves; this is known as the midsagittal plane.
3. **Coronal.** The coronal plane is a lengthwise plane running from side to side, dividing the body into anterior and posterior portions.

ABDOMINAL QUADRANTS AND REGIONS

To identify specific abdominal structures or to refer to an area of pain, the abdomen may be divided into four quadrants or nine abdominal regions.

The abdominopelvic cavity is divided into four quadrants that include the right upper quadrant (RUQ), left upper quadrant (LUQ), right lower quadrant (RLQ), and left lower quadrant (LLQ). The quadrant is determined by a midsagittal plane and a transverse plane that pass through the umbilicus.

The abdomen is commonly divided into nine regions by two vertical and two horizontal lines. The surface landmarks of the anterior abdominal wall help to define the specific abdominal regions (Figure 7-2). Each vertical line passes through the midinguinal point (i.e., the point that lies on the inguinal ligament halfway between the pubic symphysis and the anterior superior iliac spine. The upper horizontal line, referred to as the **subcostal plane,** joins the lowest point of the costal margin on each side of the body. The lowest horizontal line, the **intertubercular plane,** joins the tubercles on the iliac crests. The **transpyloric plane** is a horizontal plane that passes through the pylorus, the duodenal junction, the neck of the pancreas, and the hilum of the kidneys.

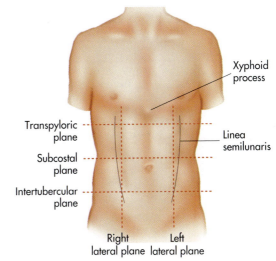

FIGURE 7-2 Surface landmarks of the anterior abdominal wall.

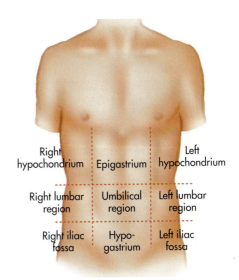

FIGURE 7-3 Regions of the abdominal wall.

The nine abdominal regions include the following: (1) upper abdomen/right hypochondrium, (2) epigastrium, (3) left hypochondrium, (4) middle abdomen/right lumbar, (5) umbilical, (6) left lumbar, (7) lower abdomen/right iliac fossa, (8) hypogastrium, and (9) left iliac fossa (Figure 7-3).

Table 7-2 provides a list of additional terms that the sonographer is likely to encounter when identifying specific body regions or structures.

BODY CAVITIES

The human body includes many cavities. These body cavities contain the internal organs, or **viscera.** The two principal body cavities are the dorsal cavity and the ventral cavity (Figure 7-4). The bony dorsal cavity may be subdivided into the *cranial cavity,* which holds the brain, and the *vertebral* or *spinal canal,* which contains

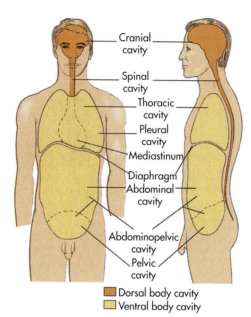

FIGURE 7-4 Body cavities. Locations and divisions of the dorsal and ventral body cavities as viewed from anterior and lateral.

TABLE 7-2	Terms for Common Body Regions and Structures
Term	**Body Region or Structure**
Abdominal	Portion of trunk below the diaphragm
Axillary	Area of armpit
Brachial	Arm
Celiac	Abdomen
Cervical	Neck region
Costal	Ribs
Femoral	Thigh; the part of the lower extremity between the hip and the knee
Groin/inguinal	Depressed region between the abdomen and the thigh
Leg	Lower extremity, especially from the knee to the foot
Lumbar	Loin; the region of the lower back and side, between the lowest rib and the pelvis
Mammary	Breasts
Pelvic	Pelvis; the bony ring that girdles the lower portion of the trunk
Perineal	Region between the anus and the pubic arch; includes the region of the external reproductive structures
Popliteal	Area behind the knee
Thoracic	Chest; the part of the trunk below the neck and above the diaphragm

the spinal cord. The ventral cavity is located near the anterior body surface and is subdivided into the *thoracic cavity* and the *abdominopelvic cavity.*

The thoracic and abdominopelvic cavities are separated by a broad muscle called the **diaphragm.** The dia-

phragm forms the floor of the thoracic cavity. Divisions of the thoracic cavity are the pleural sacs, each containing a lung, with the mediastinum between them. Within the mediastinum lie the heart, the thymus gland, and part of the esophagus and trachea. The heart is surrounded by another cavity called the *pericardial sac.*

The *retroperitoneal space* lies on the posterior abdominal wall behind the parietal peritoneum. It extends from the twelfth thoracic vertebra and the twelfth rib to the sacrum and the iliac crests.

THE ABDOMINAL CAVITY

The abdominal cavity is the upper portion of the abdominopelvic cavity, excluding the retroperitoneum and the pelvis. It is bounded superiorly by the diaphragm; anteriorly by the abdominal wall muscles; posteriorly by the vertebral column, ribs, and iliac fossa; and inferiorly by the pelvis. The abdominal cavity contains the stomach, small intestine, much of the large intestine, liver, pancreas, gallbladder, spleen, kidneys, and ureters.

Abdominal Viscera

The visceral organs within the abdominal cavity include the liver, gallbladder, spleen, pancreas, kidneys, stomach, small intestine, and part of the large intestine (Figure 7-5). Throughout the ultrasound examination, the sonographer will observe respiratory and positional variations in the abdominal viscera as they occur from patient to patient.

Liver. The liver lies posterior to the lower ribs, with most of the right lobe in the right hypochondrium and epigastrium; the left lobe lies in the epigastrium/left hypochondrium.

Gallbladder. The fundus of the gallbladder usually lies opposite the tip of the right ninth costal cartilage.

Spleen. The spleen lies in the left hypochondrium under cover of the ninth, tenth, and eleventh ribs. Its long axis corresponds to the tenth rib, and in adults it usually does not project forward of the midaxillary line.

Pancreas. The pancreas lies in the epigastrium. The head usually lies below and to the right, the neck lies on the transpyloric plane, and the body and tail lie above and to the left.

Kidneys. The right kidney lies slightly lower than the left. Each kidney moves about 1 inch in a vertical direction during full respiratory movement of the diaphragm. The hilus of the kidney lies on the transpyloric plane, about three fingerwidths from the midline.

Aorta and Inferior Vena Cava. The aorta lies anterior to the spine, slightly to the left of the midline in the abdomen. It bifurcates into the right and left common iliac arteries opposite the fourth lumbar vertebra on the intercristal plane. The inferior vena cava is formed by the confluence of the right and left common iliac veins. The inferior vena cava lies to the right of the spine.

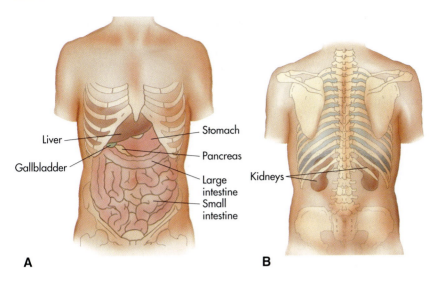

FIGURE 7-5 A, Basic abdominal landmarks and viscera viewed from anterior. **B,** Landmarks of the posterior torso.

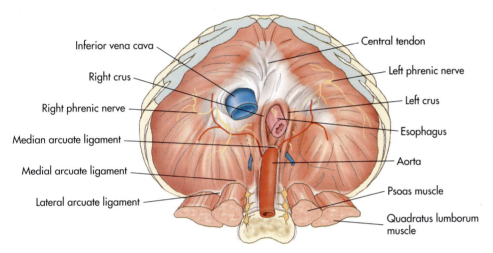

FIGURE 7-6 Inferior view of the diaphragm.

Stomach. The stomach lies in the transpyloric plane between the esophagus and the small intestine.

Small Intestine. This tubular organ extends from the pyloric sphincter to the beginning of the large intestine.

Large Intestine. The large intestine extends from the small intestine to the anal canal.

Bladder and Uterus. The bladder and uterus lie in the lower pelvis in the hypogastric plane.

Other Abdominal Structures

Diaphragm. The diaphragm is a dome-shaped muscle that separates the thorax from the abdominal cavity (Figures 7-4 through 7-6). Its muscular component arises from the margins of the thoracic outlet. The **right crus of the diaphragm** arises from the sides of the bodies of the first three lumbar vertebrae; the **left crus of the diaphragm** arises from the sides of the bodies of the first two lumbar vertebrae.

Lateral to the crura, the diaphragm arises from the medial and lateral arcuate ligaments. The **medial arcuate ligament** is the thickened upper margin of the fascia covering the anterior surface of the psoas muscle. It extends from the side of the body of the second lumbar vertebra to the tip of the transverse process of the first lumbar vertebra. The medial arcuate ligament connects the medial borders of the two crura as they cross anterior to the aorta.

The **lateral arcuate ligament** is the thickened upper margin of the fascia covering the anterior surface of the quadratus lumborum muscle. It extends from the tip of the transverse process of the first lumbar vertebra to the lower border of the twelfth rib.

The diaphragm inserts into a central tendon. The superior surface of the tendon is partially fused with the inferior surface of the fibrous pericardium. Fibers of the right crus surround the esophagus to act as a sphincter to prevent regurgitation of gastric contents into the thoracic part of the esophagus.

Abdominal Wall. Superiorly, the abdominal wall is formed by the diaphragm. Inferiorly, it is continuous with the pelvic cavity through the pelvic inlet. Anteriorly, the wall is formed above by the lower part of the thoracic

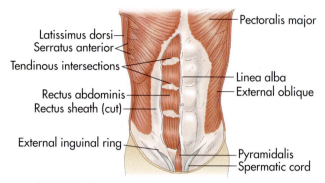

FIGURE 7-7 Anterior view of the abdominal muscles.

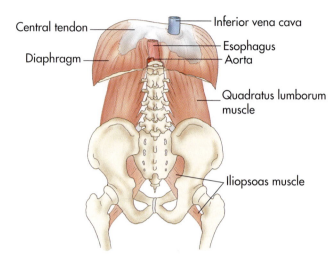

FIGURE 7-8 Posterior view of the diaphragm and abdominal muscles.

cage and below by several layers of muscles: rectus abdominis, external oblique, internal oblique, and transversus abdominis (Figure 7-7). The **linea alba** is a fibrous band that stretches from the xiphoid to the symphysis pubis. It is wider at its superior end and forms a central anterior attachment for the muscle layers of the abdomen. It is formed by the interlacing of fibers of the aponeuroses of the right and left oblique and transversus abdominis muscles.

Posteriorly, the abdominal wall is formed at the midline by five lumbar vertebrae and their disks (Figure 7-8). Posterolaterally, it is formed by the twelfth ribs, upper part of the bony pelvis, psoas muscles, quadratus lumborum muscles, and aponeuroses of the origin of the transversus abdominis muscles.

Laterally, the wall is formed above by the lower part of the thoracic wall, including the lungs and pleura, and below by the external and internal oblique muscles and the transversus abdominis muscles.

Abdominal Muscles

External Oblique Muscle. The external oblique muscle arises from the lower eight ribs and fans out to be inserted into the xiphoid process, the linea alba, the pubic crest, the pubic tubercle, and the anterior half of the iliac crest (Figure 7-9, *A*).

The **superficial inguinal ring** is a triangular opening in the external oblique aponeurosis and lies superior and medial to the pubic tubercle. The spermatic cord or the round ligament of the uterus passes through this opening.

The **inguinal ligament** is formed between the anterior superior iliac spine and the pubic tubercle, where the lower border of the aponeurosis is folded backward on itself. The lateral part of the posterior edge of the inguinal ligament gives origin to part of the internal oblique and transverse abdominal muscles.

Internal Oblique Muscle. The internal oblique muscle lies very deep to the external oblique muscle (Figure 7-9, *B*). Most of its fibers are aligned at right angles to the external oblique muscle. It arises from the lumbar fascia, the anterior two thirds of the iliac crest, and the lateral two thirds of the inguinal ligament. The muscle inserts

into the lower borders of the ribs and their costal cartilages, the xiphoid process, the linea alba, and the pubic symphysis. The internal oblique has a lower free border that arches over the spermatic cord or the round ligament of the uterus and then descends behind it to be attached to the pubic crest and the pectineal line. The lowest tendinous fibers are joined by similar fibers from the transversus abdominis to form the conjoint tendon.

Transversus Muscle. The transversus muscle lies deep to the internal oblique muscle, and its fibers run horizontally forward (Figure 7-9, *C*). The muscle arises from the deep surface of the lower six costal cartilages (interlacing with the diaphragm), the lumbar fascia, the anterior two thirds of the iliac crest, and the lateral third of the inguinal ligament. It inserts into the xiphoid process, the linea alba, and the pubic symphysis.

Rectus Sheath. The **rectus abdominis muscle** is a sheath formed by the aponeuroses of the muscles of the lateral group (Figure 7-10). The rectus muscle arises from the front of the symphysis pubis and from the pubic crest. It inserts into the fifth, sixth, and seventh costal cartilages and the xiphoid process. On contraction, the lateral margin forms a palpable curved surface, termed the **linea semilunaris,** which extends from the ninth costal cartilage to the pubic tubercle. The anterior surface of the rectus muscle is crossed by three tendinous intersections and is firmly attached to the anterior wall of the rectus sheath.

Linea Alba. The linea alba is a fibrous band stretching from the xiphoid to the symphysis pubis (see Figure 7-7). It is wider above than below and forms a central anterior attachment for the muscle layers of the abdomen. It is formed by the interlacing of the aponeuroses of the right and left oblique muscles and transversus abdominis muscles.

Back Muscles. The deep muscles of the back help to stabilize the vertebral column. They also influence the

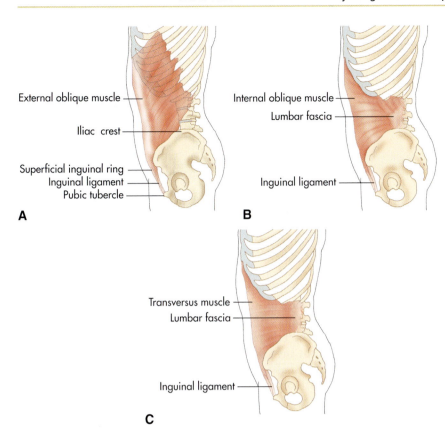

A

B

FIGURE 7-9 A, External oblique muscle of the anterior and lateral abdominal wall. **B,** Internal oblique muscle of the anterior and lateral abdominal wall. **C,** Transversus muscle of the anterior and lateral abdominal wall.

C

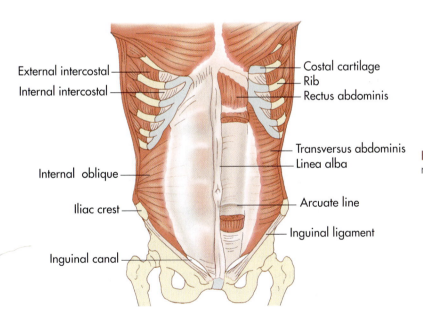

FIGURE 7-10 Anterior view of the rectus abdominis muscle and rectus sheath.

posture and curvature of the spine. These muscles have the ability to extend, flex laterally, and rotate all or part of the vertebral column.

THE RETROPERITONEUM

The retroperitoneal cavity contains the kidneys, ureters, adrenal glands, pancreas, aorta, inferior vena cava, bladder, uterus, and prostate gland. The ascending and descending colon and most of the duodenum are also located in the retroperitoneum.

Retroperitoneal Spaces

The **anterior pararenal space** (Figure 7-11) is located between the anterior surface of the renal fascia (Gerota's fascia) and the posterior area of the peritoneum. Within this area are the ascending and descending colon, the

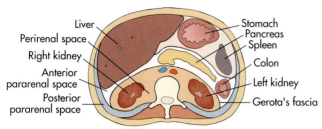

FIGURE 7-11 Transverse view of the retroperitoneum.

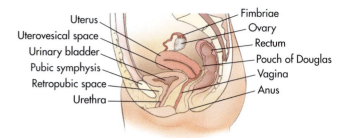

FIGURE 7-12 Midsagittal view of the female pelvis.

pancreas, and the duodenum. The **posterior pararenal space** is found between the posterior renal fascia and the muscles of the posterior abdominal wall. Only fat and vessels are found within this space. The **perirenal space** is located directly around the kidney and is completely enclosed by renal fascia. Within this space lie the kidneys, adrenal glands, lymph nodes, blood vessels, and perirenal fat.

THE PELVIC CAVITY

The lower portion of the abdominopelvic cavity is the **pelvic cavity** (see Figure 7-4). The pelvis is divided into a pelvis major (false pelvis) and a pelvis minor (true pelvis). The pelvis major is part of the abdominal cavity proper and lies between the iliac fossae, superior to the pelvic brim. The pelvis minor (which actually contains the pelvic cavity) is found inferior to the brim of the pelvis. The cavity of the pelvis minor is continuous at the pelvic brim with the cavity of the pelvis major.

The pelvic cavity contains several pelvic organs: part of the large intestine, the rectum, the urinary bladder, and the reproductive organs. In the female, the peritoneum descends from the anterior abdominal wall to the level of the pubic bone onto the superior surface of the bladder. The peritoneum covers the fundus and body of the uterus and extends over the posterior fornix and the wall of the vagina.

In the male, the peritoneum is reflected onto the upper part of the posterior surface of the bladder and the seminal vesicles, forming the rectovesical pouch. Also in the male, the pelvic cavity has a small outpocket called the **scrotal cavity,** which contains the testes.

False Pelvis

The false pelvis is bound posteriorly by the lumbar vertebrae, laterally by the iliac fossae and iliacus muscles, and anteriorly by the lower anterior abdominal wall. The sacral promontory and the iliopectineal line form the boundary between the false pelvis and the true pelvis to delineate the boundary of the abdominal and pelvic cavities.

The uterus lies anterior to the rectum and posterior to the bladder and divides the pelvic peritoneal space

into anterior and posterior pouches. The anterior pouch is termed the **vesicouterine pouch,** and the posterior pouch is called the **rectouterine pouch,** or the pouch of Douglas (Figure 7-12). The rectouterine pouch is a common location for accumulation of fluids, such as pus or blood.

The fallopian tubes extend laterally from the fundus of the uterus and are enveloped by a fold of peritoneum known as the broad ligament. This ligament arises from the floor of the pelvis and contributes to the division of the peritoneal space into anterior and posterior pouches.

True Pelvis

The true pelvis protects and contains the lower parts of the intestinal and urinary tracts and the reproductive organs. The true pelvis has an inlet, outlet, and cavity and is bounded posteriorly by the sacrum and coccyx (Figure 7-13). The anterior and lateral margins are formed by the pubis, the ischium, and a small portion of the ilium. A muscular "sling" consisting of the coccygeus and levator ani muscles forms the inferior boundary of the true pelvis and separates it from the perineum.

The true pelvis is divided into anterior and posterior compartments. The anterior compartment contains the bladder and reproductive organs. The posterior compartment contains the posterior cul-de-sac, rectosigmoid muscle, perirectal fat, and presacral space.

The walls of the pelvis are formed by bones and ligaments, which are partially lined by muscles covered with fascia and parietal peritoneum. The pelvis has anterior, posterior, and lateral walls and an inferior floor. The obturator internus muscle lines the lateral pelvic wall. These muscles are symmetrically aligned along the lateral border of the pelvis with a concave medial border (see Figure 7-13).

The psoas and iliopsoas muscles lie along the posterior and lateral margins of the pelvis major (Figure 7-14). The fan-shaped iliacus muscles line the iliac fossae in the false pelvis. The psoas and iliacus muscles merge at their inferior portions to form the iliopsoas complex. The posterior border of the iliopsoas lies along the iliopectineal line and may be used as a separation landmark of the true pelvis from the false pelvis.

The piriformis muscles form the posterior pelvic wall (Figure 7-15). The pelvic floor stretches across the pelvis and divides it into the main pelvic cavity, which contains the pelvic viscera, and the perineum below. The levator ani muscles and pubococcygeus muscles form the pelvic diaphragm. The coccygeus muscles are rounded, concave muscles that lie more posterior than the obturator internus muscles.

Perineum. The pelvic diaphragm is formed by the levatores ani and coccygeus muscles. The perineum has the following surface relationships: The pubic symphysis is anterior; posterior is the tip of the coccyx; and lateral are the ischial tuberosities. The region is divided into two triangles formed by joining the ischial tuberosities with an imaginary line. The posterior triangle is the anal triangle, and the anterior triangle is the urogenital triangle.

ABDOMINOPELVIC MEMBRANES AND LIGAMENTS

Peritoneum

The peritoneum is a serous membrane lining the walls of the abdominal cavity and clothing the abdominal viscera (Figure 7-16). The peritoneum is formed by a single layer of cells called the **mesothelium,** which rests on a thin layer of connective tissue. If the mesothelium is damaged or removed in any area (such as in surgery), the danger is that two layers of peritoneum may adhere to each other and form an adhesion. This adhesion may interfere with the normal movements of the abdominal viscera.

The peritoneum is divided into two layers. The **parietal peritoneum** is the portion that lines the abdominal wall but does not cover a viscus; the **visceral peritoneum** is the portion that covers an organ (Figure 7-17). The **peritoneal cavity** is the potential space between the

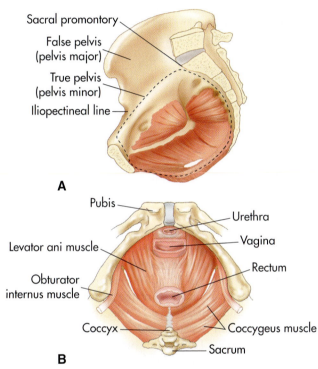

A

B

FIGURE 7-13 A, Lateral view of the pelvis, demonstrating the true pelvis and the false pelvis. **B,** Inferior view of the pelvic diaphragm muscles.

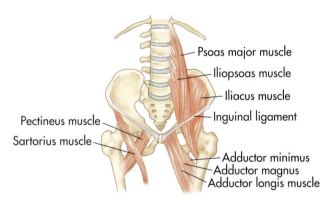

FIGURE 7-14 Anterior view of the psoas and iliopsoas muscles.

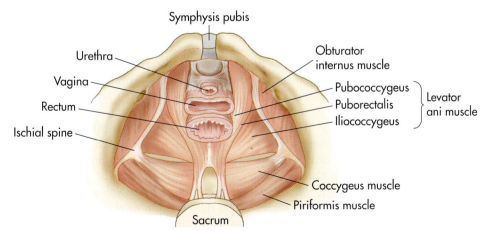

FIGURE 7-15 View of the female pelvic floor shows the levator ani, coccygeus, and piriformis muscles.

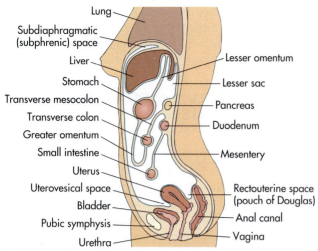

FIGURE 7-16 Lateral view of the peritoneum (*white area,* peritoneal cavity).

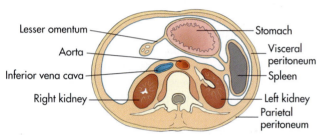

FIGURE 7-17 Axial view of the peritoneum (*white area,* peritoneal cavity).

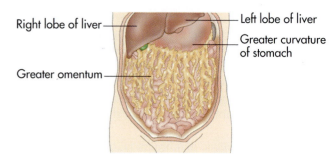

FIGURE 7-18 Anterior view of the greater omentum.

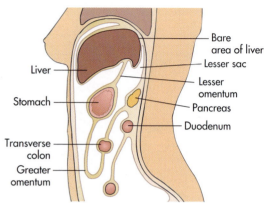

FIGURE 7-19 Sagittal view of the lesser omentum.

parietal and visceral peritonea. This cavity contains a small amount of lubricating serous fluid to help the abdominal organs move on one another without friction. With certain pathologies, the potential space of the peritoneal cavity may be distended into an actual space containing several liters of fluid. This accumulation of fluid is known as **ascites.** Other fluid substances, such as blood from a ruptured organ, bile from a ruptured duct, or fecal matter from a ruptured intestine, also may accumulate in this cavity.

The peritoneal cavity forms a completely closed sac in the male; in the female, communication with the exterior occurs through the fallopian tubes, uterus, and vagina.

Retroperitoneal organs and vascular structures remain posterior to the cavity and are covered anteriorly with peritoneum. These include the urinary system, aorta, inferior vena cava, colon, pancreas, uterus, and bladder. The other abdominal organs are located within the peritoneal cavity.

Mesentery

A mesentery is a two-layered fold of peritoneum that attaches part of the intestines to the posterior abdominal wall and includes the mesentery of the small intestine, the transverse mesocolon, and the sigmoid mesocolon.

Omentum

The omentum is a two-layered fold of peritoneum that attaches the stomach to another viscous organ. The **greater omentum** is attached to the greater curvature of the stomach and hangs down like an apron in the space between the small intestine and the anterior abdominal wall (Figure 7-18). The greater omentum is folded back on itself and is attached to the inferior border of the transverse colon. The **lesser omentum** slings the lesser curvature of the stomach to the undersurface of the liver (Figure 7-19). The gastrosplenic omentum ligament connects the stomach to the spleen.

Greater and Lesser Sacs

The peritoneal cavity may be divided into two parts known as the greater and lesser sacs. The **greater sac** is the primary compartment of the peritoneal cavity and extends across the anterior abdomen and from the diaphragm to the pelvis.

The **lesser sac** is an extensive peritoneal pouch located behind the lesser omentum and stomach (Figure 7-20). It extends upward to the diaphragm and inferior between the layers of the greater omentum. The left margin is formed by the spleen and the gastrosplenic and lienorenal ligaments. The right margin of the lesser sac opens into the greater sac through the epiploic foramen.

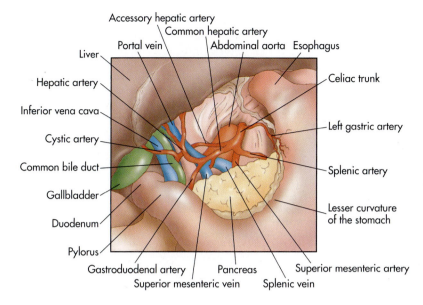

FIGURE 7-20 Upper abdominal dissection, with part of the left lobe of the liver and the lesser omentum removed to show the area of the epiploic foramen. Posterior to the foramen lie the celiac trunk, portal vein, bile duct, and related structures; this is one of the most important regions in the abdomen.

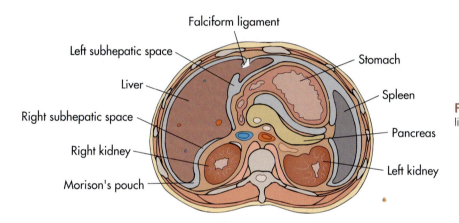

FIGURE 7-21 Transverse view of the falciform ligament.

Epiploic Foramen

The **epiploic foramen,** the opening to the lesser sac in the abdomen, includes the following boundaries: anteriorly, the free border of the lesser omentum containing the common bile duct, hepatic artery, and portal vein; posteriorly, the inferior vena cava; superiorly, the caudate process of the caudate lobe of the liver; and inferiorly, the first part of the duodenum (see Figure 7-20).

Ligament

The peritoneal ligaments are two-layered folds of peritoneum that attach the lesser mobile solid viscera to the abdominal walls. For example, the liver is attached by the **falciform ligament** to the anterior abdominal wall and to the undersurface of the diaphragm (Figure 7-21). The **ligamentum teres** lies in the free borders of this ligament. The peritoneum leaves the kidney and passes to the hilus of the spleen as the posterior layer of the **lienorenal ligament.** The visceral peritoneum covers the spleen and is reflected onto the greater curvature of the stomach as the anterior layer of the **gastrosplenic ligament.**

POTENTIAL SPACES IN THE BODY

Subphrenic Spaces

The subphrenic spaces are the result of the complicated arrangement of the peritoneum in the region of the liver (Figure 7-22). The right and left anterior subphrenic spaces lie between the diaphragm and the liver, one on each side of the falciform ligament. The sonographer should become very familiar with the right posterior subphrenic space that lies between the right lobe of the liver, the right kidney, and the right colic flexure. This is also called **Morison's pouch.** It is a frequent location for fluid collections, such as ascites, blood, and infection, to accumulate.

Peritoneal Recesses

The omental bursa normally has some empty places. Parts of the peritoneal cavity near the liver are so slitlike that they are also isolated. These areas, known as **peritoneal recesses,** are clinically important because infection may collect in them. Two common sites are where the

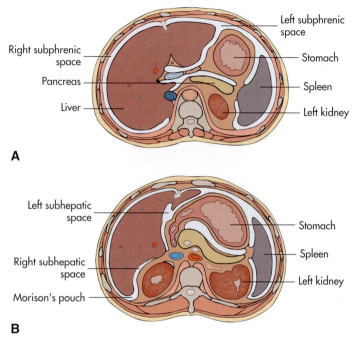

FIGURE 7-22 The supracolic compartment is located above the transverse colon and contains the right and left subphrenic spaces and the right and left subhepatic spaces. **A,** Transverse view of the subphrenic spaces. **B,** Transverse view of the subhepatic spaces.

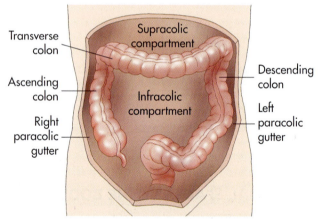

FIGURE 7-23 The infracolic compartment is found below the transverse colon. The right and left paracolic gutters are troughlike spaces located lateral to the ascending and descending colon.

duodenum becomes the jejunum and where the ileum joins the cecum.

Paracolic Gutters

The arrangement of the ascending and descending colon, the attachments of the transverse mesocolon, and the mesentery of the small intestine to the posterior abdominal wall result in the formation of four paracolic gutters (Figure 7-23). The clinical significance of these gutters is their ability to conduct fluid materials from one part of the body to another. Materials such as abscess, ascites, blood, pus, bile, or metastases may be spread through this network.

The gutters are on the lateral and medial sides of the ascending and descending colon. The right medial para-

colic gutter is closed off from the pelvic cavity inferiorly by the mesentery of the small intestine. The other gutters are in free communication with the pelvic cavity. The right lateral paracolic gutter communicates with the right posterior subphrenic space. The left lateral gutter is separated from the area around the spleen by the phrenicocolic ligament.

Inguinal Canal

The inguinal canal is an oblique passage through the lower part of the anterior abdominal wall. In the male, it allows structures to pass to and from the testes to the abdomen (Figure 7-24). In the female, it permits passage of the round ligament of the uterus from the uterus to the labium majus.

A hernia is the protrusion of part of the abdominal contents beyond the normal confines of the abdominal wall. It has the following three parts: the sac, the contents of the sac, and the coverings of the sac. The hernial sac is a diverticulum of the peritoneum and has a neck and a body. The hernial contents may consist of any structure found within the abdominal cavity and may vary from a small piece of omentum to a large viscous organ. The hernial coverings are formed from the layers of the abdominal wall through which the hernial sac passes. Abdominal hernias are classified into the following types: inguinal, femoral, umbilical, epigastric, and rectus abdominis.

PREFIXES AND SUFFIXES

The sonographer should be familiar with the prefixes and suffixes that are commonly used in medical terminology.

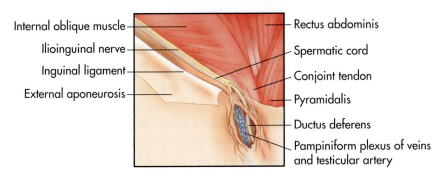

Internal oblique muscle
Ilioinguinal nerve
Inguinal ligament
External aponeurosis

Rectus abdominis
Spermatic cord
Conjoint tendon
Pyramidalis
Ductus deferens
Pampiniform plexus of veins and testicular artery

FIGURE 7-24 Right inguinal canal, spermatic cord, ductus deferens, and pampiniform plexus.

a-, an- without; away from; not

ab-, abs- from; away from; absent

ad- toward

adipo- fat

angio- blood or lymph vessels

antero- anterior; front, before

-ase enzyme

-asis, esis, iasis, -isis, -osis condition; pathologic state

-cele tumor, swelling

cephal- head

cran- helmet; *cranial:* pertaining to the portion of the skull that surrounds the brain

dextra- right

dors- back; *dorsal:* position toward the back of the body

-dynia pain

dys- difficult, bad; painful

-emia blood

end-, endo- within, inside

eryth- red

ex-, exo- out, outside of

hem-, hema-, hemato- blood

hepato- liver

homeo-, homo- same; *homeostasis:* maintenance of a stable internal environment

hydra-, hydro- hydr- water

hyp-, hyph-, hypo- less than; under

hyper- excessive

hyster- uterus

infra- below, under, beneath; inferior to; after

inter- between

intra- within

ipsi- same

-itis inflammation of

juxta- close proximity

lip-, lipo- fat

-lite, -lith, litho- stone, calculus

mega-, megalo- large, of great size

meio-, mio- less, smaller

mesio- toward the middle

meta- change; *metabolism:* chemical changes that occur within the body

necr-, necro- death; necrosis

neo- new

nephr-, nephra-, nephro- kidney

olig-, oligo- few; small

-ology study of; *physiology:* study of body functions

-oma tumor

omphal-, omphalo- navel

oophor- ovary

orchi- testicle

pariet- wall; *parietal membrane:* membrane that lines the wall of a cavity

pelv- basin; *pelvic cavity:* basin-shaped cavity enclosed by the pelvic bones

peri- around

pleur- rib; *pleural membrane:* membrane that encloses the lungs within the rib cage

-poiesis, -poietic production; formation

pre- before, in front of

pseudo- false

py-, pyo- pus

pyelo- pelvis

retro- backward, back, behind

-rhage, -rhagia rupture; profuse fluid discharge

sebo- fatty substance

-stasis standing still; *homeostasis:* maintenance of a relatively stable internal environment

sub- under; beneath

super-, supra- above; beyond; superior; on top

thrombo- blood clot; thrombus

-tomy cutting; *anatomy:* study of structure, which often involves cutting or removing body parts

trans- across, over; beyond; through

-trophin stimulation of a target organ by a substance, especially a hormone

-uria, urin- urine

vaso- vessel (blood vessel)

veno- vein

ventro-, ventr-, ventri- abdomen; anterior surface of the body

vesico- bladder; vesicle

xeno- strange, foreign

CHAPTER

8

Introduction to Abdominal Scanning: Techniques and Protocols

Sandra L. Hagen-Ansert

OBJECTIVES

On completion of this chapter, you should be able to:
- Name the scanning techniques used in abdominal scanning
- Describe how to properly label a sonogram
- List the criteria for identifying abnormalities
- Be familiar with terminology used to describe the results of ultrasound examinations
- List the criteria for an adequate scan
- Describe abdominal sectional anatomy in the transverse and longitudinal planes
- Describe the protocols included in this chapter for abdominal organs and soft tissue structures
- Describe the use of Doppler in the abdomen, including Doppler scanning techniques for abdominal vessels

OUTLINE

Before You Begin to Scan Patients
  Orientation to the Clinical Laboratory
  Scanning Techniques
  Patient Positions
  Transducer Selection
  Transducer Positions
  Initial Survey of the Abdomen
Labeling Scans and Patient Position
Criteria for an Adequate Scan
Indications for Abdominal Sonography

Medical Terms for the Sonographer
Identifying Abnormalities
Sectional Anatomy
  Transverse Plane
  Longitudinal Plane
General Abdominal Ultrasound Protocols
  Transverse Scans
  Longitudinal Scans
  Liver and Porta Hepatis Protocol
  Biliary System Protocol
  Pancreas Protocol

Spleen Protocol
Renal Protocol
Aorta and Iliac Artery Protocol
Thyroid Protocol
Parathyroid Protocol
Breast Protocol
Scrotal Protocol
Abdominal Doppler
  Doppler Scanning Techniques
  Aorta
  Inferior Vena Cava
  Portal Venous System
  Portal Hypertension

Scanning is an art that demands many talents of the sonographer: a high degree of manual dexterity and hand-eye coordination; the ability to conceptualize two-dimensional information into a three-dimensional format; and a thorough understanding of anatomy, physiology, pathology, instrumentation, artifact production, and transducer characteristics. Ultrasound equipment today is so sophisticated that producing quality images requires a greater understanding of the physical principles of sonography and computers than ever before. Moreover, sonographers should be able to incorporate Doppler techniques, color flow mapping, tissue harmonics, and three-dimensional imaging to provide an enhanced understanding of anatomy and physiology as it relates to hemodynamic blood flow and reconstruction.

Although one-on-one, hands-on training in a clinical setting is an essential part of the sonographer's experience of producing high-quality scans, this chapter will take you on a journey toward mastering the foundations of abdominal scanning. Because correlation of ultrasound images with sectional anatomy is critical for producing consistent, quality images, the chapter focuses on normal sectional anatomy and general abdominal ultrasound protocol. Specific organ protocol is discussed in the respective chapters. You may find the protocol for an abdominal scan to differ slightly between ultrasound departments; the key is to develop a protocol that is

132

Copyright © 2012, Elsevier Inc.

within the national practice guidelines and to maintain that protocol for all patients. The protocols presented here are generic and may be adapted to the particular laboratory situation. Also included in this chapter are special scanning techniques and specific applications of abdominal scanning.

BEFORE YOU BEGIN TO SCAN PATIENTS

Remember that your ultimate goal as a sonographer is to produce diagnostic images that can be interpreted by the physician to answer a clinical question. To create images that are diagnostically useful, you must be familiar with ultrasound instrumentation and the clinical considerations of the patient examination. Clinical considerations include knowing which patient position should be used for specific examinations, transducer selection and scanning techniques, patient breathing techniques, and how to perform a sonographic survey of the abdomen.

Be sure you are very familiar with various types of ultrasound equipment. Know where the operator's manual is and how to find what you need in the manual. (Every manufacturer places the power supply in a different position, so make sure you know how to turn the machine on and off!) Become familiar with the transducers available for each machine, how to activate the transducers, and how to change transducers; some of the plug-in formats take some practice to master. Know where the critical knobs are that operate the ultrasound instrumentation (e.g., time gain compensation [TGC], power, gain, depth, angle, focus, Doppler, color flow). Know where the annotate text keys are for labeling the image. If the ultrasound equipment is new to you, it may be a good idea for one sonographer to work the controls, while the other scans until you become adapted to the equipment.

It is highly recommended that the student sonographer practice in a supervised laboratory setting (away from patients) before beginning to work with patients. This way, the student sonographer can become familiar with the ultrasound equipment by scanning phantoms or even "building" his or her own phantoms to be scanned.

The next step should be for one student to scan the other students in the sonography laboratory. This allows the actual experience of feeling how "cold that gel really is" when applied to the abdomen and knowing what the probe feels like with different individual scan techniques. The student can see first hand how a *light* touch does not make as pretty an image as a moderate touch with the transducer adjacent to the skin and may experience the agony of the heavy hand as it scrapes across the rib cage. The student will also learn how much scanning gel is the right amount: If it drips down your wrist and onto your clothes, it is too much gel!

Controlled supervised scanning should also emphasize how important it is for the patient to take in a breath so the highest quality images are obtained. A recommended patient breathing technique tip is to have the patient inhale through the nose to reduce the amount of air going into the stomach. Breathing is probably the weakest learning link for the student. Careful control of respiration is critical for making a beautiful scan versus an image that is not easy to interpret.

The student sonographer should also begin to learn the specific protocols required for each examination. The protocols outlined in this chapter have been used in many laboratories across the country. You may also find nationally recognized protocols developed by the American College of Radiology (ACR) and the American Institute of Ultrasound in Medicine (AIUM) for ultrasound examinations. Likewise, the American College of OB/GYN has developed guidelines for the female patient, and the American Society of Echocardiography has developed guidelines for echocardiography. The Society for Vascular Ultrasound has established its guidelines for vascular examinations. Each of these protocols can be found on the websites of the respective organizations.

Of course, students will not completely remember all the protocols when they first begin their clinical scanning experience. Suggested building steps to help the student master the protocols are included in the workbook that accompanies this textbook.

Orientation to the Clinical Laboratory

When you arrive in the clinical ultrasound laboratory, take a few days to become familiar with the particular ultrasound department. The following points may make your entrance into the clinical world a little smoother:

- Learn the ultrasound equipment in your department. This means that every free minute should be spent with the equipment, finding the working knobs necessary to perform the examination.
- Know where the operator's manuals are for each piece of equipment so you may have a reference for troubleshooting.
- Find out what protocols are used for each examination. Most departments have a "book of protocols" for all their examinations.
- Understand how to read the patient request, find out what question the ordering physician needs to have answered, and know which items are relevant for patient identification.
- When you call for patients, be sure to check their ID bracelet, or ask them to say their name and birth date.
- Introduce yourself and explain briefly the procedure you are going to do. Also explain the procedure the department will follow to notify the patient's physician of the results of the examination.
- Keep your conversation professional.
- Discuss the case only with your mentor or with the physician responsible for interpreting the study.

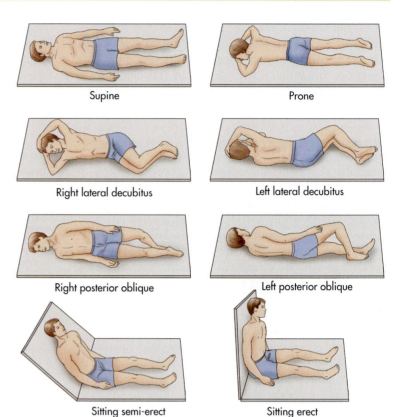

FIGURE 8-1 Various standard patient positions for the ultrasound examination.

Scanning Techniques

Ultrasound can distinguish multiple interfaces between soft tissue structures of different acoustic densities. The strength of the echoes reflected depends on the acoustic interface and the angle at which the sound beam strikes the interface. The sonographer must determine which patient "window" is best to record optimal ultrasound images, and which transducer size best fits into that window. The curved array transducer provides a large field of view but in some patients may be difficult to fit closely between the ribs to provide adequate contact for accurate reflection of the sound wave. The smaller foot-print transducer allows the sonographer to scan between intercostal spaces with the patient in a supine, coronal, decubitus, or upright position but limits the near field of view. It is not unusual to use multiple transducers on one patient to complete the examination, as transducers are available in multiple sizes and frequencies.

Patient Positions

The typical abdominal examination is done primarily in the supine position. However, the oblique, lateral decubitus, upright, and prone positions have also been used for examination of specific areas of interest (Figure 8-1). These positions will be discussed in the specific protocols.

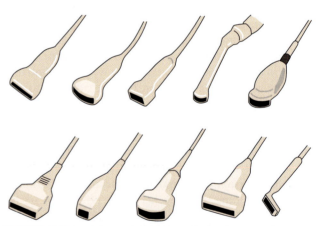

FIGURE 8-2 Transducer designs in multiple shapes and sizes are used for specific ultrasound examinations.

Transducer Selection

Know the types of transducers available for each piece of ultrasound equipment, and be familiar with which transducers are used for specific examinations (Figure 8-2). The size of the patient will influence what megahertz transducer will be used. If the transvaginal transducer is used, be familiar with the decontamination process for the transducer.

Perpendicular
The transducer is straight up and down.

Subcostal
The transducer is angled superiorly just beneath the inferior costal margin.

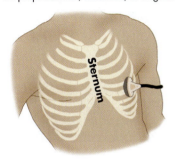

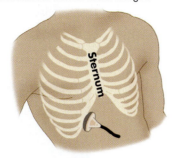

Intercostal
The transducer is between the ribs. It can be perpendicular, subcostal, or angled.

Angled
The transducer is angled superiorly, inferiorly, or right and left laterally at varying degrees.

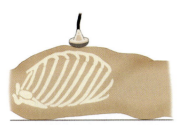

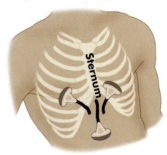

FIGURE 8-3 The sonographer must use a number of different transducer positions and angulations to complete the ultrasound examination.

Rotated
The transducer is rotated varying degrees to oblique the scanning plane.

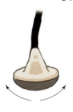

Transducer Positions

The sonographer will use multiple wrist actions throughout the study. Remember that the beam is ideally reflected when the transducer is perpendicular to the surface. However, the body has many angles, curves, and rib interferences, causing the sonographer to use intercostal spaces, subcostal windows, multiple degrees of angulation, and many rotations of the transducer to obtain anatomic images (Figure 8-3).

Initial Survey of the Abdomen

Before you begin the protocol for the specific examination, take a minute to survey the area in question. This will give you an opportunity to see how the patient images appear with "routine" instrument settings, to observe where the organs are in relationship to the patient's respiration pattern, and to see if the patient has a good "scanning window" in the supine position, or if the patient position needs to be moved into a decubitus or upright position. In a general abdominal survey, ask the patient to take in a deep breath; begin at the level of the xiphoid in the midline with the transducer angled steeply toward the patient's head, so as to be perpendicular to the diaphragm (Figure 8-4). Slowly angle the transducer inferiorly to "sweep" through the liver, gallbladder, head of pancreas, and right kidney. The transducer may then be redirected in the same manner, only angled toward the left shoulder with a gradual angulation made inferiorly, to see the stomach, spleen, pancreas, and left kidney. Likewise, a quick survey of the abdomen may be done with the transducer in the midline sagittal position (Figure 8-5). Remember to ask the patient to take in a breath and hold it in. Image the aorta first with the vertebral column posterior to the aorta. Then slowly angle the transducer to the right to image the dilated inferior vena cava and liver. Continue to angle toward the right to image the right lobe of the liver, gallbladder, and right kidney. If adequate penetration is seen with balanced TGC and overall gain adjustments, then you can proceed with the routine protocol for the abdominal study as provided later in this chapter.

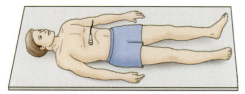

FIGURE 8-4 Most abdominal ultrasound examinations are performed initially in the supine position. The curved array probe is shown in the transverse position.

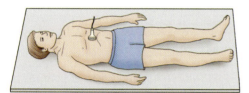

FIGURE 8-5 Longitudinal scan. The probe has now been rotated to the midline sagittal position.

LABELING SCANS AND PATIENT POSITION

Ultrasound images are labeled as *transverse* or *longitudinal* for a specific organ, such as the liver, gallbladder, pancreas, spleen, or uterus. The smaller organs that can be imaged on a single plane, such as the kidney, are labeled as *long-midline, -lateral,* or *-medial,* whereas the transverse scans are labeled as *transverse-low, -middle,* or *-high.*

All transverse supine scans are oriented with the liver on the left of the monitor; this means that the sonographer will be viewing the body from the feet up to the head ("optimistic view") (Figure 8-6). Longitudinal scans display the patient's head to the left and feet to the right of the screen and use the xiphoid, umbilicus, or symphysis to denote the midline of the scan plane (Figure 8-7).

All scans should be appropriately labeled for future reference, including the patient's name, date, and anatomic position. Body position markers are available on many ultrasound machines and may be used in the place of written labels.

The position of the patient should be described in relation to the scanning table (e.g., a right decubitus would mean the right side down; a left decubitus would indicate the left side down). If the scanning plane is oblique, the sonographer should merely state that it is an oblique view without specifying the exact degree of obliquity.

CRITERIA FOR AN ADEQUATE SCAN

With the use of real-time ultrasound, it is sometimes difficult to become oriented to all of the anatomic structures on a single image. It is therefore critical to obtain

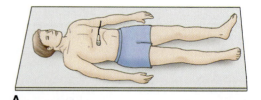

A

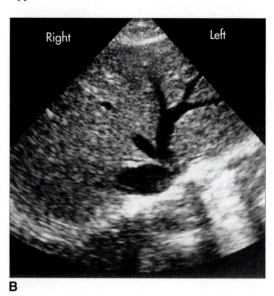

B

FIGURE 8-6 **A,** The curved array probe is held in a transverse position just under the costal margin with a steep angulation to be perpendicular to the dome of the liver. Patient is supine. **B,** All transverse supine scans are oriented as looking up from the feet, with the liver on the left side of the screen (right side of the patient is on the left of the screen).

as many landmarks of the anatomy as possible in a single image.

Make every effort to avoid rib interference to eliminate artifactual ring-down, attenuation, or reverberation noise that may distort anatomic information. As said previously, the small-footprint transducer allows the sonographer to scan in between the ribs but limits near-field visualization. Variations in the patient's respirations may also help eliminate rib interference and improve image quality. The sonographer can easily watch in real-time how much interference is caused by patient breathing and can ask the patient to take in a breath and hold it, or to stop breathing at critical points to capture particular parts of the anatomy. Watching the image form in real-time lets the sonographer see what effect respiration will have on the image.

Patients should be instructed not to eat or drink anything for 6 to 8 hours before the abdominal ultrasound procedure. This will enable the gallbladder to be distended and will prevent unnecessary bowel gas that may interfere with visualization of the smaller abdominal and vascular structures. If the left upper quadrant is not adequately imaged, the patient may be given water in an effort to fill the stomach. As the patient is rolled into a right decubitus position, the fluid flows from the body

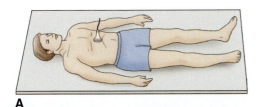

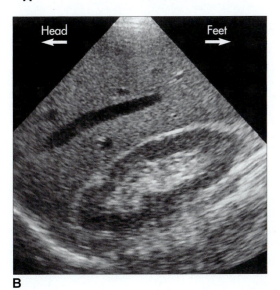

FIGURE 8-7 A, The curved array probe has been rotated 180 degrees to perform a sagittal scan of the abdomen. **B,** The longitudinal scans for the abdomen and pelvis are oriented with the patient's head toward the left of the screen and feet toward the right.

of the stomach to fill the antrum and duodenum, allowing the pancreas and great vessels to be imaged.

INDICATIONS FOR ABDOMINAL SONOGRAPHY

Multiple indications for an abdominal sonogram include, but are not limited to, the following:

- Signs or symptoms that may be referred from the abdominal and/or retroperitoneal region such as jaundice or hematuria
- Generalized abdominal, flank, or back pain
- Palpable mass or organomegaly
- Abnormal laboratory values or abnormal findings on other imaging modalities
- Follow-up of known or suspected abnormalities in the abdomen or retroperitoneum
- Search for metastatic disease or occult primary neoplasm
- Evaluation of suspected congenital abnormalities
- Trauma to the abdomen or retroperitoneum
- Pretransplant and posttransplant evaluation
- Invasive procedure localization
- Localization for free or loculated peritoneal, pleural, or retroperitoneal fluid

The request for an abdominal or retroperitoneal sonographic examination needs to provide sufficient information to demonstrate the medical necessity of the examination with allowance for proper performance and interpretation.

The documentation that must be met for medical necessity includes the following items: (1) patient signs and symptoms, and (2) previous history pertinent to the examination requested. Additional information such as the specific reason for the examination or a provisional diagnosis would be helpful and may aid in the proper performance and interpretation of the examination. This will allow the sonographer to tailor the examination to answer the question from the ordering physician.

MEDICAL TERMS FOR THE SONOGRAPHER

The sonographer is responsible for reviewing the patient's request for the ultrasound examination and for discussing any specific requests with the referring physician. Therefore, a familiarity with basic medical terminology and abbreviations is necessary. Common medical and ultrasound abbreviations are listed on the inside covers of this book for quick reference.

One of the sonographer's primary responsibilities is the identification and description of normal and abnormal anatomy. The following list of terms is universally accepted and will help the sonographer describe the results obtained from various ultrasound examinations:

anechoic or sonolucent: opposite of echogenic; without internal echoes; the structure is fluid-filled and transmits sound easily (Figure 8-8, *A*). Examples include vascular structures, distended urinary bladder, gallbladder, and amniotic cavity.

echogenic or hyperechoic: opposite of anechoic; echo-producing structure; reflects sound with a brighter intensity (Figure 8-8, *B*). Examples include gallstone, renal calyx, bone, fat, fissures, and ligaments.

enhancement, increased through-transmission: sound that travels through an anechoic (fluid-filled) substance and is not attenuated; brightness is increased directly beyond the posterior border of the anechoic structure as compared with the surrounding area—this is "enhancement" (see Figure 8-8, *A*).

fluid-fluid level: interface between two fluids with different acoustic characteristics; this level will change with patient position. An example is a dermoid with fluid level.

heterogeneous: not uniform in texture or composition (Figure 8-8, *C*). Example: Many tumors have characteristics of both decreased and increased echogenicity.

homogeneous: opposite of heterogeneous; completely uniform in texture or composition (Figure 8-8, *D*).

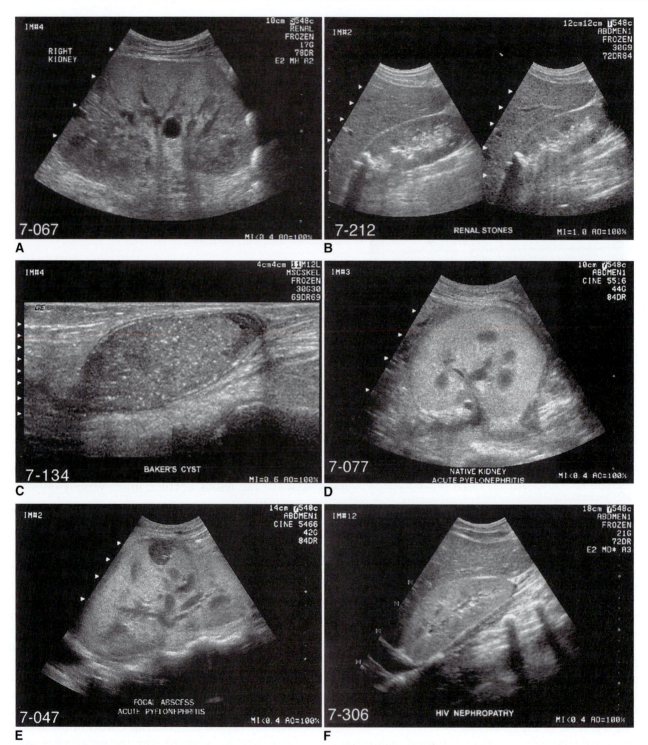

FIGURE 8-8 **A,** Anechoic (simple cyst). **B,** Echogenic (stone with shadowing). **C,** Heterogeneous (Baker cyst with mixture of fluid, debris, and bright echo reflectors). **D,** Homogeneous (renal parenchyma). **E,** Hypoechoic (hemorrhagic cyst). **F,** Infiltrating (HIV systemic disease process involving the kidney).

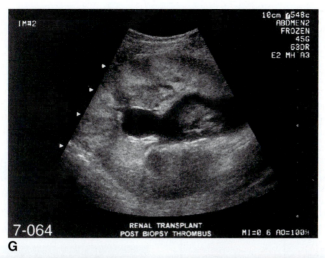

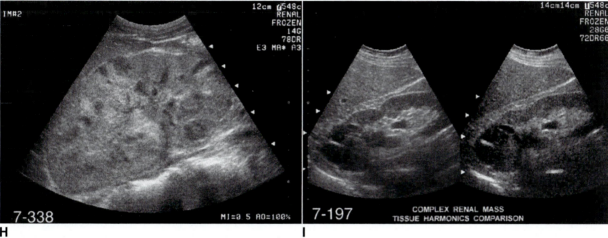

FIGURE 8-8, cont'd G, Irregular borders (thrombus within the renal pelvis). **H,** Isoechoic (one half of renal parenchyma has lower level echoes). **I,** Loculated (complex renal mass with septations).

Example: The textures of the liver, thyroid, testes, and myometrium are generally considered homogeneous.

hypoechoic: low-level echoes within a structure (Figure 8-8, *E*). An example is lymph nodes and the gastro-intestinal tract.

infiltrating: usually refers to a diffuse disease process or metastatic disease (Figure 8-8, *F*)

irregular borders: Borders are not well defined, are ill defined, or are not present (Figure 8-8, *G*). Examples include abscess, thrombus, and metastases.

isoechoic: very close to the normal parenchyma echogenicity pattern (Figure 8-8, *H*). An example is meta-static disease.

loculated mass: well-defined borders with internal echoes; the septa may be thin (likely benign) or thick (likely malignant) (Figure 8-8, *I*).

shadowing: The sound beam is attenuated by a solid or calcified object. This reflection or absorption may be partial or complete; air bubbles in the duodenum may cause a "dirty shadow" to occur secondary to reflection; a stone would cause a sharp shadow posterior to its border (see Figure 8-8, *B*).

IDENTIFYING ABNORMALITIES

Careful evaluation for the presence of pathology is incorporated into the general abdominal protocol. The sonographer needs to be able to demonstrate the normal anatomic structures, as well as the pathology that may invade or surround such structures. The abnormality is identified and evaluated according to a number of criteria (Figure 8-9), which are listed in Box 8-1.

Pathology may be further identified by the internal composition as cystic, complex, or solid (Box 8-2). This is determined by how easily the sound is able to transmit through the mass. Transmission is altered depending on what the mass is composed of pathologically. Throughout the chapters of this text, gross pathologic specimens will be included to provide the sonographer with a better understanding of these principles.

SECTIONAL ANATOMY

The sonographer must have a solid knowledge of gross and sectional anatomy and of the many anatomic variations that may occur in the body. The sonographer

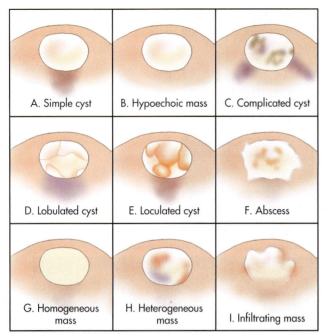

FIGURE 8-9 Ultrasound criteria for describing a mass. **A,** Simple cyst: smooth borders, anechoic, increased transmission. **B,** Hyopechoic mass: few to low-level internal echoes, smooth border, no increased transmission. **C,** Complicated cyst: mixed pattern of cystic and solid, fluid, debris, and blood; transmission may or may not increase. **D,** Lobulated cyst: well-defined with thin septa, increased transmission. **E,** Loculated cyst: well defined with thick septa. **F,** Abscess: may have irregular borders, debris within, transmission may or may not be increased. **G,** Homogeneous mass: uniform texture within. **H,** Heterogeneous mass: nonuniform texture within. **I,** Infiltrating mass: distorted architecture, irregular borders, decreased transmission.

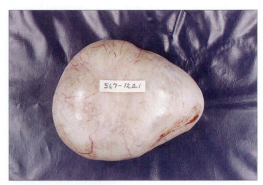

FIGURE 8-10 Gross pathology of a simple ovarian cyst showing well-defined smooth borders; straw-colored fluid was found inside the mass.

BOX 8-2	Abnormal Structures That Affect Transmission
Cyst	A cyst has smooth, well-defined borders, anechoic, increased through-transmission (Figure 8-10).
Complex	Has characteristics of both a cyst and a solid structure (Figure 8-11).
Solid	Irregular borders, internal echoes, decreased through-transmission (see Figure 8-11).

BOX 8-1	Ultrasound Criteria for Identifying Abnormal Structures
Border	Border of the structure may be smooth and well defined, or irregular.
Texture	Texture (parenchyma) of the structure may be homogeneous or heterogeneous.
Characteristic	Characteristic of an organ or of a mass is said to be anechoic, hypoechoic, isoechoic, hyperechoic, or echogenic to the rest of the parenchyma.
Transmission	Transmission of sound may be increased, decreased, or unchanged. An anechoic mass (fluid-filled cyst) will show increased transmission of sound, whereas a dermoid tumor (composed of muscle, teeth, and bone) will show decreased transmission.

should carefully evaluate organ and vascular relationships to neighboring structures, rather than memorize where in the abdomen a particular structure "should" be: It is better to recall the location of the gallbladder as anterior to the right kidney and medial to the liver than to remember that it is found 6 cm above the umbilicus.

Transverse Plane

The transverse sectional illustrations (Figures 8-12 through 8-26) are presented in descending order from the dome of the diaphragm to the symphysis pubis. The sonographer should review the relationship of each organ to its neighboring structures, while proceeding in a caudal direction. Specific detail is listed below each illustration, and a thumbnail sketch of expected anatomy is outlined below:

Dome of the liver (Figure 8-12): The **splenic artery (SA)** enters as the **splenic vein (SV)** leaves the splenic hilum. The abdominal portion of the esophagus lies to the left of the midline and opens into the stomach through the cardiac orifice. The liver extends to the left mammillary line. The **falciform ligament (FL)** extends into the diaphragm.

Level of the caudate lobe (Figure 8-13): The right **hepatic vein** enters the lateral margin of the **inferior vena cava (IVC)**. The fundus of the stomach is shown with the hepatogastric and gastrocolic ligaments. The lesser omental cavity is posterior to the stomach. The upper border of the splenic flexure of the colon is seen. The **caudate lobe** of the liver is anterior to the IVC and is demarcated by the **ligamentum venosum (LV)**. The body and tail of the pancreas are seen near the splenic hilum. The adrenal glands are lateral to the **crus of the diaphragm.**

Level of the caudate lobe and celiac axis (CA) (Figure 8-14): The **celiac axis (CA)** (branches into **left gastric**

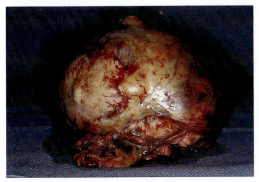

FIGURE 8-11 Gross pathology of a solid ovarian mass with irregular borders; the mass was filled with complex tissue.

artery [LGA], splenic artery, and **hepatic artery**) should be found near this section as it arises from the anterior wall of the **aorta (Ao)**. The transverse and descending colons are shown inferior to the splenic flexure. The caudate lobe of the liver is shown. The body of the pancreas is anterior to the splenic vein. Both kidneys and the adrenal glands are shown lateral to the spine and crus of the diaphragm. The IVC is shown anterior to the crus, and the aorta is posterior to the crus of the diaphragm.

Level of the superior mesenteric artery and pancreas (Figure 8-15): The **psoas major muscles** are lateral to

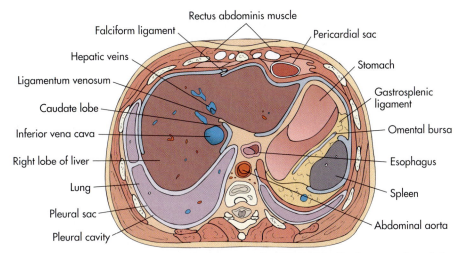

FIGURE 8-12 Cross section of the abdomen at the level of the tenth intervertebral disk. The lower portion of the pericardial sac is seen. The splenic artery enters the spleen, and the splenic vein emerges from the splenic hilum. The abdominal portion of the esophagus lies to the left of the midline and opens into the stomach through the cardiac orifice. The liver extends to the left mammillary line. The falciform ligament extends into the section above this. The spleen is shown to lie alongside the ninth rib.

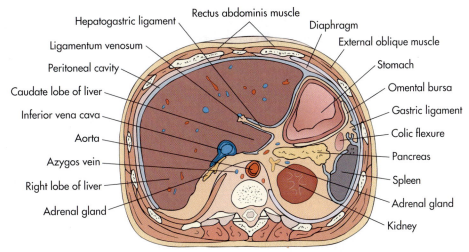

FIGURE 8-13 Cross section of the abdomen at the level of the eleventh thoracic disk. The hepatic vein is shown to enter the inferior vena cava. The renal artery and the vein of the left kidney are shown. The left branch of the portal vein is seen to arch upward to enter the left lobe of the liver. The upper part of the stomach is shown with the hepatogastric and gastrocolic ligaments. The lesser omental cavity is posterior to the stomach. The upper border of the splenic flexure of the colon is seen. The caudate lobe of the liver is in this section. The tail and body of the pancreas are shown anterior to the left kidney. The spleen is shown to lie along the left lateral border. The adrenal glands are lateral to the crus of the diaphragm.

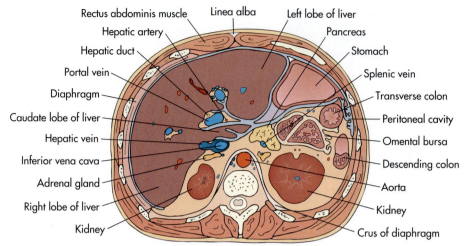

FIGURE 8-14 Cross section of the abdomen at the level of the twelfth thoracic vertebra. The celiac axis arises in the middle of this section from the anterior abdominal aorta. The right renal artery originates at this level. The hepatic vein is shown to enter the inferior vena cava. The greater curvature of the stomach and the pylorus are shown. The transverse and descending colon are shown inferior to the splenic flexure. The caudate lobe of the liver is well seen. The body of the pancreas, both kidneys, and the lower portions of the adrenal glands are shown.

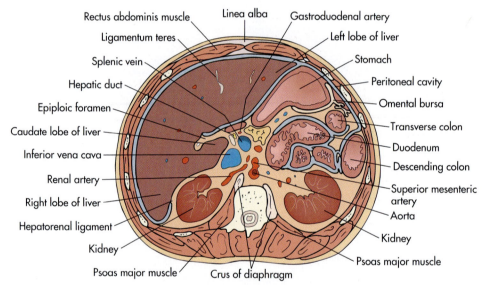

FIGURE 8-15 Cross section of the abdomen at the first lumbar vertebra. The psoas major muscle is seen. The crura of the diaphragm are shown on either side of the spine. The right renal artery is seen. The left renal artery arises from the lateral wall of the aorta. Both renal veins enter the inferior vena cava. The portal vein is seen to be formed by the union of the splenic vein and the superior mesenteric vein. The lower portions of the stomach and the pyloric orifice are seen, as is the superior portion of the duodenum. The duodenojejunal flexure and the descending and transverse colon are shown. The greater omentum is very prominent. The small, nonperitoneal area of the liver is shown anterior to the right kidney. The round ligament of the liver and the umbilical fissure, which separates the right and left lobes of the liver, are seen. The neck of the gallbladder *(not shown)* is found just inferior to this section, between the quadrate and caudate lobes of the liver. The cystic duct is cut in two places. The hepatic duct lies just anterior to the cystic duct. The cystic and hepatic ducts unite in the lower part of the section to form the common bile duct. The pancreatic duct is found within the pancreas at this level. Both kidneys are seen just lateral to the psoas muscles.

the spine. The **right renal artery** is shown posterior to the IVC. The **left renal artery** would arise from the posterolateral wall of the aorta; the **right** and **left renal veins** are inferior to the renal arteries. The **portal confluence** (also called the **confluence of the splenic and portal veins**) is formed by the splenic vein and the **superior mesenteric vein.** The superior

portion of the duodenum is shown posterior to the stomach. Part of the transverse colon is shown. The hepatic duct is anterior to the portal vein.

Level of the gallbladder and right kidney (Figure 8-16): The kidneys are lateral to the psoas muscles. The **gastroduodenal artery (GDA)** lies along the anterolateral border of the head of the pancreas, and the

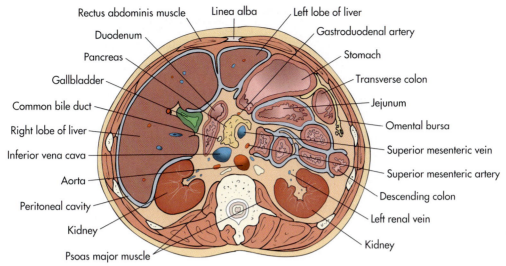

FIGURE 8-16 Cross section of the abdomen at the level of the second lumbar vertebra. The superior pancreaticoduodenal artery originates as shown in Figure 3-6 and shows some of its branches in this section. The lower portion of the stomach is found in this section, and the hepatic flexure of the colon is seen. The lobes of the liver are separated by the round ligament. The left lobe of the liver ends at this level. The head and neck of the pancreas drape around the superior mesenteric vein. Both kidneys and the psoas muscles are shown.

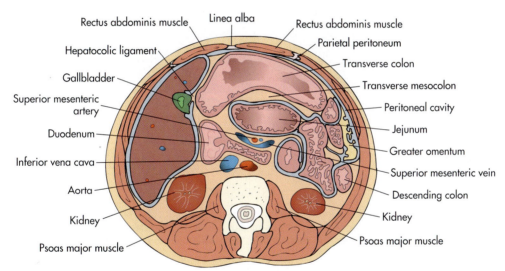

FIGURE 8-17 Cross section of the abdomen at the level of the third lumbar vertebra. The inferior mesenteric artery originates from the abdominal aorta at this level. The greater omentum is shown mostly on the left side of the abdomen. The descending and ascending portions of the duodenum lie between the aorta and the superior mesenteric artery and vein. The fundus of the gallbladder lies in the lower portion of this section. The lower poles of both kidneys lie lateral to the psoas muscles.

duodenum surrounds the lateral border. The stomach and transverse colon fill the left upper quadrant, and the liver fills the right upper quadrant. The gallbladder is medial to the liver. The common bile duct is seen along the posterior lateral border of the pancreatic head.

Level of the liver, gallbladder, and right kidney (Figure 8-17): The **inferior mesenteric artery** originates from the abdominal aorta at this level. The greater omentum is shown on the left side of the abdomen. The descending and ascending portions of the duodenum lie between the aorta and the superior mesenteric artery and vein. The gallbladder is seen along the medial border of the right lobe of the liver. Both

lower poles of the kidneys are seen lateral to the psoas muscles.

Level of the right lobe of the liver (Figure 8-18): The lower portion of the right lobe of the liver and the duodenum are shown.

Level of the bifurcation of the aorta (Figure 8-19): The psoas major muscles are lateral to the spine. The **iliac arteries** are anterior to the spine. The common **iliac veins** unite to form the inferior vena cava.

Level of the external iliac arteries (Figure 8-20): The external iliac arteries are well seen. The ileum is seen throughout this level, and the mesentery terminates at this level.

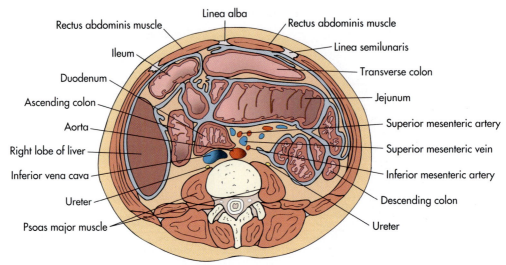

FIGURE 8-18 Cross section of the abdomen at the level of the third lumbar disk. The lower portion of the duodenum is shown. The lower margin of the right lobe of the liver is seen along the right lateral border.

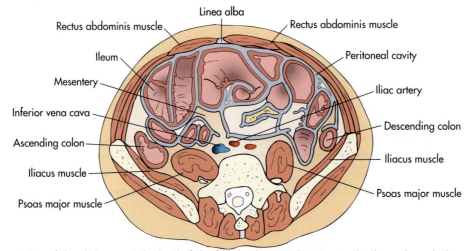

FIGURE 8-19 Cross section of the abdomen at the level of the fifth lumbar vertebra. It cuts the ileum through the upper part of the iliac fossa and passes just above the wings of the sacrum. The gluteus medius and iliacus muscles are shown. The right common iliac artery bifurcates into the external and internal iliac arteries. The common iliac veins are shown to unite to form the inferior vena cava. The lower part of the greater omentum is shown in this section.

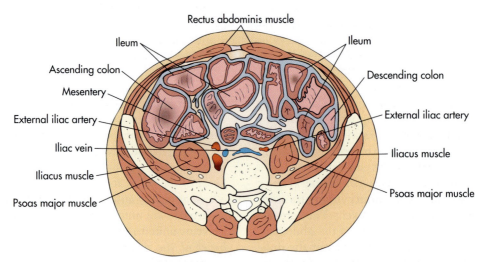

FIGURE 8-20 Cross section of the pelvis taken at the lower margin of the fifth lumbar vertebra and disk. The gluteus minimus muscle is shown on this section, as are the right external and internal iliac arteries. The left common iliac artery branches into the external and internal arteries. The ileum is seen throughout this level, and the mesentery terminates at this level.

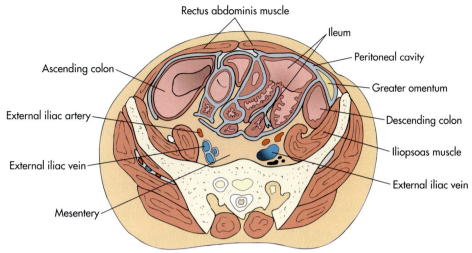

FIGURE 8-21 Cross section of the pelvis taken at the level of the sacrum and the anterior superior spine of the ilium. The gluteus maximus muscle appears on both sides. The internal and external iliac veins have united to form the common iliac vein. The ileum is seen throughout this section.

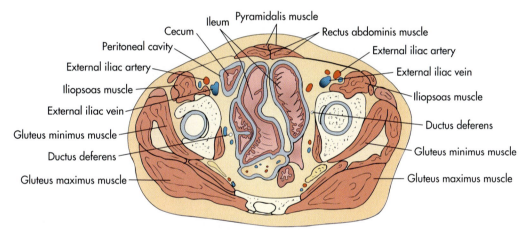

FIGURE 8-22 Cross section of the pelvis taken above the margins of the fifth anterior pair of sacral foramina and head of the femur. The external iliac arteries become the femoral arteries in this section. The femoral veins become the external iliac veins.

Level of the external iliac veins (Figure 8-21): The internal and external iliac veins have united to form the common iliac vein.

Level of the male pelvis (Figure 8-22): The external iliac arteries become the **common femoral arteries** in this section. The **femoral veins** become the external iliac veins. The cecum and rectum are seen.

Level of the male pelvis (Figure 8-23). The pelvic muscles are shown; the rectum is seen in the midline. The trigone of the bladder and urethral orifice are shown, and the seminal vesicles and the ampulla of the vasa deferentia can be identified. The ejaculatory ducts enter the urethra in the lower portion of this section.

Level of the male pelvis (Figure 8-24). The rectum, prostate gland, penis, and corpus cavernosum are seen.

Level of the female pelvis (Figure 8-25). The bladder is anterior to the uterus. The pouch of Douglas is posterior to the uterus, anterior to the rectum. The ovaries are seen along the fundal border of the uterus.

Level of the female pelvis (Figure 8-26): The pelvic diaphragm muscles are shown.

Longitudinal Plane

The longitudinal sectional illustrations (Figures 8-27 through 8-37) are presented from the right abdominal border, proceeding across the abdominal wall to the left border.

Level of the right lobe of the liver (Figure 8-27): The right lobe of the liver, diaphragm, omentum, and muscles are shown.

Level of the liver and gallbladder (Figure 8-28): The diaphragm, right lobe of the liver, gallbladder, and perirenal fat area are shown. The costodiaphragmatic recess is seen superior to the diaphragm.

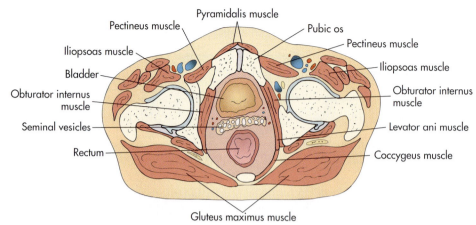

FIGURE 8-23 Cross section of the pelvis at the level of the coccyx, the spine of the ischium, the femur, and the greater trochanter. This cross section passes through the coccyx, spine of the ischium, acetabulum, head of the femur, greater trochanter, pubic symphysis, and upper margins of the obturator foramen. The gemellus inferior and superior, coccygeus, and levator ani muscles are shown. The rectum is seen in the midline. The trigone of the bladder and the urethral orifice are well shown, and the seminal vesicles and the ampulla of the vasa deferentia can be identified. The ejaculatory ducts enter the urethra in the lower portion of this section.

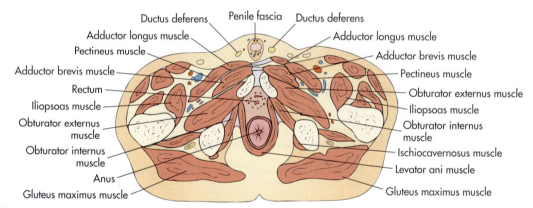

FIGURE 8-24 Cross section of the pelvis at the tip of the coccyx, inferior ramus of the pubis, and neck of the femur. This cross section passes below the tip of the coccyx, upper portion of the tuberosity of the ischium and inferior ramus of the pubis, neck of the femur, and lower portion of the greater trochanter. The rectum, penis, and corpus cavernosum are seen.

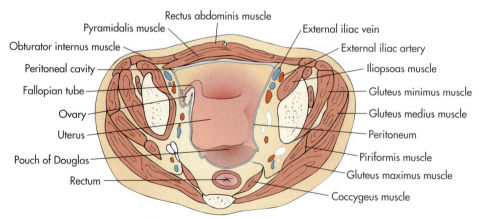

FIGURE 8-25 This cross section is a section through the female pelvis just below the junction of the sacrum and coccyx, through the anterior inferior spine of the ilium and the greater sciatic notch. The uterine artery tend vein and the ureter are shown dissected beyond the uterine wall. The bladder is anterior to the uterus. The ovaries are cut through their midsections on this level.

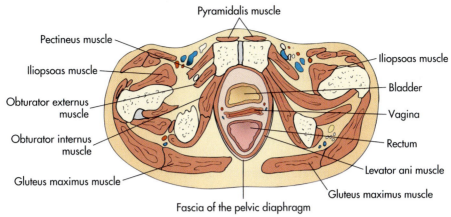

FIGURE 8-26 Cross section of the female pelvis taken through the lower part of the coccyx and the spine of the ischium. The superior gemellus muscles and the pectineus muscle appear in this section, and the coccygeus muscle terminates here. The gluteus maximus, gluteus minimus, and gluteus medius muscles all begin their insertions in the lower part of this section. The external os of the cervix is shown. The ureters empty into the bladder at the base.

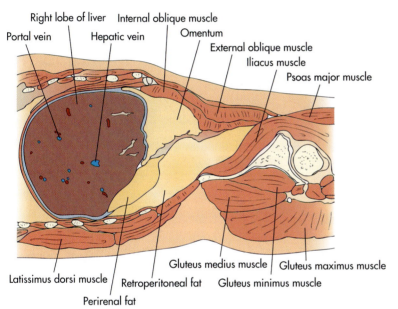

FIGURE 8-27 Sagittal section of the abdomen taken along the right abdominal border.

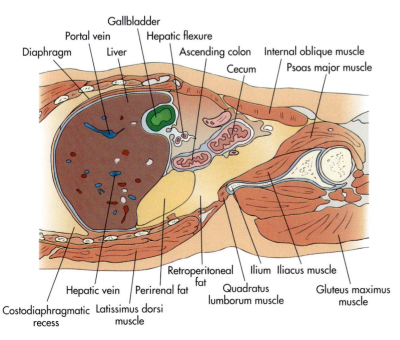

FIGURE 8-28 Sagittal section of the abdomen 8 cm from the midline.

Level of the liver, gallbladder, and right kidney (Figure 8-29): The diaphragm, right lobe of the liver, gallbladder, and right kidney are seen. The perirenal fat and fascia are shown surrounding the kidney. The caudate lobe of the liver is beginning to show.

Level of the liver, caudate lobe, and psoas muscle (Figure 8-30): The diaphragm, right lobe of the liver, caudate lobe, and neck of the gallbladder are seen. **Morison's pouch** is found anterior to the kidney and posterior to the inferior right lobe of the liver.

Level of the liver, duodenum, and pancreas (Figure 8-31): The portal vein and cystic duct are shown. The duodenum wraps around the head of the pancreas.

Level of the liver, inferior vena cava, pancreas, and gastroduodenal artery (Figure 8-32): The gastroduodenal artery is the anterior border of the head of the pancreas. The **left portal vein** is shown to enter the left lobe of the liver.

Level of the inferior vena cava, left lobe of the liver, and pancreas (Figure 8-33): The inferior vena cava is shown along the posterior border of the liver. The pancreas lies anterior to the inferior vena cava and inferior to the portal vein.

Level of the hepatic vein and inferior vena cava, pancreas, and superior mesenteric vein (Figure 8-34): The superior mesenteric vein flows anterior to the uncinate portion of the pancreas and posterior to

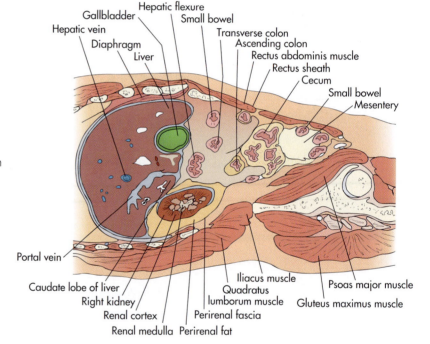

FIGURE 8-29 Sagittal section of the abdomen 7 cm from the midline.

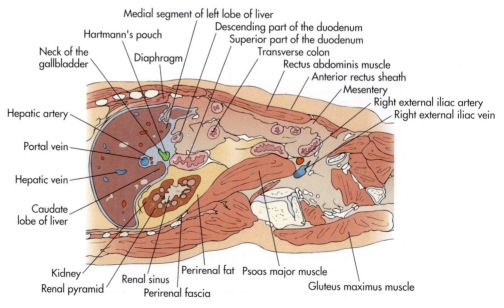

FIGURE 8-30 Sagittal section of the abdomen 6 cm from the midline.

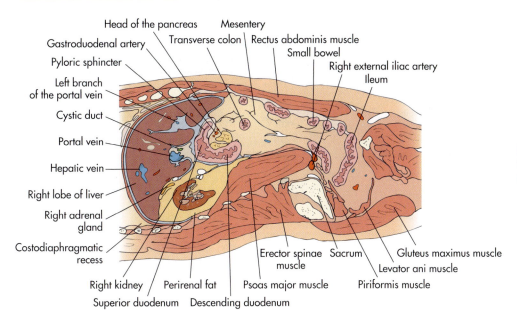

FIGURE 8-31 Sagittal section of the abdomen 5 cm from the midline.

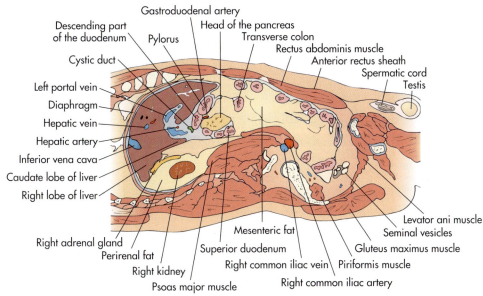

FIGURE 8-32 Sagittal section of the abdomen 4 cm from the midline.

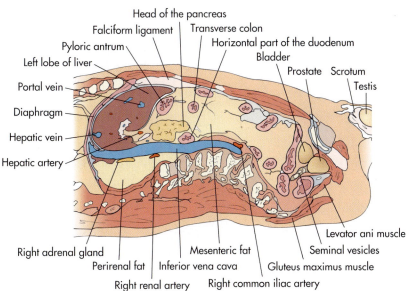

FIGURE 8-33 Sagittal section of the abdomen 3 cm from the midline.

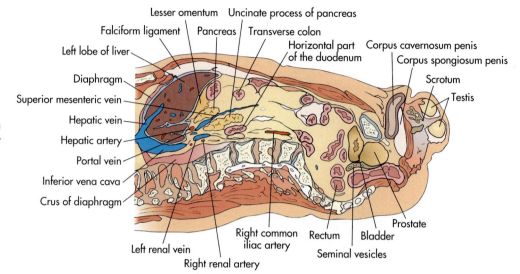

FIGURE 8-34 Sagittal section of the abdomen 2 cm from the midline.

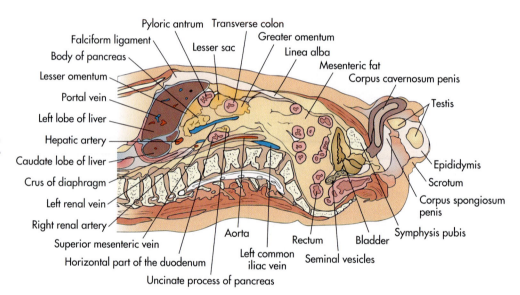

FIGURE 8-35 Sagittal section of the abdomen 1 cm from the midline.

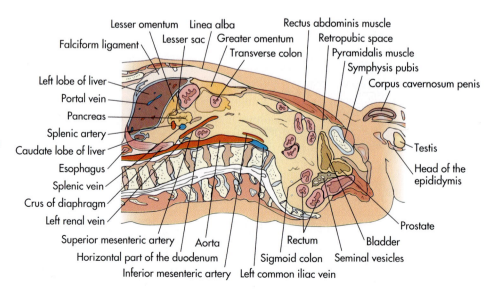

FIGURE 8-36 Midline sagittal section of the abdomen.

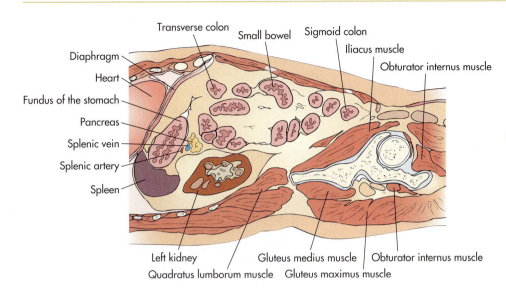

Labels (clockwise from top): Transverse colon, Small bowel, Sigmoid colon, Iliacus muscle, Obturator internus muscle, Diaphragm, Heart, Fundus of the stomach, Pancreas, Splenic vein, Splenic artery, Spleen, Left kidney, Quadratus lumborum muscle, Gluteus medius muscle, Gluteus maximus muscle, Obturator internus muscle

FIGURE 8-37 Sagittal section of the abdomen along the left abdominal border.

the body. The middle hepatic vein empties into the inferior vena cava. The falciform ligament is seen along the anterior border of the abdomen.

Level of the crus of the diaphragm and caudate lobe (Figure 8-35): The caudate lobe is seen posterior to the ligamentum venosum. The aorta is starting to come into view.

Level of the aorta and superior mesenteric artery (Figure 8-36): The **superior mesenteric artery (SMA)** arises from the anterior border of the aorta. The pancreas is seen anterior to the SMA; the splenic artery and vein form the posterior border. The left renal vein is posterior to the SMA and anterior to the aorta. The area of the lesser sac is shown.

Level of the spleen and left kidney (Figure 8-37): The spleen is shown just below the diaphragm in the left upper quadrant. The left kidney is inferior to the spleen. The tail of the pancreas lies anterior to the kidney and inferior to the **splenic hilum.**

GENERAL ABDOMINAL ULTRASOUND PROTOCOLS

It is the responsibility of the sonographer to ensure that patients are afforded the highest quality care possible during their sonographic examination. This entails identifying the patient properly, ensuring confidentiality of information and patient privacy, providing proper nursing care, and maintaining clean and sanitary equipment and examination rooms.

The upper abdomen is imaged with high-resolution real-time ultrasound equipment. The transducer selected may be a sector or curved linear array or, in many cases, a combination of the two. The frequency of the transducer used depends on the size, muscle, and fat composition of the patient. Generally, a broad-bandwidth transducer is used, with variations of 2.25 to 7.5 MHz, depending on the size of the patient and the depth of field. All organs are imaged in at least two planes: transverse and longitudinal.

Transverse Scans

The horseshoe-shaped contour of the vertebral column should be well delineated to ensure sound penetration through the abdomen without obstruction from bowel gas interference. The liver parenchyma should be evaluated for focal and/or diffuse abnormalities. The homogeneous echogenicity of the liver parenchyma should be compared with the right kidney.

With the patient in deep inspiration, the posterior border of the liver should be imaged as the transducer is angled in a cephalic-to-caudal direction from the dome of the liver to its inferior edge. This ensures that time gain compensation (TGC) is set correctly (at the posterior border of the liver). The overall gain should be adjusted to provide a smooth, homogeneous liver parenchyma throughout. If too many echoes are "outside the liver," the overall gain should be decreased. If the near gain is set too low, the anterior surface of the liver is not delineated.

The gallbladder and biliary system may require additional views to demonstrate the presence or absence of biliary stones and/or sludge. It is critical that the patient be NPO for at least 8 hours before the examination to permit adequate distention of the normally functioning gallbladder. Intrahepatic ducts may be evaluated by obtaining images of the liver and portal veins. The vascular structures, aorta, and inferior vena cava should be well seen anterior to the vertebral column as echo-free, or anechoic, structures.

The pancreas should be identified anterior to the prevertebral vessels. Oral contrast (water) may be used to outline the stomach to afford improved visualization of the pancreas.

The spleen and flow velocities in the splenic vein and artery should be assessed with the patient in a steep decubitus position. The sonographer should be aware of the fluid-filled stomach in the left upper quadrant. Bowel may be evaluated for wall thickening, dilation, hypertrophy, or other pathology. Peritoneal fluid within the abdomen may be evaluated with sonography for pericentesis.

The kidneys, adrenals, and urinary bladder are well imaged with ultrasound. The renal cortex and pelvis should be assessed, and the renal length recorded. Doppler velocities of the renal vascular structures may be assessed to identify stenosis or thrombosis.

Longitudinal Scans

The transducer should be angled from the diaphragm to the inferior border of the right lobe of the liver. The diaphragm should be well defined as a linear bright line superior to the dome of the liver. The liver parenchyma should be homogeneous and uniform throughout. If gain is adjusted to maximum without adequate uniform penetration, a lower frequency may be used to provide increased sensitivity. The larger vascular structures (aorta and inferior vena cava) should be well outlined as hollow tubular structures with the patient in deep inspiration.

The baseline upper abdominal ultrasound examination includes a survey of the liver and **porta hepatis**, vascular structures, biliary system, pancreas, kidneys, spleen, and para-aortic area. If variations in anatomy or pathology are seen, multiple views are obtained over the area of interest.

Liver and Porta Hepatis Protocol

The liver is examined as part of a comprehensive ultrasound evaluation of the abdomen (Figures 8-38 through 8-51) (Table 8-1). Abnormalities that can be evaluated include cirrhosis, fatty infiltration, hepatomegaly, portal hypertension, primary and metastatic tumors, abscess formation, and trauma. Color and pulsed wave (PW) Doppler are used to assess the hepatic vascular system.

1. Patient preparation: Nothing by mouth (NPO) for at least 6 hours.

2. Transducer selection: 2.5 to 4 MHz curvilinear/sector, or 3 to 5 MHz curvilinear. Lower frequency transducers are often necessary in patients with fatty infiltration or cirrhosis.
3. Patient position: Supine and decubitus as necessary.
4. Images and observations should include the following:
   - The echogenicity of the liver parenchyma should be compared with that of the renal parenchyma.

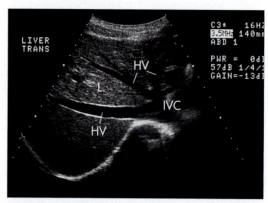

FIGURE 8-39 Transverse image at the dome of the liver (L) in full inspiration to demonstrate the hepatic veins (HV) flowing into the inferior vena cava (IVC).

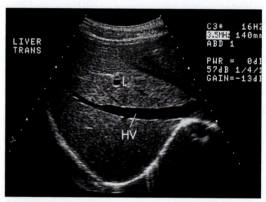

FIGURE 8-40 Transverse image of the right lobe of the liver (L) with the right hepatic vein (HV).

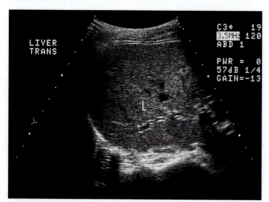

FIGURE 8-38 Transverse image at the right lobe of the liver (L) at the liver-lung interface.

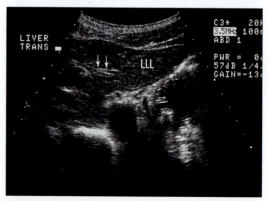

FIGURE 8-41 Transverse image of the left lobe of liver (LLL) and left portal vein (arrows).

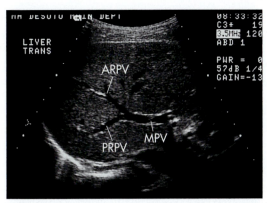

FIGURE 8-42 Transverse image of the liver, main portal vein *(MPV)*, and right portal vein with bifurcation of anterior *(ARPV)* and posterior *(PRPV)* branches.

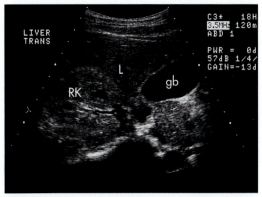

FIGURE 8-43 Transverse image of liver *(L)*, gallbladder *(gb)*, and right kidney *(RK)*.

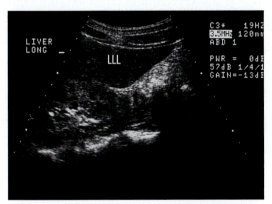

FIGURE 8-44 Longitudinal image of left lobe of liver *(LLL)*.

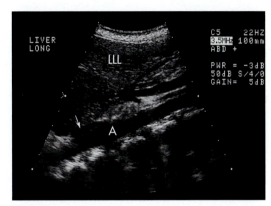

FIGURE 8-45 Longitudinal image of left lobe of liver *(LLL)*, aorta *(A)*, and superior mesenteric vein *(arrow)*.

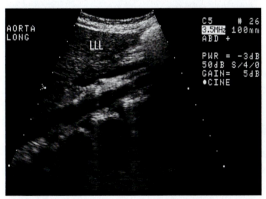

FIGURE 8-46 Longitudinal image of tip of left lobe of liver *(LLL)*.

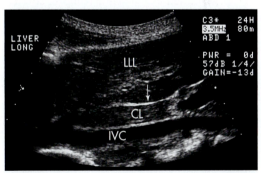

FIGURE 8-47 Longitudinal image of left lobe of liver *(LLL)*, caudate lobe *(CL)*, ligamentum venosum *(arrow)*, and inferior vena cava *(IVC)*.

- The hepatic venous, inferior vena cava, and right and left portal structures should be imaged.
- The **ligamentum teres (LT)** should be identified in the left lobe of the liver.
- The dome of the right lobe of the liver should be surveyed with the patient in deep inspiration.
- The right hemidiaphragm and right pleural gutter should be examined.
- The main lobar fissure, as it projects from the **right portal vein (RPV)** to the neck of the gallbladder, should be imaged.

- Liver size in a parasagittal scan demonstrating the diaphragm and tip of the right lobe of the liver should be recorded.
- The size of any demonstrated masses should be recorded.

The presence of ascites (including the four quadrants of the abdomen) should be evaluated and recorded.

Doppler of the vascular structures in the liver if pathology is present:

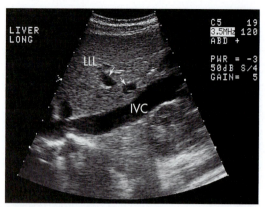

FIGURE 8-48 Longitudinal image of left lobe of liver *(LLL)*, portal vein *(arrows)*, and inferior vena cava *(IVC)*.

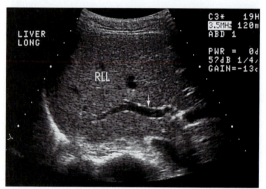

FIGURE 8-49 Longitudinal oblique image of right lobe of liver *(RLL)* and right portal vein *(arrow)*.

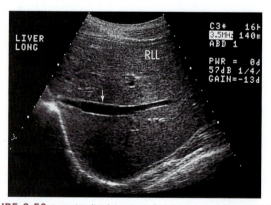

FIGURE 8-50 Longitudinal image of right lobe of liver *(RLL)* and right hepatic vein *(arrow)*. This long axis view is used to measure the long axis of the liver from the diaphragm to the tip.

- Assessment of the patency and direction of flow of the main, right, and left portal veins.
- Assessment of the patency of the right, middle, and left hepatic veins (HV).
- Assessment of the patency of the umbilical vein (recanalized umbilical vein) or other collateral vessels.
- Assessment of the patency of surgically or angiographically placed shunts.

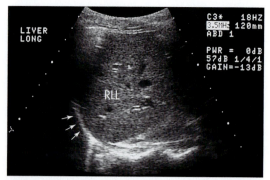

FIGURE 8-51 Longitudinal image of lateral segment of the right lobe of liver *(RLL)* and vascular structures; Diaphragm *(arrows)*.

TABLE 8-1	**Abdominal Ultrasound Protocol: Liver**	
Organ	**Scan Plane**	**Anatomy**
Liver	Trv	Rt lobe/lung
(Figures 8-38	Rt lobe/(dome)	Lt lobe/lt portal vein
to 8-51)	hepatic	Lt lobe/caudate lobe
	veins	Rt lobe/portal veins (main, rt)
		Rt lobe/gallbladder/kidney
	Long	Lt lobe/aorta
		Lt lobe/caudate lobe/IVC
		Rt lobe/dome (diaphragm)
		Rt lobe/lung
		Rt lobe/portal vein
		Rt lobe/kidney (measure rt lobe)

Lt, Left; *IVC,* inferior vena cava; *Rt,* right; *Long,* longitudinal; *Trv,* transverse.

- Performance of pulsed Doppler analysis of the hepatic artery with resistance measurements.

Biliary System Protocol

Ultrasound examinations of the gallbladder and bile ducts are performed to determine cholelithiasis, changes secondary to acute and chronic cholecystitis, obstruction, and primary or metastatic tumor involvement. The examination is performed as part of a comprehensive general abdominal evaluation (Figures 8-52 through 8-57) (Table 8-2).

1. Patient preparation: NPO for at least 6 hours.
2. Transducer selection: 2.5 to 5 MHz curvilinear.
3. Patient position: Supine and decubitus.
4. Images and observations should include the following:
   - The fundus, body, and neck should be surveyed.
   - Gallbladder wall thickness (normal is less than 3 mm) should be recorded. If thickened, the wall should be measured in the transverse plane at the

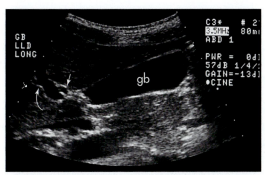

FIGURE 8-52 Longitudinal image of gallbladder *(gb)*, main lobar fissure *(arrow)*, and portal vein *(curved arrow)*.

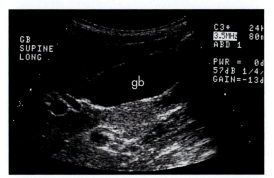

FIGURE 8-53 Longitudinal image of gallbladder *(gb)*, including neck.

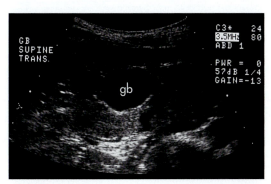

FIGURE 8-54 Transverse image of gallbladder *(gb)*.

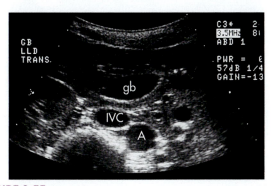

FIGURE 8-55 Transverse decubitus image of gallbladder *(gb)*, inferior vena cava *(IVC)*, and aorta *(A)*.

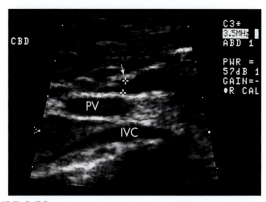

FIGURE 8-56 Longitudinal image of common bile duct *(arrow)* anterior to portal vein *(PV)* that lies anterior to the inferior vena cava *(IVC)*.

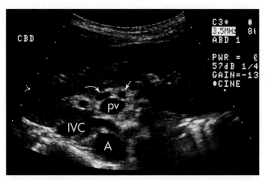

FIGURE 8-57 Transverse image of portal triad in the center of the image: portal vein *(pv)* with common bile duct *(curved arrow)* anterior and lateral; hepatic artery *(arrow)* anterior and medial; inferior vena cava *(IVC)*; and aorta *(A)*.

TABLE 8-2	**Abdominal Ultrasound Protocol: Gallbladder**	
Organ	**Scan Plane**	**Anatomy**
GB (supine and LLD) (Figures 8-52 to 8-55)	Long	Body/fundus
	Trv	Body/neck (measure wall)
		Body/neck
CBD (Figures 8-56 and 8-57)	Trv	Portal triad
	Long	Measure duct

CBD, Common bile duct; *GB,* gallbladder; *LLD,* left lateral decubitus; *Long,* longitudinal; *Trv,* transverse.

anterior wall with the transducer perpendicular to the anterior wall.

- The presence of echogenic foci (e.g., stones, polyps) within the gallbladder lumen should be evaluated. If echogenic foci are present, the sonographer should attempt to demonstrate acoustic shadowing and mobility.
- The common bile duct should be imaged in at least the oblique long-axis plane because it lies anterior

to the **main portal vein (MPV)** before coursing posterior to the head of the pancreas.

- The transverse scan of the porta hepatis may help delineate the portal vein from the common duct (anterior and to the right) and hepatic artery (anterior and to the left).
- Visualization of the intrahepatic ducts is not possible unless dilation is present. Ductal dilation may be seen as the liver is scanned, demonstrating right and left branches of the portal vein as the hepatic ducts follow a parallel course.
- To examine gallstones, the focal point of the transducer is placed at the region of the posterior gallbladder wall, and the gain reduced. This facilitates demonstration of acoustic shadowing.

Pancreas Protocol

The pancreas is examined as part of a comprehensive general abdominal study (Figures 8-58 through 8-63) (Table 8-3). Specific indications for pancreatic scanning include abdominal pain, clinically manifested acute or chronic pancreatitis, abnormal laboratory values, cholecystitis, or obstructive jaundice. The examination determines the presence of cystic and solid masses, biliary and ductal dilation, and the presence of extrapancreatic masses and fluid collections.

1. Patient preparation: NPO for at least 6 hours; may need to give water to fill the stomach as a window to image the pancreas.
2. Transducer selection: 2.5 to 5 MHz curvilinear.

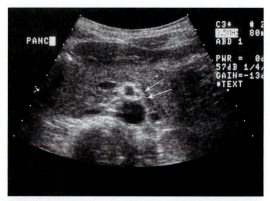

FIGURE 8-60 Transverse image of the pancreas; a sliver of splenic vein *(arrows)* lies posterior to the body and tail.

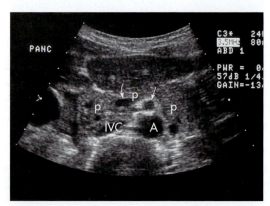

FIGURE 8-58 Transverse image of pancreas *(p)* as it lies anterior to superior mesenteric artery *(arrow)* and vein *(curved arrow)*. The aorta *(A)* and inferior vena cava *(IVC)* are anterior to the horseshoe shape of the spine.

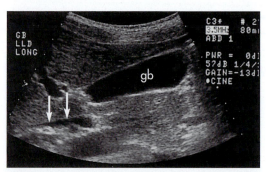

FIGURE 8-61 Longitudinal image of the pancreas (posterior to the gallbladder) with the common bile duct *(arrows)* beginning to move posterior to join the pancreatic duct.

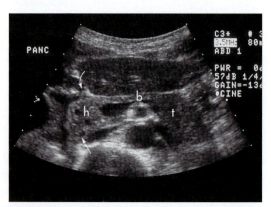

FIGURE 8-59 Transverse image of head *(h)*, body *(b)*, and tail *(t)* of the pancreas. The gastroduodenal artery *(curved arrow)* is the anterolateral border of the head; the common bile duct *(arrow)* is the posterolateral border of the head.

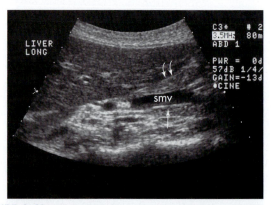

FIGURE 8-62 Longitudinal image of the superior mesenteric vein *(smv)* as it flows anterior to the uncinate process *(arrow)* and posterior to the head of the pancreas *(curved arrows)*.

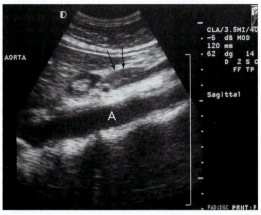

FIGURE 8-63 Longitudinal image of the body of the pancreas (*arrows*) anterior to the aorta (*A*).

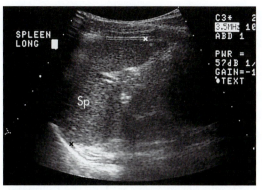

FIGURE 8-64 Longitudinal image of spleen (*Sp*). The long axis is measured from the crossbars.

TABLE 8-3	**Abdominal Ultrasound Protocol: Pancreas**	
Organ	**Scan Plane**	**Anatomy**
Pancreas (Figures 8-58 to 8-63)	Trv	Head/IVC/SMV
		Body and tail/SMV/SMA
	Long	Head/portal vein/IVC
		Body and tail/aorta

IVC, Inferior vena cava; *Long,* longitudinal; *SMA,* superior mesenteric artery; *SMV,* superior mesenteric vein; *Trv,* transverse.

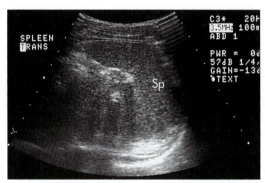

FIGURE 8-65 Transverse image of spleen (*Sp*).

3. Patient position: Supine, decubitus, or upright.
4. Images and observations should include the following:
   - The head, body, and tail should be well delineated once the celiac axis, superior mesenteric artery and vein, aorta, and inferior vena cava are identified. (Often the lie of the pancreas makes it difficult to image the gland in one plane; the tail may be seen on an image that is more superior than the head of the gland.)
   - Transverse scans along the region of the splenic vein should be performed to demonstrate the body and tail of the pancreas.
   - The pancreatic duct may be seen on the transverse scan as it courses through the body of the gland.
   - The longitudinal view of the pancreatic head lies anterior to the inferior vena cava and inferior to the portal vein.
   - The superior mesenteric vein may be seen to course anterior to the uncinate process of the head and posterior to the body.
   - The pancreatic tail may be seen, as gentle but firm pressure is applied to the abdomen to displace overlying gas in the antrum of the stomach or transverse colon. The tail may also be seen with the patient in a right decubitus position, as the transducer is angled through the spleen and left

kidney; the pancreatic tail is anterior to the left kidney.
   - The presence of dilated pancreatic or biliary ducts should be assessed and their size measured.
   - The presence of cystic or solid masses should be assessed.
   - The presence of peripancreatic nodes should be assessed.
   - The presence of peripancreatic fluid collections (e.g., pseudocysts) should be assessed.
   - The presence of any pancreatic calcifications detected should be recorded.

Spleen Protocol

Ultrasound examinations are performed to assess overall splenic architecture, to examine or detect intrasplenic masses, to examine the splenic hilum and vasculature, and to determine splenic size (Figures 8-64 and 8-65) (Table 8-4).

1. Patient preparation: NPO for at least 6 hours.
2. Transducer selection: 2.5 to 4 MHz curvilinear.
3. Patient position: Steep right lateral decubitus or right lateral.

TABLE 8-4	Abdominal Ultrasound Protocol: Spleen	
Organ	**Scan Plane**	**Anatomy**
Spleen (Figures 8-64 and 8-65)	Long	Spleen/LK (measure length)
	Trv	Splenic hilum

LK, Left kidney; *Long,* longitudinal; *Trv,* transverse.

4. Images and observations include the following:
   - Coronal scans of the long axis of the spleen should be performed.
   - The left hemidiaphragm, splenic hilus, and upper and lower borders of the spleen should be demonstrated.
   - The splenic length should be measured.
   - The texture of the spleen should be compared with that of the liver. The splenic parenchyma should be homogeneous with the liver.
   - A transverse scan of the spleen at the level of the splenic hilus should be performed. The sonographer should look for increased vascularity or splenic nodes.

Renal Protocol

Ultrasound examinations are performed to assess overall renal architecture, examine or detect intrarenal and extrarenal masses, document hydronephrosis, detect calculi, examine renal vasculature, and determine renal size and echogenicity (Figures 8-66 through 8-77) (Table 8-5). The condition of the bladder and ureters is evaluated as part of the examination protocol.

1. Patient preparation: Patient should be hydrated, unless contraindicated.
2. Transducer selection: 2.5 to 4 MHz curvilinear.
3. Patient position: Supine or decubitus.
4. Images and observations should include the following:
   - The right kidney should be demonstrated in a supine or slightly decubitus position. The liver should be used as the acoustic window.
   - The left kidney should be surveyed with the patient in a right lateral decubitus position. The spleen should be used as the acoustic window.
   - The renal cortex and medulla should be well delineated.
   - Longitudinal scans should be made through the midline and lateral and medial borders. Measurement of the long axis should be made from upper to lower poles.
   - Transverse scans should be made through the upper pole, middle section at the level of the renal pelvis, and lower pole.

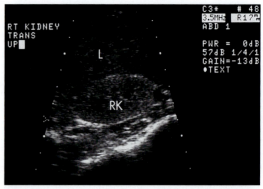

FIGURE 8-66 Transverse image of upper pole of right kidney *(RK);* liver *(L)*.

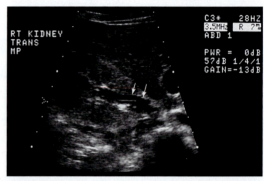

FIGURE 8-67 Transverse image of mid right kidney with the renal vein *(arrows)*.

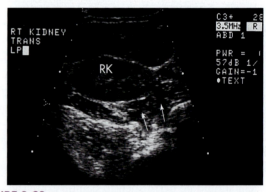

FIGURE 8-68 Transverse image of lower pole of right kidney *(RK)*. The psoas muscle is medial to the kidney *(arrows)*.

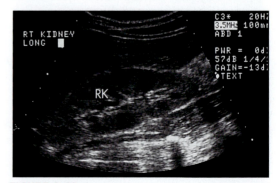

FIGURE 8-69 Longitudinal image of right kidney *(RK)*.

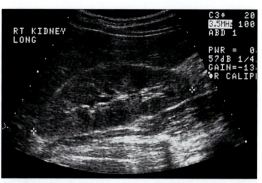

FIGURE 8-70 Longitudinal image of right kidney *(RK)* with measurements of long axis.

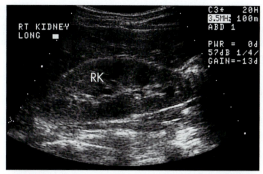

FIGURE 8-71 Longitudinal image of right kidney *(RK).*

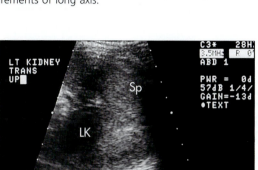

FIGURE 8-72 Transverse image of upper pole of left kidney *(LK)* and spleen *(Sp).*

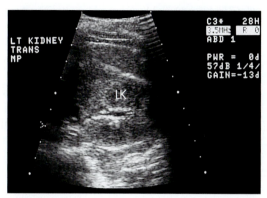

FIGURE 8-73 Transverse image of mid left kidney *(LK).*

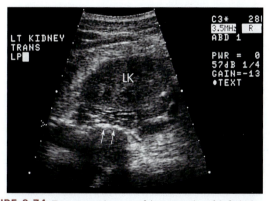

FIGURE 8-74 Transverse image of lower pole of left kidney *(LK)* and psoas muscle *(arrows).*

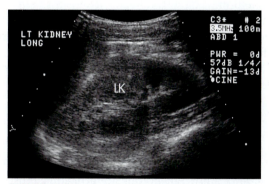

FIGURE 8-75 Longitudinal image of left kidney *(LK).*

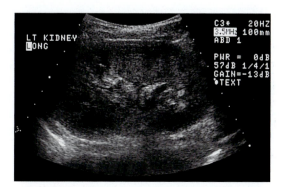

FIGURE 8-76 Longitudinal image of left kidney.

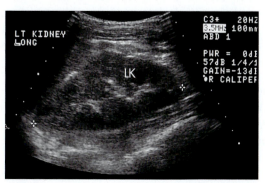

FIGURE 8-77 Longitudinal image of left kidney *(LK)* with measurement of long axis.

TABLE 8-5	Abdominal Ultrasound Protocol: Renal	
Organ	**Scan Plane**	**Anatomy**
Kidneys (Figures 8-66 to 8-77)	Trv	Upper pole Mid (at pelvis) Lower pole
	Long	Mid (measure length) Lateral Medial

Long, Longitudinal; *Trv,* transverse.

- The bladder should be imaged in a longitudinal and transverse plane.
- The bladder wall should be assessed for thickness or irregularities, and the presence of focal lesions recorded.
- If the bladder is large or if hydronephrosis is present, the evaluation of ureteral jets should be noted within the bladder (with color). Ureteral jets should also be examined in patients with renal calculus or hematuria.

Doppler flow analysis of the renal area:

- Image the origin of the renal arteries, measure resistive index and acceleration time of the pulsed waveform.
- All Doppler studies of the kidneys include pulsed Doppler tracings, with resistance measurements taken of the main, interlobar, and arcuate arteries.
- The patency of the main renal vein should be determined.

Aorta and Iliac Artery Protocol

The aorta is examined primarily to determine the presence of aneurysmal dilation (Figures 8-78 through 8-83) (Table 8-6). Aortic aneurysms are defined as those with vessel diameters greater than 3 cm or with focal dilation of the vessel. Iliac aneurysms are defined as vessels with diameters greater than 2 cm. Aneurysms larger than 5 cm and those with documented rapid rates of expansion have an increased risk of catastrophic rupture. The physician must be made aware of these patients before they leave the department.

1. Patient preparation: NPO for at least 6 hours.
2. Transducer selection: 2.5 to 4 MHz curvilinear.
3. Patient position: Supine or slightly decubitus.
4. Images and observations should include the following:
   - The aorta should be imaged in the longitudinal plane from the diaphragm to below the bifurcation at the iliac junction.

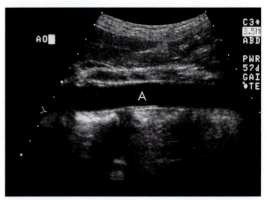

FIGURE 8-78 Longitudinal image of the proximal aorta *(A)* anterior to the spine.

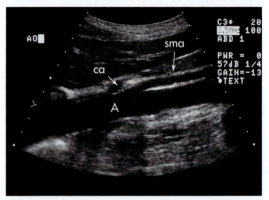

FIGURE 8-79 Longitudinal image of the aorta *(A)* with celiac axis *(ca)* and superior mesenteric artery *(sma)*.

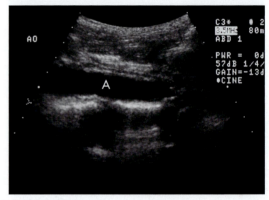

FIGURE 8-80 Longitudinal image of the distal aorta *(A)*.

- Transverse scans should be made at the level of the diaphragm, superior to the renal arteries, inferior to the renal arteries, and at the bifurcation. Scans of the iliac arteries should be made.
- Lymphadenopathy should also be evaluated because the lymph nodes lie anterior to the vessels.
- The inferior vena cava is best imaged on a longitudinal plane through the right lobe of the liver with the patient in full inspiration.
- An alternative imaging plane is the slight decubitus view. The patient rolls onto his or her left side; the

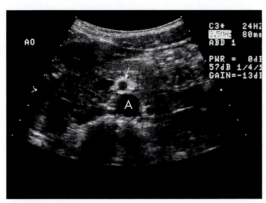

FIGURE 8-81 Transverse image of the high abdominal aorta *(A)* at the level of the superior mesenteric artery *(arrow)*.

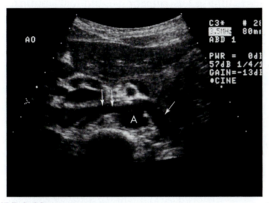

FIGURE 8-82 Transverse image of the midabdominal aorta *(A)* at the level of the renal vessels (left renal artery—*one arrow;* right renal artery—*two arrows*).

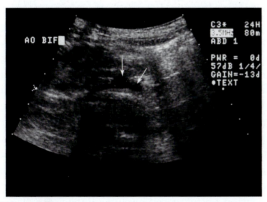

FIGURE 8-83 Transverse image of the distal aorta at the bifurcation *(arrows)*.

TABLE 8-6	Abdominal Ultrasound Protocol: Aorta	
Organ	**Scan Plane**	**Anatomy**
Aorta	Long	Prox, mid, and distal
(Figures 8-78 to 8-83)	Trv	Prox, mid, and distal

Prox, Proximal; *Long,* longitudinal; *Trv,* transverse.

transducer is longitudinal and is sharply angled from the right lobe of the liver to the left iliac wing. This allows the sonographer to image the inferior vena cava "anterior" to the aorta. It usually allows the sonographer to follow the entrance and exit of the renal veins and arteries into the great vessels and provides an excellent window to perform color flow or Doppler interrogation of the renal vessels.
- Outer to outer measurements should be taken of the aorta in the longitudinal and transverse planes.

If an aneurysm is present:
- Longitudinal scans of each iliac vessel from the bifurcation to the most distal segment should be taken.
- Transverse scans of the iliacs below the bifurcation should be taken.

Thyroid Protocol

The role of ultrasound in evaluating the thyroid is primarily limited to differentiating cystic masses from solid masses, recording the number of masses, assessing overall echogenicity and homogeneity, and evaluating the size of the gland. It is normally performed as a result of an abnormal physical examination or to correlate with nuclear medicine scans.

1. Patient preparation: None.
2. Transducer selection: 10 to 13 MHz linear.
3. Patient position: Place a rolled sheet under the shoulders to elevate the neck.
4. Images and observations should include the following:
   - Longitudinal scans of each lobe (lateral, middle, and medial portions) should be performed. Landmarks include the carotid artery laterally and the trachea medially.
   - Transverse scans of each lobe, including the most inferior, middle, and superior portions of the gland, should be performed.
   - Transverse and longitudinal scans of the thyroid isthmus should be performed.
   - The gland and any detected nodules should be measured.
   - If possible, split-screen images of the right and left lobes should be made for texture comparison.

Parathyroid Protocol

The role of ultrasound in evaluating the parathyroid is primarily to detect adenomas. The examination is normally performed as a result of abnormal calcium levels or an abnormal physical examination. There are normally four parathyroid glands, two on each side at the upper and lower aspects of the thyroid gland. It should be noted, however, that parathyroid adenomas can be positioned distinctly separate from the thyroid gland. Use the thyroid protocol.

Breast Protocol

The role of ultrasound in evaluating the breast is primarily to determine if a mass is a simple cyst or a complex or solid lesion. The patient generally has a palpable mass or an abnormal mammogram without a palpable mass, is pregnant, or has other complications that may prevent her from receiving a mammogram. Multiple approaches may be used to evaluate the breast. Please refer to the breast chapter for further delineation. This protocol is specific to evaluating a palpable breast mass.

1. Patient preparation: None.
2. Transducer selection: 8 to 12 MHz. The linear array transducer allows a larger field of view.
3. Patient position: Supine or shallow oblique is most frequently used. Steep oblique or decubitus positions are used for lesions that are more lateral.
4. Images and observations should include the following:
   - If the lesion is very superficial, an acoustically matched stand-off pad may be used with gel placed on the skin and the pad to afford adequate contact. (Stand-off pad thickness should not exceed 1.0 cm because of the elevation plane focus of the transducer.)
   - All scans should be labeled in the proper zone, including the clock position, distance from the nipple (1, 2, 3), and depth to the chest (A, B, C).
   - Scans should be made in the radial and antiradial planes over the area of interest.
   - The gain should be adjusted to note the borders, through-transmission, and internal echo pattern of the lesion. Gain settings should demonstrate breast fat as medium level gray shades.
   - The lesion should be measured.

Scrotal Protocol

High-resolution ultrasound imaging is the primary screening modality for most testicular pathology. Applications include inflammatory processes of the testes and epididymis, tumors, trauma, torsion, hydrocele, varicocele, hernias, spermatoceles, and undescended testes.

1. Patient preparation: None.
2. Transducer selection: 8 to 12 MHz linear array.
3. Patient position: Supine (Valsalva maneuver or upright position to check for varicocele).
4. Images and observations should include the following:
   - Gray scale
   - Long testicle (include medial, mid, and lateral)
   - Long epididymis

- Anteroposterior (AP) and long measurements of above anatomy
- Transverse scan of each testis (upper, mid, lower)
- Transverse scan of head of epididymis
- Include AP and transverse measurements of the middle pole of the testicles.
- If possible, a split-screen image should be obtained to compare the echogenicity of each testis.
- Images of the extratesticular area should be obtained to determine the presence of hydrocele, hernia, or other conditions.

Doppler flow analysis of the scrotal area:

- When indicated, color and pulsed Doppler analysis of intratesticular flow with resistance measurements should be obtained.
- The scanning instrument should be optimized for slow flow detection (e.g., decrease pulse repetition frequency/scale, lower filters, increase gain or power).

ABDOMINAL DOPPLER

Doppler ultrasound has been used for many decades to evaluate cardiovascular flow patterns. As in other areas of ultrasound, many improvements have been made to the technology, such as the development of pulsed wave Doppler, spectral analysis of the returning waveform, and color flow mapping. These advances in Doppler instrumentation, combined with high-resolution imaging of the vessels, have led to "duplex scanning equipment," which combines these modalities into a single probe.

Doppler is used to ascertain the presence or absence of flow. It can be used to differentiate vessels from nonvascular structures with confusingly similar images (e.g., common duct from hepatic artery, arterial aneurysm from a cyst). The determination and direction of flow may also be of diagnostic value. Once the presence and direction of flow have been determined, spectral analysis of the flow gives further information on flow velocity and turbulence. Increased velocity and poststenotic turbulence may be seen in vascular stenoses. In postoperative patients, increased turbulence alone may be present at the site of a graft anastomosis with the native vessel. Evaluation of the shape of the waveform, with comparison of the systolic and diastolic components, may yield information on increased vascular impedance, as is seen in renal transplant rejection.

Doppler Scanning Techniques

Normal, routine longitudinal, transverse, coronal, and oblique scans of vascular structures are used to produce adequate images. Doppler techniques supplement the routine examination by permitting blood flow within those vessels to be detected and characterized. Flow toward the transducer is positive, or above baseline, whereas flow away from the transducer is negative, or

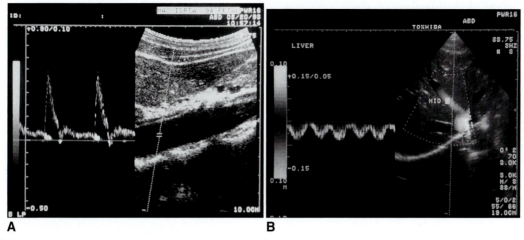

FIGURE 8-84 A, Doppler tracing of the abdominal aorta demonstrates a high systolic peak with a relatively low diastolic component on the spectral tracing. **B,** Pulsed wave (PW) Doppler tracing of the middle hepatic vein shows a continuous undulating low-flow profile representing blood flow from the hepatic vein into the inferior vena cava.

below baseline (Figure 8-84). Arterial flow pulsates with the cardiac cycle and shows its maximal peak during the systolic part of the cycle. Venous flow shows no pulsatility and has lower flow than arterial structures. A phasic pattern may be seen in the hepatic veins (near the heart) that is associated with overload of the right ventricle.

As seen in echocardiography, many abdominal vessels have characteristic waveforms. If the sample volume can be directed parallel to the flow, quantification of peak gradients can be estimated. However, given the tortuous course of most vascular structures, this can be very difficult.

Pulsed Doppler is the most common instrumentation used to evaluate abdominal flow patterns. This equipment uses combined real-time and pulsed or continuous wave Doppler. Pulsed Doppler allows placement of the small sample volume within the vascular structure of interest by means of a trackball.

Aorta

- Doppler flow in the pulsatile aorta demonstrates arterial signals in the patent lumen. If the vessel were occluded, no arterial signals would be recorded.
- Aortic dissection and pseudoaneurysms: Flow, often with two distinct patterns, can be seen in the true and false lumens by Doppler ultrasound. The development of a pseudoaneurysm as a complication of an aortic graft procedure may be difficult to determine if pulsations are present or transmitted through the aortic wall. Doppler ultrasound may be useful to detect flow within the pseudoaneurysm.

Inferior Vena Cava

- Decreased velocity: The Doppler waveform recorded in the inferior vena cava shows a lower flow than is found in arterial structures. The flow is increased in the presence of thrombus formation.

Portal Venous System

- Doppler flow patterns can be used to diagnose varices or collaterals in the **portal venous system.**
- Doppler flow patterns can be used to evaluate changes in flow patterns that occur in the course of portal hypertension.
- As liver function improves, normal hepatopetal flow is restored.
- If pressures worsen, shunting away from the liver may be increased.
- If a shunt is present in the porta hepatis, Doppler may be useful to determine the patency of the shunt.

Portal Hypertension

Portal hypertension is caused by increased resistance to venous flow through the liver. It is associated with cirrhosis, hepatic vein thrombosis, portal vein thrombosis, and thrombosis of the inferior vena cava. Ultrasound findings include dilation of the portal, splenic, and mesenteric veins; reversal of portal venous blood flow; and the development of **collateral vessels** (e.g., patent umbilical vein, gastric varices, splenorenal shunting).

The protocol for portal hypertension includes the following:

- Performing the routine abdominal imaging protocol
- Assessing for the presence of ascites
- Obtaining diameter measurements of the splenic and main portal veins on inspiration and expiration
- Assessing for the presence of collateral blood vessels (splenic hilum, porta hepatis, umbilical vein)

- Determining the flow direction of the portal veins (main, left, and right portal veins) and splenic and superior mesenteric veins
- Assessing for the presence of splenorenal shunting
- Assessing for patency of the umbilical vein
- Determining the patency and direction of flow in the IVC and hepatic veins
- Assessing and documenting the patency of surgically placed shunts

The Vascular System

Sandra L. Hagen-Ansert

Knowledge of the vascular structures within the abdomen, retroperitoneum, and pelvis is extremely useful for identifying specific organ structures. To understand the origin and anatomic variations of the major arterial and venous structures, the sonographer must be able to identify the anatomy correctly on the ultrasound image.

ANATOMY OF VASCULAR STRUCTURES

The function of the circulatory system, along with the heart and lymphatics, is to transport gases, nutrient materials, and other essential substances to the tissues, and subsequently to transport waste products from the cells to appropriate sites for excretion.

Blood is carried away from the heart by the arteries and is returned from the tissues to the heart by the veins. Arteries divide into progressively smaller branches, the smallest of which are the arterioles. These lead into the capillaries, which are minute vessels that branch and form a network where the exchange of materials between blood and tissue fluid takes place. After the blood passes

through the capillaries, it is collected in the small veins, or venules. These small vessels unite to form larger vessels that eventually return the blood to the heart for recirculation.

A typical artery in cross section consists of the following three layers (Figure 9-1):

- **Tunica intima** (inner layer), which itself consists of the following three layers: a layer of endothelial cells lining the arterial passage (lumen), a layer of delicate connective tissue, and an elastic layer made up of a network of elastic fibers
- **Tunica media** (middle layer), which consists of smooth muscle fibers with elastic and collagenous tissue
- **Tunica adventitia** (external layer), which consists of loose connective tissue with bundles of smooth muscle fibers and elastic tissue. The **vasa vasorum** comprises the tiny arteries and veins that supply the walls of blood vessels.

Specific differences exist between the arteries and the veins. The **arteries** are hollow elastic tubes that carry blood away from the heart. They are enclosed within a sheath that includes a vein and a nerve. The smaller arteries contain less elastic tissue and more smooth muscles than the larger arteries. The elasticity of the larger arteries is important in maintaining a steady blood flow. The abdominal aorta will not change in diameter with changes in respiration; however pulsation of blood flow that corresponds to the cardiac cycle will be noted.

The **veins** are hollow collapsible tubes with diminished tunica media that carry blood toward the heart. The veins appear collapsed because they have little elastic tissue or muscle within their walls. Veins have a larger total diameter than arteries, and they move blood more slowly. The veins contain special valves that prevent backflow and permit blood to flow in only one direction—toward the heart. Numerous valves are found within the extremities, especially the lower extremities, because flow must work against gravity. Venous return is also aided by muscle contraction, overflow from capillary beds, gravity, and suction from negative thoracic pressure. The sonographer may note that the inferior vena cava should dilate slightly with suspended respiration.

The **capillaries** are minute, hair-sized vessels that connect the arterial and venous systems. Their walls have only one layer. The cells and tissues of the body receive their nutrients from fluids passing through the capillary walls; at the same time, waste products from the cells

pass into the capillaries. Arteries do not always end in capillary beds; some end in anastomoses, which are end-to-end grafts between different vessels that equalize pressure over vessel length and provide alternative flow channels.

AORTA

The **aorta (Ao)** is the largest principal artery of the body. It may be divided into the following five sections: (1) root of the aorta, (2) ascending aorta and arch, (3) descending aorta, (4) abdominal aorta and abdominal aortic branches, and (5) bifurcation of the aorta into iliac arteries (Figure 9-2).

Root of the Aorta

The systemic circulation leaves the left ventricle of the heart by way of the aorta. The root of the aorta arises from the left ventricular outflow tract in the heart. The aortic root has three semilunar cusps that prevent blood from flowing back into the left ventricle. These cusps open with ventricular systole to allow blood to be ejected into the ascending aorta; the cusps are closed during ventricular diastole. The coronary arteries arise superiorly from the right and left coronary cusps to form the right and left coronary arteries, respectively. These coronary arteries further bifurcate to supply the vasculature of the cardiac structures. After the aorta arises from the left ventricle, it ascends posterior to the main pulmonary artery to form the ascending aorta.

Ascending Aorta

The ascending aorta arises a short distance from the ventricle and arches superiorly to form the aortic arch at the level of the sternoclavicular junction. Three arterial branches arise from the superior border of the aortic arch to supply the head, neck, and upper

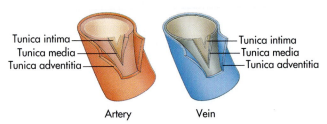

FIGURE 9-1 Cross section of an artery and vein showing the distinctions among the three layers of each vessel: tunica intima (inner layer), tunica media (middle layer), and tunica adventitia (external layer).

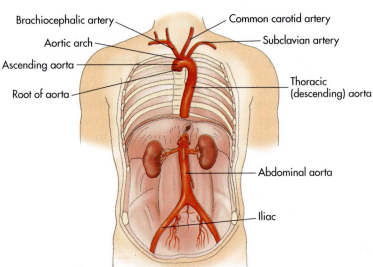

FIGURE 9-2 The aorta is divided into five sections: the aortic root, the ascending aorta, the aortic arch (brachiocephalic artery, common carotid artery, and subclavian artery), the thoracic (descending) artery, the abdominal aorta, with the bifurcation.

extremities: the brachiocephalic, left common carotid, and left subclavian arteries.

Descending Aorta

From the aortic arch, the aorta descends posteriorly along the back wall of the heart through the thoracic cavity, where it pierces the diaphragm to become the abdominal aorta. The descending (thoracic) aorta enters the abdomen through the aortic opening of the diaphragm anterior to the twelfth thoracic vertebra in the retroperitoneal space.

Abdominal Aorta

The abdominal aorta is the largest artery in the body that supplies blood to all visceral organs and to the legs. The aorta continues to flow in the retroperitoneal cavity anterior and slightly left of the vertebral column. The aorta lies posterior to the left lobe of the liver, the body of the pancreas, the gastroesophageal junction, the pylorus of the stomach, and the splenic vein (Figure 9-3). The diaphragmatic crura surround the aorta as it projects through the diaphragm into the abdominal cavity. The aorta is posterior to the superior and inferior mesenteric arteries and the left renal vein. Many branches arise from the abdominal aorta (i.e., celiac axis, superior mesenteric, inferior mesenteric, renal, suprarenal, and gonadal arteries). At the level of the fourth lumbar vertebra (near the umbilicus), the aorta bifurcates into the right and left common iliac arteries. The aorta has four branches that supply other visceral organs and the mesentery: the celiac trunk, the superior and inferior mesenteric arteries, and the renal arteries.

The diameter of the abdominal aorta measures less than 23 mm in men and less than 19 mm in women, with gradual tapering to 10 to 15 mm after it proceeds inferiorly to the bifurcation into the iliac arteries (Table

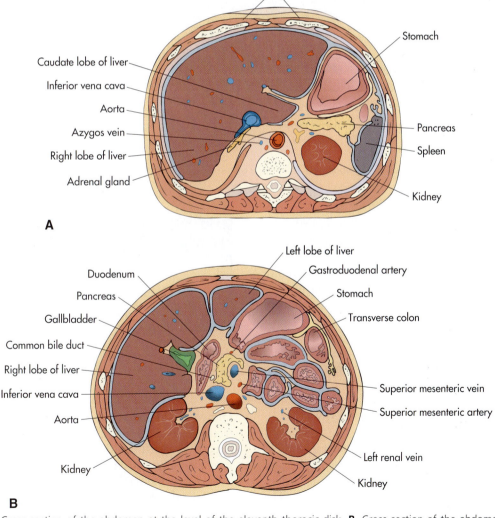

FIGURE 9-3 A, Cross section of the abdomen at the level of the eleventh thoracic disk. **B,** Cross section of the abdomen at the level of the second lumbar vertebra.

Continued

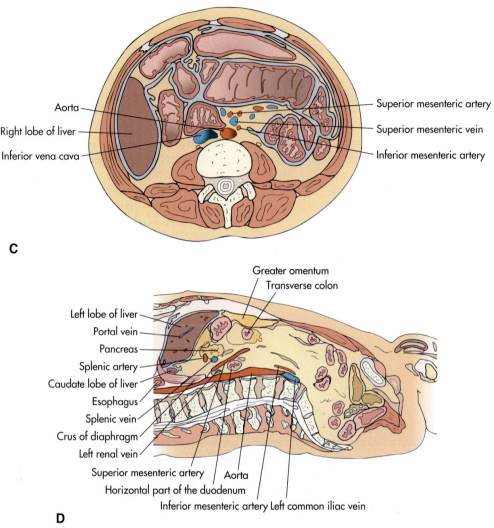

C

D

FIGURE 9-3, cont'd   C, Cross section of the abdomen at the level of the third lumbar disk. **D,** Midline sagittal section of the abdomen.

9-1). The size of the aorta will vary slightly according to body mass index; the larger the body size, the greater is the width of the aorta. It is also important to note that the aorta does change in size as we grow older; therefore an aorta in a younger adult measuring 1.8 cm may be increased to 2.27 cm by the time the adult reaches 60 years of age.

Generally speaking, a dilation (aneurysm) is considered when any abnormal bulging of the vessel is noted. The threshold for an aneurysm differs slightly for men (30 mm) and women (25.5 mm).

Abdominal Aortic Branches

The small phrenic arteries arise from the lateral walls of the aorta to supply the undersurface of the diaphragm. (Surgical intervention or trauma to the phrenic artery may cause limited movement of the diaphragm.) The celiac trunk is the first anterior branch of the aorta, arising 1 to 2 cm inferior to the diaphragm. The median arcuate ligament surrounds the aorta and has been

TABLE 9-1	Size of Abdominal Aorta and Iliac Branches	
	Men	**Women**
	Diameter ± SD, mm	**Diameter ± SD, mm**
Aorta	20.2 ± 2.5	17.0 ± 1.5
Common iliac artery	13.2 ± 2.0	12.0 ± 1.3
Common femoral artery	10.9 ± 1.5	9.6 ± 1.0

known to compress the celiac trunk. The short celiac trunk gives rise to three smaller vessels: the splenic, hepatic, and left gastric arteries (Figure 9-4). The superior mesenteric artery is the second anterior branch, arising approximately 2 cm from the celiac trunk. The right renal artery and the left renal artery are lateral branches that arise just inferior to the superior mesenteric artery. The small inferior mesenteric artery arises anteriorly near the bifurcation. The distribution of these

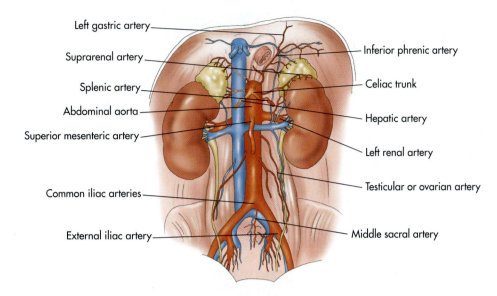

Left gastric artery

Suprarenal artery

Splenic artery

Abdominal aorta

Superior mesenteric artery

Common iliac arteries

External iliac artery

Inferior phrenic artery

Celiac trunk

Hepatic artery

Left renal artery

Testicular or ovarian artery

Middle sacral artery

FIGURE 9-4 The abdominal arterial vascular system and its tributaries.

branch arteries is to the visceral organs and the mesentery.

Common Iliac Arteries

The **common iliac arteries** arise at the bifurcation of the abdominal aorta at the fourth lumbar vertebra (near the superior sacrum). These vessels further divide into the internal and external iliac arteries. The internal iliac artery enters the pelvis anterior to the sacroiliac joint, at which point it is crossed anteriorly by the ureter. It divides into anterior and posterior branches to supply the pelvic viscera, peritoneum, buttocks, and sacral canal. The external iliac artery runs along the medial border of the psoas muscle, following the pelvic brim. The inferior epigastric and deep circumflex iliac branches branch off before they pass under the inguinal ligament to become the femoral artery. The portion of the femoral artery posterior to the knee is the popliteal artery. This artery further divides into the anterior and posterior tibial arteries.

Sonographic Findings. The abdominal aorta is usually one of the easiest abdominal structures to image with ultrasound because of the marked change in acoustic impedance between its elastic walls and blood-filled lumen. Sonography provides the diagnostic information needed to create an image of the entire abdominal aorta, to assess its diameter, and to visualize the presence of thrombus, calcification, or dissection within the walls. Multiple acoustic windows may be utilized to image the aorta. The traditional view is performed with the patient in the supine position. However, if bowel or gas is overlying the aorta, roll the patient into a right lateral decubitus and scan along the left lateral flank with the transducer directed toward the spine. (Remember, the aorta will be seen directly anterior to the spine.)

As was previously stated, the patient is routinely scanned in the supine position. Gas-filled or barium-filled loops of bowel may prevent adequate visualization of the aorta, but this can sometimes be overcome by applying gentle pressure with the transducer or by changing the angle of the transducer to move the gas out of the way. Other visualization problems encountered in the abdominal aortic ultrasound may occur with increased amounts of mesenteric fat in obese patients. Patients should not be imaged 12 to 24 hours after an endoscopic evaluation, as air may still be a residual impairment to adequate visualization.

Longitudinal scans should be made beginning at the midline with a slight angulation of the transducer to the left—from the xiphoid to well below the level of bifurcation (Figure 9-5). In the normal individual, the luminal dimension of the aorta gradually tapers as it proceeds distally in the abdomen. A low to medium gain should be used to demonstrate the walls of the aorta without "noisy" artifactual internal echoes. These weak echoes may result from increased gain, reverberation from the anterior abdominal wall fascia or musculature, or poor lateral resolution. These factors result in echoes being recorded at the same level as those from soft tissue that surround the vessel lumen, particularly if the vessels are smaller in diameter than the transducer. Try to use different techniques of breath holding to eliminate these artifactual echoes. Sometimes, increased gentle pressure may help displace bowel gas or may compress fatty tissue so that the transducer will be closer to the abdominal aorta. If the abdomen is very concave, the patient may be instructed to extend his abdomen ("push the abdomen muscle out") so as to provide a better scanning plane.

Because the aorta follows the anterior course of the vertebral column, it is important that the transducer also

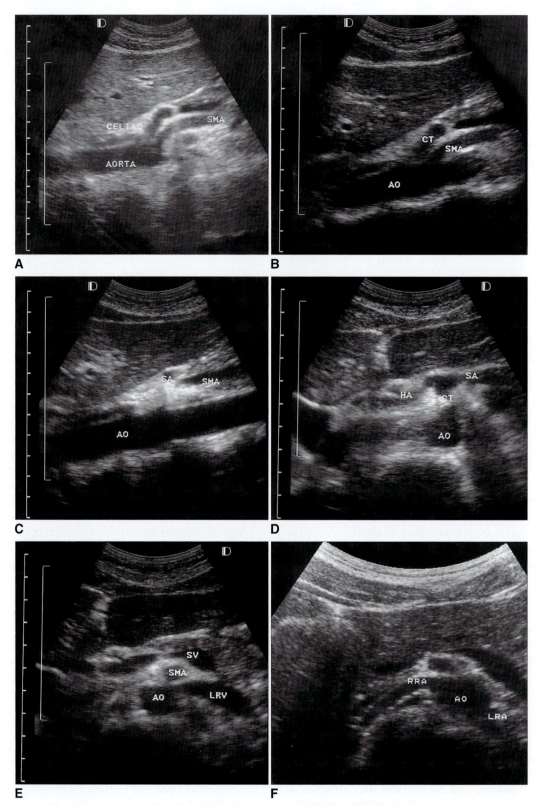

FIGURE 9-5 Normal aorta protocol. **A** through **C,** Longitudinal images. **D** through **F,** Transverse images at level of celiac trunk *(CT)*. *AO,* Aorta; *HA,* hepatic artery; *LRA,* left renal artery; *LRV,* left renal vein; *RRA,* right renal artery; *SA,* splenic artery; *SMA,* superior mesenteric artery; *SV,* splenic vein.

follow a perpendicular path along the entire curvature of the spine. The anterior and posterior walls of the aorta should be easily seen as two thin pulsatile parallel lines. This facilitates measuring the anteroposterior diameter of the aorta, which in most institutions is done from the leading outer edge of the anterior wall to the leading inner edge of the posterior wall.

In the transverse plane, the aorta is imaged as a circular structure anterior to the spine and slightly to the left of the midline. In some cases, the transverse diameter of the aorta differs from that found in longitudinal measurements; thus it is important to identify the vessel in two dimensions. Multiple scans should be made from the xiphoid to the bifurcation to record the dimensions of the aorta at the diaphragm, just above the renal vessels, just inferior to the renal vessels, and at the level of the bifurcation.

In the longitudinal plane, the aorta is imaged as a long tubular structure just anterior to the spine. The landmarks of the left lobe of the liver and the gastroesophageal junction may be seen anterior to the aorta.

If the patient has a very tortuous aorta, scans may be difficult to obtain in a single sagittal plane. During scanning in the longitudinal plane, the upper portion of the abdominal aorta may be well visualized, but the lower portion may be out of the plane of view. In this case, the sonographer should obtain a complete scan of the upper segment and then should concentrate fully on the lower segment. In some patients, the aorta may stretch from the far right of the abdomen to the far left.

Iliac Arteries. To better visualize the iliac arteries at the aortic bifurcation, use a slight lateral decubitus position. The patient should be rotated 5 to 10 degrees from the true lateral position. The patient should be examined in deep inspiration, which projects the liver and diaphragm into the abdominal cavity and provides an acoustic window in which to image the vascular structures. Slight medial to lateral angulation of the transducer may be necessary to image the bifurcation in the longitudinal plane. With the patient rolled into this oblique plane, the inferior vena cava may be visualized anterior to the aorta. This view is also useful to identify renal vessels as they project from the lateral walls of the aorta with the aid of color Doppler.

The iliac arteries should measure less than 1.2 cm in transverse anteroposterior (AP) diameter. It is common for the iliac arteries to be dilated if an aortic aneurysm is present, as most aneurysms develop inferior to the renal vessels near the bifurcation of the aorta. If the iliac artery measures greater than 3 cm, it will be considered for surgical repair.

Pathology of the Aorta

The sonographer may be asked to evaluate the abdominal aorta for several clinical reasons: pulsatile abdominal mass, abdominal pain radiating to the back, an abdomi-

nal bruit, or hemodynamic compromise in the lower legs. The arterial system may be affected by atheroma, aneurysm, connective tissue disorder, rupture, thrombosis, or infection.

The sonographer has several objectives to meet when performing a complete evaluation of the abdominal aorta. First, the entire aorta should be imaged in at least two planes (transverse and longitudinal) with appropriate measurements of the aortic diameter in the proximal, mid, and distal segments. The real advantage for the sonographer is the ability to "follow" the vessel with the transducer. If the vessel is tortuous, the transducer may be turned to follow the course of the artery. The size of the aorta increases up to 25% in the seventh and eighth decades.

It is important to distinguish between aortic ectasia and an aneurysm of the aorta. Ectasia implies the diffuse dilation of a vessel, whereas an abdominal aortic aneurysm is a region of focal enlargement. Ectasia occurs when the aorta increases both in transverse diameter and in vertical length, which causes the distal aorta to "kink," usually anterior and to the left. The aorta may be "folded," or tortuous, in its course, providing a challenge to the sonographer to follow the vessel in its entirety.

Atheromatous Disease. Arteriosclerosis, or atheroma, is a vascular wall disorder characterized by the presence of lipid deposits in the intima. Atheromatous plaque is a soft material that can break off into the lumen to create an embolus or local thrombus. Over time, these plaques build up along the weaker wall of the vessel and cause narrowing. This usually occurs inferior to the renal vessels. It is found more often in late middle-aged men than women and involves the aorta, often with extension into the common iliac arteries. The disease sometimes involves the ascending and descending aorta. When pain is present in the lower limbs, the peripheral vessels should be evaluated to rule out emboli or stenoses. Arteriosclerosis is most commonly associated with the development of an aneurysm (Figure 9-6).

Abdominal Aortic Aneurysm. An **aneurysm** is defined as a permanent localized dilation of an artery, with an

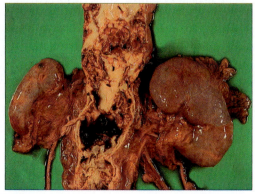

FIGURE 9-6 Atherosclerotic aneurysm with severe atherosclerosis of the aorta.

increase in diameter of greater than 1.5 times its normal diameter. Box 9-1 summarizes the features of abdominal aortic aneurysms. The normal diameter for an artery depends on several factors, including age, gender, and blood pressure. The diagnosis of an aneurysm depends on a comparison of the aortic diameter of the suspicious area versus that of the normal area of the vessel above and below that area.

Assessment is often made by physical examination of the abdomen, where a pulsatile mass slightly to the left of the midline, between the umbilicus and the xiphoid process, may be palpated.

Risk factors that contribute to the development of an aneurysm include tobacco use, hypertension, and vascular disease. Other risk factors include chronic obstructive pulmonary disease and positive family history for abdominal aortic aneurysm.

Abdominal aortic aneurysm studies suggest a 5% to 10% prevalence in men over the age of 60 in the United States. Visualization of the abdominal aorta has traditionally been an asset in diagnosing the clinical problem. Ultrasound is very capable of demonstrating abnormalities in the diameter, length, and extent of the abdominal aortic aneurysm.

A number of factors may cause the development of an aortic aneurysm:

1. Atherosclerosis
2. Trauma (following transection)
3. Congenital defects (aortic sinus, post coarctation of the aorta, ductus diverticulum)
4. Syphilis (involving the ascending aorta and arch)
5. Mycosis (fungal dissection)
6. Cystic medial necrosis (e.g., Marfan's syndrome)
7. Inflammation of media and adventitia (e.g., rheumatic fever, polychondritis, ankylosing spondylitis)
8. Increased pressure (systemic hypertension, aortic valve stenosis)
9. Abnormal volume load (severe aortic regurgitation)

Clinical Symptoms. Symptoms may vary in the patient with an abdominal aneurysm. Approximately 30% to 60% of patients with an abdominal aortic aneurysm are asymptomatic, and the enlarged vessel is found during routine physical examination or during an unrelated radiologic or surgical procedure.

Symptoms of the aortic aneurysm may result from rupture or expansion of the vessel. The enlarged vessel may produce symptoms by impinging on adjacent structures, or it may occlude a vessel by direct pressure or thrombus with resulting embolism. The large aneurysm may rupture into the peritoneal cavity or the retroperitoneum, causing intense back pain and a drop in hematocrit. Patients may present with satiety (becoming full easily) or nausea and vomiting. Abrupt onset of severe, constant pain in the abdomen, back, or flank that is unrelieved by positional changes is characteristic of rapid expansion or rupture of an aneurysm. Other complications may include dissection, thrombosis, distal embolism, infection, and obstruction and invasion of adjacent structures. Commonly, branch artery occlusions or stenoses may be seen in the inferior mesenteric artery or renal arteries.

The patient who presents with an aneurysm most likely has many other medical problems as well. It is important that the clinician be able to examine the size of the aneurysm noninvasively and follow it sequentially over a structured time period by sonography. Aneurysms that measure less than 4 cm in diameter are followed every 6 months, with intervention if the patient becomes symptomatic. It is also important in these cases to mark on the films the exact location of the aneurysm and measurements so that follow-up information will be accurate. In patients with aneurysms ranging from 4 to 5 cm in diameter, surgical intervention may be suggested if the patient is in good health. Patients with aneurysms ranging from 5 to 6 cm may benefit from surgical repair, especially if they have other factors for rupture (e.g., hypertension, smoking, chronic obstructive pulmonary disease). Patients at highest risk are those with aneurysms larger than 6 to 7 cm. The risk increases with age and other medical problems.

Surgical intervention also considers whether associated renal and iliac involvement is present, with occlusive disease or in the aneurysm process. Measuring the length of the infrarenal aortic neck is important to help determine the best surgical approach (retroperitoneal vs. transabdominal) and the location of the aortic cross clamp. Endovascular stent grafts for treatment are a less invasive approach to the repair of an aneurysm. The graft is placed through two small incisions in the abdomen.

Three primary factors are related to the growth rate of abdominal aneurysms: the initial size of the aortic aneurysm, the presence of cardiac disease, and the presence of beta-adrenergic blockade (blood pressure–lowering medications) (Box 9-2).

Another important consideration is the relationship of the aneurysm to the renal arteries. Thus not only the diameter, but also the longitudinal extent of the aneurysm as it relates to the origin of the renal vessels, should

BOX 9-2 Growth Patterns for Abdominal Aneurysms

The normal aortic lumen diameter measures less than 3 cm. With careful sonographic technique, ultrasound has an accuracy rate of 98.8% for detecting aneurysms. Aneurysms smaller than 6 cm show a very slow growth pattern (<0.2 to 0.5 cm/yr), so patients are followed at 6 months for larger aneurysms and at 12 months for smaller aneurysms. The following information has been found on follow-up study of aneurysms:

- Seventy-five percent of patients have a 1-year survival rate if the aneurysm measures less than 6 cm.
- Fifty percent of patients have a 1-year survival rate if the aneurysm is larger than 6 cm.
- Twenty-five percent of patients have a 1-year survival rate if the aneurysm is larger than 7 cm.
- A 75% risk of fatal rupture is present if the aneurysm is larger than 7 cm.
- One percent of aneurysms smaller than 5 cm rupture.
- Operative mortality before rupture is 5%, but with emergency surgery, mortality increases to 50%.

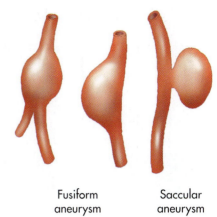

Fusiform aneurysm   Saccular aneurysm

FIGURE 9-7 Fusiform and saccular aneurysms.

be measured. Often bowel gas impairs adequate visualization of the renal arteries, and a more indirect method must be used to locate the origin of the superior mesenteric artery and renal arteries. Color Doppler may be useful for producing an image of arterial flow from the lateral margins of the abdominal aorta to the kidneys.

Classification of Aneurysms. Histologically, the aneurysm may be classified as a true aneurysm (lined by all three layers of the aorta) or as a false aneurysm (pseudoaneurysm) (not lined by all three layers). A **true aneurysm** forms when the tensile strength of the wall decreases. A small percentage of true aneurysms occur secondary to underlying diseases such as Marfan's syndrome, Ehlers-Danlos syndrome, familial aortic dissection, annulo-aortic ectasia, and intimomedial mucoid degeneration. In the pseudoaneurysm, blood escapes through a hole in the intima of the vessel wall, but is contained by the deeper layers of the aorta or by adjacent tissue. A **pseudoaneurysm** is a pulsatile hematoma that results from leakage of blood into the soft tissue abutting the punctured artery, with subsequent fibrous encapsulation and failure of the vessel wall to heal. With color Doppler, blood can be seen to flow into the protuberance during systole and out during diastole. These events can occur after trauma to the vessel as a result of accident or surgery, or after an interventional cardiac catheterization or angiography procedure.

Ultrasound evaluation of the pulsatile mass is conducted, with color Doppler showing communication between the artery and the vein. Compression of the mass with a linear transducer at 20-minute compression intervals may allow the lesion to close if the communication is small. Sometimes it takes several compressions (20 minutes on and 20 minutes off) to completely close

the communication. Color flow allows the sonographer to see whether the communication is closed. Pseudoaneurysms that are not closed require surgical intervention, as they may become a source of emboli, the site of increased chance of infection secondary to abnormal communication of blood flow, or a cause of local pressure effects. In addition, they can rupture, which may result in exsanguination.

Descriptive Terms for an Abdominal Aortic Aneurysm. An aneurysm may be described as fusiform, bulbous, saccular, or dumbbell (Figure 9-7). The idiopathic abdominal aneurysm is a true aneurysm that most commonly develops inferorenally (in more than 95% of patients). It usually begins below the renal arteries (inferior to the superior mesenteric artery) and extends to the bifurcation of the aorta at the iliac arteries (Figure 9-8).

The most common presentation of an atherosclerotic aneurysm is a **fusiform aneurysm** of the distal aorta at the aortic bifurcation (Figure 9-9). The fusiform aneurysm represents a gradual transition between normal and abnormal and extends over the length of the aorta to resemble a "football-like" shape. Sonography displays atherosclerosis of the vessel as decreased pulsations of the aortic walls, with bright echoes reflecting the degree of thickening and calcification. These aneurysms often extend into the iliac vessels in the pelvis.

The term *bulbous* describes a sharp junction between normal and abnormal. An aneurysm may be bulbous and saccular.

A s**accular aneurysm** shows a sudden transition between normal and abnormal and is somewhat spherical and larger (5 to 10 cm) than fusiform aneurysms. This type of aneurysm is connected to the vascular lumen by a mouth that varies in size but may be as large as an aneurysm. It may be partially or completely filled with mural thrombus (Figure 9-10). The sonographer must carefully follow the course of such an aneurysm to differentiate it from a retroperitoneal mass or lymphadenopathy. Pulsations are usually diminished secondary to clot formation.

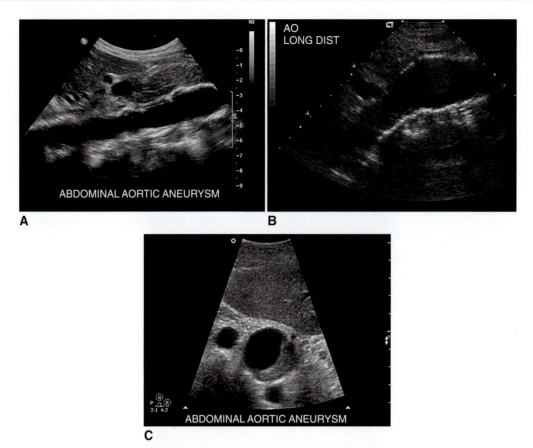

A

B

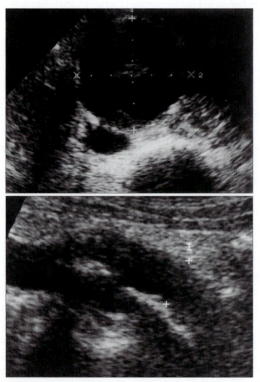

C

FIGURE 9-8 Abdominal aortic aneurysm. **A,** Longitudinal image of a small abdominal aortic aneurysm extending superior to the bifurcation. **B,** Sagittal image of a large abdominal aortic aneurysm; the largest diameter of the aneurysm should be measured. **C,** Multiple echoes within represent thrombus formation.

FIGURE 9-9 Fusiform aortic aneurysm with extension into the iliac arteries.

The term *dumbbell* applies to the figure-of-eight appearance of the aneurysm, where one may see more than one protrusion of the vessel.

The aneurysm may extend into the iliac arteries. The sonographer should examine both iliac arteries in at least two planes. At the level of the bifurcation, the iliac vessels may be seen as circular, pulsatile vessels just anterior to the spine. The oblique longitudinal scan is used to produce an image of the vessel in its entire length. Normal iliac arteries measure less than 1 cm in diameter.

Inflammatory Aortic Aneurysm. This type of aneurysm is a variant in which the wall of the aneurysm is thickened and surrounded by fibrosis and adhesions of a type similar to those found in retroperitoneal fibrosis. These patients present with a higher surgical risk. Clinically, they present with pain that may mimic a retroperitoneal hemorrhage.

Rupture of Aortic Aneurysm. The rupture of an aortic aneurysm is catastrophic, with a mortality rate of 50%. An aneurysm measuring greater than 5 cm in anteroposterior diameter has a 25% cumulative incidence of rupture over 8 years. The classic symptoms of a ruptured aortic aneurysm are excruciating abdominal pain, shock, and an expanding abdominal mass. Rupture of the aorta is a surgical emergency, and computed

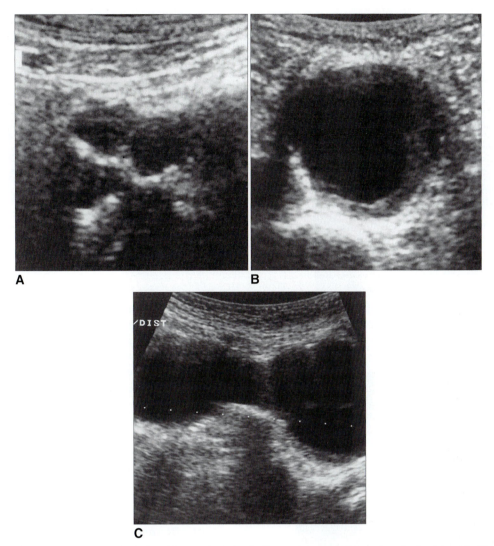

A   **B**

C

FIGURE 9-10 Saccular aneurysms are spherical and larger than the fusiform aneurysm. This patient had a "dumbbell" type of aneurysm, more typically seen in a patient with cystic medial necrosis. **A,** Sagittal view. **B,** Transverse at the umbilicus. **C,** Transverse at the umbilicus with caudal angulation.

tomography (CT) is the first choice for imaging to obtain the most information in the shortest time. CT is not hampered by bowel gas and allows a rapid overview of the abdominal pelvic structures. The operative mortality for such ruptures may exceed 40% to 60%. The rupture may extend into the perirenal space with displacement of renal hilar vessels, effacement of the aortic border, and silhouetting of the lateral psoas border at the level of the kidney. The most common site for rupture is the lateral wall inferior to the renal vessels. Hemorrhage into the posterior pararenal space accounts for loss of visualization of the lateral psoas muscle merging inferior to the kidney and may also displace the kidney.

A large aneurysm may compress its neighboring structures. Compression of the common bile duct may cause obstruction; compression of the renal artery can cause hypertension and renal ischemia. Retroperitoneal fibrosis with an aneurysm may involve the ureter, causing hydronephrosis. The left kidney is more frequently

affected than the right. The iliac aneurysm may rupture into the rectosigmoid colon, iliac vein, or ureter.

Sonographic Findings. The normal measurement for an adult abdominal aorta is less than 3 cm, with measurement taken perpendicular to the vessel from outer layer-to-outer layer walls. (This measurement correlates with the measurement made by the surgeon.) The sonographer should search for focal dilation of the abdominal aorta or lack of normal tapering distally. The anterior and posterior borders are often better imaged than the lateral borders. The adventitia is slightly echogenic, but with increased atherosclerosis, the walls may become increasingly echogenic with calcification. When an aneurysm is detected, the presence of a mural thrombus should be evaluated. A mural thrombus usually occurs along an anterior or anterolateral wall. The thrombus is often poorly attached and friable and may be a source for distal emboli. Thrombus within an aneurysm is shown ultrasonically as medium- to low-level echoes

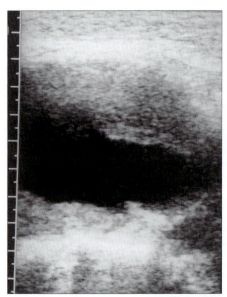

FIGURE 9-11 Longitudinal image of a large aortic aneurysm with thrombus along the anterior and posterior walls. The true lumen is anechoic.

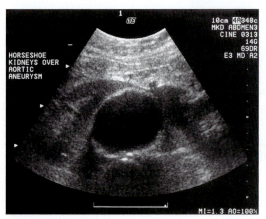

FIGURE 9-12 Transverse image of a patient with a horseshoe kidney and abdominal aortic aneurysm. The isthmus of the kidneys is shown draping anterior to the aorta.

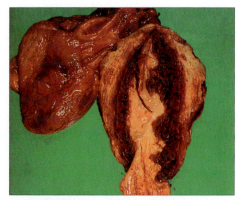

FIGURE 9-13 Dissecting aneurysm of the thoracic aorta. The blood has filled the space formed by the separation of the intima and media of the aorta.

(Figures 9-11 and 9-12). Generally, increased sensitivity is likely to highlight the low-level echoes from the thrombus. These echoes should be seen in both planes on more than one scan to be separated from low-level reverberation echoes. A chronic thrombotic clot is easier to see with sonography because of the bright calcification that appears as thick, echogenic echoes, sometimes with posterior shadowing. The amount of thrombus in a vessel has no relation to the risk of rupture.

The sonographer should note the maximum length, width, and transverse dimension of the aortic aneurysm. Documentation of the shape (fusiform, bulbous, saccular, or dumbbell) and location of the aneurysm in relation to the renal arteries is important. Extension of the aneurysm into the iliac arteries should also be noted. Measurements of length × width × height should be included in the report. A description of wall thickening,

the presence of calcification, blood flow, soft plaque, or calcified plaque should also be included in the report. Careful evaluation of the presence or absence of an aortic dissection should be noted (see below). Because the aneurysm may often affect the renal vessels, both kidneys should be analyzed. (Measure the size, and exclude pelvocaliectasis.) If hypertrophy of one or both kidneys occurs, a full Doppler evaluation of the renal vessels should be conducted to rule out renal stenosis.

A rare condition is the development of a mycotic aneurysm secondary to infection. The most common infections result from septic emboli, streptococci, staphylococci, and *Salmonella.* The infection may produce a focal abscess that appears as a complex fluid collection with irregular borders.

Aortic Dissection. A defect in the vessel intimal wall must exist along with internal weakness for a dissection to occur (Figure 9-13). Dissection of the aorta (Type II) may occur secondary to **cystic medial necrosis** (weakening of the arterial wall), to hypertension, or to the inherited disease **Marfan's syndrome.** (Individuals with this disorder are extremely tall, lanky, and double-jointed; a progressive stretching disorder exists in all arterial vessels, especially in the aorta, causing abnormal dilation, weakened walls, and eventual dissection, rupture, or both.) Color flow Doppler may be used to detect flow into the false channel.

Three classifications of aortic dissection are based on the DeBakey model (Figure 9-14). Types I and II involve the ascending aorta and the aortic arch; Type III involves the descending aorta at a level inferior to the left subclavian artery. A high incidence of mortality is associated with Type I and II dissections because of possible obstruction at the origin of the coronary arteries and possible obstruction of blood into the head and neck vessels. The lowest mortality rate is associated with the Type III dissection, which begins inferior to the left subclavian artery with possible extension into the abdominal aorta.

The Type I dissection begins at the root of the aorta and may extend the entire length of the arch, descending to the aorta and into the abdominal aorta. This is the most dangerous, especially if the dissection spirals around the aorta, cutting off the blood supply to the coronary, carotid, brachiocephalic, and subclavian vessels. The third type of dissection (Type III) begins at the lower end of the descending aorta and extends into the abdominal aorta. This may be critical if the dissection spirals around to impede the flow of blood into the renal vessels. Less than 5% of dissections occur primarily in the abdomen.

A **dissecting aneurysm** may be detected by ultrasound and usually displays one or more clinical signs and symptoms. The typical patient is 40 to 60 years old and hypertensive; males predominate over females. The patient is usually known to have an aneurysm, and sudden, excruciating chest pain radiating to the back may develop as the result of a dissection. These patients may go into shock very quickly, and CT is generally ordered to obtain the most information in the shortest amount of time. However, the patient who presents with some of these symptoms and is stable may have a slow leak aneurysm. These patients are appropriately imaged with sonography. The sonographer should look for a dissection "flap" or recent channel, with or without frank aneurysmal dilation. This flap is well demonstrated

with M-mode as a fluttering within the lumen at different phases of the cardiac cycle. The dissection of blood occurs along the laminar planes of the aortic media with formation of a blood-filled channel within the aortic wall (see Figure 9-13). Color Doppler will demonstrate flow in both channels (true and false lumens) with the flow rate differing between the channels.

When the dissection develops, hemorrhage occurs between the middle and outer thirds of the media. An intimal tear is considered if the tear is found in the ascending portion of the arch. This type of dissection extends proximally toward the heart and distally, sometimes to the iliac and femoral arteries. A small number of dissections do not have an obvious intimal tear. Extravasation may completely encircle the aorta or may extend along one segment of its circumference, or the aneurysm may rupture into any of the body cavities.

Aortic Graft. An abdominal aortic aneurysm may be surgically repaired with a flexible graft material attached to the end of the remaining aorta. The synthetic material used for a graft produces bright textured echo reflections compared with those from normal aortic walls. After surgery, the attached walls may swell at the site of attachment and form another aneurysm or pseudoaneurysm (Figures 9-15 and 9-16). Other complications of prosthetic grafts include hematoma, infection, and degeneration of graft material.

Newer surgical techniques now repair the aneurysm with an endovascular graft treatment. The graft may be anastomosed in an end-to-side or end-to-end manner. These grafts would be placed within the aorta, at the level of the aorta and iliac artery, or within the femoral artery. Further development in techniques has placed the grafts in the aortofemoral and juxtarenal positions. Complications of these grafts resulted in endoleak formations that were immediate, without outflow, and persistent. The type of graft used, the technique of graft insertion, and the aortic anatomic features all affected the rate of endoleaks.

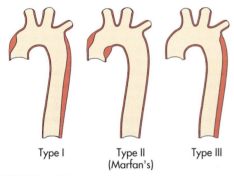

Type I   Type II (Marfan's)   Type III

FIGURE 9-14 Aortic dissection: Types I, II, and III.

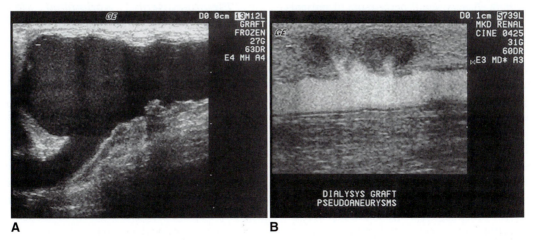

A   B

FIGURE 9-15 Complications of graft repair of aneurysms may result in new aneurysm formation **(A)** or pseudoaneurysm formation **(B)**.

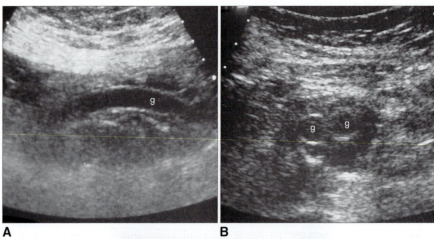

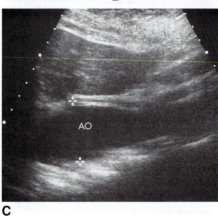

FIGURE 9-16 A through **C,** Images of a postoperative patient with an aortic graft stent in place (g).

The sonographer should carefully examine the upper and lower ends of the anastomoses with both real-time and color Doppler. During evaluation of the graft, the sonographer should look for stenosis at the ends of the graft, aneurysm formation, or pseudoaneurysm development. Doppler evaluation of the distal vessels should be conducted to ensure that adequate blood flow is available. Fluid collections (i.e., hematoma, lymphocele, seroma, or abscess formation) may develop at the graft site.

Iliac Aneurysm. A very small percentage of patients (<5%) with an abdominal aneurysm will also have an iliac aneurysm. These may occur at the bifurcation of the common iliac artery or in the external iliac just distal to the bifurcation.

Thoracic Aneurysm. If an aneurysm extends beyond the diaphragm into the thoracic aorta, it may be difficult to follow with ultrasound because of lung interference with the sound beam. Several attempts may be necessary to demonstrate this thoracic aneurysm. The transducer can be sharply angled in the longitudinal plane from the anterior abdomen at the xiphoid toward the sternal notch to allow visualization of the distal thoracic aorta. Another technique allows the sonographer to place the transducer along the left of the sternum to make a longitudinal parasternal scan over the long axis of the heart.

The thoracic aorta should be seen as the pulsatile structure posterior to the cardiac structures. A third alternative is to scan posteriorly along the patient's back to the left of the spine with the patient sitting upright or prone. The transducer should be angled slightly medially and placed in a sagittal plane along the left intercostal space. This is very effective if the thoracic aorta is deviated slightly to the left of the spine. Scalloped reverberations from the ribs will be recorded, with the luminal echoes of the thoracic aorta directly posterior.

"Pseudo-Pulsatile" Abdominal Masses. Masses other than an aortic aneurysm that can simulate a pulsatile abdominal mass include retroperitoneal tumor, huge fibroid uterus, or para-aortic nodes. Because the mass is adjacent to the aorta, pulsations are transmitted from the aorta to the mass. Next to an abdominal aneurysm, the most common cause for a pulsatile abdominal mass is enlarged retroperitoneal lymph nodes. This mass is usually the result of lymphoma in the middle-aged patient. On ultrasound, the nodes are homogeneous masses surrounding the aorta. The aortic wall may be poorly defined because of the close acoustic impedance of the nodes and the aorta. The sonographer should also look for splenomegaly.

A retroperitoneal sarcoma may present as a pulsatile mass; it may extend into the root of the mesentery and give rise to a larger intraperitoneal component. The echodensity depends on the tissue type that predominates; fatty lesions are more echodense than fibrous or myomatous lesions.

Arteriovenous Fistulas. An **arteriovenous fistula** is not a common finding with ultrasound. Most fistulas are acquired secondary to trauma. Some may develop as a complication of arteriosclerotic aortic aneurysms.

Clinical signs that the patient may have an arteriovenous fistula include low back and abdominal pain, progressive cardiac decompensation, a pulsatile abdominal mass associated with a bruit, and massive swelling of the lower trunk and lower extremities. Clinical signs are explained on the basis of the altered hemodynamics produced by a high-velocity shunt leading to increased blood volume, venous pressure, and cardiac output with cardiac failure and cardiomegaly.

If lower trunk and leg edema is present, along with a dilated inferior vena cava, an arteriovenous fistula should be suspected. If the fistula is large, the vein becomes very distended. A normal inferior vena cava measures less than 2.0 cm in its AP dimension. Right-sided heart disease or failure may also cause inferior vena cava distention.

Anterior Branches of the Abdominal Aorta

Celiac Trunk. The celiac trunk originates within the first 2 cm from the diaphragm (Figure 9-17). It is surrounded by the liver, spleen, inferior vena cava, and pancreas. After arising from the anterior wall, it immediately branches into the following three vessels: common hepatic, left gastric, and splenic arteries.

Common Hepatic Artery. The **common hepatic artery** arises from the celiac trunk and courses to the right of the abdomen at almost a 90-degree angle. At this point, it branches into the proper hepatic artery and the gastroduodenal artery. The gastroduodenal artery courses along the upper border of the head of the pancreas, behind the posterior layer of the peritoneal bursa,

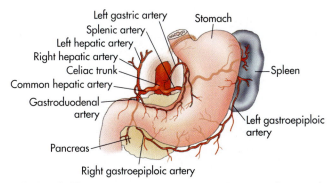

FIGURE 9-17 Celiac artery and its branches. The celiac trunk originates within the first 2 cm of the abdominal aorta and immediately branches into the left gastric, splenic, and common hepatic arteries.

to the upper margin of the superior part of the duodenum, which forms the lower boundary of the epiploic foramen. The duodenum and parts of the stomach are supplied by the **gastroduodenal artery (GDA)** and the **right gastric artery (RGA)** (see Figure 9-17). Along with the hepatic duct and the portal vein, the common hepatic artery then ascends into the liver (through the porta hepatis), which it divides into two branches: the right and left hepatic arteries.

Left and Right Hepatic Arteries. The **left hepatic artery (LHA)** is a small branch supplying the caudate and left lobes of the liver. The **right hepatic artery (RHA)** supplies the gallbladder via the cystic artery and the liver.

Left Gastric Artery. The **left gastric artery (LGA)** is a small branch of the celiac trunk, passing anterior, cephalic, and left to reach the esophagus and then descending along the lesser curvature of the stomach (see Figure 9-17). It supplies the lower third of the esophagus and the upper right of the stomach.

Splenic Artery. The **splenic artery (SA)** is the largest of the three branches of the celiac trunk (see Figure 9-17). From its origin, the artery takes a somewhat tortuous course horizontally to the left as it forms the superior border of the pancreas. At a variable distance from the spleen, it divides into two branches. One of these branches, the left gastroepiploic artery, runs caudally into the greater omentum toward the right gastroepiploic artery. The other courses in a cephalic direction and divides into the short gastric artery, which supplies the fundus of the stomach, and into a number of splenic branches, which supply the spleen.

Several smaller arterial branches originate at the splenic artery as it courses through the upper border of the pancreas: the dorsal pancreatic, great pancreatic, and caudal pancreatic arteries. The dorsal or superior pancreatic artery originates from the beginning of the splenic artery or from the hepatic artery, celiac trunk, or aorta. It runs behind and within the substance of the pancreas, dividing into right and left branches. The left branch is the transverse pancreatic artery. The right branch constitutes an anastomotic vessel to the anterior pancreatic arch and also a branch to the uncinate process.

The great pancreatic artery originates from the splenic artery farther to the left and passes downward, dividing into branches that anastomose with the transverse or inferior pancreatic artery. The caudal pancreatic artery supplies the tail of the pancreas and divides into branches that anastomose with terminal branches of the transverse pancreatic artery. The transverse pancreatic artery courses behind the body and tail of the pancreas close to the lower pancreatic border. It may originate from or communicate with the superior mesenteric artery.

The distribution of the celiac trunk vessels is to the liver, spleen, stomach, pancreas, and duodenum.

▶ **Sonographic Findings.** The celiac trunk may be visualized sonographically on transverse or longitudinal images (see Figure 9-5). It is usually seen as a small vascular structure, arising anteriorly from the abdominal aorta just below the diaphragm. Because it is only 1 to 2 cm long, it is sometimes difficult to record unless the area near the midline of the aorta is carefully examined. Sometimes the celiac trunk can be seen to extend in a cephalic rather than a caudal presentation. The superior mesenteric artery is just inferior to the origin of the celiac trunk. The superior mesenteric artery may be used as a landmark in locating the celiac trunk. Transversely, one can differentiate the celiac trunk as the "wings of a seagull," arising with its short trunk before dividing into the "wings" of the hepatic and splenic arteries (Figure 9-18).

The splenic artery may be seen to flow directly from the celiac trunk toward the spleen (Figure 9-19). Because it is so tortuous, it may be difficult to follow on the transverse scan. Generally, small pieces of the splenic artery are visible as the artery weaves in and out of the left upper quadrant.

The hepatic artery can be seen to branch anterior and to the right of the celiac trunk, where it then divides into the right and left hepatic arteries in the liver (Figure 9-20).

The left gastric artery has a very small diameter and often is difficult to visualize with ultrasound. It becomes difficult to separate from the splenic artery unless distinct structures are seen in the area of the celiac trunk branching to the left of the abdominal aorta.

Superior Mesenteric Artery. The superior mesenteric artery (SMA) arises from the anterior abdominal aortic wall approximately 1 cm inferior to the celiac trunk (see Figure 9-5). Occasionally, the SMA may have a common origin with the celiac trunk. The SMA runs posterior to the neck of the pancreas and anterior to the uncinate process, which is anterior to the third part of the duodenum; it then branches into the mesentery and colon. The right hepatic artery is sometimes seen to arise from the superior mesenteric artery.

The superior mesenteric artery has the following five main branches (Figure 9-21): inferior pancreatic artery, duodenal artery, colic artery, ileocolic artery, and intestinal artery. These branch arteries supply the small

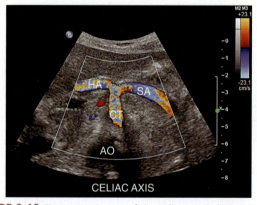

FIGURE 9-18 Transverse image of the celiac trunk (CT) as it arises from the anterior aortic wall (AO) and branches into splenic (SA) and hepatic arteries (HA).

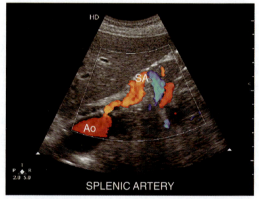

FIGURE 9-19 Transverse image of the splenic artery (SA) shown posterior to the left lobe of the liver and the tail of the pancreas. Ao, Aorta.

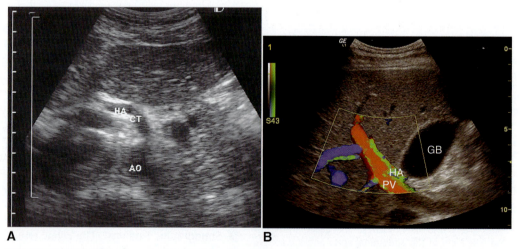

FIGURE 9-20 **A,** The common hepatic artery (HA) arises from the celiac trunk (CT) and courses toward the liver, anterior to the portal vein. AO, Aorta. **B,** Oblique transverse view of the portal triad: the portal vein (PV) is posterior, and the hepatic artery (HA) anterior and medial.

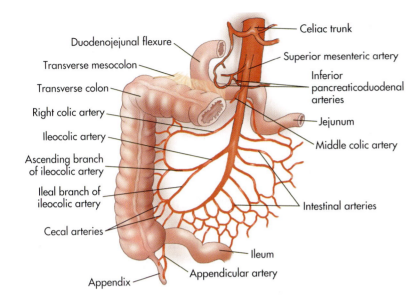

Duodenojejunal flexure
Transverse mesocolon
Transverse colon
Right colic artery
Ileocolic artery
Ascending branch of ileocolic artery
Ileal branch of ileocolic artery
Cecal arteries
Appendix
Celiac trunk
Superior mesenteric artery
Inferior pancreaticoduodenal arteries
Jejunum
Middle colic artery
Intestinal arteries
Ileum
Appendicular artery

FIGURE 9-21 The superior mesenteric artery arises anteriorly from the abdominal aorta approximately 1 cm below the celiac trunk. It supplies the proximal half of the colon and small intestine.

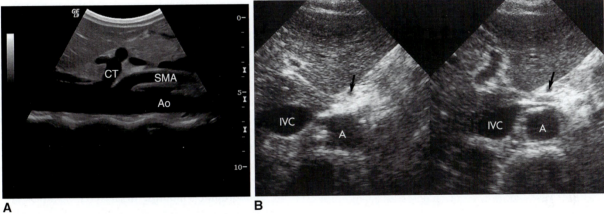

A   **B**

FIGURE 9-22 Superior mesenteric artery. **A,** Longitudinal image of the abdominal aorta (*Ao*), celiac trunk (*CT*), and superior mesenteric artery (*SMA*) arising from the anterior wall of the aorta. **B,** Transverse images show the SMA as a circle anterior to the aorta and left renal vein. The SMA is surrounded by a thick band of echogenic reflections from the mesenteric fat (*straight arrow*). *IVC,* inferior vena cava, *A,* aorta (curved arrow).

bowel; each consists of 10 to 16 branches arising from the left side of the superior mesenteric trunk. They extend into the mesentery, where adjacent arteries unite with them to form loops or arcades. Their distribution is to the proximal half of the colon (cecum, ascending, and transverse) and the small intestine.

 Sonographic Findings. The superior mesenteric artery is well seen on both transverse and longitudinal scans (Figure 9-22). As it arises from the anterior aortic wall, the SMA usually follows a parallel course along the abdominal aorta or branches off the anterior wall of the aorta at a slight angle and then follows a parallel course. Adenopathy should be considered if the angle is severe (greater than 15 degrees) (Figure 9-23).

Transversely, the artery can be seen as a separate small, circular structure anterior to the abdominal aorta and posterior to the pancreas. Characteristically, it is

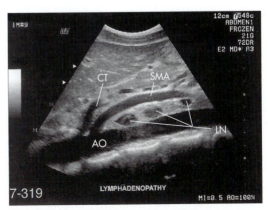

FIGURE 9-23 If the superior mesenteric artery arises at an angle steeper than 15 degrees from the aorta, lymphadenopathy should be considered, as is shown in this image with three well-defined nodes anterior to the aorta (*AO*). *CT,* celiac trunk; *LN,* enlarged lymph nodes; *SMA,* superior mesenteric artery.

surrounded by highly reflective echoes from the retroperitoneal fascia.

Inferior Mesenteric Artery. The **inferior mesenteric artery (IMA)** arises from the anterior abdominal aorta approximately at the level of the third or fourth lumbar vertebra (Figure 9-24). It proceeds to the left to distribute arterial blood to the descending colon, sigmoid colon, and rectum. It has the following three main branches: left colic, sigmoid, and superior rectal arteries. The distribution is to the left transverse colon, descending colon, sigmoid colon, and rectum.

▶ **Sonographic Findings.** The inferior mesenteric artery is more difficult to visualize using ultrasound; when it is seen, it is generally on a longitudinal scan. It is a small tubular structure inferior to the superior mesenteric artery, which originates from the anterior wall of the

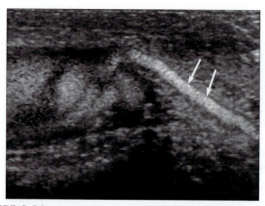

FIGURE 9-24 The inferior mesenteric artery (arrows) is well outlined with B-color (B-color is the manufacturer-specific name for the ability to detect flow velocity by assigning gray scale interpolation to flow velocity).

aorta. On transverse scans, it is difficult to separate from small loops of bowel within the abdomen.

Splanchnic Aneurysms. The splanchnic aneurysms may be atherosclerotic, posttraumatic, mycotic, congenital, or inflammatory. A small percentage of patients with chronic pancreatitis may develop these aneurysms, which may occur in the SMA, hepatic and splenic arteries, gastroduodenal arteries, or inferior mesenteric artery. They may have mural thrombus that is well demonstrated with color Doppler.

Lateral Branches of the Abdominal Aorta

Phrenic Arteries. The phrenic arteries are paired small vessels that arise from the lateral wall of the aorta to supply the undersurface of the diaphragm.

Renal Arteries. The renal arteries arise from the lateral aspect of the aorta at the level of and anterior to the first lumbar vertebra just inferior to the superior mesenteric artery (Figure 9-25). Both vessels divide into the anterior and inferior suprarenal arteries. Duplication of the renal arteries is not uncommon.

Right Renal Artery. The **right renal artery (RRA)** is a longer vessel than the left; it courses from the aorta posterior to the inferior vena cava and anterior to the vertebral column in a posterior and slightly caudal direction to enter the hilus of the right kidney. The renal artery passes posterior to the renal vein before entering the renal hilus.

Left Renal Artery. The **left renal artery (LRA)** courses from the aorta directly into the hilus of the left kidney.

▶ **Sonographic Findings.** Both renal arteries are best seen on transverse sonograms (Figure 9-26). The right

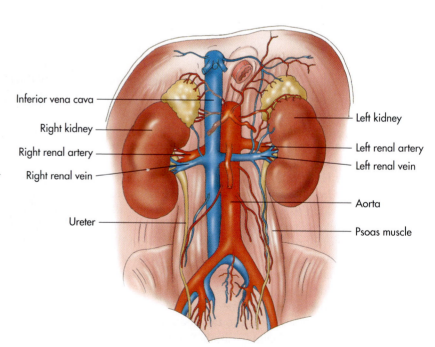

FIGURE 9-25 The kidneys and their vascular relationships.

Inferior vena cava
Right kidney
Right renal artery
Right renal vein
Ureter

Left kidney
Left renal artery
Left renal vein
Aorta
Psoas muscle

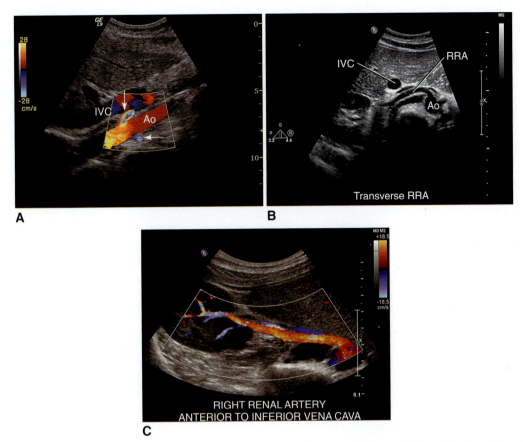

FIGURE 9-26 Renal arteries. **A,** Coronal image of both renal arteries (*arrows*) as they arise from the lateral borders of the abdominal aorta (*AO*). **B,** The right renal artery (*RRA*) may be seen posterior to the inferior vena cava (*IVC*) on the transverse image. **C,** Transverse color image of the right renal artery.

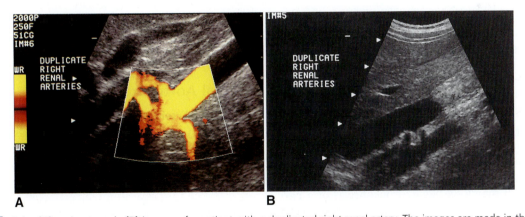

FIGURE 9-27 Color (**A**) and gray scale (**B**) images of a patient with a duplicated right renal artery. The images are made in the right coronal oblique view.

renal artery passes posterior to the inferior vena cava and anterior to the vertebral column in a posterior and slightly caudal direction. Occasionally, on longitudinal scans, a segment of the right renal artery is seen as a circular structure posterior to the inferior vena cava (Figures 9-27 and 9-28). The left renal artery takes a direct course from the aorta, anterior to the psoas muscle, to enter the renal sinus.

The coronal oblique scan of the aorta and inferior vena cava is excellent for demonstrating the origin of the renal arteries and veins (see Figure 9-27). The patient is rolled into a steep decubitus position. The transducer is directed longitudinally with its axis across the inferior vena cava and aorta in efforts to see the origin of the renal vessels. The patient should be in full inspiration to dilate the venous structures for better visualization.

Renal Artery Stenosis. Renal artery stenosis may present clinically as hypertension. The stenosis is due to atherosclerotic disease or fibromuscular hyperplasia. Color and spectral Doppler is used to investigate the

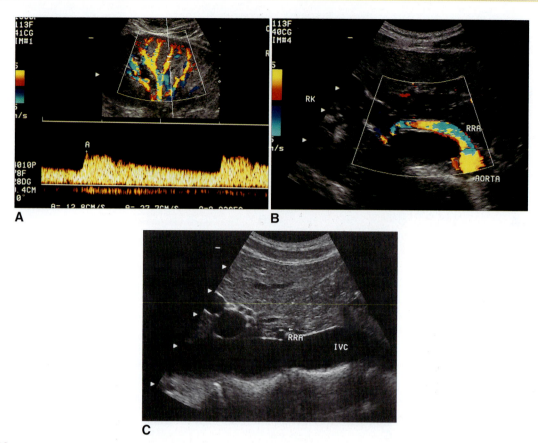

FIGURE 9-28 A through **C,** Variations in renal arteries. This patient has a right renal artery *(RRA)* that lies anterior (instead of posterior) to the inferior vena cava *(IVC).* Normal spectral flow is shown in the renal parenchyma.

renal vessels for increased velocity flow patterns representative of obstruction of flow into the kidney.

Renal Arteriovenous Fistulas. Renal arteriovenous fistulas can be congenital or acquired. Congenital arteriovenous fistulas may be of the cirsoid type or the aneurysmal type. Acquired fistulas occur secondary to trauma, surgery, or inflammation or are associated with a neoplasm, such as renal cell carcinoma.

The sonographer will find multiple anechoic tubular structures feeding the malformation with an enlarged renal artery and vein, confirming increased blood flow to the kidney. It may look like hydronephrosis or a parapelvic cyst in association with a dilated inferior vena cava. The diagnosis is made by identifying one or more channels that enter the mass, suggesting that the lesion is related to the renal vasculature. The sonographer should look for pulsations. The fistula has a characteristic sonographic appearance of a cluster of tubular anechoic structures within the kidney; it is supplied by an enlarged renal artery and is drained by a dilated renal vein. In the aneurysmal type of fistula, a vascular lesion should be suspected when the presence of a thrombus is noted in the periphery of a mass with a tubular anechoic lumen with pulsations. Occasionally, renal cell carcinoma is associated with arteriovenous shunting, resulting from invasion of larger arteries and venous structures.

Gonadal Artery. The gonadal artery arises inferior to the renal arteries and courses along the psoas muscle to the respective gonadal area.

Dorsal Aortic Branches

Lumbar Artery. Four lumbar arteries are usually present on each side of the aorta. The vessels travel lateral and posterior to supply muscle, skin, bone, and spinal cord. The midsacral artery supplies the sacrum and rectum.

INFERIOR VENA CAVA

The **inferior vena cava** (IVC) is formed by the union of the common iliac veins posterior to the right common iliac artery at the level of the fifth lumbar vertebra (Figure 9-29). The inferior vena cava ascends vertically through the retroperitoneal space on the right side of the aorta posterior to the liver, piercing the central tendon of the diaphragm at the level of the eighth thoracic vertebra to enter the right atrium of the heart. Its entrance into the lesser sac separates it from the portal vein. Caudal to the renal vein entrance, the inferior vena cava shows posterior "hammocking" through the bare area of the liver (Figure 9-30).

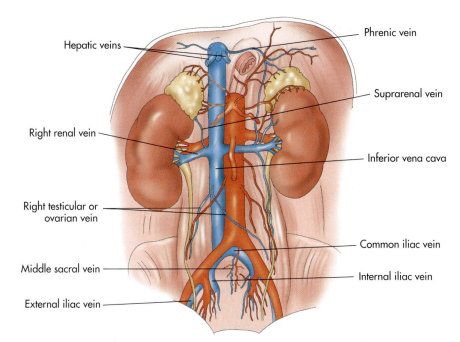

Hepatic veins

Right renal vein

Right testicular or ovarian vein

Middle sacral vein

External iliac vein

Phrenic vein

Suprarenal vein

Inferior vena cava

Common iliac vein

Internal iliac vein

FIGURE 9-29 The abdominal venous system and its tributaries.

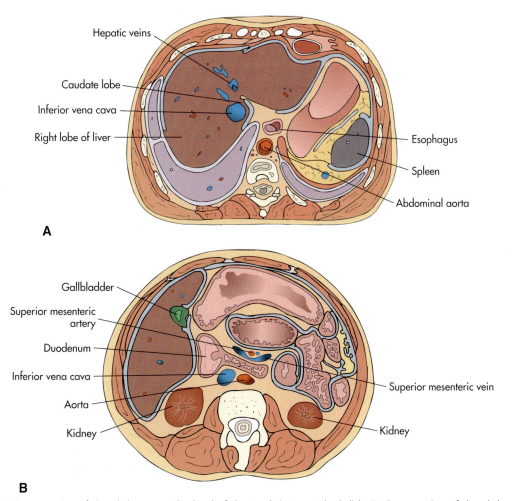

Hepatic veins

Caudate lobe

Inferior vena cava

Right lobe of liver

Esophagus

Spleen

Abdominal aorta

A

Gallbladder

Superior mesenteric artery

Duodenum

Inferior vena cava

Aorta

Kidney

Superior mesenteric vein

Kidney

B

FIGURE 9-30 A, Cross section of the abdomen at the level of the tenth intervertebral disk. **B,** Cross section of the abdomen at the first lumbar vertebra.

Continued

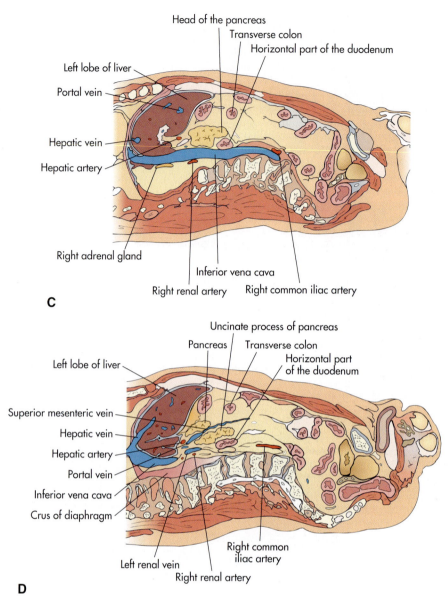

Head of the pancreas
Transverse colon
Horizontal part of the duodenum
Left lobe of liver
Portal vein
Hepatic vein
Hepatic artery
Right adrenal gland
Inferior vena cava
Right renal artery   Right common iliac artery

C

Uncinate process of pancreas
Pancreas   Transverse colon
Horizontal part
of the duodenum
Left lobe of liver
Superior mesenteric vein
Hepatic vein
Hepatic artery
Portal vein
Inferior vena cava
Crus of diaphragm
Right common
iliac artery
Left renal vein
Right renal artery

D

FIGURE 9-30, cont'd **C,** Sagittal section of the abdomen 3 cm from the midline. **D,** Sagittal section of the abdomen 2 cm from the midline.

The tributaries of the inferior vena cava include the following:

- Three anterior hepatic veins
- Three lateral tributaries: the right suprarenal vein (the left suprarenal vein drains into the left renal vein), the renal veins, and the right testicular or ovarian vein
- Five lateral abdominal wall tributaries: the inferior phrenic vein and the four lumbar veins
- Three veins of origin: the two common iliac veins and the median sacral vein

The inferior vena cava is a large, collapsible vein that returns blood from the abdomen, pelvis, and lower limbs through the system's major tributaries into the right atrium of the heart. The superior vena cava drains the head, neck, thoracic cavity, and upper extremities and will be discussed in Chapter 35. The walls of the cava are much thinner than those of the aorta because the pressure of blood flow is much lower.

Sonographic Findings. The inferior vena cava serves as a landmark for many other abdominal structures and should be routinely visualized on all examinations (Figure 9-31). The intrahepatic portion of the cava is seen by using the liver as an acoustic window. Beyond the liver border, the cava may become obscured by overlying bowel gas. The complete inferior vena cava is imaged on a sagittal scan. Beginning at the midline of the abdomen, the transducer should be angled slightly to the right with a slight oblique tilt until the entire vessel is seen. The patient should be instructed to hold his or her breath; this causes the patient to perform a slight Valsalva maneuver toward the end of inspiration, which dilates the inferior vena cava. The inferior vena cava may expand to 2 to 3 cm in diameter with this maneuver.

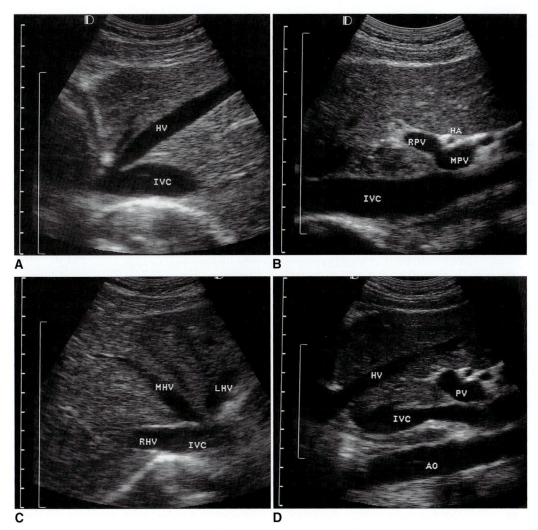

FIGURE 9-31 Normal inferior vena cava protocol. **A** and **B,** Longitudinal images. **A,** The hepatic vein *(HV)* drains into the inferior vena cava *(IVC)* at the diaphragm. **B,** The IVC is the posterior border of the portal vein. *HA,* Hepatic artery; *MPV,* main portal vein; *RPV,* right portal vein. **C,** Transverse image: The three hepatic veins are shown to drain into the IVC at the dome of the liver. *LHV,* Left hepatic vein. **D,** Oblique coronal image: The patient is rolled into a slight oblique position (right side up). The transducer is angled from the midclavicular line toward the midline of the abdomen to see the IVC "anterior" to the abdominal aorta *(AO)*.

With expiration, venous return improves, and therefore the caval diameter decreases. Both cardiac and respiratory pulsations are transmitted in the inferior vena cava to produce a phasic pattern similar to the pattern in the peripheral veins.

The pulsatile aorta is easily differentiated from the inferior vena cava as the IVC travels in a horizontal course with its proximal portion curving slightly anterior as it pierces the diaphragm to empty into the right atrial cavity. The aorta, on the other hand, follows the curvature of the spine, with its distal portion lying more posterior, before bifurcating into the iliac vessels. The lumen of the cava should be anechoic, although with slow flowing blood, the lumen becomes slightly more echogenic with swirling of the blood seen in real-time. This condition is usually seen in patients with right-sided heart failure, fluid overload, or obstruction of the inferior vena cava.

On transverse scans, the almond-shaped inferior vena cava serves as a landmark for localizing the superior mesenteric vein, which is generally found anterior and slightly to the right of or just medial to the cava. On longitudinal scans, the cava serves as a landmark for the portal vein, which is located just anterior to or midway down the anterior wall of the cava.

The diameter of the inferior vena cava will depend on the patient's age and body mass. In the adult patient, the normal cava usually measures <2.0 cm and shows respiratory variations.

The inferior vena cava is also useful in identifying the echogenic pancreas and small common bile duct. The head of the pancreas is seen just inferior to the portal vein and anterior to the inferior vena cava as it makes a slight impression or indentation on the anterior wall of the cava. The common duct is seen anterior to the portal vein as it dips posterior to enter the head of the pancreas.

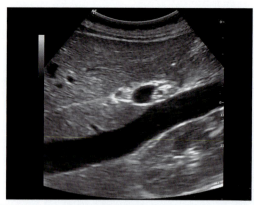

FIGURE 9-32 Sagittal scan of the dilated inferior vena cava as seen in a patient with right heart failure.

Dilation of the inferior vena cava is noted in several pathologies, including right ventricular heart failure (Figure 9-32), congestive heart disease, constrictive pericarditis, tricuspid disease, and right heart obstructive tumors. Tumor or thrombus may be found in the IVC and may cause obstruction of blood returning into the right atrium.

In patients with hepatomegaly, the IVC and hepatic veins are dilated; increased pressure is transmitted through the sinusoids, resulting in portal vein distention. If severe cirrhosis is present, the sinusoids may be unable to transmit pressure, and the portal veins will not distend.

Compression of the inferior vena cava may be seen in later stages of pregnancy as the enlarged uterus compresses the vena cava. Over time, this compression will produce edema of the ankles and feet and temporary varicose veins. Other forms of caval compression may arise from malignant retroperitoneal tumors, hepatic neoplasm, or pancreatic mass. The presence of thrombus within the vessel should be evaluated, especially in patients with a known renal tumor.

Inferior Vena Cava Abnormalities

Congenital Abnormalities. The inferior vena cava is formed by three pairs of cardinal veins in the retroperitoneum; these veins undergo sequential development and regression. The posterior cardinal veins appear at 6 weeks and form no part of the cava, but may be part of the anomalies. The subcardinal veins appear at 7 weeks to produce the prerenal segment of the inferior vena cava. The supracardinal system at 8 weeks produces the postrenal segment of the inferior vena cava. The supracardinals form the azygos and hemiazygos system above the diaphragm. The anastomosis between the subcardinal and supracardinal systems forms the renal veins. The normal left cardinal system involutes, and the right consists of the posterior infrarenal vein, supracardinal vein, renal segment, anterior suprarenal subcardinal vein, and the confluence of hepatic veins.

Double Inferior Vena Cava. Double inferior vena cava has an incidence of less than 3%. The size of the two vessels can be the same or may vary, depending on the dominant side. In the most common type, the left inferior vena cava joins the left renal vein, which crosses the midline at its normal level to join the right inferior vena cava. The left inferior vena cava does not continue above the left renal vein. Less commonly, the right inferior vena cava joins the left inferior vena cava to join the hemiazygos.

Infrahepatic Interruption of the Inferior Vena Cava. This condition results from failure of union of the hepatic veins and the right subcardinal vein, which can include azygos or, less commonly, hemiazygos continuation. The azygos veins consist of the main azygos vein, the inferior hemiazygos vein, and the superior hemiazygos vein (Figure 9-33). They drain blood from the posterior parts of the intercostal spaces, the posterior abdominal wall, the pericardium, the diaphragm, the bronchi, and the esophagus. Interruption of the inferior vena cava connection to the heart is associated with acyanotic and cyanotic congenital heart disease, abnormalities of cardiac position, and abdominal situs with asplenia and polysplenia.

Sonographic Findings. In patients with an interruption of the inferior vena cava, the azygos vein continuation is identical to or larger than the inferior vena cava, which passes along the aorta medial to the right crus of the diaphragm. The hepatic veins drain into an independent confluence that passes through the diaphragm to enter the right atrium. A membranous obstruction of the inferior vena cava may simulate infrahepatic interruption of the cava with azygos continuation. A web or membrane obstructs the inferior vena cava at the level of the diaphragm and leads to chronic congestion of the liver with centrilobular and periportal fibrosis.

The following three types of obstruction occur:

- A thin membrane at the level of the entrance to the right atrium
- An absent segment of the inferior vena cava without characteristic conical narrowing
- Complete obstruction secondary to thrombosis

Clinically, patients present in the third to fourth decade of life with portal hypertension. Ultrasound shows obstruction at the diaphragm and dilation of the azygos system. On longitudinal scans, it is very difficult to identify the presence of the inferior vena cava. The azygos system is dilated on the right side of the midline, "acting" as the inferior vena cava.

Inferior Vena Cava Dilation. In patients with right ventricular failure, the inferior vena cava does not collapse with expiration (Figure 9-34). This may result from atherosclerosis, pulmonary hypertension, pericardial tamponade, constrictive pericarditis, or atrial tumor.

Inferior Vena Cava Tumor. It is important for the sonographer to identify the entire inferior vena cava;

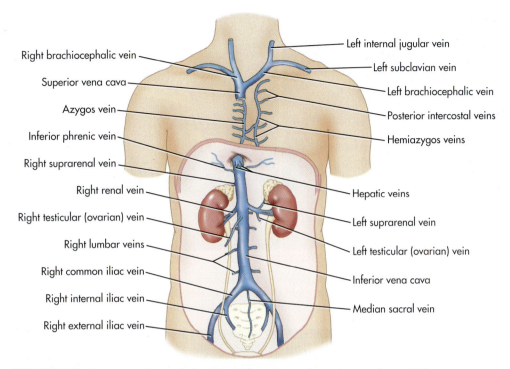

FIGURE 9-33 Illustration of the relationship of the azygos vein to the superior and inferior vena cava.

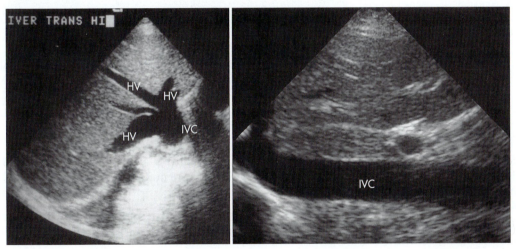

FIGURE 9-34 Transverse and sagittal scans of a patient in right ventricular heart failure show a dilated inferior vena cava *(IVC)* and hepatic veins *(HV)*.

bowel gas can make the distal cava difficult to identify.

Hepatic Portion of Inferior Vena Cava. Masses posterior to the hepatic portion of the inferior vena cava are the right adrenal, neurogenic, and hepatic. With enlargement of the liver, the cava is compressed rather than displaced. A localized liver mass would produce posterior, lateral, or medial displacement of the inferior vena cava, whereas a mass in the posterior caudate lobe and right lobe may elevate the cava.

Pancreatic Portion of the Inferior Vena Cava. The middle, or pancreatic, portion of the inferior vena cava may elevate the cava from abnormalities of the right

renal artery, right kidney, lumbar spine, or lymph node masses.

Small Bowel (Lower) Segment. Lumbar spine abnormalities or lymph nodes would elevate the inferior vena cava.

Sonographic Findings. The inferior vena cava may become obstructed by tumor formation. The ultrasound appearance of tumor is of single or multiple echogenic nodules along the wall. The cava may be distended and filled with a tumor. The most common tumor is renal cell carcinoma, usually from the right kidney. Wilms' tumor is also seen extending into the inferior vena cava and right atrium. Other less common tumors are

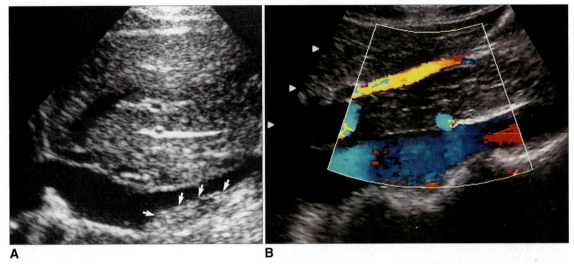

FIGURE 9-35 A, Longitudinal image of the inferior vena cava with a tumor lying along the posterior wall *(arrows)*. **B,** Color flow Doppler will delineate the patency of the inferior vena cava in the event of tumor or thrombus formation.

FIGURE 9-36 A, Longitudinal image of thrombus near the distal end of the inferior vena cava *(IVC)*. **B,** The spectral Doppler shows that flow is still patent.

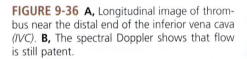

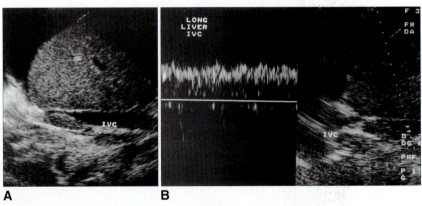

retroperitoneal liposarcoma, leiomyosarcoma, pheochromocytoma, osteosarcoma, and rhabdomyosarcoma. Benign tumors, such as angiomyolipoma, can have venous involvement.

Inferior Vena Cava Thrombosis. Complete thrombosis of the inferior vena cava is life-threatening. Patients present with leg edema, low back pain, pelvic pain, gastrointestinal complaints, and renal and liver abnormalities (Figures 9-35 and 9-36). Thrombosis within the inferior vena cava appears as a homogeneous echo mass. Color Doppler is useful to determine whether the vessel is occluded.

Inferior Vena Cava Filters. The most common origin of pulmonary emboli is venous thrombosis from the lower extremities. Surgical and angiographic placement of transvenous filters into the cava has been used to prevent recurrent embolization in patients who cannot tolerate anticoagulants (Figure 9-37). The preferred location of the filter is in the iliac bifurcation below the renal veins. The filter is a tubular wire mesh that is implanted into the IVC to trap small emboli that may cause problems in the heart or the lungs. After placement, some filters can migrate cranially or caudally and perforate the

cava, producing a retroperitoneal bleed. Filters can also perforate the duodenum, aorta, ureter, and hepatic vein.

Lateral Tributaries to the Inferior Vena Cava

Renal Veins. Five or six branches of the renal vein unite to form the main renal vein. The right and left main renal veins arise anterior to the renal artery at their respective sides of the inferior vena cava at the level of L2 (see Figure 9-29).

Left Renal Vein. The left renal vein (LRV) arises medially to exit from the hilus of the kidney (Figure 9-38). It flows from the left kidney posterior to the superior mesenteric artery and anterior to the aorta to enter the lateral wall of the inferior vena cava. Above the entry of the renal veins, the inferior vena cava enlarges because of the increased volume of blood returning from the kidneys. The left renal vein is larger than the right renal vein. It accepts branches from the left adrenal, left gonadal, and lumbar veins. The left renal vein is visualized as a circular structure coursing between the SMA and the aorta on the longitudinal image. On the

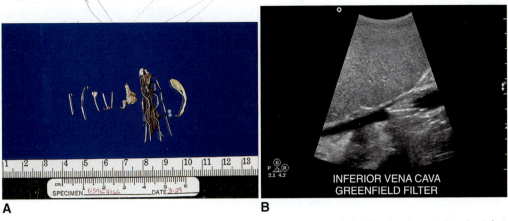

FIGURE 9-37 A, Surgical specimen of the vena cava filter. **B,** Longitudinal image of the filter in place within the inferior vena cava.

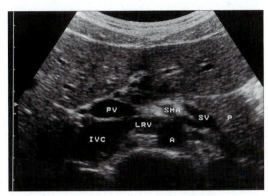

FIGURE 9-38 The left renal vein *(LRV)* is well seen as it leaves the renal hilus and flows anterior to the aorta *(A)* and posterior to the superior mesenteric artery *(SMA)* to enter the lateral wall of the inferior vena cava *(IVC)*.

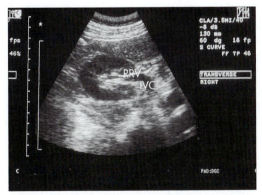

FIGURE 9-39 The right renal vein is shown as it leaves the renal hilum toward the inferior vena cava.

transverse image, the LRV is an anechoic tubular structure posterior to the SMA and anterior to the aorta.

Right Renal Vein. The **right renal vein (RRV)** is best seen on transverse images because it flows directly from the right kidney into the posterolateral aspect of the inferior vena cava (Figure 9-39). It seldom accepts tributaries; the right adrenal and right gonadal veins enter the cava directly.

Renal Vein Obstruction. Renal vein obstruction is seen in the dehydrated or septic infant. It may also be seen in adults with multiple renal abnormalities (nephrotic syndrome, shock, renal tumor, kidney transplant, or trauma). Left renal vein obstruction may result from the spread of such nonrenal malignancies as carcinoma of the pancreas or lung, or lymphoma. A retroperitoneal tumor can occlude the left renal vein by direct extension into the vein lumen or compression of the lumen by a contiguous mass.

Clinical Signs. The patient presents with flank pain, hematuria, flank mass, and proteinuria. The condition may be associated with maternal diabetes and transient high blood pressure.

Sonographic Findings. Ultrasound can be used to confirm that a palpable flank mass is kidney and to exclude hydronephrosis and multicystic kidney as causes of a nonfunctioning kidney (Figure 9-40). In infants with renal vein obstruction, enlarged kidneys without cysts are seen. Medium echoes or "clumps" of echoes may be randomly scattered within the kidney, with surrounding echo-free spaces. The parenchymal anechoic areas are the result of hemorrhage and infarcts. The renal pattern progresses to atrophy over 2 months. Late findings include increased parenchymal echoes, loss of corticomedullary junction, and decreased renal size.

Renal Vein Thrombosis. If the following are present on ultrasound, renal vein thrombosis can be diagnosed:

1. Direct visualization of thrombi in the renal vein and inferior vena cava
2. Demonstrated renal vein dilation proximal to the point of occlusion
3. Loss of normal renal structure
4. Increased renal size (acute phase)
5. Decreased flow or no flow shown on Doppler

Clinical Signs. The patient presents with pain, nephromegaly, hematuria, or thromboembolic phenomena elsewhere in the body. A variety of lesions may be associated with this abnormality.

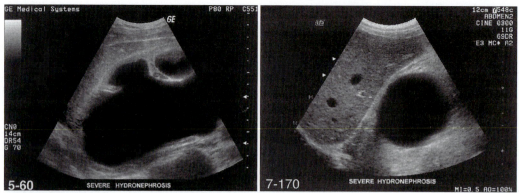

FIGURE 9-40 Hydronephrosis of the right kidney.

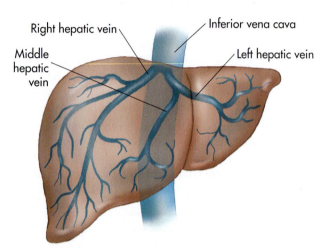

FIGURE 9-41 The hepatic veins are divided into three components: right, middle, and left. They all drain into the inferior vena cava at the level of the diaphragm.

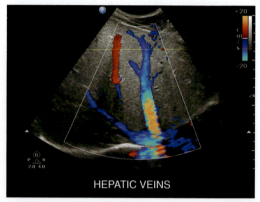

HEPATIC VEINS

FIGURE 9-42 Transverse color image at the dome of the liver with the transducer angled in a cephalad direction shows the three hepatic veins draining into the inferior vena cava.

Gonadal Veins. The gonadal veins (testicular and ovarian) course anterior to the external and internal iliac veins and continue cranially and retroperitoneally along the psoas muscle until their terminus. The left gonadal vein usually enters the left renal vein or the left adrenal vein, which empties into the inferior vena cava. The right gonadal vein enters the inferior vena cava on the anterolateral border above the entrance of the lumbar veins.

Suprarenal Veins. The right suprarenal vein arises from the suprarenal gland and usually drains directly into the inferior vena cava. The left arises from the suprarenal gland and drains into the left renal vein.

Anterior Tributaries to the Inferior Vena Cava

Hepatic Veins. The **hepatic veins (HV)** are the largest visceral tributaries of the inferior vena cava. They originate between the segments of the liver and drain posteriorly into the inferior vena cava at the level of the diaphragm (Figure 9-41). The hepatic veins return unoxygenated blood from the liver. The veins collect blood from the three minor tributaries within the liver: the right hepatic vein drains the right lobe of the liver, the middle hepatic vein drains the caudate lobe, and the left hepatic vein drains the left lobe of the liver. The middle and left hepatic veins may fuse before emptying into the inferior vena cava.

Sonographic Findings. The hepatic veins are best visualized on longitudinal scans of the liver as they drain into the inferior vena cava at the level of the diaphragm. Transverse scans obtained with a cephalic angle of the transducer at the level of the xiphoid often show at least two of the three veins draining into the inferior vena cava (Figure 9-42). The hepatic veins resemble the "bunny" or "reindeer" sign on the sonogram.

Distinguishing hepatic veins from other vascular structures requires recognition of their anatomic patterns. Hepatic veins drain cephalad toward the diaphragm and then dorsomedially toward the inferior vena cava (Figure 9-43). Hepatic veins increase in caliber as they approach the diaphragm. Unlike portal veins, they are not surrounded by bright acoustic reflections, although a slight amount of acoustic enhancement may be seen along their posterior border.

Hepatic veins demonstrate a triphasic and pulsatile flow pattern that reflects the transmitted cardiac pulsations. Patients with cirrhosis and portal hypertension will lose this pulsatile pattern, and patients in right heart failure will show increased pulsations.

PORTAL VENOUS SYSTEM

Portal Vein

The **portal vein** (**PV**) is formed posterior to the pancreas by the union of the superior mesenteric vein and splenic veins at the level of L2. Its trunk is 5 to 7 cm in length (Figure 9-44). The portal vein courses posterior to the first portion of the duodenum and then between the layers of the lesser omentum to the porta hepatis, where it bifurcates into its hepatic branches. It carries blood from the intestinal tract to the liver by means of its two main branches: the right and left portal veins. It drains blood from the gastrointestinal tract, from the lower end of the esophagus to the upper end of the anal canal, and from the pancreas, gallbladder, bile ducts, and spleen. The portal vein has an **anastomosis** with the esophageal veins, rectal venous plexus, and superficial abdominal veins. The portal venous blood traverses the liver and drains into the inferior vena cava via the hepatic veins.

The liver receives a dual blood supply from the portal vein and the hepatic artery. The portal vein supplies up to one half of the oxygen requirements of the hepatocytes because of its great flow, even though it carries incompletely oxygenated (<80%) venous blood from the intestines and spleen.

The portal triad contains branches of the portal vein, hepatic artery, and bile duct contained within a connective tissue sheath that gives the portal vein an echogenic wall as seen on liver sonographic images.

Sonographic Findings. The portal vein is clearly seen on both transverse and sagittal scans. On transverse scans, the main portal vein is a thin-walled circular structure, generally lateral and somewhat anterior to the inferior vena cava (Figure 9-45). It is often possible to record the splenic vein as it crosses the midline of the abdomen to join the superior mesenteric vein to form the main portal trunk. Thus a long section of the splenic vein can be visualized. Often the right or left portal vein can be seen branching from the portal trunk to enter the hilum of the liver.

Portal veins become smaller as they progress into the liver from the porta hepatis. Large radicles situated near or approaching the porta hepatis are portal veins, not hepatic veins. The portal veins are characterized by high-amplitude acoustic reflections that presumably arise from the fibrous tissues surrounding the portal triad as it courses through the liver substance.

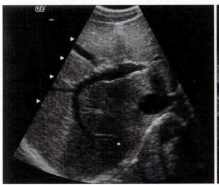

FIGURE 9-43 Longitudinal image of the hepatic vein draining the liver into the inferior vena cava. Note the thin-walled hepatic vein (HV) compared with the thicker wall of the portal vein (PV).

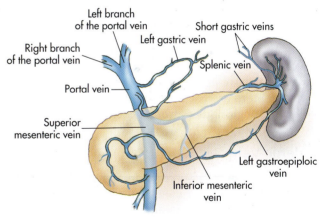

FIGURE 9-44 The superior and inferior mesenteric veins join the splenic vein to form the portal vein.

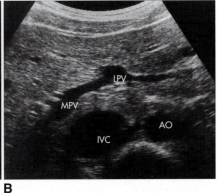

A   **B**

FIGURE 9-45 Transverse views of the portal vein. **A,** The right portal vein bifurcates into the anterior and posterior branches. **B,** The main portal vein (MPV) bifurcates into the right and left branches. This scan shows the left portal vein (LPV) as it supplies the left lobe of the liver. AO, Aorta; IVC, inferior vena cava.

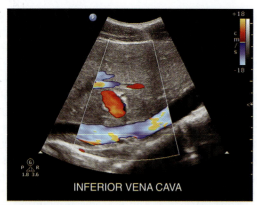

FIGURE 9-46 Longitudinal scan of the inferior vena cava *(blue)*, with the main portal vein *(red)* just anterior to its border.

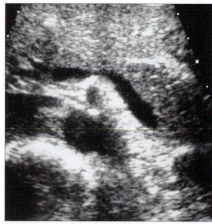

FIGURE 9-47 Transverse image of the splenic vein as it leaves the splenic hilum and courses posterior to the pancreas and anterior to the superior mesenteric artery to form the portal vein.

The right and left portal veins course transversely through the liver; thus transverse scans display their longest extent (Figure 9-46). The right portal vein is most consistently demonstrated on the sonogram. Anatomically, any intraparenchymal segment of the portal venous system lying to the right of the lateral aspect of the inferior vena cava is a branch of the right portal system. The right portal vein has an anterior branch that lies centrally within the anterior segment of the right lobe and a posterior branch that lies centrally within the posterior segment of the right lobe.

The left portal vein has a narrow-caliber trunk and may be seen coursing transversely through the left hepatic lobe from a posterior to an anterior position (see Figure 9-45, *B*). The main portal vein is well seen as a circular anechoic structure to the inferior vena cava. The portal radicle may have many different variations; therefore, it is important to become familiar with their patterns to be able to distinguish them from dilated biliary radicles.

Splenic Vein

The **splenic vein (SV)** is a tributary of the portal circulation. It begins at the hilum of the spleen, where it is formed by the union of several veins. It is subsequently joined by the short gastric and left gastroepiploic veins (see Figure 9-44). The splenic vein runs along the posteromedial border of the pancreas. It joins the superior mesenteric vein posterior to the neck of the pancreas to form the portal vein. Additional veins from the pancreas and inferior mesenteric vein drain into the splenic vein. The splenic vein drains blood from the stomach, spleen, and pancreas.

Sonographic Findings. The splenic vein is best visualized in the transverse plane as it crosses the upper abdomen from the hilum of the spleen to join the superior mesenteric vein to form the portal vein slightly to the right of midline (Figure 9-47). The splenic vein crosses anteriorly to the aorta and the inferior vena cava and generally relates to the medial and posterior borders of the pancreatic body and tail. Its course is variable, so

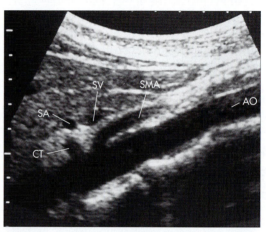

FIGURE 9-48 Longitudinal image of the splenic vein shown as a circular structure just anterior to the celiac axis. *AO,* aorta; *CT,* celiac trunk; *SA,* splenic artery; *SMA,* superior mesenteric artery; *SV,* splenic vein.

small degrees of obliquity with the transducer may be necessary to image the vein entirely. It is usually smaller than the superior mesenteric vein and the main portal vein. The larger diameter of the portal vein is the result of the influx of blood from the superior mesenteric vein. An obvious widening is demonstrated at the junction of the portal and splenic veins.

On sagittal scans, the splenic vein can be visualized posterior to the left lobe of the liver and anterior to the major vascular structures. The pancreas may be seen inferior and slightly anterior to the vein (Figure 9-48). When splenomegaly is present, it is often possible to identify the origin of the splenic vein at the splenic hilum.

Superior Mesenteric Vein

The **superior mesenteric vein (SMV)** is also a tributary to the portal vein (see Figure 9-44). It begins at the ileocolic junction and runs cephalad along the posterior abdominal wall within the root of the mesentery of the small intestine to the right of the superior mesenteric artery. The superior mesenteric vein passes anterior to the third part of the duodenum and posterior to the neck of the pancreas, where it joins the splenic vein to form the main portal vein. It also receives tributaries that correspond to the branches of the superior mesenteric artery, where it is joined by the inferior pancreaticoduodenal vein to the right gastroepiploic vein from the right aspect of the greater curvature of the stomach. The superior mesenteric vein drains blood from several smaller veins: the middle colic vein (transverse colon), the right colic vein (ascending colon), and the pancreatic duodenal vein.

◤ **Sonographic Findings.** The superior mesenteric vein is somewhat variable in its anatomic location. Generally, it is anterior to the inferior vena cava and to the right of the superior mesenteric artery. The superior mesenteric vein drains into the main portal vein (with the splenic vein); therefore, the sonographer should not be able to demonstrate these three structures together on a single transverse scan (Figure 9-49). The superior mesenteric vein is the posterior border of the neck of the pancreas and the anterior border of the uncinate process of the pancreatic head.

On sagittal scans, the vein is seen as a long, tubular structure anterior to the inferior vena cava (Figure 9-50). With correct oblique angulation of the transducer, the path of the superior mesenteric vein can be followed as it enters the portal system.

The following points help to distinguish the superior mesenteric artery from the vein:

- The superior mesenteric vein is of larger caliber than the artery.
- Real-time identification of the confluence of the superior mesenteric vein-portal vein or superior mesenteric artery is possible as the superior mesenteric artery originates directly from the anterior wall of the abdominal aorta.

Inferior Mesenteric Vein

The **inferior mesenteric vein (IMV)** drains the left third of the colon and upper colon and ascends retroperitoneally along the left psoas muscle. It begins midway down the anal canal as the superior rectal vein (see Figure 9-44). It runs cranially in the posterior abdominal wall on the left side of the inferior mesenteric artery and duodenojejunal junction to join the splenic vein posterior to the pancreas. It receives many tributaries along its way, including the left colic vein. The inferior mesenteric vein drains several tributaries: the left colic vein (descending colon), the sigmoid vein (sigmoid colon), and the superior rectal vein (upper rectum).

◤ **Sonographic Findings.** The inferior mesenteric vein is difficult to recognize on ultrasound because of its anatomic location and small diameter. It is generally covered by the small bowel and has no major vascular structures posterior to it to aid in its recognition.

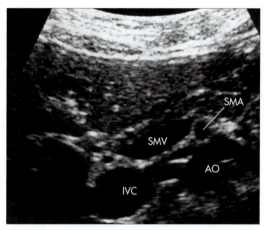

FIGURE 9-49 Transverse image of the superior mesenteric vein *(SMV)*, adjacent to the superior mesenteric artery *(SMA)* and anterior to the inferior vena cava *(IVC)* and aorta *(AO)*.

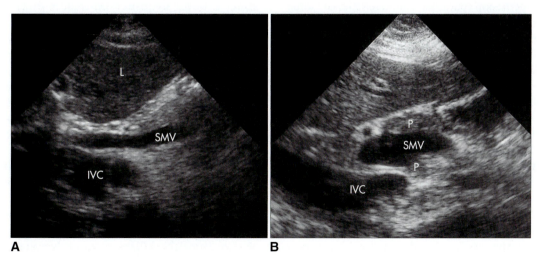

A B

FIGURE 9-50 A and **B,** Sagittal images of the superior mesenteric vein *(SMV)* as it lies anterior to the uncinate process of the pancreas *(P)* and posterior to the body. *IVC,* inferior vena cava; *L,* liver.

ABDOMINAL DOPPLER TECHNIQUES

Doppler ultrasound is a useful clinical tool for diagnosing many disease processes. The following paragraphs present an overview of abdominal applications that have been used with color flow detection and pulsed Doppler techniques. Doppler has helped detect the presence or absence of blood flow, the direction of blood flow, and flow disturbance patterns. It has also been used in tissue characterization and waveform analysis.

Blood Flow Analysis

Presence or Absence of Flow. Doppler ultrasound frequently is used to differentiate vessels from nonvascular structures. For example, to distinguish the common bile duct from the hepatic artery, look for absence of flow in the common duct; to distinguish the hepatic artery from the splenic artery, look for direction of flow; to differentiate an aneurysm from a pancreatic pseudocyst, look for slow flow in the aneurysm; to differentiate dilated intrahepatic bile ducts and prominent hepatic artery, again look for absence of flow in the bile duct.

Direction of Flow. In patients who develop **portal venous hypertension**, the portal blood flow becomes **hepatofugal** (away from the liver) instead of **hepatopetal** (toward the liver). This may occur secondary to portal venous shunts or varices. The sonographer detects a high-velocity flow pattern at the site of the shunt with a turbulent flow pattern on color Doppler.

Disturbance of Flow. A flow disturbance (increased velocity or obstruction of flow) may result from the formation of an atheroma, arteriovenous (AV) fistula, pseudoaneurysm, or aneurysmal dilation.

Tissue Characterization. Research is currently under way in the area of tissue characterization. Doppler is thought to be capable of characterizing tissue because of the specific perfusion patterns characteristic of some tissues or states of tissue activity. Hepatocellular carcinomas of the liver appear to have a specific pattern. Pseudoaneurysms of peripancreatic arteries have turbulent flow patterns. Pancreatic tumors may have specific flow patterns.

Doppler Waveform Analysis. The shape of the waveform provides information on the vascular impedance of the organ the vessel supplies. Spectral analysis tells the velocity and turbulence of blood flow.

Nonresistive Versus Resistive Vessels. Nonresistive vessels have a high diastolic component and supply organs that need constant perfusion, such as the internal carotid artery, the hepatic artery, and the renal artery. **Resistive** vessels have very little or even reversed flow in diastole and supply organs that do not need a constant blood supply, such as the external carotid and the iliac and brachial arteries.

Peak systole is compared with minimum diastole to quantify a vessel's impedance. This ratio is the **resistive index.**

Spectral display shows us the following:

x = Time is depicted on the horizontal axis.
y = Doppler shift frequency (velocity) is on the vertical axis (flow toward the transducer equals positive shift, or above baseline; flow away from the transducer equals negative shift, or below baseline).
z = Gray scale indicates the quantity of blood flowing at a given velocity. More red blood cells produce a brighter gray scale assignment.

Plug flow is a pattern of blood flow, typically seen in large arteries, in which most cells are moving at the same velocity across the entire diameter of the vessel. In other vessels, the different velocities are the result of friction between the cells and arterial walls. A "clear window" under systole is typical of plug flow. When plug flow is present, the volume of blood flow can be calculated.

Doppler Technique

Unlike visualization of the heart, in which high-velocity flows are present, visualization of abdominal vessels requires very sensitive Doppler instrumentation. Abdominal vessels generally have low velocity and flow.

Methods. Doppler is performed as part of the routine real-time examination. The patient should be fasting and should suspend respirations for the best color and pulsed **Doppler sample volume** to be obtained. The Doppler sample volume (sometimes referred to as the Doppler "gate") should be adjusted to encompass but not exceed the diameter of the vessel. If the sample volume exceeds the diameter, noise and ghost echoes may appear. This occurs because a too wide Doppler gate causes interference from surrounding vessels and structures.

The sonographer has the ability to control the velocity of the returning echoes to prevent the alias pattern by using a lower frequency transducer or changing from pulse wave to continuous wave. Another feature of Doppler is that the beam records only accurate velocity patterns when the beam is parallel to the flow (the angle of flow can be changed up to 60 degrees and still be accurate). The more perpendicular the beam is to the flow, the less signal is recorded; it falls to zero velocity when the beam is directly perpendicular to flow. Thus Doppler causes the sonographer to be creative in attempting to record accurate velocity flow patterns. The patient must be rolled into various obliquities with different angulations of the transducer to be parallel to many vascular structures.

Color Doppler is a relatively new and exciting modality that makes it easier to localize and identify smaller vessels from the biliary tree, or lymphadenopathy or other pathology. Colors are arbitrarily assigned on all equipment and refer to the direction of flow. If red is assigned as a positive flow signal, all flow toward the transducer is coded in various shades of red, depending on returning velocity. If blue is assigned a negative flow signal, the flow away from the transducer is coded in various shades of blue. The sonographer may select the particular color scheme to be used; some laboratories choose to code all positive-flow patterns red and negative-flow patterns blue. Other laboratories code all arterial flows red and venous flows blue.

Doppler Flow Patterns in the Abdominal Vessels

Box 9-3 lists Doppler flow patterns in the abdominal arteries.

Aorta. The patient should be scanned in the longitudinal plane (Figure 9-51). The flow pattern of the proximal abdominal aorta above the renal arteries shows a high systolic peak and a relatively low diastolic component. Little **spectral broadening** is evident. A clear window under systole means that plug flow is present.

BOX 9-3	Doppler Flow Patterns in Abdominal Arteries

Aorta
- Flow varies at different levels.
- Proximal aorta has high systolic/low diastolic flow.
- Distal demonstrates triphasic flow.

Celiac Axis
- Some spectral broadening
- Unchanged after meals

Hepatic Artery
- Spectral broadening
- Crucial in heart transplants

Splenic Artery
- Very turbulent flow pattern
- Very prone to aneurysm

Superior Mesenteric Artery
- Highly resistive in fasting patient
- Nonresistive in nonfasting patient

Renal Artery
- Nonresistive
- Spectral broadening

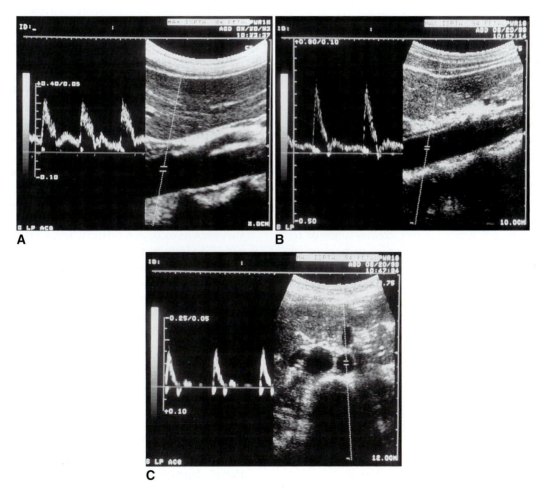

A   **B**   **C**

FIGURE 9-51 A, Sagittal scans of normal flow in the abdominal aorta. **B,** The flow pattern of the proximal aorta above the renal arteries shows a high systolic peak and a relatively low diastolic component. **C,** Transverse view.

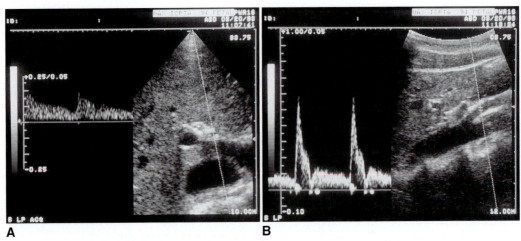

FIGURE 9-52 A, Transverse view of hepatic artery flow. More spectral broadening is seen during systole and diastole. **B,** Sagittal scan of the superior mesenteric artery flow. This vessel has high resistance in the fasting state with little flow in diastole.

The distal abdominal aorta below the renal arteries shows flow with a small reversed component present during diastole. The closer the sonographer approaches the common iliac vessels, the greater the reverse component becomes. This occurs because of the high impedance of peripheral circulation in the leg as it becomes triphasic, crossing the baseline three times.

Celiac Axis. The sonographer should scan transversely to search for the seagull sign, celiac trunk, hepatic artery, and splenic artery. If they cannot be seen, the sonographer should scan longitudinally. Typically, spectral analysis of the celiac trunk shows some window under systole with spectral broadening (turbulence) in diastole. No change in the flow pattern is observed after meals.

Hepatic Artery. The hepatic artery is the most variable of all abdominal arteries. It has been reported that 12% of the population has a replaced hepatic artery arising from the superior mesenteric artery (Figure 9-52, *A*). Two thirds of patients have a right hepatic artery that crosses posterior to the common bile duct or right hepatic duct, whereas the left hepatic artery crosses anterior to the left hepatic duct. Flow in diastole persists because of the low vascular impedance of the liver. Similar waveforms are seen in the main hepatic and intrahepatic arteries. Typically, more spectral broadening occurs during systole and diastole.

In a patient with a heart transplant, the sonographer should always document flow in the hepatic artery. Occlusion is one of the most dangerous complications, potentially resulting in death.

Splenic Artery. This splenic artery shows the greatest turbulence of all the celiac branches, probably because of its tortuosity. Aneurysms of the celiac branches have been described most commonly in the splenic branch. Patients with chronic pancreatitis are particularly prone to these. The sonographer should always apply Doppler to pancreatic pseudocysts; their appearance is very similar to that of vascular aneurysms.

Superior Mesenteric Artery. Typically, the **superior mesenteric artery (SMA)** is a highly resistive vessel (with decreased diastolic flow) in the fasting state, with little or no flow in diastole (see Figure 9-52, *B*). However, after a meal, the pattern of the superior mesenteric artery changes to a low-resistive waveform demonstrating enhanced diastolic flow. Doppler analysis of the superior mesenteric artery has the potential to diagnose mesenteric arterial occlusion and abdominal angina.

Renal Artery. The main renal artery has a low impedance (nonresistive) pattern with significant diastolic flow—usually 30% to 50% of peak systole (Figure 9-53). Continuous diastolic flow provides continuous perfusion of the kidneys. Spectral broadening occurs in systole and diastole. Segmental, interlobar, and arcuate arteries demonstrate a pattern similar to that of the main renal artery. However, the flow is progressively dampened in the periphery and shows reduced velocity patterns.

Renal Artery Stenosis. Box 9-4 lists Doppler flow patterns observed in renal disease.

It is very hard to demonstrate renal artery stenosis in a native kidney because of the difficulty involved in seeing the vessel at its origin and in its entirety (Figure 9-54). Renal artery occlusion can be declared only when the artery is unquestionably imaged. The sonographer should be careful because with complete obstruction of the native artery, collaterals may be mistaken for a patent renal artery. At least 30% of the population has multiple renal arteries, which makes it more difficult to rule out obstruction.

Renal Hydronephrosis. When even minimal separation of the renal pelvis occurs, the sonographer should use Doppler to image the area (Figure 9-55). It is surprising to note that no hydronephrosis may be found, just prominent renal vessels in the renal pelvis.

Renal Transplants. In the main renal artery, turbulence occurs near the anastomosis. Only 12% of patients have renal artery stenosis that develops after

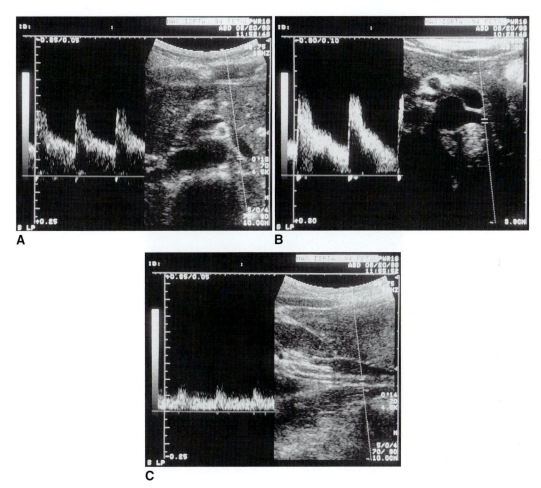

FIGURE 9-53 A and **B,** Transverse scans of the left renal artery flow. The main renal artery has a low impedance (nonresistive) pattern with significant diastolic flow, usually 30% to 50% of peak systole. **C,** Transverse scan of the right renal artery. In this view, it is much more difficult to obtain an adequate Doppler flow because the beam is perpendicular to the flow pattern. As a result, decreased velocities are obtained.

BOX 9-4	Doppler Flow Patterns in Renal Disease

Renal Artery Stenosis
- Stenoses are difficult to demonstrate.
- Collaterals may form.

Renal Hydronephrosis
- Doppler needed to rule out prominent vessels

Renal Transplants
- Turbulence near the anastomosis
- Renal artery stenosis develops in only 12% of renal transplants.
- Occlusion is easier to diagnose than in a native kidney.

Renal Transplant Rejection
- Normal flow = 30% to 50% of diastolic flow
- Impedance increases with rejection.

transplantation; it is characterized by a high-velocity jet with distal turbulence. Renal artery occlusion is easier to diagnose in transplanted kidneys than in native kidneys because no flow takes place throughout the entire transplant.

Rejection. Normal transplants have a diastolic flow that is 30% to 50% that of systole. During rejection, vascular impedance increases, resulting in a decrease in or even reversal of diastolic flow. A few methods may be used to quantify the Doppler signals.

The resistive index (RI) is the most popular method in use. An RI of 0.7 or less indicates good perfusion, whereas an RI of 0.7 to 0.9 indicates possible rejection, and greater than 0.9 indicates probable rejection.

Renal Vein. Box 9-5 lists Doppler flow patterns in renal veins and their related conditions.

The renal vein shows variable flow similar to that of the inferior vena cava (Figure 9-56). The sonographer should closely examine the renal veins in any patient with a suspected tumor or renal obstructive lesion because they may be invaded by tumor or clot (Figure 9-57). In renal transplant patients, the sonographer should always look for a patent renal vein. An occlusion backs up the whole blood supply, and the kidney acts as though it is in rejection (with elevated blood, urea, nitrogen, creatinine, and protein).

Inferior Vena Cava and Hepatic Veins. The inferior vena cava and hepatic veins present a complex

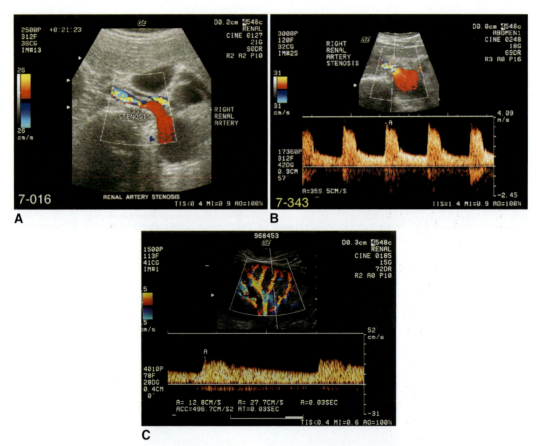

FIGURE 9-54 A, High-velocity jet shown in the right renal artery. **B,** Spectral waveform shows increased velocity of more than 4 m/sec, representing renal artery stenosis. **C,** With color Doppler, flow analysis may be made out to the peripheral renal arteries.

BOX 9-5	**Doppler Flow Patterns in Abdominal Veins**

Renal Vein
- Variable flow much like the inferior vena cava
- Evaluate with transplants.

Inferior Vena Cava and Hepatic Veins
- Vary with respiration
- Flow above and below the baseline, reflux from right atrium

Budd-Chiari Syndrome
- Thrombosis of hepatic veins
- Hepatic veins are small, with echogenic material.
- Presence of normal flow excludes Budd-Chiari syndrome.

Portal Vein
- Hepatopetal flow
- Continuous flow pattern; varies slightly with respirations

Cavernous Transformation of the Portal Vein
- Seen in patients with chronic portal vein obstruction
- Extrahepatic portal vein not visualized
- Echogenic area present in porta hepatis
- Periportal collaterals

Portal Venous Hypertension
- Determine hepatopetal versus hepatofugal flow
- Low velocity in portal vein
- Patent umbilical vein
- Loss of respiratory variation

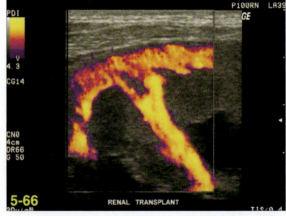

FIGURE 9-55 Doppler energy may be useful to show adequate renal artery flow in the postoperative renal transplant patient.

waveform, which flows above and below the baseline, reflecting reflux of blood from the right atrium during systole and variations with the respiratory cycle (Figure 9-58). The sonographer should always look at the cava and renal veins for tumor invasion when a renal cell carcinoma is observed.

Budd-Chiari Syndrome. A thrombosis of hepatic veins is called ***Budd-Chiari syndrome.*** Duplex Doppler

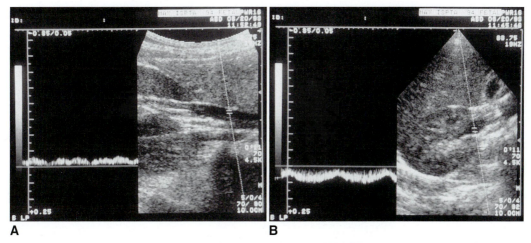

FIGURE 9-56 A and **B,** Transverse scans of right renal vein flow show variable flow similar to the pattern of the inferior vena cava.

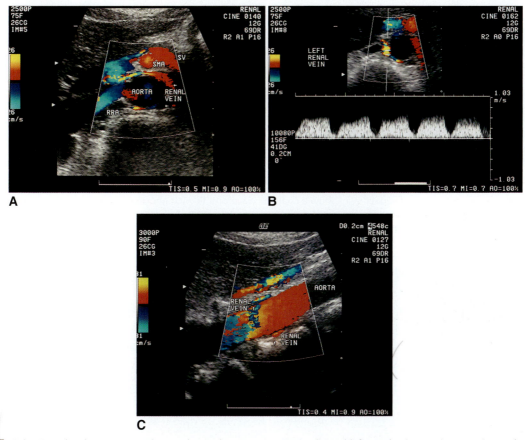

FIGURE 9-57 Color Doppler demonstrates the renal vascular anatomy. **A,** Duplicated left renal vein crossing anterior and posterior to the aorta; right renal artery leaving the lateral wall of the aorta toward the right kidney. **B,** Spectral Doppler shows increased turbulence in the posterior left renal vein. **C,** Coronal view of the association of the renal veins to the aorta.

is an effective method for screening patients suspected of having Budd-Chiari syndrome. Sonographically, hepatic veins appear reduced in size and may contain echogenic thrombotic material. The presence of "typical" blood flow in the hepatic veins permits the exclusion of Budd-Chiari syndrome. Budd-Chiari syndrome is a rare disease; 30% of cases are idiopathic. It is associated with hematologic disorders, oral contraceptives, collagen disease, echinococcus, and the periods before or after pregnancy.

Portal Vein. In the normal superior mesenteric vein and splenic vein, flow is hepatopetal (toward the liver) (Figures 9-59 and 9-60). The portal vein shows a relatively continuous flow at low velocities, which may vary slightly with respirations. Portal vein thrombosis can be easily diagnosed with sonography. A direct sign is

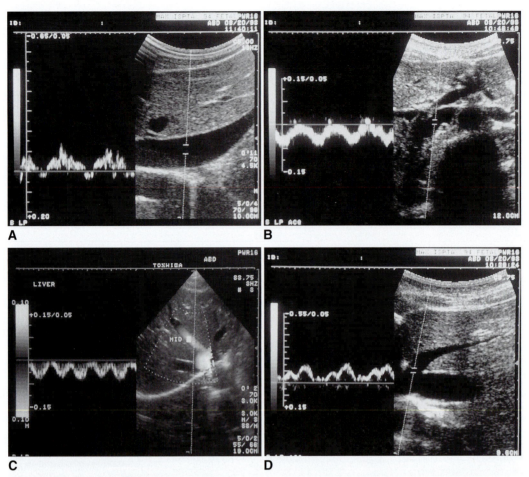

FIGURE 9-58 The inferior vena cava and hepatic veins show a complex waveform flowing above and below baseline. This reflects the reflux of blood from the right atrium during systole and variations with the respiratory cycle. **A,** Sagittal. **B,** Transverse. **C,** Transverse scan of the middle hepatic vein flow shows normal flow patterns. **D,** Sagittal scan shows the complex waveform above and below the baseline.

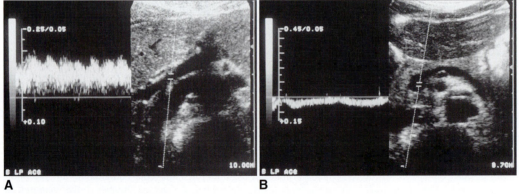

FIGURE 9-59 A, Transverse scan of the main portal vein shows positive flow as it proceeds into the liver (hepatopetal). **B,** Transverse scan of the superior mesenteric vein–portal vein flow.

visualization of a thrombus. Indirect signs include the loss of normal portal venous landmarks, dilation of the superior mesenteric vein and splenic vein, and venous collaterals in the porta hepatis (cavernous transformation of the portal vein).

Pulsed Doppler adds to these findings; lack of Doppler signals from the lumen indicates absence of blood flow.

In cirrhotic patients, thrombosis is often suspected when ascites suddenly worsens. Consequently, in these patients, special attention must be paid to the portal vein to identify a thrombus. It is often difficult to visualize the portal vein in such patients.

Cavernous Transformation of the Portal Vein. Cavernous transformation of the portal vein demonstrates periportal collateral channels in patients with chronic portal vein obstruction. Doppler analysis of the tubular structures is characteristic of portal hepatopetal venous flow hepatopetal with continuous low-velocity flow. Diagnosis can be made sonographically on the basis of the following indications:

1. Extrahepatic portal vein is not visualized.
2. High-level echoes produced by fibrosis are present in the porta hepatis.

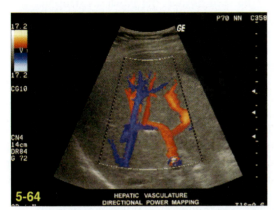

FIGURE 9-60 Color Doppler of the portal flow within the liver.

3. Multiple tubular structures are present in the porta hepatis, representing periportal collaterals.

Portal Venous Hypertension. Most portal venous hypertension is the result of intrinsic liver disease. Portal hypertension is also caused by obstruction of the portal vein, hepatic vein, or inferior vena cava, or by prolonged congestive heart failure. Doppler techniques can determine whether portal flow is hepatopetal (toward) or hepatofugal (away). In portal venous hypertension, portal blood is diverted in a hepatofugal direction via various collateral venous pathways, with the formation of multiple portosystemic anastomoses (Figure 9-61). Doppler findings include the following:

- The portal vein shows low velocity.
- A patent paraumbilical vein is the definitive diagnosis.
- Typical portal hypertensive venous flow varies.
- The condition is most frequently caused by cirrhosis and obstruction of portal venous radicles by fibrosis and regenerating nodules.
- The condition is less frequently caused by portal venous thrombosis or other obstruction.
- Respiratory variation of vessels is usually lost in portal hypertension (no collapse of veins occurs).

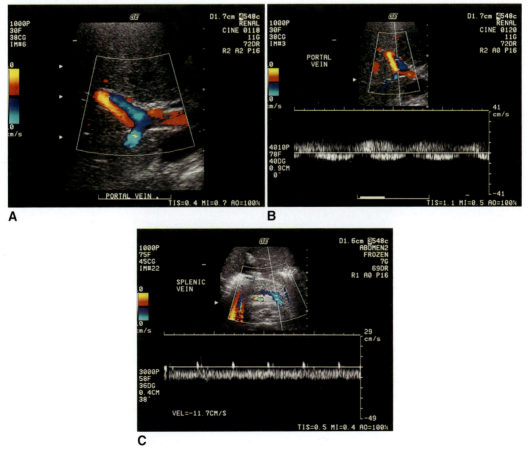

FIGURE 9-61 A, Bidirectional flow within the main portal vein. **B,** Spectral Doppler shows flow above and below baseline. **C,** Flow is reversed in the splenic vein, going away from the liver.

Sonographic findings in portal hypertension include the following:

- Dilated portal, splenic, superior mesenteric vein
- Patent paraumbilical vein
- Varices
- Splenomegaly with dilated splenic radicles
- Diminished response to respiration in portal system
- Dilated hepatic and splenic arteries
- Ascites
- Small liver with irregular surface or large liver with abnormal texture

In patients with portal hypertension, the blood flow may take one of several pathways: through coronary-esophageal varices, splenic varices, splenorenal shunts, a recanalized umbilical vein, or surgical shunts.

With splenic varices, flow in the main, right, and left portal veins is reversed (hepatofugal), as is flow in the splenic vein, and flow in the superior mesenteric vein is normal.

With splenorenal shunts, all portal flows are reversed, as are flows in the splenic vein. The superior mesenteric vein is normal.

With a recanalized umbilical vein, the main portal vein and the left portal vein show normal flow, but flow is reversed in the right portal vein. The superior mesenteric vein and splenic veins are normal.

Spontaneous Shunting. Spontaneous shunting occurs at the following four main sites:

1. *Coronary-gastroesophageal* (most common): Lower esophageal varices occur where esophageal branches of the left gastric vein form anastomoses with branches of the azygos and hemiazygos veins in the submucosa of the lower esophagus.
2. *Paraumbilical vein:* This appears as a continuation of the left portal vein and extends down the anterior abdominal wall to the umbilicus.
3. *Hemorrhoidal anastomoses:* These occur between the superior and middle hemorrhoidal veins.
4. *Retroperitoneal anastomoses:* Vascular structures within the lesser omentum may cause thickening of the omentum (especially in children). Small vessels may be seen around the pancreas. Doppler is useful in distinguishing these vessels from nodes.

Once a portosystemic shunt has been performed, shunt patency can be directly identified with Doppler. This is usually easier with direct portacaval shunts (portal vein drains into inferior vena cava) than with mesocaval (superior mesenteric vein and inferior vena cava) shunts or splenorenal (splenic vein to renal vein) shunts. If the portacaval shunt itself cannot be identified, demonstration of hepatofugal flow in the intrahepatic portal veins and hepatopetal flow in the superior mesenteric vein and splenic veins is a reliable indicator of shunt patency. In long-term follow-up after implantation of a **transjugular intrahepatic portosystemic shunt (TIPS)**, the intrashunt and portal venous Doppler velocities alone do not accurately predict elevation of the portosystemic gradient. This will be further discussed in Chapter 10.

The Liver

Sandra L. Hagen-Ansert

The liver is the largest organ in the body, weighing approximately 1500 g in the adult, and is accessible to sonographic evaluation. The parenchyma of the normal liver is used to evaluate other organs and glands in the body—that is, the kidneys are equally echogenic or less echogenic than the liver, the spleen has about the same echogenicity, and the pancreas is about as echogenic as or slightly more echogenic than the liver. The size and shape of the liver determine the quality of the sonographic examination performed. For example, the prominent left lobe of the liver facilitates visualization of the pancreas, which is situated just inferior to the border of the left lobe, whereas if the right lobe extends just below the costal margin, it may facilitate visualization of the gallbladder and right kidney.

ANATOMY OF THE LIVER

Normal Anatomy

The liver occupies almost all of the **right hypochondrium,** the greater part of the **epigastrium,** and the **left hypochondrium** as far as the mammillary line. The contour and shape of the liver vary according to the patient's habitus and lie. Its shape is also influenced by the lateral segment of the left lobe and the length of the right lobe of the liver. The liver lies inferior to the diaphragm. The ribs cover the greater part of the right lobe (usually a small part of the right lobe is in contact with the abdominal wall). In the epigastric region, the liver extends several centimeters below the xiphoid process. Most of the left lobe is covered by the rib cage.

The fundus of the stomach lies posterior and lateral to the left lobe of the liver and may frequently be seen on transverse sonograms (Figure 10-1). The remainder of the stomach lies inferior to the liver and is best visualized on sagittal sonograms. The duodenum lies adjacent to the right lobe and medial segment of the left lobe of the liver. The body of the pancreas is usually seen just inferior to the left lobe of the liver. The posterior border of the liver contacts the right kidney, inferior vena cava, and aorta. The diaphragm covers the superior border of the liver (Figure 10-2). The liver is suspended from the diaphragm and anterior abdominal wall by the falciform ligament and from the diaphragm by the reflections of the peritoneum.

Most of the liver is covered by peritoneum, but a large area rests directly on the diaphragm; this is called the **bare area** (Figure 10-3). The subphrenic space between the liver (or spleen) and the diaphragm is a common site for abscess formation. The right posterior subphrenic space lies between the right lobe of the liver, the right kidney, and the right colic flexure. The lesser sac is an enclosed portion of the peritoneal space posterior to the liver and stomach. This sac communicates with the rest of the peritoneal space at a point near the head of the

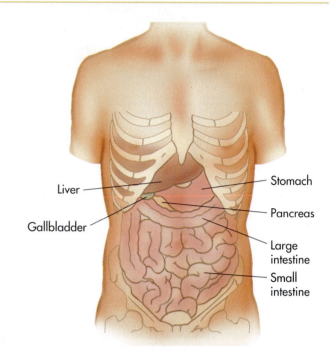

FIGURE 10-1 AP view of the abdomen shows the right lobe of the liver covered by the ribs. The left lobe of the liver lies in the midline just posterior to the tip of the sternum. The stomach lies posterior and lateral to the left lobe of the liver.

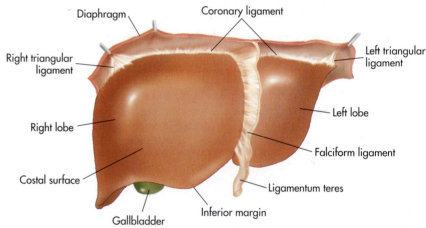

FIGURE 10-2 Anterior view of the liver. The right lobe is the largest of the four lobes of the liver.

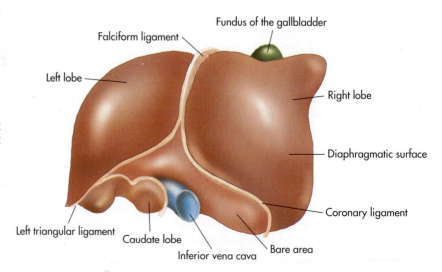

FIGURE 10-3 Superior view of the liver. The left lobe of the liver lies in the epigastric and left hypochondriac regions.

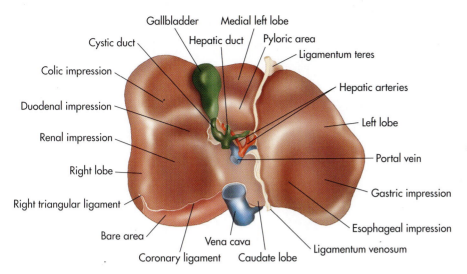

Gallbladder   Medial left lobe
Cystic duct   Hepatic duct / Pyloric area
                              Ligamentum teres
Colic impression
                              Hepatic arteries
Duodenal impression
                              Left lobe
Renal impression
                              Portal vein
Right lobe
                              Gastric impression
Right triangular ligament
                              Esophageal impression
Bare area
Vena cava   Ligamentum venosum
Coronary ligament   Caudate lobe

FIGURE 10-4 Inferior view of the visceral surface of the liver.

pancreas. It also may be a site for abscess formation. The right subhepatic space is located inferior to the right lobe of the liver and includes Morison's pouch, which lies between the posterior aspect of the right lobe and the upper pole of the right kidney.

Projections of the liver may be altered by some disease states. Tumor infiltration, cirrhosis, or a subphrenic abscess often causes inferior displacement, whereas ascites, excessive dilation of the colon, or abdominal tumors can elevate the liver. Retroperitoneal tumors may move the liver slightly anterior.

Lobes of the Liver

Right Lobe. The **right lobe of the liver** is the largest of the liver's four lobes (see Figure 10-5). It exceeds the left lobe by a ratio of 6:1. It occupies the right hypochondrium and is bordered on its upper surface by the falciform ligament, on its posterior surface by the left sagittal fossa, and in front by the umbilical notch. Its inferior and posterior surfaces are marked by three fossae: the porta hepatis, the gallbladder fossa, and the inferior vena cava fossa. A congenital variant, Riedel's lobe, can sometimes be seen as an anterior projection of the liver and may extend to the iliac crest.

Left Lobe. The **left lobe of the liver** lies in the epigastric and left hypochondriac regions (see Figure 10-3). Its upper surface is convex and molded onto the diaphragm. Its undersurface includes the gastric impression and omental tuberosity. The medial segment of the left lobe is oblong and situated on the posteroinferior surface of the left lobe (Figure 10-4). In front it is bounded by the anterior margin of the liver, behind by the porta hepatis, on the right by the fossa for the gallbladder, and on the left by the fossa for the umbilical vein. The size of the left lobe of the liver varies considerably; a more prominent left lobe will allow the sonographer to image the pancreas and vascular structures anterior to the spine.

BOX 10-1	Hepatic Segmental Anatomy

Segment I: Caudate lobe
Segments II and III: Left superior and inferior lateral segments
Segments IVa and IVb: Medial segments of the left lobe
Segments V and VI: Caudal to the transverse plane
Segments VII and VIII: Cephalad to the transverse plane

Caudate Lobe. The **caudate lobe** is a small lobe situated on the posterosuperior surface of the left lobe opposite the tenth and eleventh thoracic vertebrae (Figure 10-5). It is bounded below by the porta hepatis, on the right by the fossa for the inferior vena cava, and on the left by the fossa for the ductus venosus.

Hepatic Nomenclature. Couinaud's system of hepatic nomenclature (Box 10-1) provides the anatomic basis for hepatic surgical resections. By using this system, the radiologist may be able to precisely isolate the location of a lesion for the surgical team. The description of the liver segments is based on the portal and hepatic venous segments. There are eight segments (Figure 10-6). The right, middle, and left hepatic veins divide the liver longitudinally into four sections. Each of these sections is further divided transversely by an invisible plane through the right and left portal veins. The caudate lobe (segment I) may receive branches of both the right and left portal veins and may have one or more hepatic veins draining into the inferior vena cava.

Ligaments and Fissures. There are several important ligaments and fissures to remember in the liver: Glisson's capsule, main lobar fissure, falciform ligament, ligamentum teres (round ligament), and ligamentum venosum. These ligaments and fissures appear echogenic or hyperechoic because of the presence of collagen and fat within and around the structures.

The liver is covered by a thin connective tissue layer called Glisson's capsule. This capsule completely surrounds the liver and is thickest around the inferior vena

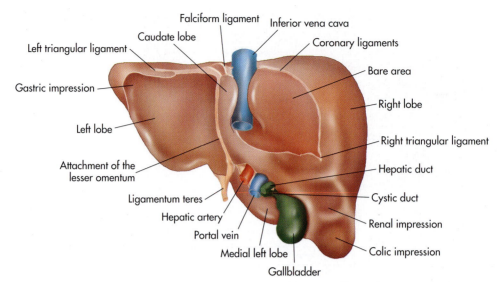

FIGURE 10-5 Posterior view of the diaphragmatic surface of the liver. The caudate lobe is located on the posterosuperior surface of the right lobe, opposite the tenth and eleventh thoracic vertebrae. The medial segment is also called the quadrate lobe.

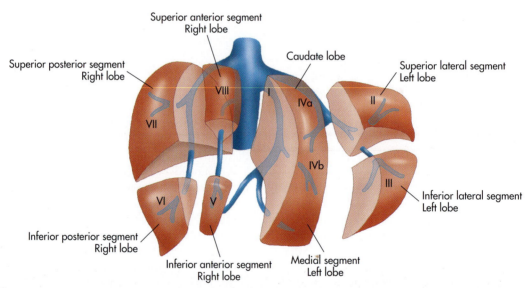

FIGURE 10-6 Couinaud's hepatic segments divide the liver into eight segments. The three hepatic veins are the longitudinal boundaries. The transverse plane is defined by the right and left portal pedicles. The caudate lobe (segment I) is situated posteriorly. Segment I includes the caudate lobe. Segments II and III include the left superior and inferior lateral segments. Segments IVa and IVb include the medial segment of the left lobe. Segments V and VI are caudal to the transverse plane. Segments VII and VIII are cephalad to the transverse plane.

cava and portal hepatis. At the porta hepatis, the main portal vein, the proper hepatic artery, and the common duct are contained within the hepatoduodenal ligament.

The **main lobar fissure** is the boundary between the right and left lobes of the liver. On the longitudinal scan, it may be seen as a hyperechoic line extending from the portal vein to the neck of the gallbladder (Figure 10-7, *A*). The sonographer uses this ligament to find the gallbladder on the longitudinal scan, especially when it is packed with stones and not well imaged.

The **falciform ligament** extends from the umbilicus to the diaphragm in a parasagittal plane and contains the ligamentum teres (Figure 10-7, *B*). In the anteroposterior

axis, the falciform ligament extends from the right rectus muscle to the bare area of the liver, where its echogenic reflections separate to contribute to the hepatic coronary ligament and attach to the undersurface of the diaphragm.

The **ligamentum teres** appears as a bright echogenic focus on the sonogram and is seen as the rounded termination of the falciform ligament (Figure 10-7, *C*). Both the falciform ligament and the ligamentum teres divide the medial and lateral segments of the left lobe of the liver.

The fissure for the **ligamentum venosum** separates the left lobe from the caudate lobe (Figure 10-8). On ultrasound, it may be seen just inferior to the dome of the

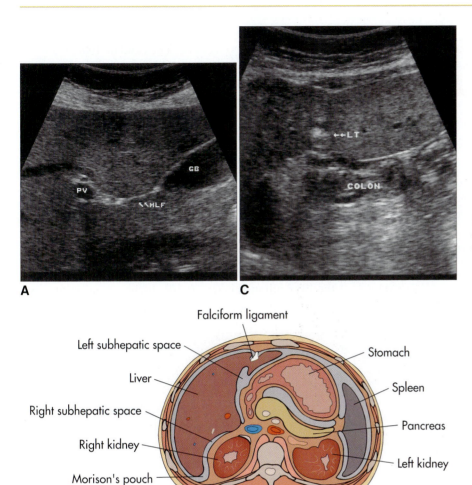

FIGURE 10-7 A, Main lobar fissure *(MLF)* extends between the long axis neck of the gallbladder *(GB)* and the main portal vein *(PV)* on the longitudinal image. **B,** Falciform ligament extends from the umbilicus to the diaphragm in a longitudinal plane. **C,** Ligamentum teres *(LT, arrows)* appears as a bright echogenic focus in the left lobe of the liver on a transverse image.

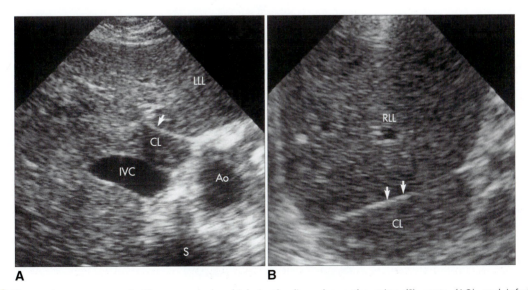

FIGURE 10-8 Ligamentum venosum. **A,** Transverse image high in the liver shows the spine *(S)*, aorta *(AO)*, and inferior vena cava *(IVC)*. The caudate lobe *(CL)* is anterior to the inferior vena cava *(IVC)* and is separated from the left lobe of the liver *(LLL)* by the ligamentum venosum *(arrow)*. **B,** Longitudinal image through the right lobe of the liver *(RLL)* shows the ligamentum venosum *(arrows)* and caudate lobe *(CL)*.

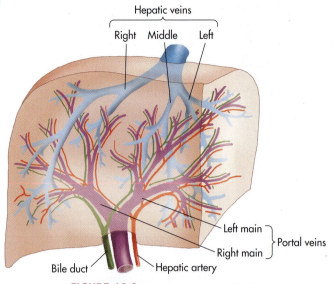

FIGURE 10-9 Vascular system of the liver.

liver as a linear horizontal line just anterior to the caudate lobe and inferior vena cava. The caudate lobe, ligamentum venosum, portal vein, and left lobe of the liver may be seen on the longitudinal plane over the area of the inferior vena cava.

Vascular Supply

Portal Venous System. The portal venous system is a reliable indicator of various ultrasonic tomographic planes throughout the liver (Figure 10-9).

Main Portal Vein. The **main portal vein** approaches the porta hepatis in a rightward, cephalic, and slightly posterior direction within the hepatoduodenal ligament. It comes in contact with the anterior surface of the inferior vena cava near the porta hepatis and serves to locate the liver hilum (Figure 10-10). It then divides into two branches: the right and left portal veins.

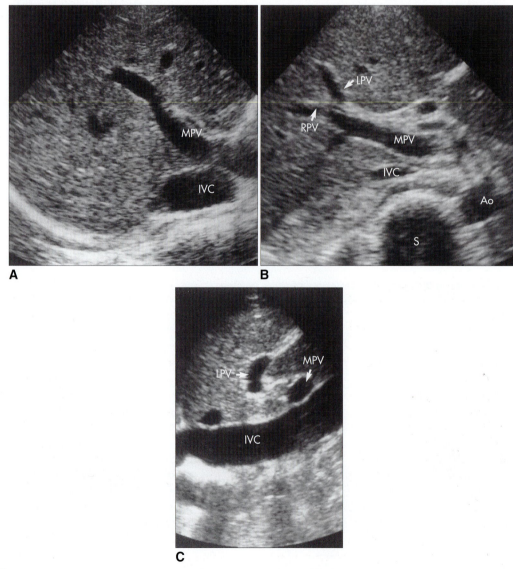

FIGURE 10-10 Main portal vein. **A,** Transverse image of the main portal vein (*MPV*) as it enters the liver. *IVC,* Inferior vena cava. **B,** Transverse image of the main portal vein (*MPV*) as it bifurcates into right (*RPV*) and left (*LPV*) branches. *AO,* Aorta; *IVC,* inferior vena cava; *S,* spine. **C,** Longitudinal image just to the right of midline shows the inferior vena cava (*IVC*), main portal vein (*MPV*), and left portal vein (*LPV*).

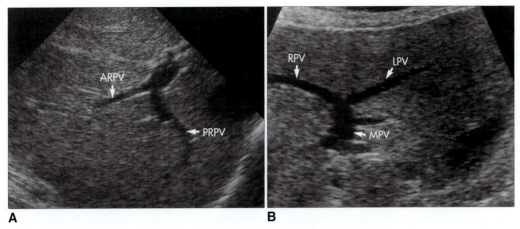

FIGURE 10-11 Right portal vein. **A,** Transverse image of the right portal vein as it bifurcates into the anterior *(ARPV)* and posterior *(PRPV)* branches. **B,** Transverse image of the main portal vein *(MPV)* as it bifurcates into right *(RPV)* and left *(LPV)* branches.

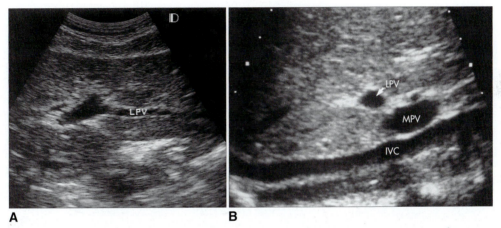

FIGURE 10-12 Left portal vein. **A,** Transverse image of the right portal vein branching into the left portal vein *(LPV)* as it flows into the left lobe of the liver. **B,** Longitudinal image just to the right of midline shows the inferior vena cava *(IVC)*, the main portal vein *(MPV)*, and the left portal vein *(LPV)*.

Right Portal Vein. The **right portal vein** is the larger of the two branches and requires a more posterior and more caudal transducer approach. It usually is possible to identify the anterior and posterior divisions of the right portal vein on sonography (Figure 10-11). The anterior division closely parallels the anterior abdominal wall.

Left Portal Vein. The **left portal vein** lies more anterior and cranial than the right portal vein. The main portal vein is seen to elongate at the origin of the left portal vein (Figure 10-12). The vessel lies within a canal containing large amounts of connective tissue, which results in the visualization of an echogenic linear band coursing through the central portion of the lateral segment of the left lobe.

Hepatic Veins. The hepatic veins are divided into three components: right, middle, and left (Figure 10-13). The right hepatic vein is the largest and enters the right lateral aspect of the inferior vena cava. The middle hepatic vein enters the anterior or right anterior surface of the inferior vena cava. The left hepatic vein, which is the smallest, enters the left anterior surface of the inferior vena cava. Often it is possible to identify a long horizontal branch of the right hepatic vein coursing between the anterior and posterior divisions of the right portal vein.

Distinguishing Characteristics of Portal and Hepatic Veins. The best way to distinguish the hepatic from the portal vessels is to trace their points of entry to the liver. The hepatic vessels flow into the inferior vena cava, whereas the splenic vein and superior mesenteric vein join to form the portal venous system. Real-time sector scanning allows the sonographer to make this assessment within a few seconds (Figure 10-14). Hepatic veins course between the hepatic lobes and segments. Hepatic veins are larger as they drain into the inferior vena cava before entering the right atrium; the portal veins are larger at their origin as they emanate from the porta hepatis. Portal veins have more echogenic borders than the hepatic veins because they have a thicker collagenous sheath.

Intrahepatic Vessels and Ducts. The portal veins carry blood from the bowel to the liver, whereas the hepatic

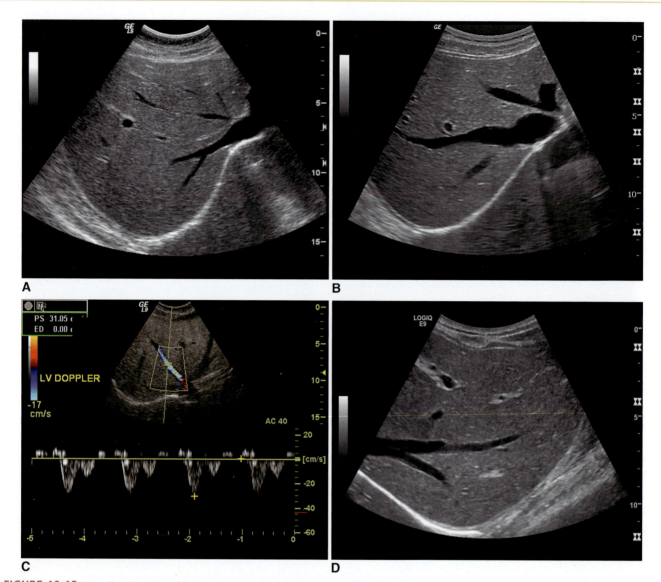

FIGURE 10-13 Hepatic veins. **A** and **B,** Transverse images at the dome of the liver show the hepatic veins as they empty into the inferior vena cava *(IVC)*. **C,** Transverse Doppler evaluation of the middle hepatic vein as it empties into the inferior vena cava. **D,** Longitudinal image of the hepatic veins draining into the inferior vena cava.

veins drain the blood from the liver into the inferior vena cava (see Figure 10-9). The hepatic arteries carry oxygenated blood from the aorta to the liver (Figure 10-15). The bile ducts transport bile, manufactured in the liver, to the duodenum.

PHYSIOLOGY AND LABORATORY DATA OF THE HEPATOBILIARY SYSTEM

The liver, bile ducts, and gallbladder constitute the hepatobiliary system, which performs metabolic and excretory functions essential to physical well-being. Sonography is an important method for detecting anatomic changes associated with hepatobiliary disease, but accurate ultrasound evaluation can be accomplished only when other diagnostic information (e.g., signs, symptoms, and laboratory results) are considered with the sonographic findings.

The task of correlating these clinical and ultrasound data falls primarily to the sonologist. However, the sonographer must also understand the entire clinical picture to be able to plan and properly perform the ultrasound examination. It is necessary, therefore, that the sonographer be aware of the normal and abnormal physiology of the hepatobiliary system. This section is intended as a primer of hepatobiliary physiology, with particular attention to physiologic alterations that commonly occur in hepatobiliary disease.

Hepatic Physiology

The liver has many functions, including metabolism, digestion, storage, and detoxification (Box 10-2). The liver is a major center of metabolism, which may be defined as the physical and chemical process whereby foodstuffs are synthesized into complex elements,

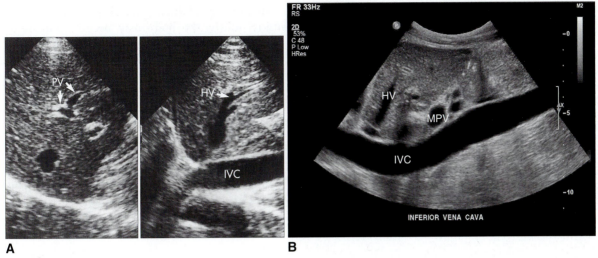

FIGURE 10-14 **A,** Portal versus hepatic veins. The portal veins *(PV)* have more echogenic borders than the hepatic veins *(HV)*. *IVC,* Inferior vena cava. **B,** Longitudinal image of the inferior vena cava with the main portal vein *(MPV)* anterior. The hepatic vein *(HV)* is not as reflective as the portal vein.

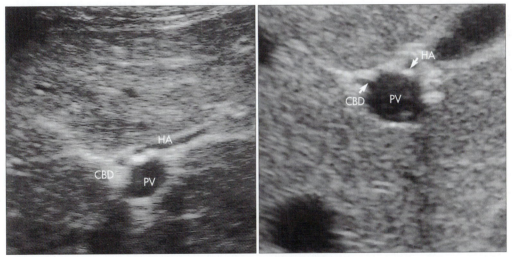

FIGURE 10-15 Hepatic artery *(HA)* may be seen anterior and medial to the portal vein on an oblique transverse image; this is known as the *portal triad. Arrow,* Hepatic artery; *CBD,* common bile duct; *PV,* portal vein.

complex substances are transformed into simple ones, and energy is made available for use by the organism. Through the process of digestion, the liver expels these waste products from the body via its excretory product, bile, which also plays an important role in fat absorption. **Bilirubin** is a pigment released when the red blood cells are broken down. The liver is a storage site for several compounds used in a variety of physiologic activities throughout the body. In hepatobiliary disease, each of these functions may be altered, leading to abnormal physical, laboratory, and sonographic findings. Finally, the liver is also a center for detoxification of the waste products of metabolism accumulated from other sources in the body and foreign chemicals (usually drugs) that enter the body.

Hepatic Versus Obstructive Disease

Diseases affecting the liver may be classified as *hepatocellular*, when the liver cells or hepatocytes are the immediate problem, or *obstructive*, when bile excretion is blocked. Viral hepatitis is an example of hepatocellular liver disease: The virus attacks liver cells and damages or destroys them, resulting in an alteration of liver function. In obstructive disorders, the flow of bile from the liver is blocked at some point, and the liver malfunctions as a secondary result of the blockage.

The differentiation between **hepatocellular disease** and **obstructive disease** is of considerable importance clinically. Hepatocellular diseases are treated medically with supportive measures and drugs; obstructive

BOX 10-2   Primary Functions of the Liver

Metabolism
- *Carbohydrate.* The liver converts glucose to glycogen and stores it; when glucose is needed, it breaks down the glycogen and releases glucose into the blood.
- *Protein.* The liver performs many important functions in metabolism of proteins, fats, and carbohydrates. It manufactures many of the plasma proteins found in the blood. The liver converts excess amino acids to fatty acids and urea. It also removes nutrients from the blood and phagocytizes bacteria and worn-out red blood cells.

Digestion
The liver secretes bile, which is important in the digestion of fats. Bilirubin, a pigment released when red blood cells are broken down, is excreted in the bile.

Storage
The liver stores iron and certain vitamins.

Detoxification
The liver detoxifies many drugs and poisons that enter the body.

disorders are usually treated surgically. In some cases the distinction between hepatocellular and obstructive disease can be made through clinical laboratory tests, but often the laboratory findings are equivocal. Sonography has been of great benefit because it allows the physician to accurately separate hepatocellular and obstructive causes of liver disease.

Hepatic Metabolic Functions

Raw materials in the form of carbohydrates (sugars), fats, and amino acids (the basic components of proteins) are absorbed from the intestine and transported to the liver via the circulatory system. In the liver, these substances are converted chemically to other compounds or are processed for storage or energy production. The following sections are brief discussions of the liver's metabolic functions and of how liver disease can disturb these functions.

Carbohydrates. Sugars may be absorbed from the blood in several forms, but only glucose can be used by cells throughout the body as a source of energy.

The liver functions as a major site for conversion of dietary sugars into glucose, which is released into the bloodstream for general use. The body requires only a certain amount of glucose at any one time, however. Excess sugar is converted by the liver to glycogen (a starch), which may be stored in the liver cells or transported in the blood to distant storage sites. When dietary sugar is unavailable, the liver converts glycogen released from stores into glucose; it can also manufacture glucose directly from other compounds, including proteins or fats, when other sources of glucose have been depleted. Thus, the liver helps to maintain a steady state of glucose in the bloodstream.

In severe liver disease, unless glucose is administered intravenously, the body may become glucose-deficient (**hypoglycemia**), with profound effects on the function of the brain and other organs. Uncontrolled increases in blood glucose (**hyperglycemia**) may occur in severe liver disease if a large dose of glucose is administered, because the liver fails to convert the excess glucose to glycogen.

Fats. The liver is also a principal site for metabolism of fats, which are absorbed from the intestine in the form of monoglycerides and diglycerides. Dietary fats are converted in the hepatocytes to lipoproteins, in which form fats are transported throughout the body to sites where they are stored or used by other organs. Conversely, stored fats may be transported to the liver and converted into energy, yielding glucose or other substances, such as cholesterol.

In severe liver disease, abnormally low blood levels of cholesterol may be noted because the liver is the principal site for cholesterol synthesis. Furthermore, failure of hepatic conversion of fat to glucose in liver disease may contribute to hypoglycemia. A striking histologic manifestation of many forms of hepatocellular disease is the so-called fatty liver. On gross pathologic examination, the fatty liver has a yellow color and feels greasy to the touch; on microscopic study, globules of fat (primarily triglycerides) crowd the hepatocytes. The cause of fat accumulation in the liver cells is poorly understood, but it is believed to result from failure of the hepatocytes to manufacture special proteins, called lipoproteins, that coat small quantities of fat, making the fat soluble in plasma and allowing for its release into the bloodstream. Fatty liver is a nonspecific finding that may be seen in a variety of conditions including viral hepatitis, alcoholic liver disease, obesity, diabetes, pregnancy, and exposure to toxic chemicals.

Proteins. The liver produces a variety of proteins, either indirectly from amino acids absorbed from the gut or directly from raw materials stored within the body. Albumin, in particular, is produced in great quantities. In the bloodstream, it functions as a transport medium for some kinds of molecules. Because it is nonionic, it also functions to draw water into the vascular system from tissue spaces; stated more technically, it helps to maintain oncotic pressure within the vascular system. When the liver is chronically diseased, clinical laboratory results may reveal a significant lowering of the serum albumin, a condition called *hypoalbuminemia*. The accompanying loss of oncotic pressure in the vascular system allows fluid to migrate into the interstitial space, resulting in edema (swelling) in dependent areas, such as the lower extremities. In patients with severe liver disease, especially advanced cirrhosis, ascites also develop. Hypoalbuminemia may account in part for the ascites, but the development of ascites is principally caused by portal hypertension.

In addition to being the primary source of albumin synthesis, the liver is the principal source of proteins

TABLE 10-1	Comparison of Laboratory Abnormalities in Hepatocellular Disease and Biliary Obstruction					
Condition	Bilirubin	Serum Albumin	AST	ALT	Alkaline Phosphatase
Hepatocellular disease	Minimal to severe increase	Decreased	Moderate to severe increase	Moderate to severe increase	Minimal to moderate increase
Obstruction	Severe increase	Normal	Mild increase	Mild increase	Severe increase

AST, aspartate aminotransferase; ALT, alanine aminotransferase.

necessary for blood coagulation, including fibrinogen (factor I), prothrombin (factor II), and factors V, VII, IX, and X. In liver disease, decreased production of these proteins may lead to inadequate blood coagulation and uncontrollable hemorrhage. Commonly such hemorrhages occur into the bowel after rupture of a dilated vein or development of an ulcer. These hemorrhages are often the immediate or contributing cause of death. Deficiencies of clotting factors II, VII, IX, and X also may result from failure of intestinal absorption of vitamin K, which is a precursor (raw material) required for synthesis of these factors. Vitamin K is a fat-soluble vitamin (as are vitamins D, A, and E) and is absorbed only from the intestine in solution with fat.

Fat absorption is severely limited in cases of bile duct obstruction because of the absence of bile salts (discussed later), which severely reduces the absorption of fat-soluble vitamins. Ultimately the deficiency of vitamin K lowers the amount of the previously mentioned factors and coagulation is retarded. Deficiency of prothrombin and other vitamin K–dependent factors can be corrected in cases of obstruction through parenteral administration of vitamin K.

In hepatocellular disease, administration of vitamin K may improve the coagulopathy but frequently does not restore normal clotting function because the primary problem is hepatocyte dysfunction.

Clotting deficiencies related to liver disease may be detected with several laboratory tests. Of particular interest are the prothrombin time (pro-time) and partial thromboplastin time (PTT) tests. The results of these tests are presented as percentages of the time required for certain coagulation steps to occur in the patient's blood compared with normal blood. Longer periods (lower percentages) indicate greater degrees of abnormality in each of these tests.

Hepatic Enzymes. Enzymes are protein catalysts used throughout the body in all metabolic processes. Because the liver is a major center of metabolism, large quantities of enzymes are present in hepatocytes, and these enzymes leak into the bloodstream when the liver cells are damaged or destroyed by disease. The presence of increased quantities of enzymes in the blood is a sensitive indicator of a hepatocellular disorder.

In hepatobiliary disease the enzymes aspartate aminotransferase (AST), alanine aminotransferase (ALT), and alkaline phosphatase are of particular interest. Serum levels of all three of these enzymes are increased in both hepatocellular disease and biliary obstruction, but the patterns of elevation may help differentiate hepatocellular from obstructive causes (Table 10-1). In biliary obstruction, elevation of AST and ALT is usually mild (serum levels typically do not exceed 300 units). However, in severe hepatocellular destruction, such as acute viral or toxic hepatitis, a striking elevation of AST and ALT may be seen (levels frequently exceed 1000 units).

Marked elevation of alkaline phosphatase, on the other hand, is typically associated with biliary obstruction or the presence of mass lesions in the liver (e.g., metastatic disease or abscesses). Low levels of alkaline phosphatase are unusual in obstruction, and high levels (greater than 15 Bodansky units) are uncommon in hepatocellular disorders. Alkaline phosphatase is such a sensitive indicator of obstruction that it may become elevated before the serum bilirubin in cases of acute obstruction. Hence, a disproportional increase of alkaline phosphatase relative to bilirubin always suggests obstruction. Elevation of serum alkaline phosphatase may be the only abnormal laboratory finding in metastatic disease.

Whereas the pattern of enzyme abnormality may strongly suggest hepatocellular disease or obstruction in some cases, it may not allow this distinction to be made in others because obstruction may be superimposed on preexisting hepatocellular disease or unrelieved obstruction may cause hepatocellular damage. Confusion in interpretation of serum enzyme abnormalities may also occur when AST, ALT, or alkaline phosphatase is released from diseased tissues other than the liver. For example, AST and ALT are increased with damage to heart and skeletal muscle, and alkaline phosphatase is elevated in bone disease and in normal pregnancies. ALT is somewhat more specific for liver disease than AST; therefore, elevation of ALT above AST suggests a hepatic cause.

Hepatic Detoxification Functions

The liver is a major location for detoxification of waste products of energy production and other metabolic activities occurring throughout the body. It is also the principal site of breakdown of foreign chemicals, such as drugs. Although these functions fall under the general definition of metabolism and could therefore be grouped in the preceding section, it is useful for instructional purposes to think of these functions as separate categories of hepatic activity.

Ammonium, a toxic product of nitrogen metabolism, is converted to nontoxic urea in the liver, which is practically the only site where this conversion occurs. Urea is subsequently eliminated from the body by the kidneys. The level of urea in the blood is measured as the **blood urea nitrogen (BUN),** and in severe liver disease (acute or chronic) the BUN may be abnormally low because of falloff of urea production. The exhaled breath of patients with severe liver disease may have a fruity or pungent odor (known as *fetor hepaticus*) because of ammonium (NH_4) accumulation. More important, the concentration of NH_4 in the blood may rise to toxic levels and cause brain dysfunction (including confusion, coordination disturbances, tremor, and coma).

Gastrointestinal hemorrhage frequently leads to the accumulation of toxic levels of NH_4 in the blood. Blood lost into the intestine is broken down by bacteria into nitrogen-containing substances, which are absorbed into the bloodstream. The failing liver may therefore be presented with a large amount of NH_4 that it cannot detoxify; coma may result and is frequently a precursor to death if the patient does not succumb to the direct effects of blood loss. Thus, failure of ammonium detoxification is a serious consequence of liver failure.

Bilirubin Detoxification. Bilirubin, the breakdown product of hemoglobin, is also an important substance detoxified in the liver. Along with detoxification, the liver also excretes bilirubin into the gut via the biliary tree. Red blood cells survive an average of 120 days in the circulatory system; they are then trapped and broken down by reticuloendothelial cells, primarily within the spleen. Hemoglobin released from the red cells is converted to bilirubin within the reticuloendothelial system and is then released into the bloodstream. The bilirubin molecules become attached to albumin in the blood and are transported to the liver, where the following metabolic steps take place in the hepatocytes:

1. *Uptake.* The bilirubin is separated from albumin, probably at the cell membrane, and is taken within the hepatocytes.
2. *Conjugation.* The bilirubin molecule is combined with two glucuronide molecules, forming bilirubin diglucuronide.
3. *Excretion.* The bilirubin molecule is actively transported across the cell membrane into the bile canaliculi, which are the microscopic "headwaters" of the biliary system. Bilirubin released from the hepatocytes passes through the bile ducts with other components of bile and is delivered to the bowel, where most bilirubin diglucuronide is excreted into the feces. (A small portion is broken down into urobilinogen by intestinal bacteria, absorbed into the portal system, and reexcreted by the liver.)

Measurement of the concentration of bilirubin in the blood is a standard laboratory test for hepatocellular disease. The following two fractions of bilirubin are measured: the direct-acting fraction, which reacts chemically in an aqueous medium and consists of conjugated bilirubin, and the indirect-acting fraction, which consists of unconjugated bilirubin released from the reticuloendothelial system. Indirect bilirubin reacts only in a nonaqueous (alcohol) medium. The total bilirubin is the sum of the direct-acting and the indirect-acting fractions and normally does not exceed 1 mg/100 ml of serum. In hematologic diseases associated with abrupt breakdown of large numbers of red blood cells (hemolytic anemias, transfusion reactions), the liver may receive more bilirubin from the reticuloendothelial system than it can detoxify. The level of indirect, or unconjugated, bilirubin therefore is elevated.

In biliary obstruction, the hepatocytes pick up bilirubin and conjugate it with glucuronide molecules but cannot dispose of it. The conjugated form is then regurgitated into the bloodstream, with resultant elevation of the direct-acting bilirubin fraction. The indirect-acting bilirubin may also rise slightly in biliary obstruction, but the direct bilirubin predominates.

The direct, or conjugated, form also predominates in hepatocellular disease. Excretion of bilirubin is the step most readily affected when the hepatocytes are damaged; therefore, the diseased hepatocytes continue to take in and conjugate bilirubin but are unable to excrete it. As in biliary obstruction, the accumulated conjugated bilirubin is regurgitated into the blood.

The direct and indirect patterns may be summarized as in Table 10-2.

Elevation of serum bilirubin results in jaundice, which is a yellow coloration of the skin, sclerae, and body secretions. Jaundice is a nonspecific finding seen in massive blood breakdown, hepatocellular disease, or biliary obstruction. Chemical separation of bilirubin into direct and indirect fractions helps to specify a hepatocellular or hematologic cause for jaundice. Furthermore, if jaundice results from liver disease, the level of bilirubin may help to separate hepatocellular disease from obstruction because it is uncommon for the total bilirubin to rise above 35 mg/100 ml of serum with obstruction.

TABLE 10-2	Direct and Indirect Patterns of Bilirubin	
Condition	Direct Bilirubin Predominates	Indirect Bilirubin Predominates
Hemolysis		X
Hepatocellular disease	X	
Biliary obstruction	X	

Hormone and Drug Detoxification. The liver breaks down several hormones that otherwise would accumulate in the body. For example, failure to metabolize estrogen in men with chronic hepatocellular disease, such as cirrhosis, causes gynecomastia (breast enlargement), testicular atrophy, and changes in body-hair patterns. Reduced detoxification of the hormone glucagon, which is an insulin antagonist, occurs in liver disease and may contribute to the fluctuations in blood sugar levels seen in severe hepatic disorders. The liver is also the primary location for breakdown of medications and other foreign chemicals administered orally or parenterally. It is of particular concern that doses of medications be reduced to compensate for the loss of this function in patients with severe liver disease; otherwise, accumulation of drugs may lead to overdosage.

Bile

Bile is the excretory product of the liver. It is formed continuously by the hepatocytes, collects in the bile canaliculi adjacent to these cells, and is transported to the gut via the bile ducts (Figure 10-16). The principal components of bile are water, bile salts, and bile pigments (primarily bilirubin diglucuronide). Other components include cholesterol, lecithin, and protein. The primary functions of bile are the emulsification of intestinal fat and the removal of waste products excreted by the liver.

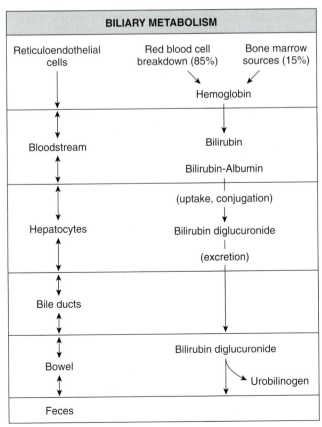

FIGURE 10-16 Biliary metabolism.

Fats are absorbed into the portal blood and intestinal lymphatics in the form of monoglycerides and triglycerides by the action of the intestinal mucosa, but efficient absorption occurs only when the fat molecules are suspended in solution through the emulsifying action of bile salts. As emulsifiers, bile salts act like nonionic detergents to suspend fats in solution within the watery medium of the intestinal contents. Both hepatocellular disease and biliary obstruction affect the amount of bile salts available for fat absorption, but obstruction generally has the more profound effect. Absence of bile salts may lead to steatorrhea (fatty stools), but a more important effect is failure of absorption of the fat-soluble vitamins (D, A, K, and E). As previously noted, vitamin K is an essential precursor for hepatic production of several clotting factors; the absence of this vitamin leads to bleeding tendencies in patients with hepatobiliary disease.

Bile Pigments. Bile pigments are the principal cause of ultrasonic scattering in echogenic bile, although cholesterol crystals may also contribute to this finding. The presence of echogenic bile indicates stasis, but this stasis is not always pathologic and may simply result from prolonged fasting.

Liver Function Tests

Liver function tests are a group of laboratory tests established to analyze how the liver is performing under normal and diseased conditions. In patients with known liver disease, a number of laboratory tests are used to help in the diagnosis, including the following:

- Aspartate aminotransferase (AST)
- Alanine aminotransferase (ALT)
- Lactic acid dehydrogenase (LDH)
- Alkaline phosphatase (alk phos)
- Bilirubin (indirect, direct, and total)
- Prothrombin time
- Albumin and globulins

Aspartate Aminotransferase. Aspartate aminotransferase (AST) is an enzyme present in tissues that have a high rate of metabolic activity, one of which is the liver. As a result of death or injury to the producing cells, the enzyme is released into the bloodstream in abnormally high levels. Any disease that injures the cells causes an elevation in AST levels. This enzyme is also produced in other high-metabolic tissues, so an elevation does not always mean liver disease is present. Significant elevations are characteristic of acute hepatitis and cirrhosis. The level is also elevated in patients with hepatic necrosis, acute hepatitis, and infectious mononucleosis.

Alanine Aminotransferase. Alanine aminotransferase (ALT) is more specific than AST for evaluating liver function. This enzyme is slightly elevated in acute cirrhosis, hepatic metastasis, and pancreatitis. There is a mild to moderate increase in obstructive jaundice.

Hepatocellular disease and infectious or toxic hepatitis produce moderate to highly increased levels. In alcoholic hepatitis, AST is higher.

Lactic Acid Dehydrogenase. Lactic acid dehydrogenase is found in the tissues of several systems including the kidneys, heart, skeletal muscle, brain, liver, and lungs. Cellular injury and death cause this enzyme to increase. This test is moderately increased in infectious mononucleosis and mildly elevated in hepatitis, cirrhosis, and obstructive jaundice. Its primary use is in detection of myocardial or pulmonary infarction.

Alkaline Phosphatase. Alkaline phosphatase is produced by the liver, bone, intestines, and placenta. It may be a good indicator of intrahepatic or extrahepatic obstruction, hepatic carcinoma, abscess, or cirrhosis. In hepatitis and cirrhosis the enzyme is moderately elevated.

Bilirubin. Bilirubin is a product of the breakdown of hemoglobin in tired red blood cells. The liver converts these by-products into bile pigments, which, along with other factors, are secreted as bile by the liver cells into the bile ducts. The following are three ways this cycle can be disturbed:

- An excessive amount of red blood cell destruction
- Malfunction of liver cells
- Blockage of ducts leading from cells

These disturbances cause a rise in serum bilirubin, which leaks into the tissues and thus gives the skin a jaundiced, or yellow, coloration.

Indirect bilirubin is unconjugated bilirubin. Elevation of this test result is seen with increased red blood cell destruction (anemias, trauma from a hematoma, or hemorrhagic pulmonary infarct).

Direct bilirubin is conjugated bilirubin. This product circulates in the blood and is excreted into the bile after it reaches the liver and is conjugated with glucuronide. Elevation of direct bilirubin is usually related to obstructive jaundice (from stones or neoplasm).

Specific liver diseases may cause an elevation of both direct and indirect bilirubin levels, but the increase in the direct level is more marked. These diseases are hepatic metastasis, hepatitis, lymphoma, cholestasis secondary to drugs, and cirrhosis.

Prothrombin Time. Prothrombin is a liver enzyme that is part of the blood clotting mechanism. The production of prothrombin depends on adequate intake and use of vitamin K. The prothrombin time is increased in the presence of liver disease with cellular damage. Cirrhosis and metastatic disease are examples of disorders that cause prolonged prothrombin time.

Albumin and Globulins. Assessment of depressed synthesis of proteins, especially serum albumin and the plasma coagulation factors, is a sensitive test for metabolic derangement of the liver. In patients with hepatocellular damage, a low serum albumin suggests decreased protein synthesis. A prolonged prothrombin time indicates a poor prognosis. Chronic liver diseases commonly show an elevation of gamma globulins.

SONOGRAPHIC EVALUATION OF THE LIVER

Evaluation of the hepatic structures is one of the most important procedures in sonography for many reasons. The normal, basically homogeneous parenchyma of the liver allows imaging of the neighboring anatomic structures in the upper abdomen. Echo amplitude, attenuation, and transmission and parenchymal textures may be physically assessed with proper evaluation of the hepatic structures. The patient should be instructed to fast for at least 6 hours to eliminate bowel gas and assure the fullness of the gallbladder. The liver is examined with the patient in a supine or right anterior oblique position, usually with deep inspiration to allow the liver to move inferior to the rib cage. The liver is then examined in a transverse, coronal, subcostal oblique, and sagittal view to completely survey the organ.

Within the homogeneous parenchyma lie the thin-walled hepatic veins, the brightly reflective portal veins, the hepatic arteries, and the hepatic duct (Figure 10-17). Color flow Doppler imaging is useful in determining the direction of flow of the portal and hepatic veins. The portal flow is shown to be **hepatopetal** (toward the liver), whereas the hepatic venous flow is **hepatofugal** (away from the liver). The portal vein serves as the landmark to locate the smaller hepatic duct and artery. Near the porta hepatis, the hepatic duct can be seen along the anterior lateral border of the portal vein, whereas the hepatic artery can be seen along the anterior medial border (Figure 10-18). With color Doppler, the hepatic artery would show flow toward the liver, whereas the ductal system would show no flow.

The system gain should be adjusted to adequately penetrate the entire right lobe of the liver as a smooth, homogeneous echo-texture pattern (Figure 10-19, *A* and *B*). Adequate sensitivity (gain) must be present to image the normal smooth liver parenchyma. If too much gain is used, the electronic "noise" or "snow" is produced that appears as low-level echoes in the background of the image (e.g., outside the liver parenchyma, above the diaphragm, or within the vascular structures). The ultrasound manufacturers have made it possible to preselect various pre -and postprocessing controls to allow the sonographer to emphasize or highlight various aspects of the liver parenchyma. This setting is automatically visible on the monitor once the equipment is turned on or the "reset" button is depressed.

The time gain compensation should be adjusted to balance the far-gain and the near-gain echo signals. The easiest way to do this is to hold the transducer over a deep segment of the right lobe of the liver. The far

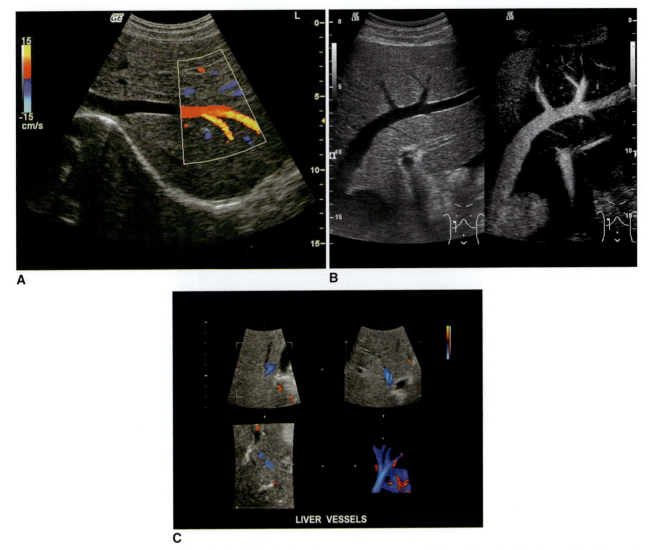

FIGURE 10-17 A, Sagittal image of the right lobe of liver shows a homogeneous texture with hepatic and portal veins scattered throughout the parenchyma. **B,** B-flow demonstrates the low flow pattern in the hepatic and portal veins. **C,** Color Doppler of the hepatic and portal venous flow.

time-gain control pods should gradually be increased with a smooth motion of the index finger until the posterior aspect of the liver is clearly visible. The near-field, time-gain controls should be adjusted (usually decreased) to image the anterior wall and musculature, the anterior hepatic capsule, and the near field of the hepatic parenchyma.

The depth should be adjusted so the posterior right lobe is positioned at the lower border of the screen (Figure 10-19, *C* and *D*). The electronic focus on the equipment is positioned near the posterior border of the liver, or the multiple focus points may be positioned equidistant throughout the liver to further enhance the hepatic parenchyma.

The multifocal technique causes the frame rate to decrease and thus causes a "slower sweep" of the real-time image (Figure 10-20). If the patient cannot take a deep breath, the sonographer may choose not to use the multiple-frequency focus with decreased frame rate. In most patients who can suspend their respiration for a variable amount of time, this multifocal technique works well because the liver is a nondynamic organ and does not need a high frame rate to obtain a quality image.

The appropriate transducer depends on the patient's body habitus and the clinical request for the ultrasound examination. The transducer frequency depends on the body habitus and size. The average adult abdomen usually requires at least a broadband 2.5- to 5-MHz frequency, whereas the more obese adult may require a lower frequency 2.25-MHz transducer. Slender adults and young children may require above a 5- to 7-MHz frequency, and the neonate may need an even higher frequency, 7.5- to 12-MHz transducer.

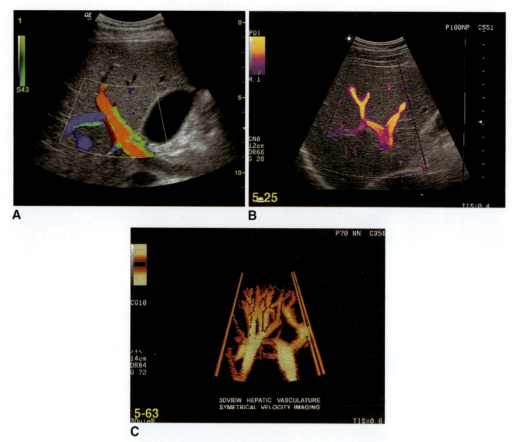

FIGURE 10-18 A, Color Doppler of the portal vein and hepatic artery shows the close relationship (anterior and medial) of the hepatic artery, seen in orange, to the portal vein. **B,** Color of the portal system within the liver in a transverse image. **C,** Three-dimensional view of the hepatic vasculature in the liver.

Generally, a wider "pie" sector or curved linear array transducer is the most appropriate to optimally image the near field of the abdomen (Figure 10-21). This transducer is especially useful in detecting liver abscesses or metastases. To image the far field better, a sector or annular array transducer with a longer focal zone is used. Often the transducers are interchanged throughout the examination to obtain the ideal image pattern.

Adequate scanning technique demands that each patient be examined with the following assessment criteria (Figures 10-22 and 10-23):

1. The size of the liver in the longitudinal plane
2. The attenuation of the liver parenchyma
3. Liver texture
4. The presence of hepatic vascular structures, ligaments, and fissures

The basic instrumentation should be adjusted in the following parameters:

1. Time gain compensation
2. Overall gain
3. Transducer frequency and type
4. Depth and focus

Normal Anatomy and Texture

The liver lies in the right upper quadrant of the abdomen, adjacent to the right hemidiaphragm. The liver is divided into four lobes: the right lobe, the left lobe, and the caudate and medial left (quadrate) lobes. The main lobar fissure separates the right lobe from the left lobe of the liver. The main lobar fissure passes through the gallbladder fossa to the inferior vena cava. The right lobe of the liver is divided further into anterior and posterior segments by the right intersegmental fissure. The left intersegmental fissure divides the left lobe into medial and lateral segments. The caudate lobe is found on the posterior aspect of the liver, with the inferior vena cava on its posterior border and the fissure for the ligamentum venosum on the anterior border. Recall the hepatic veins course between the lobes and segments (interlobar and intersegmental). The major branches of the portal veins run centrally within the segments (intrasegmental), except for the ascending portion of the left portal vein, which runs in the left intersegmental fissure.

The normal texture of the liver is homogeneous with fine, low-level echoes. When compared to the renal cortex of the kidneys, the liver texture is minimally

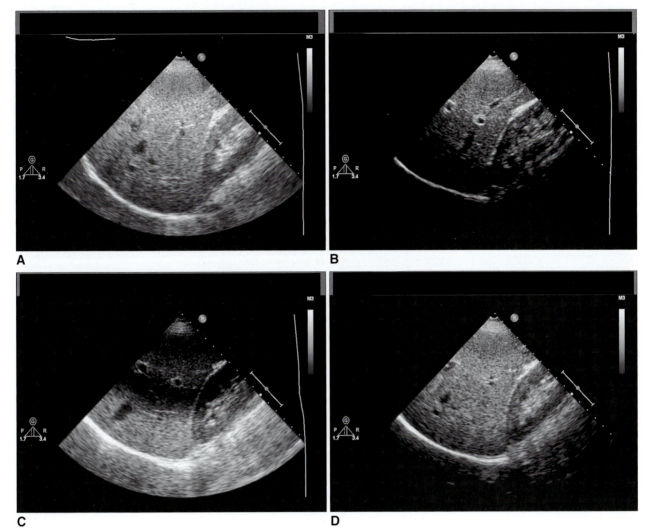

FIGURE 10-19 A, Longitudinal image of the liver shows equal distribution of echoes from anterior to posterior, which means the gain and time gain compensation settings are correct. **B,** Incorrect gain settings show the lack of echoes in the distal (posterior) lobe of the liver. **C,** Incorrect near field gain settings eliminate texture information in more than half of the liver . **D,** Depth of field set correctly at 15 cm with a balanced time gain compensation (TGC) to balance the near and far fields.

hyperechoic to isoechoic. When compared to the texture of the spleen, the liver is hypoechoic.

Sagittal Plane

The sagittal plane offers an excellent window to visualize the hepatic structures (Figure 10-24). With the patient in full inspiration, the transducer may be swept under the costal margin (with slight to medium pressure) to record the liver parenchyma from the anterior abdominal wall to the diaphragm.

Scan I. The initial scan should be made slightly to the left of the midline to record the left lobe of the liver and the abdominal aorta. The left hepatic and portal veins may be seen as small circular structures in this view (Figure 10-25, A).

Scan II. As the sonographer scans at midline or slightly to the right of midline, a larger segment of the left lobe and the inferior vena cava may be seen posteriorly. In this view, it is useful to record the inferior vena cava as it is dilated near the end of inspiration. The left or middle hepatic vein may be imaged as it drains into the inferior vena cava near the level of the diaphragm. The area of the porta hepatis is shown anterior to the inferior vena cava as the superior mesenteric vein and splenic vein converge to form the main portal vein. The common bile duct may be seen just anterior to the main portal vein. The head of the pancreas may be seen just inferior to the right lobe of the liver and main portal vein and anterior to the inferior vena cava (Figure 10-25, B).

Scan III. The next image should be made slightly lateral to this sagittal plane to record part of the right portal vein and right lobe of the liver. The caudate lobe is often seen in this view (see Figure 10-25, B).

Scans IV, V, and VI. The next three scans should be made in small increments through the right lobe of the

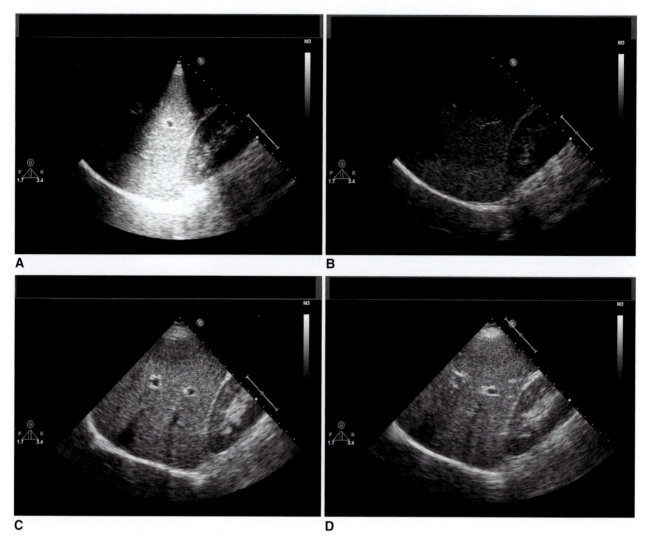

A

B

C

D

FIGURE 10-20 A through **C,** Examples of incorrect gain/focal zone settings (look at the line to the right of the image). The focal zone should be set to encompass the total area of interest or to "clean up" the far field echoes to increase sharpness. **D,** Shadowing from the portal veins or variations in breathing may cause image distortion.

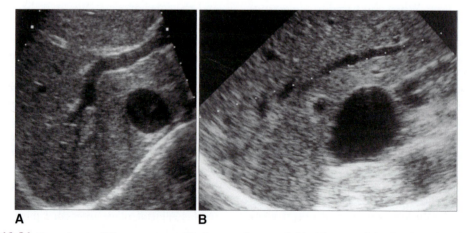

A

B

FIGURE 10-21 Curved array **(A)** versus sector **(B)** changes the near field of focus and the focal zone in the far field.

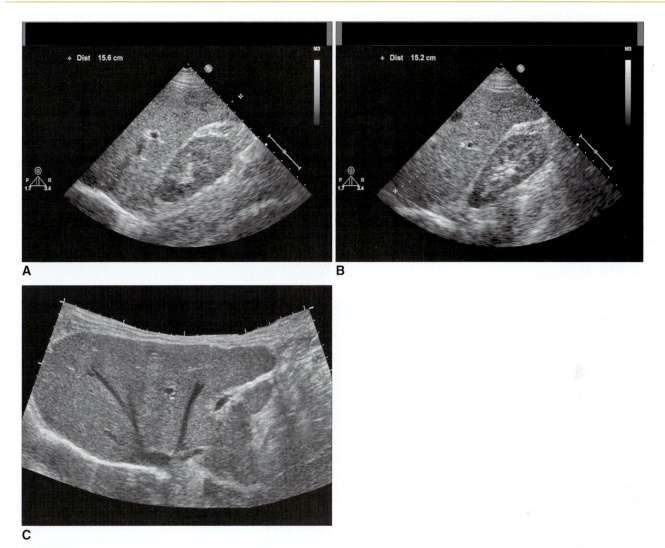

FIGURE 10-22 A-C, Longitudinal images of the right lobe of the liver are used to determine adequate gain settings and also to measure the liver from the diaphragm to its inferior border. The inferior border may be difficult to image at the same time as the diaphragm, depending on the size of the liver.

liver (Figure 10-25, *C, D,* and *E*). The last scan is usually made to show the right kidney and lateral segment of the right lobe of the liver. The liver texture is compared with the renal parenchyma. The normal liver parenchyma should have a softer, more homogeneous texture than the dense medulla and hypoechoic renal cortex. Liver size may be measured from the inferior tip of the liver to the dome at the level of the diaphragm. Generally this measurement is less than 15 cm, with 15 to 20 cm representing the upper limits of normal. Hepatomegaly is present when the liver measurement exceeds 20 cm.

Transverse Plane

Multiple transverse scans are made across the upper abdomen to record specific areas of the liver (Figure 10-26). The transducer should be angled in a steep cephalic direction to be as parallel to the diaphragm as

possible. The patient should be in full inspiration to maintain detail of the liver parenchyma, vascular architecture, and ductal structures.

Scan I. The initial transverse image is made with the transducer under the costal margin at a steep angle perpendicular to the diaphragm (Figure 10-27, *A*). The patient should be in deep inspiration to adequately record the dome of the liver. The sonographer should identify the inferior vena cava and three hepatic veins as they drain into the cava. This pattern has sometimes been referred to as the "reindeer sign" or "Playboy bunny" sign.

Scan II. The transducer is then directed slightly inferior to the point described in scan I to record the left portal vein as it flows into the left lobe of the liver (Figure 10-27, *B*).

Scan III. The porta hepatis is seen as a tubular structure within the central part of the liver. Sometimes the left or

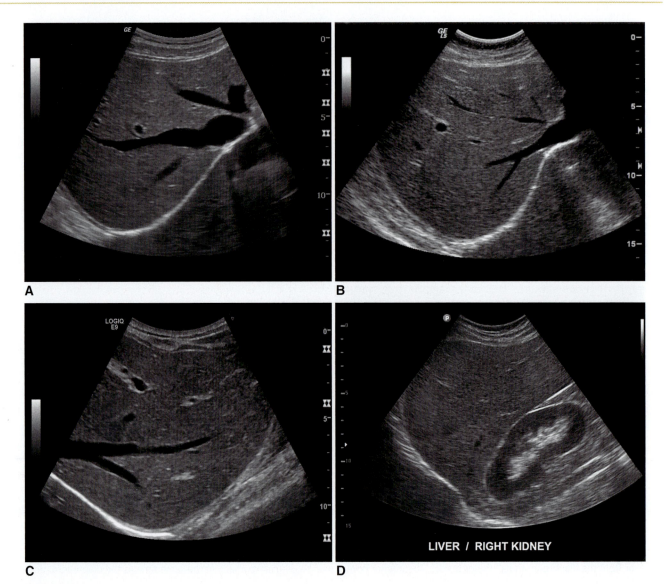

FIGURE 10-23 Transverse (**A** and **B**) and longitudinal (**C** and **D**) images should show adequate gain, time gain compensation, depth, and landmarks within the liver (ligaments, vascular structures, and spine).

right portal vein can be identified. The caudate lobe may be seen just superior to the porta hepatis; thus, depending on the angle, either the caudate lobe is shown anterior to the inferior vena cava, or, as the transducer moves inferior, the porta hepatis is identified anterior to the inferior vena cava (Figure 10-27, C).

Scan IV. The fourth scan should show the right portal vein as it divides into the anterior and posterior segments of the right lobe of the liver. The gallbladder may be seen in this scan as an anechoic structure medial to the right lobe and anterior to the right kidney (Figure 10-27, D).

Scans V and VI. These two scans are made through the lower segment of the right lobe of the liver. The right kidney is the posterior border (Figure 10-27, E). Usually intrahepatic vascular structures are not identified in these views (Figure 10-27, F).

Lateral Decubitus Plane

Left Posterior Oblique/Right Anterior Oblique. The left posterior/right anterior oblique image requires that the patient roll slightly to the left. A 45-degree sponge or pillow may be placed under the right hip to support the patient (Figure 10-28). This view allows better visualization of the lower right lobe of the liver, usually displacing the duodenum and transverse colon to the midline of the abdomen, out of the field of view. Transverse, oblique, or longitudinal scans may be made in this position.

Left Lateral Decubitus. If the previously described scans do not allow adequate visualization of the liver and vascular structures, the lateral decubitus position may be used. If the body habitus allows the transducer

Text continued on page 233

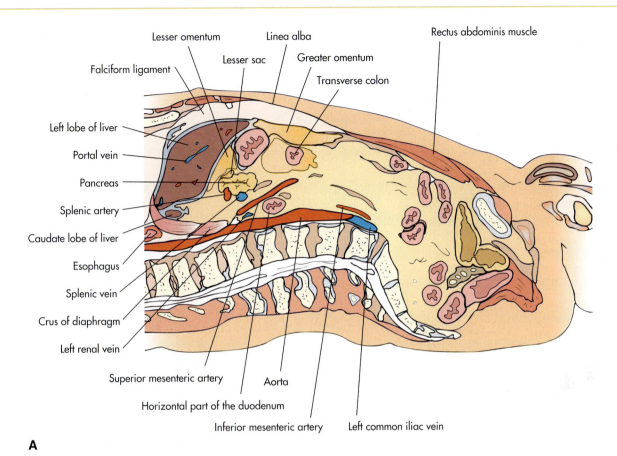

A

B

FIGURE 10-24 Longitudinal plane. **A,** Midline sagittal section of the abdomen. **B,** Sagittal section of the abdomen.

Continued

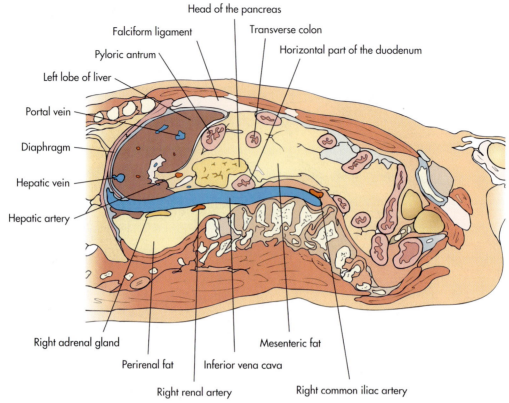

Head of the pancreas

Falciform ligament

Transverse colon

Pyloric antrum

Horizontal part of the duodenum

Left lobe of liver

Portal vein

Diaphragm

Hepatic vein

Hepatic artery

Right adrenal gland

Mesenteric fat

Perirenal fat

Inferior vena cava

Right renal artery

Right common iliac artery

C

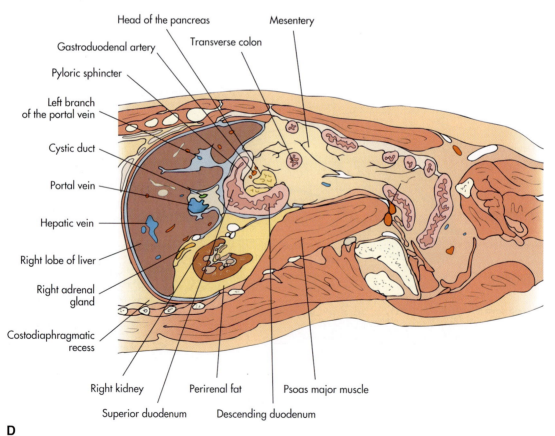

Head of the pancreas

Mesentery

Gastroduodenal artery

Transverse colon

Pyloric sphincter

Left branch of the portal vein

Cystic duct

Portal vein

Hepatic vein

Right lobe of liver

Right adrenal gland

Costodiaphragmatic recess

Right kidney

Perirenal fat

Psoas major muscle

Superior duodenum

Descending duodenum

D

FIGURE 10-24, cont'd C, Sagittal section of the abdomen 3 cm from the midline. **D,** Sagittal section of the abdomen 5 cm from the midline.

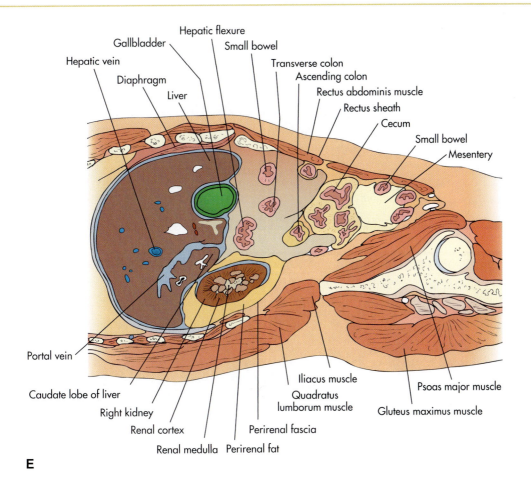

E

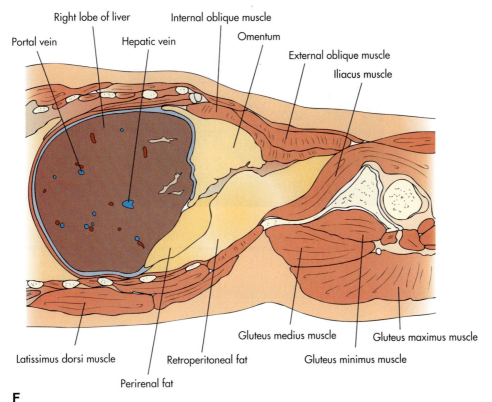

F

FIGURE 10-24, cont'd E, Sagittal section of the abdomen 7 cm from the midline. F, Sagittal section of the abdomen taken along the right abdominal border.

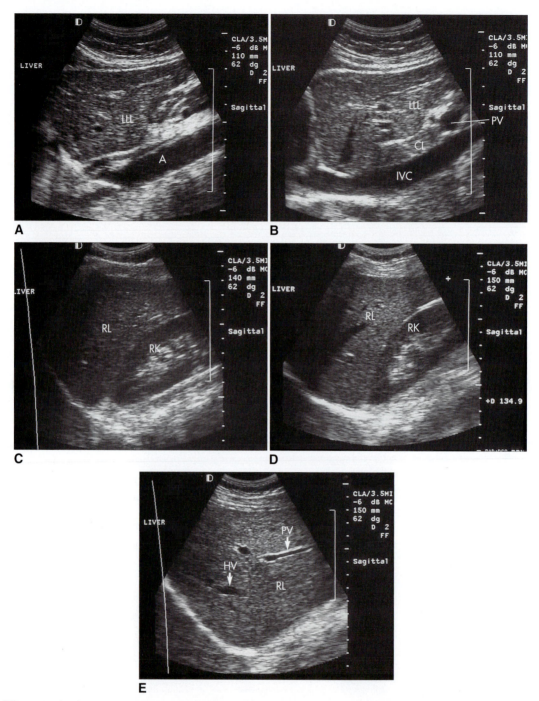

FIGURE 10-25 Longitudinal images. **A,** *Scan I:* left lobe liver, aorta. **B,** *Scan II:* left lobe liver, inferior vena cava, portal vein, caudate lobe. **C,** *Scan III:* right lobe liver, right kidney. **D,** *Scan IV:* right lobe liver, right kidney. **E,** *Scan V:* right lobe liver, portal vein, hepatic veins.

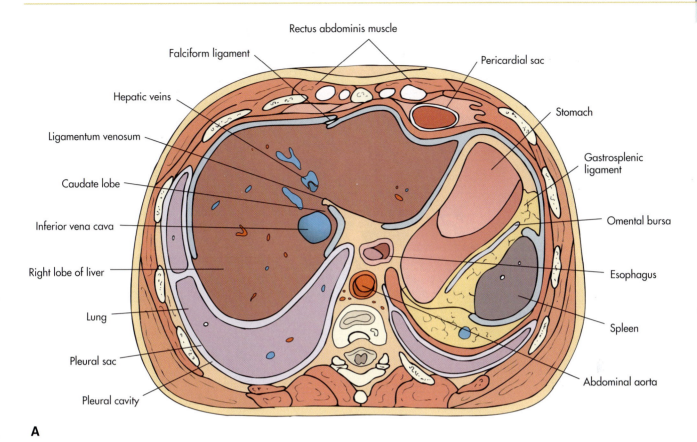

Rectus abdominis muscle

Falciform ligament

Pericardial sac

Hepatic veins

Stomach

Ligamentum venosum

Gastrosplenic ligament

Caudate lobe

Inferior vena cava

Omental bursa

Right lobe of liver

Esophagus

Lung

Pleural sac

Spleen

Pleural cavity

Abdominal aorta

A

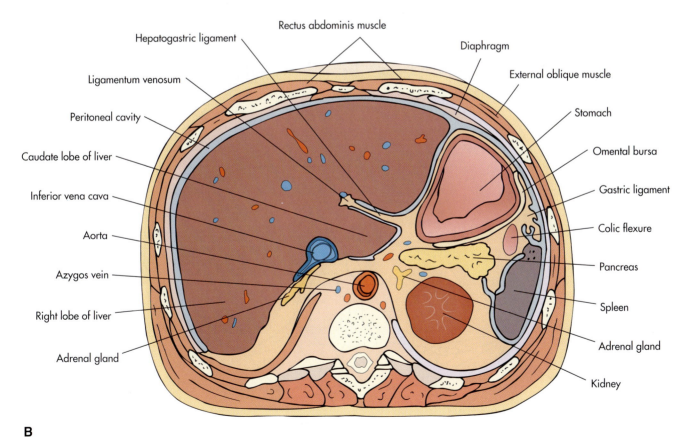

Rectus abdominis muscle

Hepatogastric ligament

Diaphragm

Ligamentum venosum

External oblique muscle

Peritoneal cavity

Stomach

Caudate lobe of liver

Omental bursa

Inferior vena cava

Gastric ligament

Aorta

Colic flexure

Azygos vein

Pancreas

Right lobe of liver

Spleen

Adrenal gland

Adrenal gland

Kidney

B

FIGURE 10-26 Transverse plane. **A,** Cross section of the abdomen at the level of the tenth intervertebral disk. **B,** Cross section of the abdomen at the level of the eleventh thoracic disk.

Continued

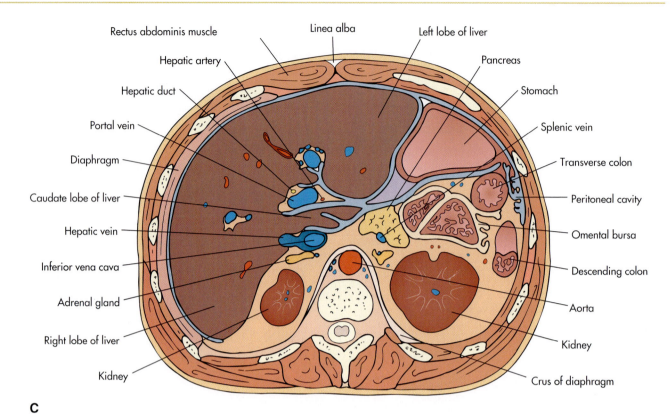

C

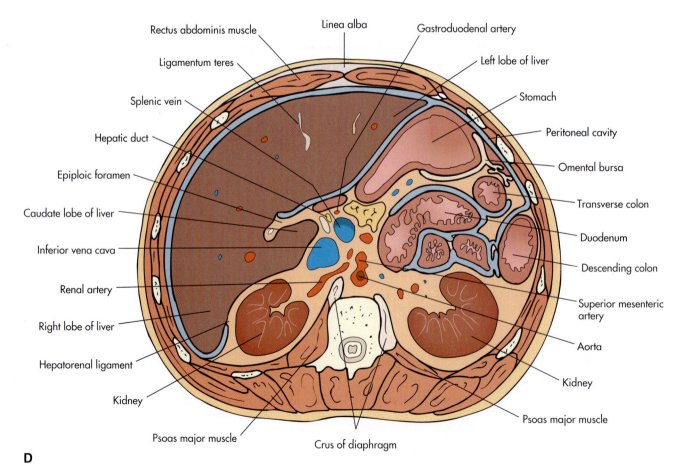

D

FIGURE 10-26, cont'd C, Cross section of the abdomen at the level of the 12th thoracic vertebra. **D,** Cross section of the abdomen at the first lumbar vertebra.

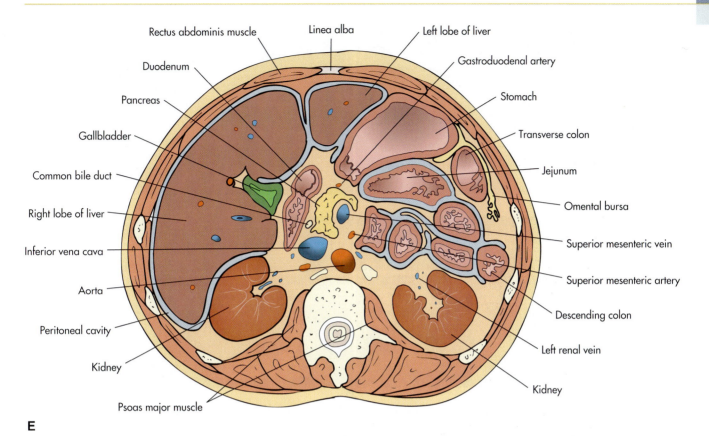

E

F

FIGURE 10-26, cont'd E, Cross section of the abdomen at the level of the second lumbar vertebra. **F,** Cross section of the abdomen at the level of the third lumbar vertebra.

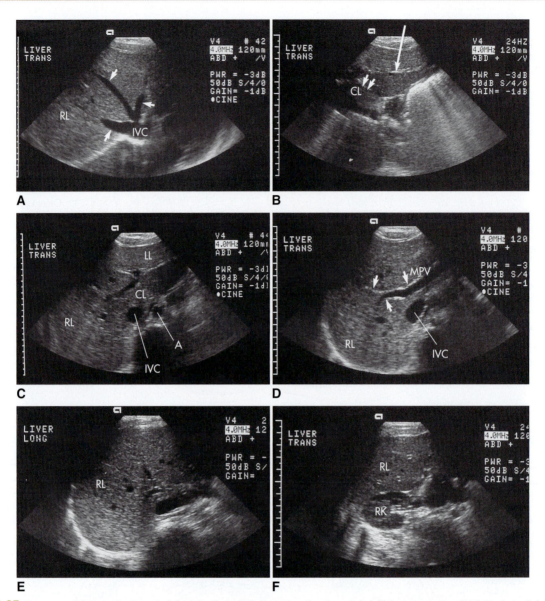

FIGURE 10-27 Transverse images. **A,** *Scan I:* right lobe liver *(RL),* hepatic veins *(arrows),* inferior vena cava *(IVC).* **B,** *Scan II:* left lobe liver, left portal vein *(arrow),* ligamentum venosum *(arrows),* caudate lobe *(CL).* **C,** *Scan III:* caudate lobe *(CL),* left lobe *(LL),* right lobe *(RL)* of liver, left and right portal veins, IVC, and aorta *(Ao).* **D,** *Scan IV:* right lobe liver *(RL),* main portal vein *(MPV),* right portal vein with branches *(RPV),* and IVC. **E,** *Scan V:* right lobe liver *(RL).* **F,** *Scan VI:* right lobe liver *(RL)* and right kidney *(RK).*

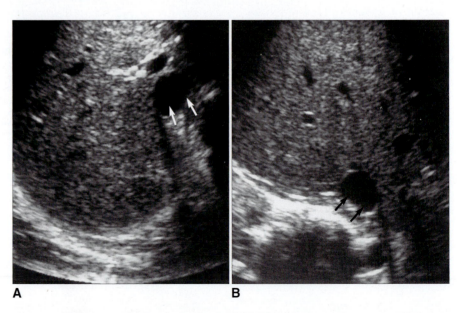

FIGURE 10-28 Oblique scans. The patient may be rolled from a supine **(A)** position into the anterior oblique position **(B).** Note the change in position of the inferior vena cava *(arrows)* as the patient is rotated.

to image between the intercostal spaces, additional views may be obtained of the dome of the liver and medial segment of the left lobe of the liver.

PATHOLOGY OF THE LIVER

Evaluation of the liver parenchyma includes the assessment of its size, configuration, homogeneity, and contour. Liver volume can be determined from serial scans in an effort to detect subtle increases in size or hepatomegaly. The development and clinical utility of three-dimensional ultrasound in determining organ volumes is currently under clinical investigation at many academic institutions.

As in other organ systems, the hepatic parenchymal pattern changes with disease processes. Hepatocellular disease affects the hepatocytes and interferes with liver function enzymes. Cirrhosis, ascites, or fatty liver patterns may be detected with the ultrasound examination. In an effort to provide a differential diagnosis for the clinician, intrahepatic, extrahepatic, subhepatic, and subdiaphragmatic masses may be outlined and their internal composition recognized as specific echo patterns.

Subsequent sections discuss the pathology of liver disease in the following categories: developmental anomalies, diffuse disease, functional disease, abscess formation, hepatic trauma and transplantation, benign disease, malignant disease, and vascular problems.

Developmental Anomalies

Agenesis. Agenesis of the liver is incompatible with life.
Anomalies of Position. The liver may be found in other locations in two conditions: situs inversus, in which the organs are reversed with the liver on the left and spleen on the right; or in a congenital diaphragmatic hernia or omphalocele, where varying amounts of liver tissue may herniate into the thorax or outside the abdominal cavity.
Accessory Fissures. True accessory fissures are uncommon and caused by infolding of peritoneum. The inferior accessory hepatic fissure is a true accessory fissure that stretches inferiorly from the right portal vein to the inferior surface of the right lobe of the liver.
Vascular Anomalies. The hepatic artery may have many variations as it arises from the celiac axis. At least 45% of patients may have the following variations: (1) replaced left hepatic artery originating from the left gastric artery, (2) replaced right hepatic artery originating from the superior mesenteric artery, and (3) replaced common hepatic artery originating from the superior mesenteric artery.

Variations in the portal venous anatomy are uncommon but include atresias, strictures, and obstructing valves. On the other hand, variations in the branching of the hepatic veins are common, with the most common

being when the accessory vein drains the superoanterior segment of the right lobe. It may empty into the middle hepatic vein or join the right hepatic vein.

Diffuse Disease

Diffuse hepatocellular disease affects the hepatocytes and interferes with liver function. The **hepatocyte** is a parenchymal liver cell that performs all the functions ascribed to the liver. This abnormality is measured through the series of liver function tests. The hepatic enzyme levels are elevated with cell necrosis. With cholestasis (i.e., interruption in the flow of bile through any part of the biliary system, from the liver to the duodenum), the alkaline phosphatase and direct bilirubin levels increase. Likewise, when there are defects in protein synthesis, there may be elevated serum bilirubin levels and decreased serum albumin and clotting factor levels.

There are many subcategories of diffuse parenchymal disease, including fatty infiltration, acute and chronic hepatitis, early alcoholic liver disease, and acute and chronic cirrhosis. See Table 10-3 for clinical findings, sonographic findings, and differential considerations for diffuse hepatic disease.

Fatty Infiltration. Fatty liver is an acquired, reversible disorder of metabolism, resulting in an accumulation of triglycerides within the hepatocytes. Fatty infiltration implies increased lipid accumulation in the hepatocytes and results from major injury to the liver or a systemic disorder leading to impaired or excessive metabolism of fat (Figure 10-29). Fatty infiltration is a benign process and may be reversible with correction of the process, although it has been shown that fatty infiltration of the liver is the precursor for significant chronic disease in a percentage of patients. The patient is usually asymptomatic; however, some patients may present with jaundice, nausea and vomiting, and abdominal tenderness or pain. Box 10-3 lists the common causes of fatty liver.

Sonographic Findings. Fatty infiltration of the liver appears in a variety of patterns that depend on the amount and distribution of fat in the liver parenchyma.

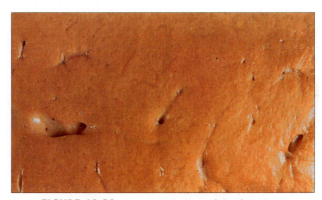

FIGURE 10-29 Gross appearance of the fatty liver.

TABLE 10-3	Liver Findings: Diffuse Disease	
Clinical Findings	**Sonographic Findings**	**Differential Considerations**
Fatty Infiltration		
Normal to ↑ hepatic enzymes ↑ Alk phos ↑ Direct bilirubin	↑ Echogenicity ↑ Attenuation Impaired visualization of borders of portal/hepatic structures (secondary to increased attenuation) Hepatomegaly May be patchy, inhomogeneous Focal sparing	Hepatitis Cirrhosis Metastases
Acute Hepatitis		
↑ AST, ALT ↑ Bilirubin Leukopenia	Nonspecific and variable Normal to slightly ↑ Echogenicity ↑ Brightness of portal vein borders Hepatosplenomegaly ↑ Thickness of gallbladder wall	Fatty liver
Chronic Hepatitis		
↑ AST, ALT ↑ Bilirubin Leukopenia	Coarse hepatic parenchyma ↑ Echogenicity ↓ Visualization brightness of portal triad Fibrosis may produce soft shadowing	Cirrhosis Fatty liver
Cirrhosis		
↑ Alk phos ↑ Direct bilirubin ↑ AST, ALT Leukopenia	Coarse liver parenchyma with nodularity ↑ Echogenicity ↑ Attenuation ↓ Vascular markings with acute cirrhosis Hepatosplenomegaly with ascites Shrunken liver with chronic cirrhosis (also ↑ nodularity) Regeneration of hepatic nodules Portal hypertension	Fatty liver Hepatitis
Glycogen Storage Disease		
Disturbance of acid-base balance	Hepatomegaly ↑ Echogenicity ↑ Attenuation von Gierke's adenoma (round, homogeneous)	Focal nodular hyperplasia Fatty liver
Hemochromatosis		
↑ Iron levels in blood	↑ Echogenicity throughout liver	Cirrhosis

Alk phos, Alkaline phosphatase; *ALT,* alanine aminotransferase; *AST,* aspartate aminotransferase.

Enlargement of the lobe affected by fatty infiltration is evident. The portal vein structures may be difficult to visualize because of the increased attenuation of the ultrasound beam. The increased attenuation also causes a decrease in penetration of the sound beam, which may be a clue for the sonographer to think of fatty liver disease. The liver is so dense that "typical" gain settings do not allow penetration to the posterior border of the liver. It thus becomes more difficult to see the outline of the portal vein and hepatic vein borders. Authors have stated that this increase in echo texture may result from increased collagen content of the liver or increase in lipid

accumulation. The following three grades of liver texture have been defined in sonography for classification of fatty infiltration:

- *Mild.* The mild form will present with minimal diffuse increase in hepatic echogenicity with normal visualization of the diaphragm and intrahepatic vascular borders (Figure 10-30, *A*).
- *Moderate.* Moderate fatty infiltration shows increased echogenicity with slightly impaired visualization of the diaphragm and intrahepatic vascular borders (Figure 10-30, *B*).

- *Severe.* The severe form presents with a marked increase in echogenicity of the liver parenchyma, decreased penetration of the posterior segment of the right lobe of the liver, and decreased to poor visualization of the diaphragm and hepatic vessels (Figure 10-30, C).

BOX 10-3	Causes of Fatty Liver

Obesity
Excessive alcohol intake (alcohol stimulates lipolysis)
Poorly controlled hyperlipidemia
Diabetes mellitus
Excess corticosteroids
Pregnancy
Total Parenteral Hyperalimentation (nutrition)
Severe Hepatitis
Glycogen Storage Disease
Cystic Fibrosis
Pharmaceutical
Chronic Illness

Focal Fatty Infiltration and Focal Fatty Sparing. Fatty infiltration is not always uniform throughout the liver parenchyma; in fact, regions of increased echogenicity are present within a normal liver parenchyma. It is not uncommon to see patchy distribution of hypoechoic masses (fat) within a dense, fatty infiltrated liver parenchyma, especially in the right lobe of the liver. It is important to note that the fat does not displace normal intrahepatic vascular architecture. The margins of the fatty tissue may appear nodular, round, or interdigitated with the normal hepatic tissue. Fatty infiltration has the ability to resolve rapidly.

The other characteristic of fatty infiltration is focal sparing. This condition should be suspected in patients who have masslike hypoechoic areas in typical locations in a liver that is otherwise increased in echogenicity. The most common areas are anterior to the gallbladder or the portal vein and the periportal region of the medial segment of the left lobe of the liver (Figure 10-31). Focal subcapsular fat may be found in diabetic patients receiving insulin in peritoneal dialysate.

Viral Hepatitis. Hepatitis is the general name for inflammatory and infectious disease of the liver, of which there

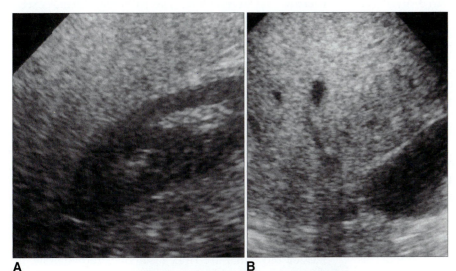

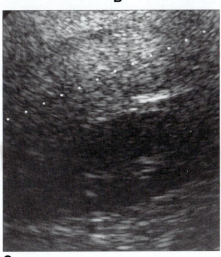

A   **B**   **C**

FIGURE 10-30 Fatty infiltration. **A,** Grade I. **B,** Grade II. **C,** Grade III.

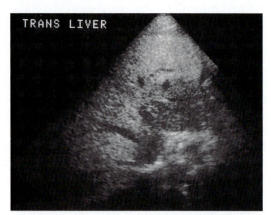

FIGURE 10-31 Focal sparing of the caudate lobe.

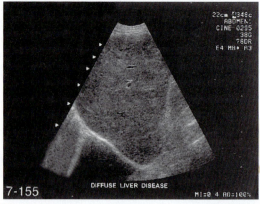

FIGURE 10-32 Hepatitis. On ultrasound examination, the liver parenchyma is coarse with increased brightness of the portal triad.

are many causes. The disease may result from a local infection (viral hepatitis), from an infection elsewhere in the body (e.g., infectious mononucleosis or amebiasis), or from chemical or drug toxicity. Mild inflammation impairs hepatocyte function, whereas more severe inflammation and necrosis may lead to obstruction of blood and bile flow in the liver and impaired liver cell function.

Hepatitis is considered to result from infection by a group of viruses that specifically target the hepatocytes. These include hepatitis A virus (HAV), hepatitis B virus (HBV), hepatitis C virus (HCV), hepatitis D virus (HDV), hepatitis E virus (HEV), and hepatitis G. In the United States, about 60% of acute viral hepatitis is type B, about 20% is type A, and about 20% is other types. Patients with acute and chronic hepatitis may initially present with flulike and gastrointestinal symptoms, including loss of appetite, nausea, vomiting, and fatigue. Viral hepatitis may be fatal with secondary acute hepatic necrosis or chronic hepatitis, which may lead to portal hypertension, cirrhosis, and hepatocellular carcinoma (HCC).

Hepatitis A is spread primarily by fecal contamination, because the virus lives in the alimentary tract. This is found worldwide. In developing countries, the disease is endemic and the infection occurs very early in life. Hepatitis A is an acute infection that leads to either complete recovery or death from acute liver failure.

Hepatitis B is caused by the type B virus, which exists in the bloodstream and can be spread by transfusions of infected blood or plasma or through the use of contaminated needles. Hepatitis B is of the greatest risk to health care workers because of the nature of transmission. This virus is also found in body fluids, such as saliva and semen, and may be spread by sexual contact.

Hepatitis C is diagnosed by the presence in blood of the antibody to HCV (anti-HCV). This disease is a major health problem in Italy and other Mediterranean countries.

Hepatitis D is entirely dependent on the hepatitis B virus for its infectivity. This is an uncommon infection in North America, occurring primarily in intravenous drug users.

Acute Hepatitis. In acute hepatitis, without complications, the clinical recovery usually occurs within 4 months. Complications of hepatitis involving damage to the liver may range from mild disease to massive necrosis and liver failure. The pathologic changes seen include the following: (1) liver cell injury, swelling of the hepatocytes, and hepatocyte degeneration, which may lead to cell necrosis; (2) reticuloendothelial and lymphocytic response with Kupffer cells enlarging; and (3) regeneration.

Sonographic Findings. On ultrasound examination the liver texture may appear normal or the sonographer may note that the portal vein borders are more prominent than usual and the liver parenchyma is slightly more echogenic than normal; attenuation may be present. Hepatosplenomegaly is present, and the gallbladder wall is thickened.

Chronic Hepatitis. Chronic hepatitis exists when there is clinical or biochemical evidence of hepatic inflammation that extends beyond 6 months. Causes include those that are viral, metabolic, autoimmune, or drug induced. In chronic active hepatitis, there are more extensive changes than in chronic persistent hepatitis, with inflammation extending across the limiting plate, spreading out in a perilobular fashion, and causing piecemeal necrosis, which is frequently accompanied by fibrosis. Patients may present with nausea, anorexia, weight loss, tremors, jaundice, dark urine, fatigue, and varicosities. Chronic persistent hepatitis is a benign, self-limiting process. Chronic active hepatitis usually progresses to cirrhosis and liver failure.

Sonographic Findings. On ultrasound examination the liver parenchyma is coarse with decreased brightness of the portal triads, but the degree of attenuation is not as great as is seen in fatty infiltration (Figure 10-32). The liver does not increase in size with chronic hepatitis. Fibrosis may be evident, which may produce "soft shadowing" posteriorly.

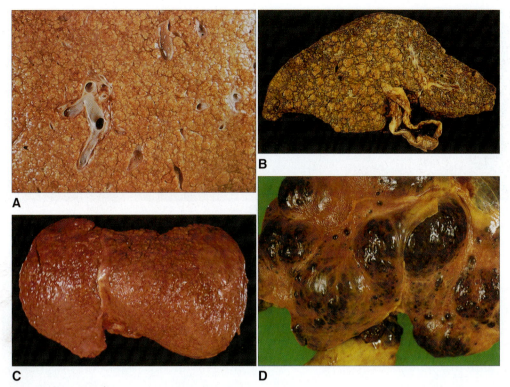

FIGURE 10-33 A, Gross pathology of alcoholic cirrhosis with high degree of fat content. **B,** Biliary cirrhosis (liver is nodular). **C,** Micronodular cirrhosis (nodules are small with uniform size). **D,** Macronodular cirrhosis.

Cirrhosis. Cirrhosis is a chronic degenerative disease of the liver in which the lobes are covered with fibrous tissue, the parenchyma degenerates, and the lobules are infiltrated with fat. The essential feature is simultaneous parenchymal necrosis, regeneration, and diffuse fibrosis resulting in disorganization of lobular architecture (Figure 10-33). Cirrhosis may be classified as micronodular (nodules 0.1 to 1 cm in diameter) or macronodular (nodules up to 5 cm in diameter). The process of cirrhosis is chronic and progressive, with liver cell failure and portal hypertension as the end stage. Micronodular cirrhosis is most commonly the result of chronic alcohol abuse, whereas macronodular cirrhosis is caused by chronic viral hepatitis or other infection. Other causes of cirrhosis include biliary cirrhosis, Wilson's disease, primary sclerosing cholangitis, and hemochromatosis.

Patients with acute cirrhosis may seem asymptomatic or may have symptoms that include nausea, flatulence, ascites, light-colored stools, weakness, abdominal pain, varicosities, and spider angiomas. The classic clinical presentation of a patient with cirrhosis is hepatomegaly, jaundice, and ascites. Chronic cirrhosis patient symptoms include nausea, anorexia, weight loss, jaundice, dark urine, fatigue, or varicosities. Chronic cirrhosis may progress to liver failure and portal hypertension.

Sonographic Findings. The sonographic diagnosis of cirrhosis may be challenging. In the early stage of cirrhosis, hepatomegaly is the first sonographic finding. As the cirrhosis becomes more severe, the liver volume decreases in the right lobe, with enlargement of the left and caudate lobes. The evaluation of the ratio of the caudate lobe width to the right lobe width (C/RL) has been used as an indicator of cirrhosis. A C/RL value of 0.65 is considered indicative of cirrhosis. (This measurement is useful if abnormal but not as sensitive when it is normal.)

Specific findings may include increased echogenicity and coarsening of the hepatic parenchyma secondary to fibrosis and nodularity (Figure 10-34). This evaluation is subjective and depends on appropriate gain settings (both time gain compensation and overall gain). Increased attenuation may be present, with decreased vascular markings. The amount of fatty infiltration will certainly influence the amount of echogenicity and attenuation. Hepatosplenomegaly may be present with ascites surrounding the liver. In addition, there may be atrophy of the right and left medial lobes of the liver.

Chronic cirrhosis may show nodularity of the liver edge, especially well demonstrated if ascites is present. The use of a higher frequency, curved array transducer may allow the sonographer to demonstrate the surface of the liver. The hepatic fissures may be accentuated. The isoechoic regenerating nodules may be seen throughout the liver parenchyma. Portal hypertension may be present with or without abnormal Doppler flow patterns. Patients who have cirrhosis have an increased incidence of hepatoma tumors within the liver parenchyma.

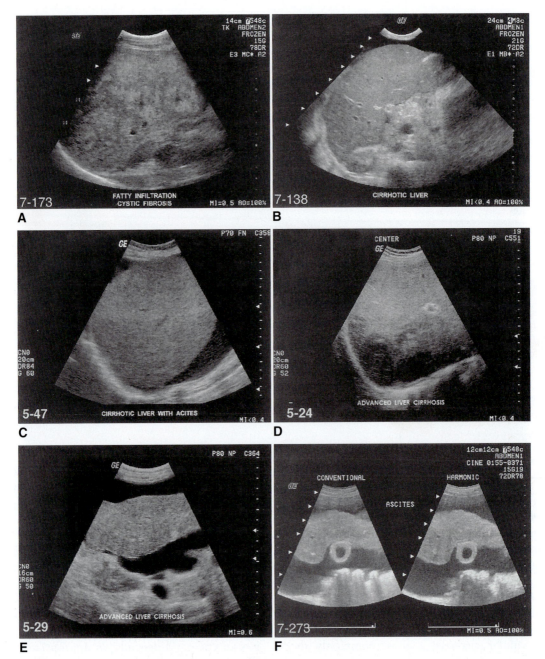

FIGURE 10-34 Diffuse liver disease. **A,** Fatty infiltration secondary to cystic fibrosis. **B,** Early stages cirrhosis: hepatomegaly, decreased vasculature. **C,** Cirrhotic liver with ascites. **D,** Advanced cirrhosis with attenuation. **E,** Late-stage cirrhosis with shrunken liver, ascites. **F,** Late-stage cirrhosis with thick gallbladder wall, ascites, shrunken liver.

Regenerating nodules represent regenerating hepatocytes surrounded by a fibrosis septa. They are "isoechoic" to the liver parenchyma and thus may be indistinguishable from normal liver texture.

Dysplastic nodules or adenomatous hyperplastic nodules are larger than the regenerating nodules and are considered premalignant. These nodules contain well-differentiated hepatocytes, portal venous blood supply, and atypical or frankly malignant cells. Color Doppler may show the portal venous blood supply.

Doppler Characteristics of Cirrhosis. Evaluation of the hepatic veins is useful to detect the presence of altered

flow dynamics. The hepatic vein velocity waveform reflects the hemodynamics of the right atrium. This is a triphasic pattern with two large antegrade diastolic and systolic waves and a small retrograde wave that corresponds to the atrial kick (from the heart). Recall that the thin walls of the hepatic veins easily receive the transfer of flow via the collaterals from the portal veins in a normal liver. In patients with compensated cirrhosis (no portal hypertension), the Doppler waveform is abnormal. Two patterns have been found in these patients with fatty infiltration of their liver: decreased amplitude of phasic oscillations with loss of reversed flow and a flattened waveform. As the cirrhosis advances, the hepatic veins develop luminal narrowing with increased velocities and turbulence of the flow patterns.

The hepatic artery waveform also shows altered flow dynamics in cirrhosis and chronic liver disease. The resistive index is blunted after a meal in patients with liver disease.

Glycogen Storage Disease. Glycogen storage disease is an inherited disease characterized by the abnormal storage and accumulation of glycogen in the tissues, especially the liver and kidneys. There are six categories of glycogen storage disease, which are divided on the basis of clinical symptoms and specific enzymatic defects. The most common is type I, or von Gierke's disease. This is a form of glycogen storage disease in which abnormally large amounts of glycogen are deposited in the liver and kidneys.

Sonographic Findings. On sonography, patients with glycogen storage disease present with hepatomegaly, increased echogenicity, and slightly increased attenuation (similar to diffuse fatty infiltration). The disease is associated with hepatic adenomas, focal nodular hyperplasia, and hepatomegaly (Figure 10-35). The adenoma presents as a well-demarcated, round, homogeneous, echogenic tumors (Figure 10-36). If the tumor is large, it may be slightly inhomogeneous.

Hemochromatosis. Hemochromatosis is a rare disease of iron metabolism characterized by excess iron deposits throughout the body. This disorder may lead to cirrhosis and portal hypertension.

Sonographic Findings. Ultrasound does not show specific findings other than hepatomegaly and cirrhotic changes. Some increased echogenicity may be seen uniformly throughout the hepatic parenchyma.

Hepatic Vascular Flow Abnormalities

Portal Venous Hypertension. Portal hypertension is defined as an increase in portal venous pressure or hepatic venous gradient. It exists when the portal venous pressure is above 10 mmHg or the hepatic venous gradient is more than 5 mmHg. Portal hypertension may be further defined by the following:

- A wedged hepatic vein pressure or direct portal vein pressure of more than 5 mmHg greater than the inferior vena cava pressure
- Splenic vein pressure of greater than 15 mmHg
- Portal vein pressure of greater than 30 cm H_2O

Portal hypertension is divided into presinusoidal and intrahepatic groups, depending on whether the hepatic vein wedged pressure is normal (presinusoidal) or elevated (intrahepatic). The development of increased

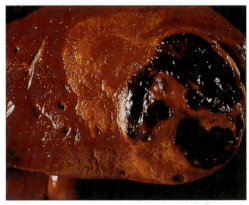

FIGURE 10-35 Gross pathology of hepatic adenoma with hemorrhage.

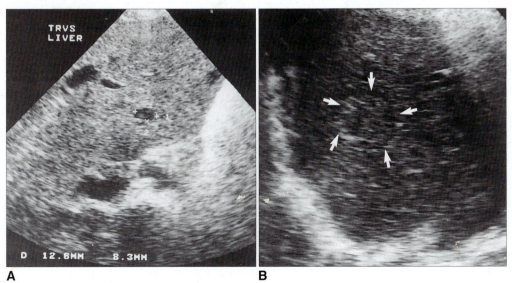

A   **B**

FIGURE 10-36 Hepatic adenoma. **A,** Patient with von Gierke's disease: hepatic adenoma is seen within the caudate lobe. **B,** A 31-year-old female with a hepatic adenoma *(arrows)* in the right lobe.

pressure in the portal-splenic venous system is the cause of extrahepatic portal hypertension. Acute or chronic hepatocellular disease can block the flow of blood throughout the liver, causing it to back up into the hepatic portal circulation. This causes the blood pressure in the hepatic circulation to increase, thus the development of portal hypertension. In an effort to relieve the pressure, collateral veins are formed that connect to the systemic veins. These are known as varicose veins and occur most frequently in the area of the esophagus, stomach, and rectum. Rupture of these veins can cause massive bleeding that may result in death.

Intrahepatic portal hypertension is the result of diseases that affect the portal zones of the liver like primary biliary cirrhosis, schistosomiasis, congenital hepatic fibrosis, or toxic drugs. Cirrhosis is the most common cause of intrahepatic portal hypertension. Diffuse metastatic liver disease may also produce portal hypertension, as the normal architecture of the liver is replaced by the distorted vascular channels that provide increased resistance to portal venous blood flow and obstruction to hepatic venous outflow. Other causes include thrombotic diseases of the inferior vena cava and hepatic veins; constrictive pericarditis or other right-sided heart failure over time will cause centrilobular fibrosis, hepatic regeneration, cirrhosis, all leading to subsequent portal hypertension.

Portal hypertension may also develop when hepatopetal flow (toward the liver) is impeded by thrombus or tumor invasion. The blood becomes obstructed as it passes through the liver to the hepatic veins and is diverted to collateral pathways in the upper abdomen. Box 10-4 lists the indications for portal hypertension.

Portal hypertension may develop along two pathways. One entails increased resistance to flow, and the other entails increased portal blood flow. The most common mechanism for increased resistance to flow occurs in patients with cirrhosis (Figures 10-37 and 10-38). The disease process of cirrhosis produces areas of micronodular and macronodular regeneration, atrophy, and fatty infiltration, which make it difficult for the blood to perfuse. This condition may be found in patients with liver disease or diseases of the cardiovascular system. Patients who present with increased portal blood flow may have an arteriovenous fistula or splenomegaly secondary to a hematologic disorder.

Collateral circulation develops when the normal venous channels become obstructed. This diverted blood flow causes embryologic channels to reopen; blood flows hepatofugally (away from the liver) and is diverted into collateral vessels. The collateral channels may be into the gastric veins (coronary veins), esophageal veins, recanalized umbilical vein, or splenorenal, gastrorenal, retroperitoneal, hemorrhoidal, or intestinal veins (Figure 10-39). The most common collateral pathways are through the coronary and esophageal veins, as occurs in 80% to 90% of patients with portal hypertension. Varices, tortuous dilations of veins, may develop because of increased pressure in the portal vein, usually secondary to cirrhosis. Bleeding from the varices occurs with increased pressure.

The most definitive way to diagnose portal hypertension is with arteriography. Ultrasound may be very useful in these patients to define the presence of ascites, hepatosplenomegaly, and collateral circulation; the cause of jaundice; and the patency of hepatic vascular channels.

BOX 10-4	Indications for Portal Hypertension

- Suspected portal hypertension secondary to liver disease
- Portal vein compression or thrombosis
- Acute onset of hepatic vein occlusion (Budd-Chiari syndrome), constrictive pericarditis, or congestive heart failure with tricuspid regurgitation
- Congenital, traumatic, or neoplastic arterioportal fistula

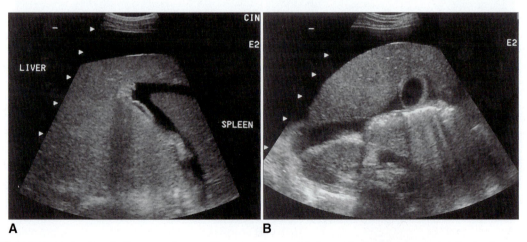

FIGURE 10-37 Portal hypertension. **A,** Transverse image of hepatosplenomegaly in a patient with advanced cirrhosis, decreased vasculature, and ascites. **B,** Transverse image of the thickened gallbladder wall, accentuated by the ascitic fluid.

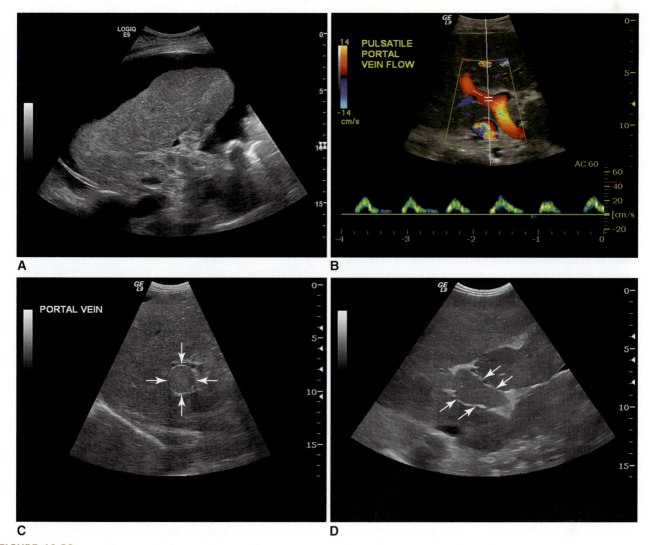

FIGURE 10-38 Portal hypertension. **A,** Hepatomegaly with massive ascites. The portal vein is filled with thrombus. **B,** The sonographer should search for hepatofugal flow in the portal vein. Note the nodular border of the liver. **C,** The portal vein is dilated and completely filled with thrombus *(arrows)*. **D,** Thrombosis of the main portal vein *(arrows)* with reduced flow.

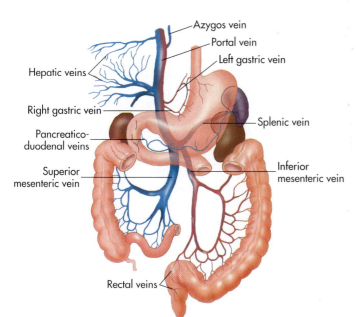

FIGURE 10-39 Collateral circulation of the extrahepatic portal circulation.

TABLE 10-4	Liver Findings: Portal Venous Hypertension	
Clinical Findings	**Sonographic Findings**	**Differential Considerations**
↑ Liver enzymes Gastrointestinal bleeding Jaundice Hematemesis	Collateral circulation/ reversal of flow Ascites Hepatosplenomegaly	Occlusion of vessels

BOX 10-5 | Major Sites of Portosystemic Venous Collaterals

- Gastroesophageal junction located between the coronary and short gastric veins and the systemic esophageal veins (may lead to fatal hemorrhage)
- Paraumbilical vein runs in the falciform ligament and connects the left portal vein to the systemic epigastric veins near the umbilicus
- Splenorenal and gastrorenal veins
- Intestinal veins
- Hemorrhoidal veins

See Table 10-4 for clinical findings, sonographic findings, and differential considerations for portal venous hypertension.

Patient Preparation and Positioning. A history should be obtained from the patient to focus on the risk factors, signs, and symptoms of hepatocellular disease. Any previous medical history relating to hepatocellular disease should be noted. Likewise, any recent surgical intervention or shunt placement within the portal venous system should be documented in the patient history worksheet. The patient is placed initially in the supine position; the patient may also be rolled into a slight left lateral decubitus position to obtain a better intercostal window. The images and Doppler evaluation may be obtained in the longitudinal, coronal, oblique, or transverse plane. Breath holding is very important in obtaining good Doppler color and spectral waveforms. Initially the sonographer should image the patient in shallow respiration to set up his or her controls and depth. Then instruct the patient to stop breathing or take in a deep breath and hold it while the Doppler images are recorded. The image may be visualized on the monitor, allowing you to see which technique works best to obtain the clearest images. It is helpful to remember that a portal vein diameter > 13 mm has been associated with portal hypertension. As portosystemic shunts develop, the diameter of the portal vein decreases. Secondary signs of splenomegaly, alterations in liver size, ascites, and portosystemic venous collaterals should be evaluated (Box 10-5).

The sonographer should keep in mind these important technical points in evaluating the patient for portal hypertension:

- Place ultrasound gel on the abdomen to ensure good transducer-to-skin contact during the abdominal Doppler imaging examination.
- The transducer's orientation marker should be pointing toward the patient's right side during the examination when a transverse scan is performed; the orientation marker is directed toward the patient's head when a longitudinal scan is performed.
- The examination is performed with both gray-scale and Doppler evaluation of the portal system, the hepatic veins, and the hepatic arteries.

- Remember, the transducer must be *parallel* to the vessel; the Doppler angle should be less than 60 degrees to obtain the maximum peak systolic velocity.
- The evaluation of the portal venous system, hepatic veins, and hepatic artery is performed during the Doppler imaging examination.
- A liver Doppler examination should also evaluate flow in the extra–hepatic-portal venous system and the inferior vena cava, as well as the size of the common bile duct, liver, kidneys, and spleen.
- The pelvic cavity, flanks, and lower quadrants should be evaluated for the presence of free fluid.

Doppler Technique. Box 10-6 summarizes Doppler technique for abdominal exams.

Color Doppler Evaluation of Collateral Circulation. The dilated venous structures near the superior mesenteric-splenic vein confluence, the main portal vein, and the gastric veins should be evaluated (Figure 10-40). As the sonographer scans in the longitudinal plane, medial to the superior mesenteric and splenic vein confluence, the right and left gastric veins may be seen as collateral circulation. If the gastric veins are serving as collateral circulation, their diameter should be enlarged to 4 to 5 mm. Remember, the Doppler signals should be obtained from the imaging plane that allows the beam to be as parallel to the vessel as possible.

The umbilical vein may become recanalized secondary to portal hypertension. This vessel is best seen on the longitudinal plane near the midline, as a tubular structure coursing posterior to the medial surface of the left lobe of the liver (Figure 10-41). On transverse scans, a bull's-eye is seen within the ligamentum teres as the enlarged umbilical vein. Color Doppler helps the sonographer identify this vascular structure. Table 10-5 on p. 245 summarizes hepatic vasculature technique.

Other vessels that may become collaterals include the esophageal vessels, which are best seen in the midline transverse plane as the transducer is angled in a cephalic direction through the left lobe of the liver. The dilated gastrorenal, splenorenal, and short gastric veins are seen in the transverse and longitudinal planes near the splenic hilum.

BOX 10-6 | Doppler Technique

- The pulse repetition frequency (PRF) allows one to record lower velocities as the PRF is lowered; as the PRF is increased, the lower velocities are filtered out to record only the higher velocity signal.
- The PRF may be changed with the scale control on the Doppler panel (look at the color bar on the left side of the monitor; the PRF will change as the "scale" on the Doppler control is changed).
- The PRF increases as imaging depth increases and decreases as depth decreases. Flow within the normal hepatic venous system is low; therefore, a lower PRF is necessary to record the flow pattern. As the flow increases beyond 40 cm/sec, the PRF should be increased to prevent aliasing. (Aliasing may also be reduced by scanning at a lower frequency.)
- The Doppler sample volume should be smaller than the diameter of the lumen. If you have difficulty finding the vessel, increase the width of the sample volume to locate the flow, and then reduce the volume width to clear up the spectral waveform.
- The Doppler angle correction should be less than 60 degrees to display the peak spectral velocity.
- Wall filters help to eliminate "noise" or low-level Doppler shifts seen within the vessel.
- Pulse wave Doppler provides quantitative information from a selected location.
- Color Doppler velocity is dependent on the direction of flow, velocity, and angle to flow. A positive Doppler shift is toward the transducer; negative shift shows flow away from the transducer. The laminar flow is distinguished from turbulent flow by varying the shades of color on the color map.
- Doppler measurements: peak systolic velocity (calculated highest velocity in cm/sec); Resistive Index (RI): subtract the end diastolic velocity from the peak systolic velocity and divide by the peak systolic velocity. Normal or low resistive RI measures <0.7.

As discussed earlier, the normal portal venous blood flows toward the liver, with the main portal vein flowing in a hepatopetal direction into the liver. Color Doppler will show this flow as a red or positive color pattern. The portal branches running posteriorly, or away from the transducer, will appear as blue, or negative, flow. Thus, the right portal vein will appear blue and the left portal vein will appear red. The normal portal vein waveform is monophasic with low velocity (15 to 18 cm/sec) and varies with the patient's respiration and cardiac pulsation. The flow should be smooth and laminar. The normal diameter of the portal vein is 1.0 to 1.2 cm. With the development of portal hypertension, the flow in the portal vein loses its undulatory pattern and becomes monophasic. With severe portal hypertension, the flow becomes biphasic and finally hepatofugal (away from the liver). At this point intrahepatic arterial-portal venous shunting may also be seen.

The superior mesenteric vein and splenic vein are more influenced by respiration and patient position; thus, if they appear larger, it may not be as a result of portal hypertension. Flow reversal is seen both with spectral waveform patterns below the baseline in the main portal vein and with reversed color direction. Obstruction of the portal venous system is recognized by turbulence within the vessel. Table 10-6 on p. 246 summarizes observations important to abdominal Doppler exams.

Doppler Interrogation. The hepatic vessels should be imaged at four anatomic locations:

1. Midline, beneath the xiphoid at the LHV, LHA, and LPV
2. Midclavicular and intercostals at the porta hepatis for the MHA and MPV
3. Lateral and intercostals at the right lobe for the RHA and RPV
4. Subcostal and midclavicular for the RHV and MHV

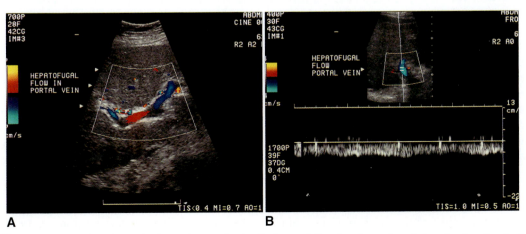

A   **B**

FIGURE 10-40 A, Flow reversal is shown in the main portal vein. **B,** Spectral Doppler shows flow below the baseline in the main portal vein.

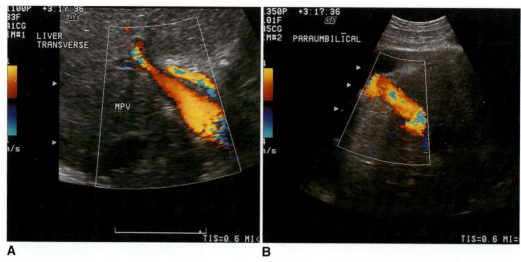

FIGURE 10-41 Hepatopetal flow in the portal vein and paraumbilical vein. **A,** Main portal vein with normal forward flow. **B,** Portal hypertension with recanalization of the paraumbilical vein.

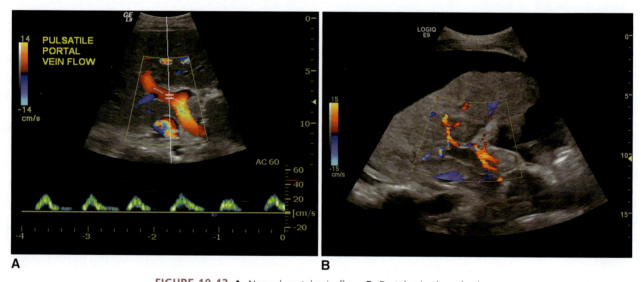

FIGURE 10-42 A. Normal portal vein flow. **B.** Portal vein thrombosis.

Portal Hypertension Secondary to Portal Vein Thrombosis. The invasion of the portal system with tumor or thrombosis may cause portal hypertension if the vessel is significantly occluded so that blood cannot flow into the liver. The clinical symptoms are very different from those of intrahepatic disease; ascites is the primary complaint. The patient does not have jaundice or a tender enlarged liver. Splenomegaly and bleeding varices may be present. Portal vein thrombosis may develop secondary to trauma, sepsis, cirrhosis, or hepatocellular carcinoma (Figure 10-42). The definitive diagnosis is made with a liver biopsy and positive findings of portal hypertension.

Sonographic Findings. Portal vein thrombosis shows absence of portal flow with echogenic thrombus within the lumen of the vein, the development of portal vein collaterals, expansion of the caliber of the vein, and cavernous transformation of the vessels. The cavernous transformation of the portal vein appears as a wormlike structure in the area of the porta hepatis that completely fills with color representing the periportal collateral circulation. Acute thrombus may appear anechoic and thus be missed by the sonographer if Doppler interrogation is not performed. Malignant thrombosis of the portal vein is closely associated with hepatocellular carcinoma and is often expansive.

Portal Vein Hypertension and Portal Caval Shunts. If portal hypertension becomes extensive, the portal system can be decompressed by shunting blood to the systemic venous system. Basically, the three types of shunts are portacaval, mesocaval, and splenorenal. It is the responsibility of the sonographer to know specifically which type of shunt the patient has in place to image the flow patterns correctly.

TABLE 10-5	Hepatic Vasculature Technique	
Vessel	**Image Plane**	**Technique**
LHV (left hepatic vein)	Transverse/longitudinal	• Locate the left lobe of the liver. • Identify the IVC and angle steeply toward the diaphragm. • The LHV and MHV should be seen as they drain into the IVC.
LPV (left portal vein) LHA (left hepatic artery)	Transverse, coronal, intercostal, decubitus Transverse	• Locate horizontal segment of LPV, adjust transducer to obtain steepest angle for Doppler (parallel to the vessel), and zoom in on the LPV. • Usually found posterior to horizontal segment of LPV. • After interrogating the LPV, look for LHA with color Doppler (expand color box to cover the LPV and adjacent liver tissue). • Place PW cursor/sample volume in area of LHA (suspend respiration); watch for "flashing" of signal as it comes in and out of view with respiration. • Look for LHA on deep inspiration. • If you cannot get the signal in the periphery of the liver, move to another location closer to the main portal vein.
Common HA (common hepatic artery)	Longitudinal—porta hepatis	• Use same technique as described for LHA. • Transplant recipient patients: usually only able to Doppler HA at the porta hepatis. • Include extrahepatic and intrahepatic segments of HA. • Difficult to image site of anastomosis.
MPV (main portal vein) IVC (inferior vena cava)	Longitudinal—porta hepatis Longitudinal, coronal—slightly to right of midline; suspend breath. Angle transducer in cephalad to caudal sweep to record flow.	• If shunt is present, anastomosis site easier to identify (more prone to thrombosis); be sure to investigate the MPV proximal, within, and distal to anastomosis. • May be difficult to obtain good angle because of horizontal location on transverse plane. • If shunt is present, evaluate site of anastomosis carefully (proximal, within, and distal). • Look carefully for presence of internal echoes that represent thrombosis. • If you suspect thrombus is present, and the Doppler signal is very "choppy" with high velocity and little phasicity, the likelihood of thrombus is good. • Be sure to follow the IVC all the way into the right atrium of the heart.
SV (splenic vein) RHA (right hepatic artery)	Transverse Transverse, anterior to right posterior portal branch	• Examine SV from the splenic hilum to the portal-splenic confluence. • Use same techniques as mentioned to Doppler the RPV and RHA. • If you are unable to locate the RHA in the periphery of the liver, move closer to the trunk of the adjacent PV. • If you cannot find the RHA at the right posterior portal branch, try looking for it at the level of the right anterior PV branch.
RPV (right portal vein)	Anterior, intercostal approach; one rib space away from window for porta hepatis	• To locate the right posterior branch of RPV, begin with the MPV at the porta hepatis. • Follow the MPV into the liver until you see the RPV. • The posterior branch extends posteriorly into the right lobe. It is easier to obtain a good Doppler angle if you use a more anterior intercostal approach.
RHV (right hepatic vein)	Transverse, subcostal	• Place the probe just below the level of the xiphoid with a steep angulation toward the diaphragm. • Locate the IVC; the RHV will be seen in the right lobe of the liver in a horizontal plane as it empties into the IVC.
MHV (middle hepatic vein)	Transverse, subcostal	• Place the probe just below the level of the xiphoid with a steep angulation toward the diaphragm. • Locate the IVC; the MHV will be seen in a vertical plane as it separates the right lobe from the left lobe of the liver as it empties into the IVC.

The portacaval shunt attaches the main portal vein at the superior mesenteric vein-splenic vein confluence to the anterior aspect of the inferior vena cava. The meso-caval shunt attaches the middistal superior mesenteric vein to the inferior vena cava (Figure 10-43). This shunt may be difficult to image if overlying bowel gas is present.

The splenorenal shunt attaches the splenic vein to the left renal vein. The shunt and connecting vessel should be documented with real-time pulsed Doppler and color Doppler to determine flow patterns and patency.

Intrahepatic shunts are created percutaneously with the use of metallic expandable stents, which can be seen

TABLE 10-6 | Doppler Observations

Hepatic Artery

- Left hepatic artery—LHA
- Right hepatic artery—RHA
- Common hepatic artery—CHA

- Low resistance waveform; forward flow in diastolic above baseline.
- Vessel is tortuous; flow may appear to move toward and away from the transducer.
- Systolic window with narrow bandwidth with parabolic flow profile.
- Spectral fill-in of systolic window because of small vessel diameter.
- High-resistance waveforms may indicate veno-occlusive disease.

Portal Venous System

- Left portal vein—LPV
- Right portal vein—RPV
- Main portal vein—MPV

- Continuous, low-velocity phasic signal (phasic means that the velocity increases and decreases with respiration, giving the signal a smooth wavelike appearance).
- Normal flow is termed *hepatopetal* (toward the liver).
- Reversed flow is *hepatofugal* (away from the liver).
- Portal venous thrombosis or postoperative anastomosis from a liver transplant can cause an abnormal portal vein signal. This results from decreased vessel lumen size, which reduces the pressure and consequently increases the velocity of flow through the narrowed region, giving a "choppy" appearance as a result of increased velocities.

Note: The hepatic artery and portal vein flow should be in the same direction, since the hepatic artery runs parallel with the portal vein.

Hepatic Venous System

- Left hepatic vein—LHV
- Right hepatic vein—RHV
- Middle hepatic vein—MHV

- Multiphasic pulsatile flow pattern secondary to proximity of the right atrium with flow above and below the baseline caused by close proximity to the right atrium, which results in hemodynamic changes.
- Right-sided heart failure may cause the hepatic veins to become pulsatile and dilated.
- Increased intrahepatic pressure or venous obstruction demonstrates a more continuous or monophasic signal.

Inferior Vena Cava

- Continuous waveform with respiratory variations; becomes more pulsatile as it empties into the right atrium.
- Best imaged with a slight cranial-caudal sweep in the longitudinal plane with the patient in deep inspiration.
- Anastomosis from surgical transplantation may alter the normal flow into the inferior vena cava.
- Thrombosis can cause the inferior vena cava waveform to appear monophasic with high velocities ("choppy" appearance). Examine for thrombus in the renal veins as well.
- If a surgical shunt is present, be sure to check the patient's history to find out if the specific type of shunt (portal/cava or mesenteric/cava) is in place.

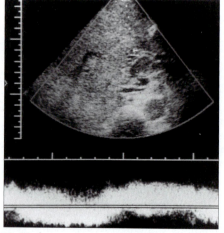

FIGURE 10-43 Mesocaval shunt. The mesocaval shunt attaches the middistal superior mesenteric vein to the inferior vena cava. This patient had thrombus at the distal end with to-and-fro flow reversal.

on ultrasound. This type of shunt is the transjugular intrahepatic portosystemic shunt (TIPS) (Figure 10-44). The TIPS shunt is easy to evaluate for patency because the liver provides an acoustic window to image the shunt. Baseline studies are performed with color and spectral Doppler so variations in flow patterns may be monitored before clinical symptoms are apparent. Stenosis may occur at the hepatic vein level or within the shunt.

Budd-Chiari Syndrome. Budd-Chiari syndrome is an uncommon, often dramatic illness caused by thrombosis of the hepatic veins or inferior vena cava. It was first described by George Budd in 1846 and by Hans Chiari in 1899. Budd-Chiari syndrome has a poor prognosis and is characterized by abdominal pain, massive ascites, and hepatomegaly. It may present acutely or as a chronic illness lasting from a few weeks to several years. Extensive hepatic vein occlusion is usually fatal within weeks or months of the onset of symptoms.

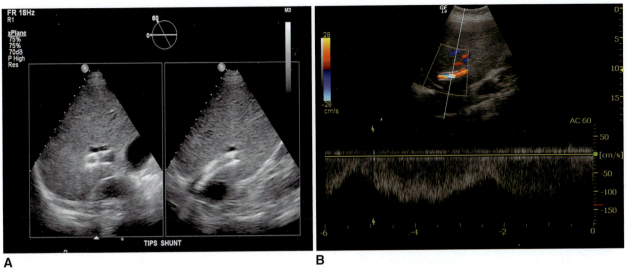

FIGURE 10-44 A and **B,** Transjugular intrahepatic portosystemic shunt (TIPS). A 50-year-old male after TIPS procedure shows patency of the stent and normal flow from the portal vein to the inferior vena cava without evidence of thrombus.

Budd-Chiari syndrome may be classified as primary or secondary on the basis of its pathophysiology. The primary type is caused by congenital obstruction of the hepatic veins or inferior vena cava by membranous webs across the upper vena cava at or just above the entrance of the left and middle hepatic veins. This lesion has been found to be most common in Asia.

The secondary type results from thrombosis in the hepatic veins or inferior vena cava. It often occurs in patients with predisposing conditions, such as polycythemia rubra vera, paroxysmal nocturnal hemoglobinuria, prolonged use of oral contraceptives, pregnancy tumors (hepatocellular carcinoma, renal cell carcinoma, adrenal carcinoma, leiomyosarcoma of the inferior vena cava), infections, and in rare cases trauma. In approximately 25% to 30% of all cases, the exact cause is never determined.

Ascites is the most characteristic clinical feature of this disease. Other symptoms are abdominal pain, hepatosplenomegaly, jaundice, vomiting, and diarrhea. Rarely, patients present with acute illness with abdominal pain, hepatomegaly, and shock. This condition often occurs in patients with an underlying disease, such as renal cell carcinoma, primary cancer of the liver, thrombophlebitis migraines, or polycythemia. More commonly, patients have a vague illness and abdominal distress weeks or months in duration, followed by the appearance of ascites and hepatomegaly. Jaundice is mild or absent. As portal hypertension increases, the spleen becomes palpable. When thrombus is found in the inferior vena cava, edema of the legs is gross and there is venous distention over the abdomen, flanks, and back. Albuminuria may be found.

Routine biochemical determinations of aminotransferases and alkaline phosphatase indicate mild or moderate impairment of hepatic function, depending on the

TABLE 10-7	Liver Findings: Budd-Chiari Syndrome	
Clinical Findings	**Sonographic Findings**	**Differential Considerations**
Ascites, right upper quadrant pain, hepatomegaly	↑ Caudate lobe Atrophy in right lobe of the liver	Portal hypertension

stage of disease. Clinically apparent jaundice is unusual. See Table 10-7 for clinical findings, sonographic findings, and differential considerations for Budd-Chiari syndrome.

Sonographic Findings. Sonography is useful in imaging patients with hepatic vein thrombosis and has proven to be diagnostic in 87% of cases. The caudate lobe of the liver, seen in longitudinal and transverse scans, has an independent vascular supply. In Budd-Chiari syndrome the caudate lobe becomes enlarged, and there is often atrophy of the right hepatic lobe, probably as a result of sparing of caudate lobe hepatic veins when there is thrombosis of the right, middle, and left hepatic veins.

The liver appears hypoechoic in the early stages of acute thrombosis; it appears hyperechoic and inhomogeneous, with fibrosis in later stages (Figure 10-45). The middle and left hepatic veins are imaged in the transverse plane at the level of the xiphoid. The transducer is angled in a cephalad position with the patient in deep inspiration. This allows the veins to be parallel to the Doppler beam. The right hepatic vein is evaluated from a right intercostal approach. With thrombosis, the hepatic veins become enlarged. In chronic cases of Budd-Chiari syndrome, the hepatic veins are usually not visualized.

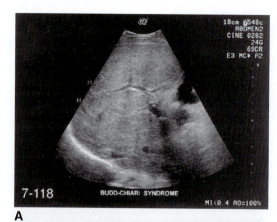

A

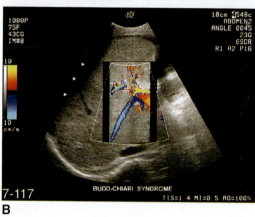

B

FIGURE 10-45 Budd-Chiari syndrome. **A,** Transverse image of the enlarged liver and thrombosis of the middle and left hepatic veins. **B,** Color Doppler shows patency of the right hepatic vein into the inferior vena cava.

Demonstration of at least one major vein may show abnormalities in the vessel suggestive of this syndrome, including stenosis, dilation, thick wall echoes, abnormal course, extrahepatic anastomoses, and thrombosis.

Doppler sonography may show altered blood-flow patterns in the hepatic veins and inferior vena cava. In normal subjects the Doppler signal in the hepatic veins is phasic in response to both the cardiac and respiratory cycles, with wide variations in flow velocity and direction. In Budd-Chiari syndrome, flow in the inferior vena cava or hepatic veins changes from phasic to absent, reversed, turbulent, or continuous. Abnormal Doppler patterns with slow, continuous flow may indicate partial obstruction. The absence of flow signals suggests subtotal or total occlusion. Turbulent flow may be observed beyond the area of stenosis. The portal venous flow pattern may also be affected with decreased velocities or reversal of flow.

Color flow Doppler is an excellent technique for evaluating the hepatic venous system. Flow direction and velocities and areas of turbulent flow can be demonstrated with color. Patency of the hepatic veins and inferior vena cava can be determined with color flow Doppler, which compares very favorably with angiography.

Treatment. The mortality rate for patients with hepatic vein thrombosis is high, but with the routine use of imaging, this syndrome has been diagnosed more often and in milder forms. Anticoagulants and streptokinase may be of value, although there is no definite evidence that this therapy promotes resolution of established thrombosis.

Surgical construction of portosystemic shunts is considered in symptomatic patients who have a patent portal vein. These include portacaval, mesocaval, and splenorenal shunts. The aim of these shunts is to decompress the congested liver and reverse portal venous flow.

Budd-Chiari syndrome may be managed with side-to-side portacaval shunting, but it is best treated by liver transplantation in patients with end-stage liver disease. Long-term anticoagulant therapy is mandatory for patients with this syndrome after liver transplantation because there is an increased risk of thrombotic complications. Membranous webs may be surgically corrected by resection. Transluminal angioplasty has also been used to dilate webs.

Nonsurgical treatments have been performed using interventional techniques. A percutaneous portacaval shunt is placed using a WallStent prosthesis and right internal jugular approach to relieve portal hypertension. This may provide an attractive alternative to surgery because many patients with Budd-Chiari syndrome are poor surgical risks.

Diagnostic Criteria for Hepatic Vascular Imaging. See Table 10-8 for the diagnostic criteria for hepatic vascular imaging, including grayscale, Doppler, and color Doppler.

Diffuse Abnormalities of the Liver Parenchyma

Abnormalities—such as biliary obstruction, common duct stones and stricture, extrahepatic mass, and passive hepatic congestion—are discussed as each lesion is seen on the ultrasound. See Table 10-9 for clinical findings, sonographic findings, and differential considerations of diffuse abnormalities of the liver parenchyma.

Biliary Obstruction: Proximal. Biliary obstruction proximal to the cystic duct can be caused by gallstones, carcinoma of the common bile duct, or metastatic tumor invasion of the porta hepatis (Figure 10-46). Clinically the patient may be jaundiced and have pruritus (itching). Liver function tests show an elevation in the direct bilirubin and alkaline phosphatase levels.

Sonographic Findings. Sonographically, carcinoma of the common duct shows as a tubular branching with dilated intrahepatic ducts best seen in the periphery of the liver (Figure 10-47). It may be difficult to image a discrete mass lesion. The gallbladder is of normal size, even after a fatty meal is administered.

Biliary Obstruction: Distal. A biliary obstruction distal to the cystic duct may be caused by stones in the common duct (Figure 10-48), an extrahepatic mass in the porta

TABLE 10-8	Diagnostic Criteria for Hepatic Vascular Imaging		
Interpretation	Gray Scale	Doppler	Color Doppler
Portal Veins			
Normal	No intraluminal echoes; bright, echogenic borders	Low-velocity signal with respiratory variation	Smooth fill-in of color
Thrombus	Enlarged or normal portal venous system with low-level echoes within the lumen; may appear isoechoic with the liver	Decreased low-velocity to absent Doppler waveform; look for hepatofugal flow	Decreased to absent color flow
Portal hypertension	Enlargement of the portal venous system Recanalization of the umbilical vein	Look for hepatofugal flow in portal venous system	Hepatofugal flow with good color fill of lumen
Cavernous transformation	Multiple vascular channels near the porta hepatis and/or splenic hilum Thrombosis of the extrahepatic portal vein (may be difficult to image) Look for recanalized umbilical vein	Continuous low-velocity flow	Color fills dilated collateral vessels; portal vein is difficult to fill with color
Hepatic Artery			
Normal	Follow course of portal vein to image hepatic artery anterior Enlarge image size to visualize artery Proximal HA best seen at level of celiac axis Distal HA seen in intercostal coronal view at level of MPV and CBD	Low-resistance waveform with systolic and diastolic component	Increase gain slightly to fill in vessel lumen with color
Thrombus	Increased low-level echoes within the lumen	Obstruction would cause increased velocity waveforms	Turbulence or absence of flow if complete obstruction is present
Inferior Vena Cava			
Normal	Low-level intraluminal echoes within the lumen returning to right atrium; changes size with respiration	Continuous triphasic waveform with respiratory variations	Color fills lumen
Thrombosis	Increased echogenicity of low-level echoes filling lumen Examine renal veins for extension of thrombus	Decreased Doppler waveform secondary to degree of thrombus	Decreased color within lumen; color will outline the area of thrombus/obstruction
Right-sided heart failure	Dilation of lumen that does not change with respiration	Multiphasic, pulsatile flow	Color fills lumen of hepatic veins and inferior vena cava
Thrombosis/Budd-Chiari	Low-level echoes within the lumen of the hepatic veins; may completely restrict blood flow into the inferior vena cava Caudate lobe enlargement may be suspicious of thrombosis of hepatic veins	Decreased flow signal	Decreased color fill-in of hepatic veins; IVC may appear collapsed with decreased blood return

hepatis, or stricture of the common duct. Clinically, common duct stones cause right upper quadrant pain, jaundice, and pruritus, as well as an increase in direct bilirubin and alkaline phosphatase.

▶ Sonographic Findings. On ultrasound examination, the dilated intrahepatic ducts are seen in the periphery of the liver (Figure 10-49). The gallbladder size is variable, usually small. Gallstones are often present and appear as hyperechoic lesions along the posterior floor of the gallbladder, with a sharp posterior acoustic shadow. Careful evaluation of the common duct may show shadowing stones within the dilated duct.

Extrahepatic Mass. An extrahepatic mass in the area of the porta hepatis causes the same clinical signs as seen in biliary obstruction.

▶ Sonographic Findings. On ultrasound examination, an irregular, ill-defined, hypoechoic, and inhomogeneous mass lesion may be seen in the area of the porta hepatis. There is intrahepatic ductal dilation, with a hydropic gallbladder. The lesion may arise from the lymph nodes,

TABLE 10-9 | Liver Findings: Diffuse Abnormalities of the Liver Parenchyma

Clinical Findings	Sonographic Findings	Differential Considerations
Biliary Obstruction: Proximal		
↑ Direct bilirubin ↑ Alk phos	Carcinoma of common bile duct shows tubular branching with dilated intrahepatic ducts Gallbladder small to normal size; gallstones	Obstruction to distal duct Extrahepatic metastases
Biliary Obstruction: Distal		
↑ Direct bilirubin ↑ Alk phos	Carcinoma of common bile duct shows tubular branching with dilated intrahepatic ducts Gallbladder small; gallstones and common duct stones	Obstruction to proximal duct Extrahepatic metastases
Extrahepatic Mass		
↑ Direct bilirubin ↑ Alk phos	Irregular, ill-defined hypoechoic, heterogeneous lesion in area of porta hepatis Intrahepatic ductal dilation Hydropic gallbladder	Proximal or distal obstruction to the cystic duct Metastases
Common Duct Stricture		
↑ Direct bilirubin ↑ Alk phos Previous cholecystectomy	Dilated intrahepatic ducts Absence of mass in porta hepatis	Extrahepatic mass Passive hepatic congestion
Passive Hepatic Congestion		
↑ LFT	↑ IVC, HV, PV	N/A

Alk phos, Alkaline phosphatase; *IVC,* inferior vena cava; *HV,* hepatic vein; *LFT,* liver function test; *N/A,* not applicable; *PV,* portal vein.

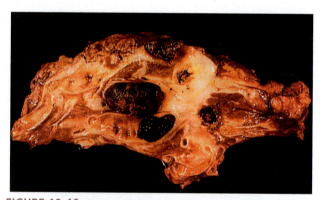

FIGURE 10-46 Gross pathology of gallstones in the hepatic duct.

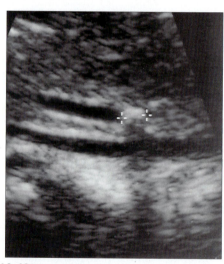

FIGURE 10-48 Obstruction distal to the cystic duct may be caused by stones in the common duct. The distal cystic duct is enlarged and obstructed by a stone at the distal end. The inferior vena cava is posterior to the duct.

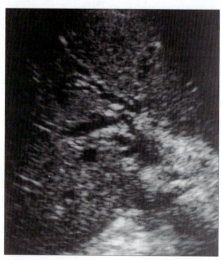

FIGURE 10-47 Obstruction proximal to the cystic duct may be secondary to pancreatic carcinoma or tumor invasion to the porta hepatis. Dilated intrahepatic ducts will result from this obstruction.

pancreatitis, pseudocyst, or carcinoma in the head of the pancreas.

Common Duct Stricture. Clinically the patient is jaundiced and has had a previous cholecystectomy. Laboratory values show an increase in the direct bilirubin and alkaline phosphatase levels.

Sonographic Findings. On ultrasound examination, common duct stricture presents as dilated intrahepatic ducts with absence of a mass in the porta hepatis.

Passive Hepatic Congestion. Passive hepatic congestion develops secondary to congestive heart failure with

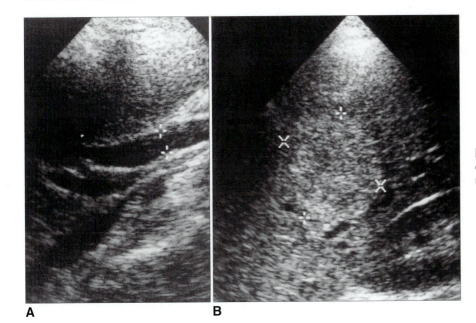

A B

FIGURE 10-49 A, Sagittal scan of the dilated common duct. **B,** Sagittal scan of a mass in the porta hepatis.

signs of hepatomegaly. Laboratory data indicate normal to slightly elevated liver function tests.

Sonographic Findings. On ultrasound examination, dilation of the inferior vena cava, superior mesenteric, hepatic, portal, and splenic veins is noted. The venous structures may decrease in size with expiration and increase with inspiration.

Focal Hepatic Disease

Few hepatic lesions have specific sonographic features. Therefore, it is important to know the patient's clinical history and the sonographic patterns associated with various lesions. The knowledge of laboratory values in liver function tests also helps determine the hepatic lesions. The differential diagnosis for focal diseases of the liver includes cysts, abscess, hematoma, primary tumor, and metastases. See Table 10-10 for clinical findings, sonographic findings, and differential considerations for focal hepatic disease.

The sonographer should be able to differentiate whether the mass is **extrahepatic** or **intrahepatic**. Intrahepatic masses may cause the following findings on ultrasound: displacement of the hepatic vascular radicles, external bulging of the liver capsule, or a posterior shift of the inferior vena cava. An extrahepatic mass may show internal invagination or discontinuity of the liver capsule, formation of a triangular fat wedge, anteromedial shift of the inferior vena cava, or anterior displacement of the right kidney.

Cystic Lesions. *Hepatic cyst* usually refers to a solitary nonparasitic cyst of the liver. The cyst may be congenital or acquired, solitary or multiple. Patients are often asymptomatic and require no treatment. Sonographic findings of a benign cyst show the lesion to be well demarcated, thin walled, and anechoic with posterior acoustic enhancement.

When the cysts become large, pain may develop as the lesion compresses the hepatic vasculature or ductal system. Fever may be present if the cyst hemorrhages and becomes infected. Once the cyst becomes infected, septations and internal echoes from the debris replace the anechoic properties. The wall may become thickened.

Cystic lesions within the liver include the following: simple or congenital hepatic cysts, traumatic cysts, parasitic cysts, inflammatory cysts, polycystic disease, and pseudocysts.

Simple Hepatic Cysts. The sonographic finding of a simple hepatic cyst is usually incidental because most patients are asymptomatic. As the cyst grows, it may cause pain or a mass effect to suggest a more serious condition, such as infection, abscess, or necrotic lesion. Hepatic cysts occur more often in females than in males.

Sonographic Findings. On ultrasound examination, the cyst walls are thin, with well-defined borders, and anechoic, with distal posterior enhancement (Figure 10-50). Infrequently, cysts contain fine linear internal septa. Complications, such as hemorrhage, may occur and cause pain (Figure 10-51). Calcification may be seen within the cyst wall and may cause shadowing.

Congenital Hepatic Cysts. A solitary congenital cyst of the liver is rare and usually is an incidental lesion. This abnormality arises from developmental defects in the formation of bile ducts.

Sonographic Findings. The mass is usually solitary and may vary in size from tiny to as large as 20 cm (Figure 10-52). The cyst is usually found on the anterior undersurface of the liver. It usually does not cause liver enlargement and is found in the right lobe of the liver more often than the left lobe.

TABLE 10-10 | Liver Findings: Focal Disease

Clinical Findings	Sonographic Findings	Differential Considerations
Simple Hepatic Cysts		
N/A	Anechoic Thin walls Well-defined borders Distal posterior enhancement May have calcification	Congenital Hematoma Necrotic tumor
Polycystic Liver Disease		
Autosomal dominant 25%–50% of patients with polycystic kidney disease have hepatic cysts 60% of patients with polycystic liver disease have associated PKD	Anechoic Well-defined borders ↑ Acoustic enhancement Multiple cysts throughout liver parenchyma	Necrotic metastasis Echinococcal cyst Hematoma Abscess Hepatic cystadenocarcinoma
Pyogenic Abscess		
↑ White cell count Abnormal LFT Anemia	Variable appearance Right central lobe most common site Hypoechoic to complex to hyperechoic when fluid level present Round to oval or irregular Complex	Amebic abscess Echinococcal cyst Hepatic candidiasis
Hepatic Candidiasis		
↑ WBC Fever	Multiple small hypoechoic masses with echogenic central core "bulls-eye" lesions "Wheel-within-wheel" pattern	Abscess Echinococcal cyst Metastases
Chronic Granulomatous Disease		
N/A	Poorly marginated Hypoechoic Posterior enhancement May have calcification/shadowing	Abscess
Amebic Abscess		
↑ Leukocytes Low fever Abdominal pain and diarrhea	Mass is variable Round or oval; lack notable borders Hypoechoic with debris	Pyogenic abscess Echinococcal cyst Hepatic candidiasis
Echinococcal Cyst		
↑ WBC History of sheep-farming exposure	Simple to complex cysts Acoustic enhancement Oval or spherical Calcification Honeycomb appearance/"water lily" sign	Polycystic liver disease Amebic abscess Pyogenic abscess

LFT, Liver function test; *N/A,* not applicable; *PKD,* polycystic kidney disease.

Peribiliary Cysts. These tiny cysts (which range in size from 0.2 to 2.5 cm) are more commonly found in patients with severe liver disease. They are located centrally within the porta hepatis at the junction of the right and left hepatic ducts. Obstruction may occur if the cyst becomes large enough to cause biliary obstruction.

▶ Sonographic Findings. These small cysts are seen as discrete, clustered tubular-appearing cysts with thin septae that parallel the bile ducts and portal veins in the central area of the liver.

Polycystic Liver Disease. Polycystic liver disease is inherited in an autosomal dominant pattern that affects 1 in 500 individuals. At least 50% to 74% of patients with polycystic renal disease have one to several hepatic cysts. Of patients with polycystic liver disease, 60% have associated polycystic renal disease. The cysts are small, less than 2 to 3 cm, and multiple throughout the hepatic parenchyma (Figure 10-53). Cysts within the porta hepatis may enlarge and cause biliary obstruction. Histologically, they appear similar to simple hepatic cysts. It may be difficult to assess an abscess formation or neoplastic lesion in a patient with polycystic liver disease. Liver function tests are usually normal.

▶ Sonographic Findings. On ultrasound examination, the cysts generally present as anechoic, well-defined borders with acoustic enhancement (Figure 10-54).

The differential diagnosis for a cystic lesion includes the following: necrotic metastasis, echinococcal cyst, hematoma, hepatic cystadenocarcinoma, and abscess. Ultrasound may be used to direct the needle if percutaneous aspiration is necessary to obtain specific diagnostic information.

Inflammatory Disease of the Liver

Hepatic abscesses occur most often as complications of biliary tract disease, surgery, or trauma. The following three basic types of abscess formation occur in the liver: intrahepatic, subhepatic, and subphrenic.

Clinically the patient presents with fever, elevated white cell count, and right upper quadrant pain. The search for an abscess must be made to locate solitary or multiple lesions within the liver or to search for abnor-

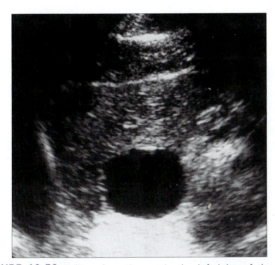

FIGURE 10-50 Solitary hepatic cyst in the left lobe of the liver shows increased through-transmission and well-defined borders.

mal fluid collections in Morison's pouch or in the subdiaphragmatic or subphrenic space. The following infectious processes are discussed: pyogenic abscess, hepatic candidiasis, chronic granulomatous disease, amebic abscess, and echinococcal disease.

Pyogenic Abscess. A **pyogenic abscess** is a pus-forming abscess. There are many routes for bacteria to gain access to the liver: through the biliary tree, the portal vein, or the hepatic artery; through a direct extension from a contiguous infection; or, rarely, through hepatic trauma. Sources of infection include cholangitis; portal pyemia secondary to appendicitis, diverticulitis, inflammatory disease, or colitis; direct spread from another organ; trauma with direct contamination; or infarction after embolization or from sickle cell anemia.

Clinically the patient presents with fever, pain, pleuritis, nausea, vomiting, and diarrhea. Elevated liver function tests, leukocytosis, and anemia are present. The abscess formation is multiple in 50% to 67% of patients. The most frequent organisms are *Escherichia coli* and anaerobes.

Sonographic Findings. The ultrasound appearance of a pyogenic abscess may be variable, depending on the internal consistency of the mass. The size varies from 1 cm to very large. The right central lobe of the liver is the most common site for abscess development. The abscess may be hypoechoic with round or ovoid margins and acoustic enhancement, or it may be complex, with some debris along the posterior margin and irregular walls (Figure 10-55). It may have a fluid level; if gas is present, it can be hyperechoic with dirty shadowing.

Hepatic Candidiasis. Hepatic candidiasis is caused by a species of *Candida*. It usually occurs in immunocompromised hosts, such as patients undergoing chemotherapy, organ transplant recipients, or individuals with human immunodeficiency infection (HIV). The candidal fungus invades the bloodstream and may affect any

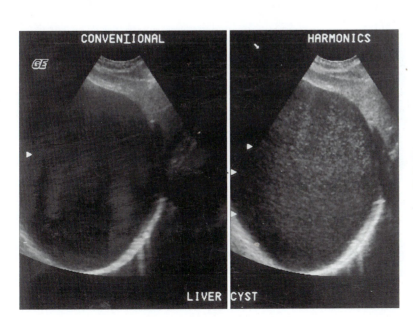

FIGURE 10-51 Simple hepatic cyst. A simple liver cyst may appear anechoic with conventional settings *(left)* and appear with low-level echoes with harmonics *(right)*.

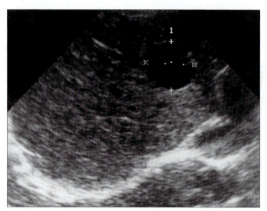

FIGURE 10-52 Simple hepatic cyst shows smooth, uniform borders and no internal echoes (anechoic).

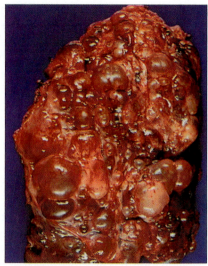

FIGURE 10-53 Gross pathology of polycystic liver disease. There are numerous large cysts throughout the liver parenchyma.

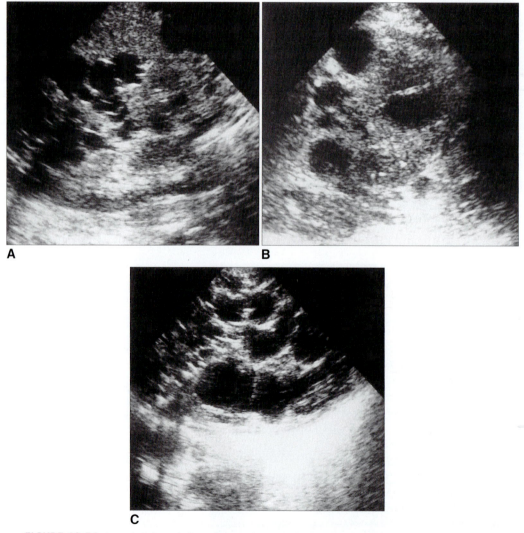

FIGURE 10-54 A to **C,** Polycystic liver disease shows multiple cysts throughout the liver and kidney.

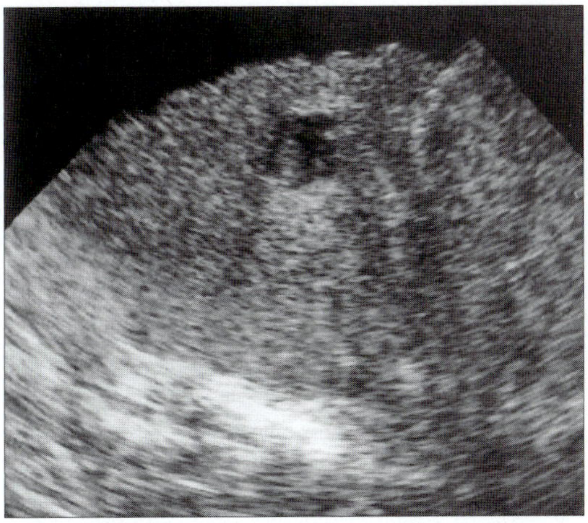

FIGURE 10-55 Pyogenic abscess is shown as a complex mass in the right lobe of the liver in a patient with cirrhosis, abdominal pain, and fever. The mass is irregular with slightly increased through-transmission.

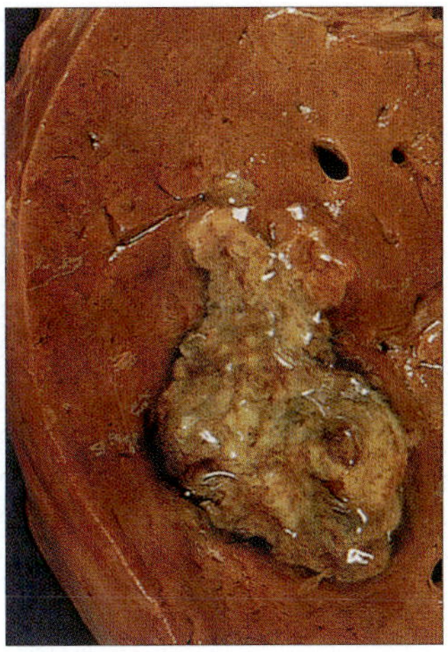

FIGURE 10-56 Gross pathology of an amebic abscess. The cavitary lesion is filled with yellow necrotic material and does not contain pus.

organ, with the more perfused kidneys, brain, and heart affected the most.

Clinically the patient may present with nonspecific findings, such as persistent fever in a neutropenic patient whose leukocyte count is returning to normal. Localized pain may also be present.

Sonographic Findings. Candidiasis within the liver may present as multiple small hypoechoic masses with echogenic central cores, referred to as **bull's-eye** or **target lesions.** The hyperechoic center (containing inflammatory cells) with a hypoechoic rim is present when the neutrophil counts return to normal. Other sonographic patterns have been described as "wheel-within-wheel" patterns, or multiple small hypoechoic lesions. A peripheral hypoechoic zone with an inner echogenic wheel and central hypoechoic focal necrosis may be found. The most common finding is uniformly hypoechoic. As scar formation develops, the pattern becomes echogenic. Specific diagnosis can only be made with fine-needle aspiration.

Chronic Granulomatous Disease. Chronic granulomatous disease is a genetic disorder in which phagocytes are unable to kill certain bacteria and fungi. It occurs mostly in children, with a more frequent occurrence in boys because it is a recessive trait. A pediatric patient may have recurrent respiratory infections.

Sonographic Findings. A poorly marginated, hypoechoic mass is seen with posterior enhancement. Calcification may be present with posterior shadowing. Aspiration is necessary to specifically classify the mass as granulomatous disease.

Amebic Abscess. Amebic abscess is a collection of pus formed by disintegrated tissue in a cavity, usually in the liver, caused by the protozoan parasite *Entamoeba histolytica* (Figure 10-56). The infection is primarily a disease of the colon, but it can also spread to the liver, lungs, and brain. The parasites reach the liver parenchyma via the portal vein. Amebiasis is contracted by ingesting the cysts in contaminated water and food. The ameba usually affects the colon and cecum, and the organism remains within the gastrointestinal tract. If the organism invades the colonic mucosa, it may travel to the liver via the portal venous system.

Patients may be asymptomatic or may show the gastrointestinal symptoms of abdominal pain, diarrhea, leukocytosis, and low fever.

Sonographic Findings. The sonographic appearance of amebic abscess is variable and nonspecific. The abscess may be round or oval and lack notable defined wall echoes. The lesion is hypoechoic compared with normal liver parenchyma, with low-level echoes at higher sensitivity. There may be some internal echoes along the posterior margin secondary to debris (Figure 10-57). Distal enhancement may be seen beyond the mass lesion. Some organisms may rupture through the diaphragm into the hepatic capsule.

Echinococcal Cyst. Hepatic echinococcosis is an infectious cystic disease common in sheep-herding areas of the world, but seldom encountered within the United States. The echinococcus is a tapeworm that infects humans as the intermediate host. The worm resides in the small intestine of dogs. The ova from the adult worm are shed through canine feces into the environment, where the intermediate hosts ingest the eggs. After entering the proximal portion of the small intestine in humans, the larvae burrow through the mucosa, enter the portal circulation, and travel to the liver.

The echinococcal cyst has two layers: the inner layer and the outer, or inflammatory, reaction layer. The smaller, daughter cysts may develop from the inner layer. The cysts may enlarge and rupture. The cysts may also impinge on the blood vessels and lead to vascular thrombosis and infarction.

Sonographic Findings. Several patterns may occur, from a simple cyst to a complex mass with acoustic

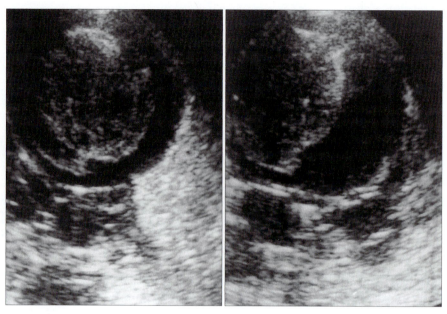

FIGURE 10-57 Amebic abscess is a complex lesion, usually in the right lobe of the liver. This patient recently returned from a vacation in Mexico and presented with right upper quadrant pain and fever for 2 weeks.

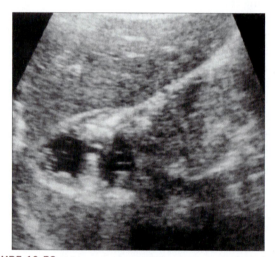

FIGURE 10-58 Echinococcal cyst. This complex mass found in the right lobe of the liver shows fluid and debris components.

enhancement. The shape may be oval or spherical, with regularity of the walls. Calcifications may occur. Septations are frequent and include honeycomb appearance with fluid collections; "water lily" sign, which shows a detachment and collapse of the germinal layer; or "cyst within a cyst." Sometimes the liver contains multiple parent cysts in both lobes of the liver; the cyst with the thick walls occupies a different part of the liver (Figure 10-58). The tissue between the cysts indicates that each cyst is a separate parent cyst and not a daughter cyst. If a daughter cyst is found, it is specific for echinococcal disease.

Pneumocystis Carinii. *Pneumocystic carinii* is the most common organism causing opportunistic infection in patients with acquired immunodeficiency syndrome. Pneumocystis pneumonia is a common life-threatening infection in patients with human immunodeficiency virus. *Pneumocystis carinii* affects patients undergoing bone marrow and organ transplantation, or patients receiving chemotherapy.

Sonographic Findings. The pattern ranges from diffuse, tiny, nonshadowing echogenic foci to extensive replacement of the liver parenchyma by various echogenic clumps of calcification.

Hepatic Tumors

A **neoplasm** is any new growth of new tissue, either benign or malignant. A benign growth occurs locally but does not spread or invade surrounding structures. It may push surrounding structures aside or adhere to them. A malignant mass is uncontrolled and is prone to metastasize to nearby or distant structures via the bloodstream and lymph nodes. Thus, it is important not only to recognize the tumor mass itself but also to appreciate which structures the malignancy may invade. See Table 10-11 for clinical findings, sonographic findings, and differential considerations for hepatic tumors.

Benign Hepatic Tumors. *Cavernous Hemangioma.* A hemangioma is a benign, congenital tumor consisting of large, blood-filled cystic spaces. Cavernous hemangioma is the most common benign tumor of the liver. The tumor is found more frequently in females. Patients are usually asymptomatic, although a small percentage may bleed, causing right upper quadrant pain. Hemangiomas enlarge slowly and undergo degeneration, fibrosis, and calcification. They are found in the subcapsular hepatic parenchyma or in the posterior right lobe more than the left lobe of the liver.

Sonographic Findings. The appearance is typically hyperechoic with acoustic enhancement (Figure 10-59). Many authors have speculated that the echo-dense

TABLE 10-11	Liver Findings: Tumors	
Clinical Findings	**Sonographic Findings**	**Differential Considerations**
Cavernous Hemangioma		
Small percentage may bleed; RUQ pain More frequent in women	Most are hyperechoic with enhancement Round or oval, well defined Larger masses may show necrosis, degeneration, calcification	Metastasis Hepatoma (HCC) Adenoma Focal nodular hyperplasia
Liver Cell Adenoma		
RUQ pain when mass bleeds	Hyperechoic with central echogenic area caused by hemorrhage Solitary or multiple Fluid may be present	Hemangioma Focal nodular hyperplasia Hepatoma (HCC)
Focal Nodular Hyperplasia		
More frequent in women <40	Multiple, well defined with hyperechoic to isoechoic patterns Frequently found in right lobe of liver	Hemangiomas Hepatoma (HCC) Metastases Adenoma
Hepatocellular Carcinoma		
70% of patients have ↑ alpha-fetoprotein level Abnormalities in liver function tests, with the indications of cirrhosis	Solitary, multiple Infiltrative, diffuse Hypoechoic, isoechoic, or hyperechoic May invade hepatic veins Thrombus	Hemangioma Metastases
Metastatic Disease		
Abnormal LFTs Jaundice Hepatomegaly Weight loss Decreased appetite	Hypoechoic or echogenic mass Diffuse distortion of bull's-eye pattern Solitary or multiple Well to ill-defined	Abscess Hemangioma Hepatoma (HCC) Adenoma
Lymphoma		
Abnormal LFT	Hypoechoic or diffuse patterns Target or echogenic lesions Intrahepatic and lucent multiple small, discrete solid lesions without enhancement	Hemangioma HCC Metastases

HCC, Hepatocellular carcinoma; *LFT,* liver function test.

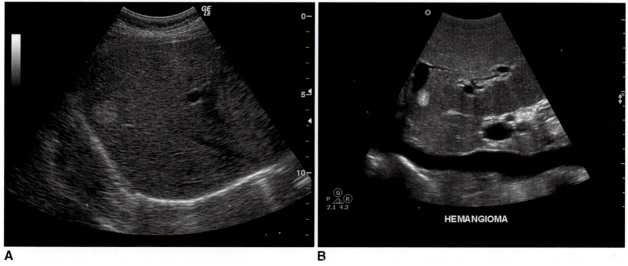

A   **B**

FIGURE 10-59 A and **B,** Cavernous hemangioma is usually found in an asymptomatic patient. The mass is irregular and echogenic secondary to the vascular component of the lesion.

pattern results from the multiple interfaces between the walls of the cavernous sinuses and blood within them. The lesions are round, oval, or lobulated with well-defined borders. The larger hemangiomas may have a mixed pattern resulting from necrosis. Hemangiomas may become more heterogeneous as they undergo degeneration and fibrous replacement. They may also project with calcifications or a complex or anechoic echo pattern. The differential considerations for hemangioma should include metastases, hepatoma, focal nodular hyperplasia, and adenoma.

Liver Cell Adenoma. An adenoma is a tumor of the glandular epithelium in which the cells of the tumor are arranged in a recognizable glandular structure. The liver cell adenoma consists of normal or slightly atypical hepatocytes, frequently containing areas of bile stasis and focal hemorrhage or necrosis. The lesion is found more commonly in women and has been related to oral contraceptive usage. Patients may present with right upper quadrant pain secondary to rupture with bleeding into the tumor. The incidence is increased in patients with type I glycogen storage disease or von Gierke's disease.

■ **Sonographic Findings.** The mass may have nonspecific findings. The echogenicity may be hyperechoic, hypoechoic, isoechoic, or mixed. With hemorrhage, a fluid component may be seen within or around the lesion. This lesion is usually hyperechoic with a central hypoechoic area caused by hemorrhage (Figure 10-60). The lesion may be solitary and well encapsulated or multiple. If the lesion ruptures, fluid should be found in the peritoneal cavity. A hepatic adenoma may be difficult to distinguish sonographically from focal nodular hyperplasia.

Focal Nodular Hyperplasia. Focal nodular hyperplasia is the second most common benign liver mass after hemangioma. It is found in women under 40 years of age. The mass is thought to arise from developmental hyperplastic lesions related to an area of congenital vascular formation. The patient is asymptomatic. The lesions occur more in the right lobe of the liver. There is typically one well-circumscribed lesion, but there may be more than one mass; many are located along the subcapsular area of the liver, some are pedunculated, and many have a central scar (Figure 10-61). The lesion consists of normal hepatocytes, Kupffer cells, bile duct elements, and fibrous connective tissue. Bands of fibrous tissue separate the multiple nodules. There may be increased bleeding within the tumors in these patients.

■ **Sonographic Findings.** Focal nodular hyperplasia is a subtle liver mass that is difficult to differentiate in echogenicity from the liver parenchyma. The sonographer may note subtle contour abnormalities and displacement of the vascular structures secondary to the mass. The central scar may be identified as a hypoechoic linear or stellate area within the center of the mass (Figure 10-62). The internal linear echoes may be seen within the lesions

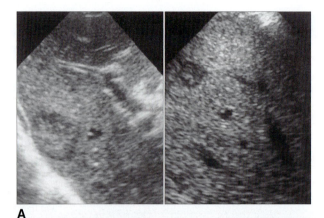
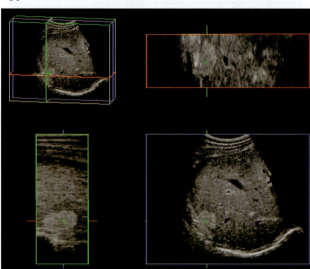

A

B

FIGURE 10-60 A, Hepatic adenoma appears as a well-defined lesion with a central hyperechoic area surrounded by a halo. **B,** Three-dimensional imaging of a hepatic mass that appears to be well defined in the dome of the right lobe of the liver. Three-dimensional technology allows one to record the image from multiple directions without moving the transducer. This most likely represents a hepatic adenoma.

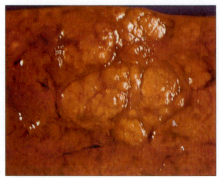

FIGURE 10-61 Gross pathology of focal nodular hyperplasia with a lobular mass with a central fibrotic scar.

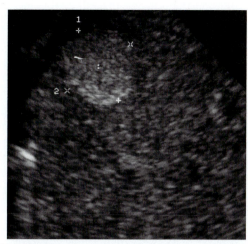

FIGURE 10-62 Focal nodular hyperplasia appears as a well-defined lesion with a hyperechoic internal texture.

if multiple nodules occur together. Color Doppler may show the well-developed peripheral and central blood vessels that feed into the focal nodular hyperplasia lesion.

Hepatic Cystadenoma. Hepatic cystadenoma contains cystic structures within the lesion. This adenoma is a rare neoplasm occurring in middle-aged women. Most have a palpable abdominal mass.

Sonographic Findings. The lesions may be multilocular with mucinous fluid.

Malignant Hepatic Neoplasms. Primary malignant tumors are relatively rare in the liver. The most common tumor is hepatocellular carcinoma. Tumors may also result from prolonged exposure to carcinogenic chemicals. Sonography has the advantage over other imaging modalities in defining liver texture in many different planes. This technique is especially useful in the diagnosis of malignant hepatic disease. A comparison of the different liver textures and patterns is shown in Figure 10-63.

The clinical signs of liver cancer are mild and general—similar to those of other hepatocellular diseases. These symptoms include nausea and vomiting, fatigue, weight loss, and hepatomegaly. Portal hypertension and splenomegaly are common.

Hepatocellular Carcinoma. As noted, hepatocellular carcinoma (HCC) is the most common primary malignant neoplasm. The prevalence varies, depending on predisposing factors such as hepatitis B and aflatoxin exposure, which contributes to the high incidence of hepatocellular carcinoma in Africa, Japan, Greece, Italy, and Southeast Asia. The incidence of HCC in the United States is low, occurring in 5 of 100,000 people.

The pathogenesis of hepatocellular carcinoma is related to cirrhosis (80% of patients with preexisting cirrhosis develop hepatocellular carcinoma), chronic hepatitis B virus infection, and hepatocarcinogens in foods. The tumor occurs more frequently in men. Clinically, patients with HCG usually present with a previous history of cirrhosis or hepatitis B and C, a palpable mass, hepatomegaly, appetite disorder, and fever.

The HCC may present in one of three patterns: solitary massive tumor, multiple nodules throughout the liver, or diffuse infiltrative masses in the liver. Pathologically the tumor may present as a focal lesion, an invasive lesion with necrosis and hemorrhage, or a poorly defined lesion (Figure 10-64). The carcinoma can be very invasive and has been known to invade the hepatic veins to produce Budd-Chiari syndrome. The portal venous system may also be invaded with tumor or thrombosis. Hepatocellular carcinoma has a tendency to destroy the portal venous radicle walls, with invasion into the lumen of the vessel.

Sonographic Findings. A variable sonographic appearance is noted with discrete lesions, either solitary or multiple, that are usually hypoechoic or hyperechoic. Sometimes the lesions may be isoechoic, and a thin, peripheral hypoechoic halo may surround the lesion (Figure 10-65). Another pattern presents as diffuse parenchymal involvement with inhomogeneity throughout the liver without distinct masses. Over time the mass becomes more complex and inhomogeneous with resulting fibrosis and necrosis. The last pattern is a combination of discrete and diffuse echoes. Hepatocellular carcinoma cannot be differentiated from metastases on ultrasound.

Internal echoes within the portal veins, hepatic veins, or inferior vena cava indicate tumor invasion or thrombosis within the vessel. The evaluation of the vascular structures with color Doppler helps to rule out the presence of clot or tumor invasion. Hepatic flow is abnormal if an obstruction is present. Obstruction of the portal vein may be present with thrombosis and well demonstrated with color Doppler.

Metastatic Disease. The most common form of neoplastic involvement of the liver is **metastatic disease**. The incidence of hepatic metastases depends on the type of tumor and its stage at initial detection. The primary sites are the colon, breast, and lung. The majority of metastases arise from a primary colonic malignancy or a hepatoma. Patients with short survival rates after initial detection of liver metastases are those with HCC and carcinoma of the pancreas, stomach, and esophagus. Patients with a more prolonged survival are those with head and neck carcinoma and carcinoma of the colon. Metastatic spread to the liver occurs as the tumor erodes the wall and travels through the lymphatic system or through the bloodstream to the portal vein or hepatic artery to the liver.

Sonographic Findings. The sonographic patterns of metastatic tumor involvement in the liver vary (Figure 10-66). It is typical to have multiple nodes throughout both lobes of the liver (Figure 10-67). The following three specific patterns have been described: (1) a well-defined hypoechoic mass, (2) a well-defined echogenic mass, and (3) diffuse distortion of the normal

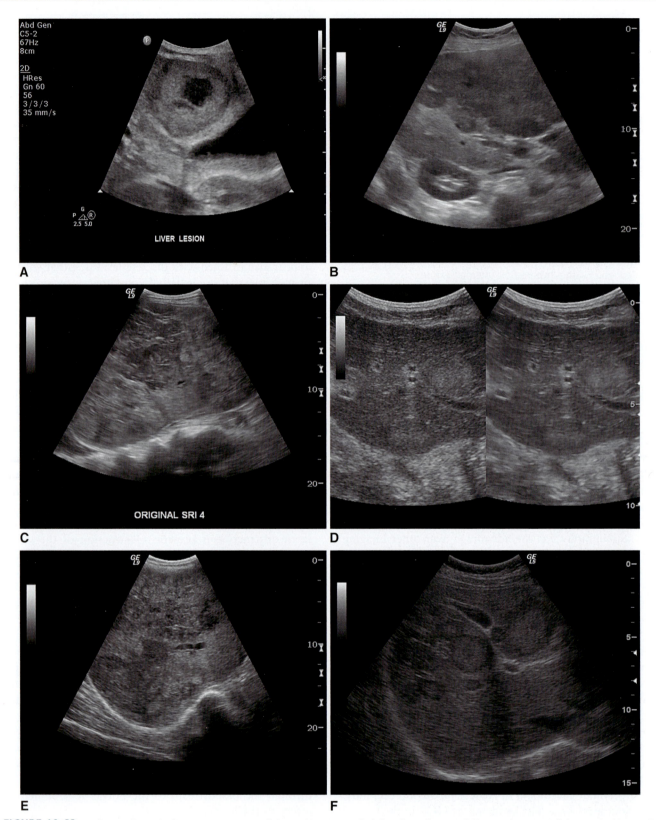

FIGURE 10-63 Malignant hepatic disease. **A,** Hepatocellular carcinoma: well-defined "Bull's-eye" lesion. **B,** Hepatocellular carcinoma: well-defined isoechoic lesion. **C,** Necrotic hepatoma: necrotic isoechoic lesion. **D,** Advanced metastases: large isoechoic lesions. **E,** Metastases: ill-defined complex necrotic lesion. **F,** Metastases: well-defined hyperechoic lesion.

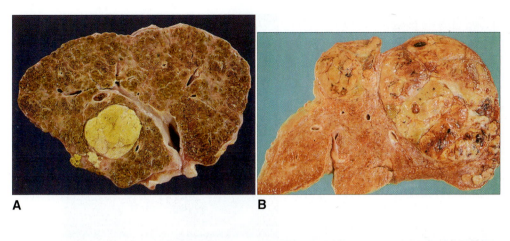

FIGURE 10-64 Gross pathology of hepatocellular carcinoma. **A,** The cirrhotic liver contains a solitary malignant nodule. **B,** The huge tumor is poorly demarcated from the remaining liver.

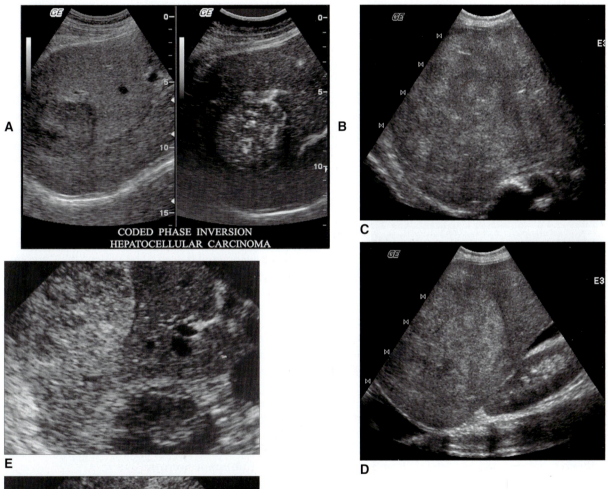

FIGURE 10-65 A and **B,** Hepatocellular carcinoma shows a discrete hypoechoic lesion in the right lobe of the liver. **C** and **D,** Transverse and sagittal images of the upper right quadrant show a large hepatocellular carcinoma in the right lobe of the liver. **E** and **F,** Hepatocellular carcinoma in a 58-year-old male shows hepatomegaly with diffuse abnormal lesions throughout the liver parenchyma.

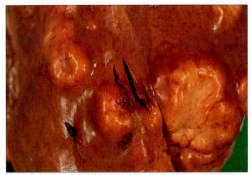

FIGURE 10-66 Metastatic carcinoma. The liver contains numerous spherical nodules, many of which show central indentation corresponding to the areas of necrosis.

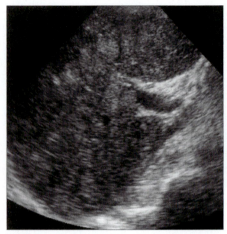

FIGURE 10-68 Lymphoma was found in this elderly male with hepatomegaly. Multiple isoechoic lesions were found throughout the liver.

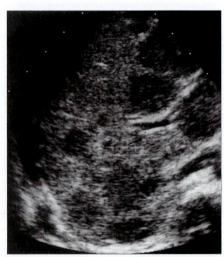

FIGURE 10-67 Metastatic disease appears as multiple, well-defined hypoechoic lesions throughout the liver.

homogeneous parenchymal pattern without a focal mass. The hypovascular lesions produce hypoechoic patterns in the liver because of necrosis and ischemic areas from neoplastic thrombosis. Most cases of hypervascular lesions correspond to hyperechoic patterns.

The common primary masses include renal cell carcinoma, carcinoid, choriocarcinoma, transitional cell carcinoma, islet cell carcinoma, and hepatocellular carcinoma. The echogenic lesions are common with primary colonic tumors and may present with calcification. Target types of metastases or bull's-eye patterns are the result of edema around the tumor or necrosis or hemorrhage within the tumor. As the nodules increase rapidly in size and outgrow their blood supply, central necrosis and hemorrhage may result.

Various combinations of these patterns can be seen simultaneously in a patient with metastatic liver disease. The first abnormality is hepatomegaly or alterations in contour, especially on the lateral segment of the left lobe. The lesions may be solitary or multiple, be variable in size and shape, and have sharp or ill-defined margins. Metastases may be extensive or localized to produce an inhomogeneous parenchymal pattern.

Ultrasound may be useful to follow patients after surgery. After a baseline hepatic ultrasound has been performed, the sonographer can assess any regression or progression of tumor and change in parenchymal pattern.

Lymphoma. Lymphomas are malignant neoplasms involving lymphocyte proliferation in the lymph nodes. The two main disorders, Hodgkin's lymphoma and non-Hodgkin's lymphoma, are differentiated by lymph node biopsy. No specific cause is known. Patients with lymphoma have hepatomegaly with a normal or diffuse alteration of parenchymal echoes. A focal hypoechoic mass is sometimes seen. The patient may present with enlarged, nontender lymph nodes, fever, fatigue, night sweats, weight loss, bone pain, or an abdominal mass. The presence of splenomegaly or retroperitoneal nodes may help confirm the diagnosis of lymphadenopathy.

Sonographic Findings. Hodgkin's lymphoma shows up as diffuse parenchymal changes in the liver. Non-Hodgkin's lymphoma may appear with target hypoechoic mass lesions. Burkitt's lymphoma lesions may appear intrahepatic and lucent. Patients with leukemia have multiple small, discrete hepatic masses that are solid with no acoustic enhancement (Figure 10-68). A bull's-eye appearance with a dense central core may be present as a result of tumor necrosis.

In the pediatric population, the most common malignancies are neuroblastomas, Wilms' tumor, and leukemia. The neuroblastoma presents as a densely reflective echo pattern with liver involvement similar to that of a hepatoma. In patients with a Wilms' tumor, metastases generally invade the lung; however, the liver may be a secondary site. These lesions present as a densely reflective pattern with lucencies resulting from necrosis.

Hepatic Trauma

The liver is the third most common organ injured in the abdomen after the spleen and kidney. Laceration of the liver occurs in 3% of trauma patients and is frequently associated with other injured organs. The need for surgery is determined by the size of the laceration, the amount of hemoperitoneum, and the patient's clinical status. The right lobe is affected more often than the left. The degree of trauma can vary, with a small laceration, large laceration with a hematoma, subcapsular hematoma, or capsular disruption.

■ **Sonographic Findings.** Computed tomography is used more often than ultrasound to localize the extent of the laceration within the liver and surrounding areas. Ultrasound does not clearly distinguish small lacerations in the dome of the right lobe of the liver. Intraperitoneal fluid should be assessed along the flanks and into the pelvis. Intrahepatic hematomas are hyperechoic in the first 24 hours and hypoechoic and sonolucent thereafter because of the resolution of the blood within the area. Septations and internal echoes develop 1 to 4 weeks after the trauma (Figure 10-69). A subcapsular hematoma may appear as anechoic, hypoechoic, septated lenticular, or curvilinear. It may be differentiated from ascitic fluid in that it occurs unilaterally, along the area of laceration. The degree of homogenicity depends on the age of the laceration.

Liver Transplantation

Liver transplantation is performed in patients with end-stage liver disease to eliminate irreversible disease when more conservative medical and surgical treatments have failed. The most common indications for transplantation in adults is hepatitis C, followed closely by alcoholic liver disease, and cryptogenic cirrhosis (especially secondary to chronic active hepatitis), fulminant active hepatitis, congenital metabolic disorders, sclerosing cholangitis, Budd-Chiari syndrome, and unresectable hepatoma. Many centers consider transplantation only in patients with early stage HCC, or, on the rare occasion, neuroendocrine metastases. The guidelines for HCC patients to receive a transplant use the Milan criteria of no lesion greater than 5 cm in diameter or no more than three lesions of greater than 3 cm in diameter. Improvements in posttransplant survival have been attributed to a combination of better donor-recipient matching, improved immunosuppressive therapy, advanced surgical techniques, and early recognition of transplant complications.

Contraindications for liver transplantation include compensated cirrhosis without complications,

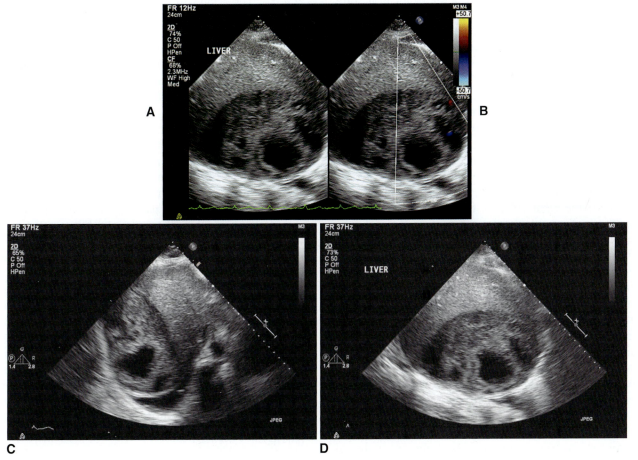

FIGURE 10-69 Hepatic trauma. **A-D,** A complex mass was found in the right lobe of the liver in a patient who had been in an automobile accident. A large complex subcapsular hematoma was seen.

extrahepatic malignancy, cholangiocarcinoma, active untreated sepsis, advanced cardiopulmonary disease, active alcoholism or substance abuse, or an anatomic abnormality precluding the surgical procedure. The presence of portal vein thrombosis is a predictor of a higher risk in these transplant patients.

Surgical Technique. The surgical procedure of the recipient includes hepatectomy and replacement with a cadaveric allograft, revascularization of the new liver (hepatic artery, hepatic veins, portal venous system, and subhepatic and infrahepatic inferior vena cava), hemostasis, and biliary reconstruction.

The hepatic artery is reconstructed with an anastomosis between the donor celiac artery and either the bifurcation of the right and left hepatic arteries or the branch point of the gastroduodenal and proper hepatic artery of the recipient. If the native hepatic artery is very small, a donor iliac artery interposition graft may be anastomosed directly to the supraceliac or infrarenal aorta.

The portal vein anastomosis is end-to-end between the donor and the recipient portal vein. If there is portal vein thrombosis in the recipient, a venous jump graft from the donor portal vein or the iliac vein is used. If that fails, an anastomosis between the portal vein and hepatic artery of the donor and the arterial vessels of the recipient is performed.

Usually the inferior vena cava of the recipient is transected above and below the intrahepatic portion. The donor IVC is anastomosed with two end-to-end suprahepatic and infrahepatic anastomoses.

The donor and recipient common bile duct are anastomosed in an end-to-end manner, after a cholecystectomy. A T-tube may be left in place for other biliary procedures. If the recipient common hepatic duct is diseased, too short, or too narrow, a choledochojejunostomy is performed.

Many centers have performed living related donor transplantations because of the lack of available cadaveric donor organs. This technique replaces the recipient liver with the right lobe of the living donor. In the pediatric patient, the lateral segment of the left lobe or the entire left lobe has been used with success. For living related transplants, the donor surgery removes the gallbladder, right lobe of the liver, and right hepatic vein.

Normal Sonographic Liver Transplant. Sonography can play an important role in the preoperative and postoperative evaluation of hepatic transplantation. The primary function of the sonographic examination is to evaluate the portal venous system, the hepatic artery, the inferior vena cava, and the liver parenchymal pattern. The vascular structures should be assessed for size and patency in the preoperative evaluation. The liver parenchyma should be examined to rule out the presence of hepatic architecture disruption. The sonographer should also evaluate the biliary system, to look for dilation, and the portosystemic collateral vessels.

In the pediatric patient, the most common reason for liver transplantation is biliary atresia and associated anomalies of the spleen, hepatic vasculature, and kidneys. Therefore, in addition to the examination described previously, both kidneys and the spleen must be examined.

The normal liver transplant should have a homogeneous or slightly heterogeneous echotexture on sonography. Right after surgery there may be a small amount of free intraperitoneal fluid or small periphepatic seroma/hematoma, which usually resolves within a week. The biliary tree should also appear normal with the anechoic lumen and thin walls. If a choledochojejunostomy has been performed, a pneumobilia may be seen, causing the shadowing of the structures in the area of the bile duct. This air may be confused with small biliary stones or adjacent hepatic arterial calcifications, as they appear identical on sonography.

Vascular patency of the transplanted vessels is assessed by narrowing of the diameter and the presence of thrombus within the vessel lumen. The hepatic artery is examined with Doppler and color flow ultrasound in the area of the porta hepatis. The normal hepatic artery flow produces a rapid systolic upstroke with an acceleration time of less than 100 m/sec. There is continuous flow throughout diastolic with a resistive index between 0.5 and 0.7. The hepatic artery flow is a low-resistance arterial signal. Thrombosis may be detected when this signal is absent. In the adult patient, collateral vessels in the region of the hepatic artery have not developed. However, collateral hepatic arterial circulation may have developed in children. Thus, the scans should be made within 24 hours after surgery, 48 hours after surgery, and weekly thereafter to assess for changes in the velocity flow pattern. The portal veins show continuous hepatopetal flow with mild velocity variations as a result of respiration. The normal Doppler appearance of the hepatic veins shows a phasic waveform reflecting physiologic changes in blood flow during the cardiac cycle.

Complications. Complications of transplantation include rejection, thrombosis or leak, biliary stricture or leak, infection, and neoplasia. Rejection is the most common cause of hepatic dysfunction that is confirmed by clinical diagnosis and liver biopsy.

Vascular complications include thrombosis, stricture, and arterial anastomotic pseudoaneurysms. Vascular thrombosis may affect the hepatic artery, the portal vein, or, less commonly, the inferior vena cava (more common in Budd-Chiari patients). During the postoperative period, hepatic artery thrombosis is the most serious complication of liver transplantation. Color Doppler may show an absence of flow in the area of the porta hepatis. Occasionally, a tardus parvus arterial waveform (RI < 0.5, AT > 100 ms) may be obtained within the hepatic parenchyma.

The development of anastomotic stenoses is another problem in the transplant patient. The sonographer may note direct visualization of the vessel narrowing. Color Doppler is useful to detect a focal region of color aliasing within the hepatic artery, which would indicate the presence of high-velocity turbulent flow produced by the stenotic segment. This velocity flow pattern may exceed 2 or 3 m/sec with distal turbulent flow. This flow pattern is a turbulent, high-velocity signal indicative of hepatic arterial stenosis. Indirect evidence of hepatic artery stenosis includes a tardus parvus arterial waveform (RI < 0.5, AT > 100 ms) anywhere within the hepatic artery. Hepatic artery pseudoaneurysms are another complication of transplantation, usually occurring at the site of the anastomosis.

Portal vein stenosis or thrombosis may also occur in the postoperative period (Figure 10-70). Doppler interrogation shows a focal region of color aliasing that reflects the high-velocity turbulent flow at the area of stenosis. Portal vein thrombosis presents as an echogenic solid material within the portal vein lumen. In the acute state, the thrombus may be anechoic or softly echogenic. Air in the portal vein may be seen as brightly echogenic moving targets within the portal venous system. A fatal complication is hepatic necrosis associated with thrombosis of the hepatic artery or portal vein. Massive necro-

sis produces gangrene of the liver and air in the hepatic parenchyma.

Compromise of the inferior vena cava is another complication of transplantation. It is rare to find stenosis at the level of the inferior vena cava, but occasionally this may occur either at the suprahepatic or infrahepatic anastomosis. Thrombosis of the inferior vena cava also occurs on an occasional basis. The thrombus may be well seen as a slightly echogenic mass within the IVC. If hepatocellular carcinoma has recurred, the tumor or thrombus extension may extend from the hepatic veins into the IVC.

Biliary complications, stricture, and leakage affect a small percentage of transplant patients. Because the hepatic artery is the sole supply of blood to the bile ducts in transplant patients, identification of a stricture of the bile duct is an indication for assessment of hepatic artery patency. Hepatic arterial occlusion, pretransplant primary sclerosing cholangitis, choledochojejunostomy, cholangitis at liver biopsy, and young age are greatly associated with biliary strictures. Patients with biliary strictures may be asymptomatic, present with painless jaundice, or manifest with abnormalities in liver function tests. Anastomotic strictures are the most common cause

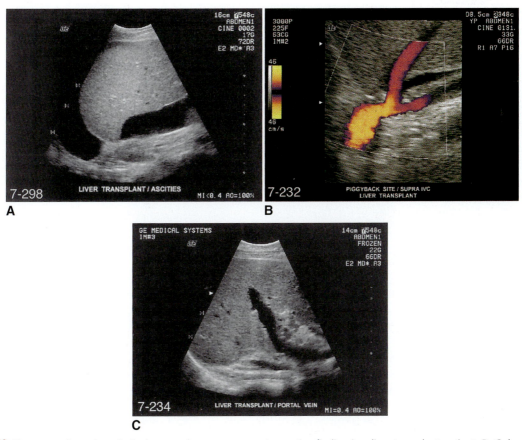

FIGURE 10-70 Liver transplantation. **A,** Ascites may be seen as a postoperative finding in a liver transplant patient. **B,** Color can define the site of the piggyback anastomosis of the suprahepatic inferior vena cava (IVC) to the intrahepatic IVC. **C,** Patency of the portal vein can be assessed by gray scale and color Doppler.

of biliary obstruction after transplantation. Intrahepatic strictures occur proximal to the anastomosis and may be either unifocal or multifocal. Other complications of the biliary system include sclerosing cholangitis, biliary sludge and stones, and dysfunction of the sphincter of Oddi.

Periphepatic fluid collections and ascites are frequently observed after transplantation. As discussed previously, it is not uncommon to find a small amount of free fluid or right pleural effusion postsurgery. Fluid collections and hematomas are common in the areas of vascular anastomosis. Fluid may also accumulate at the bare area of the liver, the falciform ligament, and ligamentum venosum secondary to the ligation of the transplantation. Other fluid collections found in the postoperative state may include abscess, hematomas, or infarct.

The Gallbladder and the Biliary System

Sandra L. Hagen-Ansert

Together with the liver and pancreas, the biliary system plays a role in the digestive process. The gallbladder serves as a reservoir for bile that is drained from the hepatic ducts in the liver. Sonographic evaluation of the gallbladder and biliary system is used as a primary diagnostic tool and has proven to be effective in diagnosing various types of gallbladder disease, including the more common problems of cholelithiasis, cholecystitis, and dilation of the ductal system.

ANATOMY OF THE BILIARY SYSTEM

Normal Anatomy

The biliary apparatus consists of the right and left hepatic ducts, the common hepatic duct, the common bile duct, the pear-shaped gallbladder, and the cystic duct (Figure 11-1).

Hepatic Ducts. The right and left hepatic ducts emerge from the right lobe of the liver in the **porta hepatis** and unite to form the common hepatic duct, which then passes caudally and medially. The hepatic duct runs parallel with the portal vein. Each duct is formed by the union of bile canaliculi from the liver lobules.

The common hepatic duct is approximately 4 mm in diameter and descends within the edge of the lesser omentum. It is joined by the cystic duct to form the common bile duct. The **common hepatic duct** is the bile duct system that drains the liver into the common bile duct.

Common Bile Duct. The normal **common bile duct** has a diameter of up to 6 mm. The first part of the duct lies in the right free edge of the lesser omentum (Figure 11-2). The second part of the duct is situated posterior to the first part of the duodenum. The third part lies in

a groove on the posterior surface of the head of the pancreas. It ends by piercing the medial wall of the second part of the duodenum about halfway down the duodenal length. There the common bile duct is joined by the main pancreatic duct, and together they open through a small ampulla (the **ampulla of Vater**) into the duodenal wall. The end parts of both ducts (common bile duct and main **pancreatic duct**) and the ampulla are surrounded by circular muscle fibers known as the **sphincter of Oddi.**

The proximal portion of the common bile duct is lateral to the hepatic artery and anterior to the portal vein. The duct moves more posterior after it descends behind the duodenal bulb and enters the pancreas. The distal duct lies parallel to the anterior wall of the vena cava.

Within the liver parenchyma, the bile ducts follow the same course as the portal venous and hepatic arterial branches. The hepatic and bile ducts are encased in a common collagenous sheath, forming the portal triad.

Cystic Duct. The **cystic duct** is about 4 cm long and connects the neck of the gallbladder with the common hepatic duct to form the common bile duct. It is usually somewhat S-shaped and descends for a variable distance in the right free edge of the lesser omentum.

Gallbladder. The **gallbladder** is a pear-shaped sac in the anterior aspect of the right upper quadrant, closely related to the visceral surface of the liver. It is divided into the fundus, body, and neck. Representative transverse (Figure 11-3) and sagittal (Figure 11-4) anatomy demonstrates the relational anatomy to the gallbladder and biliary system. The rounded fundus usually projects below the inferior margin of the liver, where it comes into contact with the anterior abdominal wall at the level of the ninth right costal cartilage. The body generally lies in contact with the visceral surface of the liver and is directed upward, backward, and to the left. The neck becomes continuous with the cystic duct, which turns

Text continued on page 273

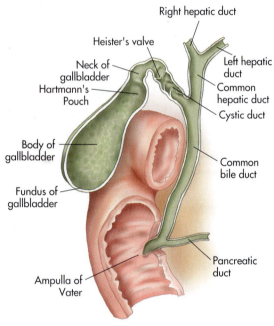

FIGURE 11-1 Gallbladder and biliary system.

Right hepatic duct
Heister's valve
Neck of gallbladder
Hartmann's Pouch
Left hepatic duct
Common hepatic duct
Cystic duct
Body of gallbladder
Common bile duct
Fundus of gallbladder
Pancreatic duct
Ampulla of Vater

FIGURE 11-2 Relationships within the porta hepatis.

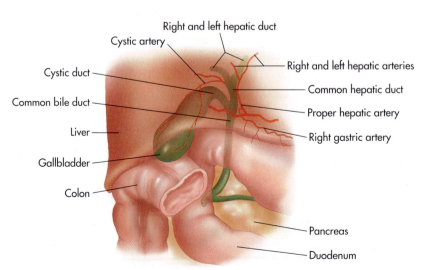

Right and left hepatic duct
Cystic artery
Cystic duct
Right and left hepatic arteries
Common hepatic duct
Common bile duct
Proper hepatic artery
Liver
Right gastric artery
Gallbladder
Colon
Pancreas
Duodenum

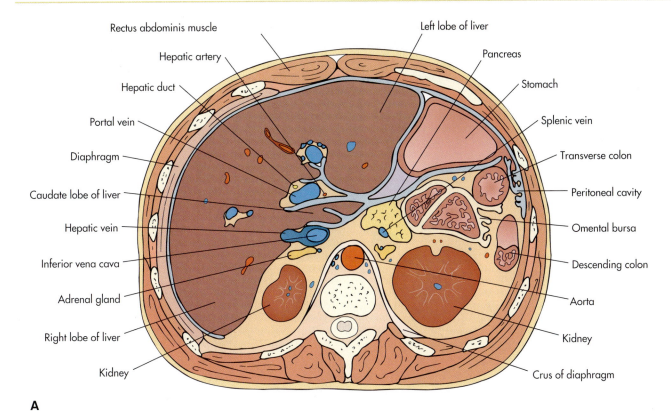

A

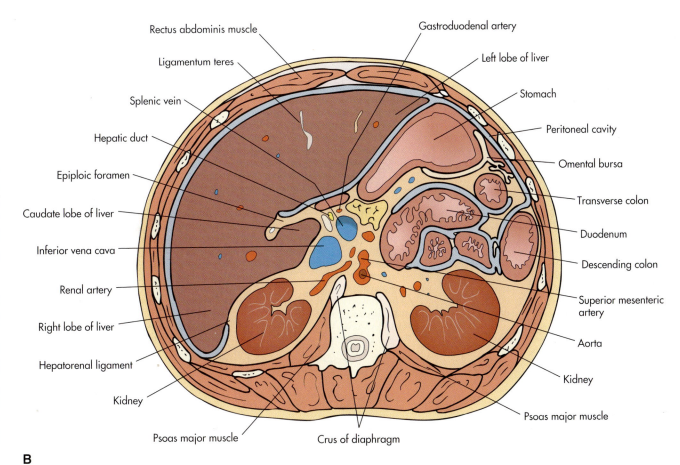

B

FIGURE 11-3 Transverse views of the right upper quadrant to include the biliary system, beginning at the level of the caudate lobe and proceeding in a caudal direction. **A,** Cross section of the abdomen at the level of the 12th thoracic vertebra. **B,** Cross section of the abdomen at the first lumbar vertebra.

Continued

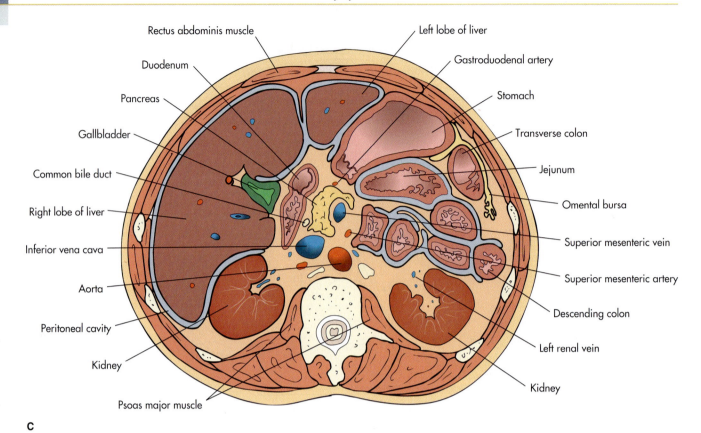

C

D

FIGURE 11-3, cont'd C, Cross section of the abdomen at the level of the second lumbar vertebra. **D,** Cross section of the abdomen at the level of the third lumbar vertebra.

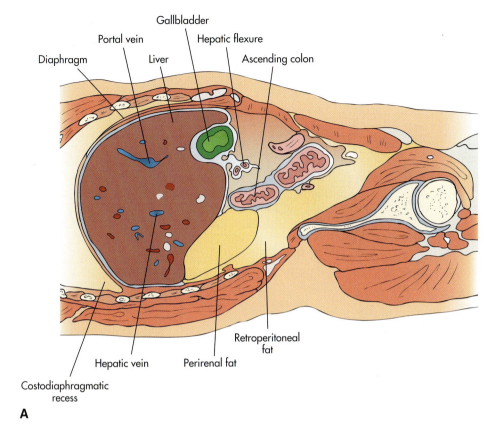

Gallbladder

Portal vein   Hepatic flexure

Diaphragm   Liver   Ascending colon

Retroperitoneal
fat

Hepatic vein   Perirenal fat

Costodiaphragmatic
recess

A

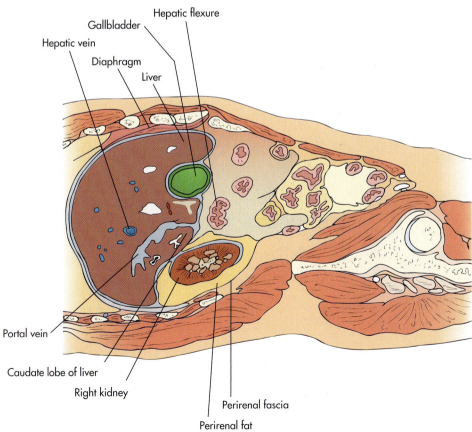

Hepatic flexure

Gallbladder

Hepatic vein

Diaphragm

Liver

Portal vein

Caudate lobe of liver

Right kidney

Perirenal fascia

Perirenal fat

B

FIGURE 11-4 Sagittal views of the right upper quadrant to include the biliary system beginning near the midclavicular line and moving toward the midline. **A,** Sagittal section of the abdomen 8 cm from the midline. **B,** Sagittal section of the abdomen 7 cm from the midline.
Continued

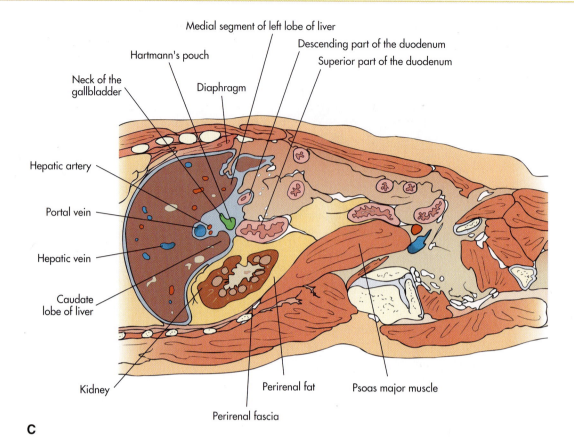

C

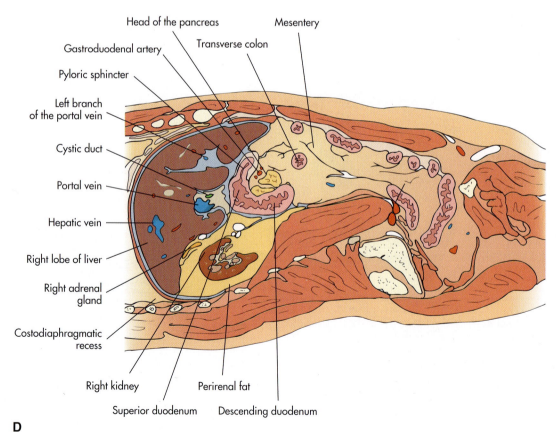

D

FIGURE 11-4, cont'd C, Sagittal section of the abdomen 6 cm from the midline. **D,** Sagittal section of the abdomen 5 cm from the midline.

into the lesser omentum to join the right side of the common hepatic duct to form the common bile duct.

The neck of the gallbladder is oriented posteromedially toward the porta hepatis. The fundus is situated lateral, caudal, and anterior to the neck. Occasionally the gallbladder lies in an intrahepatic or other anomalous location, and it may be difficult to detect by sonography if the entire upper abdomen is not examined.

The size and shape of the gallbladder are variable. Generally the normal gallbladder measures about 2.5 to 4 cm in diameter and 7 to 10 cm in length. The walls are less than 3 mm thick. Dilation of the gallbladder is known as **hydrops**.

Several anatomic variations may occur within the gallbladder to give rise to its internal echo pattern on the sonogram. The gallbladder may fold back on itself at the neck, forming **Hartmann's pouch** (see Figure 7-1). Other anomalies include partial septation, complete septation (double gallbladder), and folding of the fundus (**Phrygian cap**) (Figure 11-5).

With a capacity of 50 ml, the gallbladder serves as a reservoir for bile. It also has the ability to concentrate the bile. To aid this process, its mucous membrane con-

tains folds that unite with each other, giving the surface a honeycomb appearance. **Heister's valve** in the neck of the gallbladder helps to prevent kinking of the duct (see Figure 11-1).

The gallbladder lies in the intrahepatic position, but as it migrates to the surface of the liver during development it acquires a peritoneal covering over most of its surface. The remainder of the gallbladder surface is covered with adventitial tissue that merges with the connective tissue with the liver. This potential space between the liver and the gallbladder is an area for infection or inflammation to collect. If this migration does not occur, the gallbladder remains intrahepatic or it may be enveloped in the visceral peritoneum, hanging into the lower abdomen. The gallbladder has been found to lie in various ectopic positions (suprahepatic, suprarenal, within the anterior abdominal wall, or in the falciform ligament).

Failure of the gallbladder to develop is rare; this is known as agenesis of the gallbladder. These patients may still have the biliary ductal system, which can become inflamed or filled with stones.

Vascular Supply

The arterial supply of the gallbladder is from the cystic artery, which is a branch of the right hepatic artery. The cystic vein drains directly into the portal vein. Smaller arteries and veins run between the liver and the gallbladder.

PHYSIOLOGY AND LABORATORY DATA OF THE GALLBLADDER AND BILIARY SYSTEM

The primary functions of the extrahepatic biliary tract are (1) the transportation of bile from the liver to the intestine and (2) the regulation of its flow. This is an important function as the liver secretes approximately 1 to 2 liters of bile per day.

When the gallbladder and bile ducts are functioning normally, they respond in a fairly uniform manner in various phases of digestion. Concentration of bile in the gallbladder occurs during a state of fasting. It is forced into the gallbladder by an increased pressure within the common bile duct, which is produced by the action of the sphincter of Oddi at the distal end of the gallbladder.

During the fasting state, very little bile flows into the duodenum. Stimulation produced by the influence of food causes the gallbladder to contract, resulting in an outpouring of bile into the duodenum. When the stomach is emptied, duodenal peristalsis diminishes, the gallbladder relaxes, the tonus of the sphincter of Oddi increases slightly, and thus very little bile passes into the duodenum. Small amounts of bile secreted by the liver are retained in the **common duct** and forced into the

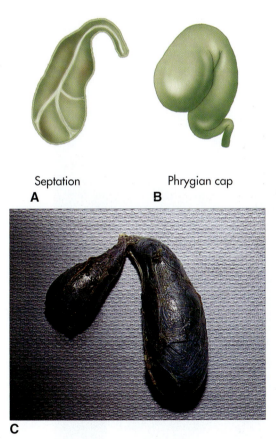

Septation   Phrygian cap
A   B

C

FIGURE 11-5 A, Septations may be found in the gallbladder. Changes in patient position will show the septation to remain in the same position in the gallbladder. **B,** A Phrygian cap is a variant in which part of the fundus of the gallbladder is bent back on itself. **C,** The double gallbladder is seen infrequently; the recognition of two distinct sacs will confirm the diagnosis.

gallbladder. The contracted gallbladder appears as a thick-walled structure with a slit for the bile. It is nearly impossible to see luminal or wall abnormalities when the gallbladder is contracted.

Removal of the Gallbladder

When the gallbladder is removed, the sphincter of Oddi loses tonus, and pressure within the common bile duct drops to that of intraabdominal pressure. Bile is no longer retained in the bile ducts but is free to flow into the duodenum during fasting and digestive phases. Dilation of the extrahepatic bile ducts (usually less than 1 cm) occurs after **cholecystectomy.**

Secretion is largely caused by a bile salt–dependent mechanism, and ductal flow is controlled by secretion. Bile salts form micelles, solubilize triglyceride fat, and assist in its absorption and that of calcium, cholesterol, and fat-soluble vitamins from the intestine.

Bile is the principal medium for excretion of **bilirubin** and cholesterol. The products of steroid hormones are also excreted in the bile, as are drugs and poisons (e.g., salts of heavy metals). The bile salts from the intestine stimulate the liver to make more bile. Bile salts activate intestinal and pancreatic enzymes.

SONOGRAPHIC EVALUATION OF THE BILIARY SYSTEM

Gallbladder

To ensure maximum dilation of the gallbladder, the patient should be given nothing to eat for at least 4 to 6 hours before the ultrasound examination. The patient is initially examined in the supine position in full inspiration. Transverse (Figure 11-6), sagittal (Figure 11-7), and oblique (Figure 11-8) scans are made over the upper abdomen to identify the gallbladder, biliary system, liver, right kidney, and head of the pancreas. The patient should also be rolled into a steep decubitus or upright position (to ensure there are no stones within the gallbladder) in an attempt to separate small stones from the gallbladder wall or cystic duct.

The gallbladder may be identified as a sonolucent oblong structure located anterior to the right kidney, lateral to the head of the pancreas and duodenum. The

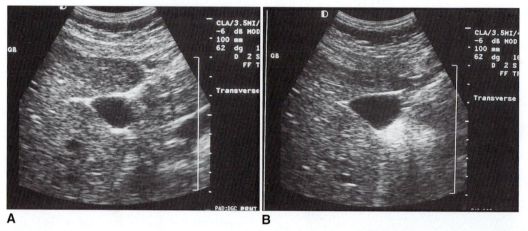

FIGURE 11-6 A and **B,** Transverse images of the gallbladder as it lies anterior to the kidney within the right lobe of the liver.

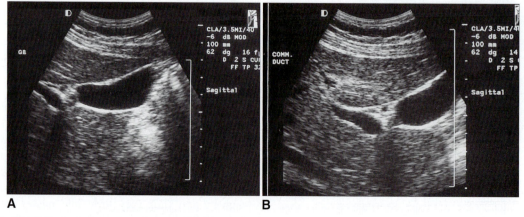

FIGURE 11-7 A and **B,** Sagittal images of the gallbladder from the neck to the fundus. The portal vein is seen off the neck of the gallbladder.

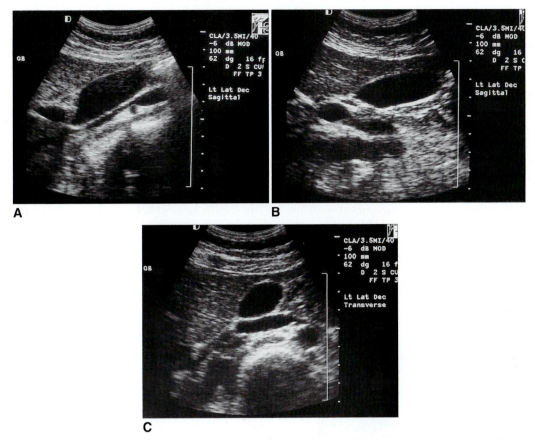

FIGURE 11-8 A and **B,** As the patient is rolled into a slight decubitus position and the transducer angled toward the midline of the abdomen, the gallbladder is seen anterior to the inferior vena cava and aorta in the sagittal plane. **C,** Transverse image of the gallbladder in the decubitus position.

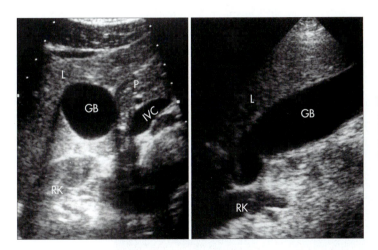

FIGURE 11-9 The gallbladder *(GB)* is identified as a sonolucent oblong structure located anterior to the right kidney *(RK)* and inferior vena cava *(IVC),* lateral to the head of the pancreas *(P)* and duodenum, and indenting the inferior to medial aspect of the right lobe of the liver *(L).*

gallbladder fossa shows a slight indentation on the posterior surface of the medial aspect of the right lobe of the liver (Figure 11-9). The sagittal scans show the right kidney posterior to the gallbladder. The fundus is generally oriented slightly more anterior and, on sagittal scans, often reaches the anterior abdominal wall. Box 11-1 lists the sonographic characteristics of the normal gallbladder.

BOX 11-1	Sonographic Characteristics of the Normal Gallbladder

- Size: ≤ 4 cm transverse; ≤ 12 cm longitudinal
- Wall thickness: < 3 mm
- Lumen: anechoic
- Landmarks: right upper quadrant, between right and left lobes of liver, right kidney, main lobar fissure, and portal vein

The middle hepatic vein lies in the same anatomic plane and may prove to be a useful landmark in locating the gallbladder. The interlobar fissure (a structure that separates the two hepatic lobes), is seen as a bright linear echo within the liver connecting the gallbladder fossa and the right portal vein (Figure 11-10). The neck of the gallbladder usually comes into contact with the main segment of the portal vein near the origin of the left portal vein. The gallbladder commonly resides in a fossa on the medial aspect of the liver. Because of fat or fibrous tissue within the main lobar fissure of the liver (which lies between the gallbladder and the right portal vein), this bright linear reflector is a reliable indicator of the location of the gallbladder. The gallbladder lies in the posterior and caudal aspect of the fissure. The caudal aspect of the linear echo "points" directly to the gallbladder.

A small echogenic fold has been reported to occur along the posterior wall of the gallbladder at the junction of the body and infundibulum. It may be very small (3 to 5 mm) but may give rise to an acoustic shadow in the supine position. It is not duplicated in the oblique position. The cause for such a **junctional fold** is the indentation between the body and infundibulum or Heister's valve, which is a spiral fold beginning in the neck of the gallbladder and lining the cystic duct (see Figure 11-1). This is called a **Phrygian cap**.

A prominent gallbladder may be normal in some individuals secondary to their fasting state (Figure 11-11). A large gallbladder has been detected in patients with diabetes, patients bedridden with protracted illness or pancreatitis, and patients taking anticholinergic drugs. A large gallbladder may even fail to contract after a fatty meal or intravenous **cholecystokinin;** other studies may be needed before making a diagnosis of obstruction.

If a gallbladder appears too large, a fatty meal may be administered and further sonographic evaluation made to detect whether the enlargement is abnormal or normal. If the gallbladder fails to contract during the examination, the pancreatic area should be investigated further. Courvoisier's sign indicates an extrahepatic mass compressing the common bile duct, which can produce an enlarged gallbladder (Figure 11-12). In addition, the liver should be carefully examined for the presence of dilated bile ducts.

In a well-contracted gallbladder, the wall changes from a single to a double concentric structure with the following three components: (1) a strongly reflective outer contour, (2) a poorly reflective inner contour, and (3) a sonolucent area between both reflecting structures.

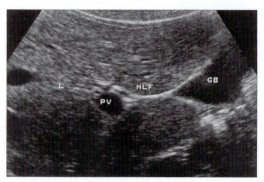

FIGURE 11-10 The main lobar fissure *(MLF)* is seen as an echogenic linear echo within the liver *(L)* connecting the right portal vein *(PV)* to the neck of the gallbladder *(GB)*.

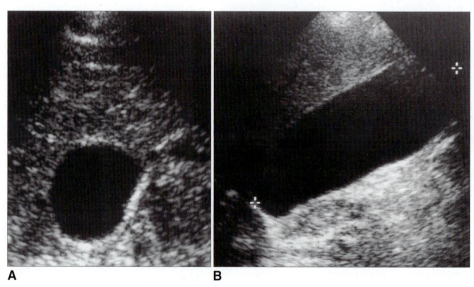

FIGURE 11-11 A, Transverse and **B,** longitudinal scans of the distended gallbladder. The gallbladder size may be quite variable from patient to patient. A good rule of thumb is to compare the size of the gallbladder with the transverse view of the right kidney. The width should always be smaller, ≤4 cm.

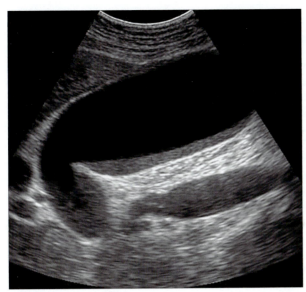

FIGURE 11-12 Distention (hydrops) of the gallbladder may be found in patients who have been on intravenous fluids for several days or may be secondary to a mass or enlarged lymph nodes compressing the common bile duct.

Bile Ducts

Sonographically, the common duct lies anterior and to the right of the portal vein in the region of the porta hepatis and gastrohepatic ligament. The hepatic artery lies anterior and to the left of the portal vein. On a transverse scan, the common duct, hepatic artery, and portal vein have been referred to as the portal triad or "Mickey Mouse sign" (Figure 11-13). The portal vein serves as Mickey's face, with the right ear the common duct and the left ear the hepatic artery. To obtain such a cross section, the transducer must be directed in a slightly oblique path from the left shoulder to the right hip.

On sagittal scans, the right branch of the hepatic artery usually passes posterior to the common duct (Figure 11-14). The common duct is seen just anterior to the portal vein before it dips posteriorly to enter the head of the pancreas. The patient may be rotated into a slight (45-degree) or steep (90-degree) right anterior oblique position, with the beam directed posteromedially to visualize the duct. This enables the examiner to avoid cumbersome bowel gas and to use the liver as an acoustic window.

When the right subcostal approach is used, the main portal vein may be seen as it bifurcates into the right and left branches. As the right branch continues into the right lobe of the liver, it can be followed laterally in a longitudinal plane. The portal vein appears as an almond-shaped sonolucent structure anterior to the inferior vena cava. The common hepatic duct is seen as a tubular structure anterior to the portal vein. The right branch of the hepatic artery can be seen between the duct and the portal vein as a small circular structure.

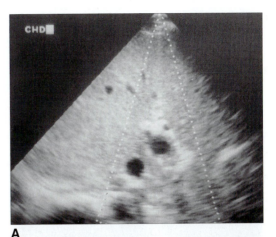

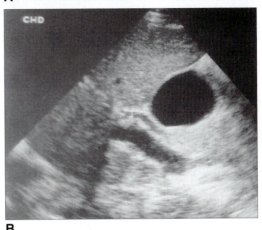

FIGURE 11-13 Transverse **(A)** and sagittal **(B)** views of the common bile duct. The transverse view shows the portal triad with the portal vein posterior, the common duct anterior and lateral, and the hepatic artery anterior and medial. The sagittal view shows the common duct anterior to the main portal vein.

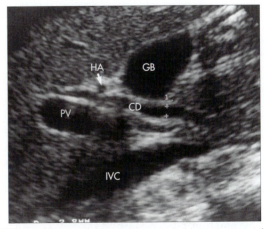

FIGURE 11-14 On this sagittal image, the hepatic artery (HA) is shown anterior to the common duct (CD). The portal vein (PV) is anterior to the inferior vena cava (IVC). GB, Gallbladder.

The small cystic duct is generally not identified. Because this landmark is necessary to distinguish the common hepatic duct from the common bile duct, the more general term *common duct* is used to refer to these structures (Figure 11-15).

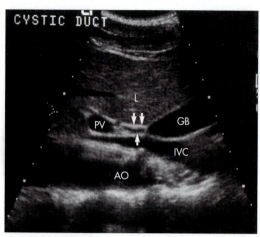

FIGURE 11-15 The cystic duct is sometimes seen to arise from the neck of the gallbladder *(arrows)*. This coronal decubitus view shows the aorta *(AO)*, inferior vena cava *(IVC)*, gallbladder *(GB)*, portal vein *(PV)*, and liver *(L)*.

PATHOLOGY OF THE GALLBLADDER AND BILIARY SYSTEM

See Table 11-1 for clinical findings, sonographic findings, and differential considerations for gallbladder and biliary diseases and conditions.

Clinical Symptoms of Gallbladder Disease

Pain. The most classic symptom of gallbladder disease is right-upper-quadrant abdominal pain, usually occurring after ingestion of greasy foods. Nausea and vomiting sometimes occur and may indicate the presence of a stone in the common bile duct. A gallbladder attack may cause pain in the right shoulder, with inflammation of the gallbladder often causing referred pain in the right shoulder blade.

TABLE 11-1	The Gallbladder and the Biliary System	
Clinical Findings	**Sonographic Findings**	**Differential Considerations**
Sludge		
May be asymptomatic	Low-level internal echoes layering in dependent part of GB Prominent gallbladder size Changes with patient position	Pseudosludge Empyema of GB Hemobilia Neoplasm
Acute Cholecystitis		
↑ Serum amylase Abnormal LFTs	Dilation and rounding of GB + Murphy's sign Thick GB wall with irregular wall (edema) Stones Pericholecystic fluid	Chronic cholecystitis Nonfasting GB Acute pancreatitis GB carcinoma
Chronic Cholecystitis		
↑ Serum amylase Abnormal LFTs RUQ pain–transient	Contraction of GB Stones WES sign	Cholelithiasis Nonfasting GB Acute pancreatitis GB carcinoma
Acalculous Cholecystitis		
↑ Serum amylase Abnormal LFTs	Dilation of GB + Murphy's sign Thick GB wall with irregular wall (edema) Sludge Pericholecystic fluid Subserosal edema	Chronic cholecystitis Nonfasting GB Acute pancreatitis GB carcinoma
Emphysematous Cholecystitis		
Gas-forming bacteria in GB Abnormal LFTs	Bright echo in area of GB with ring down or comet tail artifact May appear as WES	Chronic cholecystitis GB carcinoma
Gangrenous Cholecystitis		
Abnormal LFTs	Medium to coarse echogenic densities that fill GB lumen in absence of duct obstruction No shadow Not gravity dependent Does not layer	GB carcinoma

TABLE 11-1	The Gallbladder and the Biliary System—cont'd	
Clinical Findings	**Sonographic Findings**	**Differential Considerations**
Cholelithiasis		
Check bilirubin levels	Dilated GB with thick wall	Duodenal gas
Acute ↑ amylase	Hyperechoic intraluminal echoes with posterior acoustic	Porcelain GB
Abnormal LFTs	shadowing	Sludge
(increased alkaline phosphatase);	WES sign	
AST and ALT may be normal	Gravity-dependent calcifications in GB	
Choledochal Cysts		
Jaundice	True cysts in RUQ with or without communication with biliary	Hepatic cyst
Possibly increased bilirubin	system	Hepatic artery aneurysm
	Classified by anatomy:	Pancreatic pseudocyst
	1. Localized dilated cystic CBD	
	2. Diverticulum of CBD	
	3. Invagination of CBD into duodenum	
	4. Dilated CBD and CHD	
Adenoma of the Gallbladder		
	Occurs as flat elevations located in the body of the GB, almost	Adenomyomatosis
	always near the fundus	
	Does not change with position	
	No shadow produced	
Adenomyomatosis of the Gallbladder		
	Papillomas may occur singly or in groups and may be scattered	Adenoma
	over a large part of the mucosal surface of the GB	
	Does not move with position changes.	
	"Comet-tail" artifact	
Porcelain Gallbladder		
Female predominance	Gallbladder wall is thickly calcified with shadowing	Gallstones with emphysematous
Found in patients over 60		cholecystitis
Choledocholithiasis		
Increased direct bilirubin	Echogenic structure in extrahepatic duct	Surgical clips
Abnormal liver enzymes	Dilated biliary tree	Artifact from right hepatic artery
Leukocytosis		Cystic duct remnant
Increased alkaline phosphatase		

Jaundice. Jaundice is characterized by the presence of bile in the tissues with resulting yellow-green color of the skin. It may develop when a tiny gallstone blocks the bile ducts between the gallbladder and the intestines, producing pressure on the liver and forcing bile into the blood.

Sludge

Sludge, or thickened bile, frequently occurs from bile stasis. This may be seen in patients with prolonged fasting or hyperalimentation therapy and with obstruction of the gallbladder. Some gallbladders may be so packed with this thickened bile that the gallbladder is isoechoic and difficult to separate from the liver parenchyma. Occasionally sludge is also found in the common duct. Sludge is gravity dependent. With alterations in a patient's position, the sonographer may be able to separate sludge from occasional artifactual echoes found in the gallbladder. Sludge should be considered an abnormal finding because either a functional or a pathologic abnormality exists when calcium bilirubin or cholesterol precipitates in bile.

▶ **Sonographic Findings.** Occasionally a patient presents sonographically with a prominent gallbladder containing low-level internal echoes, which may be attributed to thick or inspissated bile. The source of echoes in biliary sludge is thought to be particulate matter (predominantly pigment granules with lesser amounts of cholesterol crystals). The viscosity does not appear to be important in the generation of internal echoes in fluids. The particles can be small and still produce perceptible echoes (Figure 11-16). Sludge may also be seen in combination with cholelithiasis, cholecystitis, and other biliary diseases.

Wall Thickness

The normal wall thickness of the gallbladder is less than 3 mm. Biliary causes of gallbladder wall thickening

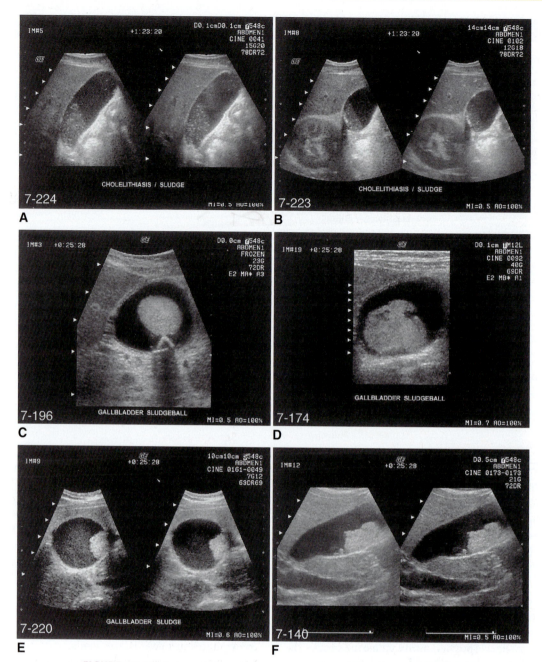

FIGURE 11-16 A through **F,** Multiple patterns of sludge within the gallbladder.

include cholecystitis, adenomyomatosis, cancer, acquired immunodeficiency syndrome, cholangiopathy, and sclerosing cholangitis (Box 11-2). Nonbiliary causes include diffuse liver disease (cirrhosis and hepatitis), pancreatitis, portal hypertension, and heart failure. A thickened wall is a nonspecific sign and is not necessarily related to gallbladder disease. It may also be found in the following conditions, along with those previously discussed: hepatitis, gallbladder tumor, or severe hypoalbuminemic states.

Sonographic Findings. The gallbladder wall thickness should be measured when the transducer is

BOX 11-2	Common Causes of Thickening of the Gallbladder Wall (≥3 mm)
Intrinsic	**Extrinsic**
Cholecystitis	Hepatitis/cirrhosis
Gallbladder perforation	Hypoalbuminemia
Sepsis	Renal failure
Hyperplastic cholecystosis	Right heart failure
Gallbladder carcinoma	Ascites
AIDS cholangiography	Multiple myeloma
Sclerosing cholangitis	Portal node lymphatic obstruction

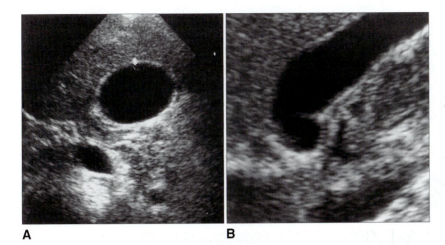

FIGURE 11-17 A, The gallbladder wall should be measured on the transverse image at the anterior wall that is perpendicular to the transducer (see markings). **B,** The sagittal image of the gallbladder is often at an angle to the transducer and may be used to measure the wall thickness when the sonographer can achieve a perpendicular angle.

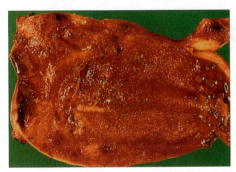

FIGURE 11-18 Gross pathology of acute cholecystitis. The gallbladder contained stones. The gallbladder wall was thick and swollen.

perpendicular to the anterior gallbladder wall. This is usually done in the transverse plane, but in some cases the longitudinal plane allows a better alignment. The gain should be reduced and the focal zone brought up to the gallbladder area to clearly demarcate the anterior wall. The anterior wall is measured from outer to outer margins. The normal wall thickness should be less than 3 mm. Sonographically the gallbladder wall may be underestimated when the wall has extensive fibrosis or is surrounded by fat (Figure 11-17).

Cholecystitis

Cholecystitis is an inflammation of the gallbladder that may have one of several forms: acute or chronic, acalculous, emphysematous, or gangrenous.

Acute Cholecystitis. The most common cause of acute cholecystitis is gallstones. When stones become impacted in the cystic duct or in the neck of the gallbladder (Hartmann's pouch), it results in obstruction with distention of the lumen, ischemia, and infection (cholecystitis) with eventual necrosis of the gallbladder (Figure 11-18). In the majority of patients obstructed with an impacted stone, the stone will spontaneously disimpact. This condition is found three times more frequently in females than in males over 50, but it has a similar incidence at

higher age groups. Clinically the patient with acute cholecystitis presents with acute right-upper-quadrant pain (positive **Murphy's sign**—inspiratory arrest upon palpation of gallbladder area; may be false positive in a small percentage of patients), fever, and leukocytosis; increased serum bilirubin and alkaline phosphatase levels may be present. Complications of acute cholecystitis may be serious to include empyema, emphysematous or gangrenous cholecystitis, and perforation.

Sonographic Findings

- Gallbladder wall > 3 mm
- Distended gallbladder lumen > 4 cm
- Gallstones
- Impacted stone in Hartmann's pouch or cystic duct
- Positive Murphy's sign
- Increased color Doppler flow
- Pericholecystic fluid collection

The sonographic appearance of acute cholecystitis is identified as a gallbladder with an irregular outline of a thickened wall (Figure 11-19). A sonolucent area probably caused by edema has been found within the thickened wall. Thick gallbladder walls often indicate disease. Some walls will be thicker because of a pericholecystic abscess. Occasionally a thickened gallbladder wall is seen in normal individuals. It seems to be related to the degree of contraction of a normal gallbladder (Figure 11-20). Color Doppler should demonstrate increased flow surrounding the gallbladder wall.

The sonographic Murphy's sign is positive when tenderness is demonstrated over the area of the gallbladder when the sonographer touches the right upper quadrant with the transducer and gentle compression is applied. When the patient takes in a deep breath, the gallbladder is displaced below the protective costal margin. This positive sign may not be present if the patient has been given analgesics before the study or if the condition has been prolonged with resultant gangrenous cholecystitis.

Color Doppler with low PRF is increased in the cystic artery, which feeds into the gallbladder. Power Doppler

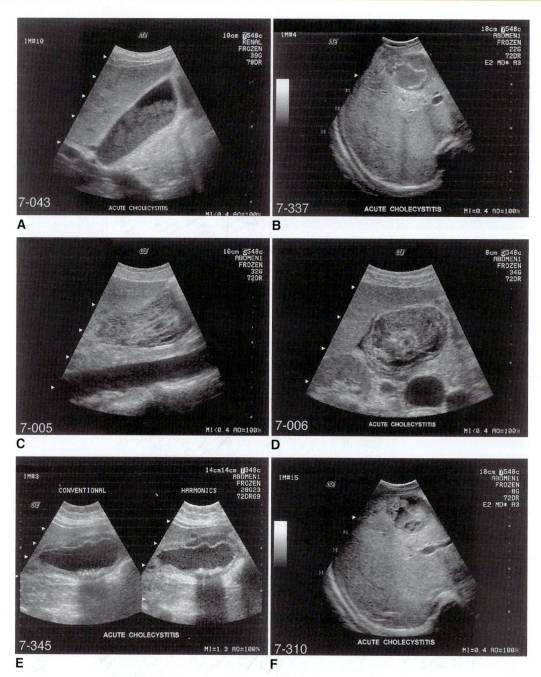

FIGURE 11-19 A through **F,** Multiple patterns of acute cholecystitis.

may better demonstrate this increased flow because the transducer does not need to be parallel to flow as it does with color Doppler.

The sonographer should assess the presence or absence of pericholecystic fluid (Figure 11-21). The wall may become inflamed and edematous with subsequent leakage into the pericholecystic space surrounding the gallbladder.

If the thickened wall is localized and irregular, an abscess, cholecystosis, or carcinoma of the gallbladder should be considered.

Cholelithiasis

Cholelithiasis is the most common disease of the gallbladder. In cholelithiasis there may be a single large gallstone or hundreds of tiny ones (Figure 11-22). The tiny stones are the most dangerous because they can enter the bile ducts and obstruct the outflow of bile. After a fatty meal, the gallbladder contracts to release bile; if gallstones block the outflow tract, pain results. As the bile is being stored in the gallbladder, small crystals of bile salts precipitate and may form gallstones

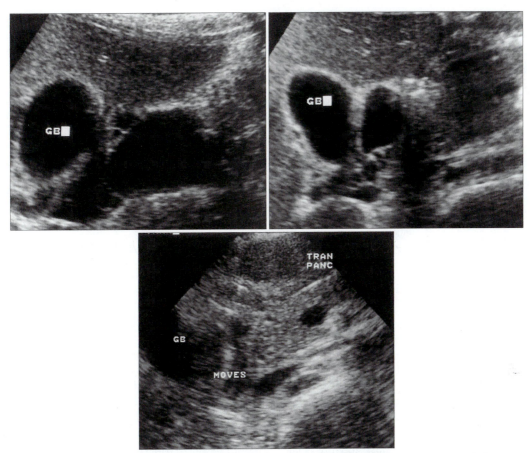

FIGURE 11-20 The sonographer should observe other fluid collections in the right upper quadrant for signs of change, or peristalsis, as illustrated in these images. The large collection of fluid was in the antrum and duodenum; with time, the fluid collection changed shape and distinct peristaltic movement could be seen with real-time imaging. *GB,* Gallbladder.

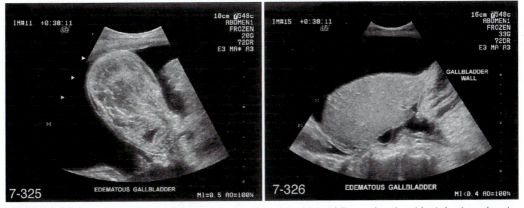

FIGURE 11-21 Swollen, edematous gallbladder was found in this middle-aged male with cirrhosis and ascites.

varying from pinhead size to the size of the organ itself. Gallstones may also consist of cholesterol.

Clinically the patient falls under the so-called five F's: fat, female, forty, fertile, and fair. In addition, many other factors lead to the development of gallstones that include pregnancy, diabetes, oral contraceptive use, hemolytic diseases, diet-induced weight loss, and total parenteral nutrition. Patients may be asymptomatic until a stone lodges in the cystic or common duct. Right-upper-quadrant pain with radiation to the shoulder after a high-fat meal is a typical presentation for cholelithiasis. Epigastric pain, nausea, and vomiting are present when the symptoms become acute.

Sonographic Findings. The evaluation of gallstones with real time has proven to be an extremely useful procedure in patients who show symptoms of

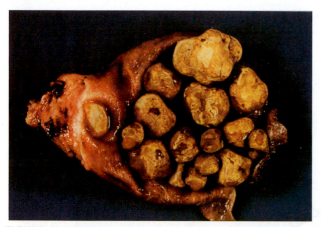

FIGURE 11-22 Gross pathology of multiple gallstones within the gallbladder.

cholelithiasis. The gallbladder is evaluated for increased size, wall thickness, presence of internal reflections within the lumen, and posterior acoustic shadowing (Figure 11-23). Frequently, patients with gallstones have a dilated gallbladder lumen. Stones that are less than 1 to 2 mm may be difficult to separate from one another by ultrasound evaluation and thus are reported as gallstones without comment on the specific number that may have been seen on the scan (Figure 11-24). A high-frequency transducer should be used to better delineate the stones and their shadowing characteristics. The curved array probe will allow a broader view of the near field to image the gallbladder.

When the gallbladder is completely packed full of stones, the sonographer will only be able to image the anterior border of the gallbladder, with the stones casting a distinct acoustic shadow known as the **wall echo shadow (WES) sign** (Figure 11-25).

The patient's position should be shifted during the procedure to demonstrate the presence of movement of the stones. Patients should be scanned in the left decubitus, right lateral, or upright position. The stones should shift to the most dependent area of the gallbladder. In some cases, the bile has a thick consistency and the stones remain near the top of the gallbladder. Thus, the density of the stones and the posterior shadow will be the sonographic evidence for stones.

With regard to acoustic shadowing, scattered reflections do not affect shadowing as much as specular reflections. The factors that produce a shadow are attributed to acoustic impedance of the gallstones; refraction through them or diffraction around them; their size, central or peripheral location, and position in relation to the focus of the beam; and the intensity of the beam (Figure 11-26).

All stones cast acoustic shadows regardless of the specific properties of the stones. The size of the stone is important. Stones greater than 3 mm always cast a shadow. It has been shown that any stone scanned two or more times with the same transducer and machine

settings may or may not generate a shadow even when the scans are made within seconds of each other. The shadow is highly dependent on the relationship between the stone and the acoustic beam. If the central beam is aligned on the stone, a shadow can be seen. Thus, some critical ratio between the stone diameter and the beam width must be achieved before shadowing is seen.

Some stones are seen to float ("floating gallstones") when contrast material from an oral cholecystogram is present because the contrast material has a higher specific gravity than the bile. The gallstones seek a level at which their specific gravity equals that of the mixture of bile and contrast material (Figure 11-27).

Complications of Acute Cholecystitis

Emphysematous Cholecystitis. This is a rare complication of acute cholecystitis appearing in less than 1% of all cases of acute cholecystitis, but it is rapidly progressive and fatal in 15% of patients. This occurs more frequently in men than in women, 50% of patients are diabetic, and gallstones may not be present in 30% to 50% of patients. This disease is associated with the presence of gas-forming bacteria in the gallbladder wall and lumen with extension into the biliary ducts. As many as 50% of patients with emphysematous cholecystitis have diabetes, and less than 50% have gallstones. Gangrene with associated perforation is a complication. This condition is a surgical emergency.

Sonographic Findings. The sonographic appearance will depend on the amount of gas within the wall of the gallbladder. If the gas is intraluminal, the sonographer should look for a prominent bright echo along the anterior wall with ring down or comet-tail artifact directly posterior to the echogenic structure. If a large amount of gas is present, the appearance may simulate a packed bag or WES sign with a curvilinear echogenic area with complete posterior fuzzy shadowing.

Gangrenous Cholecystitis. Another serious painful complication of acute cholecystitis that may lead to perforation is gangrenous cholecystitis. This process occurs after a prolonged infection, which causes the gallbladder to undergo necrosis. The gallbladder wall may be thickened and edematous, with focal areas of exudate, hemorrhage, and necrosis. In addition, there may be ulcerations and perforations resulting in pericholecystic abscesses or peritonitis. Gallstones or fine gravel occur in 80% to 95% of patients.

Sonographic Findings. The common echo features of gangrene are the presence of diffuse medium to coarse echogenic densities filling the gallbladder lumen in the absence of bile duct obstruction. This echogenic material has the following three characteristics: (1) it does not cause shadowing, (2) it is not gravity dependent, and (3) it does not show a layering effect (Figure 11-28). The lack of layering is attributed to increased viscosity of the bile. In addition, the gallbladder wall becomes irregular,

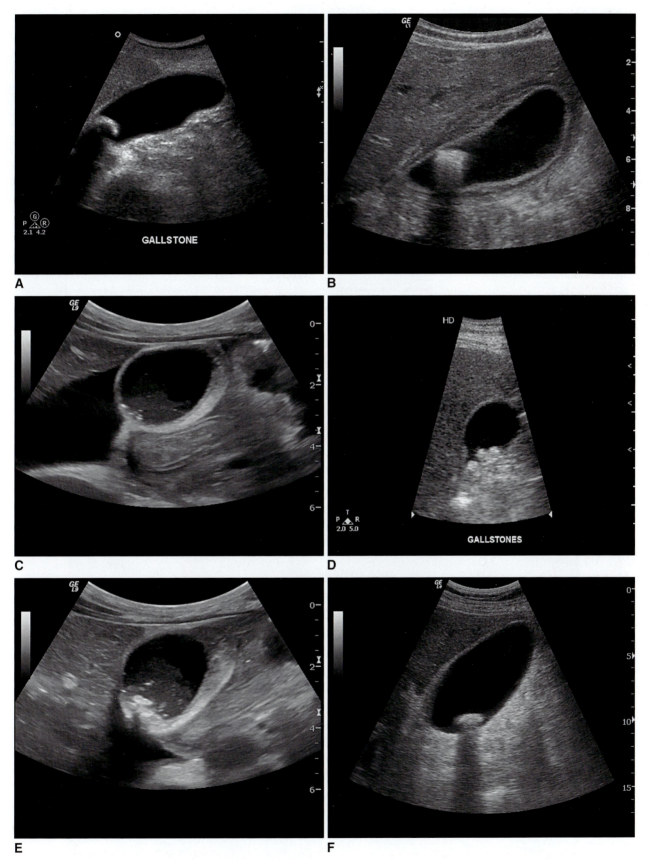

FIGURE 11-23 A, A single large gallstone is lodged into the neck of the distended gallbladder. Note the sharply defined shadow. **B,** A single large gallstone near the neck of the gallbladder. Note the thickening of the gallbladder wall. **C,** Tiny gallstones are seen within the sludge layered along the posterior margin of the gallbladder. **D,** Several medium-sized stones (without a shadow) are seen along the posterior margin of the gallbladder. The patient should be rolled into a decubitus position to watch the movement of these stones. **E,** Multiple stones with posterior shadow. **F,** Solitary stone with posterior shadow.

FIGURE 11-24 A, Multiple small stones are layered along the posterior wall of the gallbladder. These bright echogenic foci give acoustic shadowing beyond. **B,** A higher-frequency transducer would outline the stones and the shadowing even more clearly.

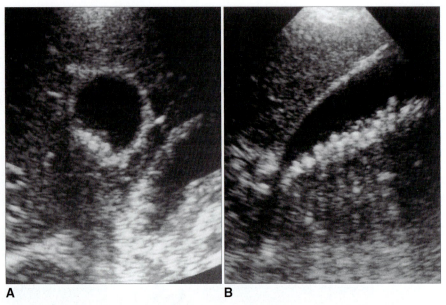

A

B

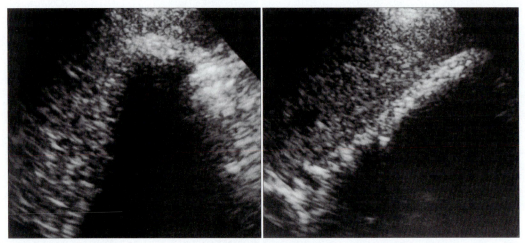

FIGURE 11-25 A 45-year-old female with right-upper-quadrant pain and distention. The "wall echo shadow" (WES) sign was visualized and indicated that the gallbladder was a packed bag. Note the sharp posterior shadow. This appearance is different from that of the porcelain gallbladder because the anterior wall is not as bright or echogenic.

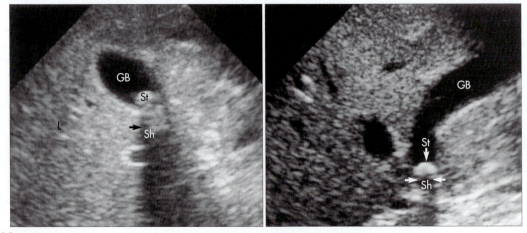

FIGURE 11-26 A 45-year-old female with right-upper-quadrant pain and increased bilirubin. Large echogenic calculus *(St)* is seen in the dependent neck of the gallbladder *(GB)*. Acoustic shadowing *(Sh)* is present beyond the stone.

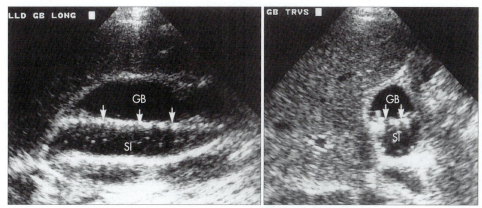

FIGURE 11-27 Longitudinal and transverse scans of the gallbladder *(GB)*, with a layer of stones "floating" *(arrows)* along the thick bile layer of sludge *(SI)*.

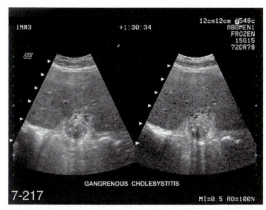

FIGURE 11-28 A 52-year-old female presented with fever and right-upper-quadrant pain for the previous 2 weeks. At surgery, the patient was found to have gangrenous cholecystitis. Multiple tiny gas pockets are seen within the gallbladder, causing posterior shadowing.

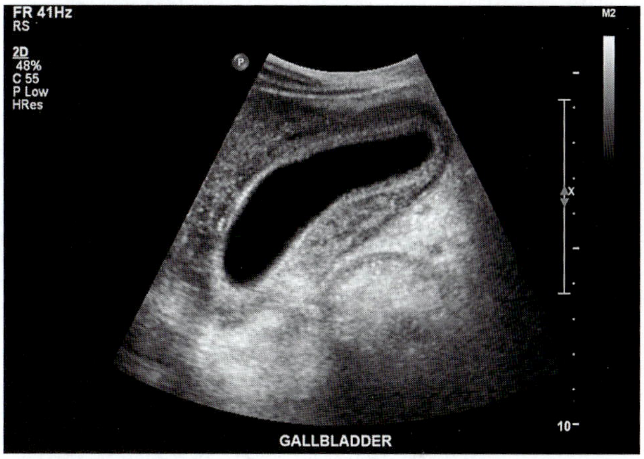

FIGURE 11-29 Acute cholecystitis with thickening of the gallbladder wall secondary to edema and inflammation.

with edematous pockets within the wall representing hemorrhage or abscess collections. The wall may become so inflamed with hemorrhage that a hemorrhagic cholecystitis develops. Pericholecystic fluid may be present in the area surrounding the gallbladder bed.

Acalculous Cholecystitis. This uncommon condition is an acute inflammation of the gallbladder in the absence of cholelithiasis. It is most likely caused by decreased blood flow through the cystic artery. Conditions that produce depressed motility (trauma, burns, postoperative patients, HIV, etc.) may prelude the development of acalculous cholecystitis. Extrinsic compression of the cystic duct by a mass or lymphadenopathy may also cause this condition. Clinically the patient has a positive Murphy's sign.

Sonographic Findings. The gallbladder wall is extremely thickened (greater than 4 to 5 mm), and echogenic sludge is seen within a dilated gallbladder. Look for the presence of pericholecystic fluid within ascites or subserosal edema (Figure 11-29).

Torsion of the Gallbladder

Torsion of the gallbladder is a rare condition that is found more in elderly females and is associated with a mobile gallbladder with a long suspensory mesentery. Symptoms present typical of acute cholecystitis.

Sonographic Findings. The gallbladder becomes massively inflamed and distended. The cystic artery and cystic duct may also become twisted. If the gallbladder becomes twisted more than 180 degrees, the risk of gangrene may develop. Surgical intervention is the treatment for this condition.

Chronic Cholecystitis

Chronic cholecystitis is the most common form of gallbladder inflammation. This is the result of numerous attacks of acute cholecystitis with subsequent fibrosis of the gallbladder wall (Figure 11-30). Clinically the patients may have some transient right-upper-quadrant pain, but not the tenderness as experienced with acute cholecystitis.

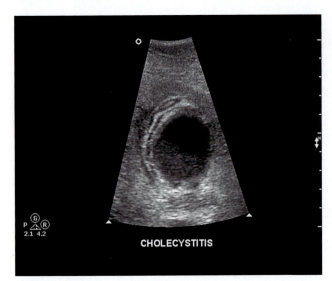

FIGURE 11-30 Transverse image of acute cholecystitis with wall edema and sludge.

Sonographic Findings. Cholelithiasis, or gallstones in the gallbladder, is frequently found in a contracted gallbladder with coarse gallbladder wall thickening. The WES sign (wall, echo, shadow) is described as a contracted bright gallbladder with posterior shadowing caused by a packed bag of stones.

Porcelain Gallbladder

A **porcelain gallbladder** is a rare occurrence that is defined as calcium incrustation of the gallbladder wall. It is associated with gallstones in the majority of patients and may represent a form of chronic cholecystitis. It occurs more often in older female patients. The patient is generally asymptomatic and the diagnosis is generally made as an incidental finding or when a mass is found on physical examination. A finding of porcelain gallbladder is significant in that 25% of those patients will develop cancer on the gallbladder wall.

Sonographic Findings. On ultrasound examination, a bright echogenic echo is seen in the region of the gallbladder with shadowing posterior. The differential will include a packed bag or WES sign. A small percentage of these patients with a porcelain gallbladder may go on to develop carcinoma of the gallbladder.

Hyperplastic Cholecystitis

Hyperplastic cholecystitis is represented by a variety of degenerative and proliferative changes of the gallbladder characterized by hyperconcentration, hyperexcitability, and hyperexcretion. The incidence is found in 30% to 50% of all cholecystectomy specimens and is found more commonly in females. Cholesterolosis and adenomyomatosis of the gallbladder are two types of this condition.

It is important to differentiate the common benign polyp from the rare malignant polyp. The benign polyp may be multiple and small in size (less than 10 mm). It does not change size when followed serially. Malignancy is suspected when the polyp is singular and measures greater than 10 mm, the patient is older than 60 years, gallbladder disease is present, there has been a rapid change in size upon follow-up sonography, and there is a sessile morphology.

Cholesterolosis. Cholesterolosis is a condition in which cholesterol is deposited within the lamina propria of the gallbladder. The disease process is associated with cholesterol stones in 50% to 70% of patients (although these stones are not demonstrable on radiography). It is often referred to as a "strawberry gallbladder" because the mucosa resembles the surface of a strawberry.

Most patients with cholesterolosis do not show thickening of the gallbladder wall on imaging studies; a small percentage of patients with this condition will show cholesterol polyps, which may be detected with ultrasound. **Polyps of the gallbladder** are small, well-defined soft tissue projections from the gallbladder wall. The cholesterol polyp is a small structure covered with a single layer of epithelium and is attached to the gallbladder with a delicate stalk. These polyps usually are found in the middle third of the gallbladder and are less than 10 mm in diameter.

Cholesterol polyp is the most common pseudotumor of the gallbladder. Other masses that occur are mucosal hyperplasia, inflammatory polyps, mucous cysts, and granulomata (resulting from parasitic infections).

Sonographic Findings. Cholesterol polyps are small, smooth ovoid wall projections seen to arise from the gallbladder wall (Figure 11-31). The polyps usually are multiple, do not shadow, and remain fixed to the wall with changes in patient position. The comet-tail artifact may be present, emanating from the cholesterol polyps, and this may be indistinguishable from adenomyomatosis.

Adenoma. Adenomas are benign neoplasms of the gallbladder with a premalignant potential much lower than colonic adenomas. This condition usually occurs as a solitary lesion. The smaller lesions are pedunculated, whereas the larger lesions may contain foci of malignant transformation. The adenomas tend to be homogeneously hyperechoic but become more heterogeneous as they grow. If the gallbladder wall is thickened adjacent to the adenoma, then malignancy should be suspected.

Adenomyomatosis. Adenomyomatosis is a hyperplastic change in the gallbladder wall. Papillomas may occur alone or in groups and may be scattered over a large part of the mucosal surface of the gallbladder. These papillomas are not precursors to cancer.

On the oral cholecystogram, the tumor is better seen after partial contraction of the gallbladder. Various patient positions and compression show the lesion to be immobile within the gallbladder.

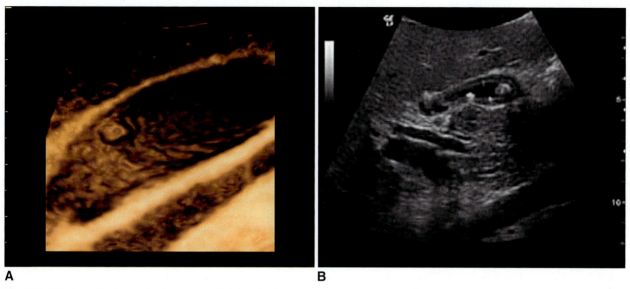

FIGURE 11-31 A, B, Cholesterol polyps are well-defined echogenic structures that arise from the gallbladder wall. They do not alter their position with changes in body movement.

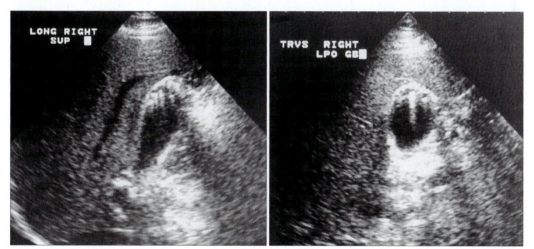

FIGURE 11-32 Adenomyomatosis is a hyperplastic change in the gallbladder wall. Multiple papillomas are seen along the anterior wall of this gallbladder, causing a "ring down" of echoes to occur.

Sonographic Findings. Benign tumors appear as small elevations in the gallbladder lumen. These elevations maintain their initial location during positional changes and are the cause for a "comet tail." No acoustic shadow is seen posterior to this papillomatous elevation (Figure 11-32).

Gallbladder Carcinoma

Primary carcinoma of the gallbladder is rare and is nearly always a rapidly progressive disease, with a mortality rate approaching 100%. It is associated with cholelithiasis in about 80% to 90% of cases (although there is no direct proof that gallstones are the carcinogenic agent). Patients with a porcelain gallbladder have an increased incidence of gallbladder cancer. It is twice as common as cancer of the bile ducts and occurs most frequently in women 60 years of age and older.

The tumor arises in the body of the gallbladder or rarely in the cystic duct (Figure 11-33). The tumor infiltrates the gallbladder locally or diffusely and causes thickening and rigidity of the wall. The adjacent liver is often invaded by direct continuity extending through tissue spaces, the ducts of Luschka, the lymph channels, or some combination of these.

Obstruction of the cystic duct results from direct extension of the tumor or extrinsic compression by involved lymph nodes (this obstruction occurs early).

The gallbladder tumor is usually columnar cell adenocarcinoma, sometimes mucinous in type. Squamous cell carcinoma occurs but is unusual. Metastatic carcinoma in the gallbladder may occur secondary to melanoma. It

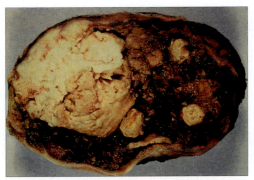

FIGURE 11-33 Carcinoma of the gallbladder shows the gallbladder partially filled and infiltrated with neoplastic tissue.

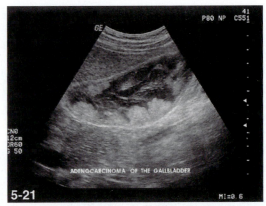

FIGURE 11-34 Sagittal image of a patient with adenocarcinoma of the gallbladder shows invasion of the gallbladder wall with the tumor.

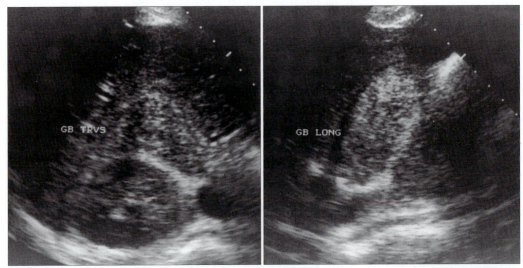

FIGURE 11-35 The most frequent sonographic finding in gallbladder *(GB)* carcinoma is a large, irregular, fungating mass that contains low-intensity echoes within the gallbladder, causing obscurity of the gallbladder wall.

usually is accompanied by liver metastases. Most patients have no symptoms that relate to the gallbladder unless there is complicating acute cholecystitis.

Sonographic Findings. The global shape of malignant gallbladder masses is similar to that of the gallbladder. The mass has a heterogeneous solid or semisolid echo texture. The gallbladder wall is markedly abnormal and thickened (Figures 11-34 and 11-35). The adjacent liver tissue, in the hilar area, is often heterogeneous because of direct tumoral spread. There may be dilated biliary ducts within the liver parenchyma, causing the "shotgun" sign (a "double-barrel" appearance of portal veins and dilated ducts) (Figure 11-36).

Carcinoma of the gallbladder is almost never detected at a resectable stage. Obstruction of the cystic duct by the tumor or lymph nodes occurs early in the course of the disease and causes nonvisualization of the gallbladder on oral cholecystogram.

PATHOLOGY OF THE BILIARY TREE

Choledochal Cysts

Choledochal cysts are an unusual, diverse group of diseases that may manifest as congenital, focal, or diffuse cystic dilatation of the biliary tree. The choledochal cyst may be the result of pancreatic juices refluxing into the bile duct because of an anomalous junction of the pancreatic duct into the distal common bile duct, causing duct wall abnormality, weakness, and outpouching of the ductal walls. These cysts are rare; the incidence is more common in females than males (4:1), with an increased incidence in infants (the condition may occur in less than 20% of adults). Choledochal cysts may be associated with gallstones, pancreatitis, or cirrhosis. The patient presents with an abdominal mass, pain, fever, or jaundice. The diagnosis may be confirmed with a nuclear

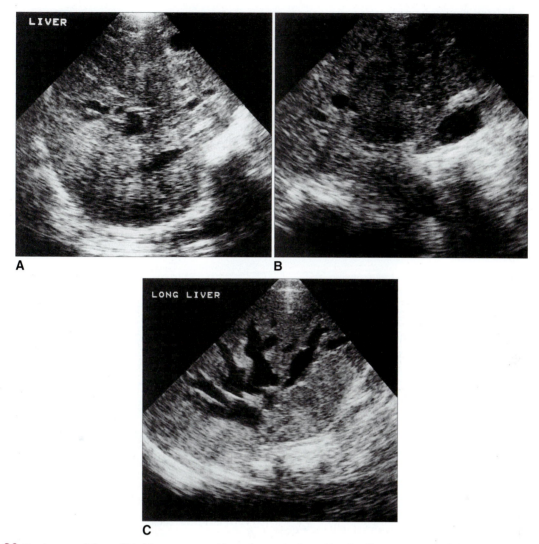

FIGURE 11-36 Carcinoma of the gallbladder may extend into the cystic duct either by direct extension of the tumor or by extrinsic compression by the involved lymph nodes. **A,** A transverse scan of the liver shows dilated ducts with an inhomogeneous liver parenchyma. **B,** A transverse scan of the inhomogeneous liver parenchyma. **C,** A transverse scan of the dilated ducts within the liver.

medicine hepatobiliary scan. The majority of cases are thought to be congenital and result from bile reflux. The mass presents as a cystic dilation of the biliary system.

The classification of choledochal cysts is divided into five types. Type I, a fusiform dilatation of the common bile duct, is the most common, along with type IVa. These are associated with a long common channel (> 20 mm) between the distal bile duct and the pancreatic duct. The rare type II cysts are true diverticula of the bile ducts. Type III cysts (choledochoceles) are confined to the intraduodenal portion of the CBD. Type IVa cysts are multiple intra- and extrahepatic biliary dilations. Type IVb cysts are confined to the extrahepatic biliary tree. Type V cysts have been classified as Caroli's disease (discussed later).

Sonographic Findings. Choledochal cysts appear as true cysts in the right upper quadrant with or without an apparent communication with the biliary system (Figure 11-37). The cystic structure may contain internal

sludge, stones, or solid neoplasm. If the cyst is very large, the connection to the bile duct may be difficult to distinguish on sonography.

The cysts are classified by anatomy as follows:

- Localized cystic dilation of the common bile duct
- Diverticulum from the common bile duct
- Invagination of the common bile duct into the duodenum
- Dilation of the entire common bile duct and the common hepatic duct

Caroli's Disease

Caroli's disease is a rare congenital abnormality that is most likely inherited in an autosomal recessive fashion. This condition is a communicating cavernous ectasia of intrahepatic ducts characterized by congenital segmental saccular cystic dilation of major intrahepatic bile ducts.

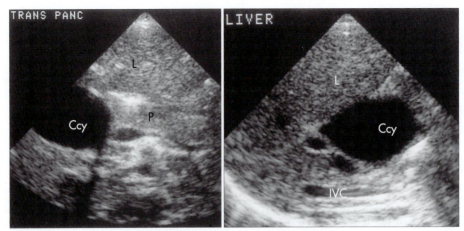

FIGURE 11-37 Transverse and longitudinal scans of a young patient with a choledochal cyst *(Ccy)* in the right upper quadrant. *IVC,* Inferior vena cava; *L,* liver; *P,* pancreas.

It is found in the younger adult or pediatric population and may be associated with renal disease or congenital hepatic fibrosis. Patient symptoms include recurrent cramplike upper abdominal pain secondary to biliary stasis, ductal stones, cholangitis, and hepatic fibrosis. Cystic disease of the kidney (medullary sponge kidney) is strongly associated with Caroli's disease.

There are two types of Caroli's disease: the simple classic form, and the more common form that is associated with periportal hepatic fibrosis.

▶ **Sonographic Findings.** On ultrasound examination, multiple cystic structures in the area of the ductal system converge toward the porta hepatis. These masses may be seen as localized or diffusely scattered cysts that communicate with the bile ducts. The differential will include polycystic liver disease. In addition to the abnormality in the porta hepatis, the ducts may show a beaded appearance as they extend into the periphery of the liver. Ectasia of the extrahepatic and common bile ducts may be present. In addition, sludge or calculi may reside in the dilated ducts.

Dilated Biliary Ducts

The small size of the intrahepatic bile ducts implies that sonography cannot image the ducts routinely until their size dilates to greater than 4 mm. Evaluation of the portal structures will allow the sonographer to search for the dilated ducts as they parallel the course of the portal veins. The common hepatic duct has an internal diameter of less than 4 mm. A duct diameter of 5 mm is borderline, and one of 6 mm requires further investigation. A patient may have a normal-size hepatic duct and still have distal obstruction. The distal duct is often obscured by gas in the duodenal loop. The common bile duct has an internal diameter slightly greater than that of the hepatic duct. Generally a duct more than 6 mm in diameter is considered borderline and more than 10 mm is dilated (Figure 11-38).

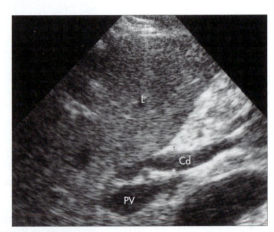

FIGURE 11-38 Sagittal scan of a prominent common bile duct *(Cd)* as it runs anterior to the portal vein *(PV)* and posterior to the head of the pancreas. *L,* Liver.

Biliary Obstruction

The most common cause of biliary ductal system obstruction is the presence of a tumor or thrombus within the ductal system. The process may be found in the extrahepatic or intrahepatic ductal pathway. Obstruction of the biliary ductal system is diagnosed by ultrasound when the sonographer finds the presence of ductal dilation. This finding has been termed on sonography as "too many tubes" or "shotgun" sign when intrahepatic ducts are dilated.

Bile ducts expand centrifugally from the point of obstruction. Therefore, extrahepatic dilation occurs before intrahepatic dilation. In patients with obstructive jaundice, isolated dilation of the extrahepatic duct may be present. Fibrosed or infiltrative disease of the liver may prevent intrahepatic dilation because of lack of compliance of the hepatic parenchyma.

Clinically the elevation of cholestatic liver parameters may present as jaundice. Painful jaundice is seen with

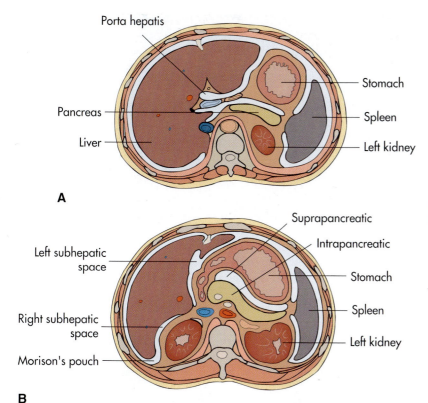

A

B

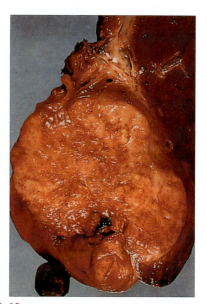

FIGURE 11-39 Levels of obstruction. **A,** Porta hepatic. **B,** Intrapancreatic and suprapancreatic.

acute obstruction or infection that may invade the biliary tree.

Extrahepatic Biliary Obstruction. The job of the sonographer is to localize the level and cause of the obstruction. There are three primary areas for obstruction to occur: (1) intrapancreatic, (2) suprapancreatic, and (3) porta hepatic (Figure 11-39).

Intrapancreatic Obstruction. There are three important conditions that cause the majority of biliary obstruction at the level of the distal duct and cause the extrahepatic duct to be entirely dilated: (1) pancreatic carcinoma, (2) choledocholithiasis, and (3) chronic pancreatitis with stricture formation.

Suprapancreatic Obstruction. This obstruction originates between the pancreas and the porta hepatis. The head of the pancreas, the intrapancreatic duct, and pancreatic duct are normal with ultrasound. The most common cause for this obstruction is malignancy or adenopathy at this level.

Porta Hepatic Obstruction. This area of obstruction is usually due to a neoplasm. In patients with obstruction at the level of the porta hepatis, ultrasound will show intrahepatic ductal dilation and a normal common duct. Hydrops of the gallbladder may be present.

Other Causes of Obstruction. Cholangiocarcinoma is a rare malignancy that originates within the larger bile ducts (usually the common duct or common hepatic duct) (Figure 11-40). A **Klatskin's tumor** is a specific type of cholangiocarcinoma that can occur at the bifurcation of the common hepatic duct, with involvement of both

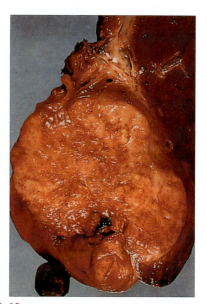

FIGURE 11-40 Gross pathology of cholangiocellular carcinoma.

the central left and right duct. The most suggestive sonographic feature to indicate cholangiocarcinoma is isolated intrahepatic duct dilation. Even though the obstructing mass may not be imaged, a nonunion of the right and left ducts is characteristic for a Klatskin's tumor.

Mirizzi syndrome is an uncommon cause for extrahepatic biliary obstruction resulting from an impacted stone in the cystic duct, which creates extrinsic mechanical

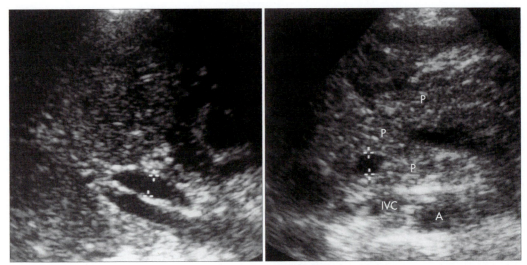

FIGURE 11-41 Inflammation of the pancreas may cause the common duct to dilate. This patient had acute pancreatitis *(P)* and dilation of the common duct *(crossbars)*. *A,* Aorta; *IVC,* inferior vena cava.

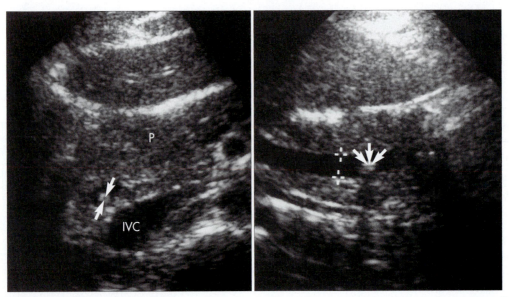

FIGURE 11-42 Stones within the common duct are seen if the duct is dilated. The small echogenic focus *(arrows)* is well seen within the duct in this transverse view. *IVC,* Inferior vena cava; *P,* pancreas.

compression of the common hepatic duct. The patient presents with painful jaundice. This stone may penetrate into the common hepatic duct or the gut, which results in a cholecystobiliary or cholecystenteric fistula. In this case, the cystic duct inserts unusually low into the common hepatic duct, and thus the two ducts have parallel alignment, which allows for the development of this syndrome. Using sonography, an intrahepatic ductal dilation is seen with a normal-size common duct and a large stone in the neck of the gallbladder or cystic duct.

Tumors arising from the common bile duct and ampullar carcinoma have the same ultrasonic features as pancreatic tumors. A specific pattern exists when the ampulloma bulges inside a dilated common bile duct. Cancer of the biliary convergence or of the hepatic duct

usually infiltrates the ductal wall without bulging outside. It may be difficult to image these tumors; the diagnosis is indirect and based on biliary dilation above the tumor.

▶ **Sonographic Findings.** Minimal dilation may be seen in nonjaundiced patients with gallstones or pancreatitis or in jaundiced patients with a common duct stone or tumor (Figures 11-41 and 11-42). However, a diameter of more than 11 mm suggests obstruction by stone or tumor of the duct or pancreas or some other source (Figure 11-43). One study reported measurement of the common duct at 7.7 mm in nonjaundiced patients who had undergone cholecystectomy.

Dilated ducts may also be found in the absence of jaundice. The patient may have biliary obstruction involving one hepatic duct, an early obstruction

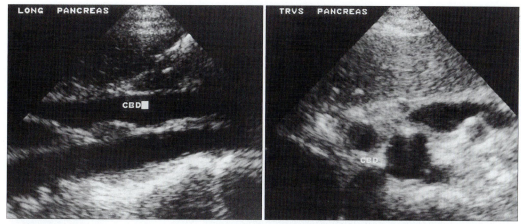

FIGURE 11-43 Carcinoma of the head of the pancreas with obstruction of the common bile duct *(CBD)*.

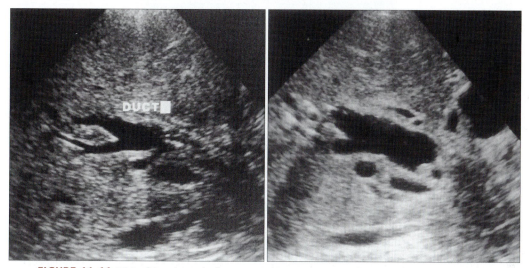

FIGURE 11-44 Dilated intrahepatic ducts secondary to a mass in the area of the porta hepatis.

secondary to carcinoma, or gallstones causing intermittent obstruction resulting from a ball-valve effect (Figures 11-44 and 11-45).

The following five characteristics traditionally distinguish bile ducts from other intrahepatic structures (parasagittal scans provided the best visualization of the ducts):

- *Alteration in the anatomic pattern adjacent to the main (right) portal vein segment and the bifurcation.* This is more pronounced in individuals who display greater degrees of dilation of the intrahepatic bile ducts.
- *Irregular walls of dilated bile ducts.* As the intrahepatic biliary system dilates, the course and caliber of ducts become increasingly tortuous and irregular.
- *Stellate confluence of dilated ducts.* This is noted at the points where the ducts converge. Dilated ducts look like spokes of a wheel.
- *Acoustic enhancement by dilated bile ducts.* Both portal veins and ducts are surrounded by high-amplitude reflections.

- *Peripheral duct dilation.* It is normally unusual to visualize hepatic ducts in the liver periphery, whereas dilated bile ducts may be observed.

Choledocholithiasis

Choledocholithiasis is classified into primary and secondary forms. Primary choledocholithiasis is the *de novo* formation of calcium stones in the bile duct. These stones may result from disease causing strictures or dilation of the bile ducts leading to stasis, that is, sclerosing cholangitis, Caroli's disease, parasitic infections, chronic hemolytic diseases, and prior biliary surgery. The secondary form denotes that the majority of stones in the common bile duct have migrated from the gallbladder. Common duct stones are usually associated with calculous cholecystitis (Figure 11-46).

Sonographic Findings. Stones tend to become impacted in the ampulla of Vater and may project into the duodenum. This is the reason it is important for the surgeons to check the common bile duct when removing

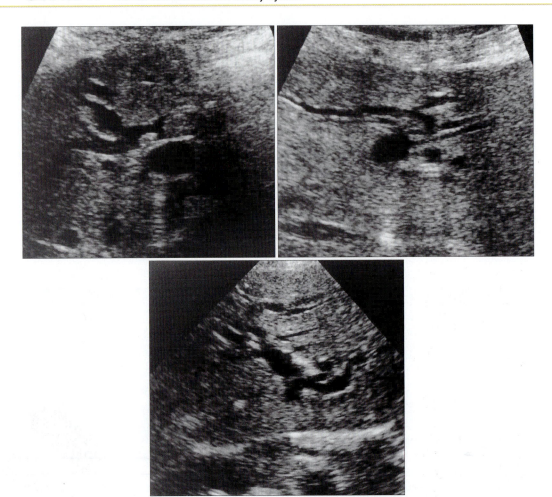

FIGURE 11-45 A 60-year-old female with a history of cholecystectomy several years previously. The patient was known to have had previous hepatic calculi and now has right-upper-quadrant pain. Moderate diffuse dilation of the right and left intrahepatic ducts is present. Echogenic ovoid structures seen in the distal right hepatic and left hepatic ducts represent calculi or sludge balls. The intrahepatic duct was minimally dilated.

the gallbladder. The sonographer should look for a dilated duct with a bright echogenic mass (stone) casting a posterior shadow.

Other Causes of Shadowing. The sonographer should be aware that structures or conditions other than stones may lead to attenuation of the ultrasound beam or shadowing. Calcifications of the small vascular structures within the right upper quadrant may cause shadowing to occur in the area of the gallbladder and be misinterpreted as stones. Air or gas within the duodenum may also give rise to a dirty shadow in the right upper quadrant. Intrabiliary gas is sometimes difficult to separate from stones, although the gas usually produces a brighter reflection with a ring down artifact and dirtier shadow versus the clean sharp shadow from a stone.

◤ **Sonographic Findings.** Another cause of shadowing in the right upper quadrant is gas in the biliary tree. This is a spontaneous occurrence resulting from the formation of a biliary enteric fistula in chronic gallbladder disease (Figure 11-47).

Hemobilia

Biliary trauma secondary to percutaneous biliary procedures or liver biopsies accounts for the majority of hemobilia cases. Other causes include cholangitis, cholecystitis, vascular malformations, abdominal trauma, and malignancies. The usual clinical findings are pain, bleeding, and jaundice. The sonographic appearance of blood in the biliary tree will depend on the length of time the blood has been present. Acute hemorrhage will appear as fluid with low-level internal echoes. Look for blood clots that may move in the duct with extension into the gallbladder.

Pneumobilia

Pneumobilia is air within the biliary tree secondary to biliary intervention, biliary-enteric anastomoses, or common bile duct stents. In the patient with an acute abdomen, pneumobilia may be caused by emphysematous cholecystitis, inflammation from an impacted stone

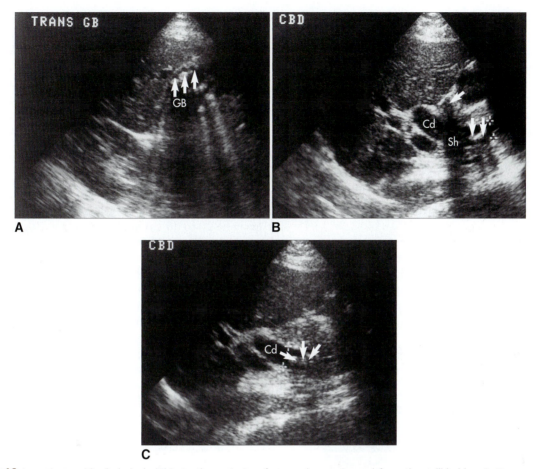

FIGURE 11-46 In patients with choledocholithiasis, the majority of stones have migrated from the gallbladder. **A,** Transverse: gallstones *(arrows)*. *GB,* gallbladder. **B,** Longitudinal. *Arrows,* stone; *Cd,* common duct; *Sh,* shadow; *single arrow,* gallstone. **C,** Longitudinal: dilated common duct with stone *(arrows)*.

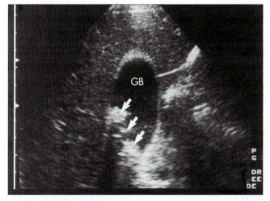

FIGURE 11-47 Gas in the right upper quadrant may cause shadowing in the area of the gallbladder *(GB, arrows)*.

in the common bile duct, or prolonged acute cholecystitis, which may lead to erosion of the bowel. On sonography, the air in the bile ducts presents as bright, echogenic linear structures that follow the portal triads. The posterior dirty shadow and reverberating artifact is seen. The sonographer should look for the movement of tiny air bubbles with a change in the patient's position.

Cholangitis

Cholangitis is an inflammation of the bile ducts (Figure 11-48). It may present as acute bacterial cholangitis, recurrent pyogenic cholangitis, or primary sclerosing cholangitis. The cause of cholangitis is dependent on the type of disease, but the obstruction may include ductal strictures, parasitic infestation, bacterial infection, stones, choledochal cysts, or neoplasm.

Cholangitis may be identified as oriental sclerosing cholangitis (seen more frequently in the United States with immigration). Other forms of cholangitis include AIDS cholangitis and acute obstructive suppurative cholangitis. Clinically the patient presents with malaise and fever, followed by sweating and shivering. There may be right-upper-quadrant pain and jaundice. In severe cases, the patient is lethargic, prostrate, and in shock. Elevated lab values show leukocytosis as well as elevation of serum alkaline phosphatase and bilirubin.

Cholangitis is a medical emergency as it develops increasing pressure in the biliary tree with pus accumulation. Decompression of the common bile duct is necessary. More than half of the patients with sclerosing cholangitis have ulcerative colitis. Both sclerosing and

AIDS cholangitis can have intrahepatic biliary changes that are nearly identical on ultrasound.

▶ **Sonographic Findings.** The sonographer needs to determine the cause and level of obstruction as well as exclude other diseases such as cholecystitis or hepatitis. The biliary tree is dilated and the common bile duct wall may show a smooth or irregular thickening (Figure 11-49). There may be choledocholithiasis with sludge. Actually the ductal wall may be so thickened that it is difficult to recognize on sonography without careful evaluation. Cholangitis usually involves the bile duct in a more generalized manner. Careful evaluation of the liver parenchyma should also be made to look for hepatic abscesses.

The subcostal oblique imaging of the porta hepatis to image the portal venous system is the landmark to find the biliary tree. The common bile duct may or may not be enlarged, but the walls may become slightly irregular and thickened. The stones are usually lodged in the distal common bile duct or must be mobile to cause intermittent obstruction.

In patients with oriental cholangitis, the lateral segment of the left lobe of the liver is most often involved.

In the acute septic phase, the patient may need urgent percutaneous biliary decompression or surgery. Atrophy of the affected duct develops with chronic stasis and inflammation followed by biliary cirrhosis and cholangiocarcinoma. Ultrasound is excellent for following these patients. As the biliary tree dilates, the internal lumen may be hypoechoic or echogenic with stones; these stones may not shadow, especially if they are tiny.

Ascariasis

This is a parasitic roundworm *(Ascaris lumbricoides)* that uses a fecal-oral route of transmission. The worm may be 20 to 30 cm long and 6 cm in diameter. It grows in the small bowel before entering the biliary tree through the ampulla of Vater. These worms cause acute biliary obstruction and are dramatic when seen on sonography. Clinically the patient may be asymptomatic or present with biliary colic, pancreatitis, or biliary symptoms.

▶ **Sonographic Findings.** On sonography the sonographer may denote an enlarged duct with a moving "tube" or parallel echogenic lines within the biliary ducts. As the transducer is rotated into the transverse position, the worm is surrounded by the duct wall and gives a target appearance. If the transducer is held in place over the area, small discrete movements may be seen on the image. The worm may fold over itself, or there may be multiple worms that present as an amorphous echogenic filling defect in the right upper quadrant.

Intrahepatic Biliary Neoplasms

Changes in the intrahepatic biliary ducts occur secondary to extrahepatic bile duct obstruction in most cases. Occasionally intrahepatic lesions are responsible for the changes in the duct.

Intrahepatic biliary tumors are rare and are primarily limited to cystadenoma and cystadenocarcinoma. The tumors are more frequently found in middle-aged women who clinically present with abdominal pain or mass or

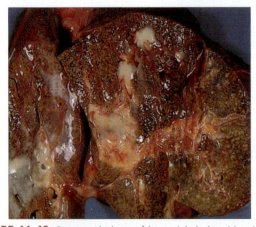

FIGURE 11-48 Gross pathology of bacterial cholangitis with pus in the bile ducts.

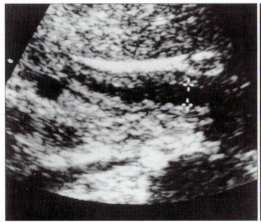 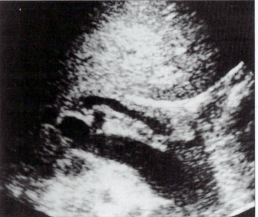

FIGURE 11-49 Sclerosing cholangitis appears as dilated ducts with thickened walls. This may be seen in patients with severe or prolonged infections, such as acquired immunodeficiency syndrome (AIDS).

jaundice (if the mass is near the porta hepatis). The sonographic appearance is a cystic mass with multiple septa and papillary excrescences. The mass may show variations in this pattern and present as unilocular, calcified, or multiple. The lesion may be associated with dilation of the intrahepatic ducts. The differential includes a hemorrhagic cyst or infection, echinococcal cyst, abscess, or cystic metastasis.

Cholangiocarcinoma

This neoplasm may arise from any portion of the biliary tree. The incidence is uncommon and the frequency increases with age. The most common risk factor in the Western world is primary sclerosing cholangitis. The classification of the tumor is based on the anatomic location: intrahepatic (peripheral), hilar (Klatskin's), and distal. Most cholangiocarcinomas are adenocarcinomas, followed by squamous carcinomas. The tumors are further divided into subtypes: sclerosing, nodular, and papillary. Nodular sclerosing tumors are the most common. Hilar cholangiocarcinoma is a nodular sclerosing tumor, a firm mass surrounding and narrowing the affected duct with a nodular intraductal component. Papillary cholangiocarcinomas are found in the distal common bile duct.

Intrahepatic Cholangiocarcinoma. Although this is the least common location for cholangiocarcinomas, it represents the second most common primary malignancy of the liver. An increased incidence of this tumor has risen over the past two decades secondary to an increasing number of patients with liver cirrhosis and hepatitis C infection. These tumors are often unresectable, with a poor prognosis.

> **Sonographic Findings.** On sonography, a large hepatic mass may be seen. The appearance is varied, from hypoechoic to hyperechoic. There may be a heterogeneous texture or hypovascular solid mass. Biliary ductal dilatation is associated with these obstructive masses in one third of cases. Uncommonly, an intrahepatic cholangiocarcinoma presents as one or more polypoid intraductal masses. Another uncommon form may present as a solid mass within a cystic structure that represents a tumor within a very dilated duct that does not communicate with the biliary tree.

Hilar Cholangiocarcinoma. This tumor is challenging for most imaging modalities. The patient clinically presents with jaundice, pruritus, and elevated cholestatic liver parameters. This disease usually begins in the right or left bile duct and then extends into the proximal duct and distally into the common hepatic duct and contralateral bile ducts. The tumor may extend outside the ducts to involve the adjacent portal vein and arteries. Chronic obstruction leads to atrophy of the involved lobe. The nodal disease originates in the porta hepatis and extends to the celiac axis with subsequent metastases to the liver. Although surgical resection is utilized, the majority of patients die within a year of diagnosis.

With sonography, careful attention is directed to the porta hepatis region. The sonographer should assess the level of the obstruction, the presence of a mass, lobar atrophy, and the patency of main, right, and left portal veins; the sonographer should also evaluate the encasement of the hepatic artery and look for local and distant adenopathy and metastases.

If the ducts are dilated, the sonographer should follow their course centrally toward the hepatic hilum to determine which order of branching is involved with the tumor. Resection is precluded once the tumor extension is found in the segmental ducts.

Evaluation of the portal system is critical. The narrowing of the right or left portal vein leads to compensatory increased flow in the hepatic artery. Tumor narrowing or encasing that obliterates the main portal vein or proper hepatic artery makes the tumor unresectable.

Distal Cholangiocarcinoma. This tumor is difficult to distinguish from hilar cholangiocarcinoma, although progressive jaundice is seen in the majority of patients. The tumor mass may be sclerosing or polypoid. Evaluation of tumor spread in the superior ductal system and extrahepatic area should be carefully evaluated. The tumor may extend into the adjacent lymph nodes.

> **Sonographic Findings.** On sonography, the sclerosing tumor is nodular with focal irregular ductal constriction and wall thickening. The tumor is hypoechoic and hypovascular with poorly defined margins. The more common polypoid tumor is seen as a hypovascular well-defined mass found within the distal ductal system.

Metastases to the Biliary Tree. The most common tumor sites that can spread to the biliary system are from the breast, colon, or melanoma. These metastases can affect the intrahepatic and extrahepatic ductal system. On sonography, the appearance of metastases is similar to that of cholangiocarcinoma.

The Pancreas

Sandra L. Hagen-Ansert

The pancreas continues to be a technical challenge for the sonographer because this gland is located in the retroperitoneal cavity posterior to the stomach, duodenum, and proximal jejunum of the small bowel. In addition, the transverse colon may obstruct visualization of the pancreas because it runs horizontally across the abdominal cavity.

Other noninvasive procedures were unsuccessful in visualization of the pancreas before the development of computed tomography (CT), magnetic resonance imaging (MRI), and ultrasound. Plain film of the abdomen may lead to a diagnosis of pancreatitis if calcification is visible in the pancreatic area, but calcification does not occur in all cases. Localized **ileus**, dilated loops of bowel without peristalsis ("paralyzed gut") caused by gas and fluid accumulation near the area of inflammation may be shown on the plain radiograph in patients with pancreatitis. The upper gastrointestinal test series provides indirect information about the pancreas when the widened duodenal loops are visualized. Other diagnostic methods—such as hypotonic duodenography, isotope examination, arteriography, fiberoptic gastroscopy, and intravenous cholangiography—all provide indirect information about the pancreas or prove limited in their diagnostic ability.

CT and MRI have become the primary modalities to image the patient with pancreatic disease because of their improved resolution of the retroperitoneal structures. However, the normal pancreas can be visualized in the majority of gas-free patients with sonography by using the neighboring organs and vascular landmarks to aid in localization. The gland appears sonographically

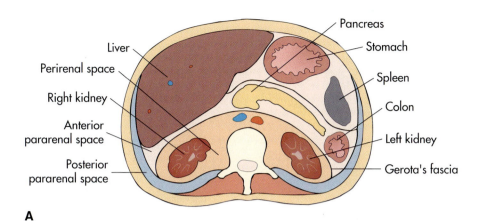

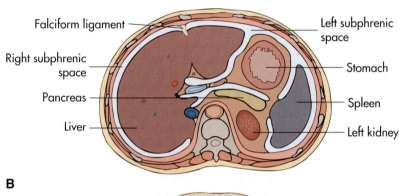

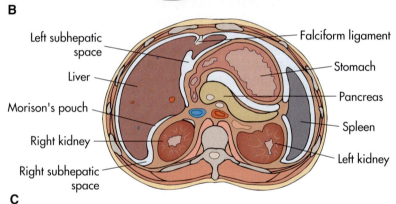

FIGURE 12-1 A, The pancreas lies in the anterior pararenal space. **B,** The stomach is anterior to the body and tail of the gland, whereas the aorta and inferior vena cava, superior mesenteric artery, and vein lie posterior to the gland. **C,** The head of the pancreas lies in the lap of the duodenum.

isoechoic to more hyperechoic than the hepatic parenchyma. Variations in patient positioning or ingestion of water to fill the stomach (that serves as a window to image the pancreas) are used routinely in many laboratories to further aid in visualizing the entire gland. In addition, clinicians performing the endoscopic retrograde cholangiopancreatography (ERCP) examination of the pancreatic duct are incorporating endoscopic ultrasound as an aid in visualizing the detailed anatomy of the pancreatic area.

Sonography is readily accessible and less expensive than the other imaging modalities. The primary task of the sonographer is to distinguish the normal gland from an abnormal process, to image the ductal system, and to separate inflammation of the gland from malignancies. Sonography may also aid in percutaneous fine needle aspiration when a lesion is found.

ANATOMY OF THE PANCREAS

Normal Anatomy

The pancreas lies anterior to the first and second lumbar bodies located deep in the epigastrium and left hypochondrium, behind the lesser omental sac (Figure 12-1). The major posterior vascular landmarks of the pancreas are the aorta and inferior vena cava. The pancreas most commonly extends in a horizontal oblique lie from the second portion of the duodenum to the splenic hilum. Other variations in the lie of the pancreas include transverse, horseshoe, sigmoid, L-shaped, and inverted V. When this occurs, it may be more difficult to obtain a single image of the pancreatic gland, as the tail will be in a different plane than the body and the head.

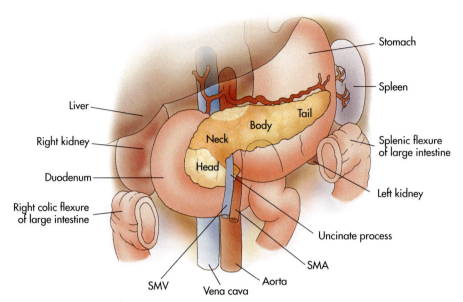

FIGURE 12-2 The aorta and inferior vena cava are the posterior landmarks of the pancreas; the stomach is the anterior border. The tail of the pancreas is directed toward the upper pole of the left kidney and hilum of the spleen. The body and head lie anterior to the prevertebral vessels. The four major areas of the pancreas are the head (with the uncinate process), the neck, the body, and the tail. The superior mesenteric vein *(SMV)* is anterior to the uncinate process. The superior mesenteric artery *(SMA)* is posterior to the neck/body.

It may be surprising that the majority of the pancreas lies within the retroperitoneal cavity, with the exception of a small portion of the head that is surrounded by peritoneum (Figure 12-2). The gland occupies the anterior pararenal space and lies obliquely between the C-loop of the duodenum and splenic hilum. Posterior to the pancreas are the connective prevertebral tissues, the portal-splenic confluence, the superior mesenteric vessels, the aorta, the inferior vena cava, and the lower border of the diaphragm. The stomach, duodenum, and transverse colon form the superior and lateral borders of the pancreas, which makes visualization of the pancreas by ultrasound difficult (air and gas interference).

The pancreas is divided into the following four areas: head, neck, body, and tail (see Figure 12-2). Each area is discussed as it relates to its surrounding anatomy. The reader is referred to the multiple cross-sectional drawings (Figures 12-3 and 12-4) to gain a relational understanding of the adjacent anatomy to the pancreas.

Head. The **head of the pancreas** is the most inferior portion of the gland. It lies anterior to the inferior vena cava, to the right of the portal-splenic confluence, inferior to the main portal vein and caudate lobe of the liver, and medial to the duodenum as it "lies in the lap" of the **C-loop of the duodenum** (see Figure 12-2). The splenic vein drains the spleen and forms the posterior medial border of the pancreas, where it is joined by the **superior mesenteric vein** (that drains the small bowel and proximal colon) to form the main portal vein, thus forming the **portal-splenic confluence** (Figure 12-5). The superior mesenteric vein crosses anterior to the uncinate process of the head of the gland and posterior to the neck and body of the pancreas. The **uncinate process** is the small,

curved tip at the end of the head of the pancreas. It lies anterior to the inferior vena cava and posterior to the superior mesenteric vein. As Figure 12-6 shows, the common bile duct passes through the first part of the duodenum and courses through a groove posterior to the pancreatic head, whereas the gastroduodenal artery (a branch of the hepatic artery rising from the celiac axis) forms the anterolateral border.

Neck. The **neck of the pancreas** is found directly anterior to the portal-splenic confluence or superior mesenteric vein. The portal vein is formed posterior to the neck by the junction of the superior mesenteric vein and the splenic vein (see Figure 12-5). The neck is located between the pancreatic head and body, and often it is included as "part of the body" of the gland.

Body. The **body of the pancreas** is the largest section of the pancreas. It lies anterior to the aorta and celiac axis (splenic artery, hepatic artery, and LGA), left renal vein, adrenal gland, and kidney. The tortuous splenic artery is the superior border of the gland (see Figure 12-4). The anterior border is the posterior wall of the antrum of stomach. The neck of the pancreas forms the right lateral border. The splenic vein courses across the posteromedial surface of the pancreas to join the main portal vein.

Tail. The **tail of the pancreas** is more difficult to image because it lies anterior to the left kidney and posterior to the left colic flexure and transverse colon. The tail begins to the left of the lateral border of the aorta and extends toward the splenic hilum (see Figure 12-5). The splenic vein is the posterior border of the body and tail. The splenic artery forms the superior border of the tail, whereas the stomach is the anterior border.

Text continued on page 308

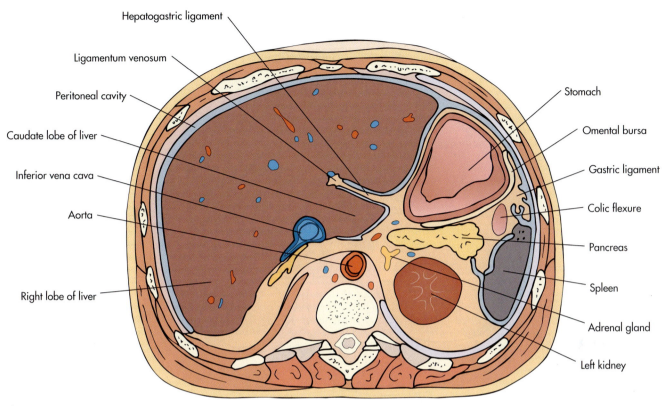

A,

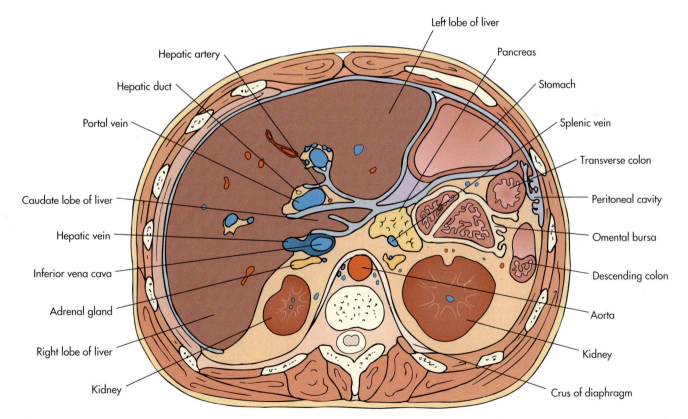

B,

FIGURE 12-3 Transverse planes of the pancreas. **A,** Note the relationship of the tail of the pancreas to the spleen, left kidney and adrenal gland, stomach, and colic flexure. **B,** The body of the pancreas is adjacent to the left lobe of the liver, the stomach, the omental bursa, and the left kidney.

Continued

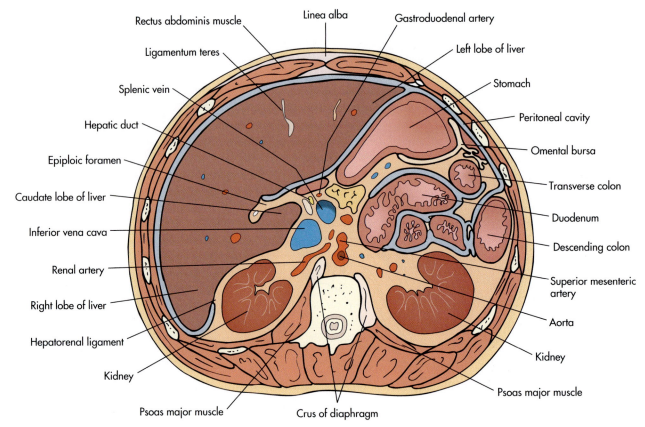

C

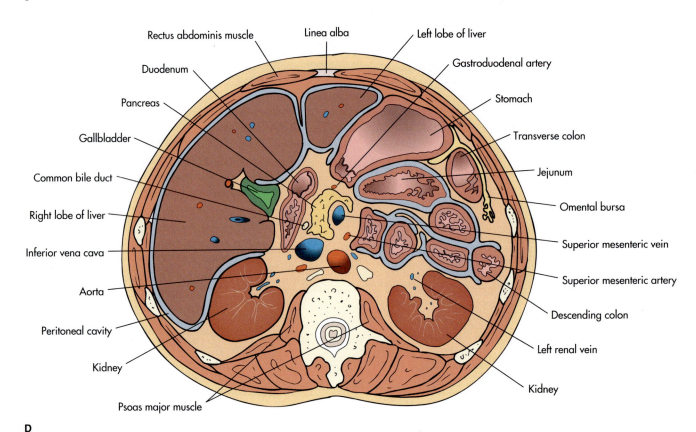

D

FIGURE 12-3, cont'd **C,** The size of the left lobe of the liver helps to push the stomach away from the pancreatic area for better visualization. **D,** The head of the pancreas is adjacent to the duodenum, superior mesenteric vessels, inferior vena cava, and aorta.

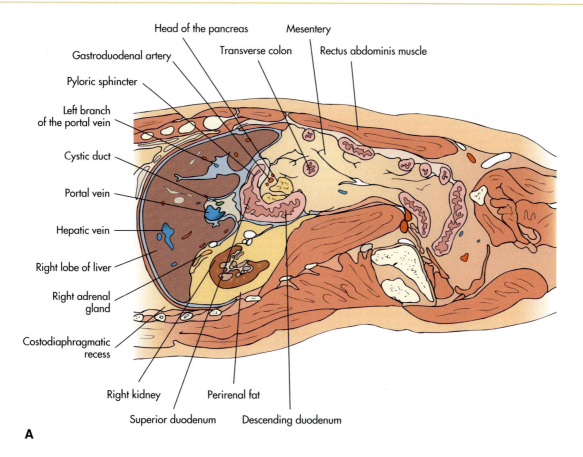

Head of the pancreas
Gastroduodenal artery
Pyloric sphincter
Left branch of the portal vein
Cystic duct
Portal vein
Hepatic vein
Right lobe of liver
Right adrenal gland
Costodiaphragmatic recess

Mesentery
Transverse colon
Rectus abdominis muscle

Right kidney
Superior duodenum
Perirenal fat
Descending duodenum

A

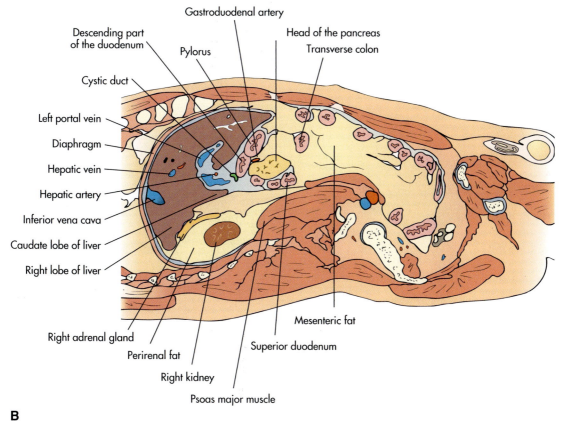

Descending part of the duodenum
Cystic duct
Left portal vein
Diaphragm
Hepatic vein
Hepatic artery
Inferior vena cava
Caudate lobe of liver
Right lobe of liver

Gastroduodenal artery
Pylorus
Head of the pancreas
Transverse colon

Mesenteric fat
Superior duodenum
Psoas major muscle

Right adrenal gland
Perirenal fat
Right kidney

B

FIGURE 12-4 Sagittal planes of the pancreas. **A,** The head of the pancreas lies in the lap of the duodenum. The gastroduodenal artery is the anterior lateral border of the head. **B,** The head of the pancreas may be obscured by mesenteric fat and air in the duodenum.

Continued

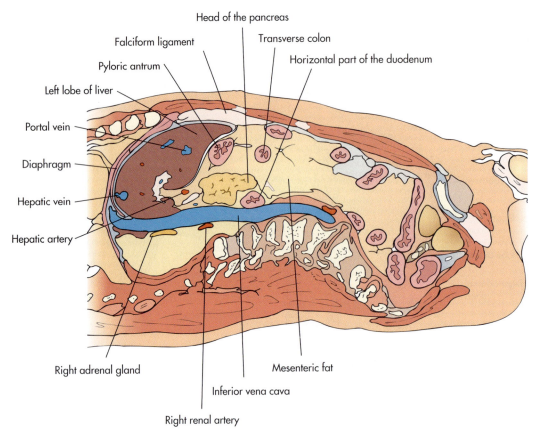

Head of the pancreas

Falciform ligament

Transverse colon

Pyloric antrum

Horizontal part of the duodenum

Left lobe of liver

Portal vein

Diaphragm

Hepatic vein

Hepatic artery

Right adrenal gland

Mesenteric fat

Inferior vena cava

Right renal artery

C

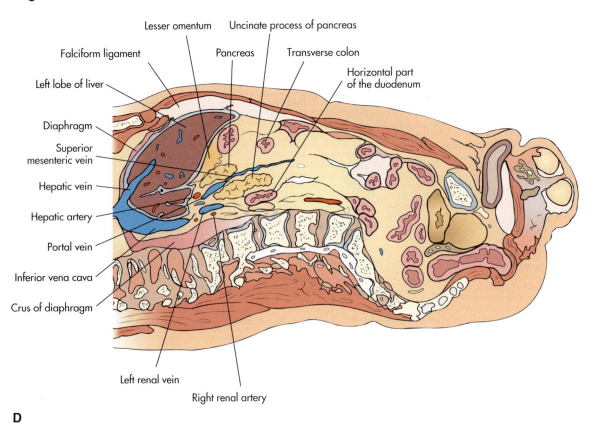

Lesser omentum

Uncinate process of pancreas

Falciform ligament

Pancreas

Transverse colon

Left lobe of liver

Horizontal part
of the duodenum

Diaphragm

Superior
mesenteric vein

Hepatic vein

Hepatic artery

Portal vein

Inferior vena cava

Crus of diaphragm

Left renal vein

Right renal artery

D

FIGURE 12-4, cont'd C, The head of the pancreas lies anterior to the inferior vena cava and inferior to the portal vein. **D,** Note the adjacent relationship of the lesser omentum to the pancreas. The superior mesenteric vein is posterior to the neck and anterior to the uncinate process.

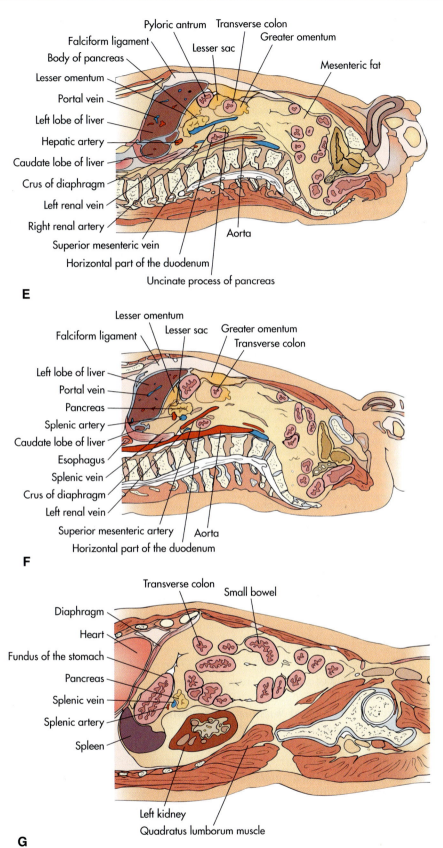

E,

Pyloric antrum   Transverse colon
Falciform ligament   Greater omentum
Body of pancreas   Lesser sac
Lesser omentum   Mesenteric fat
Portal vein
Left lobe of liver
Hepatic artery
Caudate lobe of liver
Crus of diaphragm
Left renal vein
Right renal artery
Superior mesenteric vein   Aorta
Horizontal part of the duodenum
Uncinate process of pancreas

F,

Lesser omentum
Falciform ligament   Lesser sac   Greater omentum
Transverse colon
Left lobe of liver
Portal vein
Pancreas
Splenic artery
Caudate lobe of liver
Esophagus
Splenic vein
Crus of diaphragm
Left renal vein
Superior mesenteric artery   Aorta
Horizontal part of the duodenum

G,

Transverse colon   Small bowel
Diaphragm
Heart
Fundus of the stomach
Pancreas
Splenic vein
Splenic artery
Spleen
Left kidney
Quadratus lumborum muscle

FIGURE 12-4, cont'd E, Note the relationship of the lesser omentum, pyloric antrum, lesser sac, transverse colon, and superior mesenteric vein to the body of the pancreas. **F,** Note the intimate relationship of the splenic vein and artery, superior mesenteric artery, aorta, and left lobe of the liver to the pancreas. **G,** The tail of the pancreas is more difficult to image on the sagittal plane secondary to the adjacent colon and small bowel. Occasionally a fluid-filled stomach, prominent spleen, or left kidney may help to localize the tail of the pancreas.

FIGURE 12-5 The portal venous system is the posterior border of the pancreas. The splenic vein lies along the posterior border, the superior mesenteric vein crosses anterior to the uncinate process and posterior to the neck, and the main portal vein is the posterior border to the head of the pancreas. The tortuous splenic artery is the superior border to the body and tail of the pancreas. The hepatic artery gives rise to the gastroduodenal artery, which serves as the anterolateral border to the head of the pancreas. The splenic artery branches into the magna pancreatic artery and dorsal pancreatic artery. The celiac axis rises from the anterior abdominal aorta just below the diaphragm and serves as the superior border of the pancreas.

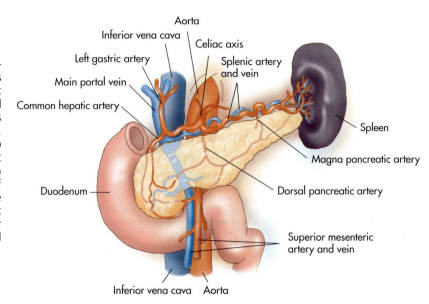

FIGURE 12-6 The head of the pancreas lies in the C-loop of the duodenum. The common bile duct passes through the first part of the duodenum and courses through a groove posterior to the pancreatic head, where it meets the pancreatic duct to enter the duodenum through the ampulla of Vater. This opening is guarded by the sphincter of Oddi.

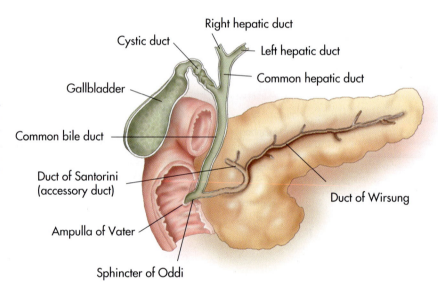

Pancreatic Duct. Two ducts are seen within the pancreas, the duct of Wirsung and the duct of Santorini. To aid in the transport of pancreatic fluid, the ducts have smooth muscle surrounding them. The **duct of Wirsung** is a primary duct extending the entire length of the gland (see Figure 12-6). It receives tributaries from lobules at right angles and enters the medial second part of the duodenum with the common bile duct at the ampulla of Vater (guarded by the sphincter of Oddi). The **duct of Santorini** is a secondary duct that drains the upper anterior head. It enters the duodenum at the minor papilla about 2 cm proximal to the ampulla of Vater.

The duct of Wirsung is easier to visualize as it courses through the midline of the body of the gland. It appears as an echogenic line or lucency bordered by two echogenic lines. The duct should measure less than 2 mm, with tapering as it reaches the tail. Color Doppler imaging may help distinguish the dilated pancreatic duct from the vascular structures (splenic vein and artery) in the area.

Common Bile Duct. The common bile duct runs inferiorly in the free edge of the lesser omentum to the level of the duodenum. Then it travels posterior to the first portion of the duodenum and the head of the pancreas to the right of the main pancreatic duct. The common bile duct opens into the duodenum after forming a common trunk with the pancreatic duct.

Size of the Pancreas

The normal length of the pancreas (head to tail) is about 15 cm, with the range extending between 12 and 18 cm. The head is the thickest part of the gland, measuring 2 to 3 cm in its anterior-to-posterior dimension. The neck measures 1.5 to 2.5 cm, the body measures 2 to 2.5 cm, and the tail measures 1 to 2 cm. The sonographer should evaluate the total size, contour, and texture of the gland to determine enlargement. The gland appears larger or thicker in children than in adults and decreases in size with advancing age.

Vascular Supply

The blood supply for the pancreas is the splenic artery and **pancreaticoduodenal arteries** (see Figure 12-5). The anterior and inferior pancreaticoduodenal arteries supply the head and part of the duodenum. The splenic artery supplies the body and tail of the pancreas through four smaller branches: (1) suprapancreatic (rises from the celiac axis/splenic artery), (2) pancreatic, (3) prepancreatic (before leaving the pancreas), and (4) prehilar (before leaving the spleen) and hepatic artery (gastroduodenal artery). The **dorsal pancreatic artery** rises from the suprapancreatic section, the pancreatica magna artery rises from the pancreatic section, and the **caudal pancreatic artery** rises from the prepancreatic or prehilar section. Venous drainage is through tributaries of the splenic and superior mesenteric veins.

Vascular and Ductal Landmarks to the Pancreas

Celiac Axis and Branches. The celiac axis originates from the anterior abdominal aorta and serves as the superior border of the pancreas. It gives rise to three branches: the left gastric, common hepatic, and splenic arteries (see Figure 12-5).

Splenic Artery. The splenic artery follows a tortuous course along the superior border of the pancreatic body and tail as it crosses horizontally toward the splenic hilum.

Common Hepatic Artery. The common hepatic artery rises from the celiac axis and courses along the superior margin of the first portion of the duodenum to divide into the proper hepatic artery and gastroduodenal artery, usually when it crosses anterior to the portal vein. The **common hepatic artery** forms the right superior border of the body and head of the gland and gives rise to the gastroduodenal artery. In some patients the right hepatic artery rises from the superior mesenteric artery and courses posterior to the medial portion of the splenic vein.

Gastroduodenal Artery. The gastroduodenal artery is seen along the anterolateral border of the pancreas as it travels a short distance along the anterior aspect of the pancreatic head just to the right of the neck before it divides into the superior pancreaticoduodenal branches; they join with the inferior pancreaticoduodenal branches, which rise from the superior mesenteric artery.

Superior Mesenteric Artery. The **superior mesenteric artery** rises from the aorta inferior to the celiac axis and

posterior to the lower portion of the pancreatic body and courses anterior to the third portion of the duodenum to enter the small bowel mesentery (see Figure 12-5).

Portal Vein and Tributaries. The main portal vein is formed posterior to the neck of the pancreas by the junction of the superior mesenteric vein and splenic vein (see Figure 12-5). The splenic vein runs from the splenic hilum along the posterior aspect of the pancreas. The superior mesenteric vein runs posterior to the neck of the pancreas and anterior to the uncinate process, which forms the small, curved tip of the pancreatic head.

Common Bile Duct. The common bile duct crosses the anterior aspect of the portal vein to the right of the proper hepatic artery. The portal vein is anterior to the inferior vena cava. The duct passes along the anterior border of the portal vein and travels posterior to the first portion of the duodenum to course inferior and somewhat posterior in the parenchyma of the head of the pancreas (see Figure 12-6). It joins the pancreatic duct close to the ampulla of Vater.

Congenital Anomalies

Congenital abnormalities of the pancreas are uncommon. The following abnormalities are presented: agenesis, pancreas divisum, ectopic pancreatic tissue, and annular pancreas.

Agenesis. Agenesis of the body and tail, with hypertrophy of the pancreatic head, is a congenital defect.

Pancreas Divisum. This rare condition is caused by the lack of fusion of the dorsal and ventral pancreatic buds. The drainage of the dorsal pancreas is through the minor papilla, with the ventral part draining through the major papilla. On sonography, this diagnosis is challenging. A persistent dorsal pancreatic duct in the head may be identified, but communication with the ventral duct is difficult to ascertain with sonography.

Ectopic Pancreatic Tissue. Ectopic pancreatic tissue is the most common pancreatic anomaly, usually in the form of intramural nodules. The ectopic tissue may be found in various places in the gastrointestinal tract. Frequent sites are the stomach, duodenum, small bowel, and large bowel. On palpation these lesions may seem polypoid, and they characteristically have a central dimple. They consist of elements of the pancreas, usually the acinar and ductal structures and less frequently the islets of Langerhans. They are generally small (0.5 to 2 cm), and acute pancreatitis or tumor may occur within these elements.

Annular Pancreas. Annular pancreas is a rare anomaly in which the head of the pancreas surrounds the second portion of the duodenum (Figure 12-7). It is more common in males than in females, and all grades (from an overlapping of the posterior duodenal wall to a complete ring) may be found. It may be associated with complete or partial atresia of the duodenum and is susceptible to any of the diseases of the pancreas.

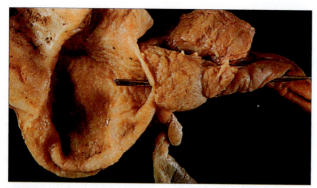

FIGURE 12-7 Gross pathology of the annular pancreas in which the head surrounds the second portion of the duodenum.

TABLE 12-1	Pancreatic Exocrine Function	
Enzymes of Pancreatic Juice		**Digestive Action**
Lipase		Fats
Amylase		Carbohydrates
Trypsin, chymotrypsinogen, carboxypeptidase		Proteins
Nucleases		Nucleic acids

PHYSIOLOGY AND LABORATORY DATA OF THE PANCREAS

Physiology

The pancreas is both a digestive (**exocrine**) and hormonal (**endocrine**) gland. The primary exocrine function is to produce pancreatic juice, which enters the duodenum together with bile. The exocrine secretions of the pancreas and those of the liver, which are delivered into the duodenum through duct systems, are essential for normal intestinal digestion and absorption of food. Pancreatic secretion is under the control of the vagus nerve and two hormonal agents, secretin and pancreozymin, that are released when food enters the duodenum. The endocrine function controls the secretion of glucagons and insulin into the blood. Failure of the pancreas to furnish sufficient insulin leads to diabetes mellitus.

Exocrine Function. Exocrine function is performed by **acini cells** of the pancreas, which can produce up to 2L of pancreatic juice per day. These cells are arranged in saclike clusters (acini) connected by small intercalated ducts to larger excretory ducts. The excretory ducts converge into one or two main ducts, which deliver the exocrine secretion of the pancreas into the duodenum. The enzymes of the pancreatic juice that aid in digestion include **lipase,** which digests fats; **amylase,** which digests carbohydrates; carboxypeptidase, trypsin, and chymotrypsinogen, which digest proteins; and nucleases, which digest nucleic acids (Table 12-1).

Pancreatic juice is the most versatile and active of the digestive secretions. Its enzymes are capable of nearly completing the digestion of food in the absence of all other digestive secretions. Because the digestive enzymes that are secreted into the lumen of the small intestine require an almost neutral pH for best activity, the acidity of the contents entering the duodenum must be reduced. Thus, the pancreatic juice contains a relatively high concentration of sodium bicarbonate, and this alkaline salt is largely responsible for the neutralization of gastric acid.

The nervous secretion of pancreatic juice is thick and rich in enzymes and proteins. The chemical secretion, resulting from pancreozymin activity, also is thick, watery, and rich in enzymes. Pancreatic juice is alkaline and becomes more so with increasing rates of secretion. This is because of a simultaneous increase in bicarbonates and decrease in chloride concentration.

The proteolytic enzyme trypsin may hydrolyze protein molecules to polypeptides. Chymotrypsinogen is activated by trypsin. Amylase causes hydrolysis of starch with the production of maltose, which is further hydrolyzed to glucose. Lipase is capable of hydrolyzing some fats to monoglycerides and some to glycerol and fatty acids. Although lipases are also secreted by the small intestine, what is secreted by the pancreas accounts for 80% of all fat digestion. Thus, impaired fat digestion is an important indicator of pancreatic dysfunction.

Partially digested food, or chyme, in the duodenum stimulates the release of hormones that act on pancreatic juice formation. These hormones include gastrin, cholecystokinin, acetylcholine (all digestive enzymes), and secretin (stimulates production of sodium bicarbonate).

The pancreatic juice enters the duodenum through the duct of Wirsung. This duct joins the common bile duct as it drains bile from the liver and both enter the duodenum through the ampulla of Vater. The sphincter of Oddi is a muscle surrounding the ampulla of Vater that relaxes to allow pancreatic juice and bile to empty into the duodenum.

Endocrine Function. The endocrine function is located in the **islets of Langerhans** in the pancreas. Specialized cells within the islets are called *alpha, beta,* and *delta* cells. The beta cells are most prevalent and produce **insulin,** a hormone that causes glycogen formation from glucose in the liver. It also enables cells within insulin receptors to take up glucose (to decrease blood sugar). Alpha cells produce **glucagon,** a hormone that causes the cells to release glucose to meet the energy needs of the body. Glucagon stimulates the liver to convert glycogen to glucose to increase sugar levels. Delta cells are the smallest composition of endocrine tissue and produce somatostatin. This hormone inhibits the production of both insulin and glucagon. All the hormones are released into the bloodstream (Table 12-2).

TABLE 12-2	Pancreatic Endocrine Function	
Pancreatic Hormone	**Cell Type**	**Action**
Insulin	Beta	Glucose to glycogen
Glucagon	Alpha	Glycogen to glucose
Somatostatin	Delta	Alpha and beta inhibitor

TABLE 12-3	Laboratory Values for Pancreatic Disease
Condition	**Amylase Level**
Acute pancreatitis	Twice normal
Chronic pancreatitis	No change
Mumps, ischemic bowel disease, pelvic inflammatory disease	↑
Condition	**Lipase Level**
Acute pancreatitis	↑
Carcinoma of the pancreas	↑
Condition	**Blood Glucose Level**
Severe diabetes	↑
Chronic liver disease	↑
Overactive endocrine glands	↑
Tumor in islet of Langerhans	↓

↑, Increased; ↓, decreased.

Laboratory Tests

There are specific enzymes of the pancreas that may become altered in pancreatic disease, namely amylase and lipase. Increased glucose levels may indicate abnormalities of the pancreas (Table 12-3).

Amylase. Amylase is a digestive enzyme for carbohydrates. It is secreted by the pancreas, parotid glands, gynecologic system, and bowel. In certain types of pancreatic disease, the digestive enzymes of the pancreas escape into the surrounding tissue, producing necrosis with severe pain and inflammation. Under these circumstances there is an increase in **serum amylase.** A serum amylase level of twice normal usually indicates acute pancreatitis.

Other conditions that may cause an increase in amylase include chronic pancreatitis, obstruction of the pancreatic duct, perforated peptic ulcer, acute cholecystitis, and alcohol poisoning. Less common conditions include mumps, ischemic bowel disease, and pelvic inflammatory disease.

Urine Amylase. Urine amylase may be elevated in pancreatitis. Diseases not affecting the pancreas may cause the elevation of serum amylase without elevation of urine amylase.

Lipase. Lipase is an enzyme that is excreted specifically by the pancreas and that parallels the elevation in amylase levels. The lipase test is performed to assess damage to the pancreas. The pancreas secretes lipase, and small amounts pass into the blood. The lipase level rises in acute pancreatitis and in carcinoma of the pancreas. Both amylase and lipase rise at the same rate, but the elevation in lipase concentration persists for a longer period. Lipase may also be elevated with obstruction of the pancreatic duct, pancreatic carcinoma, and acute cholecystitis.

Glucose. Glucose controls the blood sugar level in the body. The glucose tolerance test is performed to discover whether there is a disorder of glucose metabolism. An increased blood glucose level is found in severe diabetes, chronic liver disease, and overactivity of several of the endocrine glands. There may be a decreased blood sugar level in tumors of the islets of Langerhans in the pancreas.

SONOGRAPHIC EVALUATION OF THE PANCREAS

The pancreas is one of the most difficult abdominal organs to image with sonography because it lies posterior to the stomach and sometimes the transverse colon. To help visualize the pancreas, the patient should fast 6 to 8 hours; this decreases the amount of air and fluid in the stomach and colon that may impede visualization. It also promotes dilation of the gallbladder and ducts. If fluid is administered to better visualize the gland, real-time visualization of peristaltic movement of food particles within the duodenum and stomach can be a useful landmark to help outline the head, body, and tail of the pancreas. This will be discussed in more detail later in the chapter.

Normal Pancreatic Texture

The echogenicity of the pancreas is discussed in terms of how it relates to the liver's homogeneous soft echo pattern. The normal pancreas has an echo pattern that is slightly more hyperechoic and finer in texture than that of the surrounding retroperitoneum. The echo intensity of the pancreas is usually slightly less than that of surrounding soft tissue and slightly greater than that of the liver.

The parenchymal texture of the pancreas depends on the amount of fat between the lobules and to a lesser extent on the interlobular fibrous tissue. The internal echoes of the pancreas consist of closely spaced elements of the same intensity with uniform distribution throughout the gland.

Fat is strongly echogenic, and the extensive fatty infiltrations of the pancreas are difficult to visualize by ultrasound because the pancreas blends in with the surrounding retroperitoneal fat. A lesser degree of fatty infiltration may not render the pancreas invisible but may raise the amplitude of returning pancreatic echoes, resulting in the clinical observation that the pancreas returns stronger echoes than the liver. Fibrous tissue may also account for the portion of increased echogenicity. Box 12-1 lists the sonographic characteristics of the normal pancreas.

Sonographic Scan Technique

The patient is usually examined in the supine, oblique, and sometimes upright positions. Sonographic techniques vary according to the patient's body habitus. For adult patients, use at least 3- to 5-megahertz (MHz) broadband transducer with a midfocal zone; for pediatric patients, use at least a 5- to 7.5-MHz transducer. The curved linear array transducer allows for a better near field of view than the sector transducer allows. The time gain compensation and overall gain should be adjusted so that the pancreatic tissue has the same echo brightness or slightly greater than the normal liver. The texture of the pancreas will appear coarser than the liver depending on the amount of fibrous/fatty tissue interfaces within the gland. The younger pediatric patients tend to have less echogenicity of the pancreas than the older patients do (i.e., more fatty interfaces in the gland of the older patient). The diabetic patient may be challenging to image through the fatty liver texture; therefore, a lower frequency transducer may be useful. With the patient in deep inspiration, gentle pressure on the abdomen with the transducer allows the sonographer to get as close as possible to the pancreatic tissue to improve visualization.

Box 12-2 summarizes the normal pancreatic landmarks. The sonographer should identify the head, neck, body, and tail in the transverse and longitudinal planes (Figures 12-8 and 12-9). The sonographer should evaluate the shape, contour, lie, and texture of the pancreas (as compared with the liver parenchyma). The oblique or upright position of the patient may improve visualization of the pancreas and peripancreatic region. The following surrounding structures should be identified: superior mesenteric artery and vein, portal and splenic veins, aorta and inferior vena cava, common bile duct, gastroduodenal artery, left renal vein, duodenal bulb, posterior wall of the stomach, and pancreatic duct.

Windows for Visualization. Difficulties in visualization of the pancreas may result from bowel gas, a transverse stomach obscuring the anatomy, or a small left lobe of the liver (Figure 12-10). A left lobe measuring at least 2 to 2.5 cm makes an excellent sonic window for imaging

the pancreatic area. The subcostal view can be used with a slight caudal angle of the transducer (15 to 20 degrees) as the transducer is directed from the midabdomen (at the level of the xiphoid process), through the left lobe of the liver, and angled through the pancreatic area with the prevertebral vessels demarcating its posterior border.

The patient should be in full inspiration to image the pancreas well. This causes the liver to be inferiorly displaced and provides a better scanning window. If the patient has a concave abdomen, ask the patient to take in a deep breath and push out the abdomen to provide a better scanning window.

If the sonographer is unable to image the pancreas, the water ingestion technique may be an effective window to image the gland. The initial scans of the biliary system should be made before asking the patient to drink 32 to 300 ml of fluid through a straw (to prevent swallowing of air) in the erect or right lateral decubitus position. In the upright position, the stomach can be used as a window; if the patient is unable to sit up, the examination can be done in the decubitus position. This water method fills the body and antrum of the stomach initially to help outline the body and tail of the pancreas (Figure 12-11). The fluid then fills the duodenal cap to outline the lateral margin of the head of the pancreas. The upright position allows the air to move from the gastric antrum to the fundus of the stomach and causes the upper viscera to move downward for a better sonic window. The upright position also results in distention of the venous structures, which further aids in the localization of the pancreas (see Box 12-2).

Transverse Plane. Generally the pancreas is imaged first in the transverse plane. The patient should be in full inspiration to distend the venous structures that serve as posterior landmarks to visualize the pancreas. As previously mentioned, the sonographer should use the left lobe of the liver at the level of the xiphoid and angle the transducer slightly toward the feet to image the aorta and celiac axis. This is near the superior border of the pancreas (remember that the tortuous splenic artery may be seen rising from the celiac axis to demarcate the superior border of the pancreas) (Figure 12-12). The body and tail of the gland should be imaged as the transducer

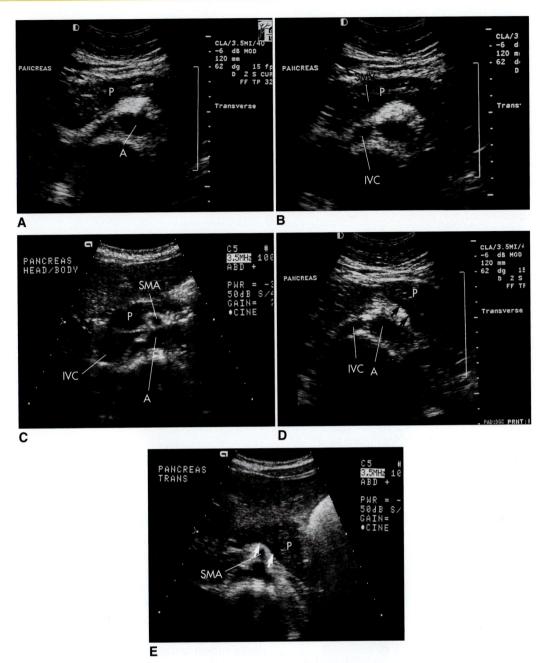

FIGURE 12-8 Transverse images of the pancreas *(P)*. **A,** Body and tail of the pancreas drape anterior to the aorta *(A)*. **B,** Head, body, and tail of the pancreas shown anterior to aorta, superior mesenteric vein *(SMV)*, and inferior vena cava *(IVC)*. **C,** The superior mesenteric artery *(SMA)*, aorta *(A)*, and inferior vena cava *(IVC)* are posterior borders to the pancreas. **D,** The splenic vein outlines the posterior border of the tail of the pancreas *(arrows)*. **E,** The SMA and splenic vein *(arrows)* outline the posterior border of the tail of the pancreas.

is slowly angled inferiorly from the celiac axis. Visualization of the superior mesenteric vessels, left renal vein, and inferior vena cava also helps delineate the borders of the body of the pancreas (Figure 12-13). The stomach may be seen as the walls are collapsed because it lies anterior to the pancreas (Figure 12-14). The duodenum, gastroduodenal artery, and common bile duct are useful landmarks in identifying the lateral margin of the pancreatic head (Figure 12-15). The sonographer may watch for peristalsis or fluid to pass through the second part of

the duodenum as it forms the C-loop around the lateral border of the head.

Sagittal Plane. The initial scan should be made slightly to the right of midline with the patient in full inspiration. The dilated inferior vena cava is seen as the posterior border (Figure 12-16). The main portal vein or right branch of the portal vein is the next landmark seen anterior to the cava. The pancreas lies just inferior to the portal vein and anterior to the inferior vena cava. As the pancreas enlarges, a slight indentation is apparent on

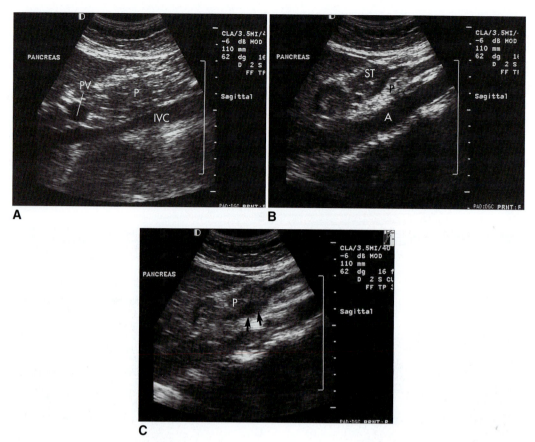

FIGURE 12-9 Sagittal images of the pancreas *(P)*. **A,** The pancreas lies inferior to the portal vein *(PV)* and anterior to the inferior vena cava *(IVC)*. **B,** The stomach *(ST)* is anterior to the pancreas. The aorta *(A)* is the posterior border. **C,** A small segment of the superior mesenteric vein *(arrows)* is seen along the posterior border of the neck of the pancreas.

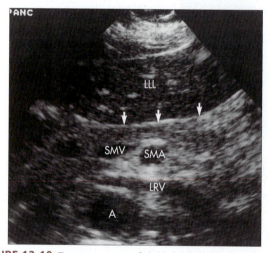

FIGURE 12-10 Transverse scan of the left lobe of liver *(LLL)*. If the left lobe measures at least 2 to 3 cm, it may serve as an ideal window to visualize the pancreas posterior *(arrows)*. *A,* Aorta; *LRV,* left renal vein; *SMA,* superior mesenteric artery; *SMV,* superior mesenteric vein.

the anterior border of the cava. This view is also good for visualizing the common bile duct because it lies anterior to the portal vein before dropping posterior to enter the head of the pancreas (Figure 12-17). The hepatic artery is sometimes visible as a circular tube when the

common duct is seen (Figure 12-18). The use of color Doppler may help the sonographer separate the hepatic artery from the common duct.

Subsequent scans are made slightly to the left of the midline to image the aorta and superior mesenteric artery and vein because they form the posterior border of the body of the pancreas. The superior mesenteric vein flows cephalad to join the portal vein and may be seen as a long, tubular structure posterior to the neck of the pancreas and anterior to the uncinate process (Figure 12-19). The tail of the pancreas is more difficult to see, but it may be imaged as the sonographer angles slightly to the left of the aorta. The patient may be rolled into a steep right decubitus position to image the tail of the gland as it lies in the hilum of the spleen near the left kidney.

The antrum of the stomach appears as a collapsed bull's-eye and may be identified anterior and slightly caudal to the body of the pancreas (Figure 12-20). The splenic vein is a circular sonolucent structure posterior to the cephalic portion of the gland (Figure 12-21). The left renal vein is a slitlike sonolucency between the aorta and the superior mesenteric artery.

Pancreatic Duct. The main pancreatic duct may be visualized best on the transverse image as it courses through the body of the gland (Figure 12-22). The sonographer should be sure to identify pancreatic tissue

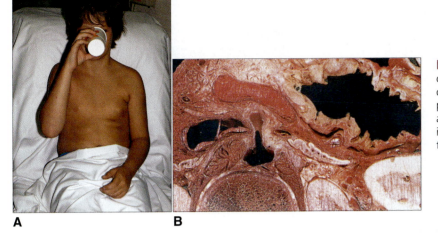

FIGURE 12-11 A, To better visualize the pancreas, the patient should drink more than 16 ounces of water and be imaged in the semiupright position. **B,** Gross anatomy of the midepigastrium at the level of the SMA. The body of the pancreas is clearly seen anterior to the SMA and posterior to the stomach.

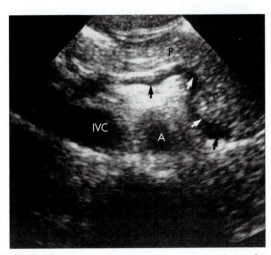

FIGURE 12-12 The tortuous splenic artery *(arrows)* rises from the celiac axis. The pancreas is usually inferior to the splenic artery; however, in this patient the gland is shown anterior to the vessel. *A,* Aorta; *IVC,* inferior vena cava; *P,* pancreas.

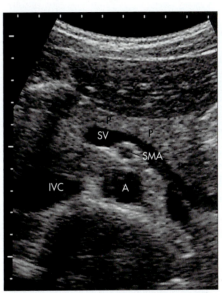

FIGURE 12-13 Transverse scan of the normal pancreas and its vascular landmarks. *A,* Aorta; *IVC,* inferior vena cava; *P,* pancreas; *SMA,* superior mesenteric artery; *SV,* splenic vein.

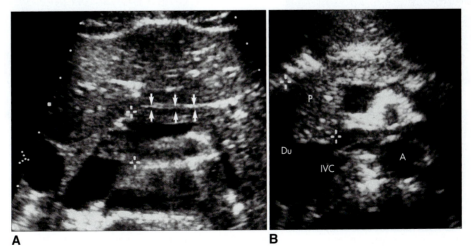

FIGURE 12-14 A, The collapsed wall of the stomach *(arrows)* may be seen as two parallel lines anterior to the body of the pancreas. **B,** The fluid-filled duodenum *(Du)* marks the lateral border of the head of the pancreas *(P)*. *A,* Aorta; *IVC,* inferior vena cava.

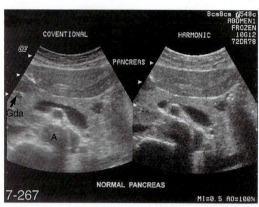

FIGURE 12-15 The small gastroduodenal artery *(Gda)* is the anterolateral border of the head of the pancreas. *A,* Aorta.

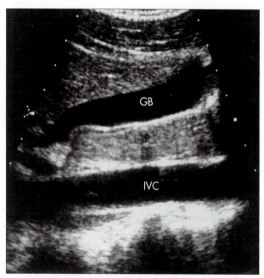

FIGURE 12-16 Sagittal oblique scan of the dilated inferior vena cava *(IVC)* as it demarcates the posterior border of the pancreas *(P).* The gallbladder *(GB)* is seen anterior.

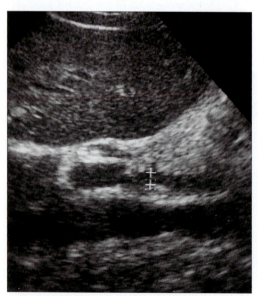

FIGURE 12-17 The common bile duct *(markers)* is seen along the posterior border of the pancreas with the patient in a decubitus position.

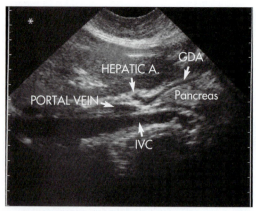

FIGURE 12-18 Sagittal scan of the pancreas and its surrounding vascular landmarks. *GDA,* Gastroduodenal artery; *IVC,* inferior vena cava.

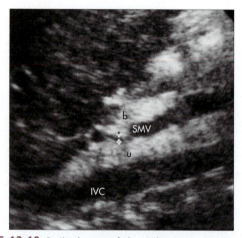

FIGURE 12-19 Sagittal scan of the right upper quadrant shows the superior mesenteric vein *(SMV)* as it flows anterior to the uncinate process *(u)* and posterior to the body *(b)* of the pancreas. *IVC,* Inferior vena cava.

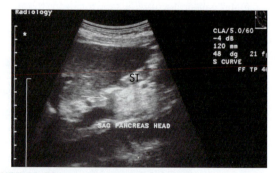

FIGURE 12-20 The collapsed antrum of the stomach *(ST)* is seen as a target lesion anterior to the body of the pancreas.

on both sides of the duct so as not to confuse it with vascular structures that may lie near it. The splenic vein is usually too posterior and the hepatic artery too anterior to be confused with the duct. Color Doppler may be used to help distinguish a dilated duct from vascular structures. The duct appears as an echo-free area sharply

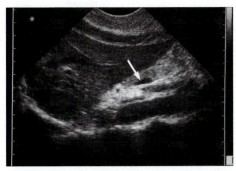

FIGURE 12-21 The splenic vein is seen as a circle on the sagittal plane as it flows along the posteromedial border of the pancreas *(arrow)*.

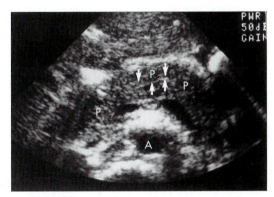

FIGURE 12-22 The pancreatic duct is seen as two parallel lines *(arrows)* within the center of the pancreas *(P)*. *A,* Aorta.

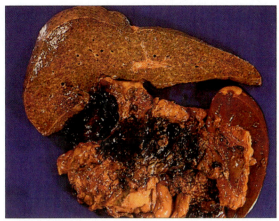

FIGURE 12-23 Gross pathology of acute hemorrhagic pancreatitis. The pancreas has been completely obliterated by blood.

marginated by two parallel echogenic lines. A thin strip of retroperitoneal fat may underlie the anterior aspect of the pancreas. This sonolucent linear pattern should not be mistaken for duct. On transverse scans, the posterior wall of the antrum can be seen overlying the pancreas. Care should be taken to distinguish the antrum of the collapsed stomach from the small pancreatic duct.

PATHOLOGY OF THE PANCREAS

Pancreatitis

Pancreatitis is inflammation of the pancreas. It may be chronic or acute. Pancreatitis occurs when the pancreas becomes damaged and malfunctions as a result of increased secretion and blockage of ducts. When this occurs, the pancreatic tissue may be digested by its own enzymes. Pancreatitis may be classified as acute or chronic with a further subdescription of mild to severe. In patients with acute pancreatitis, ultrasound may not always be the first imaging performed because often ileus is associated with this condition. Therefore, the optimal imaging procedure is the dynamic intravenous and oral contrast-enhanced computed tomography. See Table 12-4 for clinical findings, sonographic findings, and differential considerations for pancreatitis.

Acute Pancreatitis. Acute pancreatitis is an inflammation of the pancreas caused by the inflamed acini releasing pancreatic enzymes into the surrounding pancreatic tissue. Normally these enzymes do not become active until they reach the duodenum where they enable the breakdown of food in the system. The acute process of pancreatitis usually does not last more than several days. The patient may be at risk for abscess and hemorrhage secondary to the pancreatitis (Figure 12-23).

An acute attack of pancreatitis is commonly related to biliary tract disease and alcoholism. The most common cause of pancreatitis in the United States is biliary tract disease. Gallstones are present in 40% to 60% of patients, and 5% of patients with gallstones have acute pancreatitis. Gallstone pancreatitis causes a relatively sudden onset of constant biliary pain. As the pancreatic parenchyma is further damaged, the pain becomes more severe and the abdomen becomes rigid and tender.

Alcohol abuse is the second most common cause of pancreatitis. Other less common causes include trauma, inflammation from adjacent peptic ulcer or abdominal infection, pregnancy, mumps, tumors, congenital causes, vascular thrombosis or embolism, and drugs.

The laboratory analysis of pancreatic enzymes (protease, lipase, and elastase) is the key to pancreatic destruction (see Table 12-4).

Acute pancreatitis may be mild to severe (Figure 12-24). Damage to the acinar tissue and ductal system results either in exudation of pancreatic juice into the gland's interstitium, leakage of secretions into the peripancreatic tissues, or both. After the acini or duct disrupts, the secretions migrate to the surface of the gland. The common course is for fluid to break through the pancreatic connective tissue layer and thin posterior layer of the peritoneum and enter the lesser sac. The mild form of pancreatitis demonstrates interstitial edema within the gland with little or no peripancreatic inflammation. There may be small areas of acinar cell necrosis within the pancreas. As the process becomes more severe,

TABLE 12-4	Pancreatitis Findings		
Clinical Findings	**Sonographic Findings**		**Differential Considerations**
Acute Pancreatitis			
• Sudden onset of moderate to severe abdominal pain with radiation to back • Nausea and vomiting • History of gallstones (localized) or alcoholism • Mild fever • ↑ Pancreatic enzymes in blood (amylase, lipase) • Leukocytosis (↑ white blood cells) • Abdominal distention	• Ranges from normal size to focal/diffuse enlargement • Hypoechoic texture (edema) • Borders distinct but irregular • Enlargement of head causes depression on inferior vena cava • 40% to 60% have gallstones • Pancreatic duct may be enlarged • Parapancreatic fluid collections		• Hemorrhagic pancreatitis • Pancreatic neoplasm • Lymphoma • Retroperitoneal neoplasm
Hemorrhagic Pancreatitis			
• ↓ Hematocrit and serum calcium level • Intense, severe pain radiating to back, with subsequent shock and ileus • Hypotension despite volume replacement, with metabolic acidosis and adult respiratory distress syndrome	• Depends on age of hemorrhage • Well-defined homogeneous mass in area of pancreas		• Chronic hemorrhage
Phlegmonous Pancreatitis			
See *Acute pancreatitis*	• Hypoechoic, ill-defined mass		• Chronic hemorrhage
Pancreatic Abscess			
• Fever, chills • ↑ Leukocytosis • Hypotension • Tender abdomen	• Hypoechoic mass with smooth borders • Thick walls • Echo-free to echogenic		• Acute pancreatitis • Chronic pancreatitis
Chronic Pancreatitis			
• Severe abdominal pain radiating to back • Malabsorption • Fatty stools • Signs of diabetes • Weight loss • Jaundice • ↑ Amylase and lipase	• Gland is small and fibrotic • Irregular borders • Mixed echogenicity • Dilated pancreatic duct (string of pearls sign with dilated duct) • Look for calculi within duct		• Acute pancreatitis • Thrombosis of portal system • Pancreatic pseudocyst • Dilated common bile duct
Pancreatic Pseudocyst			
• Asymptomatic unless large enough to put pressure on other organs • ↑ Amylase and lipase • ↑ Alkaline phosphatase if obstruction develops	• Well-defined mass, usually in area of pancreas • ↑ Through-transmission • Variable size (round or oval) • May have debris at bottom		• True cyst • Fluid-filled cystadenoma

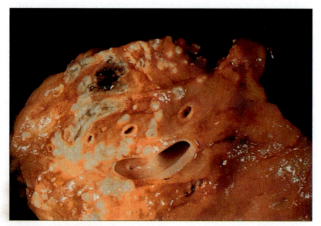

FIGURE 12-24 Gross pathology of acute pancreatitis. The foci of fat necrosis appear as white opaque patches.

fat necrosis, parenchymal necrosis, and necrosis of the blood vessels develops with subsequent hemorrhage and peripancreatic inflammation within 1 to 2 days. With time, this necrotic tissue is replaced by diffuse or focal fibrosis, calcifications, and irregular ductal dilations. The formation of a pseudocyst may develop secondary to acute pancreatitis.

The pancreatic juice enters the anterior pararenal space by breaking through the thin layer of the fibrous connective tissue, or the fluid may migrate to the surface of the gland and remain within the confines of the fibrous connective tissue layer.

Collections of fluid in the peripancreatic area generally retain communication with the pancreas. A dynamic equilibrium is established so that fluid is continuously

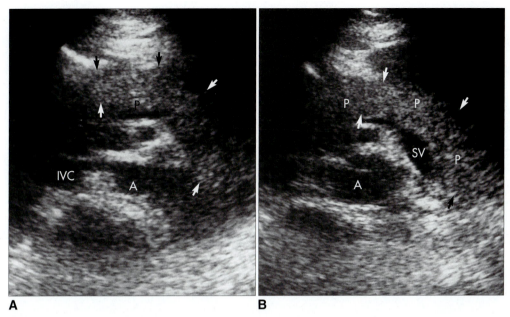

FIGURE 12-25 A 45-year-old male presented with midepigastric pain, elevated amylase and lipase levels, and tenderness. The pancreas is diffusely enlarged representing acute pancreatitis. **A, B,** Transverse scans over the upper abdomen show the inflamed pancreatic tissue. *A,* Aorta; *IVC,* inferior vena cava; *P,* pancreas; *SV,* splenic vein.

absorbed from the collection and replaced by additional pancreatic secretions. The drainage of juices may cease as the pancreatic inflammatory response subsides and the rate of pancreatic secretions returns to normal. The collections of extrapancreatic fluid should be reabsorbed or, if drained, should not recur with recovery of proper drainage through the duct.

The symptoms begin with severe pain that usually occurs after a large meal or alcohol binge. The serum amylase value increases within 24 hours, whereas the serum lipase value increases within 72 to 96 hours and remains elevated for a period of time. (Note that the serum lipase takes a longer time to elevate but remains elevated longer than the serum amylase value.) The disease may be mild and respond to medical therapy or it may progress to multisystem failure. Patients with acute pancreatitis may go on to develop other complications, such as pseudocyst formation (10%), phlegmon (18%), abscess (1% to 9%), hemorrhage (5%), or duodenal obstruction.

Sonographic Findings. The sonographic description of acute pancreatitis may be defined by distribution (focal or diffuse) and by severity (mild, moderate, or severe). In the early stages of acute pancreatitis the gland may not show swelling on sonography (Figure 12-25). When swelling does occur, the gland is hypoechoic to anechoic and is less echoic than the liver because of the increased prominence of lobulations and congested vessels (Figure 12-26). The borders may be somewhat indistinct but smooth. On a longitudinal scan, the anterior compression of the inferior vena cava by the swollen head of the pancreas may be apparent. Thus pancreatic

enlargement and decreased pancreatic echogenicity are sonographic landmarks for acute pancreatitis.

If localized enlargement is present, it may be difficult to separate from neoplastic involvement of the gland (Figure 12-27). Analysis of patient history and laboratory values should enable the clinician to make the distinction. If the serum amylase level is normal and the patient is asymptomatic, the mass is likely to represent a neoplasm. However, if the patient has severe abdominal pain, tender to the touch, this focal hypoechogenicity is more likely caused by pancreatitis than by a neoplastic growth. If the mass has calcification within an enlarged ductal system, a neoplasm is more likely suspected. The evaluation by ERCP may provide better resolution of the pancreatic head and ductal system to further delineate neoplastic growth from pancreatitis.

The pancreatic duct may be obstructed in acute pancreatitis as a result of inflammation, spasm, edema, swelling of the papilla, or pseudocyst formation. The detection of biliary obstruction is important as so many of the patients have coexisting liver disease. Obstruction of the biliary system may be due to stricture in the distal common duct or to compression of the common bile duct by a pseudocyst or inflammation of the head of the pancreas.

The alteration in the size and echogenic texture of the pancreas may be subtle; therefore, the diagnosis of pancreatitis may be based on the visualization of peripancreatic fluid collections in a patient with abnormal pancreatic enzymes and clinical history suggestive of pancreatitis. Fluid collections around the pancreatic bed, along the pararenal spaces, within Morison's pouch, and

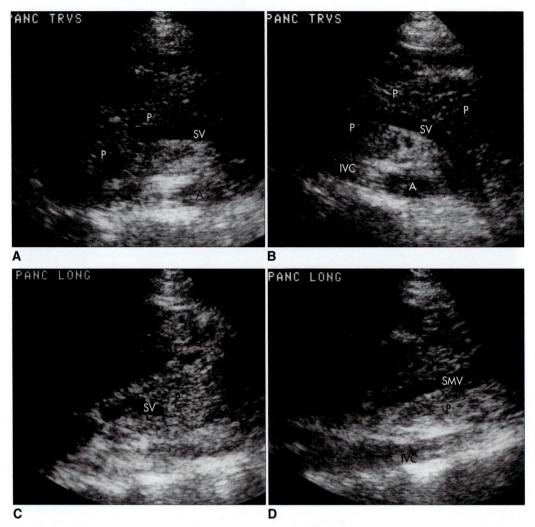

FIGURE 12-26 A 29-year-old female presented with back pain, nausea, and vomiting for 1 week, and elevated lipase. The pancreas was found to be diffusely enlarged with decreased echogenicity representing pancreatitis. **A, B,** Transverse images. *A,* Aorta; *IVC,* inferior vena cava; *P,* pancreas; *SV,* splenic vein. **C, D,** Sagittal images. *IVC,* Inferior vena cava; *P,* pancreas; *SMV,* superior mesenteric vein; *SV,* splenic vein.

around the duodenum may be present in a patient with acute pancreatitis.

In diffuse pancreatitis, the pancreas enlarges and the texture becomes hypoechogenic when compared with the "normal" liver texture. Because alcohol is a frequent cause of pancreatitis, the development of a hyperechoic diffuse fatty liver makes this comparison invalid. As the disease progresses, the decreased echogenicity and enlargement are readily seen secondary to increased fluid content in the interstitium caused by the inflammation. The pancreas may be diffusely inhomogeneous. The pancreatic duct may be either compressed by the edema or dilated (from the focal pancreatic inflammation or obstruction of the stone or tumor).

Sonography is not as effective as CT in the early stages of pancreatitis, as CT is more specific in its ability to demonstrate the detail of the pancreas and the retroperitoneal structures, regardless of bowel interference. CT can detect necrosis and acute fracture of the pancreas. Sonographic detection of pancreatitis is effective when

ileus is not present to obstruct the visualization of the pancreatic area.

Complications of acute pancreatitis include hemorrhage, pseudocyst formation, inflammatory mass, and intrapancreatic and extrapancreatic fluid collections. Sonography may directly guide the interventionalist for needle aspiration to help differentiate between an infected and noninfected inflammatory mass and pseudocyst collection.

Acute Pancreatitis in Children. The pediatric pancreas is more easily seen because there is less body fat to interfere with visualization (Figure 12-28). Often the left lobe of the liver is more prominent and the gland is more isotonic than hyperechoic. In acute pancreatitis, the gland is increased in size with a hypoechoic pattern and an indistinct outline.

Extrapancreatic Fluid Collections and Edema. The findings of fluid collections and edema are frequent in patients with severe acute pancreatitis. The most common sites for fluid collection are found in the lesser sac,

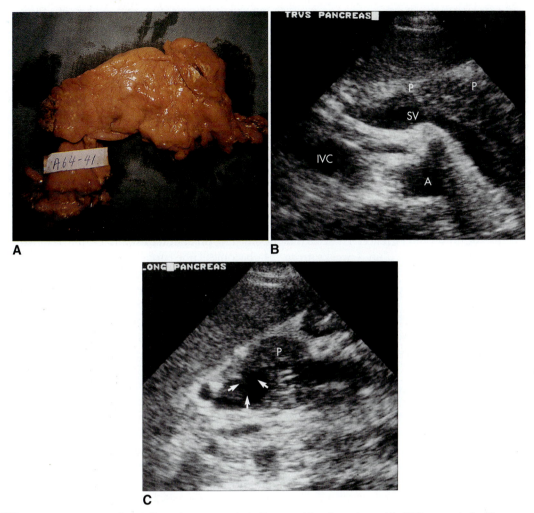

FIGURE 12-27 A, Gross specimen of an inflamed pancreas. **B,** A 37-year-old male patient with AIDS presented with pancreatitis, hepato-splenomegaly, and peripancreatic adenopathy. The pancreas is enlarged and slightly hypoechoic. *A,* Aorta; *IVC,* inferior vena cava; *P,* pancreas; *SV,* splenic vein. **C,** Sagittal scan of the enlarged pancreas *(P)* with adenopathy *(arrows).*

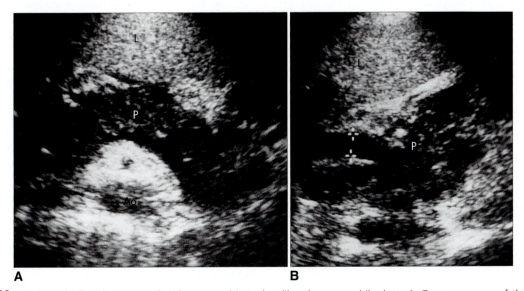

FIGURE 12-28 A 9-year-old female presented with pancreatitis and a dilated common bile duct. **A,** Transverse scan of the pancreas *(P),* liver *(L),* and aorta *(Ao).* **B,** Sagittal scan of the dilated common bile duct *(calipers)* as it enters the pancreas *(P). L,* Liver.

anterior pararenal spaces, mesocolon, perirenal spaces, and peripancreatic soft tissue spaces. For the sonographer, the fluid in the lesser sac that is found between the stomach and the pancreas is easily imaged. Fluid in the superior recess of the lesser sac is seen to surround the caudate lobe with visualization of the gastrohepatic ligament. Fluid that lies in the perirenal space may also be demonstrated on sonography. As fluid collects in the anterior pararenal space, it is best demonstrated on the sagittal sonographic image. The fluid may be anechoic or contain fine linear lines within that represent septations secondary to infection or hemorrhage. The more solid composition of the retroperitoneal or intraperitoneal fluid collections is most difficult to image with sonography because of bowel interference. These extrapancreatic fluid collections occur within 4 weeks from the acute onset of the pancreatitis and may resolve spontaneously. The formation of a pseudocyst occurs when the fluid collection develops into a well-defined, walled-off fluid collection of amylase. Other sonographic findings may include ascites, thickened wall of the gallbladder, and thickening of the adjacent gastrointestinal tract.

Complications of Pancreatitis

Pancreatic Pseudocysts. Pancreatic and parapancreatic fluid collections are most often complications of pancreatitis. These fluid collections may resolve spontaneously, but those that do not are recognized as pseudocysts on imaging studies when the well-defined wall becomes visible. Pseudocysts are always acquired; they result from trauma to the gland or acute or chronic pancreatitis (see Table 12-4). In approximately 10% to 20% of patients with acute pancreatitis, a pseudocyst develops. A **pseudocyst** may be defined as a collection of fluid that arises from the loculation of inflammatory processes, necrosis, or hemorrhage (Figure 12-29). The pseudocyst usually develops over four to six weeks after the onset of pancreatitis. The pancreatic enzymes that escape the ductal system cause enzymatic digestion of the surrounding tissue and pseudocyst development. The walls of the pseudocyst form in the various potential spaces in which the escaped pancreatic enzymes are found.

A **pancreatic pseudocyst** develops when pancreatic enzymes escape from the gland and break down tissue to form a sterile abscess somewhere in the abdomen. Its walls are not true cyst walls; hence the name *pseudo-*, or false, cyst. Pseudocysts generally take on the contour of the available space around them and therefore are not always spherical, as are normal cysts. There may be more than one pseudocyst, so the sonographer should search for daughter collections.

The pseudocyst usually creates few symptoms until it becomes large enough to cause pressure on the surrounding organs. Pseudocysts usually develop through the lesser omentum, displacing the stomach or widening the duodenal loop. Although the most common association of pseudocyst development is in patients with alcoholic or biliary disease, it may also develop after blunt trauma or secondary to pancreatic malignancy. Clinically the patient may present with a history of pancreatitis, persistent pain, and elevated amylase levels.

Locations of a Pseudocyst. The most common location of a pseudocyst is in the lesser sac anterior to the pancreas and posterior to the stomach. The second most common location is in the anterior pararenal space (posterior to the lesser sac, bounded by Gerota's fascia). The spleen is the lateral border of the anterior pararenal space on the left. Fluid occurs more commonly in the left pararenal space than the right. Sometimes the posterior pararenal space is fluid-filled; fluid spreads from the anterior pararenal space to the posterior pararenal space on the same side. Fluid may enter the peritoneal cavity via the foramen of Winslow or by disrupting the peritoneum in the anterior surface of the lesser sac. It may extend into the mediastinum by extending through the esophageal or aortic hiatus, or it may extend into small bowel mesentery or down into the retroperitoneum into the pelvis and groin.

Sonographic Findings. Sonographically, pseudocysts usually appear as well-defined masses with essentially sonolucent, echo-free interiors. Debris seen within the collection may occur from complications of infection or hemorrhage; scattered echoes may be seen at the bottom of the cysts, and increased through-transmission is present (Figure 12-30). The borders are very echogenic, and the cysts usually are thicker than other simple cysts. Calcification may develop within the walls of the pseudocyst. When a suspected pseudocyst is located near the stomach, the stomach should be drained so the cyst is not mistaken for a fluid-filled stomach. If the patient has been on continual drainage before the ultrasound examination, this problem is eliminated.

Unusual Sonographic Patterns. A series of pseudocysts have been found to contain unusual internal echoes

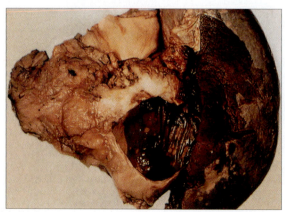

FIGURE 12-29 Gross pathology of pancreatic pseudocyst filled with hemorrhagic fluid in the tail with extension into the hilum of the spleen.

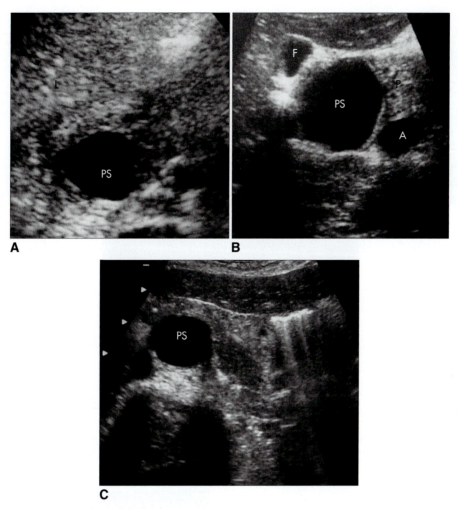

FIGURE 12-30 A-C, Ultrasound patterns of a typical pancreatic pseudocyst. *A*, Aorta; *F*, fluid; *L*, liver; *P*, pancreas; *PS*, pseudocyst.

(Figure 12-31). There were three classifications: (1) septated, which presents with multiple internal septations; (2) excessive internal echoes, caused by an associated inflammatory mass, hemorrhage, or clot formation; and (3) pseudocyst, with absence of posterior enhancement caused by the rim of calcification.

Spontaneous Rupture of a Pseudocyst. Spontaneous rupture is the most common complication of a pancreatic pseudocyst, occurring in 5% of patients. In 3% of these patients, drainage is directly into the peritoneal cavity. Clinical symptoms are sudden shock and peritonitis. The mortality rate is 50%. **Pancreatic ascites** occurs when the pancreatic pseudocyst ruptures into the abdomen. Pancreatic ascites that develops as a consequence of spontaneous rupture may be differentiated from pancreatic ascites associated with cirrhosis in patients who have known rupture of a pseudocyst by analysis of the fluid for elevated amylase and protein content (Figure 12-32).

In 2% of patients, the rupture is into the gastrointestinal tract. Such patients may present a confusing picture sonographically. The initial scan shows a typical pattern for a pseudocyst formation, but the patient may have

intense pain develop secondary to the rupture, and consequent examination shows the disappearance of the mass.

Other complications may include erosion of the pseudocyst into adjacent vascular structures with resultant intracystic hemorrhage or formation of a pseudoaneurysm. Hemorrhage may occur with a subsequent pancreatic abscess and severe necrotizing pancreatitis without pseudocyst formation.

Hemorrhagic Pancreatitis. Hemorrhagic pancreatitis is a rapid progression of acute pancreatitis with rupture of pancreatic vessels and subsequent hemorrhage (see Table 12-4). In hemorrhagic pancreatitis, there is diffuse enzymatic destruction of the pancreatic substance caused by a sudden escape of active pancreatic enzymes into the glandular parenchyma (Figure 12-33). These enzymes cause focal areas of fat necrosis in and around the pancreas, which leads to rupture of pancreatic vessels and hemorrhage. Nearly half of these patients have sudden necrotizing destruction of the pancreas after an alcoholic binge or an excessively large meal.

Sonographic Findings. Specific sonographic findings depend on the age of the hemorrhage. A well-defined

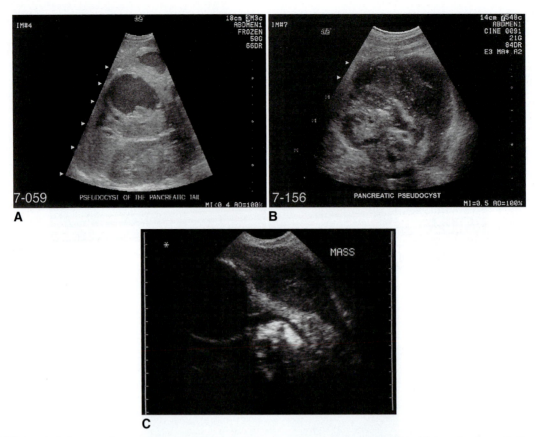

A 7-059 PSEUDOCYST OF THE PANCREATIC TAIL

B 7-156 PANCREATIC PSEUDOCYST

C

FIGURE 12-31 Atypical ultrasound patterns of a pancreatic pseudocyst. **A,** Septations with low-level internal echoes. **B,** Excessive internal echoes. **C,** Calcification around the rim.

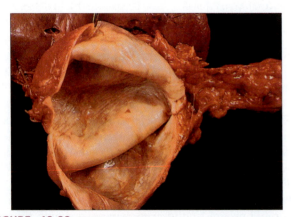

FIGURE 12-32 Gross pathology of a pancreatic pseudocyst rupture.

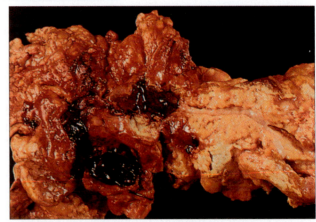

FIGURE 12-33 Gross pathology of acute hemorrhagic pancreatitis. Hemorrhagic fat necrosis and a pseudocyst filled with blood are seen on cross section.

homogeneous mass in the area of the pancreas may be seen with areas of fresh necrosis (Figure 12-34). Foci of extravasated blood and fat necrosis are also seen. Further necrosis of the blood vessels results in the development of hemorrhagic areas referred to as Grey Turner's sign (discoloration of the flanks). At 1 week, the mass may appear cystic with solid elements or septation. After several weeks the hemorrhage may appear cystic.

Phlegmonous Pancreatitis. A phlegmon is an inflammatory process that spreads along fascial pathways, causing localized areas of diffuse inflammatory edema of soft tissue that may proceed to necrosis and suppuration. Extension outside the gland occurs in 18% to 20% of patients with acute pancreatitis.

▶ **Sonographic Findings.** The phlegmonous tissue appears hypoechoic with good through-transmission (Figure 12-35). The phlegmon usually involves the lesser

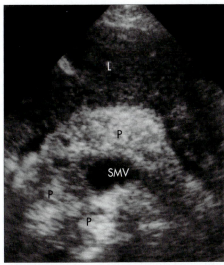

FIGURE 12-34 Pancreatitis with hemorrhage. The gland is enlarged and echogenic secondary to freshly clotted blood. *L,* Liver; *P,* pancreas; *SMV,* superior mesenteric vein.

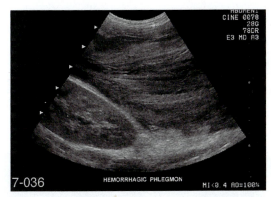

FIGURE 12-35 Hemorrhagic phlegmon is a complication of pancreatitis. The phlegmon is ill defined as it lies anterior to the kidney.

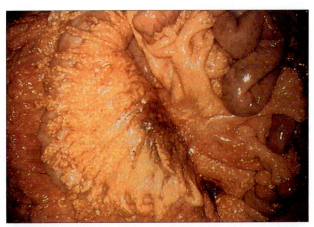

FIGURE 12-36 Gross pathology of peritonitis complicating acute pancreatitis. The mesentery shows foci of fat necrosis and hemorrhage. Bloody ascites has already been removed.

sac, left anterior pararenal space, and transverse mesocolon. Less commonly, it involves the small bowel mesentery, lower retroperitoneum, and pelvis. See Table 12-4 for sonographic findings and differential considerations for phlegmonous pancreatitis.

Pancreatic Abscess. Pancreatic abscess has a low incidence, although it is a serious complication of pancreatitis; the condition is related to the degree of tissue necrosis (see Table 12-4). The majority of patients develop abscess secondary to pancreatitis that develops from postoperative procedures. A very high mortality rate is associated with this condition if left untreated. An abscess may rise from a neighboring infection, such as a perforated peptic ulcer, acute appendicitis, or acute cholecystitis. A pancreatic abscess may be unilocular or multilocular and can spread superiorly into the mediastinum, inferiorly into the transverse mesocolon, or down the retroperitoneum into the pelvis (Figure 12-36). Acute peritonitis may develop as the pseudocyst ruptures into the peritoneal cavity.

Sonographic Findings. A pancreatic abscess is imaged on ultrasound as a poorly defined hypoechoic mass with smooth or irregular thick walls, causing few internal echoes; it may be echo-free to echodense. The sonographic appearance depends on the amount of debris present. If air bubbles are present, an echogenic region with a shadow posterior is imaged. A pseudocyst that forms during acute necrotizing pancreatitis has a higher likelihood of spontaneous regression, whereas a pseudocyst that forms secondary to chronic pancreatitis and develops calcification in its walls usually does not resolve on its own.

Chronic Pancreatitis. Chronic pancreatitis results from recurrent attacks of acute pancreatitis and causes continuing destruction of the pancreatic parenchyma (see Table 12-4). It generally is associated with chronic alcoholism or biliary disease, although patients with **hypercalcemia** (elevated calcium levels) and **hyperlipidemia** (elevated fat levels) are more predisposed to chronic pancreatitis. In chronic alcoholic pancreatitis, the alcoholic intake causes increased pancreatic protein secretion with subsequent ductal obstruction resulting in chronic calcifying pancreatitis. The fibrous connective tissue rapidly grows around the ducts and between the lobules with resultant scarring that leads to a nodular, irregular surface of the pancreas. The pancreatic ducts become obstructed with a build-up of protein plugs with resultant calcifications along the duct. The less common type is chronic obstructive pancreatitis with a nonlobular distribution, less ductal epithelial damage, and rarely calcified stones. This form is usually caused by stenosis of the sphincter of Oddi by cholelithiasis or pancreatic tumor.

Patients with chronic pancreatitis may have pseudocysts (25% to 40%), a dilated common bile duct, or thrombosis of the splenic vein with extension into the portal vein. Patients with chronic pancreatitis have an increased risk of developing pancreatic cancer.

On pathologic examination, the pancreas shows an increase in the interlobular fibrous tissue and chronic inflammatory infiltration changes. Stones of calcium carbonate may be found inside the ductal system, and pseudocysts are common (Figure 12-37). There is calcification of the gland in 20% to 40% of the patients.

◀ Sonographic Findings. Chronic pancreatitis on ultrasound appears as a mixed pattern. The tissue may appear as a diffuse or localized involvement of the gland (Figure 12-38). Echogenicity of the pancreas is increased beyond normal because of fibrotic and fatty changes, with a mixture of hypoechoic (from inflammation) and hyper-echoic foci. The size of the gland is reduced and the borders are irregular, and the pancreatic duct may be irregular and dilated secondary to stricture or as the result of an extrinsic stone moving from a smaller pancreatic duct into a major duct. The classic sonographic finding is calcifications. With pancreatic ductal lithiasis, shadowing may be present, with the most common site of obstruction at the papilla. Generally speaking, chronic pancreatitis is more highly suspected when the duct contains calcification and no obstructing mass lesion is seen, whereas carcinoma is suggested when a parenchymal mass lesion is identified at the site of obstruction of the pancreatic duct.

A focal mass or enlargement may be seen in the pancreas secondary to perilobular scarring with edema and inflammation. The presence of calcification is useful to differentiate such focal enlargements from neoplasms. Pseudocysts over 5 cm in size that persist beyond 6 weeks require decompression with significant risk of complications. Decompression may also be required in smaller pseudocysts that compress adjacent structures to cause persistent symptoms or if significant complications arise such as infection, hemorrhage, or perforation.

Cystic Lesions of the Pancreas

A wide variety of cystic lesions of the pancreas may be seen on imaging studies of the abdomen, but pseudocysts

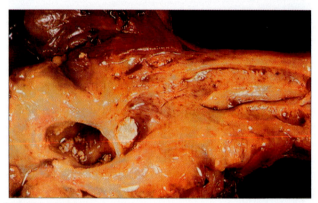

FIGURE 12-37 Gross pathology of chronic pancreatitis. The main pancreatic duct is dilated and contains calculi. The pancreatic acini have been replaced by fibrous tissue.

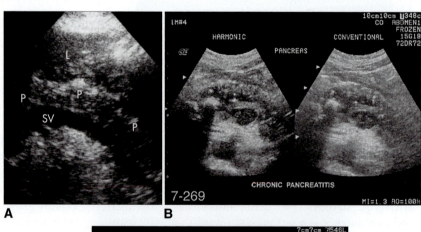

FIGURE 12-38 Ultrasound patterns in chronic pancreatitis. **A,** Calcifications are seen along the body of the pancreas *(P)*. *L,* Liver; *SV,* splenic vein. **B,** The pancreas is shrunken in size. **C,** The pancreatic duct is enlarged.

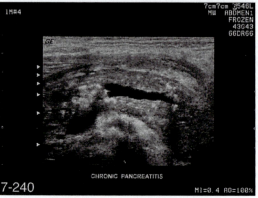

TABLE 12-5 | **Congenital Pancreatic Lesions**

Clinical Findings	Sonographic Findings	Differential Considerations
Autosomal Dominant Polycystic Kidney Diseases		
• Asymptomatic, often found in patients with polycystic renal disease	• Well-defined mass with serous fluid • Size varies from microscopic to several centimeters	• Pseudocyst • Other cystic lesions of the pancreas
Von Hippel-Lindau Disease		
• Asymptomatic • Patients may have central nervous system and retinal hemangioblastomas, visceral cysts, pheochromocytomas, and renal cell carcinoma	• Well-defined mass with thick fluid; calcifications • Single or multiple • Size varies from microscopic to several centimeters	• Pseudocyst • Other cystic lesions of the pancreas
Cystic Fibrosis		
• Asymptomatic	• Well-defined mass with serous fluid • Size varies from microscopic to several centimeters	• Pseudocyst • Other cystic lesions of the pancreas
True Pancreatic Cysts		
• Asymptomatic, often found in infants	• Well-defined mass with serous fluid • Unilocular or multilocular	• Pseudocyst • Other cystic lesions of the pancreas

are the most common. Cystic neoplasms may be misdiagnosed as pseudocysts if careful analysis of the clinical history is not obtained. Ultrasound, CT, MRI, and ERCP are imaging modalities that are used to help narrow the differential diagnosis to aid the clinician in arriving at a diagnosis when correlated with clinical, pathologic, and laboratory findings. See Table 12-5 for clinical findings, sonographic findings, and differential considerations for pancreatic cysts.

Multiple Pancreatic Cysts

Autosomal Dominant Polycystic Disease. Extrarenal cysts are most commonly found in the liver, but they may also be found in the pancreas, spleen, endometrium, ovaries, seminal vesicles, epididymis, and thyroid gland. The incidence of cysts increases with age. These cysts vary from microscopic to several centimeters in diameter and have an epithelial lining.

Von Hippel-Lindau Syndrome. Von Hippel-Lindau syndrome is an autosomal dominant condition characterized by central nervous system and retinal hemangioblastomas, visceral cysts, pheochromocytomas, and renal cell carcinoma. Pancreatic cysts are found in 75% of cases at autopsy. Cysts vary in size from millimeters to centimeters. Other pancreatic lesions include microcystic adenomas, islet cell tumors, angiomas, and vascular neoplasms.

Congenital Cystic Lesions of the Pancreas. Most congenital pancreatic cysts are multiple, and nearly all are associated with underlying congenital diseases that primarily affect other organ systems. Solitary congenital cysts are rare. Congenital cysts of the pancreas result from the anomalous development of the pancreatic ducts. They are usually multiple in number and range from small to 3 to 5 cm in size (Figure 12-39).

Cystic Fibrosis. Cystic fibrosis is a hereditary disease that causes excessive production of thick mucus by the endocrine glands. The most common pancreatic abnormality found is fatty replacement of the pancreas, sometimes with calcifications. The cysts develop from inspissated mucin that obstructs the pancreatic ducts. The cysts are either single or multiple. Most are microscopic, but they can also be several centimeters in diameter.

Fibrocystic Disease of the Pancreas. Fibrocystic disease of the pancreas is a hereditary disorder of the exocrine glands seen frequently in children and young adults. The pancreas is usually firm and of normal size. Cysts are very small but may be present in the advanced stages. The acini and ducts are dilated. The acini are usually atrophic and may be totally replaced by fibrous tissue in many of the lobules. Nausea and vomiting may also occur, leading to malnourishment. The pancreatic secretion is gradually lost. With advancing pancreatic fibrosis, jaundice may develop from common duct obstruction. Diabetes is a late manifestation. Grossly the pancreas is found to be somewhat nodular and firm. There may be edema and fat necrosis, but gradually fibrous replacement will occur throughout the parenchyma. The pancreatic duct may enlarge and contain calculi.

Solitary Pancreatic Cysts.
This category includes true cysts and lymphoepithelial cysts.

True Cysts. True cysts are microscopic sacs that may be congenital or acquired. Congenital cysts are the result of anomalous development of the pancreatic duct and may be single, but they are usually multiple and without septation. True pancreatic cysts rise from within the gland, more commonly in the head first, then in the body and tail. They have a lining epithelium, which may be lost with inflammation. The cysts contain pancreatic enzymes or may be found to be continuous with the pancreatic duct. Both true cysts and pseudocysts may protrude anteriorly in any direction, although the true cyst is generally associated directly with the pancreatic area.

Lymphoepithelial Cysts. These are rare, usually found in middle-aged to elderly males. Lesions vary from 1 to 17 cm, have a squamous lining, and contain keratinous material.

Neoplasms of the Pancreas

See Table 12-6 for clinical findings, sonographic findings, and differential considerations for pancreatic tumors.
Exocrine Pancreatic Tumors.

Adenocarcinoma. The most common primary neoplasm of the pancreas is adenocarcinoma. This fatal tumor involves the exocrine portion of the gland (ductal epithelium) and accounts for greater than 90% of all malignant pancreatic tumors (Figure 12-40). Pancreatic carcinoma accounts for approximately 5% of all cancer

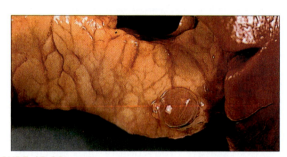

FIGURE 12-39 Gross pathology of a small congenital cyst of the pancreas.

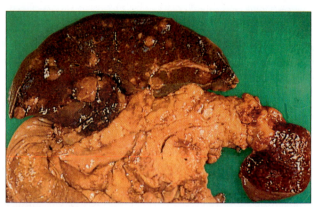

FIGURE 12-40 Carcinoma of the body of the pancreas. The tumor has metastasized to the liver.

TABLE 12-6	Pancreatic Tumor Findings	
Clinical Findings	**Sonographic Findings**	**Differential Considerations**
Adenocarcinoma		
• Depends on size and location of tumor (Symptoms occur late if located in body or tail) • Weight loss • Decreased appetite • Nausea, vomiting • Stool changes • Pain radiating to back • Painless jaundice if tumor is located in the head (hydrops of GB—Courvoisier's sign) • Metastasizes to lymph nodes, liver, lungs, bone, duodenum, peritoneum, and adrenal glands	• Loss of normal pancreatic parenchyma • Hypoechoic poorly defined mass • Focal mass with irregular borders • Enlargement of pancreas • If mass is located in head of pancreas, look for hydrops, compression of IVC, and dilated ducts	• Pseudocyst • Cystadenoma • Lymphoma
Cystadenoma		
• ↑ Amylase	• Anechoic mass with posterior enhancement • May have internal septa • Thick walls • Small size of tumor makes it difficult to image • Single or multiple • Occur in body and tail • Hypoechoic	• Pseudocyst • Metastases
Cystadenocarcinoma		
• Epigastric pain or palpable mass • Abdominal pain	• Irregular lobulated cystic tumor • Thick walls • Hypoechoic mass	• Pseudocyst • Cystadenoma • Adenocarcinoma • Islet cell tumor

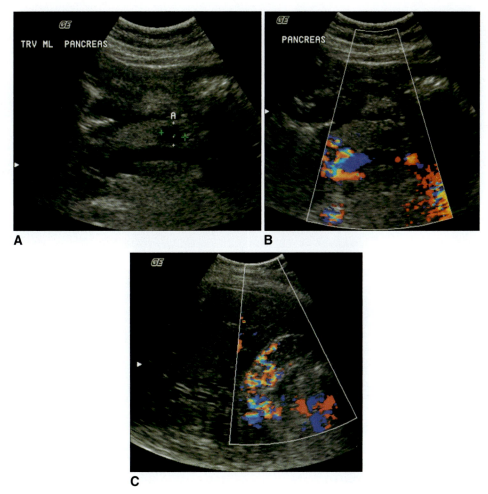

FIGURE 12-41 Fifty-two-year-old female with mucinous adenoma of the appendix with increased alkaline phosphatase. **A, B,** Transverse images of the pancreas demonstrate a rounded hypoechoic lesion within the body of the gland. This lesion may represent a metastatic focus to the gland. Color Doppler shows no sign of flow to the lesion. **C,** The gallbladder is markedly heterogeneous with a thickened wall. This may represent metastatic tumor.

deaths and is the fourth most common cause of cancer-related mortality, after lung, breast, and colon cancer. Carcinoma of the pancreas is rare before the age of 40; the majority of patients present after the age of 60. The prognosis is poor with a median survival time of 2 to 3 months and a 1-year survival of only 8%.

Clinical symptoms depend on the location of the tumor. Tumors in the pancreatic head present symptoms early, causing obstruction of the common bile duct with subsequent jaundice and hydrops of the gallbladder (**Courvoisier's sign**). A palpable, nontender gallbladder accompanied by jaundice is present in 25% of patients with pancreatic carcinoma. Tumors in the body and tail of the gland present with less specific symptoms, most commonly weight loss, pain, jaundice, and vomiting as the gastrointestinal tract becomes invaded by tumor. The tumors in the body and tail are more frequently larger in size and tend to invade the adjacent organs such as the stomach, transverse colon, spleen, and adrenal gland. These organs tend to present with metastases more often than tumors in the head. Metastases to the liver, regional lymph nodes, lungs, peritoneum, and adrenal glands have been reported. Peripancreatic, gastric, mesenteric, omental, and portohepatic nodes have been identified with adenocarcinoma.

On pathology, nearly all adenocarcinomas of the pancreas originate in the ductal epithelium, with less than 1% arising in the acini. The tumor may be either mucinous or nonmucinous. The most frequent site of occurrence is in the head of the gland (60% to 70%), with 20% to 30% in the body and 5% to 10% in the tail (Figure 12-41). One fifth of the tumors are diffuse.

Sonographic Findings. The sonographic appearance of adenocarcinoma is the loss of the normal pancreatic parenchymal pattern (Figures 12-42 and 12-43). The most common finding on sonography is a poorly defined mass in the region of the pancreas. The lesion represents localized change in the echogenicity of the pancreas texture. The echo pattern is hypoechoic or isoechoic, with a texture less dense than the pancreas or liver. (The hypoechoic or isoechoic ill-defined tumor is better

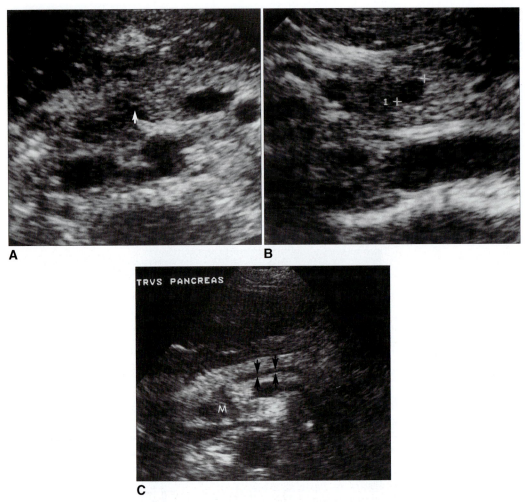

FIGURE 12-42 Adenocarcinoma of the pancreas. **A,** Transverse image; arrow points to the hypoechoic abnormal tissue in the head of the pancreas. **B,** Sagittal image of the dilated pancreatic duct *(crossbars)*. **C,** Transverse image of a dilated pancreatic duct *(arrows)* measuring more than 3 mm in a patient with a large mass *(M)* in the head of the gland.

identified when the pancreatic texture is more echogenic). Rarely, necrosis will be seen as a cystic area within the mass. The borders of the gland become irregular and the pancreas may be enlarged. There may be secondary enlargement of the common duct resulting from edema or tumor invasion of the pancreatic head. If the mass causes obstruction of the duct, look for dilation of the pancreatic duct (>2 to 3 mm). If the tumor is located within the head, look for biliary duct dilation. Remember the level of the obstruction may be in the head, above the head, or in the porta hepatis, depending on the size of the lesion. The distinction of echogenic sludge within the common bile duct may be difficult to separate from tumor extension. Dilatation of both the pancreatic and common bile duct may be seen in chronic pancreatitis as well as pancreatic adenocarcinoma.

There may be expansion or compression of the adjacent structures. The formation of a pseudocyst secondary to associated pancreatitis may be seen adjacent to the carcinoma. A diffuse spread of the tumor throughout the pancreas may appear as edematous pancreatitis. The

sonographer should carefully evaluate the gland for the vague appearance of a lobulated mass and correlate with clinical symptoms.

The sonographer should look for metastatic spread into the liver, para-aortic nodes (abnormal displacement of the superior mesenteric artery), or portal venous system. The superior mesenteric vessels may be displaced posteriorly by the pancreatic mass; anterior displacement is present when the carcinoma is in the uncinate process, and posterior displacement is present when the tumor is in the head or body. A soft tissue thickening caused by neoplastic infiltration of perivascular lymphatics may be seen surrounding the celiac axis or superior mesenteric artery; this occurs more with carcinoma of the body and tail.

Most patients have **obstructive jaundice** and anterior wall compression of the inferior vena cava when the tumor involves the head of the pancreas. A tumor in the tail can compress the splenic vein, producing secondary splenic enlargement. A tumor may displace or invade the splenic or portal vein or produce thrombosis. Atrophy

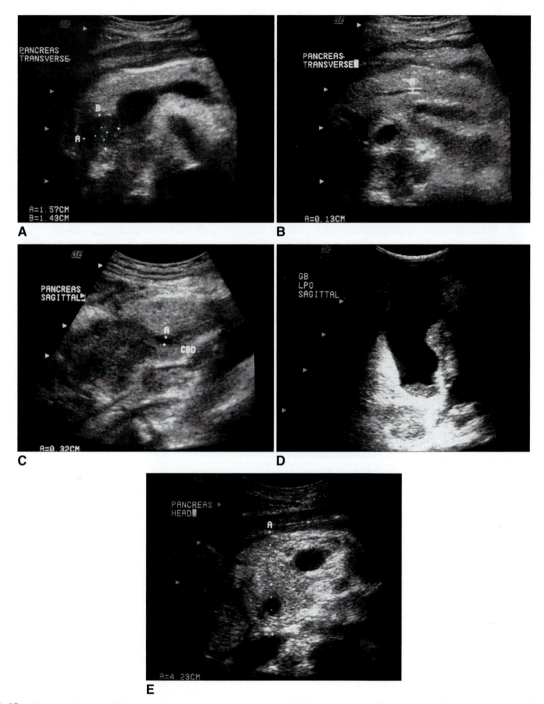

FIGURE 12-43 Adenocarcinoma of the pancreas. **A,** Transverse image of the pancreas with a hypoechoic mass in the head (*A* marks first caliper measurement; *B* marks second caliper measurement). **B,** The pancreatic duct is prominent; the mass is still present in the head of the pancreas. The common bile duct is dilated, measuring 13 mm. **C,** Sagittal image of the dilated common duct as it flows posterior to the head of the pancreas. *A,* Aorta. **D,** Dilated gallbladder with sludge. **E,** Magnified transverse image of the head of the pancreas and the dilated common bile duct. *A,* Aorta.

of the gland proximal to an obstructing mass in the head may appear hypoechoic or hyperechoic.

Doppler patterns feature characteristics of other malignant lesions with increased velocity and diminished flow impedance. The increased velocity is most likely from arteriovenous shunting and the diminished impedance to vascular spaces that lack muscular walls.

Significance of Sonography in Staging Pancreatic Tumors. Sonography may play an important role not only in identifying the pancreatic tumor mass but also in assessing the possibility of tumor resection. Surgery remains the treatment of choice in carcinomas that are considered resectable, but it comes with a high rate of mortality and morbidity. The ability to identify the

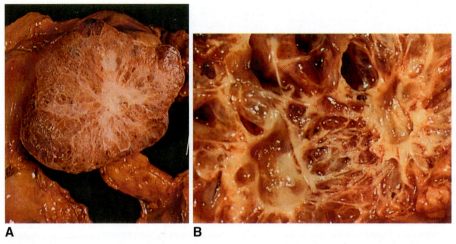

A   **B**

FIGURE 12-44 Gross pathology of serous cystadenoma. **A,** Well-circumscribed tumor. **B,** Tumor appears microcystic.

extension of the carcinoma beyond the border of the pancreas—including invasion of the carcinoma into the lymph nodes, surrounding venous structures and organs, retroperitoneal fat, and liver metastases—precludes the feasibility of surgery. The demonstration of these structures by sonography will be determined by the adequate image quality. The retroperitoneal structures are often precluded by bowel gas interference and thus inadequate image quality results. However, if the pancreas can be adequately imaged in its entirety and has a normal appearance, pancreatic carcinoma can be excluded with a high degree of certainty.

The sonographer should strive to carefully evaluate the vascular structures surrounding the pancreas. The gland lies in the middle of a significant vascular highway, and if a mass is present in the pancreas it may easily travel to adjacent organs. It may be difficult to distinguish compression and invasion of the venous structures. Secondary signs should be noted, such as interruption of a vein, organomegaly, or collateral formation in the peripancreatic and periportal region and along the stomach wall. Enlargement of the lymph nodes in the pancreatic area may lead to encasement of the celiac axis or superior mesenteric artery.

Differential Diagnosis for Pancreatic Carcinoma. The primary differential diagnosis of pancreatic carcinoma is focal pancreatitis or a focal mass associated with chronic pancreatitis. Calcification may be seen in patients with pancreatitis to help delineate the gland. However, it is possible to have concurrent neoplastic growth in the presence of pancreatitis. Comparative imaging with CT and ERCP may be necessary to evaluate the texture of the gland and retroperitoneal area and to further assess the pancreatic duct.

Enlarged lymph nodes in the peripancreatic area may be differentiated from pancreatic cancer by identifying the echogenic septa between each of the hypoechoic nodes. The absence of jaundice in the presence of a mass

near the head of the pancreas favors the presence of lymphadenopathy over pancreatic carcinoma.

Ampullary adenocarcinomas have a better prognosis than pancreatic adenocarcinoma when lesions are less than 2 cm. Endoscopic ultrasound has allowed the visualization of the pancreatic duct to stage this neoplastic growth. Dilation of the pancreatic and common duct is common with the ampullary tumor.

Cystic Pancreatic Neoplasms

The cystic neoplasms of the pancreas account for between 10% and 15% of all pancreatic cysts and less than 1% of all pancreatic malignancies. There are two types of cystic neoplasms: microcystic (serous) adenoma and macrocystic (mucinous) adenoma. Microcystic adenoma (serous cystadenoma) is a rare, benign disease found more often in elderly females. The tumor is well circumscribed and usually consists of a large mass with multiple tiny cysts (Figure 12-44). Macrocystic adenoma (mucinous cystadenoma/cystadenocarcinoma) may be either malignant or benign with a malignant potential. It occurs predominantly in both middle- and old-aged females, usually in the body or tail. It typically comprises well-defined cysts containing thick mucinous fluid, internal septations, or mural nodules. Clinically, patients present with nonspecific abdominal symptoms, weight loss, abdominal mass, or jaundice.

Microcystic Adenoma (Cystadenoma, Serous Adenoma, Glycogen-Rich Adenoma). Microcystic adenoma is a rare benign lesion of the pancreas that is found most frequently in elderly women over 60 years of age. The microcystic adenoma is one of the pancreatic lesions found in von Hippel-Lindau disease. The cysts can be either single or multiple, and it can involve any part of the pancreas. The cysts vary in size from 1 mm to 20 mm in diameter.

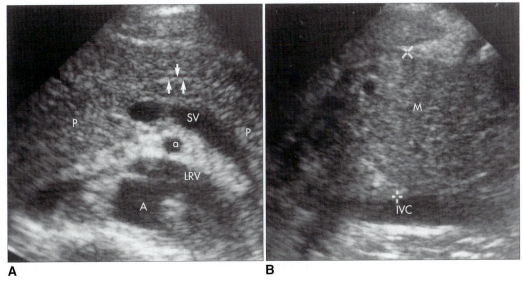

FIGURE 12-45 A 65-year-old patient with cystadenoma in the head of the pancreas that is not causing obstruction of the pancreatic duct. **A,** Transverse image of the pancreas *(P)*, pancreatic duct *(arrows)*, splenic vein *(SV)*, superior mesenteric artery *(a)*, left renal vein *(LRV)*, and aorta *(A)*. **B,** Large mass *(M)* in the head of the pancreas seen compressing the inferior vena cava *(IVC)*.

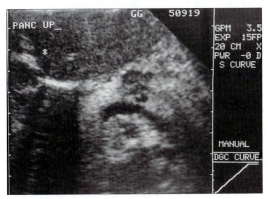

FIGURE 12-46 Pancreatic cystadenoma was found in the body of the pancreas in this 53-year-old female.

▶ **Sonographic Findings.** The microcystic adenomas are well-defined tumors with external lobulation. The sonographic appearance depends on the number and size of the cysts. The lesions may appear cystic, solid, or even echogenic if the cysts are very small and more numerous along the periphery. The coarsely lobulated cystic tumors sometimes present sonographically with cyst walls thicker than the membranes between multilocular cysts (Figures 12-45 and 12-46). A minority of the cysts have an echogenic central stellate scar that may have calcification. The pseudocapsule and septa of the mass tends to be hypervascular and seen well with color Doppler. The mass usually does not cause obstruction of the pancreatic duct. It is difficult to differentiate a benign microcystic adenoma from a malignant mucinous cystic tumor without pathologic confirmation.

Macrocystic Adenocarcinoma (Mucinous Cystadenoma or Cystadenocarcinoma). Macrocystic adenocarcinoma is an uncommon, slow-growing tumor that rises from the ducts as a cystic neoplasm. It consists of a large cyst (greater than 2 cm) with or without septations and has a significant malignant potential. The overall survival if the lesion is intact is better than with adenocarcinoma. These lesions are unilocular or multilocular. The mass occurs more commonly in the tail and body, with 60% in the tail, 35% in the body, and 5% in the head of the pancreas. Frequently, foci of calcification may be seen within the pancreas. Patients present with epigastric pain or a palpable mass. Many patients have concurrent diseases: diabetes, calculous disease of biliary tract, or arterial hypertension.

▶ **Sonographic Findings.** This lesion presents as well-circumscribed, smooth-surfaced, thin- or thick-walled, unilocular or multilocular cystic lesions of variable sizes (usually more than 20 mm in diameter and less than six in number) on sonography. The macrocystic neoplasms may be further classified into four types: hypoechoic cysts, echogenic cysts containing debris, cysts with solid mural vegetations, or completely filled or solid-looking cysts.

Intraductal Papillary Mucinous Tumor (IPMT). The intraductal papillary mucinous tumor is a form of mucinous cystic neoplasm. The tumor originates from the main pancreatic duct or its branches. This slow-growing lesion affects both men and women in the sixth and seventh decades. The histology ranges from benign to malignant. Clinical symptoms of abdominal pain are accompanied by an elevated serum amylase level, so pancreatitis is a differential. The ductal tumors demonstrate four primary patterns on imaging. The main pancreatic duct type presents as segmental or diffuse dilatation of the duct with or without side branch dilatation. The branch type shows a single or multicystic mass with a microcystic or macrocystic appearance. Careful demonstration of the mass should show communication with the pancreatic duct, usually best seen with ERCP. The tumors may present as nonvascular nodules within the dilated ducts. The presence of vascular nodules and a thick wall differentiates the mass benign from malignant.

Differential Diagnoses. The sonographer is not able to pathologically identify the type of tumor, but specific findings may help identify the differential diagnosis of pancreatic tumors. Adenocarcinoma presents as an irregular, poorly defined homogeneous or heterogeneous hypoechoic mass. Microcystic lesions are defined by their well-demarcated tiny cysts. The mucinous cystic tumor presents with a multilocular mass with septa and solid components. A choledochal cyst may mimic a cystic neoplasm in the head of the pancreas; however, the choledochal cyst may be seen to communicate with the common bile duct.

Endocrine Pancreatic Neoplasms

These endocrine tumors rise from the islet cells of the pancreas. There are several types of islet cell tumors; they may be functional or nonfunctional. The tumors may be classified as benign adenomas or malignant tumors. Nonfunctioning islet cell tumors comprise one third of all islet cell tumors, with 92% being malignant. The growth rate is very slow and they usually do not spread beyond the regional lymph nodes and the liver.

The most common functioning islet cell tumor is insulinoma (60%) followed by gastrinoma (18%). The tumor size is small (1 to 2 cm), and they are well encapsulated with a good vascular supply (Figure 12-47). A large percentage of insulinoma tumors occur in patients with hyperinsulinism and hypoglycemia. Most gastrinomas are malignant, with up to 40% appearing with metastatic disease at the time of diagnosis.

These endocrine tumors may be isolated or associated with the multiple endocrine neoplasia syndrome type 1 (MEN 1), which is characterized by the triad of parathyroid, pituitary, and pancreatic lesions. The lesions may be solitary, multiple, or diffuse. Necrosis, hemorrhage,

and calcification are seen more frequently in the larger malignant type of islet-cell tumors. These tumors are further classified into functioning or nonfunctioning tumors.

Insulinoma (B-Cell Tumor). Insulinoma is the most common functioning islet cell tumor. The clinical triad is found in patients in their fourth to sixth decades of life with hypoglycemic symptoms with immediate relief of symptoms after the administration of IV glucose. Clinical symptoms include palpitations, headache, confusion, pallor, sweating, slurred speech, and coma. This tumor is usually benign. A small percent of insulinomas are multiple, 10% are malignant, and 10% of patients have hyperplasia rather than neoplasia. Most of the insulinomas are small, well encapsulated, and hypervascular. Some of the lesions contain calcification.

Gastrinoma (G-Cell Tumor). Gastrinoma is the second most common functioning islet cell tumor and produces the Zollinger-Ellison syndrome. This condition is caused by non-insulin-secreting pancreatic tumors, which secrete excessive amounts of gastrin. This stimulates the stomach to secrete great amounts of hydrochloric acid and pepsin, which in turn leads to peptic ulceration of the stomach and small intestine. These lesions usually affect young adults who have peptic ulcer disease (when ulcers are recurrent, intractable, multiple, or in unusual locations). Diarrhea is common because of the increased gastrin on the small bowel. Gastrinomas are frequently multiple, extrapancreatic, difficult to locate, and 60% are malignant. Total gastrectomy and local excision of the pancreatic tumor may be performed if metastases have not appeared. Most gastrinomas are found in the pancreas with a small amount (10% to 15%) arising in the duodenum.

Rare Islet-Cell Tumors. The rare functioning islet-cell tumors include glucagonoma, lipoma, somatostatinoma, and carcinoid and multihormonal tumors. The highest incidence of malignancy is found in glucagonomas and vipomas. Vipomas is also associated with gallbladder dilation, fluid-filled distended bowel loops, and excessive secretion of fluid and electrolytes. Thickening of the gastric wall may also be present.

Nonfunctioning Islet-Cell Tumors. These tumors comprise 33% of all islet-cell neoplasms. They have a tendency to present as large tumors in the head of the pancreas with a high incidence of malignancy.

Sonographic Findings. Sonographically, islet cell tumors are difficult to image because of their small size. The ability to adequately image the pancreatic area is further impeded by the obese size of the patients secondary to their overeating for fear of hypoglycemic episodes. The greatest success is when they are located in the head of the pancreas. The tumors may be multiple and occur mostly in the body and tail, where there is the greatest concentration of Langerhans islets (Figure 12-48). Endoscopic ultrasound (EUS) has increased the visualization of these smaller tumors as they present as well-defined

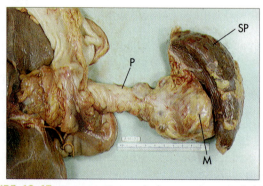

FIGURE 12-47 Gross specimen of a pancreatic mass *(M)* in the tail of the gland. *P,* Pancreas; *SP,* spleen.

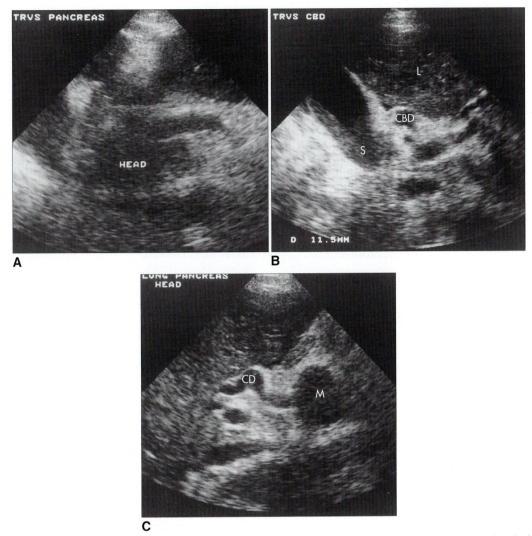

FIGURE 12-48 A 46-year-old female presents with sweating and insulin shock. An ill-defined mass is seen in the head of the pancreas, compressing the common bile duct. This was an islet cell tumor of the pancreas. **A,** Transverse scan of the head of the pancreas shows the irregularly margined mass. **B,** The dilated common bile duct *(CBD)* measures 11.5 mm. The distended gallbladder is half filled with sludge *(S). L,* Liver. **C,** Sagittal scan of the distended common duct *(CD)* and mass *(M)* in the head of the pancreas.

hypoechoic tumors without calcification. Those tumors that present as isoechoic are more difficult to distinguish; however, careful evaluation of the contour changes in the pancreas may increase the suspicion. The larger tumors may present as irregular with either hypoechoic or echogenic with calcification and necrosis (more likely to be irregular).

Intraoperative ultrasound has enabled the demonstration of the small islet-cell tumors with improved accuracy. The demonstration of the tumor in relation to the pancreatic or common bile duct may be clearly identified.

Metastatic Disease to the Pancreas

Generally speaking, metastasis to the pancreas is uncommon but has been reported to be found in 10% of patients with cancer. Primary tumors that can metasta-

size to the pancreas include melanomas, breast, gastrointestinal, and lung tumors.

Parapancreatic Neoplasms

Lymphomas are malignant neoplasms that rise from the lymphoid tissues. They are the most frequent parapancreatic neoplasm. It may be difficult to separate a parapancreatic lymphadenopathy from a primary lesion in the pancreas. An intraabdominal lymphoma may appear as a hypoechoic mass or with necrosis, a cystic mass in the pancreas (Figure 12-49). The superior mesenteric vessels may be displaced anterior instead of posterior as seen with a primary pancreatic mass. Multiple nodes are seen along the pancreas, duodenum, porta hepatis, and superior mesenteric vessels; they may be difficult to distinguish from a pancreatic mass. The enlarged nodes appear hypoechoic and well defined.

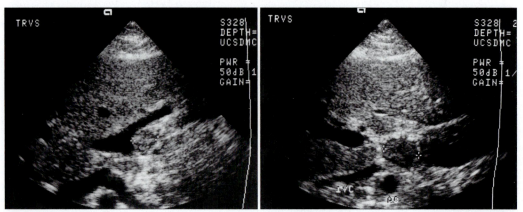

FIGURE 12-49 Patient with lymphoma who presented with epigastric pain. Multiple nodes *(calipers)* were seen in the peripancreatic area. *AO,* Aorta; *IVC,* inferior vena cava.

Other types of retroperitoneal neoplasms that may appear as a cystic lesion near the area of the pancreas include lymphangiomas, paragangliomas, cystic teratomas, and metastases. The lymphangiomas are most often thin-walled, homogeneous, small cysts, but they have also been seen to have septa, thick walls, calcification, and internal debris. The paragangliomas are usually found near the inferior mesenteric artery or near the kidney. The cystic teratomas are found more frequently in children and young adults. Their appearance is a mixed sonographic pattern of cystic, solid, fat, and calcifications.

The Gastrointestinal Tract

Sandra L. Hagen-Ansert

OBJECTIVES

On completion of this chapter, you should be able to:
- Describe the anatomy and relational landmarks of the gastrointestinal system
- Discuss the size of wall thickness and diameters of the gastrointestinal tract
- Describe the sonographic technique used to image the gastrointestinal tract and appendix
- Differentiate the sonographic appearances of the pathologies covered in this chapter

OUTLINE

The gastrointestinal tract may be difficult to image with ultrasound in most patients unless they ingest fluids or some other acoustic transmittable contrast agent. Many laboratories have begun to investigate various contrast agents in pursuit of the ideal medium for imaging the stomach, duodenum, small bowel, and colon.

ANATOMY OF THE GASTROINTESTINAL TRACT

Normal Anatomy

The digestive tract, also known as the **alimentary tract,** is a long tube (about 8 m long) extending from the mouth to the anus (Figure 13-1). The gastrointestinal tract is that part of the digestive system below the diaphragm. The sequential parts of the digestive system include the mouth, pharynx, esophagus, stomach, small intestine (duodenum, jejunum, and ileum), and large intestine (cecum, ascending colon, transverse colon, descending colon, and rectum). Three types of accessory digestive glands—the salivary glands, liver, and pancreas—secrete digestive juices into the digestive system.

Esophagus. The esophagus extends from the pharynx through the thoracic cavity, then passes through the diaphragm and empties into the stomach (see Figure 13-1). The lower end of the esophagus is a circular muscle that acts as a sphincter, constricting the tube so that the entrance to the stomach, at the **cardiac orifice,** is generally closed. This helps to prevent gastric acid from moving up into the esophagus.

Stomach. The stomach is a large, smooth, muscular organ that has two surfaces: the lesser curvature and the greater curvature (Figure 13-2). The stomach is divided into three parts: The *fundus* is found in the superior aspect, the *body* makes up the major central axis, and the *pylorus* is the lower aspect. The pylorus is further subdivided into the antrum, the pyloric canal, and the pyloric sphincter. The **pyloric canal** is a muscle that connects the stomach to the proximal duodenum.

Supporting ligaments of the greater curvature of the stomach include the **greater omentum,** the **gastrophrenic ligament,** the **gastrosplenic ligament,** and the **lienorenal ligament.** Ligaments that support the lesser curvature of the stomach include the **gastrohepatic ligament** of the **lesser omentum.** Folds of the **mucosa** and **submucosa** are called **rugae.**

Small Intestine. The small intestine is a long, coiled tube about 5 m long by 4 cm in diameter (see Figure 13-1). The first 22 cm is the duodenum, which is curved like the letter C. The duodenum is subdivided into four

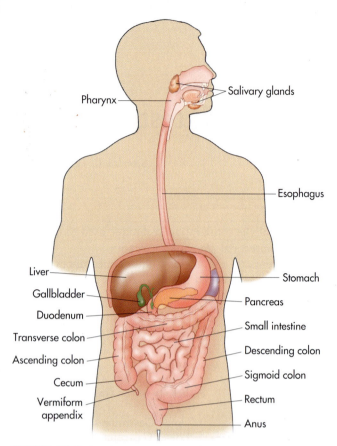

FIGURE 13-1 The digestive system includes the mouth, pharynx, esophagus, stomach, small intestine, large intestine, rectum, and anus.

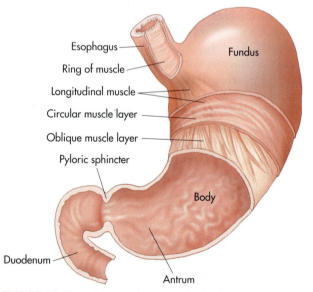

FIGURE 13-2 Food enters the stomach after leaving the esophagus through the gastroesophageal junction at the level of the diaphragm. The three parts of the stomach (fundus, body, and antrum) are shown. Food leaves the stomach through the pylorus and pyloric sphincter to enter the duodenum.

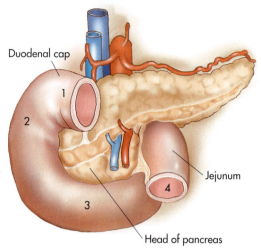

FIGURE 13-3 The duodenal cap is an excellent landmark for the head of the pancreas. The duodenum is divided into four sections. See text for explanation. (The fourth part of the duodenum is posterior to the jejunum.)

segments: (1) superior, (2) descending, (3) transverse, and (4) ascending (Figure 13-3). The first part of the duodenum is not attached to the mesentery; the remainder of the small intestine, including the rest of the duodenum, is attached to the mesentery. The **mesentery** projects from the parietal peritoneum and attaches to the small intestine to anchor it to the posterior abdominal wall.

The first part of the duodenum begins at the pylorus and terminates at the neck of the gallbladder, posterior to the left lobe of the liver and medial to the gallbladder. The **duodenal bulb** is peritoneal, supported by the hepatoduodenal ligament, and passes anterior to the common bile duct, gastroduodenal artery, common hepatic artery, hepatic portal vein, and head of the pancreas.

The second part (descending) of the duodenum is retroperitoneal and runs parallel, posterior, and to the right of the spine. The transverse colon crosses anterior to the middle third of the descending duodenum. The pancreatic head is medial to the duodenum at this point. The common bile duct joins the pancreatic duct to enter the ampulla of Vater.

The third part (transverse) of the duodenum begins at the right of the fourth lumbar vertebra and passes anterior to the aorta, inferior vena cava, and crura of the diaphragm. The superior mesenteric vessels course anterior to the duodenum.

The fourth part (ascending) of the duodenum ascends superiorly to the left of the spine and aorta to the second lumbar vertebra, where it joins the proximal jejunum (duodenojejunal flexure). This portion lies on the left crus of the diaphragm. It is held in place by the ligament of Treitz (which courses from the left toward the right crus of the diaphragm).

As the tube turns downward, it is called the jejunum; the jejunum extends for about 2 m before becoming the

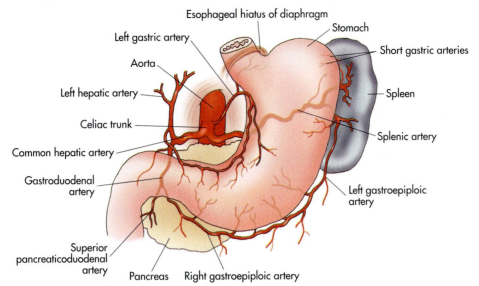

FIGURE 13-4 Vascular supply to the stomach is received from the branches of the celiac axis. The left gastric artery supplies the lower third of the esophagus and the upper right part of the stomach. The right gastric artery supplies the lower right part of the stomach. The short gastric arteries supply the fundus. The left gastroepiploic artery supplies the upper part of the greater curvature of the stomach, and the right gastroepiploic artery supplies the lower part of the greater curvature of the stomach.

ileum. The inner wall of the small intestine is marked by circular folds of the mucous membrane, **villi.** The **valvulae conniventes** are large folds of mucous membrane that project into the lumen of the bowel and help retard the passage of food to provide greater absorption. The lower part of the small intestine is the ileum. The ileocecal orifice marks the entry into the large intestine and prevents food from reentering the small intestine.

Large Intestine. The large intestine is larger in diameter and shorter in length than the small intestine. The vermiform appendix; cecum; ascending, transverse, and descending colon; rectum; and anus all make up the large intestine (see Figure 13-1). The colon is divided into segments called **haustra.** The ascending colon extends from the cecum vertically to the lower part of the liver. It turns horizontally at the **hepatic flexure** and moves to become the transverse colon. On the left side of the abdomen, at the **splenic flexure,** it then descends vertically to become the descending colon and eventually the sigmoid colon, which empties into the rectum. The rectum is 12 cm long, terminating at the anus.

The mucosa of the large intestine lacks villi and produces no digestive enzymes. The surface epithelium consists of cells specialized for absorption and goblet cells that secrete mucus.

Vascular Anatomy

Esophagus. The arteries that supply the esophagus rise from the high, mid, and lower sections of this muscular tube. The inferior thyroid branch of the subclavian artery supplies the upper esophagus, the descending thoracic aorta supplies the midesophagus, and the gastric branch of the celiac axis and the left inferior phrenic artery of the abdominal aorta supply the lower end of the esophagus. Varices may be seen to rise from the gastroesophageal arteries (Figure 13-4).

Stomach. The vascular supply to the stomach is provided by the right gastric arterial branch, pyloric and right gastroepiploic branches of the hepatic artery, left gastroepiploic branch and vasa brevia of the splenic artery, and left gastric artery (see Figure 13-4). The venous system of the stomach is parallel to the arterial vessels, which drain into the portal venous system.

Small Intestine. The mesentery outlines the small intestine and contains superior mesenteric vessels, nerves, lymphatic glands, and fat between its two layers. The celiac axis supplies the duodenum through its right gastric, gastroduodenal, and superior pancreaticoduodenal branches (Figure 13-5). The superior mesenteric artery has multiple branches to the small bowel, which include the inferior pancreaticoduodenal, jejunal, and ileal arteries. The venous system parallels the arterial system and empties into the portal venous system.

Large Intestine. The celiac, superior mesenteric, and inferior mesenteric arteries supply both the small and the large intestine. The superior mesenteric arterial branches include the ileocolic, right colic, and middle colic arteries (see Figure 13-5). The inferior mesenteric artery supplies the intestine from the left border of the transverse colon to the rectum, rising from the anterior surface of the abdominal aorta at the level of the third lumbar vertebra and descending retroperitoneally (Figure 13-6). Branches of the inferior mesenteric artery include the left colic, sigmoid, and superior rectal arteries. The venous system parallels the arterial system and empties into the portal venous system.

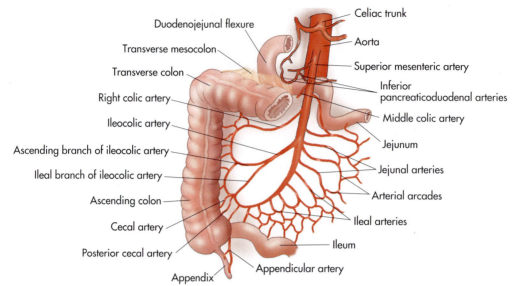

FIGURE 13-5 The superior mesenteric artery supplies the gut from halfway down the second part of the duodenum to the distal third of the transverse colon.

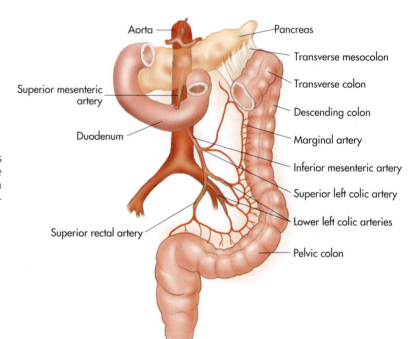

FIGURE 13-6 The inferior mesenteric artery supplies the large bowel from the distal third of the transverse colon to halfway down the anal canal. It forms an anastomosis with the middle colic branch of the superior mesenteric artery.

PHYSIOLOGY AND LABORATORY DATA OF THE GASTROINTESTINAL TRACT

Digestion and absorption are the primary functions of the gastrointestinal tract. In fact, the gastrointestinal tract is the largest endocrine organ in the body.

Food is ingested through the mouth, chewed, and swallowed. The molecules of food must be further digested, or mechanically broken down, and chemically split into small molecules. The chemical digestion of food breaks down long-chain organic molecules (i.e., polysaccharides or proteins). Each reaction is carried on with the help of a specific enzyme produced by cells of the digestive tract or its accessory glands. When these particles are small enough, nutrient molecules pass through the wall of the intestine into the blood or lymph system by **absorption.**

Nutrients are transported to the liver after they are absorbed by the blood; the liver processes and stores nutrients. Remaining nutrients in the blood are transported to cells throughout the body. Undigested and unabsorbed food is eliminated from the digestive tract by the process of defecation.

When food enters the stomach, the rugae gradually smooth out, causing the stomach to stretch and increase its capacity for food intake. Contractions of the stomach help to mix the food. The three layers of smooth muscle in the wall enable the stomach to mash and churn food and move it along through **peristalsis.** Large amounts of mucus are secreted in the stomach. Gastric glands secrete gastric juice containing hydrochloric acid and enzymes.

Over a 3- to 4-hour period, food is converted into chyme. This soupy mixture is moved toward the pylorus and into the small intestine. Small quantities of water, salts, and lipid-soluble substances, such as alcohol, are absorbed through the stomach mucosa, with little absorption taking place in the stomach. The pyloric sphincter is a strong band of muscle that relaxes at the time necessary to release the food.

Villi within the small intestine increase its surface area for digestion and absorption of nutrients; otherwise, food would move quickly through the intestine without time for absorption. The intestinal glands are found between the villi and secrete large amounts of fluid that serve as a medium for digestion and absorption of nutrients. The hormone **gastrin,** which is released by the stomach mucosa, stimulates the gastric glands to secrete. Most digestion occurs within the duodenum. Bile and enzymes from the liver and pancreas are secreted into the duodenum to act on the chyme and break down the food particles for absorption. The intestinal glands are stimulated to release their fluid mainly by local reflexes initiated when the small intestine is distended by chyme.

Other gastrointestinal hormones include **cholecystokinin** and **secretin.** Cholecystokinin is released by the presence of fat in the intestine and regulates gallbladder contraction and gastric emptying. Secretin is released from the small bowel to stimulate the secretion of bicarbonate to decrease the acid content of the intestine.

A period of 1 to 3 days or longer may be required for the journey through the large intestine. Bacteria within the large intestine devour the chyme and in turn produce vitamins that can be absorbed and used by the body. Most of the absorption process of sodium and water occurs in the cecum. Sodium is absorbed by active transport, and water follows by osmosis.

The most common laboratory data the sonographer may come across in a patient with gastrointestinal disease relate to the presence of blood in the stool. Anemia may be present as a result of chronic blood loss. Blood in the stool indicates the presence of a bleed somewhere in the gastrointestinal system. Infection would show elevation of the white blood count. An increase in the carcinoembryonic antigen is found in patients with inflammatory bowel disease.

Clinical signs and symptoms of nausea, vomiting, and diarrhea are common with gastrointestinal problems. Abdominal pain and fever may also be present with gastrointestinal conditions, such as colitis, bowel **abscess,** acute diverticulitis, and appendicitis.

> **BOX 13-1 | Layers of Bowel**
>
> 1. **Mucosa:** directly contacts the intraluminal contents; lined with epithelial folds; echogenic
> 2. **Submucosa:** contains blood vessels and lymph channels
> 3. **Muscularis:** contains circular and longitudinal bands of fiber
> 4. **Serosa:** thin, loose layer of connective tissue
> 5. **Mesothelium:** covers intraperitoneal bowel loops

SONOGRAPHIC EVALUATION OF THE GASTROINTESTINAL TRACT

Visualization of the gastrointestinal tract with ultrasound may be difficult because intraluminal air produces an echogenic shadow, which prevents the sound beam from penetrating structures posteriorly. The scattering and reflection effect of gas in the gastrointestinal tract often produces an incomplete or mottled distal acoustic shadow. The rim of lucency represents the wall (i.e., intima, media, and serosa), and its periserosal fat produces the outer echogenic border of the tract wall.

The bowel wall consists of five layers (Box 13-1). The odd-numbered walls (first, third, and fifth) are echogenic, and the even-numbered walls (second and fourth) are hypoechoic, with an average total thickness of 3 mm if distended and 5 mm if undistended.

The technique used to observe the upper gastrointestinal tract is for the patient to drink 10 to 40 oz of water through a straw after a baseline ultrasound study of the upper abdomen is completed. The straw helps prevent ingestion of excess air when the water is consumed. The patient should be in an upright position for the examination; this causes air in the stomach to rise to the fundus of the stomach and not interfere with the ultrasound beam (Figure 13-7). The lower gastrointestinal tract requires no preparation. When imaging the lower colon, it may be useful to give the patient a water enema to better delineate the colon.

Stomach

The gastroesophageal junction is seen on the sagittal scan to the left of the midline as a bull's eye or target-shaped structure anterior to the aorta, posterior to the left lobe of the liver, and inferior to the hemidiaphragm (Figure 13-8). The left lobe of the patient's liver must be large enough to allow imaging of the gastroesophageal junction.

The gastric antrum can be seen as a target shape in the midline (Figure 13-9). The remainder of the stomach usually is not visualized well unless dilated with fluid (Figures 13-10 and 13-11).

When pathology is present, the serosal layer of the normal gastric wall is seen running toward the serous side of a tumor, which allows differentiation of intramural from extraserosal tumors. If a serosal bridging layer

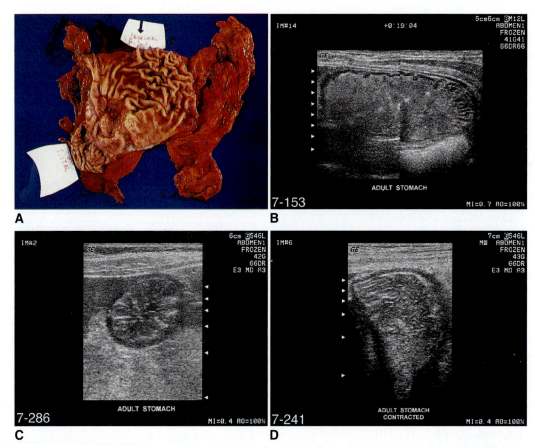

FIGURE 13-7 A, Gross specimen of the stomach showing the internal rugae of the wall. **B,** Sagittal image of the fluid-filled stomach. Rugae may be seen along the peripheral margins of the wall. **C,** Transverse image of the prominent stomach and rugae. **D,** Contracted stomach after fluid has passed through the pylorus.

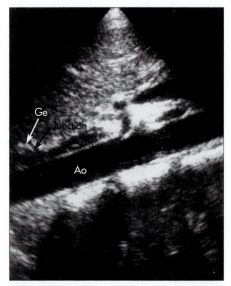

FIGURE 13-8 Sagittal image of the gastroesophageal *(Ge)* junction, which is shown as a small bull's eye shape anterior to the aorta *(Ao)* and posterior to the left lobe of the liver, inferior to the hemidiaphragm.

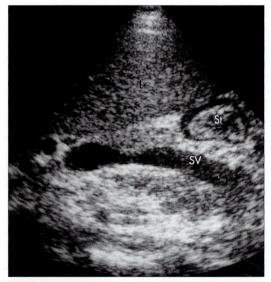

FIGURE 13-9 Transverse view of the left lobe of the liver *(L).* The antrum of the stomach *(St)* is seen posterior to the liver and anterior to the splenic vein *(SV).*

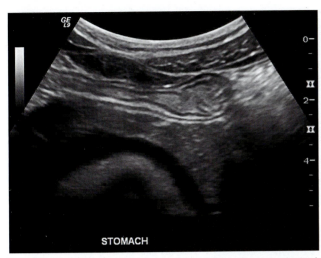

FIGURE 13-10 Transverse image of the collapsed empty stomach anterior to the pancreas and splenic vein.

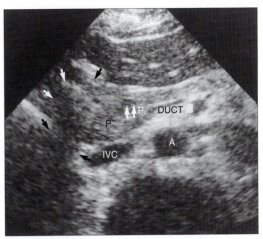

FIGURE 13-12 The duodenum, when filled with a small amount of fluid (arrows), serves as an excellent landmark for the head of the pancreas (P). A, Aorta; IVC, inferior vena cava.

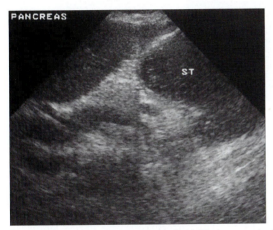

FIGURE 13-11 Transverse view of the fluid-filled stomach. Real-time imaging shows movement throughout the stomach (ST).

(three layers are seen on the mucosal side of the tumor, and at least two of them are continuous with the first and second layers of normal gastric wall) is present, the tumor lies within the gastric wall. If mucosal bridging is continuous with the mucosal layers of the normal gastric wall, is intramucosal, or is deeply infiltrated, carcinoma can be excluded. The sonographer should orient the transducer vertical to the area of transition between the lesion and the stomach wall to show their relationship.

Cystic Mass in the Left Upper Quadrant. If a patient has a cystic mass in the left upper quadrant, several measurements can be taken to determine whether the mass is the fluid-filled stomach or another mass arising from adjacent organs. The sonographer may give the patient a carbonated drink to see bubbles in the stomach, ask the clinician to place a nasogastric tube for drainage, watch for a change in the shape or size of the "stomach" mass with ingestion of fluids, alter the patient's position by scanning in an upright or left or right lateral decubitus

position, watch for peristalsis, or ask the patient to drink water to see the swirling effect.

Duodenum

Usually, only the gas-filled duodenal cap is seen to the right of the pancreas. The duodenum is divided into the following four portions (see Figure 13-3):

1. A superior portion that courses anteroposteriorly from the pylorus to the level of the neck of the gallbladder
2. A sharp bend in the duodenum into the descending portion that runs along the inferior vena cava at the level of L4
3. A transverse portion that passes right to left with a slight inclination upward in front of the great vessels and crura
4. An ascending portion that rises to the right of the aorta and reaches the upper border at L2, where at the duodenojejunal flexure, it turns forward to become the jejunum (usually not seen with ultrasound)

The duodenum can be outlined easily with water ingestion or a change in position (Figure 13-12). Generally, the right lateral decubitus position allows the fluid to drain from the antrum of the stomach into the duodenum. Observation of peristalsis is useful to delineate the duodenum.

Small Bowel

The sonographer usually cannot see the small bowel with sonography; the valvulae conniventes may be seen as linear echo densities spaced 3 to 5 mm apart (Figure 13-13). This is called the "keyboard sign" and can be seen in the duodenum and jejunum. The ileum is smooth walled, and the small bowel wall is less than 3 mm thick.

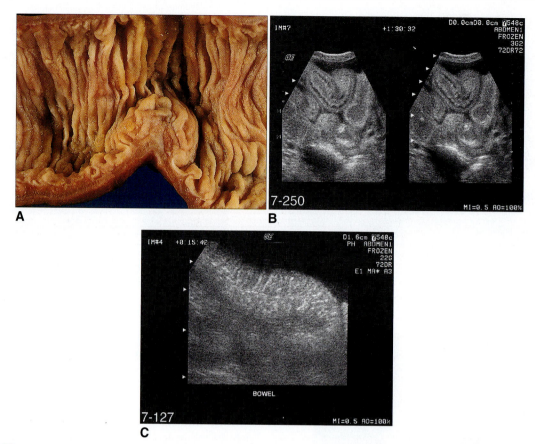

FIGURE 13-13 A, Gross specimen showing the valvulae conniventes within the small bowel lumen. **B** and **C,** Ultrasound images of prominent small bowel with valvulae conniventes.

The small bowel is more difficult to image unless contrast or fluid is present. When fluid is present in the bowel loops, the sonographer may be able to look for peristalsis, air movement, or movement of intraluminal fluid contents to rule out obstruction.

Appendix

The vermiform appendix is a remnant of what was originally the apex of the cecum. It is a long, tubular structure extending from the cecum in one of several directions; it may lie superiorly behind the cecum, medially behind the ileum and mesentery, or downward and medial into the true pelvis (see Figure 13-1). The appendix is located on the abdominal wall under McBurney's point. **McBurney's point** is located by drawing a line from the right anterosuperior iliac spine to the umbilicus. At approximately the midpoint of this line lies the root of the appendix.

The appendix varies from 1 to 9 inches in length, averaging 3 inches. It is retained in position by a fold of the peritoneum that forms a mesentery for it, which is derived from the left leaf of the mesentery. This triangular structure covers two thirds of the appendix, leaving the distal one third completely uncovered by peritoneum.

A branch of the ileocolic artery, the artery of the appendix, lies between the layers of this mesentery (see Figure 13-5). This artery runs the entire length of the appendix.

The small canal of the appendix communicates with the cecum by an orifice that is below and behind the ileocecal opening. The cellular layers that make up the appendix are the serosa or adventitia, muscularis propria, submucosa, and mucosa—the same layers as in the intestine. An abundant amount of retiform tissue is found in the mucosa layer, especially in younger ages. The appendix has no known physiologic significance.

Colon

A prominent fluid-filled colon may present as a mass (Figures 13-14 and 13-15). The water enema technique should be used to help delineate if the mass is within the colon, separate from the colon, or just the colon itself. The patient should have a full bladder when scanned to help push the small bowel out of the pelvis. The water in the enema should be lukewarm and the patient rolled into the left lateral decubitus position. Only a small amount of water needs to be given as the sonographer follows the rectum and rectosigmoid colon. The normal

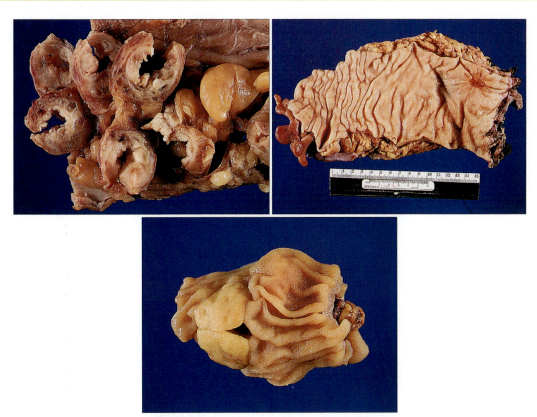

FIGURE 13-14 Gross specimens of the colon.

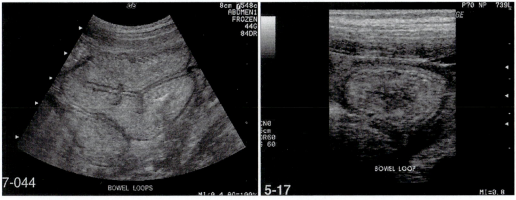

FIGURE 13-15 Target or bull's eye sign. Ultrasound images of the prominent colon.

wall thickness measures 4 mm. The colon consists of five layers: From innermost to outermost, the first two layers are mucosa, the third is submucosa, the fourth is muscularis propria, and the fifth is subserosal fatty tissue.

If the colon is dilated, the sonographer should measure from the fluid to the outside of the wall. Distention is considered adequate if the stomach diameter is greater than 8 cm, the small bowel is larger than 3 cm, and the lower bowel is larger than 5 cm; the entire halo should measure less than 2 cm (target sign).

PATHOLOGY OF THE GASTROINTESTINAL TRACT

Upper Gastrointestinal Tract

Table 13-1 lists the clinical findings, sonographic findings, and differential considerations for upper gastrointestinal tract diseases and conditions.

Duplication Cyst. Duplication cysts are embryologic mistakes. They may cause symptoms, depending on their size, location, and histology (see Table 13-1). The criteria

TABLE 13-1	Upper Gastrointestinal Tract Findings	
Clinical Findings	**Sonographic Findings**	**Differential Considerations**
Duplication Cysts		
↓ Hematocrit with hemorrhage	Anechoic mass with thin inner echogenic rim Wide outer hypoechoic rim	Mesenteric or omental cyst Pancreatic cyst Enteric cyst Renal cyst Splenic cysts Hepatic cyst in LLL
Gastric Bezoar		
Nausea Vomiting Pain	Complex mass with internal mobile components Hyperechoic curvilinear dense strip at anterior margin	Tumor Cyst
Polyps		
Abdominal pain	Echogenic Heterogeneous	Leiomyoma
Leiomyomas		
N/A	Hypoechoic and contiguous with muscular layer of stomach Solid with cystic areas (necrosis)	Carcinoma Polyp
Gastric Carcinoma		
↑ LFTs Abdominal pain	Target or pseudokidney sign Gastric wall thickening	Leiomyoma Lymphoma Metastatic disease
Lymphoma		
Nausea, vomiting Weight loss	Large, hypoechoic mass Thickened gastric walls Spoke-wheel pattern	Gastric carcinoma Leiomyosarcoma Metastatic disease
Leiomyosarcoma		
N/A	Target lesion with variable pattern Irregular echoes Cystic cavity	Lymphoma Gastric carcinoma Metastatic disease
Metastatic Disease		
Secondary to other cancers	Target pattern Circumscribed thickening Uniform widening of wall without layering	Lymphoma Gastric carcinoma Leiomyosarcoma

LFTs, Liver function tests; *LLL*, left lobe of the liver; *N/A*, not applicable.

for a duplication cyst are as follows: (1) The cyst is lined with alimentary tract epithelium, (2) the cyst has a well-developed muscular wall, and (3) the cyst is contiguous with the stomach. These cysts may come from the pancreas or duodenum and occur more often in females than in males. They usually are found on the greater curvature of the stomach. Clinical symptoms include high intestinal obstruction-distention, vomiting, and abdominal pain; **hemorrhage** and fistula formation may also occur. Differential considerations include mesenteric or omental cyst, pancreatic cyst or pseudocyst, enteric cyst, renal cyst, splenic cyst, congenital cyst of the left lobe of the liver, and gastric distention.

Sonographic Findings. On ultrasound examination, duplication cysts appear anechoic with a thin inner echo-

genic rim (mucosa) and a wider outer hypoechoic rim (muscle layer).

Gastric Bezoar. Bezoars are divided into the following three categories: (1) trichobezoars—hair balls in young women, (2) phytobezoars—vegetable matter (e.g., unripe persimmons), and (3) concretions—inorganic materials (e.g., sand, asphalt, shellac).

Gastric bezoars are movable intraluminal masses of congealed ingested materials that are seen on upper gastrointestinal radiographs. Clinically, patients present with nausea, vomiting, and pain (see Table 13-1). Their symptoms may simulate those of a tumor.

Sonographic Findings. A complex mass is seen on sonography with internal mobile echogenic components. In the fasting patient, the sonographer would see a broad band of high-amplitude echoes or a hyperechoic curvilinear dense strip at the anterior margin.

Benign Tumors

Polyp. A **polyp** is a small, tumor-like growth that projects from a mucous membrane surface. A gastric polyp is an outgrowth of tissue from the gastric wall. Patients are asymptomatic when the polyp is small. As the polyp grows, abdominal pain may be present. See Table 13-1 for clinical findings, sonographic findings, and differential considerations for upper gastrointestinal tract polyps.

Sonographic Findings. Polyps are seen with fluid distention of the stomach and appear as solid masses that adhere to the gastric wall. The polyp has variable echogenicity. A large polyp may be inhomogeneous; its contours may be sharply defined, depending on the nature of the surface; a pedicle may be detected.

Leiomyomas. Leiomyoma is the most common tumor of the stomach. Leiomyoma is seen as a mass similar to carcinoma; it is usually small and asymptomatic for the patient (see Table 13-1). It is often associated with other gastrointestinal abnormalities, such as cholelithiasis, peptic ulcer disease, adenocarcinoma, and leiomyosarcoma.

Sonographic Findings. On sonography, the mass is seen as hypoechoic and continuous with the muscular layer of the stomach (Figure 13-16). It may also be seen as a circular or oval space-occupying lesion with a homogeneous echo pattern and hemispheric bulging into the lumen, frequently separated from the lumen by two or three layers continuous with those of normal wall. The mass may appear as a solid with cystic areas that represent necrosis.

Malignant Tumors

Gastric Carcinoma. At least 90% to 95% of malignant tumors of the stomach are carcinomas. Gastric carcinoma is the sixth leading cause of death; it occurs more frequently in older males. One half of these tumors occur in the pylorus, and one fourth occur in the body and fundus of the stomach. The lesions may be ulcerated, diffuse, polypoid, superficial, or some combination of these (see Table 13-1) (Figure 13-17).

Sonographic Findings. The sonographer should look for the target or pseudokidney sign; the patient may have gastric wall thickening.

Lymphoma. **Lymphoma** can occur as a primary tumor of the gastrointestinal tract (3% of stomach tumors). In patients with disseminated lymphoma, a primary tumor occurs as a multifocal lesion in the gastrointestinal tract. The stomach has enlarged and thickened mucosal folds, multiple submucosal nodules, ulceration, and a large extraluminal mass. Clinical symptoms include nausea and vomiting with weight loss (see Table 13-1).

Sonographic Findings. The sonographer will note a large and poorly echogenic (hypoechoic) mass, thickening of the gastric walls, and a spoke-wheel pattern within the mass.

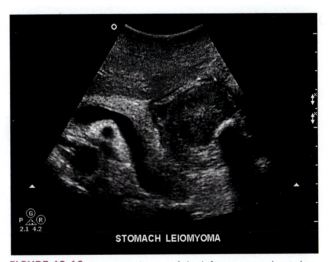

STOMACH LEIOMYOMA

FIGURE 13-16 Transverse image of the left upper quadrant demonstrates a complex tumor in the region of the stomach, which was diagnosed as a leiomyoma.

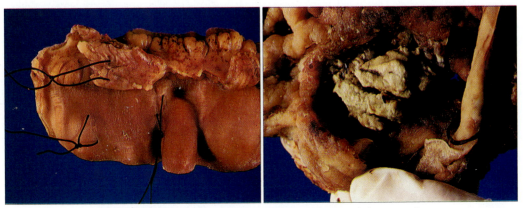

FIGURE 13-17 Gross specimen of adenocarcinoma of the stomach.

Leiomyosarcoma. The second most common malignant tumor is the leiomyosarcoma gastric sarcoma (1%–5% of tumors). It occurs in the fifth to sixth decade of life. The mass is generally globular or irregular; it may become huge, outstripping its blood supply, with central necrosis leading to cystic degeneration and cavitation (see Table 13-1).

Sonographic Findings. A target-shaped lesion is visible on sonography. Although the pattern is variable, hemorrhage and necrosis may occur, causing irregular echoes or a cystic cavity.

Metastatic Disease. Metastatic disease to the stomach is rare; it may result from a melanoma or lung or breast cancer. The tumor is found in the submucosal layer, forming circumscribed nodules or plaques (see Table 13-1).

Sonographic Findings. A target pattern with circumscribed thickening or uniform widening of the stomach wall without layering is visible.

Lower Gastrointestinal Tract

Table 13-2 lists the clinical findings, sonographic findings, and differential diagnoses for lower gastrointestinal tract diseases and conditions.

Obstruction and Dilation. A small-bowel obstruction is associated with dilatation of the bowel loops proximal to the site of obstruction (Figure 13-18). In 6% of cases, the dilated loops are fluid-filled and can be mistaken for a soft tissue mass on x-ray examination (see Table 13-2).

Sonographic Findings. The dilated loops have a tubular or round echo-free appearance. In adynamic ileus, the dilated bowel has normal to somewhat increased peristaltic activity and less distention than in dynamic ileus. In dynamic ileus, the loops are round, with minimal deformity at the interfaces with adjacent loops of distended bowel; valvulae conniventes and peristalsis are seen. The fluid loops are not always associated with obstruction; they can occur with gastroenteritis and

TABLE 13-2	Lower Gastrointestinal Findings	
Clinical Findings	**Sonographic Findings**	**Differential Considerations**
Obstruction and/or Dilatation		
Epigastric pain	Tubular, round, echo-free lesion Compressibility of bowel	Appendicitis
Acute Appendicitis		
Pain rebound tenderness over McBurney's point Diarrhea Fever Nausea, vomiting	Thickened muscular wall and ↑ appendiceal diameter (6 mm) Lack of peristalsis Not compressible ↑ Blood flow (Doppler)	Ruptured ectopic pregnancy Fluid-filled colon Inflammation of Meckel's diverticulum
Mucocele		
↑ Leukocytes RLQ pain Asymptomatic	Variable: anechoic, hypoechoic, complex	Appendicitis
Meckel's Diverticulitis		
Rectal bleeding Tenderness	Loop pattern	Acute appendicitis
Crohn's Disease		
Diarrhea Fever RLQ pain	Symmetrically swollen bowel Target pattern with preserved parietal layers around stenotic and hyperdense lumen ↑ Wall thickening Rigidity to pressure Peristalsis absent or sluggish	Appendicitis Meckel's diverticulum Diverticulitis
Lymphoma		
Abdominal pain Palpable mass Weight loss Blood loss	Large, discrete mass Exoenteric pattern	Pseudokidney Leiomyosarcoma
Leiomyosarcoma		
Abdominal pain Palpable mass	Large, solid mass Contained in necrotic areas	Lymphoma

RLQ, Right lower quadrant.

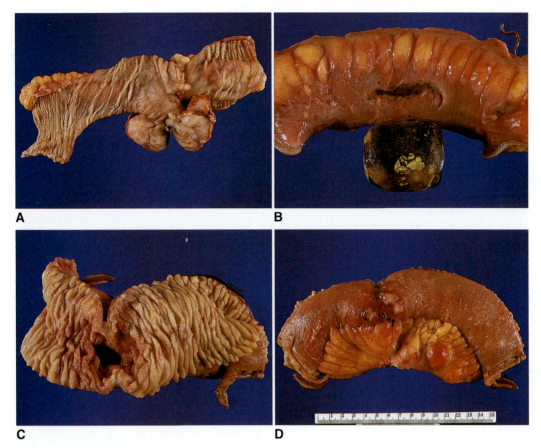

FIGURE 13-18 **A,** Gross specimen example of small-bowel obstruction. **B,** Small-bowel obstruction secondary to gallstones. **C** and **D,** Small-bowel adenocarcinoma. The tumor may cause obstruction of the small bowel.

paralytic ileus, or in dilated, fluid-filled bowel loops without peristalsis. The sonographer should demonstrate pliability and compressibility of the bowel wall (Figure 13-19, *A* through *D*).

With volvulus (closed-loop obstruction), the involved loop is doubled back on itself abruptly, so that a U-shaped appearance is seen on sagittal scan, and a C-shaped anechoic area with a dense center is seen on transverse scan. The dense center represents medial bowel wall and mesentery.

Abnormalities of the Appendix

Acute Appendicitis. Acute appendicitis is the result of luminal obstruction and inflammation, leading to ischemia of the vermiform appendix (Figure 13-20). This may produce necrosis, perforation, and subsequent abscess formation and peritonitis.

The appendix lumen may be obstructed by fecal material, a foreign body, carcinoma of the cecum, stenosis, inflammation, kinking of the organ, or even lymphatic hypertrophy resulting from systemic infection. Obstruction results in edema, which can compromise the vascular supply to the appendix. Subsequently, the permeability of the mucosa increases, and bacterial invasion of the wall of the appendix results in infection and inflammation. Increased intraluminal pressure may cause occlusion of the appendicular end artery. If the condition

persists, the appendix may necrose, leading to gangrene, rupture, and subsequent local or generalized peritonitis. Periappendiceal abscess or peritonitis does not necessarily mean perforation; the organism may permeate the wall in the absence of perforation to cause these extra-appendiceal complications.

The symptoms of acute appendicitis are pain and rebound tenderness, which is usually localized over the right lower quadrant (**McBurney's sign**). Typically, the pain is followed by nausea and vomiting, diarrhea, and systemic signs of inflammation, such as leukocytosis and fever (see Table 13-2). Acute appendicitis can occur at any age but is more prevalent at younger ages.

Progression of acute appendicitis to frank perforation is more rapid in the younger child, sometimes occurring within 6 to 12 hours. The rate of perforation in the preschool child can be as high as 70% compared with the overall figure of 30% for children and 21% to 22% for adults. Women aged 20 to 40 years are at high risk for misdiagnosis of the condition on initial physical examination.

Diagnosis of even the classic case of appendicitis is complicated by the fact that many disorders present with a similar clinical picture of an acute condition in the abdomen. Differential diagnosis may include the following: (1) acute gastroenteritis, (2) mesenteric

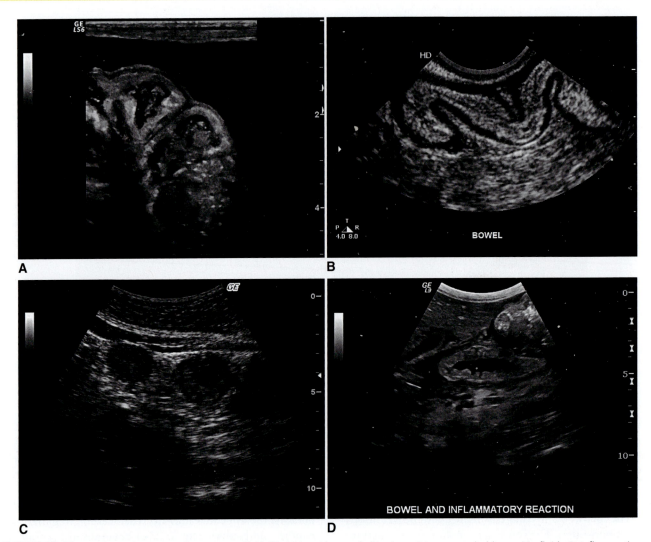

FIGURE 13-19 A, Transverse image of prominent fluid-filled bowel loops. **B,** The bowel is surrounded by ascitic fluid. **C,** Inflammation of the bowel demonstrates prominent dilated loops of bowel shown as circular bull's eye or target structures in the lower abdomen. **D,** Inflammatory reaction of the bowel.

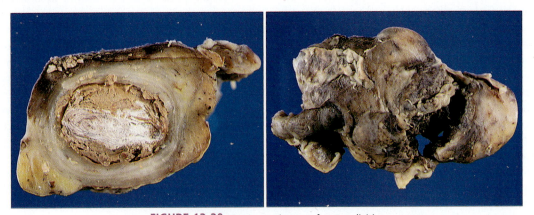

FIGURE 13-20 Gross specimens of appendicitis.

lymphadenitis in children, (3) ruptured ectopic pregnancy, (4) mittelschmerz, (5) inflammation of Meckel's diverticulum, (6) regional enteritis, and (7) right ovarian torsion.

🔖 **Sonographic Findings.** The normal appendix occasionally can be visualized with gradual compression

sonography. The maximal outer diameters of the normal appendix can measure up to 6 mm. The inflamed appendix will show edema of the wall measuring greater than 2 mm thick; perforation may be present when asymmetrical wall thickening is seen. In inflamed specimens, both the integrity and the stratification of wall layers are

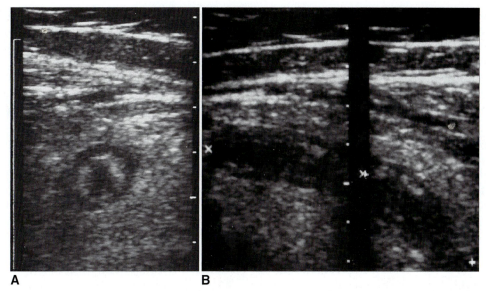

FIGURE 13-21 Appendicitis. Transverse **(A)** and sagittal **(B)** images of the inflamed appendix, which was not compressed with the linear-array transducer.

altered. The distinction of layers is impaired, and each layer is sonographically inhomogeneous.

Wall appearance should not be the only criterion for confirmation of appendicitis. The ultrasound pattern of acute appendicitis is characterized by a target-shaped appearance of the appendix in transverse view. Views of the appendix in the transverse plane should demonstrate a thickened muscular wall and increased appendiceal diameter (Figure 13-21). The typical target-shaped lesion consists of a hypoechoic, fluid-distended lumen, a hyperechoic inner ring representing mainly the mucosa and the submucosa, and an outer hypoechoic ring representing the **muscularis** externa. The inflamed appendix is further characterized by lack of peristalsis and compressibility, and by demonstration of its "blind end tip." It is important to carefully survey the entire length of the appendix to prevent a false-negative examination.

Retrocecal appendicitis is seen in approximately 28% of pediatric appendicitis patients and is easy to diagnose by ultrasound. No bowel loops are interposed between the appendix and the lateral wall of the abdomen. The inflamed appendix is identified on cross section as a **target sign** underneath the abdominis muscle. The incidence of complex masses is greater in retrocecal appendicitis, reflecting a higher incidence of perforation. The sonographic appearance of an appendiceal abscess is a complex mass. Sometimes the sonographer can recognize the appendix inside the mass. The omentum wrapping the appendix is seen as an echogenic band and bowel loops.

The initial inflammatory changes in appendicitis are more pronounced in the distal half of the appendix and may be focally confined to the appendiceal tip. Ulcerations and necrosis may cause loss of the echogenic submucosal layer in the tip of the appendix. The appendix should be compressed to the tip and visualized longitudinally and transversely to its blind termination. **Appendicoliths** are fecaliths or calculi in the appendix. They are seen as intraluminal foci of high-amplitude echoes with acoustic shadowing.

In infancy and childhood, the appendix frequently becomes decompressed after perforation, and the inflammatory process may not wall off or form a well-defined abscess, as is typically seen in adults. With perforation and decompression and an abnormally thickened wall, a collapsed appendix may still be identified. In some patients, however, no appendix may be found, and only questionable remnants remain. Supplemental findings, such as free abdominal fluid with debris or thickening of the adjacent abdominal wall, may suggest the diagnosis. However, the possibility of appendicitis cannot be ruled out even in a patient who lacks an abnormal appendix or a well-defined abscess. Radiographic contrast studies may help diagnosis.

Gas collections within the appendix may be a pitfall in ultrasound evaluation. Gas within the appendix is diagnosed on the basis of sonographic findings of high-amplitude echogenic foci, causing distal reverberation artifacts (i.e., "comet-tails" or "dirty" acoustic shadowing). Although this is a relatively rare finding, its importance lies in the fact that it may be misconstrued as a normal bowel loop or a gas-forming appendiceal abscess. Gas collections from within the bowel loops should be distinguished from an inflamed appendix. The inflamed appendix is noncompressible and demonstrates other specific anatomic features.

Graded compression ultrasound is an alternative technique for diagnosing appendicitis; it has a sensitivity of 88% and a specificity of 96%. Color Doppler ultrasound imaging can be used to detect increased flow, demonstrating hyperperfusion associated with inflammation. Vessels can be seen coursing through the periphery of the dilated appendix. Addition of color Doppler alone does not increase the sensitivity for detecting appendicitis compared with ultrasound alone. Color Doppler is a simple means of confirming gray scale sonographic findings.

Mucocele. Mucocele of the appendix is a rare pathologic entity. This term designates gross enlargement of the appendix from accumulation of mucoid substance within the lumen. It was recognized in 0.2% to 0.3% of 45,000 appendectomies. Scarring or **fecalith** after an appendectomy is the most common cause of mucocele, although proximal obstruction of the lumen by inflammatory fibrosis, cecal carcinoma, carcinoid polyp, and even endometriosis has been reported. Mucoceles have been classified into three distinct entities: mucosal hyperplasia (an innocuous hyperplastic process), mucinous cystadenoma (a benign neoplasm), and mucinous cystadenocarcinoma (a malignant tumor).

Several classifications of mucoceles are known. If the tumor remains encapsulated and no malignant cells are present, this lesion is called a mucocele. If the mucus spreads through the abdominal cavity without evidence of malignant cells, this condition is called pseudomyxoma peritonei. Pseudomyxoma assumes a malignant potential only when epithelial cells occur within the gelatinous peritoneal fluid in association with carcinoma.

Appendiceal mucoceles reportedly show a female-to-male predominance of 4:1, with an average age at presentation of 55 years. The most common clinical complaint is right lower quadrant pain (see Table 13-2). About 25% of cases are asymptomatic. Other symptoms include right iliac fossa mass, sepsis, and urinary symptoms. Bloating of the abdomen is specific to patients with pseudomyxoma peritonei. Laboratory values show an increased erythrocyte sedimentation rate and an elevated leukocyte count. Also, elevated levels of carcinoembryonic antigen have been reported. Pseudomyxoma peritonei significantly decreases survival of patients with appendiceal cystadenocarcinomas.

Preoperative diagnosis of mucocele is helpful. If a mucocele is suspected, needle aspiration is not advised. Careful surgical mobilization may reduce the possibility of rupture, peritoneal contamination, and development of pseudomyxoma peritonei. Radiographically, a mucocele is seen as a soft tissue mass, typically with a rimlike, curvilinear calcification of the mucocele wall. A barium enema examination classically describes nonfilling of the appendix and an extrinsic or submucosal mass at the cecal tip with intact overlying mucosa.

▶ **Sonographic Findings.** The sonographer should locate the appendix in the right lower quadrant, referencing the psoas muscle and iliac vessels. The image varies according to the content of the mucocele, which may be anechoic when mucoid material is more fluid.

The following patterns have been defined: (1) a purely cystic lesion with anechoic fluid; (2) a hypoechoic mass containing fine internal echoes; and (3) a complex mass with high-level echoes (Figure 13-22). As it enlarges, inspissation of the mucoid material creates this internal echo pattern. This mass has an irregular inner wall caused by mucinous debris with varying degrees of epithelial hyperplasia. Calcification of the rim can produce acoustic shadowing. Internal, thin septations have been seen along with variable degrees of mucosal atrophy and ulceration.

Pseudomyxoma peritonei is seen as septated **ascites** (fluid in the abdomen) with numerous suspended echoes that do not mobilize as the patient changes position. When combined with ultrasound, paracentesis may accurately establish the diagnosis of gelatinous ascites.

Meckel's Diverticulitis. A **diverticulum** is a pouchlike herniation through the muscular wall of a tubular organ that occurs in the stomach, the small intestine, or, most commonly, the colon. **Meckel's diverticulum** is located on the antimesenteric border of the ileum, approximately 2 feet from the ileocecal valve. It is present in 2% of the population. In Meckel's diverticulitis, adults may present with intestinal obstruction, rectal bleeding, or diverticular inflammation (see Table 13-2). Acute appendicitis and acute Meckel's diverticulitis may not be distinguished clinically.

▶ **Sonographic Findings.** The wall of Meckel's diverticulum consists of mucosal, muscular, and serosal layers. Noncompressibility of the obstructed, inflamed diverticulum indicates that intraluminal fluid is trapped. The area of maximal tenderness is evaluated along with its distance from the cecum.

Crohn's Disease. Crohn's disease is regional enteritis, a recurrent granulomatous inflammatory disease that affects the terminal ileum, colon, or both at any level (Figures 13-23 through 13-25). The reaction involves the entire thickness of the bowel wall. Clinical symptoms include diarrhea, fever, and right lower quadrant pain (see Table 13-2).

▶ **Sonographic Findings.** A symmetrically swollen bowel target pattern with preserved parietal layers around the stenotic and echogenic lumen is seen on sonography. Findings are most prominent in ileocolonic disease, with uniformly increased wall thickness involving all layers, especially the mucosa and submucosa. A matted-loop pattern is found in late stages. Patients with Crohn's disease show rigidity to pressure exerted with the transducer. Peristalsis is absent or sluggish.

Tumors of the Colon

Lymphoma. Lymphoma is a tumor that usually occurs late in life, near the sixth decade; it is also the most common tumor of the gastrointestinal tract in children younger than 10 years of age. Intraperitoneal masses frequently involve the mesenteric vessels that encase them. Clinical signs include intestinal blood loss, weight loss, anorexia, and abdominal pain (see Table

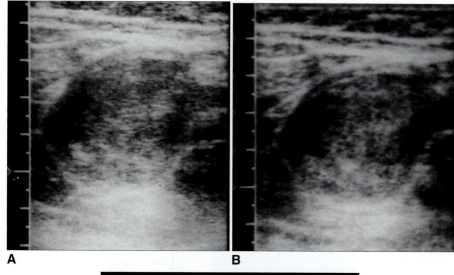

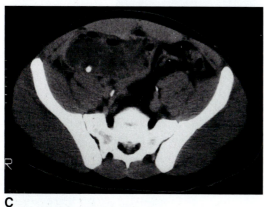

FIGURE 13-22 A and **B,** Ultrasound images of a mucocele. This patient shows a complex mass with high-level echoes. **C,** Computed tomographic image of the mucocele.

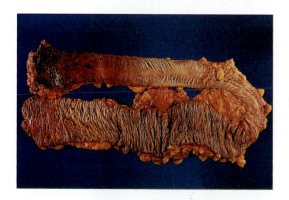

FIGURE 13-23 Gross specimen of ulcerative colitis.

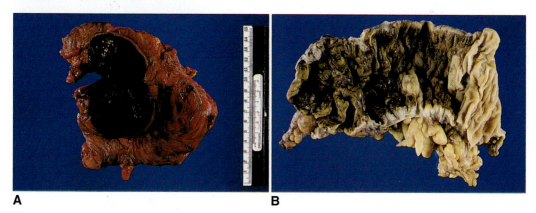

FIGURE 13-24 Gross specimens show complications of colitis. **A,** Hematoma in the colon. **B,** Gangrenous colon.

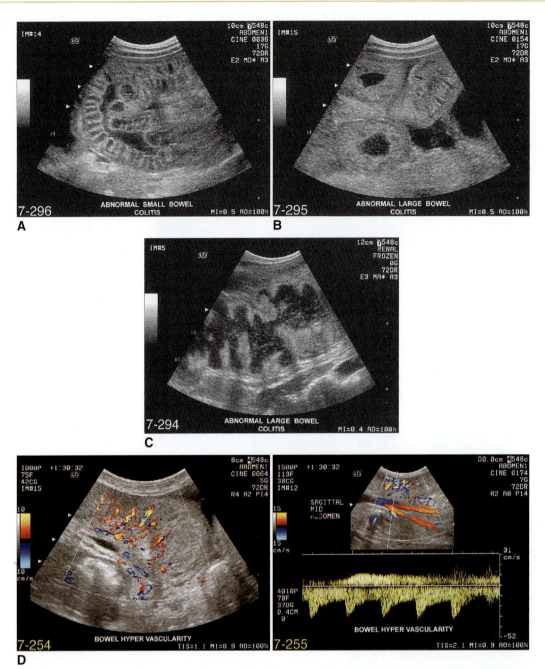

FIGURE 13-25 Ulcerative colitis. **A,** Small-bowel colitis. **B** and **C,** Dilated colon with colitis. **D,** Prominent colon with increased vascularity.

13-2). The patient may have an intestinal obstruction or a palpable mass.

◗ **Sonographic Findings.** The sonographer may see a large, discrete mass with a target pattern, an exoenteric pattern with a large mass on the mesenteric surface of bowel, and a small anechoic mass representing subserosal nodes or mesenteric nodal involvement.

Lymphomatous involvement of the intestinal wall may lead to pseudokidney or hydronephrotic pseudokidney. The lumen may be dilated with fluid and may demonstrate lack of peristalsis. The bowel wall is uni-

formly thickened, with homogeneous low echogenicity between the well-defined mucosal and serosal surfaces that contain a persistent, echo-free, wide, and long lumen.

Leiomyosarcoma. Leiomyosarcoma represents 10% of primary small-bowel tumors. Approximately 10% to 30% of these occur in the duodenum, 30% to 45% in the jejunum, and 35% to 55% in the ileum. Patients are in their fifth to sixth decade of life.

◗ **Sonographic Findings.** A large solid mass containing necrotic areas anterior to solid viscus may be found.

The Urinary System

Kerry Weinberg and Shpetim Telegrafi

OBJECTIVES

On completion of this chapter, you should be able to:
- Discuss normal anatomic location, function, and sonographic appearance of urinary system organs
- Discuss normal physiology of the urinary system
- Describe the sonographic scanning technique to image the urinary system
- Define and discuss the pathologies discussed in this chapter
- Identify and define the sonographic appearance of pathologies included in this chapter
- Discuss the role and limitations of sonography in postrenal transplant patients
- Describe the clinical signs and symptoms of urinary tract problems and the laboratory tests that are used to evaluate them

OUTLINE

The urinary system has two principal functions: excreting wastes and regulating the composition of blood. Blood composition must not be allowed to vary beyond tolerable limits, or the conditions in tissue necessary for cellular life will be lost. Regulating blood composition involves not only removing harmful wastes but also conserving water and metabolites in the body.

ANATOMY OF THE URINARY SYSTEM

Normal Anatomy

Kidneys. The urinary system is located posterior to the peritoneum lining the abdominal cavity in an area called the **retroperitoneum.** The kidneys lie in the retroperitoneal cavity near the posterior body wall, just below the diaphragm (Figure 14-1). The lower ribs protect both kidneys. The right kidney lies slightly lower than the left kidney because the large right lobe of the liver pushes it inferiorly. The kidneys move readily with respiration; on deep inspiration, both kidneys move downward approximately 1 inch.

The kidneys are dark red, bean-shaped organs that measure 9 to 12 cm long, 5 cm wide, and 2.5 cm thick. The outer **cortex** of the kidney is darker than the inner **medulla** because of the increased perfusion of blood. The inner surface of the medulla is folded into projections called *renal pyramids,* which empty into the renal pelvis. The **arcuate arteries** are located at the base of the pyramids and separate the medulla from the cortex. Numerous collecting tubules bring the urine from its sites of formation in the cortex to the pyramids. The renal tubules, or **nephrons,** are the functional units of the kidney.

On the medial surface of each kidney is a vertical indentation called the **renal hilum,** where the renal

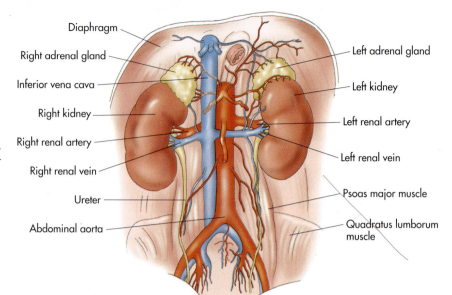

FIGURE 14-1 Relationships of the kidneys, suprarenal glands (adrenal), and vascular structures to one another.

vessels and ureter enter and exit. Within the **hilus** of the kidney are other vascular structures, a ureter, and the lymphatics. The renal artery is the most posterior and superior structure. The two branches of the renal vein are anterior to the renal artery (Figure 14-2). The **ureter** is located slightly inferior to the renal artery. When present, the third branch of the renal artery may be seen to arise from the hilus. The lymph vessels and sympathetic fibers also are found within the renal hilus.

A fibrous capsule called the true capsule surrounds the kidney. Outside of this fibrous capsule is a covering of perinephric fat. The perinephric fascia surrounds the perinephric fat and encloses the kidneys and adrenal glands. The perinephric fascia is a condensation of areolar tissue that is continuous laterally with the fascia transversalis. The renal fascia, known as **Gerota's fascia,** surrounds the true capsule and perinephric fat.

Anterior to the right kidney are the right adrenal gland, liver, **Morison's pouch,** second part of the duodenum, and right colic flexure (Figure 14-3). Anterior to the left kidney are the left adrenal gland, spleen, stomach, pancreas, left colic flexure, and coils of jejunum.

Posterior to the right kidney are the diaphragm, costodiaphragmatic recess of the pleura, twelfth rib, psoas muscle, quadratus lumborum, and transversus abdominis muscles. The subcostal (T12), iliohypogastric, and ilioinguinal (L1) nerves run downward and laterally. Posterior to the left kidney are the diaphragm, costodiaphragmatic recess of the pleura, eleventh and twelve ribs, psoas muscle, quadratus lumborum, and transversus abdominis muscles. The same nerves are seen near the left kidney as in the right.

Within the kidney, the upper expanded end of the ureter, known as the **renal pelvis** of the ureter, divides into two or three **major calyces,** each of which divides further into two or three **minor calyces** (see Figure 14-2). The apex of a medullary pyramid, called the renal

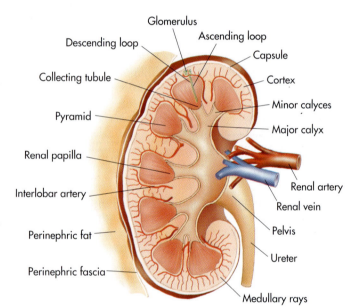

FIGURE 14-2 The kidney cut longitudinally to show the internal structure.

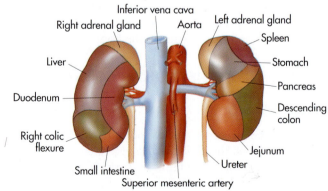

FIGURE 14-3 Anatomic structures related to the anterior surfaces of the kidneys.

papilla, indents each minor **calyx.** The kidney consists of an internal medullary portion and an external cortical substance. The medullary substance consists of a series of striated conical masses, called the *renal pyramids.* The pyramids vary from 8 to 18 in number, and their bases are directed toward the outer circumference of the kidney. Their apices converge toward the **renal sinus,** where their prominent papillae project into the lumina of the minor calyces. Spirally arranged muscles surround the calyces and may exert a milking action on these tubes, aiding in the flow of urine into the renal pelvis. As the pelvis leaves the renal sinus, it rapidly becomes smaller and ultimately merges with the ureter.

Nephron. A nephron consists of two main structures—a renal corpuscle and a renal tubule. Nephrons filter the blood and produce urine. Blood is filtered in the renal corpuscle. The filtered fluid passes through the renal tubule. As the filtrate moves through the tubule, substances needed by the body are returned to the blood. Waste products, excess water, and other substances not needed by the body pass into the collecting ducts as urine.

The **renal corpuscle** consists of a network of capillaries called the **glomerulus,** which is surrounded by a cuplike structure known as **Bowman's capsule.** Blood flows into the glomerulus through a small **afferent arteriole** and leaves the glomerulus through an **efferent arteriole.** This arteriole conducts blood to a second set of capillaries, the peritubular capillaries, which surround the renal tubule.

Filtrate passes into the renal tubule through an opening in the bottom of Bowman's capsule. The first part of the renal tubule is the coiled proximal convoluted tubule. After passing through the proximal convoluted tubule, filtrate flows into the **loop of Henle** and then into the distal convoluted tubule. Urine from the distal convoluted tubules of several nephrons drains into a collecting duct. A portion of the distal convoluted tubule curves upward and contacts the afferent and efferent arterioles. Some cells of the distal convoluted tubule and some cells of the afferent arteriole are modified to form the juxtaglomerular apparatus, a structure that helps regulate blood pressure in the kidney.

The renal corpuscle, the proximal convoluted tubule, and the distal convoluted tubule of each nephron are located within the renal cortex. The loops of Henle dip down into the medulla.

Ureter. The **ureter** is a 25 cm tubular structure whose proximal end is expanded and continuous with the funnel shape of the renal pelvis. The renal pelvis lies within the hilus of the kidney and receives major calyces. The ureter emerges from the hilus of the kidney and runs vertically downward behind the parietal peritoneum along the psoas muscle, which separates it from the tips of the transverse processes of the lumbar vertebrae. It enters the pelvis by crossing the bifurcation of the common iliac artery anterior to the sacroiliac joint. The ureter courses along the lateral wall of the pelvis to the region of the ischial spine and turns forward to enter the lateral angle of the bladder. The ureter from the ureteropelvic junction to the bladder is not routinely visualized on a sonogram. The superior and distal ends of the ureters are more readily visualized than the midsection. The ureters are located in the retroperitoneal cavity and are obscured by bowel gas.

Three constrictions are seen along the ureter's course: (1) where the ureter leaves the renal pelvis, (2) where it is kinked as it crosses the pelvic brim, and (3) where it pierces the bladder wall.

Urinary Bladder. The **urinary bladder** is a large muscular bag. It has a posterior and lateral opening for the ureters and an anterior opening for the urethra. The interior of the bladder is lined with highly elastic transitional epithelium. When the bladder is full, the lining is smooth and stretched; when it is empty, the lining is a series of folds. In the middle layer, a series of smooth muscle coats distend as urine collects and contract to expel urine through the urethra. Urine is produced almost continuously and accumulates in the bladder until the increased pressure stimulates the organ's nervous receptors to relax the urethra's sphincter and urine is released from the urinary bladder. The urinary bladder is visualized sonographically when it is distended with fluid.

Urethra. The **urethra** is a membranous tube that passes from the anterior part of the urinary bladder to the outside of the body. It includes two sphincters: the internal sphincter and the external sphincter. The urethra is not routinely visualized sonographically.

Vascular Supply

The arterial supply to the kidney is provided through the main renal artery. This vessel is a lateral branch of the aorta and rises just inferior to the superior mesenteric artery (Figure 14-4). Each artery is divided into three branches to enter the hilus of the kidney—two anterior and one posterior to the pelvis of the ureter. The branches

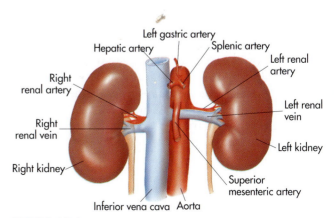

FIGURE 14-4 Vascular relationships of the great vessels and their tributaries to the kidneys.

of the renal artery may vary in size and number. In most cases, the renal artery is divided into two primary branches: a larger anterior and a smaller posterior. These arteries break down into smaller segmental arteries, then into interlobar arteries, and finally into tiny arcuate arteries.

Five to six veins join to form the main renal vein. This vein emerges from the renal hilus anterior to the renal artery. The renal vein drains into the lateral walls of the inferior vena cava (see Figure 14-4).

The lymphatic vessels follow the renal artery to the lateral aortic lymph nodes near the origin of the renal artery. Nerves originate in the renal sympathetic plexus and are distributed along the branches of the renal vessels.

Blood supply to nephrons begins at the renal artery. The artery subdivides within the kidneys. A small vessel (afferent arteriole) enters Bowman's capsule, where it forms a tuft of capillaries, the glomerulus, which entirely fills the concavity of the capsule. Blood leaves the glomerulus via the efferent arteriole, which subdivides into a network of capillaries that surround the proximal and distal tubules and eventually unite as veins, which become the renal vein.

The renal vein returns the cleansed blood to the general circulation. Movements of substances between the nephron and the capillaries of the tubules change the composition of the blood filtrate moving along in the tubules. From the nephrons, the fluid moves to collecting tubules and into the ureter, leading to the bladder, where urine is stored.

The arterial supply to the ureter is provided by the following three sources: the renal artery, the testicular or ovarian artery, and the superior vesical artery.

PHYSIOLOGY AND LABORATORY DATA OF THE URINARY SYSTEM

The urinary system consists of two kidneys, which remove wastes from the blood and produce urine, and two ureters, which act as tubal ducts leading from the hilus of the kidneys and drain into the urinary bladder. The bladder collects and stores urine, which is eventually discharged through the urethra. The urinary system is located posterior to the peritoneum lining the abdominal cavity in an area called the retroperitoneum.

The function of the kidneys is to excrete urine. More than any other organ, the kidneys adjust the amounts of water and electrolytes leaving the body so that these equal the amounts of substances entering the body. The formation of urine involves the following three processes: glomerular filtration, tubular reabsorption, and tubular secretion.

Excretion

Cells in the body continually carry on metabolic activities that produce waste products. If permitted to accumulate, metabolic wastes eventually reach toxic concentrations and threaten **homeostasis.** To prevent this, metabolic wastes must be quickly excreted. The process of excretion entails separating and removing substances harmful to the body. The skin, lungs, liver, large intestine, and kidneys carry out excretion.

The principal metabolic waste products are water, carbon dioxide, and nitrogenous wastes (including urea, uric acid, and **creatinine [Cr]**). Nitrogen is derived from amino acids and nucleic acids. Amino acids break down in the liver, and the nitrogen-containing amino group is removed. The amino group is then converted to ammonia, which is chemically converted to urea. Uric acid is formed from the breakdown of nucleic acids. Both urea and uric acid are carried away from the liver into the kidneys by the vascular system. Creatinine is nitrogenous waste produced from phosphocreatine in the muscles.

Laboratory Tests for Renal Disease

The clinical symptoms of a patient with specific renal pathology may be nonspecific. A patient's history of infection, previous urinary tract problems (renal stones), or hypertension or family history of renal cystic disease is useful information. A patient with a renal infection or disease process may present with any of the following symptoms: flank pain, hematuria, polyuria, oliguria, fever, urgency, weight loss, or general edema.

A patient who presents with symptoms of renal infection, renal insufficiency, or disease may undergo a number of laboratory tests to help the clinician determine the cause of the problem.

Urinalysis. Urinalysis is essential to detect urinary tract disorders in patients whose renal function is impaired or absent. Most renal inflammatory processes introduce a characteristic exudate for a specific type of inflammation into the urine. The presence of an acute infection causes hematuria, or red blood cells in the urine; pyuria is pus in the urine.

Urine pH. Urine pH is very important in managing diseases such as bacteriuria and renal calculi. The pH refers to the strength of the urine as a partly acidic or alkaline solution. The abundance of hydrogen ions in a solution is called pH. If urine contains an increased concentration of hydrogen ions, the urine is acidic. The formation of renal calculi depends in part on the pH of urine. Other conditions, such as renal tubular acidosis and chronic renal failure, are associated with alkaline urine.

Specific Gravity. The **specific gravity** is the measurement of the kidney's ability to concentrate urine. The concentration factor depends on the quantity of dissolved waste products. Excessive intake of fluids or decreased perspiration may cause a large output of urine and a decrease in the specific gravity. Low fluid intake, excessive perspiration, or diarrhea can cause the output of urine to be low and the specific gravity to increase. The specific gravity is especially low in cases of renal failure, glomerular nephritis, and pyelonephritis. These diseases cause renal tubular damage, which affects the ability of the kidneys to concentrate urine.

Blood. Hematuria is the appearance of blood cells in the urine; it can be associated with early renal disease. An abundance of red blood cells in the urine may suggest renal trauma, neoplasm, calculi, pyelonephritis, or glomerular or vascular inflammatory processes, such as acute glomerulonephritis and renal infarction.

Leukocytes may be present whenever inflammation, infection, or tissue necrosis originates from anywhere in the urinary tract.

Hematocrit. The hematocrit is the relative ratio of plasma to packed cell volume in the blood. Decreased hematocrit occurs with acute hemorrhagic processes secondary to disease or blunt trauma.

Hemoglobin. Hemoglobin is present in urine whenever extensive damage or destruction of the functioning erythrocytes occurs. This condition injures the kidney and can cause acute renal failure.

Protein. When glomerular damage is evident, albumin and other plasma proteins may be filtered in excess, allowing the overflow to enter the urine, which lowers the blood serum albumin concentration. Albuminuria is commonly found with benign and malignant neoplasms, calculi, chronic infection, and pyelonephritis.

Creatinine Clearance. Specific measurements of creatinine concentrations in urine and blood serum are considered an accurate index for determining the glomerular filtration rate. Creatinine is a by-product of muscle energy metabolism; it is normally produced at a constant rate as long as the body muscle mass remains relatively constant. Creatinine normally goes through complete glomerular filtration without being reabsorbed by the renal tubules. Decreased urinary creatinine clearance indicates renal dysfunction because creatinine blood levels are constant, and only decreased renal function prevents the normal excretion of creatinine.

Blood Urea Nitrogen. The **blood urea nitrogen (BUN)** is the concentration of urea nitrogen in blood and is the end product of cellular metabolism. Urea is formed in the liver and is carried to the kidneys through the blood to be excreted in urine. Impairment of renal function and increased protein catabolism result in BUN elevation that is relative to the degree of renal impairment and the rate of urea nitrogen excretion by the kidneys.

Serum Creatinine. Renal dysfunction also results in serum creatinine elevation. Blood serum creatinine levels are said to be more specific and more sensitive in determining renal impairment than BUN.

SONOGRAPHIC EVALUATION OF THE URINARY SYSTEM

Kidneys

Sonographic evaluation of the kidneys is a noninvasive, relatively inexpensive, reproducible diagnostic test used to evaluate renal problems. Until recently, an intravenous pyelogram (IVP) was the initial diagnostic test performed on patients who presented with renal colic (flank pain). In patients who present with renal colic without a history of renal stones, a noncontrast computed tomography (NCCT) is typically performed. NCCT requires no patient preparation and is not operator or patient dependent. The main disadvantages of NCCT are cost and the use of ionizing radiation. Patients who present with a history of renal stones require a plain film x-ray, and a renal sonogram with Doppler is usually the first diagnostic test performed. In many areas where computed tomography (CT) is not readily available, an IVP is performed if the patient can tolerate the contrast agent used and does not have an allergic reaction to it.

Magnetic resonance imaging (MRI) using magnetic resonance urography (MRU) is currently being investigated for diagnosing renal disease. MRU can assess renal function, similarly to an IVP, in addition to diagnosing obstructive uropathy. MRI can assess other abdominal organs for disease.

A renal sonogram is able to demonstrate the acoustic properties of a mass, delineate an abnormal lie of a kidney resulting from an extrarenal mass, or determine whether hydronephrosis is secondary to renal stones. In addition, sonography can define perirenal fluid collections, such as a hematoma or abscess, determine renal size and parenchymal detail, detect dilated ureters and **hydronephrosis**, and image renal congenital anomalies.

Normal Texture and Patterns. The kidneys are imaged by sonography as organs with smooth outer contours surrounded by reflected echoes of perirenal fat. The renal parenchyma surrounds the fatty central renal sinus, which contains the calyces, infundibula, pelvis, vessels, and lymphatics (Figure 14-5). Because of the fat interface, the renal sinus is imaged as an area of intense echoes with variable contours. If two separate collections of renal sinus fat are identified, a double collecting system should be suspected.

Generally, patients are given nothing by mouth before a sonogram or other imaging examinations are performed. This state of dehydration causes the infundibula and renal pelvis to be collapsed and thus indistinguishable from the echo-dense renal sinus fat. If, on the other hand, the bladder is distended from rehydration, the intrarenal collecting system also will become distended. An extrarenal pelvis may be seen as a fluid-filled structure medial to the kidney on transverse scans. The normal variant from obstruction is differentiated by

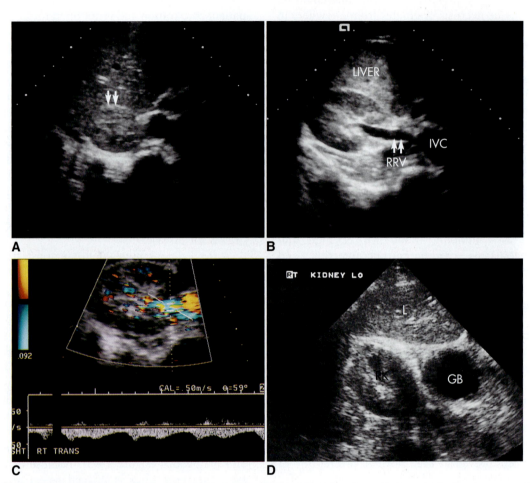

FIGURE 14-5 Transverse section of the abdominal cavity through the epiploic foramen.

Inferior vena cava

Aorta

Right kidney

Subserous fascia

Peritoneum

Lesser sac

Left kidney

Lienorenal ligament

Diaphragm

FIGURE 14-6 A and **B,** Transverse scan of the normal upper pole of the right kidney imaged through the homogeneous liver. Scans are made from the upper pole, from the mid pole to include the right renal vein *(RRV),* and from the inferior vena cava *(IVC)* to the lower pole. **C,** Normal blood flow is seen through the right renal vein to the IVC. **D,** A slight decubitus position allows the liver *(L)* to roll anterior to the right kidney *(RK)* and gallbladder *(GB)* for better visualization.

noting the absence of a distended intrasinus portion of the renal pelvis and infundibula. Dilation of the collecting system has also been noted in pregnant patients. (The right kidney is generally involved with a mild degree of hydronephrosis. This distention returns to normal shortly after delivery.)

Patient Position and Technique. The most efficient way to examine the kidneys is to use the liver as a window to image the right kidney (Figures 14-6 and

14-7) or through the spleen for the left kidney (Figure 14-8). The patient should be in a supine and/or decubitus position. Several alternative scanning windows can be used to image the kidney. These include the right posterior oblique, right lateral decubitus, and left lateral decubitus views. Having the patient take in a deep breath will move the liver and spleen distally, which may create a better window to enhance visualization of the kidneys. A subcostal or intercostal transducer approach may be

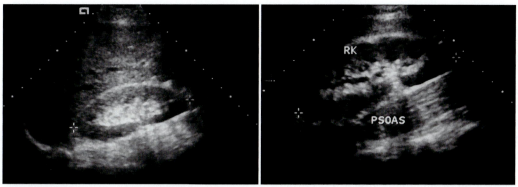

FIGURE 14-7 Longitudinal scans through the long axis of the right kidney *(RK)* and psoas muscle. Measurements are made along the maximum length of the right kidney from upper pole to lower pole.

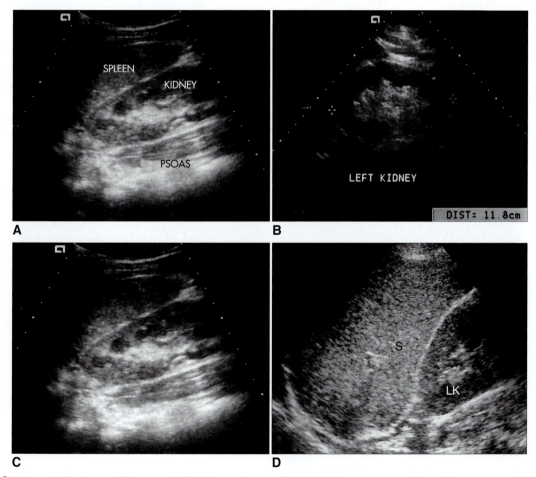

FIGURE 14-8 **A,** Longitudinal scan of the normal left kidney as imaged through the homogeneous spleen. The psoas muscle is the posterior medial border of the kidney. **B,** Measurements are made along the maximum length of the kidney from the upper pole to the lower pole. **C,** The patient may be rolled into a right lateral decubitus position for better visualization of the renal medullary pyramids and parenchyma. **D,** Splenomegaly *(S)* aids in visualization of the upper pole of the left kidney.

used for visualization of the upper and lower poles of the kidneys.

Proper adjustment of time gain compensation (TGC) with adequate sensitivity settings allows a uniform acoustic pattern throughout the image. The renal cortical echo amplitude should be compared with the liver paren-chymal echo amplitude at the same depth to effectively set the TGC and sensitivity.

If the patient has a substantial amount of perirenal fat, a high-frequency transducer may not provide the penetration necessary to optimally visualize the area. The deeper areas of the kidney may appear hypoechoic.

Renal detail may also be obscured if the patient has hepatocellular disease, gallstones, rib interference (Figures 14-9 and 14-10), or other abnormal collections between the liver and kidney. The use of harmonic imaging or tissue contrast enhancement technology (TCE) (Figure 14-11) may help to optimize visualization of the kidneys.

Renal Parenchyma. The parenchyma is the area from the renal sinus to the outer renal surface (Figure 14-12). The arcuate arteries and interlobar vessels are found within and are best demonstrated as intense specular echoes in cross section or oblique section at the cortico-medullary junction.

The cortex generally is echo producing (Figure 14-13) (although its echoes are less intense than those from normal liver), whereas the medullary pyramids are hypoechoic (Figure 14-14). The two are separated from each other by bands of cortical tissue, called columns of Bertin, which extend inward to the renal sinus.

Diseases of the renal parenchyma are those that accentuate cortical echoes but preserve or exaggerate the corticomedullary junction (type I) and those that distort the normal anatomy, obliterating the corticome-dullary differentiation in a focal or diffuse manner (type II).

Criteria for type I changes include the following: (1) The echo intensity in the cortex must be equal to or greater than that in the adjacent liver or spleen, and (2) the echo intensity in the cortex must be equal to that in the adjacent renal sinus. Minor signs would include the

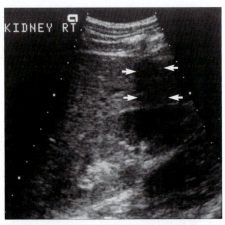

FIGURE 14-9 The ribs may interfere with uniform visualization of the kidney. Variations in respiration help the sonographer find the best window through which to image the renal parenchyma without rib interference.

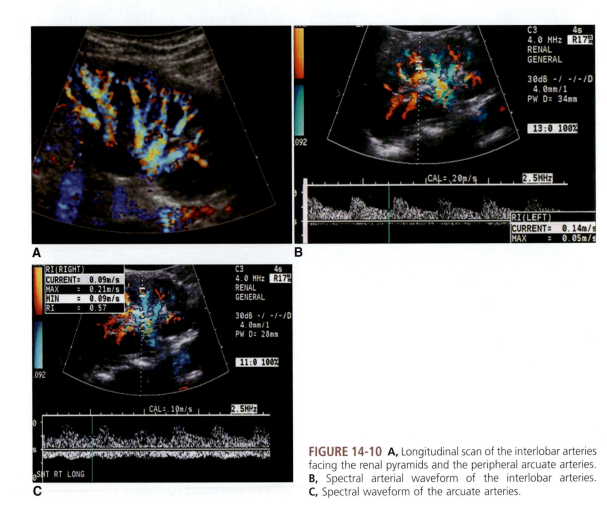

FIGURE 14-10 A, Longitudinal scan of the interlobar arteries facing the renal pyramids and the peripheral arcuate arteries. **B,** Spectral arterial waveform of the interlobar arteries. **C,** Spectral waveform of the arcuate arteries.

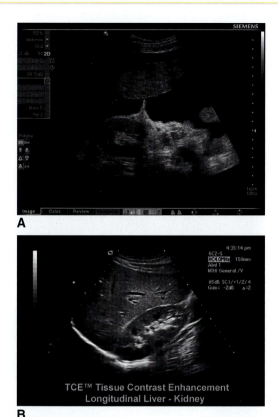

A

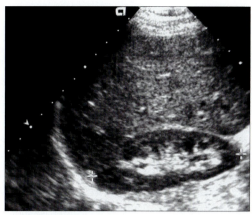

FIGURE 14-13 Sagittal scan of the normal kidney. The cortex is the brightest of the echoes within the renal parenchyma. The medullary pyramids are echo free. The pyramids are separated from the cortex by bands of cortical tissue and the columns of Bertin that extend inward to the renal sinus. *(Courtesy Joseph Yee, New York University.)*

TCE™ Tissue Contrast Enhancement
Longitudinal Liver - Kidney

B

FIGURE 14-11 A, Transverse view of right kidney with ascites in Morison's pouch. **B,** Sagittal view of normal liver/kidney using tissue contrast enhancement technology (TCE). *(Courtesy Siemens Medical Solutions USA, Inc.)*

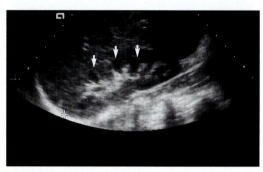

FIGURE 14-14 Longitudinal image of a neonatal left kidney with normal hypoechoic renal pyramids.

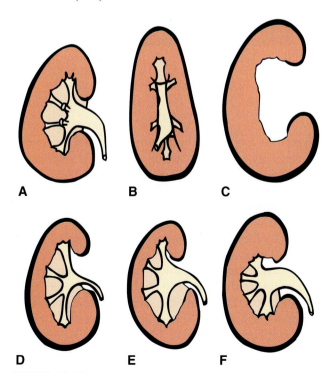

FIGURE 14-12 Thickness of the renal substance. **A,** Maximal in the polar regions, medium in the middle zone. **B,** Medial plane showing the pelvis emerging through the hilum and minimal thickness anteriorly and posteriorly. **C,** Hypertrophy. **D,** Normal adult proportions of the renal substance. **E,** Senile atrophy. **F,** Normal appearance in a 2-year-old child.

loss of identifiable arcuate vessels and the accentuation of corticomedullary definition.

Type II changes can be seen in focal disruption of normal anatomy with any mass lesion, including cysts, tumors, abscesses, and hematomas.

Renal Vessels. The arteries are best seen with the supine and left lateral decubitus views. The right renal artery extends from the lateral wall of the aorta to enter the central renal sinus (Figure 14-15). On the longitudinal scan, the right renal artery can be seen as a round anechoic structure posterior to the inferior vena cava (Figure 14-16). The right renal vein extends from the central renal sinus directly into the inferior vena cava (Figure 14-17). Both vessels appear as tubular structures in the transverse plane.

The renal arteries have an echo-free central lumen with highly echogenic borders that consist of a vessel wall and surrounding retroperitoneal fat and connective tissue. They lie posterior to the veins and can be demonstrated with certainty if their junction with the aorta is seen.

The left renal artery flows from the lateral wall of the aorta to the central renal sinus (Figure 14-18). The left

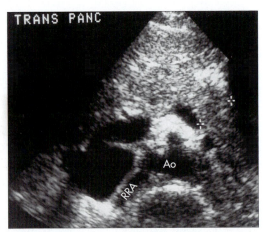

FIGURE 14-15 Transverse image of the right renal artery *(RRA)* as it extends from the posterior lateral wall of the aorta *(Ao)* to enter the central renal sinus.

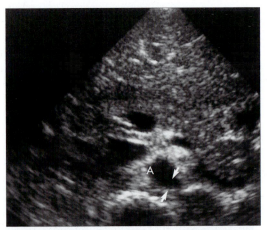

FIGURE 14-18 The left renal artery *(arrows)* flows from the posterior lateral wall of the aorta *(A)* to the central renal sinus.

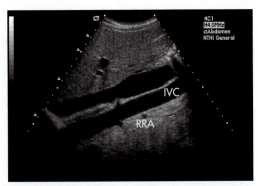

FIGURE 14-16 On longitudinal scan of the IVC and aorta at renal bifurcation, the right renal artery *(RRA)* can be seen as a circular structure posterior to the inferior vena cava *(IVC)*.

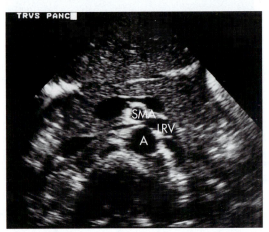

FIGURE 14-19 The left renal vein *(LRV)* flows from the central renal sinus, anterior to the aorta *(A)* and posterior to the superior mesenteric artery *(SMA)*, to join the inferior vena cava.

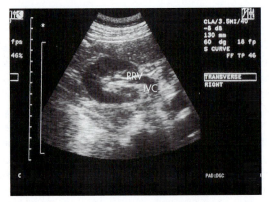

FIGURE 14-17 The right renal vein *(RRV)* extends from the central renal sinus directly into the inferior vena cava *(IVC)*.

renal vein flows from the central renal sinus, anterior to the aorta and posterior to the superior mesenteric artery, to join the inferior vena cava (Figure 14-19). It is seen as a tubular structure on the transverse scan.

The diaphragmatic crura run transversely in the paraaortic region. The crura lie posterior to the renal arteries and should be identified by their lack of pulsations and

absence of Doppler flow (Figure 14-20). They vary in echogenicity, depending on the amount of surrounding retroperitoneal fat. They may appear hypoechoic, as lymph nodes do.

Renal Medulla. The renal medulla consists of hypoechoic pyramids dispersed in a uniform distribution, separated by bands of intervening parenchyma that extend toward the renal sinus. The pyramids are uniform in size, shape (triangular), and distribution. The apex of the pyramid points toward the sinus, and the base lies adjacent to the renal cortex. The interlobar arteries lie alongside the pyramids, and arcuate vessels lie at the base of the pyramids (see Figures 14-2 and 14-10).

Renal Variants

Renal variants include slight alterations in anatomy that may lead the sonographer to suspect an abnormality is present when it really is a normal variation. See Table 14-1 for a description of renal variants and anomalies.

Columns of Bertin. The **columns of Bertin** are prominent invaginations of the cortex located at varying depths within the medullary substance of the kidneys. Hypertrophied columns of Bertin contain renal pyramids and may be difficult to differentiate from an avascular renal neoplasm. The columns are most exaggerated in patients with complete or partial duplication (Figure 14-21).

▶ **Sonographic Findings.** Sonographic features of a renal mass effect produced by a hypertrophied column of Bertin include the following: a lateral indentation of the renal sinus, a clear definition from the renal sinus, or a maximum dimension that does not exceed 3 cm. Contiguity with the renal cortex is evident, and overall echogenicity is similar to that of the renal parenchyma.

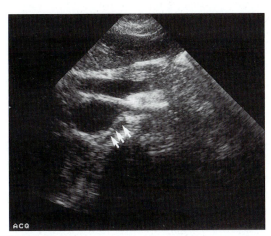

FIGURE 14-20 The crura of the diaphragm lie posterior to the renal arteries and should be identified by their lack of pulsations and lack of Doppler flow *(arrows)*.

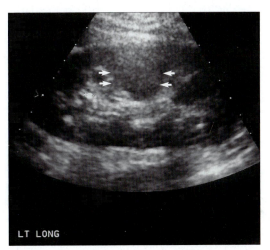

FIGURE 14-21 Longitudinal scan of the kidney with prominent column of Bertin.

TABLE 14-1	**Renal Anomalies and Variants**			
Type	**Location**	**Sonographic Appearance**	**Differential Considerations**	**Distinguishing Characteristics**
Column of Bertin	Medulla	Indentation of the renal sinus	Renal mass effect	Similar to renal parenchyma; contiguous with cortex
Dromedary hump	Lateral border of the kidney	Identical to the renal cortex	Mass effect	Usually seen on the left kidney
Junctional parenchymal defect	Upper pole of renal parenchyma	Echogenic triangular area	Mass effect	Best seen on sagittal scans
Fetal lobulation	Surface of the kidney	Indentations between the calyces	Mass effect	Best seen on sagittal scans
Lobar dysmorphism	Middle and upper calyces	Elongation of upper and middle calyces	Column of Bertin	Best seen on sagittal scans
Duplex collecting (complete) system	Central renal sinus	Two echogenic regions separated by moderately echogenic parenchymal tissue	Mass effect	"Faceless"; no echogenic renal pelvis seen on transverse view at the level of the midpole
Bifid renal pelvis (incomplete duplication)	Central renal sinus	Middle calyces, two echogenic regions	Pseudomass effect	One ureter entering the bladder on each side of the bladder
Extrarenal pelvis	Long renal pelvis that extends outside the renal border	Central cystic region that extends beyond the medial renal border	Renal aneurysm, dilated proximal ureter	Best seen on a transverse view at the level of the midpole
Horseshoe kidney	Kidneys seen more medial and anterior to the spine	Fusion of the polar region, usually the lower poles	Inferior poles lie more medial, associated with pyelocaliectasis, anomalous extrarenal pelvis, urinary calculi	

Dromedary Hump. A dromedary hump is a bulge of cortical tissue on the lateral surface of a kidney (usually the left), resembling the hump of a dromedary camel. It is seen in persons whose spleen or liver presses down. It is a normal variant but may resemble a renal neoplasm.

▐ **Sonographic Findings.** On sonography, the echogenicity is identical to the rest of the renal cortex, and a renal pseudotumor needs to be considered (Figure 14-22).

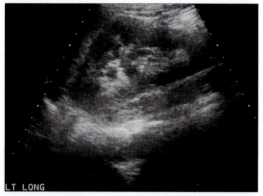

FIGURE 14-22 Coronal view of the left kidney. The dromedary hump is a cortical bulge that occurs on the lateral border of the kidney, typically on the left more than on the right.

Junctional Parenchymal Defect. A junctional parenchymal defect is a triangular, echogenic area typically located anteriorly and superiorly. It is a result of partial fusion of two embryonic parenchymal masses called renunculi during normal development (Figure 14-23).

▐ **Sonographic Findings.** Junctional parenchymal defects are best demonstrated on sagittal scans and must not be confused with pathologic processes such as parenchymal renal scars and angiomyolipoma. A lobar dysmorphism is a lobar fusion variant in which malrotation of the renal lobe occurs. The middle and upper calyces may be splayed and displaced, and the lower calyx is deviated posteriorly. The dysmorphic lobe may resemble a mass or prominent column of Bertin on a sonogram (Figure 14-24).

Fetal Lobulation. Fetal lobulation is developmental variation that is usually present in children up to 5 years old, and may be persistent in up to 51% of adults. The surfaces of the kidneys are generally indented in between the calyces, giving the kidneys a slightly lobulated appearance (Figure 14-25).

Sinus Lipomatosis. Sinus lipomatosis is a condition characterized by deposition of a moderate amount of fat in the renal sinus with parenchymal atrophy (Figure 14-26). In sinus lipomatosis, the abundant fibrous

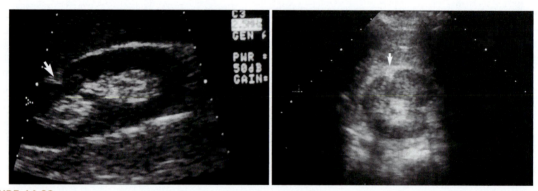

FIGURE 14-23 The junctional parenchymal defect *(arrows)* is a triangular area in the upper pole of the renal parenchyma.

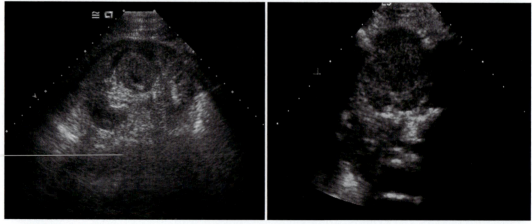

FIGURE 14-24 **A,** Longitudinal scan of lobar dysmorphism. **B,** Transverse view of lobar dysmorphism.

tissue may cause enlargement of the sinus region with increased echogenicity and regression toward the center of the parenchymal. Occasionally, a fatty mass is localized in only one area; this is called lipomatosis circumscripta.

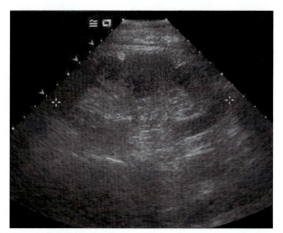

FIGURE 14-25 Remnant fetal renal lobulations (an irregularly shaped renal border).

Extrarenal Pelvis. The normal renal pelvis is a triangular structure. Its axis points inferiorly and medially. The intrarenal pelvis lies almost completely within the confines of the central renal sinus. This is usually small and foreshortened. The extrarenal pelvis tends to be larger with long major calyces.

◢ **Sonographic Findings.** On sonography, the pelvis appears as a central cystic area that may be partially or entirely beyond the confines of the bulk of the renal substance. Transverse views are best for viewing continuity with the renal sinus. The dilated extrarenal pelvis will usually decompress when the patient is placed in the prone position (Figure 14-27).

Renal Anomalies

Renal anomalies comprise abnormalities in number, size, position, structure, or form (Figures 14-28 and 14-29) (see Table 14-1). Anomalies in number include agenesis, dysgenesis (defective embryonic development of the kidney), and supernumerary kidney. Supernumerary kidney is an additional kidney to the number usually

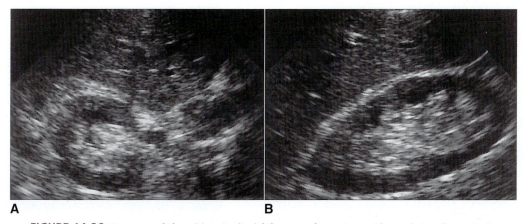

FIGURE 14-26 Transverse **(A)** and longitudinal **(B)** scans of a patient with renal sinus lipomatosis.

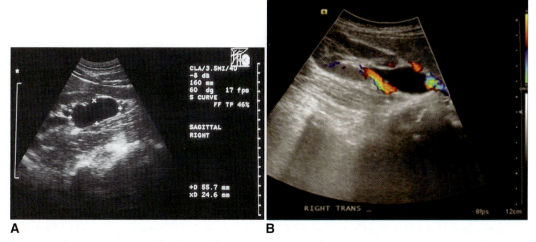

FIGURE 14-27 Extrarenal pelvis. **A,** Scan of the right kidney with an extrarenal pelvis appearing as a cystic area that extends beyond the confines of the renal borders. **B,** Color Doppler confirming the extrarenal pelvis.

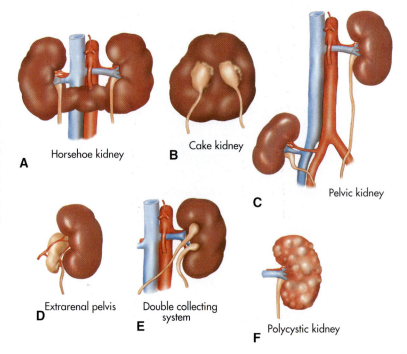

FIGURE 14-28 Variations of renal anatomy, position within the retroperitoneal cavity, and pathology. **A,** Horseshoe kidney shown as two kidneys connected by an isthmus anterior to the great vessels and inferior to the inferior mesenteric artery. **B,** Cake kidney with a double collecting system. **C,** Pelvic kidney with one kidney in the normal retroperitoneal position. **D,** Extrarenal pelvis. **E,** Double collecting system in a single kidney. **F,** Polycystic kidney.

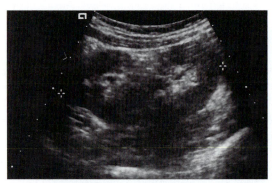

FIGURE 14-29 Longitudinal view of a malrotated right kidney, with the renal pelvis facing anteriorly.

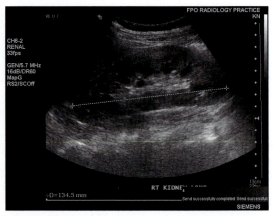

FIGURE 14-30 Enlarged solitary kidney with unilateral renal agenesis.

present, which is two. In some cases, separation of the reduplicated organ is incomplete (fused supernumerary kidney). *Bifid* means *cleft,* or *split into two parts.* Bifid renal pelvis is a common anomaly and is considered a normal variant. The renal pelvis may appear to be more prominent on sonography. A pseudotumor is an overgrowth of cortical tissue that indents the echogenic renal sinus and may be mistaken for a renal tumor on sonography.

Renal Agenesis. Renal agenesis is absence of the kidney or failure of the kidney to form; it may be bilateral or unilateral. Bilateral renal agenesis is very rare—0.3% of newborns—and is incompatible with life. Unilateral renal agenesis results in a solitary kidney. Congenital absence of one kidney is rare, with a 1/1000 birth incidence, and is commonly associated with other congenital anomalies such as seminal vesical cyst, vaginal agenesis, or bicorn uterus. Renal compensatory hypertrophy

(enlargement) generally occurs with a solitary kidney (Figure 14-30).

Renal hypoplasia is incomplete development of the kidney, usually with fewer than five calyces. Functionally and morphologically, the kidney is normal and should be differentiated from a shrunken kidney secondary to pyelonephrosis or renal artery stenosis. Usually, the pyelonephritic kidney is scarred and echogenic, and the small kidney that results from renal artery stenosis has abnormal Doppler parameters (tardus and parvus waveform).

Incomplete Duplication. Incomplete, or partial, duplication is the most frequently occurring congenital anomaly in the neonate. Duplication consists of two collecting systems and two ureters, with a single ureter entering into the urinary bladder. The two ureters join

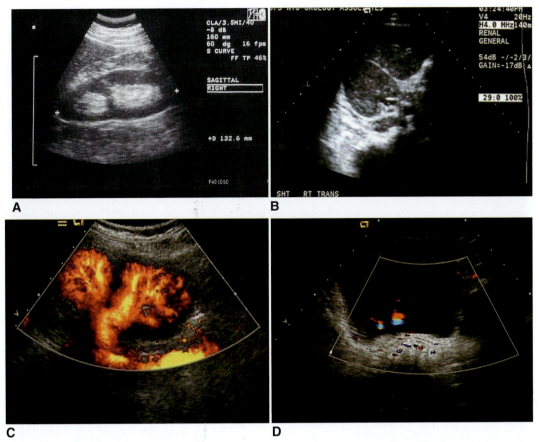

FIGURE 14-31 A, Complete duplex collecting system. The central sinus appears as two echogenic regions separated by a cleft of moderate hypoechoic tissue similar to the normal renal parenchyma. **B,** Transverse view of the echogenic tissue that separates the renal sinus ("faceless"). **C,** Power Doppler of duplex collecting system. **D,** Double right ureteral jets confirm a complete duplex collecting system.

and form a single ureter anywhere between the kidney and the bladder.

Complete Duplication. Complete duplication is the rare condition of a duplex collecting system. This anomaly results in two separate collecting systems, each with its own ureter that enters the bladder. In cases of double ureter, the ureter from the upper pole of the kidney usually opens below and medial to the one from the lower pole (rule of Weigert-Meyer). The ureter of the lower calyx inserts into the bladder more superiorly and laterally to the normal location of the vesicoureteral orifice, with a short intramural portion. This short intramural portion of the ureter increases the chance of a prevesicoureteral reflux. The ureter from the upper pole calyx inserts into the bladder medially and distally to the normal location of the vesicoureteral orifice. The low insertion of the ureter into the bladder causes an ectopic posterior insertion of the urethra with posterior displacement of the vagina, which increases the chance of urethral obstruction by a stricture or ureterocele, vesicoureteral reflux, or both.

Sonographic Findings. The way to confirm a complete collecting system is to demonstrate two ureteral jets entering the bladder on the same side. The duplex kidney is usually enlarged with smooth margins. The central

renal sinus appears as two echogenic regions separated by a cleft of moderately echogenic tissue similar in appearance to the normal renal parenchyma. On the transverse view, the area separating the renal pelvis is called "faceless" because the tissue is homogenous, with no central echogenic renal pelvis. Hydronephrosis of the upper pole with a ureterocele, or hydronephrosis of the upper pole and lower pole calyces, may be present (Figures 14-31 and 14-32).

Renal Ectopia. Renal ectopia (ectopic kidney) describes a kidney that is not located in its usual position. It results when the kidney fails to ascend from its origin in the true pelvis or from a superiorly ascended kidney located in the thorax. Pelvic kidney, also called sacral kidney, is the most common renal ectopia and should not be misdiagnosed as a primary pelvic tumor. It is almost always malrotated; the renal pelvis faces anteriorly and is predisposed to reflux, infection, ureteropelvic junction (UPJ) obstruction, and stone formation (Figure 14-33). Pelvic kidney may be bilateral, but this is very rare. A thoracic kidney migrates through the diaphragm into the thoracic cavity. It is a rare finding and is not easily diagnosed with ultrasound. Other renal ectopias include intrathoracic kidney and abdominal (iliac crest) kidney.

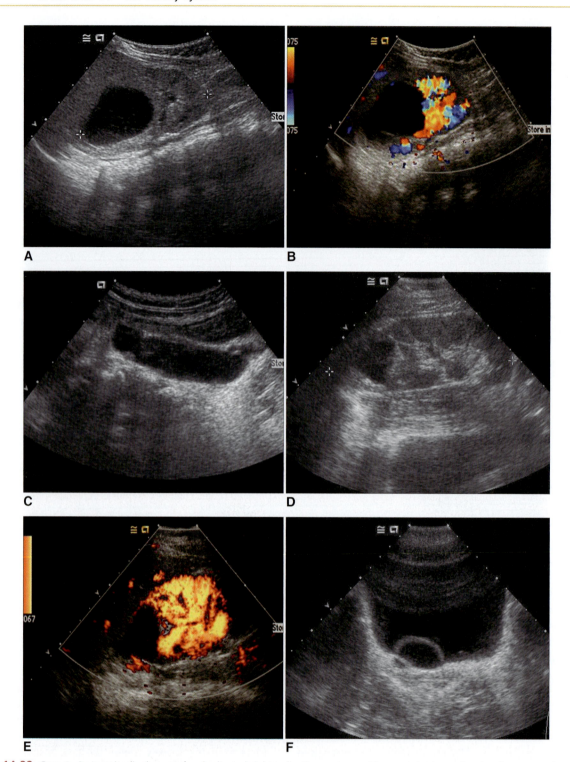

FIGURE 14-32 *Case 1*: **A,** Longitudinal scan of a duplicated right collecting system with severe hydronephrosis of upper moiety. **B,** Color Doppler demonstrates good renal perfusion on the lower moiety. **C,** Ectopic right distal ureter. *Case 2*: **D,** Longitudinal scan of a duplicated right collecting system with moderate hydronephrosis of the upper moiety. **E,** Power Doppler shows good renal perfusion on the lower moiety. **F,** Ureterocele of the distal right ureter ("rule of Weigert-Meyer").

Two types of crossed renal ectopia can occur: fused and nonfused. Both are associated with malrotation. Fused crossed renal ectopia occurs eight times more frequently than nonfused and most often on the right side. In most cases of crossed renal ectopia, the ureters are not ectopic. Cystoscopy reveals a normal trigone, and the incidence of associated congenital anomalies is low. Renal calculi are the most common complication. Sonography shows both kidneys located on the same side, with most demonstrating fusion (Figure 14-34).

Horseshoe Kidney. **Horseshoe kidney** is the most common renal anomaly, occurring in approximately 1/400 births. Fusion of the lower poles occurs in 96% of cases, with ureters passing anterior to the renal parenchyma. The isthmus, or connecting bridge, typically consists of renal parenchymal tissue; rarely is it fibrotic

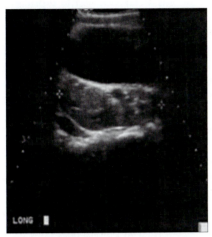

FIGURE 14-33 Ectopic kidney found in the pelvis, just posterior to the distended urinary bladder.

tissue. Horeseshoe kidney is associated with kidney malrotation and predisposition to stone formation, hydronephrosis, and infection. The isthmus of the kidney lies anterior to the spine and may simulate a solid pelvic mass or enlarged lymph nodes (Figure 14-35).

Evaluation of a Renal Mass

Before starting the sonographic examination for the evaluation of a renal mass, the sonographer should review the patient's chart, including the laboratory findings and previous diagnostic examinations, which may include a plain radiograph of the abdomen, CT, or MRI. Whenever possible, these films should be obtained before the sonogram is done, so the examination can be tailored to address the clinical problem. The sonographer should evaluate the sonographic images to determine the shape and size of the kidney and the location of the mass lesion, to observe distortion of the renal or ureter structure, and to look for calcium stones or gas within the kidney.

Renal masses are categorized as cystic, solid, or complex by a sonographic evaluation. A cystic mass sonographically displays several characteristic features: (1) smooth, thin, well-defined border; (2) round or oval

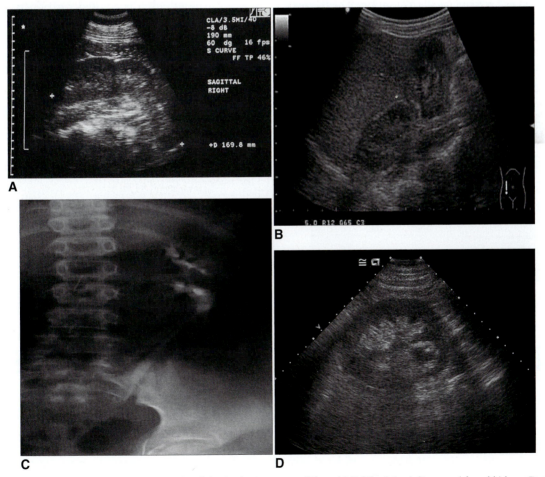

FIGURE 14-34 A, Crossed kidney on the right side of the body. Sonogram **(B)** and IVP **(C)** of the left crossed fused kidney. **D,** Cake kidney
(Courtesy Nexhmi Hyseni, M.D., University Clinical Center of Prishtina.)

shape; (3) sharp interface between the cyst and the renal parenchyma; (4) no internal echoes (anechoic); and (5) increased posterior acoustic enhancement.

A solid lesion projects as a nongeometric shape with irregular borders, a poorly defined interface between the mass and the kidney, low-level internal echoes, a weak posterior border caused by increased attenuation of the mass, and poor through-transmission.

Areas of necrosis, hemorrhage, abscess, or calcification within the mass may alter the classification and cause the lesion to fall into the complex category. This means the mass shows characteristics associated with both cystic and solid lesions.

Sonography allows the sonographer to carefully evaluate the renal parenchyma in many stages of respiration. If the mass is very small, respiratory motion may cause it to move in and out of the field of view. Careful evaluation of the best respiratory phase combined with use of the cine-loop feature will allow the sonographer to adequately image most renal masses to determine their characteristic composition.

Aspiration of Renal Masses

Most renal masses that have met the criteria for a simple cystic mass do not require needle aspiration. The Bosniak classification of cysts is used to determine the appropriate workup for a cystic mass (Table 14-2). A needle

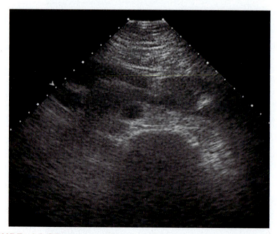

FIGURE 14-35 Transverse scan of the horseshoe kidney with isthmus connecting each pole.

aspiration may be recommended to obtain fluid from the lesion to evaluate its internal composition.

The patient should be placed in a prone position with sandbags or rolled sheets under the abdomen to help push the kidneys toward the posterior abdominal wall and provide a flat scanning surface. Sterile technique is used for aspiration and biopsy procedures. The transducer must be gas sterilized. Sterile lubricant is used to couple the transducer to the patient's skin.

The renal mass should be located in the transverse and longitudinal planes, with scans performed at mid-inspiration. Hold the transducer lightly over the scanning surface so as not to compress the subcutaneous tissue. The depth of the mass should be noted from its posterior to anterior borders, so the exact depth can be given to aid in placement of the needle. Compression of the subcutaneous tissue results in an inaccurate depth measurement. When the area of aspiration is outlined on the patient's back, the distance is measured from the posterior surface to the middle of the lesion.

A beveled needle causes multiple echoes within the walls of the lesion. If the needle is slightly bent, many echoes appear until the bent needle is completely out of the transducer's path. The larger the needle gauge, the stronger the reflection.

The patient's skin is painted with tincture of benzalkonium (Zephiran), and sterile drapes are applied. A local anesthetic agent is administered over the area of interest, and the sterile transducer is used to relocate the lesion. The needle is inserted into the central core of the cyst. The needle stop helps ensure that the needle does not go through the cyst. The fluid is then withdrawn according to volume calculations. The volume of the cyst may be determined by measuring the radius of the mass and using the following formula: $V = 4/3\pi r^3$

The diameter of the mass can be applied to this formula:

$$V = d^3/2$$

Lower Urinary Tract

Ureters

Stricture. Ureteral narrowing due to fibrosis is a common form of ureteral stricture. Ureteral strictures

TABLE 14-2	Bosniak Cyst Categories, Criteria, and Workup	
Category	**Criteria**	**Workup**
Simple cyst (I)	Thin smooth wall, anechoic, round or oval in shape; increased through-transmission	None
Mildly complex cyst (II)	Thin septation or calcified wall	2–3 month follow-up with CT or sonogram
Mildly complex (IIF)	Atypical features; does not fall into category II	6–12 month follow-up
Indeterminate lesion (III)	Multiple septa, thickened septa, internal echoes	Biopsy or partial nephrectomy—increased risk for malignancy
Malignant lesion (IV)	Solid component, irregular walls	Nephrectomy

may also result from inflammatory disease, tuberculosis, localized periureteral fibrosis, impacted ureteral stone, schistostomiasis, iatrogenic ureteral injury, or radiation therapy. Other causes include amyloidosis, adjacent malignancies, metastases, extrinsic compression due to primary retroperitoneal tumors, enlarged lymph nodes, and medial lower pole renal masses (Box 14-1).

Ureterocele. A ureterocele is a cystlike enlargement of the lower end of the ureter (Figure 14-36) caused by congenital or acquired stenosis of the distal end of the ureter. Ureteroceles are usually small and asymptomatic, although they may cause obstruction and infection of the upper urinary system. If large, a ureterocele may cause bladder outlet obstruction. Ureteroceles are found more often in adults than in children and may be unilateral or bilateral. On sonography, a *cobra head* appearance is seen in sagittal view.

Sonographic Findings. A large ureterocele may fill the urinary bladder and have the same sonographic appearance as diverticula. If the patient can partially empty the bladder, a better diagnostic-quality image will be produced, as the ureterocele will be empty. Alternate filling and emptying of the ureterocele as the result of peristalsis may be demonstrated with sonographic imaging. Calculi may also be present.

Ectopic Ureterocele. Ectopic ureteroceles are rare and are found more commonly in children and young adults, especially in females. They usually are associated with complete ureteral duplication. The ureter, which empties the upper pole, inserts low in the bladder by the bladder neck, urethra, or lower genital tract. The ectopic ureter may become stenotic and cause ureteral obstruction, which is associated with hydroureter and hydronephrosis. The ureterocele sac may obstruct the bladder outlet or may prolapse through the urethra.

Sonographic Findings. An ectopic ureterocele appears on sonography as a round, thin-walled cystic structure that may contain debris protruding into the bladder.

Bladder

Ultrasound is not the imaging modality of choice to examine the bladder. Cystoscopy is usually used to examine the bladder because of its ability to diagnose early neoplasms. Transabdominal sonography will allow visualization of most lesions greater than 5 mm. A transurethral intravesicular sonographic approach has been used to evaluate bladder tumors.

The urinary bladder should be examined at the same time as the upper urinary tract. A complete review of the patient's chart, including previous diagnostic imaging procedures, should be conducted before a sonographic examination of the bladder is begun.

A sonogram of the bladder is obtained with a distended bladder. The patient lies in a supine position. A right or left decubitus position may be used to demonstrate movement of calculi. Proper adjustment of the TGC allows for minimization of anterior wall reverberations and anechoic bladder, with posterior acoustic enhancement. The depth of the image should be set to

BOX 14-1	Causes of Narrowing of the Ureter

Internal causes
   Fibrosis
   Inflammatory disease
   Tuberculosis
   Localized periureteral fibrosis
   Impacted ureteral stone
   Schistosomiasis
   Iatrogenic ureteral injury
   Radiation therapy
   Amyloidosis
Extrinsic compression
   Adjacent malignancies
   Metastases
   Primary retroperitoneal tumors
   Enlarged lymph nodes
Medial lower renal pole mass

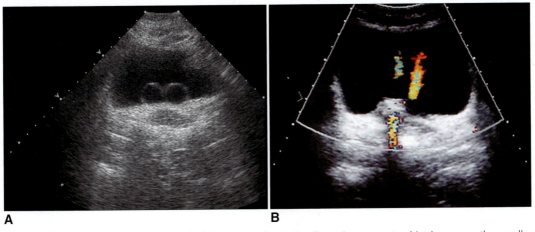

FIGURE 14-36 **A,** Longitudinal scan of a double ureterocele. **B,** Small continuous ureteral jet known as the candle sign.

BOX 14-2	Conditions That Cause Incomplete Emptying of Bladder

Bladder calculi
Diabetes mellitus
Foley catheter
Inflammation
Neoplasms—benign or malignant
Neurogenic bladder
Postsurgical intervention
Pregnancy
Radiation therapy
Rectal or vaginal fistulas
Renal disease
Sexual intercourse
Trauma (blood clot)
Tuberculosis (lower ureteric stricture)
Urethral stricture

BOX 14-3	Signs and Symptoms of Renal Disease

Renal Cystic Disease
Inflammatory or necrotic cysts
- Flank pain
- Hematuria
- Proteinuria
- White blood cells in urine
- ↑ Protein

Renal subcapsular hematoma
- Hematuria
- ↓ Hematocrit

Renal Inflammatory Processes
Abscess
- Acute onset of symptoms
- Fever
- Palpable mass
- ↑ White blood cell count
- Pyuria

Acute focal bacterial nephritis
- Fever
- Flank pain
- Pyuria
- ↑ Blood urea nitrogen
- ↑ Albumin
- ↑ Total plasma proteins

Acute tubular necrosis
- Moderate to severe intermittent flank pain (caused by renal calculi)
- Vomiting (caused by renal calculi)
- Hematuria
- Infection
- Leukocytosis with infection

Chronic renal failure
- ↑ Concentration of urea in blood
- High urine protein excretion
- ↑ Creatinine
- Presence of granulocytes

Renal cell carcinoma
- Erythrocytosis may occur.
- Leukocytosis
- Red blood cells in urine
- Pyuria
- ↑ Lactic acid dehydrogenase

visualize any structure that may lie posterior or caudal to the bladder. A 3.5 MHz transducer is usually used. In very thin patients, a 5 MHz transducer may be used. If evaluation of the anterior bladder wall is indicated, a high-frequency, curved linear-array transducer will give a larger field of view than a sector transducer.

The transducer should be placed in the middle of the filled urinary bladder and angled laterally, inferiorly, and superiorly. The bladder walls should be smooth and thin (3–6 mm). The bladder should be midline and should not be deviated to either side or have any irregular or asymmetrical indentations.

Sonography is used to evaluate residual bladder volume in patients with outflow obstruction. The post-void bladder is scanned in two planes: anteroposterior and transverse. Measurements are obtained in three planes: anterior-posterior, transverse, and longitudinal. Images and measurements are obtained at the largest dimensions. Because bladder shape varies, any volume measurement can be used to approximate volume. A residue of less than 20 ml of urine is considered normal in an adult.

Ureteral jets should be identified as flashes of Doppler color entering the bladder from the lateral posterior border of the bladder and coursing superior and medial.

An enlarged prostate, enlarged uterus, pelvic mass, or filled loop of bowel may indent and displace the urinary bladder. Box 14-2 lists the conditions under which the bladder may not empty completely.

PATHOLOGY OF THE URINARY SYSTEM

See Table 14-3 for clinical findings, sonographic findings, and differential considerations for various renal diseases and conditions. Box 14-3 lists the main signs and symptoms of common renal diseases.

Renal Cystic Disease

Simple renal cystic disease encompasses a wide range of disease processes, which may be typical, complicated, or atypical. The disease may be acquired (nongenetic) or inherited (genetic) (e.g., von Hippel-Lindau disease, tuberous sclerosis). Cystic disease may occur in the renal cortex, medulla, or renal sinus (see Table 14-3).

Simple Renal Cyst. The most common renal mass lesion is a simple cortical renal cyst. Although the origin is unknown, these cysts are considered acquired lesions, probably arising from obstructed ducts or tubules. It

Text continued on page 379

TABLE 14-3	Renal Findings	
Clinical Findings	**Sonographic Findings**	**Differential Considerations**
Simple Cysts		
Usually asymptomatic Usually normal laboratory findings	Found anywhere in the kidney, but usually in cortex Round or ovoid in shape, anechoic Thin, well-defined walls No color flow or Doppler in mass	Hemorrhagic cyst, infected cyst, necrotic cyst, malignant cyst, obstruction of upper pole, calyceal diverticula, pseudoaneurysm, arteriovenous malformation
Parapelvic Cysts		
Usually asymptomatic May present with hypertension or obstruction (hilum cyst) Pain Usually normal laboratory findings	Found in the renal hilum or renal sinus Well-defined sonolucent mass with regular or irregular borders Good through-transmission Not connected to the renal collecting system	Hydronephrosis
von Hippel-Lindau Cysts		
Flank pain General discomfort Involves many body systems Usually presents in third to fifth decade Initial clinical symptoms caused by cerebellar or spinal cord hemangioblastomas, not abdominal If renal involvement occurs, there is an ↑ chance of renal carcinoma No hypertension or renal failure	Bilateral cysts and masses Other organs are affected Masses may develop within the cysts Hyperplastic linings of cysts Pancreatic cysts	Multiple cysts Renal adenoma
Tuberous Sclerosis		
Involves several body systems Patient usually presents with mental retardation, seizures, and cutaneous lesions	Multiple cysts or angiomyolipomas Multiple organs involved Multiple angiomyolipomas that may become large	Angiomyolipomas
Acquired Cystic Disease of Dialysis		
Usually occurs in patients on renal dialysis for ≥3 yr Flank pain	Found in cortex Simple cysts Atypical because of hemorrhage Normal or small echogenic kidneys with ↓ in corticomedullary distinction with simple or atypical cysts	Renal cyst Adenoma Renal cell carcinoma
Adult Polycystic Kidney Disease		
Hypertension Renal failure Abdominal, flank pain Fever, chills (infection) Uremia Palpable mass Polycythemia Hematuria	Bilateral enlarged kidneys with multiple cysts of varied size Kidneys lose their reniform shape; in the late stages, no normal renal parenchyma may be identified Cysts may be atypical because of infection or hemorrhage Cysts may be found in liver, spleen, testes, pancreas	Cortical cysts Localized hydronephrosis Renal tuberculosis Multilocular cyst
Infantile Polycystic Kidney Disease		
May be seen in utero Renal insufficiency Lung hypoplasia, usually fatal depending on the amount of renal function In juvenile form: Portal hypertension Hepatic fibrosis GI hemorrhage	Bilateral enlarged echogenic kidneys Cysts too small to be seen No distinction between the corticomedullary region	In utero—ADPKD, dysplasia, glomerulocystic kidney disease

Continued

TABLE 14-3   Renal Findings—cont'd

Clinical Findings	Sonographic Findings	Differential Considerations
Multicystic Dysplastic Kidney		
Most common palpable mass in neonates Restricted growth in children Polyuria Hypertension Infection Usually unilateral; bilateral is incompatible with life	Multiple cysts of varying size No renal parenchyma surrounding the cyst Enlarged kidneys in children Small kidneys in adults Absence of renal vascularity	Hydronephrosis
Medullary Sponge Kidney		
Usually asymptomatic unless calculus is present, then hematuria and infections Pain Hydronephrosis Infection	Normal or small kidneys with echogenic parenchyma (cysts too small to be resolved on a sonogram) or Small cysts in medulla and corticomedullary region with ↑ echogenicity	Papillary necrosis Nephrocalcinosis Renal cystic disease Pyelonephritic cysts
Medullary Cystic Disease		
Normal renal function Anemia Salt loss Progressive azotemia Polyuria Pain Infection	Normal or small echogenic kidneys with Widening of the renal sinus after 2 cm in the medulla or corticomedullary junction	Medullary sponge kidney small cysts under 2 cm
Renal Cell Carcinoma		
Hematuria Weight loss Fatigue Fever Flank pain Palpable mass Hypertension	Cystic or complex mass that may have areas of calcifications May displace renal pyramids and invade renal architecture Irregular margins Hypervascular Renal vein or IVC thrombosis	Angiomyolipoma Transitional cell carcinoma Lymphoma Oncocytoma Column of Bertin Renal vein or IVC thrombus
Transitional Cell Carcinoma		
Hematuria Weight loss Fatigue Fever Flank pain	Solid hypoechoic mass Not well defined within the renal sinus May be multiple	Squamous cell tumor Renal cell carcinoma Adenoma Blood clot Fungus ball
Squamous Cell Carcinoma		
Gross hematuria History of chronic irritation Palpable kidney if severe hydronephrosis is present	Large bulky mass Invasion of the renal vein and IVC	Transitional cell carcinoma
Renal Lymphoma		
Not a primary site; usually caused by adjacent lymph involvement More common in patients with non-Hodgkin lymphoma Usually no renal symptoms Asymptomatic Pain Hematuria	Hypoechoic mass may be bilateral Enlarged kidney	Renal cell carcinoma Cyst
Wilms' Tumor		
Palpable abdominal mass in children Abdominal pain Nausea and vomiting Hematuria	Usually unilateral, may be bilateral Heterogeneous Look for extension into renal vein and inferior vena cava	Nephroblastoma Renal cell carcinoma Mesoblastoma Multicystic kidney Retroperitoneal sarcoma

TABLE 14-3	Renal Findings—cont'd	
Clinical Findings	**Sonographic Findings**	**Differential Considerations**
Benign Renal Tumor		
Usually asymptomatic May cause painless hematuria	Well-defined mass—hyperechoic to hypoechoic	Angiomyolipoma Transitional cell carcinoma Oncocytoma Lymphoma Column of Bertin
Adenoma		
Asymptomatic	Well-defined mass with calcifications	Renal cell carcinoma
Angiolipoma		
Usually asymptomatic Possible flank pain Normal laboratory values Hematuria if tumor hemorrhages	Usually echogenic homogeneous mass with well-defined borders Hemorrhagic neoplasm	Oncocytoma Renal cell carcinoma
Lipoma		
Usually asymptomatic Normal laboratory values	Well-defined echogenic mass	Fibromas Adenoma
Oncocytoma		
Asymptomatic	Well-defined mass with spoke-wheel patterns of enhancement and central scar	Renal abscess
Acute Glomerulonephritis		
Nephrotic syndrome Hypertension Anemia Peripheral edema	↑ Cortical echoes	Chronic glomerulonephritis Acute tubular nephrosis AIDS Lupus nephritis Acute interstitial nephritis
Acute Interstitial Nephritis		
Uremia Hematuria Rash Fever Eosinophilia	Enlarged kidneys with ↑cortical echoes	Acute glomerulonephritis Chronic glomerulonephritis Acute tubular necrosis AIDS Lupus nephritis
Lupus Nephritis		
Hematuria Proteinuria Renal vein thrombus Renal insufficiency	↑ Cortical echoes and renal atrophy	Acute glomerulonephritis Chronic glomerulonephritis Acute tubular necrosis AIDS Acute interstitial nephritis
Acquired Immunodeficiency Syndrome (AIDS)		
Renal dysfunction	Kidneys are normal or enlarged Echogenic parenchyma ↑ Cortical echoes	Acute glomerulonephritis Chronic glomerulonephritis Acute tubular necrosis Lupus nephritis Acute interstitial nephritis
Sickle Cell Nephropathy		
Hematuria Renal vein thrombosis	Varies—*patients with acute renal vein thrombosis*: Enlarged kidneys with ↓ echogenicity *Subacute*: Enlarged kidneys with ↑cortical echogenicity	Lupus nephritis
Hypertensive Nephropathy		
Uncontrolled hypertension	Small kidneys with smooth borders may have distortion of intrarenal anatomy	Hypoplasia

Continued

TABLE 14-3	Renal Findings—cont'd	
Clinical Findings	**Sonographic Findings**	**Differential Considerations**
Papillary Necrosis		
Hematuria Flank pain Hypertension Dysuria Acute renal failure	Fluid-filled spaces at the corticomedullary junction Round or triangular Mimics calculi	Congenital megacalyces Hydronephrosis Postobstruction atrophy
Renal Atrophy		
Renal failure	Small echogenic kidneys	Renal hypoplasia Chronic renal failure
Renal Sinus Lipomatosis		
Asymptomatic	Enlarged kidneys with ↑ echogenicity of renal sinus Hyperechoic areas ↓ Renal parenchyma	Infection Atrophy Hydronephrosis
Acute Renal Failure		
Renal insufficiency ↓ Urine output	Hydronephrosis Enlarged hypoechoic kidneys Renal artery stenosis	Prerenal, renal, or postrenal causes
Obstructive Hydronephrosis		
Renal insufficiency ↓ Urine output Hypertension	Fluid-filled renal collecting system Thin parenchyma Hydroureter ↓ or absent ureteral jets	Extrarenal collecting system Parapelvic cyst Reflux Renal artery aneurysm Transient diuresis Congenital megacalyces Papillary necrosis Arteriovenous malformation
Renal Infarction		
Asymptomatic	Irregular triangle masses in the renal parenchyma Lobulated renal contour	Renal lobulations Dromedary hump
Acute Tubular Necrosis		
Renal insufficiency Hematuria	Bilaterally enlarged kidneys with hyperechoic pyramids	Nephrocalcinosis
Chronic Renal Failure		
Renal failure Hypertension	Bilateral small echogenic kidneys	Multiple causes AIDS Chronic parenchymal infection
Pyonephrosis		
Renal insufficiency Hematuria	Dilated collecting system with low-level echoes or ↓ through-transmission	Hydronephrosis Hemorrhage Blood clot Uroepithelial tumors
Xanthogranulomatous Pyelonephritis		
Multiple infections Nonfunctioning kidneys	"Staghorn appearance" Destruction of renal parenchyma ↑ Echogenicity ↑ Renal size Dilated calyces	Hydronephrosis Renal calculi

↑, Increase; ↓, decrease; *GI,* gastrointestinal; *IVC,* inferior vena cava.

is estimated that they occur in 50% of the population older than 50 years of age. Most patients with a simple cyst are asymptomatic, and the cyst is detected as an incidental finding in the kidney. A renal simple cyst can be solitary or multiple, involving one or both kidneys. Rarely, several simple cysts may involve only one kidney or a localized portion of a kidney. In rare cases, a large lower pole cyst may obstruct the collecting system and cause hydronephrosis and/or hypertension. Local pain and hematuria may be caused by distention of the cyst wall or spontaneous bleeding into the cyst. Occasionally, a simple cyst can be complicated by hemorrhage, infection, or calcification, which causes it to become a complex cyst. Renal cysts are unusual in children, with an overall frequency of less than 1%. A cyst in a child must be examined carefully to differentiate a benign cyst from a cystic form of nephroblastoma (Wilms' tumor).

Sonographic Findings. Sonography is the most efficient imaging modality for confirming the presence of a simple cyst that is poorly seen during CT and/or MRI. Classical sonographic criteria used to diagnose a simple renal cyst include a round or oval shape, anechoic, thin imperceptible walls, and posterior acoustic enhancement. If all of these sonographic findings are present, no further evaluation is required (Figure 14-37).

Complex Cyst. If a renal cyst does not meet the criteria for a simple cyst, it is termed *complex* and must be con-sidered malignant until otherwise proven. Complex cysts may contain septations, thick walls, calcifications, internal echoes, and mural nodularity.

Sonographic Findings. Thick walls: Anything thicker than 1 mm is considered abnormal, and the cystic form of a renal carcinoma often presents in this manner (Figure 14-38). Most of the time, internal echoes within a cyst are the result of protein content, hemorrhage, and/or infection. Any irregularity at the base of the cyst should be considered a malignant growth (see Box 14-4). Thin septations can be detected by sonography, and their presence alone does not suggest malignancy. If irregularity of septa (thicker than 1 mm) showing vascularity on color or power Doppler is seen, the lesion must be presumed malignant. Fine, thin linear calcification in the cyst wall or in a septum without associated soft tissue mass or enhancement on CT likely represents a complex cyst, rather than a malignancy.

Bosniak classification of cysts was introduced in 1986, before CT/MRI was used for diagnosing renal cystic disease. In 2005, Bosniak classification was updated from four categories—I, II, III, and renal cyst IV—to five categories:

- **Category I** lesions are simple benign cysts: anechoic, thin walls, no calcifications or septations; no atypical features and no further evaluation needed

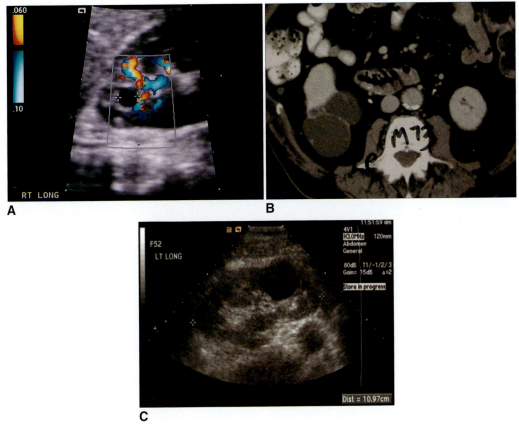

FIGURE 14-37 A, Upper pole renal cyst with no blood flow to the cyst. **B,** CT scan of the lower pole complicated cyst. **C,** Sagittal view of the left kidney with a cystic mass. *(B and C courtesy Joseph Yee, New York University.)*

- **Category II** lesions are cystic lesions with one or two thin (≤1 mm thick) septations, fine calcifications in the walls or septa (wall thickening >1 mm advances the lesion into surgical category III), and hyperdense benign cysts with all features of category I cysts, except for being homogeneously hyperechoic. A benign category II lesion must be 3 cm or less in diameter, must have one quarter of its wall extending outside the kidney so the wall can be assessed, and must show no vascularity (must be nonenhancing after contrast material is administered on CT) on color Doppler.

- **Category IIF** comprises minimally complicated cysts that need follow-up. This is a group not well defined by Bosniak, but it consists of lesions that do not fall neatly into category II. These lesions have some atypical features and are most likely benign. Six months to 1 year follow-up is required.

- **Category III** consists of true indeterminate cystic masses showing uniform wall thickening, nodularity (especially in the base of the cyst), thick or irregular peripheral calcification, or a multilocular nature with multiple vascular (enhancing) septa. These cysts cannot be distinguished from malignancies and require

a biopsy and/or surgery for evaluation. The distinction between some categories, especially IIF and III, is not clear, and variability in how the cysts in these two categories are classified may occur.

- **Category IV** cysts have diffuse wall thickening and may include areas with increased vascularity, or large nodules in the wall, or clearly solid vascular components in the cystic lesion—all features that strongly suggest malignancy. The cystic masses are presumed to be renal cell carcinoma and the same treatment is followed, typically a nephrectomy.

Sonographically, it is difficult to differentiate between a septated cyst and small, adjacent cortical cysts known as "kissing" cysts (Figure 14-39). A cyst may also have a cyst or mass within it (Figure 14-40). Sometimes small sacculations or infoldings of the cystic wall produce wall irregularity; a cyst puncture or aspiration may be recommended to ascertain the pathology of the fluid within the mass.

Low-level echoes within a renal cyst may be artifacts (sensitivity too high or transducer frequency too low) or may result from infection, hemorrhage (Figures 14-41 and 14-42), or a necrotic cystic tumor, or, in rare cases, malignancy.

Renal Sinus Parapelvic Cysts. The parapelvic cyst originates from the renal sinus and is most likely lymphatic in origin. These small cysts do not communicate with the collecting system. Most often, patients with parapelvic cysts are asymptomatic. Clinical symptoms are infrequent, but occasionally, the cyst may cause pain, hematuria, hypertension, or obstruction.

▶ **Sonographic Findings.** The sonogram shows a well-defined mass with no internal septations. The cyst can have irregular borders because it may compress adjacent renal sinus structures. Parapelvic cysts (especially those located in the medial lower portion of the kidney) may cause obstruction; peripelvic cysts do not. The sonographer should be able to differentiate the

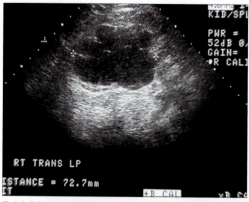

FIGURE 14-38 Transverse view of lower pole with a complex cyst.

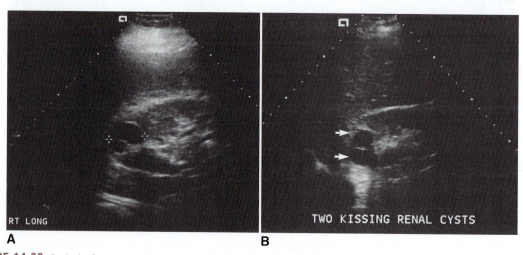

FIGURE 14-39 A, A single upper-pole cortical cyst with a thin septation. **B,** Two small adjacent renal cysts ("kissing" cysts).

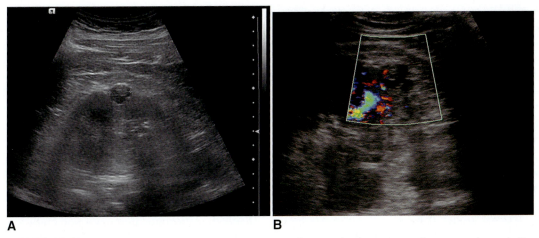

FIGURE 14-40 A, A small 15 mm mass within a cyst. **B,** Color Doppler demonstrates intratumoral vascularity.

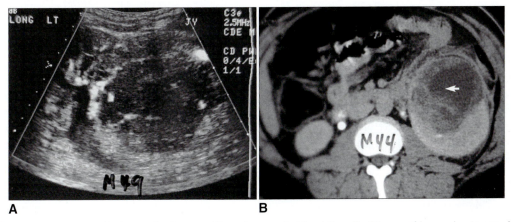

FIGURE 14-41 A, Transverse scan of a hemorrhagic cyst with no increase in blood flow. **B,** CT scan of hemorrhagic cyst. *(Courtesy Joseph Yee, New York University.)*

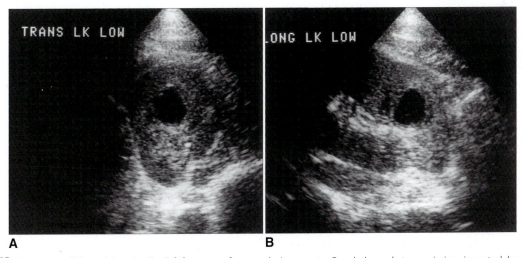

FIGURE 14-42 Transverse **(A)** and longitudinal **(B)** scans of a renal sinus cyst. Good through-transmission is noted beyond the renal parenchyma.

parapelvic cyst from hydronephrosis by trying to connect the dilated renal pelvis centrally. A transverse view is very useful. The dilated renal pelvis may present a cauliflower appearance, whereas the parapelvic cyst is more spherical in appearance.

Renal Cysts Associated With Renal Neoplasms

von Hippel-Lindau (VHL). Von Hippel-Lindau disease is an autosomal dominant genetic disorder. Several areas of the body may be affected. Predominant abnormalities include retinal angiomas, cerebellar hemangioblastomas, and a variety of abdominal cysts and tumors, including renal and pancreatic cysts, renal adenomas, and frequent multiple and bilateral renal adenocarcinoma tumors. Renal cell carcinoma in patients with this disease is multifocal and bilateral. A high incidence of renal cysts is found in patients with VHL, usually of cortical origin.

Tuberous Sclerosis. Tuberous sclerosis is an autosomal dominant genetic disorder characterized by mental retardation, seizures, and adenoma sebaceum. Associated renal lesions include multiple renal cysts or angiomyolipomas and/or cutaneous, retinal, and cerebral hamartomas. This disease may be difficult to separate from adult polycystic kidney disease.

Acquired Cystic Kidney Disease (ACKD). This condition is found in native kidneys of patients with renal failure who need to undergo renal dialysis or peritoneal dialysis. Patients with this condition have been shown to have a slightly increased incidence of renal cysts, adenomas, and renal carcinoma. It is theorized that epithelial hyperplasia caused by tubular obstruction that occurs as a result of toxic substances plays a role in the development of these masses. Incidence increases with time, particularly after the first 3 years of dialysis. It increases up to 90% after 5 years of dialysis. Renal cysts can show spontaneous bleeding and hemorrhage, causing pain and flank discomfort. Solid tumors, including adenomas, oncocytomas, and renal cell carcinomas, are seen in up to 7% of patients.

Sonographic Findings. On a sonogram, the native kidneys are small and echogenic with several small cysts. In a patient with chronic renal failure, three to five cysts in each kidney are diagnostic. The incidence of hemorrhage into the renal cysts is increased; this will reveal internal echoes within the cyst or hyperechoic cysts. Renal masses with internal echoes, mural nodularities, and increased vascularity on color Doppler, with no posterior acoustic enhancement, are likely to be renal carcinoma.

Polycystic Kidney Disease. Polycystic renal disease may present in one of two forms: the infantile autosomal recessive form and the adult autosomal dominant form.

Autosomal Recessive Polycystic Kidney Disease. Autosomal recessive polycystic kidney disease (ARPKD), also called infantile polycystic disease, is a fairly rare genetic disorder. The gene that causes this disorder has been located on chromosome 6. Dilatation of the renal collecting tubules causes renal failure, and in later forms of the disease, liver involvement is seen. Four forms of ARPKD are classified according to the age of the patient at the onset of clinical signs: perinatal, neonatal, infantile, and juvenile. The perinatal form is found in utero and usually progresses to renal failure, causing pulmonary hypoplasia and intrauterine demise. On the perinatal sonogram, oligohydramnios, hypoplastic lungs, and massively enlarged echogenic kidneys may be visualized.

The juvenile form may present with hypertension, renal insufficiency, nephromegaly, hepatic cysts, bile duct proliferation, Caroli's disease, which may be associated with periportal fibrosis, which causes portal hypertension and esophageal varices. Renal function is usually decreased secondary to hepatic problems when ARPKD appears later in life. In older children, the kidneys are enlarged with an echogenic cortex and medulla and lack of corticomedullary differentiation. Microscopic or small cysts (1 to 2 mm) may be located in the medulla, often associated with hepatic fibrosis and splenomegaly.

Autosomal Dominant Polycystic Kidney Disease. Autosomal dominant polycystic kidney disease (ADPKD) (previously known as *adult polycystic renal disease*) is a common genetic disease that occurs in both men and women. The severity of the disease varies depending on the genotype. The most common type is ADPKD1 (located on the short arm of the 16th chromosome), which affects the kidneys more severely than ADPKD2 (located on the long arm of the fourth chromosome). A number of people have no known genetic disposition to ADPKD, but it may result from spontaneous mutations. It is a bilateral disease that is characterized by enlarged kidneys with multiple asymmetrical cysts varying in size and location in the renal cortex and medulla. The cysts may be asymmetrical. The disease is progressive and does not usually clinically manifest until the fourth or fifth decade when hypertension or hematuria develops. By the age of 60, approximately 50% of patients will have end-stage renal disease (ESRD). Clinical symptoms include pain (common complaint), hypertension, palpable mass, hematuria, headache, urinary tract infection, and renal insufficiency. Complications may include infection, hemorrhage, stone formation, rupture of cyst, and renal obstruction.

Associated abnormalities include cysts in the liver, spleen, pancreas, thyroid, ovary, testes, breast, cerebral berry aneurysm, and abdominal aortic aneurysm. Patients who are on renal dialysis have an increased incidence of renal cell carcinoma.

Sonographic Findings. The sonographic appearance of ADPKD is similar to the autosomal recessive form of polycystic disease. In the neonate, sonography demonstrates diffusely enlarged kidneys, due to multiple interfaces of the small cysts. This appearance is not unique to ADPKD, but further screening is warranted when noted on prenatal sonographic examination. Diagnosis is based on family history and tissue sampling.

In the adult patient, bilateral renal enlargement occurs with multiple asymmetrical cysts of varying size in both cortex and medulla. In the most advanced cases, the normal renal parenchyma is replaced bilaterally with multiple cysts (Figures 14-43 and 14-44) and the kidneys lose their reniform shape. The cysts may grow large enough to obliterate the renal sinus. They may become

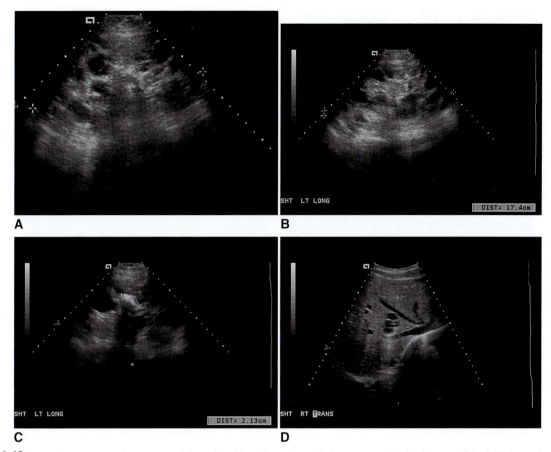

FIGURE 14-43 **A** and **B,** Images of a young adult male with polycystic renal disease. Longitudinal scans of both kidneys show enlarged kidneys (right kidney [RK] 15.2 cm and left kidney [LK] 17.4 cm) with a variety of cyst sizes. **C,** Polycystic kidney with stone. **D,** About one third of patients with polycystic renal disease also have cysts on the liver or other organs.

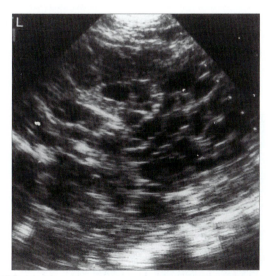

FIGURE 14-44 A 30-year-old male with a solitary left polycystic kidney and hematuria was sent to rule out obstruction. It is very difficult to rule out obstruction with so many small cysts.

infected or hemorrhagic, which is characterized sonographically by internal debris within the cysts or thickened walls. The walls of the cysts may be calcified, or stones may form. A complicated cyst may result in spontaneous bleeding, causing flank pain for the patient (see Table 14-3).

Multicystic Dysplastic Kidney. Multicystic dysplastic kidney (MCDK) disease is a common nonhereditary renal dysplasia that usually occurs unilaterally, with the kidney functioning poorly, if at all. MCDK is the most common form of cystic disease in neonates and is believed to be the consequence of early in utero urinary tract obstruction. Dysplastic changes usually involve the entire kidney but, rarely, may be segmental or focal. Bilateral MCDK is incompatible with life. Complications arising from a multicystic dysplastic kidney that is not removed include hypertension, hematuria, infection, and flank pain. A slightly increased risk of malignant transformation can occur if the kidney is not removed.

Sonographic Findings. In neonates and children, the kidneys are multicystic, with absence of renal parenchyma, renal sinus, and atretic renal artery. In adults, the kidneys may be small (atrophic and calcified) and echogenic. Other possible findings include ureteral atresia (failure of the ureter to develop from the calyceal system), contralateral ureteropelvic obstruction (in 30% of patients) (development of the ureter from the bladder with retrograde filling), and a nonfunctioning kidney.

Medullary Cystic Disease

Medullary Sponge Kidney. Medullary sponge kidney (MSK) is a development anomaly that occurs in the medullary pyramids and consists of cystic or fusiform dilatation of the distal collecting ducts (ducts of Bellini), causing stasis of urine and stone formation. Because the medullary sponge kidney is an anatomic rather than a metabolic defect, the pathologic process may be unilateral or segmental. The cause is unknown. Many patients remain asymptomatic, but patients with hematuria, infection, and renal stones should be evaluated for medullary sponge kidney.

MSK may be associated with a variety of other congenital and inherited disorders, including Beckwith-Wiedemann syndrome, polycystic kidney disease (PKD) (about 3% of patients with autosomal dominant polycystic kidney disease have evidence of MSK), Caroli's disease, and congenital hepatic fibrosis.

Medullary Cystic Disease and Nephronophthisis. Nephronophthisis and medullary cystic kidney disease are inherited disorders that eventually lead to end-stage renal disease. They are grouped together because they share many features. Pathologically, they cause cysts restricted to the renal medulla or corticomedullary border, as well as a triad of tubular atrophy, tubular basement membrane disintegration, and interstitial fibrosis.

Medullary cystic kidney disease (MCKD) is very similar to the childhood disease familial juvenile nephronophthisis (NPH). Both lead to scarring of the kidney and formation of fluid-filled cavities (cysts) in the deeper parts of the kidney. In these conditions, the kidneys do not concentrate the urine enough, leading to excessive urine production and loss of sodium and other chemical changes in the blood and urine.

MCKD occurs in older patients and is inherited in an autosomal dominant pattern. NPH occurs in young children and is usually due to autosomal recessive inheritance.

Sonographic Findings. The patient presents with small echogenic kidneys, with loss of corticomedullary differentiation, and multiple medullary small cysts (smaller than 2 cm). With MSK, sonography shows hyperechoic calyces, with or without stones (Figures 14-45 and 14-46).

Renal Neoplasms

The sonographic appearance of most renal masses is nonspecific. Usually, an abnormal renal contour is the first finding that a mass may be present and may require further investigation. Very often, the sonographic characteristic patterns of benign and malignant tumors cannot be differentiated from one another. In most outpatient clinical settings, a sonogram is usually the first step in the discovery of a renal mass. If a solid mass is detected, renal cell carcinoma, oncocytoma, angiomyolipoma, transitional cell carcinoma, or secondary neoplasms (e.g., metastasis, lymphoma) must be considered (Box 14-4).

Renal Cell Carcinoma. Renal cell carcinoma (RCC), also called hypernephroma, or Grawitz's tumor, is the most common of all renal neoplasms and represents 85% of all kidney tumors. It is twice as common in males as in females, usually in the sixth to seventh decade of life. The classical clinical presentation is nonspecific; however, the patient may report hematuria, flank pain, and a palpable mass. The tumor appears bilaterally in 0.1% to 1.5% of patients, and is multifocal in 13% of cases. An association with von Hippel-Lindau disease, acquired cystic disease (dialysis patients), and tuberous sclerosis is reported. Regardless of histologic subtype, the sonographic appearance of most RCCs is solid with

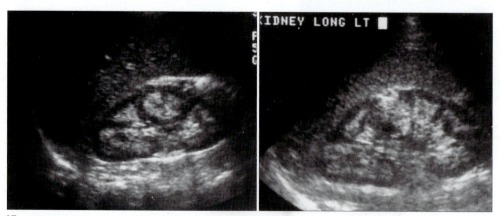

FIGURE 14-45 Longitudinal scans of a young patient with medullary sponge kidney show nephrocalcinosis and stone formation.

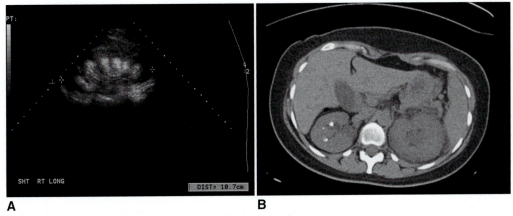

FIGURE 14-46 A, Longitudinal view of the right kidney with hyperechoic calyces and stones. **B,** Tiny medullary calculi are detected on CT.

BOX 14-4	What to Do When a Renal Mass Is Discovered

- If the renal mass is solid, it must be considered malignant, unless fat is present within the mass.
- The presence of calcifications in a renal mass is always a sign of malignancy.
- If a cystic renal mass does not meet the sonographic criteria for a simple renal cyst, it must be considered malignant.
- A renal pseudotumor needs to be considered when a renal mass is discovered.
- 10%–15% metastasis at time of diagnosis

Sonographic Considerations
- Evaluate the renal vein and inferior vena cava into the right atrium to look for thrombus/tumor.
- Evaluate the contralateral kidney, liver, and retroperitoneum for metastases.

no predilection for left or right kidney or location in the organ. One to two percent of RCCs are predominantly cystic, and very rarely the tumor may be entirely cystic. ▶ **Sonographic Findings.** Most RCCs are isoechoic, but they may also present as hyperechoic (Figure 14-47). Usually, the bigger the tumor, the more hetereogeneous is its echotexture, caused by intratumoral hemorrhage and necrosis. Small tumors (less than 3 cm in diameter) are usually hyperechoic, and it is difficult to distinguish them with sonography from echogenic fat-containing tumors, such as angiomyolipomas. A hypoechoic rim, which represents a vascular pseudocapsule on color Doppler, may be very helpful in making the diagnosis of RCC. The presence of intratumoral calcifications is considered specific for RCC. In cases in which renal cell carcinoma is represented as cystic, a variety of types, such as unilocular, multilocular, completely necrotic, and tumor originating in a cyst, may be demonstrated on sonography.

Use of color Doppler for the detection of tumor vascularity shows high sensitivity for malignant renal

tumors, especially renal cell carcinoma. In RCC, tumor vascularity can be demonstrated in up to 92% of cases, and the most common vascular patterns include a "basket sign" and/or "vessels within the tumor." High systolic and high end-diastolic arterial flow with low resistive index (RI) is the most typical flow pattern in spectral Doppler waveforms. Renal vein (RV) and inferior vena cava (IVC) invasion occurs from 5% to 24% of RCCs at the time of diagnosis, and metastasis from renal malignancies is seen in lungs, mediastinum, other nodes, liver, bone, adrenal, and the opposite kidney. CT and MRI with contrast are the most sensitive radiographic examinations for the detection and characterization of renal masses (Figures 14-48 to 14-50). Box 14-5 summarizes the sonographic characteristics of malignant renal tumors.

Transitional Cell Carcinoma. Transitional cell carcinoma (TCC) accounts for 90% of malignancies that involve the renal pelvis, ureter, and bladder, and for up to 7% to 10% of all renal tumors. The tumor is often multifocal, with a 40% to 80% incidence. TCC occurs twice as often in men as in women, with a peak occurrence in the seventh decade. TCC of the renal pelvis is two to three times more common than ureteral neoplasm, and is almost 50 times less common than TCC of the urinary bladder. The TCC may be papillary or flat. Papillary TCCs are more common, with an exophytic polypoid appearance attached to mucosa. They usually are low-grade malignancies and tend to have a more benign course. Small TCCs tend to be flat and are difficult to detect with any type of imaging. Small TCCs are generally high-grade malignancy tumors and metastasize easily to the other tissues and organs. Clinically, the patient may present with gross or microscopic hematuria and flank pain. The differential diagnosis includes other tumors of the renal pelvis, such as squamous cell tumor, adenoma, a blood clot, or a fungus ball (see Table 14-2). ▶ **Sonographic Findings.** The typical appearance is that of a hypoechoic mass within the collecting system, with low vascularity on color Doppler and, extremely rarely, calcifications. TCC may invade adjacent renal

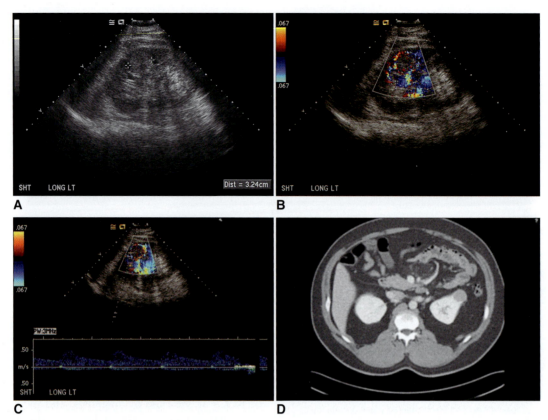

FIGURE 14-47 A, Longitudinal view of a small hyperechoic renal cell carcinoma. **B** and **C,** Color Doppler demonstrates peripheral vascularity of the tumor ("basket sign"). **D,** Contrast CT confirms a small enhancing renal tumor; pathology confirmed cell carcinoma.

BOX 14-5	Sonographic Characteristics of a Malignant Renal Tumor

- Renal cell carcinomas (RCCs) less than 2–3 cm in diameter are always hyperechoic.
- The bigger the tumor, the more heterogeneous is its echotexture.
- Hypoechoic rim represents a vascular pseudocapsule.
- In up to 92% of RCCs, peripheral (basket sign) and/or central (vessel within the tumor) vascularity can be demonstrated on color Doppler.
- Invasion of renal vein and/or inferior vena cava (IVC) occurs in 5%–24% of cases.

In Cases with Cystic Appearance
- Thick wall >1 mm
- Irregularity at the base of the cyst
- Septations
- Calcifications
- Presence of vascularity in the septa and/or cystic wall

parenchyma and form an infiltrating mass, which usually preserves the renal contour.

Squamous Cell Carcinoma. Squamous cell carcinoma is a rare, highly invasive tumor with a poor prognosis. Clinically, the patient usually presents with a history of chronic irritation and gross hematuria, with a palpable kidney secondary to severe hydronephrosis.

Sonographic Findings. The sonographic finding is usually a large mass in the renal pelvis. Obstruction from kidney stones may also be present (Figures 14-51 and 14-52).

Renal Lymphoma. Primary lymphomatous involvement of the kidneys is rare, with a 3% occurrence. The secondary form is more common. This form of lymphoma may occur as a hematogenous spread (90%) or as direct extension via the retroperitoneal lymphatic channels with a contiguous spread from the retroperitoneum (see Table 14-2). Non-Hodgkin lymphoma is more common than Hodgkin. Lymphoma is more common as a bilateral invasion with multiple nodules.

Sonographic Findings. The kidneys are enlarged and hypoechoic relative to the renal parenchyma (the mass may simulate a renal cyst without acoustic enhancement). The mass rarely demonstrates a sonographic halo of hypoechoic mass in the perinephric regions (Figure 14-53). The sonographer should be careful of highly hypoechoic renal tumors with poorly defined margins without posterior enhancement, as they may be mistaken initially for "renal cysts."

Secondary Malignancies of the Kidneys. Metastases to the kidneys are relatively common, occurring late in the course of the disease. Secondary malignancies are bilateral in one third of cases and multiple in more than 50%. The most common primary malignancies that metastasize to the kidneys include carcinoma of the lung

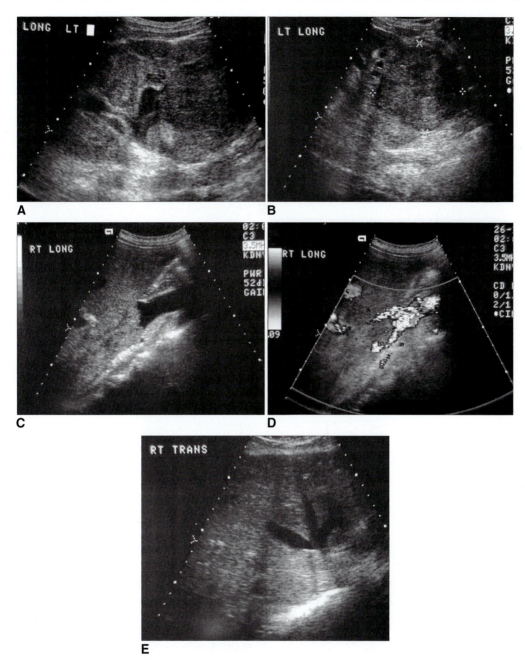

FIGURE 14-48 Stage III renal cell carcinoma with invasion into the inferior vena cava. **A,** Longitudinal scan shows lower pole mass with no normal renal parenchyma. **B,** Measurement of the lower pole mass. **C,** Longitudinal scan demonstrating the thrombus-filled inferior vena cava (IVC). **D,** Longitudinal scan of IVC with color flow showing obstruction. **E,** Transverse view of the dome of the liver with patent hepatic veins and nonvisualization of the IVC. *(Courtesy Joseph Yee, New York University.)*

or breast and renal cell carcinoma of the contralateral kidney. On sonography, the lesion usually presents as multiple, poorly marginated hypoechoic masses. Renal enlargement without a discrete mass also may occur.

Sonographic Findings. The tumor may spread beyond the **renal capsule** and invade the venous channel, with tumor cells extending into the inferior vena cava and right atrium and with eventual metastasis into the lungs. The tumor may be multifocal in a small percentage of patients.

Nephroblastoma. Nephroblastoma, or Wilms' tumor, is the most common abdominal malignancy in children (7.8/100,000 younger than age 15) and the most common solid renal tumor in pediatric patients 1 to 8 years old. Peak incidence is seen at 2.5 to 3 years of age; 90% of patients are younger than 5 years old, and 70% are younger than 3 years old. Nephroblastoma is two to eight times more common in patients with horseshoe kidney. Clinical signs may include abdominal flank mass, hematuria, fever, and anorexia.

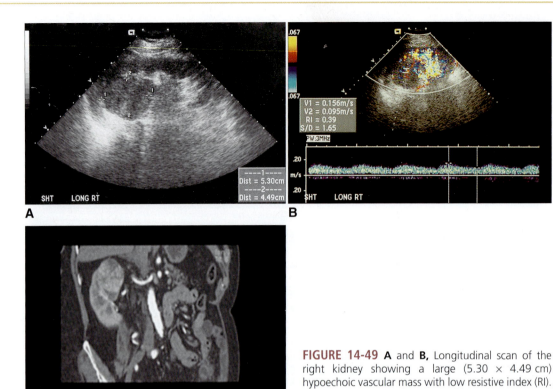

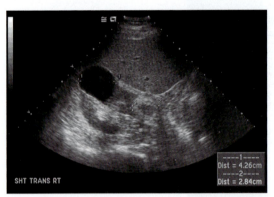

FIGURE 14-49 A and **B,** Longitudinal scan of the right kidney showing a large (5.30 × 4.49 cm) hypoechoic vascular mass with low resistive index (RI). **C,** Contrast CT confirms a highly enhancing renal tumor; pathology confirmed renal cell carcinoma.

FIGURE 14-50 A transverse view of the right kidney demonstrating a cyst and a small hyperechoic mass, which is consistent with renal cell carcinoma.

Sonographic Findings. The sonographer is able to determine whether the mass is cystic or solid, and to confirm if it is renal in origin. The mass varies from hypoechoic to moderately echogenic. A 5% to 10% incidence of bilateral tumors has been reported, so careful evaluation of both kidneys is crucial. Up to 40% of patients with Wilms' tumor have renal vein thrombosis and/or vena cava or atrial thrombus by the time of diagnosis. Venous obstruction may result, with findings of leg edema, varicocele, or Budd-Chiari syndrome (Figures 14-54 to 14-56).

Benign Renal Tumors. Benign renal tumors are rare. All renal tumors are treated as malignant until proven otherwise. The patient usually is asymptomatic and

presents with flank pain only if the mass is large, or if hemorrhage from the mass occurs. Adenomas and oncocytomas are two common benign renal tumors (see Table 14-3).

Renal Angiomyolipoma. Renal angiomyolipoma (AML) is the most common benign renal tumor. It is composed of varying proportions of fat, muscle, and blood vessels. Angiomyolipoma has an incidence of 0.07% to 0.3% in the general population; 80% of cases occur in females, and 80% in the right kidney. The tumor is found in 80% of patients with tuberous sclerosis. Tumor size varies between 1 and 20 cm and may be multifocal.

Sonographic Findings. The echo pattern of AML is usually hyperechoic, depending on the proportions of fat, muscle, and vessels within the mass. Intratumoral hemorrhage and organ displacement are the primary complications. Differential diagnosis is made with small (less than 3 cm) renal cell carcinomas, which are also hyperechoic in echotexture and may simulate AML in up to 33% of cases. A hypoechoic rim, presented as a basket sign on color Doppler, favors renal cell carcinoma. Color Doppler shows no intratumoral vascularity. On angiography, the tumor is highly vascular; CT is determinant in the diagnosis of AML because of its sensitivity in detecting intratumoral fat (Figures 14-57 and 14-58).

Renal Adenomatous Tumors. Renal adenomatous tumors can be seen as nephrogenic adenofibroma or embryonal adenoma. Patients are usually asymptomatic. Incidental findings may be noted if the mass is large, or

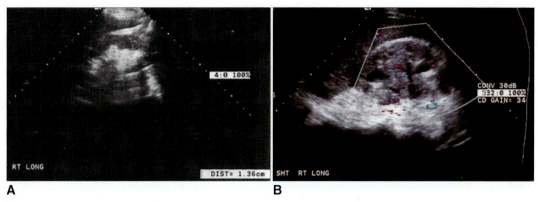

FIGURE 14-51 A, Longitudinal scan of the right kidney with a small hypoechoic mass (transitional cell carcinoma [TCC]) in the mid upper collection system and a 1.36 cm nonobstructing stone in the lower pole. **B,** A large vascular hypoechoic mass occupying most of the collecting system and causing an obstruction *(arrows)*.

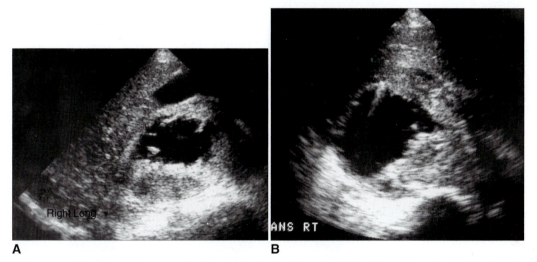

FIGURE 14-52 Sixty-year-old patient with metastatic disease. **A,** Sagittal image of right kidney shows irregularly shaped mass filling the renal sinus. **B,** Transverse image of the squamous cell carcinoma.

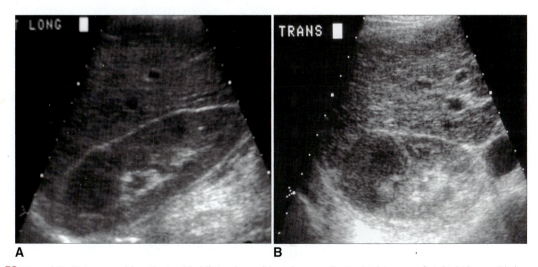

FIGURE 14-53 A and **B,** Sixty-year-old patient with bilateral renal lymphomas. **A,** Sagittal image of right kidney with hypoechoic upper pole mass. **B,** Transverse image of upper pole of right kidney with hypoechoic lymphoma.

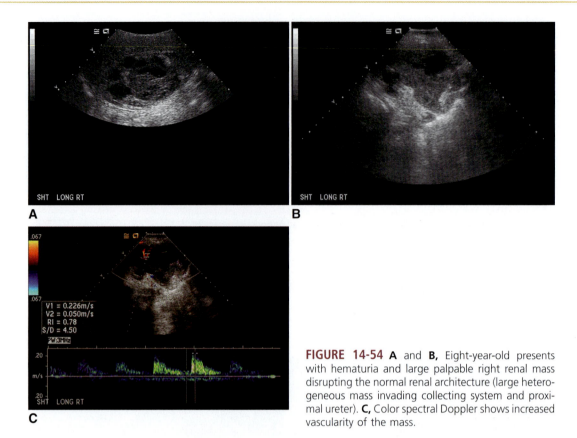

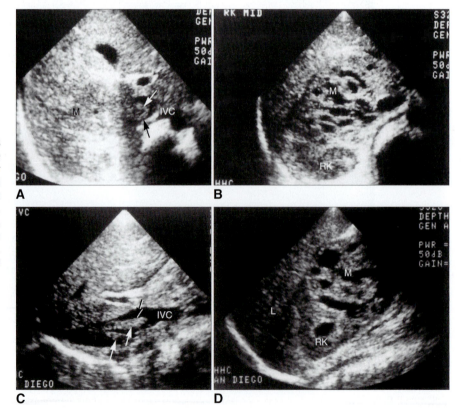

FIGURE 14-54 A and **B,** Eight-year-old presents with hematuria and large palpable right renal mass disrupting the normal renal architecture (large heterogeneous mass invading collecting system and proximal ureter). **C,** Color spectral Doppler shows increased vascularity of the mass.

FIGURE 14-55 A, One of the complications of a Wilms' tumor *(M)* is spread beyond the renal capsule into the renal vein and inferior vena cava *(IVC)*. **B,** This 18-month-old child had a large, complex tumor with extension into the inferior vena cava *(IVC, arrows)*. *RK,* Right kidney. **C** and **D,** Longitudinal scan, showing the dilated inferior vena cava with tumor echoes along the posterior border. The tumor may extend into the right atrium of the heart. *L,* Liver; *RK,* right kidney.

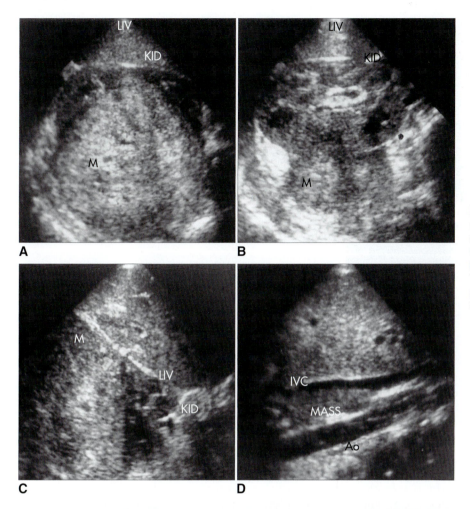

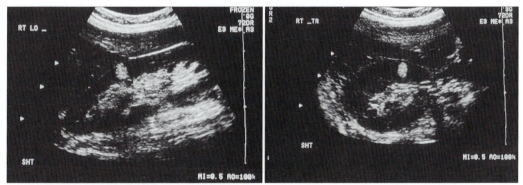

FIGURE 14-56 A through **D,** A 14-month-old child with a large Wilms' tumor *(M)* extending from the right kidney *(KID)* into the inferior vena cava *(IVC)*. On coronal scan **(D),** the tumor mass is seen within the IVC. The patient is rolled into a slight decubitus position for better imaging of the IVC and aorta *(Ao). LIV,* Liver.

FIGURE 14-57 Angiomyolipoma appears as an echogenic focal mass in the renal parenchyma.

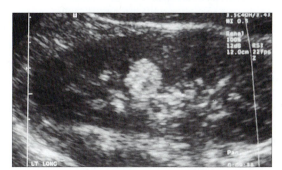

FIGURE 14-58 Angiolipomas are common benign tumors that usually appear as unilateral solitary or multiple echogenic masses in middle-aged women. Renal function is normal.

if intratumoral hemorrhage occurs. In some cases, these tumors may cause hematuria.

Sonographic Findings. These tumors appear as solid masses on sonography, are hyperechoic to hypoechoic in echotexture, and are hypovascular on color Doppler (Figure 14-59). As with oncocytomas, renal adenomatous tumors may be indistinguishable from renal cell carcinoma.

Oncocytoma. Oncocytoma is another uncommon renal tumor that is usually benign. Incidence is increased in the middle-aged or elderly patient. This lesion represents 3.1% to 6% of all renal tumors. Tumor size varies,

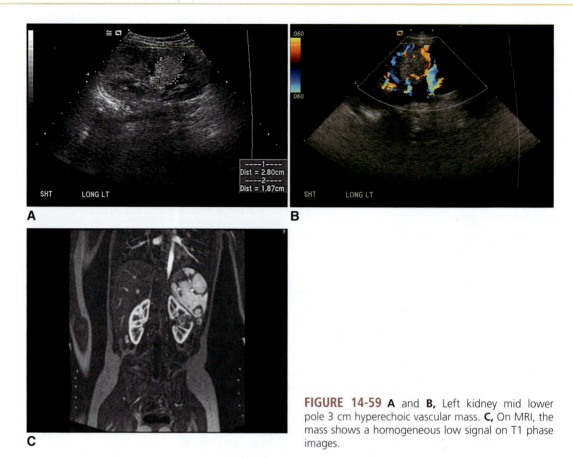

FIGURE 14-59 A and **B,** Left kidney mid lower pole 3 cm hyperechoic vascular mass. **C,** On MRI, the mass shows a homogeneous low signal on T1 phase images.

with an average size of 6 cm. The patient is typically asymptomatic, but the tumor may cause pain and hematuria.

▶ **Sonographic Findings.** In more than 50% of cases, the mass is hypoechoic in echotexture. Oncocytomas resemble "spoke-wheel" patterns of enhancement with a central scar. It is practically impossible to differentiate them from renal cell carcinoma; 5% of oncocytomas are initially diagnosed as RCC (Figure 14-60).

Lipomas. A lipoma consists of fat cells and is the most common of the mesenchymal type of tumors. This tumor is found more often in females than in males. The patient is typically asymptomatic, but the tumor has been reported to cause hematuria.

▶ **Sonographic Findings.** Lipomas appear as well-defined echogenic masses within the kidney (Figure 14-61).

Renal Disease

Intrinsic renal disease can be identified by examining the renal parenchyma with ultrasound. Two classifications of disease processes have been described. One group produces a generalized increase in cortical echoes, believed to result from deposition of collagen and fibrous tissue. This group includes interstitial nephritis, acute tubular necrosis, amyloidosis, diabetic nephropathy, systemic lupus erythematosus, and myeloma. The second group of diseases may cause loss of normal anatomic detail, resulting in inability to distinguish the cortex and medullary regions of the kidneys. This group of diseases includes chronic pyelonephritis, renal tubular ectasia, and acute bacterial nephritis (see Table 14-3).

The end stage of many of these disease processes is renal atrophy, which can be identified on a sonogram by measuring renal length and cortical thickness. Some acute renal disorders produce exactly the opposite findings—decreased parenchymal echogenicity and renal enlargement. Examples include acute renal vein thrombosis, acute pyelonephritis, and acute renal transplant rejection. Interstitial edema is believed to be the most likely cause of these findings.

Acute Glomerulonephritis. In acute glomerulonephritis, necrosis or proliferation of cellular elements (or both) occurs in the glomeruli. The vascular elements, tubules, and interstitium become secondarily affected; the end result is enlarged, poorly functioning kidneys.

▶ **Sonographic Findings.** Different forms of glomerulonephritis, including membranous, idiopathic, membranoproliferative, rapidly progressive, and post-streptococcal, can be associated with abnormal echo patterns from the renal parenchyma on a sonogram (Figure 14-62). Increased cortical echoes probably result from changes within the glomerular, interstitial, tubular, and vascular structures. Patients have many symptoms,

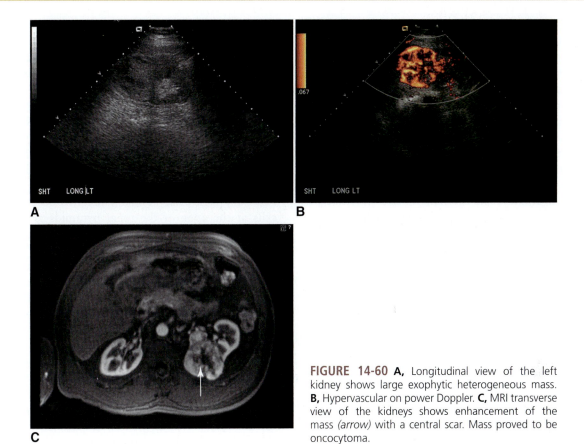

A

B

C

FIGURE 14-60 **A,** Longitudinal view of the left kidney shows large exophytic heterogeneous mass. **B,** Hypervascular on power Doppler. **C,** MRI transverse view of the kidneys shows enhancement of the mass *(arrow)* with a central scar. Mass proved to be oncocytoma.

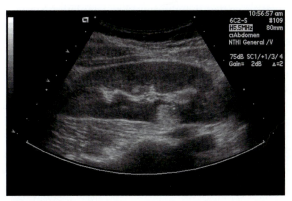

FIGURE 14-61 Sagittal view of left kidney with lipoma. *(Courtesy Siemens Medical Solutions USA, Inc.)*

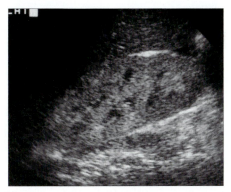

FIGURE 14-62 Acute glomerulonephritis may be suspected when the echogenicity of the renal parenchyma exceeds that of the liver.

including nephrotic syndrome, hypertension, anemia, and peripheral edema.

Acute Interstitial Nephritis. Acute interstitial nephritis has been associated with the infectious processes of scarlet fever and diphtheria. It may be a manifestation of an allergic reaction to certain drugs. Patient signs and symptoms include uremia, proteinuria, hematuria, rash, fever, and eosinophilia.

Sonographic Findings. The kidneys are enlarged and mottled. On a sonogram, renal cortical echogenicity is increased. The increase in echogenicity is greatest in cases of diffuse active disease. This increase is less apparent in diffuse scarring.

Lupus Nephritis. Systemic lupus erythematosus is a connective tissue disorder believed to result from an abnormal immune system. Females are affected more often than males, and incidence peaks between 20 and 40 years of age. The kidneys are involved in more than 50% of patients. Renal manifestations include hematuria, proteinuria, hypertension, renal vein thrombosis, and renal insufficiency.

Sonographic Findings. Sonography shows increased cortical echogenicity and renal atrophy (Figure 14-63).

Acquired Immunodeficiency Syndrome. Acquired immunodeficiency syndrome (AIDS) is a highly contagious disease, spread mainly by unprotected sexual activity or infected needles. The virus destroys T cells and then replicates rapidly within the body. It affects many organs. Patients have various symptoms (see Table 14-2).

Unexplained uremia or azotemia may indicate renal dysfunction resulting from AIDS; it is usually a late finding. Causes of renal dysfunction in AIDS patients include acute tubular necrosis, nephrocalcinosis, interstitial nephritis, and focal segmental glomerulosclerosis.

▶ **Sonographic Findings.** An echogenic parenchymal pattern is evident on a sonogram. Cortical echogenicity is increased. Kidneys are normal in size or enlarged (Figures 14-64 to 14-66). If AIDS-related lymphoma or Kaposi's sarcoma occurs, the kidneys appear enlarged and hypoechoic on a sonogram.

Sickle Cell Nephropathy. Renal involvement is common in patients with sickle cell disease. Abnormalities include glomerulonephritis, renal vein thrombosis, and papillary necrosis. Hematuria is common.

▶ **Sonographic Findings.** The sonographic appearance depends on the type of disorder. In acute renal vein thrombosis, the kidneys are enlarged with decreased echogenicity secondary to edema. In patients with subacute cases, renal enlargement is present with increased cortical echoes.

Hypertensive Nephropathy. Uncontrolled hypertension can lead to progressive renal damage and azotemia.

▶ **Sonographic Findings.** Sonographically, the kidneys are small with smooth borders. Superimposed scars of pyelonephritis or lobar infarction may distort the intrarenal anatomy. Bilateral small kidneys occur secondary to end-stage disease as a result of hypertension, inflammation, or ischemia.

Papillary Necrosis. Papillary necrosis occurs when the cells at the apex of the renal pyramids are destroyed. Many conditions (e.g., analgesic abuse, sickle cell disease, diabetes, obstruction, pyelonephritis, renal transplant) can lead to papillary necrosis. Necrosis may develop within weeks or months after transplantation. Patients previously treated for rejection and those with cadaveric kidney are at greatest risk. Ischemia is believed to have an important role in necrosis.

Symptoms suggest calculus or an inflammatory process. Complaints include hematuria, flank pain, dysuria, hypertension, and acute renal failure. Differential considerations include congenital megacalyces, hydronephrosis, and postobstructive atrophy.

▶ **Sonographic Findings.** Sonographic findings include one or more fluid spaces at the corticomedullary junction that correspond to the distribution of the renal pyramids. The cystic spaces may be round or triangular. Sometimes the arcuate vessels are seen.

Renal Atrophy. Renal atrophy results from numerous disease processes. Intrarenal anatomy is preserved with uniform loss of renal tissue. Renal sinus lipomatosis occurs secondary to renal atrophy. More severe lipomatosis results from a tremendous increase in renal sinus fat content in cases of marked renal atrophy caused by hydronephrosis and chronic calculus disease.

▶ **Sonographic Findings.** The kidneys appear enlarged with a highly echogenic, enlarged renal sinus and a thin

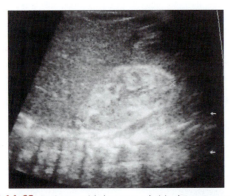

FIGURE 14-63 Patients with lupus nephritis demonstrate a highly echogenic renal parenchymal pattern compared with the liver. Renal atrophy is usually present.

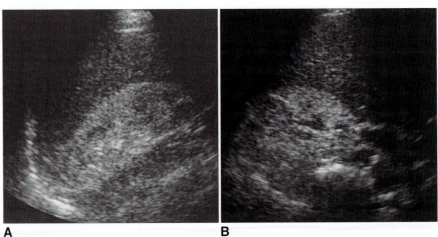

FIGURE 14-64 Longitudinal **(A)** and transverse **(B)** scans in a patient with acquired immunodeficiency syndrome (AIDS) show cortical echogenicity with normal to slightly increased renal size.

A   B

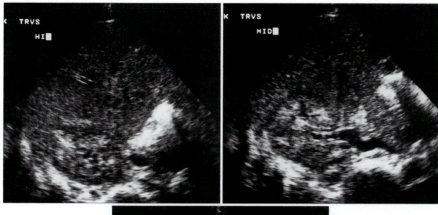

FIGURE 14-65 Transverse scans of a young male with acquired immunodeficiency syndrome (AIDS) show a mildly echogenic renal parenchyma.

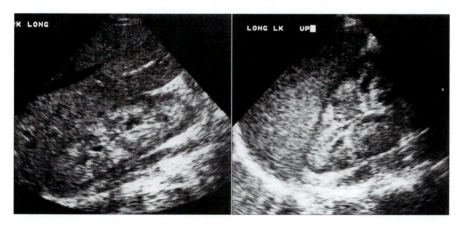

FIGURE 14-66 Longitudinal scans of a 26-year-old male with acquired immunodeficiency syndrome (AIDS).

cortical rim. Renal sinus fat is easily seen on a sonogram as highly echogenic reflections (Figure 14-67).

Renal Failure

The excretory and regulatory functions of the kidneys are decreased in acute and chronic renal failure. Acute renal failure (ARF) is a common medical condition that can be caused by numerous medical diseases or pathophysiologic mechanisms. ARF is typically an abrupt transient decrease in renal function often heralded by oliguria. Pathophysiologic states that cause varying degrees of renal malfunction have been categorized as prerenal, renal, and postrenal (Box 14-6). Decreased

BOX 14-6	Causes of Renal Failure
Prerenal	
Hypoperfusion	
Hypotension	
Congestive heart failure (CHF)	
Renal	
Infection	
Nephrotoxicity	
Renal artery occlusion	
Renal mass or cyst	
Postrenal	
Lower urinary tract obstruction (ureter, bladder)	
Retroperitoneal fibrosis	

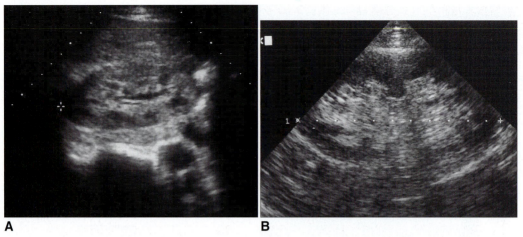

A   **B**

FIGURE 14-67 A, A 73-year-old man with chronic renal disease. Small echogenic kidney with inability to distinguish the medulla from the cortex region of the kidney. **B,** Renal sinus lipomatosis appears as enlarged kidneys with an echogenic, enlarged renal sinus and a thin cortical rim. Renal sinus fat is easily seen on ultrasound as highly echogenic reflections.

perfusion of the kidneys can cause prerenal failure (e.g., renal vein thrombus, congestive heart failure [CHF], renal artery occlusion) and can be diagnosed by clinical and laboratory data and also by color Doppler. Renal causes of acute azotemia include parenchymal disease (e.g., acute glomerulonephritis, acute interstitial nephritis, acute tubular necrosis) and hydronephrosis. Major postrenal causes of acute renal failure include bladder, pelvic, or retroperitoneal tumor and calculi. Prompt diagnosis and treatment of postrenal failure is crucial; the condition is potentially reversible.

Chronic renal failure may be caused by obstructive nephropathies, parenchymal diseases, renovascular disorders, or any process that progressively destroys nephrons. See Table 14-3 for clinical findings, sonographic findings, and differential considerations for malfunctioning kidney conditions.

Numerous studies have previously documented that sonography is extremely sensitive in diagnosing hydronephrosis. Patients for whom laboratory test results indicate compromised renal function should receive rule-out obstruction studies. Most agree that sonography is the initial procedure of choice in evaluating all patients with known or suspected renal failure. See Table 14-3 for clinical findings, sonographic findings, and differential considerations for renal failure.

Acute Renal Failure. Acute renal failure may occur in prerenal, renal, or postrenal failure stages (see Box 14-6). The prerenal stage is secondary to hypoperfusion of the kidney. The renal stages may be caused by parenchymal diseases (i.e., acute glomerulonephritis, acute interstitial nephritis, or acute tubular necrosis). They may also be caused by renal vein thrombosis or renal artery occlusion. In postrenal failure, radiologic imaging plays a major role. This condition is usually the result of outflow obstruction and is potentially reversible. Postrenal failure is usually increased in patients with malignancy of the

bladder, prostate, uterus, ovaries, or rectum. Less frequent causes include retroperitoneal fibrosis and renal calculi.

Sonographic Findings. The cause of acute renal disease urinary outflow obstruction can be differentiated from parenchymal disease. The kidneys may appear normal in size or enlarged and may be hypoechoic with parenchymal disease. Obstruction is responsible for approximately 5% of cases of acute renal failure. The most important issue is the presence or absence of urinary tract dilatation. The degree of dilatation does not necessarily reflect the presence or severity of an obstruction. A sonographer should try to determine the level of obstruction. A normal sonogram does not totally exclude urinary obstruction. In the clinical setting of acute obstruction secondary to calculi, a nondistended collecting system can be present.

Acute Tubular Necrosis. Acute tubular necrosis (ATN) is the most common medical renal disease to produce acute renal failure, although it can be reversible.

Sonographic Findings. The sonogram shows bilaterally enlarged kidneys with hyperechoic pyramids; this can revert to a normal appearance. Differential considerations include nephrocalcinosis. In pediatric patients, the renal pyramids are highly echogenic without shadowing. The calculi may be too small to cause dilatation and shadowing of the pyramids (Figure 14-68). As renal function improves, echogenicity decreases. This can occur in the medulla or the cortex. If the condition reverses, it is probably acute tubular necrosis.

Chronic Renal Disease. Chronic renal disease is the loss of renal function as a result of disease, most commonly parenchymal disease. Three primary types of chronic renal failure are known: nephron, vascular, and interstitial abnormalities. Glomerulonephritis, chronic pyelonephritis, renal vascular disease, and diabetes are a few of the diseases that lead to renal failure.

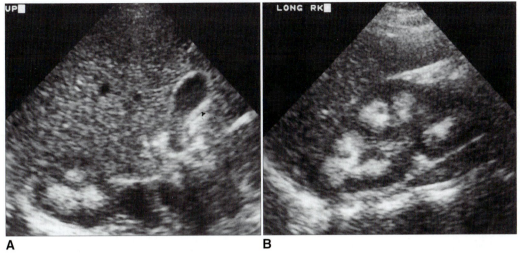

FIGURE 14-68 Transverse **(A)** and longitudinal **(B)** scans of the pediatric patient with acute tubular necrosis and nephrocalcinosis. The echogenic renal pyramids are well seen.

<table>
<tr><td colspan="2">BOX 14-7 | Causes of Hydronephrosis</td></tr>
</table>

Acquired
Bladder tumors
Calculi
Carcinoma of the cervix
Neurogenic bladder
Normal pregnancy
Pelvic mass
Prostatic enlargement
Retroperitoneal fibrosis

Intrinsic
Bladder neck obstruction
Calculus
Congenital
Inflammation
Posterior urethral valves
Pyelonephritis
Stricture
Ureterocele
Ureteropelvic junction (UPJ) obstruction

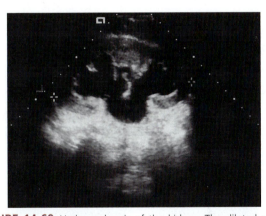

FIGURE 14-69 Hydronephrosis of the kidney. The dilated pyelo-caliceal system appears as separation of the renal sinus echoes by fluid-filled areas that conform anatomically to the infundibula, calyces, and pelvis.

🔺 **Sonographic Findings.** Chronic renal disease is a diffusely echogenic kidney with loss of normal anatomy. It is a nonspecific sonographic finding; chronic renal disease can have multiple causes (AIDS can produce echogenic kidneys). If chronic renal disease is bilateral, small kidneys are identified. This may result from hypertension, chronic inflammation, or chronic ischemia.

Hydronephrosis

Hydronephrosis–Urinary Tract Obstruction (UTO).
Hydronephrosis is the separation of renal sinus echoes by interconnected fluid-filled calyces. Box 14-7 lists the causes of hydronephrosis. Dilatation of the pelvocalyceal system is called hydronephrosis. In 1988, the Society for Fetal Urology proposed the following classification of grading hydronephrosis:

- Grade 1: small fluid-filled separation of the renal pelvis
- Grade 2: dilatation of some but not all of the calyces; calyx orientation still concave
- Grade 3: complete pelvocaliectasis; calyx orientation changed in convex; echogenic line separating collecting system from renal parenchyma can be demonstrated (Figure 14-69)
- Grade 4: prominent dilatation of the collecting system, thinning of renal parenchyma, and no differentiation between collecting system and renal parenchyma

Urinary tract obstruction is not synonymous with dilatation; in almost 35% of cases with acute urinary obstruction, no dilatation is seen. Nonobstructive dilation is also seen in childhood during vesicoureteral reflux (see Box 14-7).

Sonographic Findings. Whenever the renal collecting system is dilated, the ureters and bladder are scanned to locate the level of obstruction. It is possible to identify the site of obstruction by using sonography. A congenital obstruction of the ureteropelvic junction can be seen in utero and in infants. The collecting system will be dilated without dilation of the ureter. Localized hydronephrosis occurs as a result of strictures, calculi, focal masses, or a duplex collecting system (Figures 14-70 and 14-71). Hydronephrosis with a dilated ureter indicates obstruction of the ureterovesical junction; hydroureteronephrosis with a dilated bladder indicates obstruction of the posterior urethra (posterior urethral valves).

A mildly distended collecting system can be caused by overhydration, a normal variant of extrarenal pelvis, or by a previous urinary diversion procedure (Figure 14-72). Postvoid scanning techniques are helpful in preventing these errors.

If hydronephrosis is suspected, the sonographer should examine the bladder. If it is full, a postvoid longitudinal scan of each kidney should be done to show that hydronephrosis has disappeared or remains the same. At the level of obstruction, the sonographer should sweep the transducer back and forth in two planes to see if a mass or stone can be distinguished. The sonographer must be able to rule out a parapelvic cyst (septations may be numerous) or a crossing renal vessel in the peripelvic area (color flow Doppler is extremely useful). An extrarenal pelvis would protrude outside of the renal area, and the sonographer probably would not confuse this pattern with hydronephrosis.

In evaluating the patient for hydronephrosis, the sonographer must be sure to look for a dilated ureter, an enlarged prostate (which may cause the ureter to become obstructed), or an enlarged bladder (which may occur secondary to an enlarged prostate). Bladder carcinoma may obstruct the pathway of the urethra, causing urine to back into the ureter and renal pelvis. A ureterocele may also block urine output. This condition occurs when the ureter inserts into the bladder wall. The ureter can turn inside out and obstruct the orifice.

Obstructive Hydronephrosis. Dilatation of the renal pelvis is just one factor present in patients with obstructive hydronephrosis. (See Table 14-3 for clinical findings, sonographic findings, and differential considerations for obstructive hydronephrosis.)

Sonographic Findings. In cases of acute urinary tract obstruction (UTO), the RI (resistive index) of the interlobar and arcuate intrarenal vessels may be greater than 0.70, starting 6 hours after acute onset and up to 72 hours (Figure 14-73). The RI returns to normal value after 120 hours of obstruction. The value of the RI may be higher than 0.70 in some normal conditions, as in neonates and infants up to 6 years old and in elderly patients, and in some pathologic conditions related to intrinsic renal disease, diabetes, and/or hypertension. Use of nonsteroidal anti-inflammatory drugs may lower the value of the RI on the affected side, which decreases the sensitivity of Doppler ultrasound in identifying UTO. Level of obstruction is another important factor in

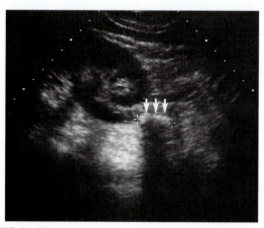

FIGURE 14-70 Slight dilatation of the collecting system is seen. A longitudinal left kidney scan with dilatation of the proximal ureter caused by a stone *(arrows)*.

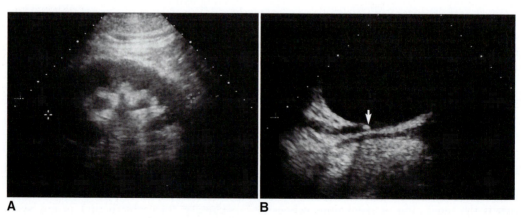

FIGURE 14-71 **A,** Mild hydronephrosis is seen. **B,** A longitudinal scan of the bladder shows a distended distal ureter with a small stone *(arrow)*.

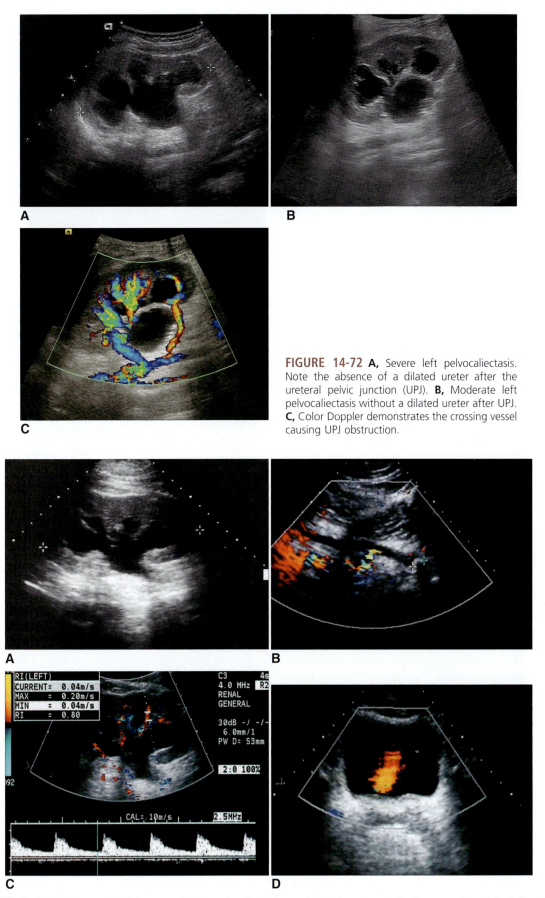

FIGURE 14-72 A, Severe left pelvocaliectasis. Note the absence of a dilated ureter after the ureteral pelvic junction (UPJ). **B,** Moderate left pelvocaliectasis without a dilated ureter after UPJ. **C,** Color Doppler demonstrates the crossing vessel causing UPJ obstruction.

FIGURE 14-73 A, Grade 2 to grade 3 left uretero-hydronephrosis. **B,** 1 cm obstructing stone in the lower portion of the left ureter. **C,** High resistive index (RI = 0.80) documenting an acute urinary obstruction. **D,** Absence of the left ureteral jet.

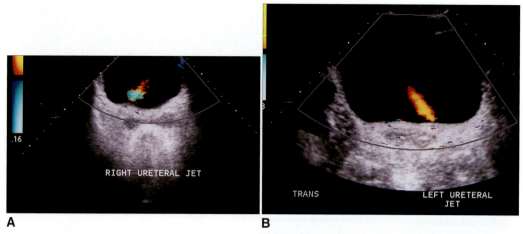

FIGURE 14-74 Normal right **(A)** and left **(B)** ureteral jets seen in the fluid-filled bladder.

elevation of the RI value. The resistive index is greater in patients with an obstruction in the proximal ureter or in the distal intramural ureteral portion.

It is very important to measure and compare the resistive index in both kidneys, because a ΔRI is more useful for diagnosis of UTO than a solid value for RI. No ureteral jet will be seen on the affected side if the obstruction is complete, or the jet may be noted if obstruction is partial.

Classical sonographic findings in the diagnosis of UTO include the following: Grade I or II hydronephrosis; Doppler showing elevated RI or difference of ΔRI; absence of the respective ureteral jet; and visualization of the dilated ureter and/or stone. Sonography can be normal in up to 50% of cases in the first 6 hours after acute onset, which means that the normal sonogram does not exclude acute urinary obstruction, and a noncontrast CT will be necessary.

Ureteral Jet Phenomenon. The ureteral jet phenomenon picked up by gray scale or color Doppler is caused by the difference in density between urine in the bladder and urine coming from the ureter (kidney). The frequency and size (velocity) of the ureteral jet range from 0.2 m/sec to 1.7 m/sec. Duration of the jets is 0.6 to 4.1 seconds, with a 30 second interval jet time. The jets are directed upward and toward the contralateral side, and the shape of the spectral Doppler curve varies with the amount of urine produced. Complete obstruction shows absence of the respective ureteral jet; partial obstruction may show a low-level jet on the side of obstruction and/or asymmetry of the ureteral jets.

Urine fills the bladder at a rate of up to 2 ml/min. Patients who have voided before the renal examination and are rehydrated may have a false-positive absence of ureteral jets. This occurs because the concentration of urine in the recently distended bladder is similar in density to that of urine entering the bladder. Comparison of the two ureteral jets is necessary to confirm that nonvisualization of the symptomatic side is not related to

<table>
<tr><td>**BOX 14-8**</td><td>**Conditions That Mimic Hydronephrosis**</td></tr>
</table>

Arteriovenous malformation
Congenital megacalyces
Extrarenal pelvis
Papillary necrosis
Parapelvic cysts
Persistent diuresis
Reflux
Renal artery aneurysm

the fact that the density of urine in the ureter is similar to that in the bladder (Figure 14-74 and 14-75).

Nonobstructive Hydronephrosis. Dilatation of the renal pelvis does not always mean that obstruction is present. Several other factors, such as reflux, infection, large extrarenal pelvis, high flow states (polyuria), distended renal bladder, atrophy after obstruction, or pregnancy dilatation, may cause the renal pelvis to be dilated. (The enlarged uterus can compress the ureter; this usually occurs more frequently on the right during the third trimester, causing the so-called "hydronephrosis of pregnancy" with normal RI.)

False-Positive Hydronephrosis. Many conditions may mimic hydronephrosis (Box 14-8); these include extrarenal pelvis, parapelvic cyst, reflux, multicystic kidney, central renal cyst, transient diuresis, congenital megacalyces, papillary necrosis, renal artery aneurysm (color can help distinguish that this enlargement, not the renal pelvis, is vascular), or an arteriovenous malformation (color can distinguish this abnormality).

Localized hydronephrosis may occur secondary to strictures, calculi, or focal masses (transitional). It may also be seen in a duplex system when one of the systems can be obstructed by an ectopic insertion of the ureter. In females, the ureter can insert below the external urinary sphincter, causing dribbling.

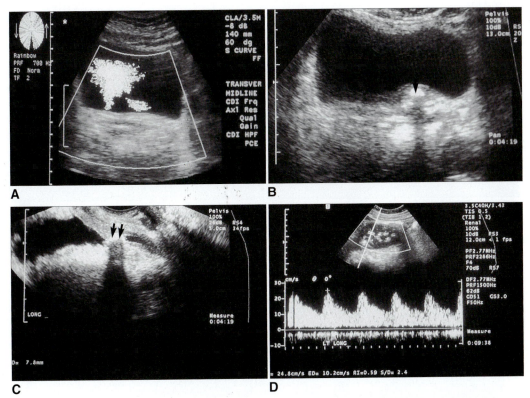

FIGURE 14-75 A, Transverse scan of a fluid-filled bladder with a normal right ureteral jet. A partially obstructed left ureter with decreased flow. **B,** Transverse scan of a partially obstructed distal left ureter. *Arrows* indicate the stone and shadowing posterior to the stone. **C,** Transvaginal scan of the dilated distal ureter with a ureteral stone. **D,** Normal resistive index (RI) of 0.59 for left kidney.

False-Negative Hydronephrosis. A dilated renal pelvis may be distinguished from other conditions by the use of other techniques. In patients with retroperitoneal fibrosis or necrosis, give liquids to see if the renal pelvis dilates. In patients with distal calculi, no obstruction can be seen unless the calculi have been there for several days. A staghorn calculus can mask an associated dilatation.

The conditions of adult polycystic disease and multicystic renal disease with severe hydronephrosis may be confused. In patients with severe hydronephrosis, the image shows dilated calyces as they radiate from a larger central fluid collection in the renal pelvis. The kidney usually retains a normal shape. The sonographer sees fluid-filled sacs in a radiating pattern or cauliflower configuration. In patients with adult polycystic renal disease or multicystic renal disease, the renal cysts are randomly distributed, the contour is disturbed, and the cysts are variable in size. Once obstruction has been ruled out, consider renal medical disease, which is the leading cause of acute renal failure.

Renal Infections

A spectrum of severity is possible in renal infection. The disease can progress from pyelonephritis to focal bacterial nephritis to an abscess. An abscess can be transmitted through the parenchyma into the blood. Most renal infections stay in the kidney and are resolved with antibiotics. A perirenal abscess may occur from direct extension. (See Table 14-3 for clinical findings, sonographic findings, and differential considerations for renal infections.)

Pyonephrosis. Pyonephrosis occurs when pus is found within the collecting renal system. It is often associated with severe urosepsis and represents a true urologic emergency that requires urgent intravenous (IV) antibiotherapy and/or percutaneous drainage. It usually occurs secondary to long-standing ureteral obstruction resulting from calculus disease, stricture, or a congenital anomaly.

▶ **Sonographic Findings.** Sonographic findings include the presence of low-level echoes with a fluid-debris level (Figures 14-76 and 14-77). The sonographer should be aware that an anechoic dilated system may be found. (Sonographic guided aspiration or CT may be necessary.)

Emphysematous Pyelonephritis. Emphysematous pyelonephritis occurs when air is present in the parenchyma (diffuse gas-forming parenchymal infection). It may be caused by *Escherichia coli* bacteria. When this occurs in diabetic patients, they become very sick. It generally is found unilaterally and may be cause for an emergency nephrectomy.

▶ **Sonographic Findings.** On a sonogram, the enlarged kidneys appear hypoechoic and inflamed.

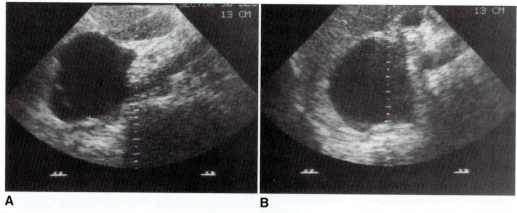

A   **B**

FIGURE 14-76 Renal infection. This patient presented with an elevated white blood cell count and spiking fever. **A,** Supine sagittal scan reveals a homogeneous, slightly irregular mass arising from the upper pole of the right kidney. **B,** Transverse scan of the renal abscess. Note the decreased through-transmission posterior to the abscess wall.

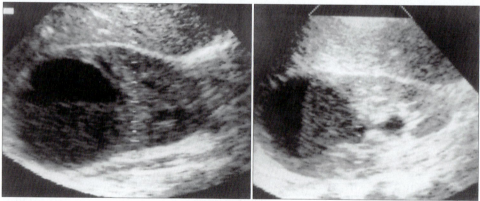

FIGURE 14-77 Other findings in a patient with pyonephrosis include a fluid and/or debris level within a well-defined mass lesion.

Xanthogranulomatous Pyelonephritis. Xanthogranulomatous pyelonephritis is an uncommon renal disease associated with chronic obstruction and infection. It involves destruction of renal parenchyma and infiltration of lipid-laden histiocytes. Clinically, the patient presents with a large nonfunctioning kidney, staghorn calculus, and multiple infections (Figure 14-78). The disease is more common in females and is poorly understood. It is thought to represent an impaired host response to infection in a chronically obstructed and infected kidney.

Sonographic Findings. The sonographic appearance may show bright echogenicity from the staghorn calculus. (Peripelvic fibrosis can prevent the staghorn from shadowing.) The renal parenchyma is replaced by cystic spaces. Overall renal size is increased. The disease process may be diffuse or segmental.

Urinary Tract Calcifications

Renal Calcifications. Renal calcifications may be seen as localized parenchymal calcifications, resulting from scar tissue caused by bacterial infection, renal abscess, infected hematoma, urinoma, lymphocele, tuberculosis, or infarction, or post percutaneous renal procedures. Malignant solid and/or cystic masses often demonstrate calcifications, but benign renal masses may also calcify. Linear vascular calcifications commonly are associated with renal artery atherosclerosis and/or vascular malformation.

Most of the intraluminal renal calcifications seen on sonography are renal calculi. Milk of calcium cyst and obstructed calyceal diverticulum are rare conditions with suspension of small calcified crystals and/or small stones layers within the renal cystic structure.

Medullary Sponge Kidney. As was previously discussed, medullary sponge kidney (MSK), or intratubular renal calcification is a developmental anomaly that occurs in the medullary pyramids and consists of cystic or fusiform dilatation of the distal collecting ducts (ducts of Bellini), causing stasis of the urine and stone formation. Because MSK is an anatomic rather than a metabolic defect, the pathologic process may be unilateral or segmental. The cause is unknown. Many patients

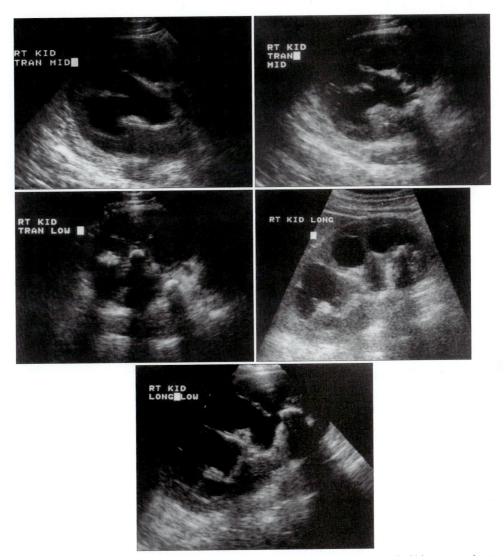

FIGURE 14-78 Patient with xanthogranulomatous pyelonephritis shows a large, nonfunctioning right kidney secondary to a stone. Multiple areas of shadowing are seen within the renal parenchyma from the renal stones.

remain asymptomatic, but patients with hematuria, infection, and renal stones should be evaluated for MSK. Sonographically, MSK appears as hyperechoic calyces, with or without stones (Figure 14-79).

Nephrocalcinosis. Nephrocalcinosis, or parenchymal calcification, involves diffuse foci of calcium deposits, which usually are located in the medulla but infrequently can be seen in the renal cortex. Both kidneys are affected. Calcification may be dystrophic from devitalized tissues, ischemia, and/or necrosis, or from hypercalcemic states, hyperparathyroidism, renal tubular acidosis, and renal failure.

Metastatic nephrocalcinosis is based on location and is classified as cortical or medullary. Cortical nephrocalcinosis is most commonly seen with chronic

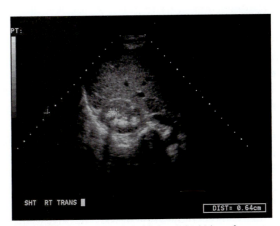

FIGURE 14-79 Transverse view of the right kidney for measuring the renal stone.

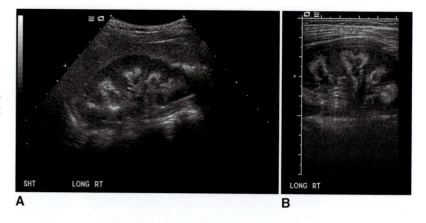

FIGURE 14-80 A and **B,** Longitudinal scans of the right kidney show hyperechoic pyramids, consistent with nephrocalcinosis.

glomerulonephritis, chronic hypercalemic states, sickle cell disease, and rejected renal transplants. Medullary nephrocalcinosis occurs more often with disorders such as hyperparathyroidism (40%), renal tubular acidosis (20%), medullary sponge kidney, chronic pyelonephritis, hyperthyroidism, sickle cell disease, and renal papillary necrosis.

▶ **Sonographic   Findings.** Sonographically, cortical nephrocalcinosis appears as increased cortical echogenicity with spared pyramids (Figure 14-80). In cases of medullary nephrocalcinosis, the pyramids become more echogenic than the adjacent cortex. A combination corticomedullary form exists, which shows both renal cortex and medulla as echogenic.

Renal Artery Stenosis

Renal artery stenosis (RAS) is the most common correctable cause of hypertension. Only 1% to 5% of hypertensive patients have a renovascular origin; most patients have essential hypertension. Renovascular hypertension is renin mediated and occurs as a response to renal ischemia, and later as a response to high circulating levels of angiotensin II. The most common causes of renal artery stenosis are atherosclerosis and fibromuscular dysplasia (Box 14-9).

Atherosclerosis is associated with hypertension, which is more common in older patients, and accounts for one third of cases of RAS. It occurs more frequently in males. Atherosclerosis usually occurs within the first 2 cm of the renal artery, and because this is a generalized process, it may be multifocal, or both renal arteries may be affected.

Fibromuscular dysplasia accounts for approximately two thirds of renal artery stenosis cases and is seen in younger patients. Fibromuscular dysplasia may involve any layer of the renal artery wall and is classified as intimal, medial, or adventitial, creating a smooth stenosis, usually in the midportion of the renal artery. Involvement of the medial layer is seen in the most common subtype of fibromuscular dysplasia, accounting for more than 90% of cases. Medial dysplasia consists of the

---

BOX 14-9 | Sonographic Characteristics of Renal Artery Stenosis

Kidney smaller than contralateral side
Absence of early systolic peak (ESP)
Overall waveform shape: "tardus and parvus" waveform
Delayed systolic rise time: $\Delta T < 0.1$ sec
Peak systolic velocity: PSV > 160/180 cm/sec

$$\text{Resistive index: } RI = \frac{(S-D)}{S} \geq 0.70$$

---

replacement of smooth muscle by collagen, forming thick ridges and alternating with areas of small aneurysm formation, which results in the classic "string of beads" appearance on arteriography or CT angiography. Fibromuscular dysplasia is most commonly seen in young women. It is progressive and may be seen not only in renal arteries but also in cephalic, visceral, and peripheral arteries.

▶ **Sonographic Findings.** Selective renal arteriography is the gold standard for visualizing renal artery stenosis. Color Doppler sonography was developed as a noninvasive alternative to detect RAS in hypertensive patients. Direct evaluation of the main renal artery and indirect evaluation via the arcuate and intralobar renal arteries are the two methods used. Accuracy rate depends on operator hand, patient body habitus, and adequacy of the technique.

The most reliable signs for diagnosing renal artery stenosis (RAS) using the main renal artery are (1) increased velocity through the stenotic area greater than 150 to 190 cm/sec and (2) turbulence distal to the narrowing. Use of peak systolic velocity (PSV) has not proved accurate because of overestimation caused by suboptimal angles of incidence. The use of frequency ranges has been shown to be of little value because of the tortuosity of the renal artery, which causes varied frequencies throughout the vessel.

A problem that occurs when the main renal artery is used to evaluate renal blood flow is that more than one renal artery may be found. The main renal artery may have normal blood flow and a stenotic accessory renal artery, causing hypertension. Evaluating the entire course of the main renal arteries is a long and tedious study and one that sonographers and sonologists try to avoid. Several technical factors (body habitus, tortuosity of the vessel, overlying bowel gas, respiratory motion, and underlying arteriosclerotic disease) may prohibit visualization of the entire length of the renal artery. The proximal portion of the renal arteries may be difficult to evaluate because of cardiac or aortic pulse frequencies.

Evaluating the segmental and intralobar renal vessels is an indirect method of evaluating for RAS. They are easier to see than the main renal artery with the use of convergent color or power color (Figure 14-81 to Figure 14-83). It is very difficult to obtain a 60 degree angle of the renal vessels. Convergent color and power color are not angle dependent.

Studies have used various Doppler parameters to assist in the evaluation of RAS. The normal intrarenal Doppler signal has a rapid systolic upstroke and an early systolic peak (ESP) (Figures 14-84 and 14-85). The absence of early systolic peak and a prolonged systolic upstroke or acceleration time (AT), together with decreased peak systole and dampening of the distal waveform, are indications of RAS. The term *tardus-*

parvus is used to describe the decreased acceleration time and the decreased peak (Figure 14-86).

Clinical studies with contrast agents are continuing to improve the use of sonography and Doppler for evaluation of renal vascularity. The use of three-dimensional (3D) imaging to demonstrate the renal vasculature is also being investigated (Figure 14-87).

Renal Infarction

A renal infarction occurs when part of the tissue undergoes necrosis after cessation of the blood supply, usually as a result of artery occlusion. Renal function is usually normal. This may result from a thrombus, a tumor infiltration, or obstruction, or it may be iatrogenic. (See Table 14-3 for clinical findings, sonographic findings, and differential considerations for renal infarction.)

Sonographic Findings. Infarcts within the renal parenchyma appear as irregular areas, somewhat triangular in shape, along the periphery of the renal border. The renal contour may be somewhat "lumpy-bumpy." Remember that lobulations in the pediatric patient may be normal, except for the dromedary hump variant. In the adult patient, the renal contour should be smooth. In a patient with a renal infarct, the irregular area may be slightly more echogenic than the renal parenchyma.

Arteriovenous Fistulas and Pseudoaneurysm

Arteriovenous fistulas (AVFs) are most often acquired rather than congenital. AVFs may be due to renal biopsies, complications from partial nephrectomies, or trauma. Gray-scale sonography shows no abnormalities in the kidney, but color Doppler easily depicts the arteriovenous malformation. The diagnosis is based on detection of a perivascular artifact that reflects local tissue vibration produced by the arteriovenous shunt. Because power Doppler usually demonstrates a larger, artifactual area of uniform color signal that is more pronounced than on conventional color Doppler imaging, it has the potential to facilitate detection of small, low-

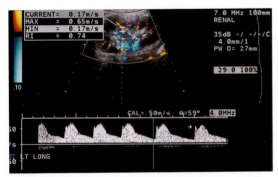

FIGURE 14-81 Normal resistive index (RI) of 0.74 in a 4-year-old female. The *arrow* indicates an early systolic peak.

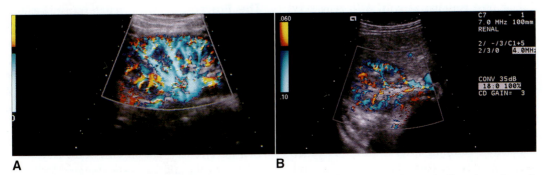

FIGURE 14-82 Longitudinal **(A)** and transverse **(B)** color Doppler of normal intrarenal vessels with vascular flow throughout the renal cortex.

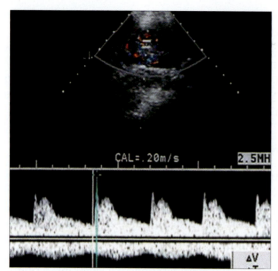

FIGURE 14-83 Normal renal spectral waveform taken at the interlobar arteries.

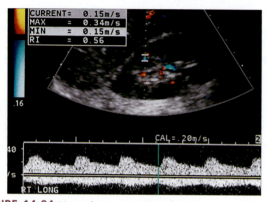

FIGURE 14-84 Normal arcuate vessel Doppler spectral signal. A rapid systolic rise with a resistive index (RI) of 0.56. A gradual decrease into diastole.

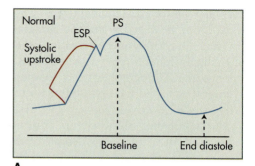

A

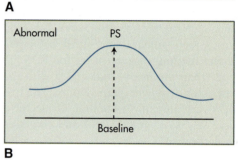

B

FIGURE 14-85 A, Diagram of a normal renal artery spectral waveform with early systolic peak *(ESP)* and a rapid systolic upstroke followed by peak systole *(PS)* and a gradual decrease into diastole. **B,** Diagram of an abnormal renal artery spectral waveform with absence of early systolic peak and a long systolic upstroke.

flow AVF. No abnormalities or small cystic lesions are evident on gray scale. Spectral Doppler shows increased flow velocities, decreased resistive indexes, and arterialization of the draining vein, regardless of the cause of arteriovenous malformation.

Pseudoaneurysm may develop following graft anastomosis, renal biopsy, or intratumoral hemorrhage (angiomyolipomas), or it may occur post renal surgery (partial nephrectomies) or post trauma; as with AVF, it is very rarely congenital. Color flow Doppler sonographic patterns associated with pseudoaneurysm have been well described in the literature. Sonography shows a round hypoechoic or cystic mass in the renal parenchyma that fills with color signal on color flow Doppler imaging. Spectral analysis performed at the level of the communicating channel shows a typical pattern known as the to-and-fro sign, which signifies both systolic feeding arterial flow and diastolic draining arterial flow—in other words, bidirectional flow occurs (Figures 14-88 and 14-89).

Renal Transplant

Renal transplantation and dialysis are currently used to treat chronic renal failure or end-stage renal disease. Sonography has emerged as an excellent tool for monitoring such transplant patients and may complement nuclear medicine and laboratory values in distinguishing the course of rejection. Because the sonogram does not rely on the function of the kidney, serial studies can be readily incorporated to determine the diagnosis and to select the treatment to be administered.

Complications that may arise after transplantation include rejection, acute tubular necrosis (ATN), obstructive nephropathy, extraperitoneal fluid collections, hemorrhage or infarction, recurrent glomerulonephritis, graft rupture, and renal emphysema. Decreased renal function is commonly the main indication for ultrasonic evaluation.

The Procedure. Most renal transplant patients have had long-standing renal failure without obstructive nephropathy. Before the procedure, patient risk factors to be considered are age, primary diagnosis, secondary medical complications, and transplant source. It has been found that recipients between 16 and 45 years of age with primary renal disease are at lowest risk for morbidity and mortality.

The major problem encountered with transplantation is graft rejection. The success of the transplant is directly related to the source of the donated kidney. Living relatives and cadavers are the two donor types.

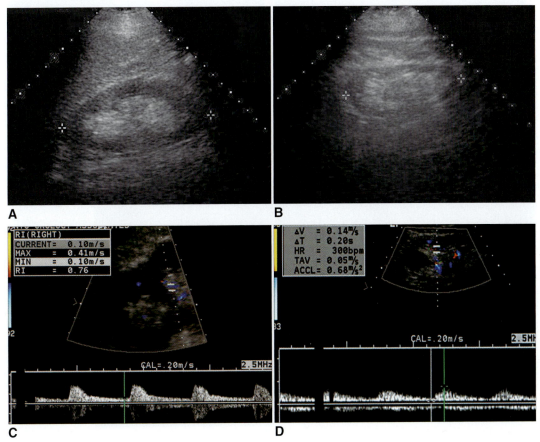

FIGURE 14-86 A, Longitudinal scan of normal size of right kidney. **B,** Longitudinal scan of small (shrunken) left kidney with cortical atrophy. **C,** Normal spectral waveform right kidney. **D,** Parvus-tardus (delayed SRT) left kidney consistent with renal artery stenosis.

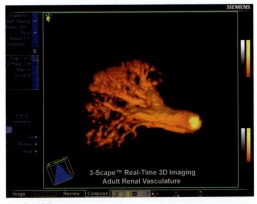

FIGURE 14-87 Adult renal vasculature demonstration using 3-Scape real-time three-dimensional imaging. *(Courtesy Siemens Medical Solutions USA, Inc.)*

The surgical procedure begins with removal of the donor's left kidney, which is then rotated and placed in the recipient's right iliac fossa or groin region. The renal artery is attached by an end-to-end anastomosis with the common or external iliac artery (Figure 14-90). The ureter is inserted into the bladder above the normal ureteral orifice through a submucosal tunnel in the bladder wall. The tunnel creates a valve in the terminal ureter to prevent reflux of urine into the transplanted kidney.

Although the kidney is more vulnerable to trauma when it is placed in the iliopelvic region, this has rarely been a problem. The advantage of such a location is its observation accessibility. Complications may arise after transplantation, however, so a variety of examinations may be incorporated to detect and follow the transplant. Useful information may be accumulated through laboratory tests, nuclear medicine, sonography, intravenous pyelography, and renal arteriography.

Sonographic Evaluation. As early as 48 hours after surgery, a baseline sonographic examination is performed to identify renal size, calyceal pattern, and extrarenal fluid collections (Figures 14-91). Hydronephrosis can be easily recognized sonographically with calyceal dilatation. Perirenal fluid collections (hematoma, abscess, lymphocele, or urinoma) can be diagnosed reliably and differentiated from acute rejection. Serial scans may be done at 3 to 6 month intervals to detect fluid collections at an early, asymptomatic stage. The patient should be examined at the first sign of tenderness in the graft area or mass development.

Technique for Sonographic Examination. To locate the kidney precisely by ultrasound, transverse

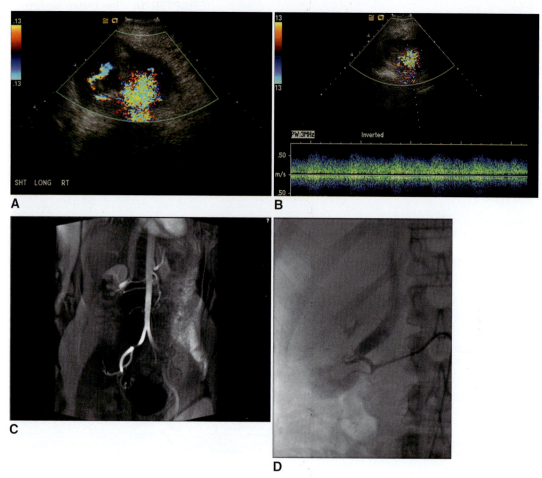

FIGURE 14-88 **A,** Color duplex Doppler with a pulsating vascular malformation in the right renal hilum. **B,** Arterialization of renal venous flow. **C,** MRI coronal view with simultaneous visualization of the renal artery (aorta) and the inferior vena cava (IVC) consistent with an arteriovenous (AV) fistula. **D,** Renal angiogram shows early visualization of the IVC.

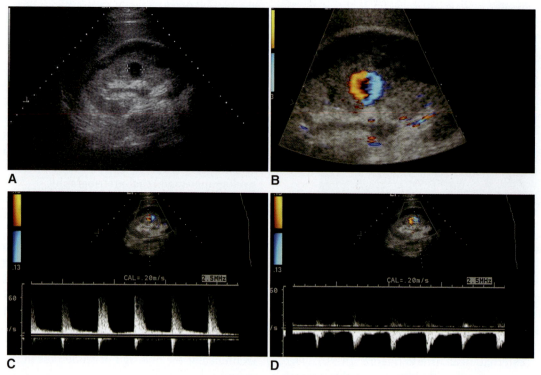

FIGURE 14-89 **A,** Longitudinal scan of the right kidney 1 week post ureteroscopic laser treatment for a mid calyx stone with a perinephric fluid collection and a newly discovered 1.8 cm cystic structure. **B,** Color Doppler shows a typical "yin-yang" or swirling appearance consistent with a renal artery pseudoaneurysm. **C** and **D,** Spectral arterial waveform demonstrates clean bidirectional arterial blood flow above and below baseline, consistent with a renal pseudoaneurysm.

supine scans are made from the pubic symphysis to above the level of the graft. Longitudinal and transverse scans are made parallel with and perpendicular to the long axis of the kidney. From these scans, accurate measurements of renal length, width, and anteroposterior dimensions can be taken (Figure 14-92).

Sonographic Findings. The normal transplant should appear as a smooth structure surrounding the homogeneous parenchymal pattern. A dense band of echoes in

the midportion of the transplant represents the renal pelvis, calyces, blood vessels, and fatty fibrous tissues. The medullary pyramids are discrete sonolucent structures surrounded by the homogeneous grainy texture of the cortex (Figure 14-93). The psoas appears as parallel linear echoes posterior to the kidney transplant (Figure 14-94). The Doppler flow pattern for a healthy transplant kidney is the same as for a normally functioning native kidney (Figure 14-95).

A sonolucent appearance of the anterior portion of the kidney and, at times, an increased echogenic band across the anterior kidney are seen on some scans because of inaccurate settings in the near field. Decreased amplification of the near gain in the first few centimeters of the slope obliterates decreased echoes of the near field and allows better fill-in of the anterior portion of the kidney. This difference in anterior structure delineation is probably a result of attenuation of sound by subcutaneous fat, muscle thickness, skin texture, and scarring, or the fact that some patients transmit the sound frequency more readily than others.

The opposite is true for the problem of increased echoes in the near field. Following decreases in near gain, suppression of echoes in the near field yields an image with uniform texture. Thus it is important to maintain

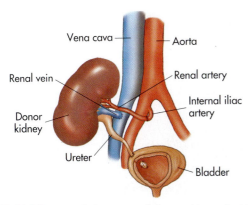

FIGURE 14-90 Surgical placement of the renal transplant into the iliac fossa.

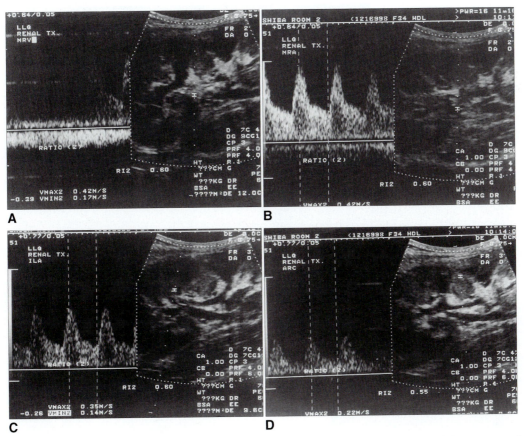

FIGURE 14-91 Normal evaluation of the renal transplant includes evaluation of size, renal parenchyma, and the presence of abnormal fluid collections, as well as Doppler assessment of the renal vessels. **A,** Main renal vein flow. **B,** Main renal artery flow. **C,** Interlobar arterial flow. **D,** Arcuate artery flow.

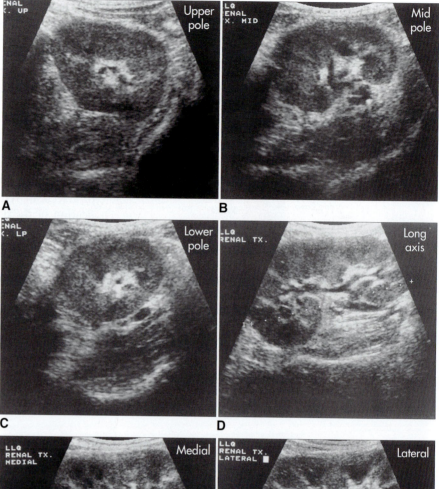

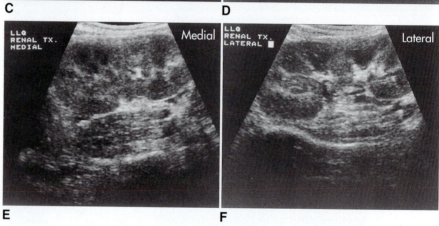

FIGURE 14-92 A through **C,** Multiple transverse scans of the renal transplant taken in the transverse planes at the upper, middle, and lower segments. **D** through **F,** Longitudinal scans should be made along the longest axis of the kidney in the midline, medial, and lateral planes.

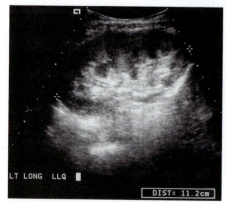

FIGURE 14-93 A 41-year-old female with a kidney transplant. The medullary pyramids are discrete sonolucent structures surrounded by homogeneous grainy texture of the cortex.

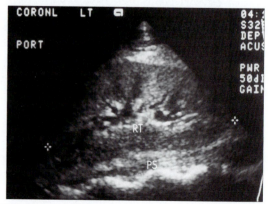

FIGURE 14-94 The psoas muscle *(PS)* is posterior to the renal transplant *(RT)* and appears as parallel linear echoes along the posterior border.

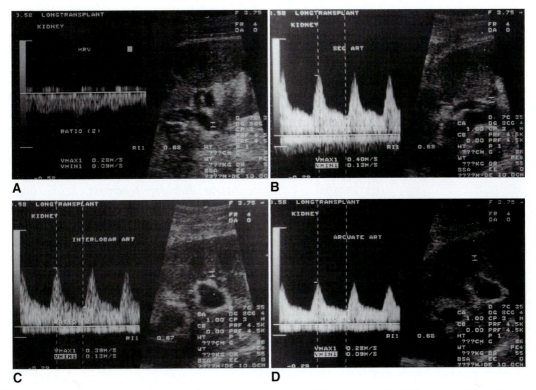

FIGURE 14-95 Normal flow patterns in a recent renal transplant patient. **A,** Main renal vein. **B,** Main segmental renal artery. **C,** Interlobar artery. **D,** Arcuate artery.

proper penetration and delineation of internal structures with a good outline of adjacent musculature.

To record echoes from the parenchyma and distinguish the cortex from the medulla, the sonographer should scan the patient with low-gain and high-gain settings. These scans should include both kidneys and the pararenal area (i.e., iliac wing and iliopsoas).

Complications of Renal Transplantation

Renal Transplant Rejection. Rejection has been the most difficult of the medical complications to accurately diagnose without percutaneous needle biopsy. No single imaging method permits accurate diagnosis with sufficient specificity and sensitivity to totally obviate the need for renal biopsy.

Four types of rejection have been identified: hyperacute, acute, immunologic, and chronic. Hyperacute rejection occurs within hours of transplantation and is caused by vasculitis leading to thrombosis and usually loss of the graft. Acute rejection occurs within days to months after transplant. Causes of immunologic rejection include pre-formed antibodies, immune complexes, and cell-mediated responses. Pathologically, acute rejection is separated into vascular and interstitial forms. Without aggressive therapy, the graft can be lost. Last, chronic rejection can occur months after transplantation with gradual onset. It tends to be secondary to mononuclear infiltration and fibrosis. Steroid therapy and antilymphocyte serum are of little benefit in improving renal function and can lead to opportunistic infection.

Sonographic Findings. Sonography can be useful in the diagnosis of rejection. Care must be taken to observe the size and shape of the kidneys; the appearance of the pyramids, cortex, and parenchyma; and the presence of any surrounding fluid collections. The following five changes in the renal parenchymal echo pattern have been observed during the process of rejection:

1. Enlargement and decreased echogenicity of the pyramids. This appearance is not at all uniform, and only a few pyramids may appear as such (Figure 14-96).
2. Hyperechogenic cortex. The swollen, sonolucent pyramids stand out against the background of increased echogenicity of the outer and interpyramidal cortex (Figure 14-97).
3. A localized area of renal parenchyma, including both the cortex and the medulla presenting an anechoic appearance, is very difficult to fill in even when high sensitivity and TGC settings are used. This is usually seen in polar regions.
4. Distortion of the renal outline caused by localized areas of swelling involving both the cortex and the pyramids. The renal sinus echoes may appear compressed and displaced (Figure 14-98).
5. Patchy sonolucent areas involving both cortex and medulla with coalescence on follow-up studies. These areas can become quite extensive, affecting a large portion of the renal parenchyma.

In long-standing rejection, two patterns have been observed: (1) a normal-size renal transplant with very little differentiation between parenchymal and renal sinus echoes, and (2) a small kidney with irregular margins and an irregular parenchymal echo pattern.

These sonographic appearances correlate with pathologic occurrences. When swelling is present with increased internal echoes within the cortex, rejection can be diagnosed. Edema, congestion, and hemorrhage of the

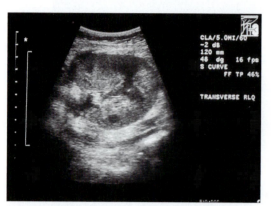

FIGURE 14-96 Transverse view of a chronic renal transplant rejection. Enlargement and decreased echogenicity of the pyramids caused by edema and congestion with hemorrhage of the interstitial tissue. Ischemia and cellular infiltration (fibrosis) result in hyperechogenicity of the cortex.

interstitium produce swelling of the pyramids, which appears as decreased echogenicity. Ischemia and cellular infiltration produce increased echogenicity of the cortex. Increased areas of sonolucency may occur in the cortex as a result of necrosis and infarction. These areas are usually seen in the polar regions of the transplant. If actual necrosis begins, the affected part appears as an area of decreased echogenicity, which suggests partial liquefaction. Irregular parenchymal echo patterns may result from parenchymal atrophy with fibrosis and shrinkage resulting from long-standing renal rejection.

Acute Tubular Necrosis. Acute tubular necrosis (ATN) is a common cause of acute posttransplant failure. Some degree of the disorder occurs in almost every transplant patient, and it has been suggested that as many as 50% of recipients of cadaveric kidneys experience ATN after transplantation. The incidence of ATN is usually higher in cadaveric transplants than in donor-relative transplants or in kidneys that undergo warm ischemia or prolonged preservation, kidneys with multiple renal arteries, or kidneys obtained from elderly donors. ATN usually occurs as a medical complication after loss of blood supply to the transplant tissue. This can occur in the donor before the kidney is harvested; during the process of harvesting, preserving, and transportation; during surgery; or as a result of poor circulation after

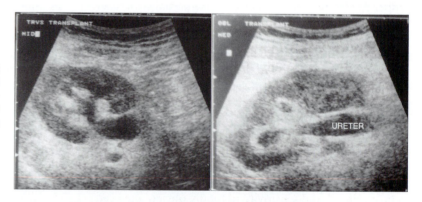

FIGURE 14-97 The hyperechogenic cortex appears as swollen sonolucent pyramids against a background of increased echogenicity of the outer and interpyramidal cortex. In addition, this patient had obstruction near the distal ureter, causing mild dilation of the renal pelvis and ureter.

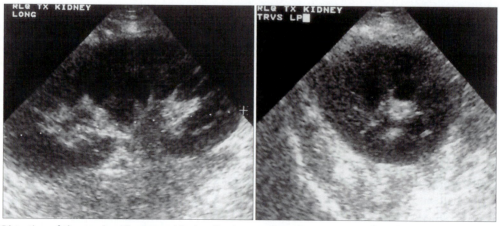

FIGURE 14-98 Distortion of the renal outline caused by localized areas of swelling involving both the cortex and the pyramids. The renal sinus echoes may appear compressed and displaced.

the transplant. ATN is associated with prolonged severe ischemia; therefore, the likelihood that it may occur after any incidence of cardiac arrest cannot be ruled out. This pertains to both the donor and the recipient.

ATN usually resolves early in the postoperative period. Uncomplicated ATN is often reversible and can be treated by immediate use of diuretics and satisfactory hydration. It is important to recognize uncomplicated ATN and to distinguish it from acute rejection because therapy for the two conditions is very different.

Clinically, ATN may present a variety of different patterns. Urine volumes may be good initially, followed by oliguria or anuria, or urine output may be low from the time of transplantation. The serum creatinine level is always elevated. If urine output remains low and BUN and creatinine remain elevated, ATN may be difficult to distinguish from rejection. Other indications of rejection (e.g., hematuria, elevated eosinophil counts, pain over the transplant) are helpful but may be late signs.

Sonographic Findings. Sonographically, no changes are usually seen within the renal parenchyma. In the initial postoperative period, the kidney may enlarge slightly as a result of secondary hypertrophy. This is believed to be a normal physiologic response of the newly transplanted kidney, or it may be caused by swelling that often regresses within a week. However, if swelling persists, ATN or rejection should be considered. With ATN, the renal parenchymal pattern remains unchanged, in contrast to the earlier description of parenchymal changes that occur during rejection. If these changes are lacking and the transplant fails to function, the cause is most likely ATN, provided that radionuclide evaluation has confirmed the patency of the vascular supply to the transplant.

Cyclosporine Toxicity. Cyclosporine (cyclosporin, ciclosporin, cyclosporine A) is an immunosuppressant drug used to prevent rejection of kidney allogenic transplants. It is toxic to the kidneys, especially in high doses. Renal biopsy is currently the best diagnostic procedure for toxicity.

Malignancy. Malignancy is a newly discovered delayed complication that is now becoming prevalent as the life of transplants has improved. A total of 55% of renal transplant recipients in a long-term (17 year) study developed at least one malignancy. The two major types of neoplasms found in transplant patients are non-Hodgkin lymphoma and skin cancer. Research on the incidence of occurrence of these malignancies has shown a strong correlation with the immunosuppressive drug used to maintain the transplant. A cyclosporine regimen has shown an increased incidence of non-Hodgkin lymphoma (38% over azathioprine). Azathioprine produces an increased incidence of skin and lip tumors (40% over cyclosporine A). Cases have been documented of a neoplasm from a transplant primary, but this is uncommon. Even so, prescreening donor kidneys may reduce this occurrence.

BOX 14-10	Fluid Collections Associated With Renal Transplant

HAUL (Order of Postoperative Occurrence)
Hematoma
Abscess
Urinoma
Lymphocele

Extraperitoneal Fluid Collections. Numerous extraperitoneal fluid collections may occur after transplantation, including lymphocele and lymph fistula, urinary fistula and urinoma, and hematoma and perinephric abscess (Box 14-10). These collections consist of lymph, blood, urine, and, if infected, pus. A sign common to several of these complications is a decrease in renal function manifested by increased creatinine values.

Sonographic Findings. Sonographically, the fluid collections may appear as round or oval structures with irregular and slightly thickened walls, often with thin multiseptations. Usually clinical or laboratory correlation suggests the origin of the fluid. Because the transplant is superficial, scans can be made easily, and, if necessary, sonographic guidance can be rendered for aspiration of the contents for further analysis (Figure 14-99).

Hematoma. A hematoma may develop shortly after surgery. One of the major indications for a sonogram may be a drop in the hematocrit value. Other clinical findings pertinent to hematomas include signs of bleeding, perinephric hemorrhage, a palpable mass, hypertension, and impaired renal function. The hematoma may be an incidental finding during scanning.

Sonographic Findings. Hematomas appear as walled-off, well-defined areas whose sonolucent echo production depends on the age or stage of the hematoma. Hematoma may appear sonolucent while the blood is fresh and may be difficult to distinguish from a lymphocele or urinoma. As the clot becomes organized, the hematoma may tend to fragment, and low-level internal echoes may develop. The mass then appears complex and eventually solid. After a time, it may revert to a sonolucent mass and form a seroma.

Perinephric Abscess. Perinephric infections can be very hazardous to the transplant patient undergoing immunosuppressive therapy. It is an uncommon complication reported as early as 12 days or many months after transplantation. If the patient has a fever of unknown origin, care must be taken to rule out abscess formation.

Sonographic Findings. Sonographically, an abscess may appear with septa in it. Edema and inflammation may be present around the mass, making the borders appear less distinct than those found with lymphoceles and hematomas.

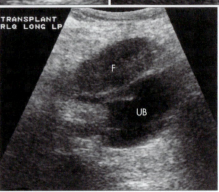

FIGURE 14-99 A 29-year-old male with a right lower quadrant renal transplant. Two fluid collections *(F)* were noted, one adjacent to the lower pole of the renal transplant and another within the anterior abdominal wall at the incision site. *UB,* Urinary bladder.

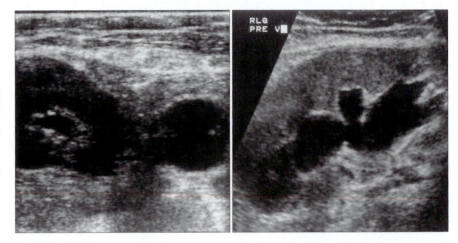

FIGURE 14-100 A 30-year-old female with a renal transplant performed 14 years previously presented with right upper quadrant and midabdominal pain. She had rigors and chills, but was afebrile. A tender cystic collection of fluid located above and to the right of the umbilicus and anterior to the inferior vena cava represented an infected lymphocele. She also had mild to moderate hydronephrosis.

Lymphocele. Lymphoceles are a common complication of transplantation, occurring in approximately 12% of all transplant patients. The source of the lymph collection is probably vessels severed during the preparation of recipient vessels, or it may be the kidney itself, in the form of leakage from injured capsular and hilar lymphatics. The lymph drains into the peritoneal cavity, provoking a fibrous reaction and eventually walling itself off. Primary clinical signs include deterioration of renal function (usually within 2 weeks to 6 months of transplantation), development of painless fluctuant swelling over the transplant, ipsilateral leg edema, and wound drainage of lymph cells. If an IVP was performed, a mass indenting the bladder, ureteral deviation, ureteral obstruction, or kidney deviation will be seen.

Sonographic Findings. Sonographically, the lymphocele is a well-defined anechoic area, occasionally with numerous septations (Figure 14-100). Urinomas may appear similar to lymphoceles, although usually they appear early, whereas lymphoceles are more common chronically. If the mass is complex with solid components, hematoma or abscess must be considered. Percutaneous aspiration and drainage with sonography or CT guidance has a success rate of 80%, with little risk of urinoma or abscess. Lymphoceles often recur after catheter drainage, and further surgery may be required.

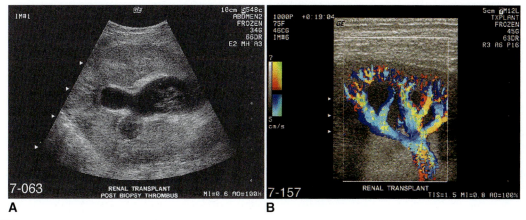

FIGURE 14-101 A, Renal transplant with mild hydronephrosis and thrombus after a biopsy procedure. **B,** Normal color flow image in a renal transplant patient.

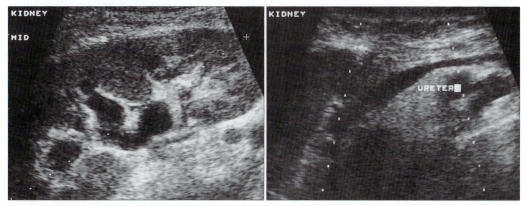

FIGURE 14-102 In the early postoperative stages, the ureter may be compressed by extrarenal fluid collections, mass effect, or kinks within the ureter. The result is mild obstruction, extending into the renal ureter.

Obstructive Nephropathy. Early signs of obstruction include anuria or severe oliguria in a patient with satisfactory renal volumes. Numerous conditions, such as ureteral necrosis, abscess, lymphocele, fungus ball, retroperitoneal fibrosis, stricture at the ureterovesical junction, ureteral calculus, and hemorrhage into the collecting system with obstruction from clots, may cause obstruction.

▶ **Sonographic Findings.** Obstruction can be identified sonographically as hydronephrosis. Obstruction after renal transplantation has many causes. In the early postoperative period, edema at the ureteric implantation site can cause temporary mild obstruction (Figure 14-101), or extrinsic mass effect from perinephric fluid collections can impinge on and impair ureteral drainage (Figure 14-102). In the later postoperative period, rejection or vascular insufficiency may predispose to distal ureteric stricture. Ureteric blood clots or calculi can also cause the obstruction. A very common benign form of pelvic dilatation of the collecting system, pyelocaliectasis, can mimic obstruction. Analysis of laboratory values and increased RI help to rule this out. Finally, the sonographer should be wary of functional obstruction caused

simply by an overdistended urinary bladder. Have the patient void, and rescan to confirm.

Vascular insufficiency in the form of arterial stenosis or venous thrombus can best be diagnosed with color and duplex Doppler imaging. When trying to rule out renal artery stenosis, look for a high-velocity jet with distal turbulence.

Graft Rupture. Graft rupture can occur in the first 2 weeks after surgery, presenting with an abrupt onset of pain and swelling over the graft, oliguria, and shock.

▶ **Sonographic Findings.** Sonographically, graft rupture appears as a gross distortion of the graft contour and a perinephric or paranephric hematoma.

Improvement of RI Specificity. Perhaps the most confusing and frustrating problem presently involves use of the RI to accurately determine and specify transplant disease. Because many transplant complications exhibit increased RI, is there a way to help limit the differentials with time since transplant? Given that many transplant complications tend to surface at particular times after surgery, a more holistic approach to interpretation of increased RIs may be the answer at present.

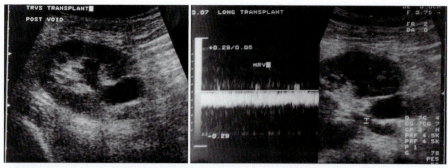

FIGURE 14-103 Observation of renal vein patency is very important after renal transplantation. This patient showed a normal renal vein flow pattern.

Sonographic Findings. If renovascular impedance is high immediately after surgery, patency of the renal vein must be tested. With the use of color and pulsed Doppler imaging, renal thrombosis displays a distinctive spectral pattern with a plateau-like reversal of diastolic flow (accentuated at end diastole) (Figure 14-103). Renal artery stenosis exhibits a high-velocity jet with distal turbulence. After venous patency has been established, the sonographer must question whether the RI increase is caused by extrarenal compression (e.g., an adult allograft in a child is a common initial cause of extrarenal compression; for evaluation, the child's position should be changed to alleviate vascular compromise).

Although ATN does not commonly become abnormal until 24 hours after reperfusion of the graft, this is still a possible cause of increased RI immediately after surgery (Figures 14-104 and 14-105). Percutaneous biopsy will confirm ATN or rejection (hyperacute or acute). If an abnormally high renovascular impedance is seen within the first few days after surgery (after a previous normal sonogram), obstructive uropathy should be suspected. The renal transplant should be evaluated with color (lack of color confirms hydronephrosis). Pyelocaliectasis is common, and its appearance of hydronephrosis can lead to a false-positive diagnosis of ureteral obstruction.

Clinically, the patient should next be examined for pyelonephritis, pyuria, and extrarenal compression. At this later period, fluid collection can be the cause of extrarenal compression. The patient should be examined for periallograft fluid collections.

When renovascular impedance is increased in the second week after surgery, rejection is by far the most common cause, especially if rejection has a vascular component. Biopsy is necessary to confirm rejection and determine whether rejection has resulted from a vascular or interstitial pathologic cause.

Finally, if creatinine levels increase in the first weeks after transplant, if RIs reveal increased renovascular impedance, and if no evidence of obstruction, compression, or infection can be found, the most common cause by far is acute rejection, which can be confirmed by biopsy.

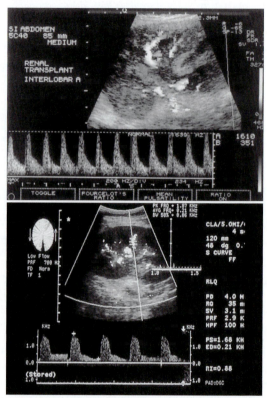

FIGURE 14-104 Color flow and Doppler of a normal flow pattern with good perfusion versus an abnormal flow pattern with high resistive index (RI), as seen in a patient with chronic rejection.

Color and Doppler Imaging. Vascular malformations such as pseudoaneurysm or arteriovenous (AV) fistula can be readily seen using color Doppler imaging (see Figure 14-89). The color shows turbulent flow in the affected area in cases of AV malformation and a typical "to-and-fro" appearance in cases of pseudoaneurysm. Power Doppler used in conjunction with color Doppler improves the evaluation of vessels. Power Doppler is not angle dependent and has greater sensitivity to detect blood flow; it has the potential to increase the detection rate for intrarenal AV fistulas. Convergent color, which is not angle dependent and can detect the direction of blood flow, may be the color imaging modality of the future.

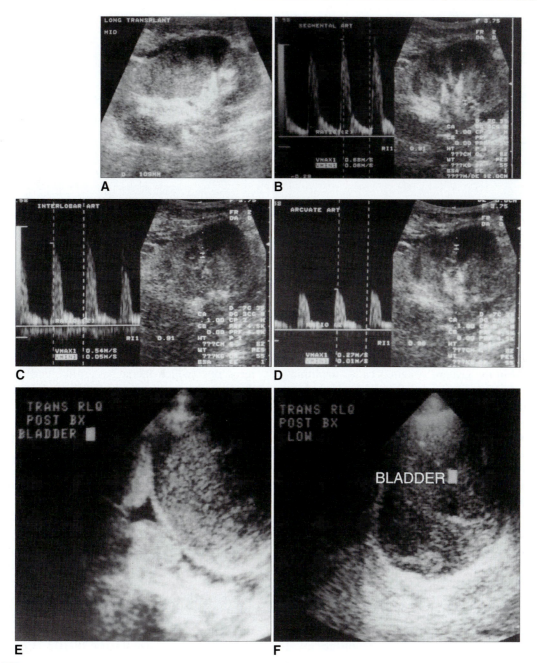

FIGURE 14-105 Abnormal flow patterns in a patient with rejection. **A,** Large, hypoechoic area along the anterior border of the kidney with compression of the calyceal system. **B,** Abnormal flow pattern in the segmental artery with decreased diastolic flow and increased resistive index (RI) to 0.9. **C,** Abnormal flow in the interlobar artery. **D,** Abnormal flow in the arcuate artery. **E** and **F,** The patient had a renal biopsy; status after biopsy shows fine, stippled echoes throughout the bladder indicating hematoma within the bladder. Before and after biopsy, scans should be made routinely to search for hematoma collections around the kidney or within the bladder.

Heart rate has a statistically significant effect on the RI in renal arteries. By increasing the heart rate of patients and taking measurements at paced rate intervals (70, 80, 90, 100, and 120 beats per minute), researchers have found that RI decreased with increasing heart rate in six of eight patients. This suggests that when RI renal arteries are interpreted, the actual heart rate must always be considered.

Many factors must be considered when the meaning of increased RI in the transplanted kidney is interpreted.

Knowledge of the different complications and their relation to postoperative time, patient history, donor history, and clinical findings plays an integral part in enhancing understanding and finding the cause of increased RI.

Contrast Agents. The use of contrast agents for visualization of renal arteries is not Food and Drug Administration (FDA) approved. Some research studies have used contrast agents to visualize the main renal arteries. The results have been encouraging: Improved

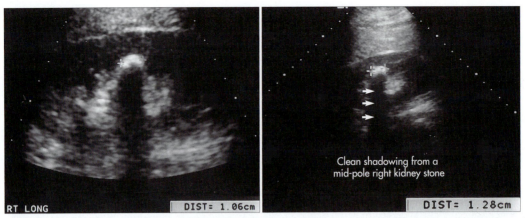

RT LONG   DIST= 1.06cm

Clean shadowing from a
mid-pole right kidney stone

DIST= 1.28cm

FIGURE 14-106 A 69-year-old male presented with right flank pain. A midpole echogenic structure with indicating posterior shadowing *(arrows),* representative of a renal stone.

visualization of normal renal arteries and decreased scanning time have resulted from the use of contrast agents.

Kidney Stone (Urolithiasis)

A stone located in the urinary system is called **urolithiasis.** Most urinary tract stones are formed in the kidney and course down the urinary tract. Stones consist of a combination of chemicals that precipitate out of urine. The most common chemical found in stones is calcium, along with oxalate or phosphate. Uric acid, cystine, and xanthine can also be found in kidney stones. Kidney stones are one of the most common kidney problems that can occur; they may cause obstruction, and this obstruction can be extremely painful. Most kidney stones are small and can travel through the urinary system without treatment or with increased hydration. Stones that are large and fill the renal collecting system are called staghorn calculi. Kidney stones that travel down the urinary system may obstruct the ureter in constricted areas.

The number of people with kidney stones in the United States has increased in the past 20 years. Kidney stones are more common in men. Some people are more likely to form kidney stones than others, and once a kidney stone has formed, the person is at increased risk of getting stones in the future. Kidney stones are associated with renal acidosis (a rare hereditary disorder); people taking the protease inhibitor indinavir are at increased risk for developing kidney stones. The initial clinical sign of a kidney stone is extreme pain, typically followed by cramping on the side on which the stone is located; nausea and vomiting may also occur. The pain may subside while the stone is traveling down the ureter.

Treatment for stones that cause obstruction varies depending on the size and location of the stone. Treatment can include extracorporeal shockwave lithotripsy (ESWL), percutaneous nephrolithotomy, and ureteroscopic stone removal. Extracorporeal shockwave lithotripsy uses ultrasound or x-ray to locate the stone, and

shock waves are used to break up the stone into smaller particles, which can readily pass through the urinary system. Percutaneous nephrolithotomy is a surgical procedure in which an opening is made in the kidney, and a nephroscope is used to remove the stone from the kidney. For mid and lower urinary tract stones, a ureteroscope (which has a basket-like end) can be placed through the urethra and bladder and guided up to the level of the stone to capture and remove the stone. Early treatment of stones that cause obstruction is important to reverse any renal damage that the obstruction may cause.

▶ **Sonographic Findings.** Renal stones are highly echogenic foci with posterior acoustic shadowing (Figure 14-106). When searching for renal stones, the sonographer should scan along the lines of renal fat; usually, stones smaller than 3 mm may not shadow with the use of traditional B-mode. Prominent renal sinus fat, mesenteric fat, and bowel have high attenuation and may appear as an indistinct echogenic focus with questionable posterior acoustic shadowing, making it difficult to differentiate from stones. The use of tissue harmonics can demonstrate the shadowing of small stones measuring millimeters in size (Figure 14-107). Color and power Doppler have increased the sensitivity of confirming the presence of stones. Color and power Doppler cause a twinkling artifact posterior to the stone. This artifact is referred to as the *twinkling sign* and is imaged as a rapidly changing mixture of red and blue colors posterior to the stone (Figure 14-108). Color and power Doppler are more sensitive when an "all-digital" processing technology is used because of its increased color sensitivity and acoustic power.

If the stone causes obstruction, hydronephrosis will be noted, and depending on the location of the stone, the ureter may be dilated superior to the level of obstruction (Figure 14-109). The ureter—from the ureteropelvic junction to the bladder—is not routinely visualized on a sonogram unless dilated. The superior and distal ends of the ureters are more readily visualized than the midsection. The ureters lie in the retroperitoneal cavity and are obscured by bowel gas. Stones can also be imaged when the urinary bladder is distended with fluid (Figures 14-110 and 14-111).

Bladder Diverticulum

A bladder diverticulum is a herniation of the bladder wall. These outpouchings may be singular or multiple and are thinner than the normal bladder wall (Figure

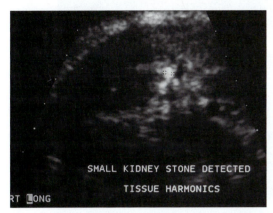

FIGURE 14-107 A small (3.1 mm) right renal stone detected using tissue harmonics.

14-112). Diverticula can be congenital or acquired. An acquired bladder diverticulum is an outpouching of bladder mucosa between muscle bundles caused by increased intravesical pressure. A diverticulum lacks a muscular layer and has a neck, which usually is narrow. Acquired diverticula are commonly associated with calculi and are more prevalent in patients with chronic bladder outlet obstruction or neurogenic bladder.

Congenital bladder diverticula are rare. They originate at the posterior angle of the bladder trigone and contain all components of the bladder wall.

Sonographic Findings. The sonographic finding is a neck of varying size connecting the adjacent fluid-filled structure to the bladder. The diverticulum may still be filled with fluid after the patient empties the bladder. Urine stasis leads to recurrent infection and stone formation (Figure 14-113).

Bladder Inflammation (Cystitis)

Inflammation of the bladder has several infectious and noninfectious causes. Cystitis is usually secondary to another condition that causes stasis of urine in the bladder. Conditions that cause incomplete emptying of the bladder include urethral stricture, benign and

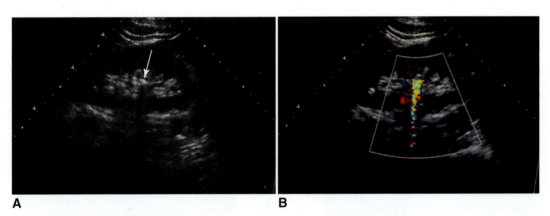

A   **B**

FIGURE 14-108 **A,** Small stone in the renal sinus *(arrow).* **B,** Color Doppler. A twinkle effect.

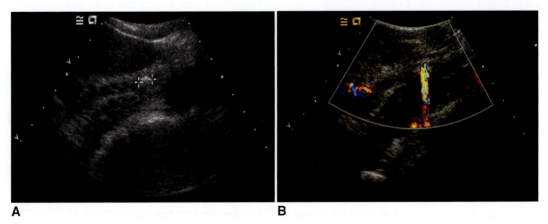

A   **B**

FIGURE 14-109 **A,** An 8 mm right midpole obstructing ureteral stone. **B,** Color Doppler shows twinkle sign.

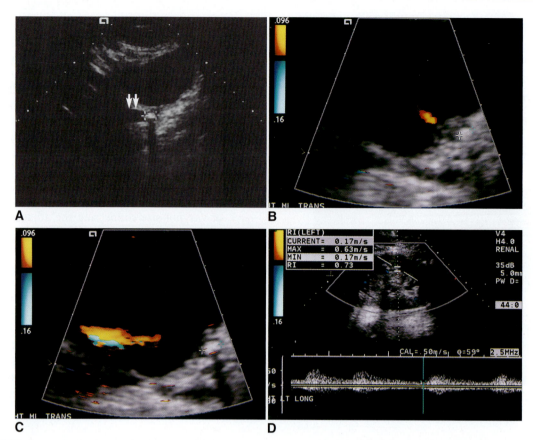

FIGURE 14-110 A, Longitudinal scan of a 65-year-old man with a stone in the distal left ureter *(arrows).* **B,** Partial obstruction of left ureter with decreased ureteral jet. **C,** Transverse scan of bladder with left ureteral stone measuring 8 mm and normal right ureteral jet. **D,** Increased left intrarenal resistive index (RI) of 0.73.

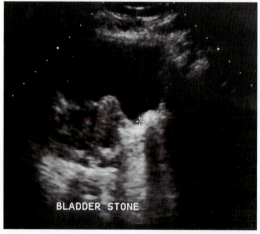

FIGURE 14-111 Transverse scan of the bladder stone with shadowing measuring 1.21 cm.

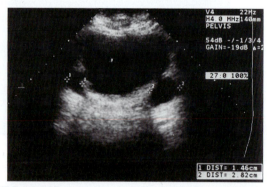

FIGURE 14-112 Transverse scan of two bladder diverticula, one on either side.

malignant neoplasms, bladder calculi, trauma (blood clot), tuberculosis (lower ureteric strictures), pregnancy, neurogenic bladder, and radiation therapy. Other causes of cystitis include Foley catheter, common rectal or vaginal fistulas, renal disease, sexual intercourse, poor hygiene, diabetes mellitus, and inflammation following surgical intervention.

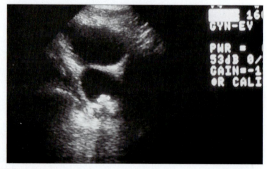

FIGURE 14-113 Transverse scan of the urinary bladder with a stone in the diverticulum.

Sonographic Findings. Sonographically, the bladder wall may appear normal in the early stages of inflammatory disease. As the duration of inflammation increases, the smooth bladder wall will become diffuse or nondiffuse with hypoechoic thickening. As the inflammatory process progresses, the bladder wall will become fibrotic and scarred. The bladder wall will appear more echogenic on a sonogram.

Bladder Tumors

Most bladder tumors in adults (95%) are transitional cell carcinoma (TCC). Bladder tumors usually are not detected until they have become advanced. Patients usually present with gross hematuria and may also present with dysuria, urinary frequency, or urinary urgency. Sonography cannot distinguish between benign and malignant masses. A cystoscopy or a biopsy may allow differentiation between a benign and a malignant neoplasm. The bladder may be the secondary site of malignancy. The most common site is the prostate. Invasion of the bladder may result from colon, uterine, or ovarian carcinoma or endometriosis.

Sonographic Findings. The sonographic appearance of bladder masses varies; they commonly appear as a focal bladder wall thickness. Sonography, CT, or MRI may be used to perform staging of bladder carcinoma. A transabdominal sonographic approach can detect intravesical lesions as small as 3 to 4 mm. Sonography

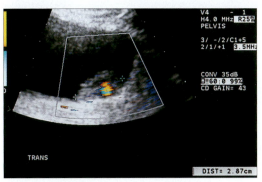

FIGURE 14-114 Carcinoma of the urinary bladder with blood flow seen within the mass.

is limited and is unable to detect a perivesical extension and pelvic wall involvement. A transrectal approach can be used to detect intravesicular involvement.

Benign tumors are typically hypoechoic when compared with malignant bladder tumors, but they may have the same echogenicity. All primary bladder tumors—squamous cell carcinoma, adenocarcinoma, and rhabdomyosarcoma in children—have the same sonographic appearance: an irregular echogenic mass that projects into the lumen of the bladder. Color Doppler can be used to determine increased vascularity (Figure 14-114). Any bladder mass may cause outflow obstruction, and the kidneys should be evaluated for hydronephrosis.

The Spleen

Sandra L. Hagen-Ansert

OBJECTIVES

On completion of this chapter, you should be able to:
- List the normal anatomy and relational landmarks of the spleen
- Discuss the size and primary functions of the spleen
- Describe the normal sonographic pattern of the spleen
- Discuss the sonographic findings and differential diagnoses for the pathologies discussed in this chapter

OUTLINE

The spleen is the largest single mass of lymphoid tissue in the body. It is part of the **reticuloendothelial** system and has a role in the synthesis of blood proteins. The spleen is active in blood formation (**hematopoiesis**) during the initial part of fetal life. This function decreases gradually by the fifth or sixth month, when the spleen assumes its adult characteristics and discontinues its hematopoietic (blood-producing) activities. The spleen plays an important role in the defense of the body. Although it is often affected by systemic disease processes, the spleen is rarely the primary site of disease.

The left upper quadrant may be rapidly assessed with sonography in patients with palpable **splenomegaly** or trauma to the left upper quadrant. The advantage that sonography has over other imaging modalities is the portability of the equipment, which allows the sonographer to rapidly evaluate the anatomy at the patient's bedside. The normal texture of the spleen is very homogeneous (slightly more echogenic than the texture of the liver); therefore pathology or blood collection secondary to a splenic rupture is usually easily identified.

ANATOMY OF THE SPLEEN

Normal Anatomy

The spleen lies in the **left hypochondrium,** with its axis along the shaft of the tenth rib (Figure 15-1). Its lower pole extends forward as far as the midaxillary line. The spleen is an **intraperitoneal** organ covered with peritoneum over its entire extent, except for a small area at its hilum, where the vascular structures and lymph nodes are located (Figure 15-2). The spleen lies in the posterior left hypochondrium between the fundus of the stomach and the diaphragm. The inferomedial surface of the spleen comes into contact with the stomach, left kidneys, pancreas, and splenic flexure. The peritoneal ligament that attaches the spleen to the stomach and the kidney is called the splenorenal ligament. This ligament is in contact with the posterior peritoneal wall, the phrenicocolic ligament, and the gastrosplenic ligament. The gastrosplenic ligament is significant in that it is composed of the two layers of the dorsal mesentery that separate the lesser sac posteriorly from the greater sac anteriorly. A protective capsule covers the spleen with peritoneum.

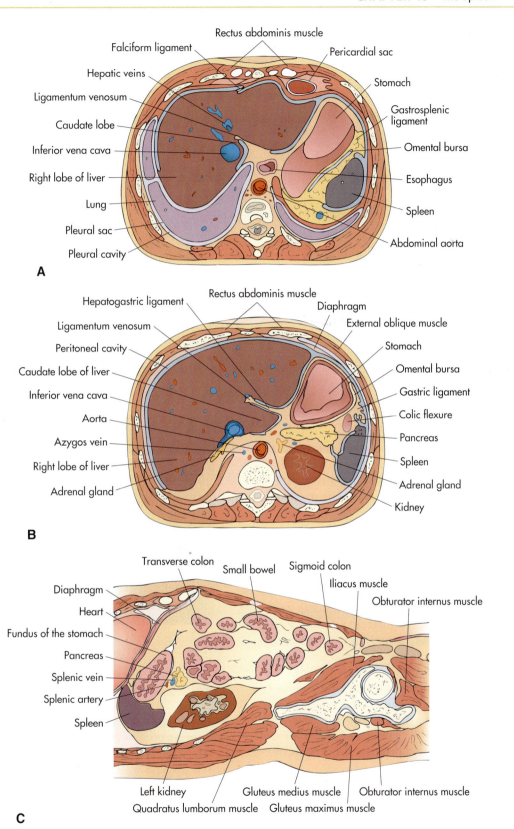

FIGURE 15-1 A, Transverse plane of the upper abdomen shows the posterior position of the spleen in the left upper quadrant. **B,** Transverse plane of the spleen. **C,** Sagittal plane of the spleen and left kidney.

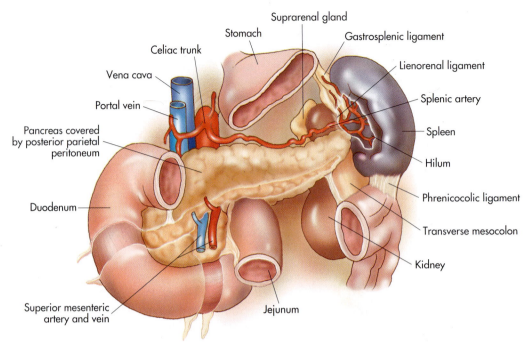

FIGURE 15-2 Anterior view of the spleen as it lies in the left hypochondrium. Note the relational anatomy, ligament attachments, and vascular landmarks.

In most adults, a portion of the splenic capsule is firmly adherent to the fused dorsal mesentery anterior to the upper pole of the left kidney, which produces a "bare area" of the spleen. This bare area can be helpful in distinguishing intraperitoneal from pleural fluid collections.

Size

The spleen is of variable size and shape (e.g., "orange segment," tetrahedral, triangular) but generally is considered to be ovoid with smooth, even borders and a convex superior and concave inferior surface (Figure 15-3). The spleen is normally measured with ultrasound on a longitudinal image from the upper margin (near the diaphragm) to the inferior margin at the long axis. Normal measurements for the average adult should be 8–13 cm in length, 7 cm in width, and 3 to 4 cm in thickness. The spleen decreases slightly in size with advancing age. The size of the spleen may vary in size in accordance with the nutritional status of the body.

Vascular Supply

Blood is supplied to the spleen by the tortuous **splenic artery** that travels horizontally along the superior border of the pancreas (see Figure 15-2). Upon entering the **splenic hilum,** the splenic artery immediately branches into six smaller arteries to supply the organ with oxygenated blood to profuse the splenic parenchyma. Color Doppler imaging allows the sonographer to image the vascularity of the spleen; gray-scale imaging will show

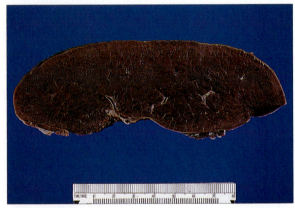

FIGURE 15-3 Gross specimen of the spleen demonstrates its homogeneous texture and shape.

small echogenic lines throughout the spleen that represent the arterial system. The splenic arteries are subject to **infarction** because adequate anastomoses between the vessels are lacking.

The **splenic vein** is formed by multiple branches within the spleen and leaves the hilum in a horizontal direction to join the superior mesenteric vein. The superior mesenteric vein returns unoxygenated blood from the bowel to form the main portal vein (Figure 15-4). The splenic vein travels along the posteromedial border of the pancreas.

The **lymph** vessels emerge from the splenic hilum, pass through other lymph nodes along the course of the splenic artery, and drain into the celiac nodes. The nerves

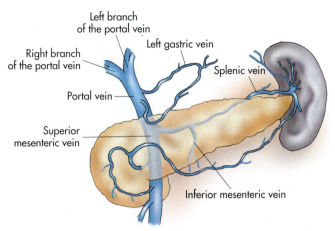

Left branch of the portal vein
Left gastric vein
Right branch of the portal vein
Splenic vein
Portal vein
Superior mesenteric vein
Inferior mesenteric vein

FIGURE 15-4 The splenic vein leaves the hilum of the spleen to join the main portal vein posterior to the head of the pancreas.

to the spleen accompany the splenic artery and are derived from the celiac plexus.

Relational Anatomy

The spleen lies between the left hemidiaphragm and the stomach. The diaphragm may be seen as a bright, curvilinear, echogenic structure close to the proximal superolateral surface of the spleen. Posteriorly, the diaphragm, left pleura, left lung, and ribs (eighth to eleventh) are in contact with the spleen. The medial surface is related to the stomach and lesser sac. The fundus of the stomach may contain gas or fluid, which may cause confusion in the left upper quadrant during attempts to demonstrate the spleen. Alteration in the patient position or ingestion of fluids may help to separate stomach from splenic tissue. The tail of the pancreas lies posterior to the stomach and lesser sac as it approaches the hilum of the spleen and splenic vessels. The spleen may serve as a great window to image the tail of the pancreas. The left kidney lies inferior and medial to the spleen (see Figure 15-2).

Displacement of the Spleen

The spleen is held in place by the **lienorenal, gastrosplenic,** and **phrenocolic ligaments** (see Figure 15-2). These ligaments are derived from the layers of peritoneum that form the greater and lesser sacs. A mass in the left upper quadrant may displace the spleen inferiorly. Caudal displacement may occur secondary to a subclavian abscess, splenic cyst, or left pleural effusion. Cephalic displacement may result from volume loss in the left lung, left lobe pneumonia, paralysis of the left hemidiaphragm, or a large intra-abdominal mass. A normal spleen with medial lobulation between the pancreatic tail and the left kidney may be confused with a cystic mass in the tail of the pancreas.

Wandering Spleen

The term **wandering spleen** describes a spleen that has migrated from its normal location in the left upper quadrant. It is the result of an embryologic anomaly of the dorsal mesentery that fails to fuse with the posterior peritoneum without supporting ligaments of the spleen. The patient may present with an abdominal or pelvic mass, intermittent pain, and volvulus (splenic torsion). The sonographer should use color Doppler to map the vascularity within the spleen. When torsion is complete, the vascular pattern shows decreased velocity.

Congenital Anomalies

Splenic Agenesis. Complete absence of the spleen (asplenia), or **splenic agenesis,** is rare and by itself causes no difficulties. However, it may occur as part of a major congenital abnormality. Visceral heterotaxy is the common name that consists of a spectrum of anomalies. Asplenic or **polysplenia** syndromes are associated with complex cardiac malformations, bronchopulmonary abnormalities, or visceral heterotaxis (anomalous placement of organs or major blood vessels, including a horizontal liver, malrotation of the gut, and interruption of the inferior vena cava with azygos continuation). The normal arrangement of asymmetrical body parts is called *situs solitus.* The mirror image condition is called *situs inversus.* The term *situs ambiguous* is used when the anatomy falls in between these two conditions.

Patients with polysplenia may have bilateral left-sidedness (two morphologic left lungs, left-sided azygous continuation of an interrupted inferior vena cava, biliary atresia, absence of the gallbladder, gastrointestinal malrotation, and cardiovascular abnormalities). On the other hand, patients with asplenia may have bilateral right-sidedness (two morphologic right lungs, midline location of the liver, reversed position of the abdominal aorta and inferior vena cava, anomalous pulmonary venous return, and horseshoe kidneys). Patients with agenesis of the spleen have major problems with serious infection, as their immune response is absent.

Splenic agenesis may be ruled out by demonstrating a spleen on ultrasound. The sonographer should be careful not to confuse the spleen with the bowel, which may lie in the area normally occupied by the spleen. Color Doppler helps determine the splenic vascular pattern and thus helps to separate it from the colon.

Accessory Spleen. An **accessory spleen,** or splenunculus, is a more common congenital anomaly that may be found in up to 30% of patients (Figure 15-5). The accessory spleen may be difficult to demonstrate by sonography if it is very small. However, when it is seen, it appears as a homogeneous pattern similar to that of the spleen. It usually is found near the hilum or inferior border of the spleen but has been reported elsewhere in the abdominal cavity. Lesions affecting the normal spleen

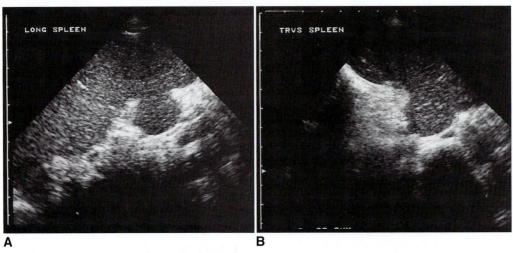

FIGURE 15-5 Accessory spleen. Long **(A)** and transverse **(B)** images of the small accessory spleen as it projects from the hilum of the spleen.

would also affect the accessory spleen. An accessory spleen results from failure of fusion of separate splenic masses forming on the dorsal mesogastrium; it is most commonly located in the splenic hilum or along the splenic vessels or associated ligaments. The location of the accessory spleen has been reported anywhere from the diaphragm to the scrotum, and it is usually solitary. It usually remains small and does not present as a clinical problem. The accessory spleen may simulate enlarged lymph nodes in the area of the spleen, or a tumor of the pancreatic, suprarenal, or retroperitoneal structures. As the spleen enlarges, so does the accessory spleen.

PHYSIOLOGY AND LABORATORY DATA OF THE SPLEEN

The spleen is part of the reticuloendothelial system and is rarely the site of primary disease. It is commonly involved in metabolic, hematopoietic, and infectious disorders. Blunt abdominal trauma to the spleen may result in splenic laceration and rupture. The spleen is active in the body's defense against disease; its major function is to filter the peripheral blood.

The spleen is a soft organ with elastic properties that allow it to distend as blood fills the venous sinuses. These characteristics are related to the function of the spleen as a blood reservoir. Within the lobules of the spleen are tissues called *pulp*. Two components are found within the spleen: red pulp and white pulp.

White pulp is distributed throughout the spleen in tiny islands. This tissue consists of splenic nodules, which are similar to those found in lymph nodes and contain large numbers of lymphocytes. Red pulp fills the remaining spaces of the lobules and surrounds the venous sinuses. The pulp contains relatively large numbers of red blood cells, which are responsible for its color, along with many lymphocytes and macrophages.

The **red pulp** of the spleen consists of **splenic sinuses** alternating with splenic cords. The blood capillaries within the red pulp are quite permeable. Red blood cells can squeeze through the pores in these capillary walls and enter the venous sinuses. The older, more fragile red blood cells may rupture as they make this passage, and the resulting cellular debris is removed by phagocytic macrophages located within the splenic sinuses. The macrophages engulf and destroy foreign particles, such as bacteria, that may be carried in the blood as it flows through the sinuses. The lymphocytes of the spleen help to defend the body against infection.

The blood that leaves the splenic sinuses to enter the reticular cords passes through a complex filter. The venous drainage of the sinuses and cords is not well defined, but it is assumed that tributaries of the splenic vein connect with sinuses of the red pulp.

The **white pulp** of the spleen consists of the **malpighian corpuscles,** small nodular masses of lymphoid tissue attached to the smaller arterial branches. Extending from the splenic capsule inward are the trabeculae, which contain blood vessels and lymphatics. The lymphoid tissue or malpighian corpuscles have the same structure as the follicles in the lymph nodes; however, they differ in that the splenic follicles surround arteries, so that on cross section, each contains a central artery. These follicles are scattered throughout the organ and are not confined to the peripheral layer or cortex, as are lymph nodes.

As part of the reticuloendothelial system, the spleen plays an important role in the defense mechanisms of the body and is also implicated in pigment and lipid metabolism. It is not essential to life and can be removed with no ill effects. The functions of the spleen may be classified under two general headings: those that reflect the functions of the reticuloendothelial system and those that are characteristic of the organ itself (Box 15-1).

BOX 15-1 | Functions of the Spleen

Functions of the Spleen as an Organ of the Reticuloendothelial System
Production of lymphocytes and plasma cells
Production of antibodies
Storage of iron
Storage of other metabolites

Functions Characteristic of the Spleen
Maturation of the surface of erythrocytes
Reservoir
Culling
Pitting function
Disposal of senescent or abnormal erythrocytes
Functions related to platelet and leukocyte life span

The role of the spleen as an immunologic organ involves the production of cells capable of making antibodies (lymphocytes and plasma cells); however, antibodies are also produced at other sites.

Phagocytosis of **erythrocytes** and the breakdown of **hemoglobin** occur throughout the entire reticuloendothelial system, but roughly half the catabolic activity is localized in the normal spleen. In splenomegaly, the major portion of hemoglobin breakdown occurs in the spleen. The iron that is liberated is stored in the splenic phagocytes. In anomalies such as the hemolytic anemias, the splenic phagocytes become engorged with **hemosiderin** when erythrocyte destruction is accelerated.

In addition to storing iron, the spleen is subject to storage diseases such as Gaucher's disease and Niemann-Pick disease. Abnormal lipid metabolites accumulate in all phagocytic reticuloendothelial cells but may also involve the phagocytes in the spleen, producing gross splenomegaly.

Functions of the spleen that are characteristic of the organ relate primarily to the circulation of erythrocytes through it. In a normal individual, the spleen contains only about 20 to 30 ml of erythrocytes. In splenomegaly the reservoir function is greatly increased, and the abnormally enlarged spleen contains many times this volume of red blood cells. Transit time is lengthened, and the erythrocytes are subject to destructive effects for a long time. In part, ptosis causes consumption of glucose, on which the erythrocyte depends to maintain normal metabolism, and the erythrocyte is destroyed. Selective destruction of abnormal erythrocytes is also accelerated by splenic pooling.

As erythrocytes pass through the spleen, the organ inspects them for imperfections and destroys those it recognizes as abnormal or senescent. **Pitting** is the process of removing the nuclei from the red blood cells. **Culling** is the process by which the spleen removes abnormal red blood cells. The normal function of the spleen keeps the number of circulating erythrocytes with inclusions at a minimum.

The spleen also pools platelets in large numbers. Entry of platelets into the splenic pool and their return to the circulation are extensive. In splenomegaly, the splenic pool may be so large that it produces thrombocytopenia. Sequestration of leukocytes in the enlarged spleen may produce **leukopenia.**

Laboratory data include the following:

- **Hematocrit.** The hematocrit indicates the percentage of red blood cells per volume of blood. Abnormally low readings indicate hemorrhage or internal bleeding within the body.
- **Bacteremia.** The test for bacteremia indicates the presence of bacteria within the body. The term *sepsis* indicates bacteria in the bloodstream. Typical symptoms of fever and chills, along with other medical conditions, may indicate the presence of an infection.
- **Leukocytosis.** An increase in the number of white cells present in the blood is usually a typical finding in infection. This finding may also occur after surgery, in malignancies, or in the presence of leukemia.
- **Leukopenia.** Abnormal decrease in white blood corpuscles may be secondary to certain medications or bone marrow disorder.
- **Thrombocytopenia.** Thrombocytopenia is an abnormal decrease in platelets, which may be due to internal hemorrhage.

SONOGRAPHIC EVALUATION OF THE SPLEEN

Normal Texture and Patterns

Sonographically, the splenic parenchyma should have a fine uniform homogeneous mid- to low-level echo pattern, as is seen within the liver parenchyma (Figure 15-6). The texture of the spleen is actually considered to be more echogenic than that of the liver. As the spleen enlarges, echogenicity further increases. The shape of the spleen has considerable variation. The spleen has two components joined at the hilum: a superomedial component and an inferolateral component. On transverse scans, it has a "crescent" inverted comma appearance, usually with a large medial component and a thin component extending anteriorly. This part of the spleen may be seen to indent the fundus of the stomach. Moving inferiorly, only the lateral component is imaged. On longitudinal scans, the superior component extends more medially than the inferior component. The superomedial component or the inferolateral component may enlarge independently. The irregularity of these components makes it difficult to assess mild splenomegaly accurately.

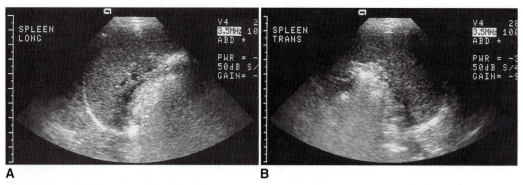

FIGURE 15-6 Normal spleen. Long **(A)** and transverse **(B)** images of the normal spleen. The parenchyma is homogeneous throughout except for the area of the hilum where the vascular structures enter and leave the spleen.

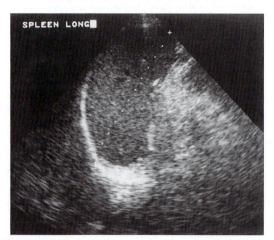

FIGURE 15-7 Splenic size. The spleen is measured in the long axis and should be 8 to 13 cm in length.

Size

The spleen is normally measured along its long axis (Figure 15-7). The normal spleen measures 8 to 13 cm in length, 7 cm in anteroposterior diameter, and less than 5 cm in thickness. In children, the formula for splenic length is $5.7 + 0.31 \times$ age (in years). The length of the spleen usually measures greater than the length of the kidney. Splenomegaly is diagnosed when the spleen measures more than 13 cm in the adult patient, or more than normal length in the respective child.

Patient Position and Technique

The left upper quadrant may be imaged as the sonographer carefully manipulates the 2.5 MHz curvilinear transducer between costal margins to image the left kidney, spleen, and diaphragm. The sector transducer may fit between the intercostal margins better than the larger curved-array transducer. The spleen generally lies in an oblique pathway in the posterior left upper quadrant; therefore, the transducer may be placed in the intercostal margin and with a slow anterior to posterior sweep may demonstrate the long axis of the spleen.

When the patient is lying supine, the problem of overlying air-filled stomach or bowel anterior to the spleen may interfere with adequate visualization; thus the patient should be rotated into a steep right decubitus position to permit better transducer contact between the ribs without as much bowel interference. The patient should be instructed to raise his or her left arm over his or her head to further open up the intercostal spaces to allow the transducer better access to the spleen. The right lateral decubitus, or axillary, position enables the sonographer to scan in an oblique fashion between the ribs. If the ultrasound laboratory has a cardiac bed with a dropleaf component, the patient should be rolled onto his or her left side and the transducer directed along the left intercostal margin to image the spleen. Excellent visualization is achieved because the spleen will lie flush against the patient's abdominal wall.

Variations in patient respiration may also facilitate imaging of the spleen; deep inspiration causes the lungs to expand with air and displaces the diaphragm; the lungs may expand so fully that the costophrenic angle is obscured and visualization of the spleen is impeded. The sonographer should observe the patient's breathing pattern and modify the amount of inspiration to adequately image the spleen without interference from the air-filled lungs.

In a routine abdominal examination, the spleen should be surveyed to ensure that the parenchyma is uniform with a homogeneous texture, except for the splenic hilum, which shows normal tubular vascular structures. At least two images of the spleen should be recorded in the longitudinal and transverse planes (see Figure 15-6). The longitudinal plane should demonstrate the left hemidiaphragm, the superior and inferior margins of the spleen, and the upper pole of the left kidney. The sonographer should look at the left pleural space superior to the diaphragm to see if fluid is present in the lower costal margin. The long axis of the spleen is measured from its superior-to-inferior border.

After the longitudinal oblique scan is completed, the transducer is rotated 90 degrees to survey the spleen in a transverse plane. The sonographer should obtain at least one transverse image at the hilum of the spleen. The sonographer should observe the flow of the splenic artery and vein with color Doppler. Forward (positive to the baseline) arterial flow should be seen entering the main splenic artery as it bifurcates into multiple branches to supply the splenic parenchyma (Figure 15-8). Conversely, returning flow (negative to the baseline) from the multiple splenic venous branches enters into the splenic vein. The splenic vein leaves the hilum of the spleen to transverse horizontally across the abdomen before joining the superior mesenteric vein, which leads into the main portal vein anterior to the inferior vena cava (Figure 15-9).

Increased hypoechoic structures in the area of the splenic hilum may indicate portal hypertension with collateral vessels or enlarged lymph nodes. A correlation has been noted between the caliber of splenic arteries and the size of the spleen in cirrhotic patients with esophageal varices. The splenic artery is larger in patients with splenomegaly (patients with cirrhosis with esophageal varices and patients with hematologic malignancies). The use of color Doppler imaging will help the sonographer determine whether the structures are vascular or nonvascular in composition (Figure 15-10).

Care should be taken when hepatomegaly is present with a prominent left lobe of the liver. The homogeneous texture of the liver may be confused as spleen, especially if the left lobe extends to the left upper quadrant. The sonographer should evaluate the patient in multiple planes in an effort to separate the splenic tissue from the hepatic structures.

Nonvisualization of the Spleen

The inability to image the spleen in its normal location may be a result of one of several conditions (e.g., asplenia syndrome, polysplenia syndrome, traumatic fragmentation of the spleen, wandering spleen).

Atrophy. Atrophy of the spleen may be found in normal individuals. It may also occur in wasting diseases. Chronic hemolytic anemias, particularly sickle cell anemia, involve excessive loss of pulp, increasing fibrosis, scarring from multiple infarcts, and encrustation with iron and calcium deposits. In the final stages of atrophy, the spleen may be so small that it is hardly recognizable. Advanced atrophy is sometimes referred to as autosplenectomy.

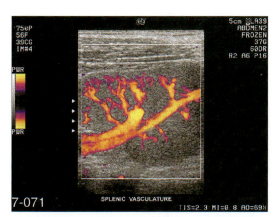

FIGURE 15-8 Color Doppler shows the splenic arterial system within the spleen.

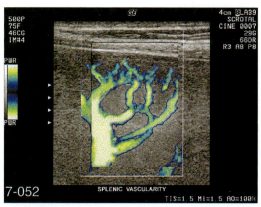

FIGURE 15-9 The splenic venous system is well demarcated with color Doppler.

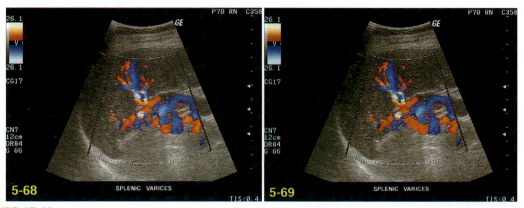

FIGURE 15-10 Color Doppler shows the dilated splenic vessels that may be seen with portal hypertension and varices.

PATHOLOGY OF THE SPLEEN

Table 15-1 lists the clinical findings, sonographic findings, and differential considerations for selected splenic diseases and conditions.

Splenomegaly

As the largest unit of the reticuloendothelial system, the spleen is involved in all systemic inflammations and generalized hematopoietic disorders and many metabolic disturbances (Table 15-2 and Box 15-2). It is rarely the primary site of disease. Whenever the spleen is involved in systemic disease, splenic enlargement, or **splenomegaly,** usually develops (Figure 15-11).

Obvious gross splenomegaly is easily defined with sonography. If mild splenomegaly is present, sonographic findings may be more difficult to obtain. Volume measurements of the spleen are necessary to determine the exact size. Although splenomegaly is the most common disease process encountered by the sonographer when evaluating this organ, careful evaluation of splenic contour and homogeneity should be undertaken to determine whether a disease process involves the spleen. Evaluation of the splenic parenchyma and vascular patterns may demonstrate changes in the size, texture, and

TABLE 15-1	Splenic Findings	
Clinical Findings	**Sonographic Findings**	**Differential Considerations**
Splenomegaly		
Depends on cause	Long axis ≥13 cm Look for liver anomalies (e.g., cirrhosis, diffuse disease)	
Splenic Abscess		
Fever Leukocytosis	Splenomegaly Irregular, ill-defined borders May have internal septa	Hematoma Necrotic neoplasm Lymphoma Leukemia
Splenic Infarction		
Related to primary diagnosis	Acute: wedge-shaped, hypoechoic area Chronic: wedge-shaped, echogenic area (base points to periphery) Look for splenic atrophy	Infection Hemorrhage Neoplasm Lymphoma
Splenic Trauma		
↓ Hematocrit	Spleen may appear enlarged Hematoma may form later along subcapsular area or internally	
Splenic Cysts		
Asymptomatic	Solitary Anechoic↑ Transmission Well-defined walls Look for tissue compression	Hematoma Lymphangioma Echinococcal cyst
Primary Tumors		
Depends on primary	Splenomegaly May be diffuse, single, or multiple Hypoechoic to hyperechoic	Infection

TABLE 15-2	Sonographic-Pathologic Classification of Splenic Disorders				
Uniform Splenic Sonodensity			**Focal Defects**		
Normal Sonodensity	**Low Sonodensity**	**Sonodense**	**Sonolucent**	**Perisplenic Defects**
Erythropoiesis (including myeloproliferative disorders) Reticuloendothelial Congestion Hyperactivity	Granulocytopoiesis (excluding myelo disorders) Lymphopoiesis Other (multiple myeloma) Congestion	Nonspecific (metastasis)	Nonspecific (benign primary neoplasm, cyst, abscess, malignant neoplasm [lymphopoietic])	Nonspecific (hematoma)

From Mittelstaedt CA, Partain CL: Radiology 134:697, 1980.

BOX 15-2	Pathologic Classification of Splenic Disorders

Hematopoiesis
Granulocytopoiesis
   Reactive hyperplasia to acute and chronic infection (low sonodensity)
Noncaseous granulomatous inflammation
Myeloproliferative syndromes (normal)
Chronic myelogenous leukemia
Acute myelogenous leukemia
Lymphopoiesis (low sonodensity or focal sonolucent)
Chronic lymphocytic leukemia
   Lymphoma
   Hodgkin's disease
Erythropoiesis (normal)
Sickle cell disease
   Hereditary spherocytosis
   Hemolytic anemia
   Chronic anemia
   Myeloproliferative syndrome
Other
   Multiple myeloma (low sonodensity)

Reticuloendothelial Hyperactivity (Normal)
Still's disease
Wilson's disease
Felty's syndrome
Reticulum cell sarcoma

Congestion (Normal or Low Sonodensity)
Hepatocellular disease

Nonspecific
Neoplasm-metastasis (focal sonodense)
Cyst (focal sonolucent)
Abscess (focal sonolucent)
Malignant neoplasm (focal sonolucent)
   Hodgkin's disease
   Lymphoma
Benign neoplasm (focal sonolucent)
   Lymphangiomatosis
Hematoma (perisplenic)

TABLE 15-3	Causes of Splenomegaly	
Degree of Splenomegaly	**Possible Causes**	
Mild to moderate	Infection Portal hypertension AIDS	
Moderate	Leukemia Lymphoma Infectious mononucleosis	
Massive	Myelofibrosis	
Focal lesions	Lymphomatous involvement Metastatic disease Hematomas	

Congestion of the Spleen

Two types of splenic congestion are known: acute and chronic. In acute congestion, active hyperemia accompanies the reaction in the moderately enlarged spleen. In chronic venous congestion, diffuse enlargement of the spleen occurs. The venous congestion may be of systemic origin, caused by intrahepatic obstruction to portal venous drainage or by obstructive venous disorders in the portal or splenic veins. Systemic venous congestion is found in cardiac decompensation involving the right side of the heart. It is particularly severe in tricuspid or pulmonary valvular disease and in chronic cor pulmonale.

The most common causes of striking congestive splenomegaly are the various forms of cirrhosis of the liver. It is also caused by obstruction to the extrahepatic portal or splenic vein (e.g., spontaneous portal vein thrombosis) (Box 15-4).

Storage Disease

Amyloidosis. In systemic diseases leading to **amyloidosis,** the spleen is the most frequently involved organ.

Sonographic Findings. The spleen may be of normal size or decidedly enlarged, depending on the amount and distribution of amyloid. Two types of involvement are seen: nodular and diffuse. In the nodular type, amyloid is found in the walls of the sheathed arteries and within the follicles, but not in the red pulp (see Figure 15-11). In the diffuse type, the follicles are not involved, the red pulp is prominently involved, and the spleen is usually greatly enlarged and firm.

Gaucher's Disease. All age groups can be affected by Gaucher's disease. About 50% of patients are younger than 8 years of age, and 17% are younger than 1 year of age. Clinical features follow a chronic course, with bone pain and changes in skin pigmentation.

Sonographic Findings. On ultrasound examination, splenomegaly, diffuse inhomogeneity, and multiple splenic nodules (well-defined hypoechoic lesions) are seen. These nodules may be irregular, hyperechoic, or

vascularity of the organ, which could be helpful in the patient's clinical evaluation to rule out the presence of a diffuse disease process or focal lesion. The spleen may grow to enormous size with extension into the iliac fossa. The medial segment may cross the midline of the abdomen to mimic a mass inferior to the left lobe of the liver. Splenomegaly has multiple causes (Box 15-3). Table 15-3 lists possible causes, depending on the degree of enlargement.

Clinical signs of splenomegaly may include left upper quadrant pain (secondary to stretching of the splenic capsule or ligaments) or fullness. Enlargement of the spleen may encroach upon surrounding organs, such as the left kidney, pancreas, stomach, and intestines.

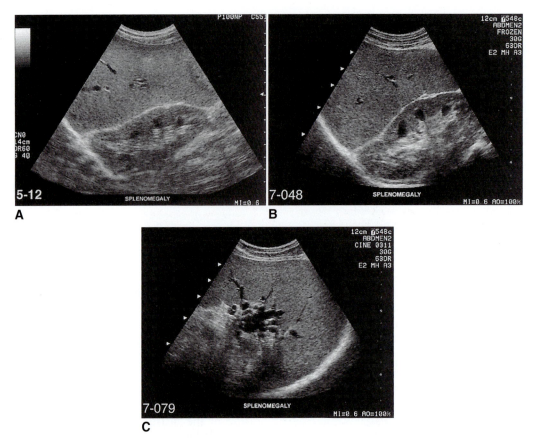

FIGURE 15-11 Patterns of splenomegaly. **A** and **B,** The tip of the spleen covers the lower pole of the kidney in patients with splenomegaly. **C,** The dilated splenic hilum is secondary to portal hypertension. Both the liver and the spleen are enlarged.

BOX 15-3	Causes of Splenomegaly

Collagen-vascular disease
Congestion
Extramedullary hematopoiesis
Hemolytic anemia
Infection
Neoplasm
Storage disease
Trauma

BOX 15-4	Causes of Congestive Splenomegaly

Acute splenic sequestration crisis of sickle cell disease
Cirrhosis
Cystic fibrosis
Heart failure
Portal hypertension
Portal or splenic vein thrombosis

mixed. They represent focal areas of Gaucher's cells associated with fibrosis and infarction.

Niemann-Pick Disease. Niemann-Pick disease is a rapidly progressing fatal disease that predominantly affects female infants. Clinical features consist of hepatomegaly, digestive disturbances, and lymphadenopathy.

Diffuse Disease

Erythropoietic abnormalities include the following: sickle cell, hereditary spherocytosis, hemolytic anemia, chronic anemia, polycythemia vera, thalassemia, and myeloproliferative disorders. On ultrasound, they tend to produce an isoechoic pattern.

Sickle Cell Anemia. In the earlier stage of **sickle cell anemia,** as seen in infants and children, the spleen is enlarged with marked congestion of the red pulp. Later, the spleen undergoes progressive infarction and fibrosis and decreases in size until, in adults, only a small mass of fibrous tissue may be found (autosplenectomy). It is generally believed that these changes result when sickle cells plug the vasculature of the splenic substance, effectively producing ischemic destruction of the spleen.

Sonographic Findings. On ultrasound examination, sickle cell disease has different sonographic appearances, depending on its disease state (Figure 15-12). An acute **sickle cell crisis** commonly occurs in children with homozygous sickle cell disease with splenomegaly and a sudden decrease in hematocrit. In addition, these patients may develop a subacute hemorrhage that appears as a hypoechoic area in the periphery of the spleen.

Congenital Spherocytosis. In congenital or hereditary **spherocytosis,** an intrinsic abnormality of the red cells gives rise to erythrocytes that are small and spheroid

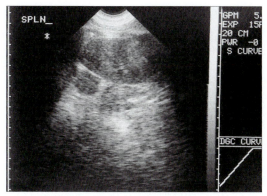

FIGURE 15-12 Sickle cell crisis. Patient with sickle cell anemia demonstrated a small spleen with progressive infarction and fibrosis, as seen in autosplenectomy.

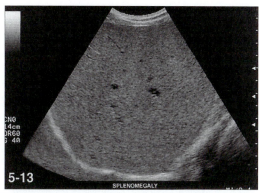

FIGURE 15-13 A patient with thalassemia major shows a huge spleen extending into the lower abdominal cavity.

rather than normal, flattened, biconcave disks. The two results of this disease are production by the bone marrow of spherocytic erythrocytes and increased destruction of these cells in the spleen. The spleen destroys spherocytes selectively.

▌ **Sonographic Findings.** The spleen may be enlarged.

Hemolytic Anemia. **Hemolytic anemia** is the general term applied to anemia linked to decreased life of the erythrocytes. When the rate of destruction is greater than what the bone marrow can compensate for, anemia results.

Autoimmune Hemolytic Anemia. **Autoimmune hemolytic anemia** can occur in its primary form without underlying disease, or it may be seen as a secondary disorder in patients already suffering from some disorder of the reticuloendothelial or hematopoietic system, such as lymphoma, leukemia, or infectious **mononucleosis.**

▌ **Sonographic Findings.** In its secondary form, splenic changes are dominated by the underlying disease; in its primary form, the spleen is variably enlarged.

Polycythemia Vera. Polycythemia is an excess of red blood cells. **Polycythemia vera** is a chronic disease of unknown cause that involves all bone marrow elements. It is characterized by an increase in red blood cell mass and hemoglobin concentration. Clinical symptoms include weakness, fatigue, vertigo, tinnitus, irritability, splenomegaly, flushing of the face, redness and pain in the extremities, and blue-and-black spots.

▌ **Sonographic Findings.** In polycythemia vera, the spleen is variably enlarged, rather firm, and blue-red. Infarcts and thromboses are common in polycythemia vera.

Thalassemia. The spleen is severely involved in **thalassemia.** This hemoglobinopathy differs from the others in that an abnormal molecular form of hemoglobin is not present. Instead, suppression of synthesis of beta or alpha polypeptide chains occurs, resulting in deficient synthesis of normal hemoglobin. Not only are the erythrocytes deficient in normal hemoglobin, they are also abnormal in shape; many are target cells, whereas others

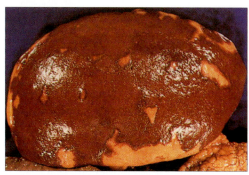

FIGURE 15-14 Chronic myeloid leukemia shows infarcts in a gross specimen with splenomegaly.

vary considerably in size and shape. Their life span is short because they are destroyed by the spleen in large numbers. The disease ranges from mild to severe.

▌ **Sonographic Findings.** Changes in the spleen are greatest in the severe form, called thalassemia major (Figure 15-13). The spleen is very large, often seeming to fill the entire abdominal cavity.

Myeloproliferative Disorders. Myeloproliferative disorders include acute and chronic myelogenous leukemias, polycythemia vera, myelofibrosis, megakaryocytic leukemia, and erythroleukemia (Figure 15-14).

▌ **Sonographic Findings.** An isoechoic ultrasound pattern is seen because the parenchyma is hypoechoic compared with the liver (Figure 15-15).

Granulocytopoietic Abnormalities. Granulocytopoietic abnormalities include reactive hyperplasia resulting from acute or chronic infection (e.g., splenitis sarcoid, tuberculosis).

▌ **Sonographic Findings.** On ultrasound examination, splenomegaly is seen with a diffusely hypoechoic pattern (less dense than the liver). Patients who have had a previous granulomatous infection have bright echogenic lesions on ultrasound, with or without shadowing. Histoplasmosis and tuberculosis are the most common causes; sarcoidosis is rare. The sonographer may also find calcium in the splenic artery.

Reticuloendotheliosis. Diseases characterized by reticuloendothelial hyperactivity and varying degrees of lipid

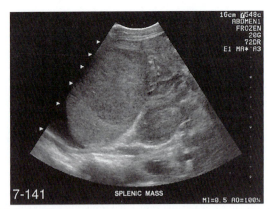

FIGURE 15-15 Patient with acute myelogenous leukemia shows a large mass within the splenic parenchyma and enlarged nodes in the hilum.

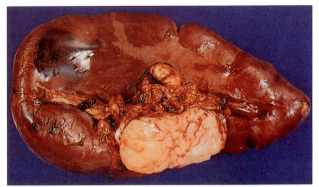

FIGURE 15-16 Lymphoblastic lymphoma. Tumor cells form a discrete mass in the spleen.

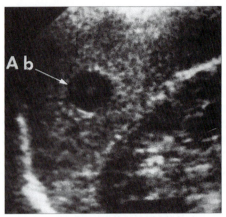

FIGURE 15-17 Splenic abscess *(Ab)*. A small, well-defined hypoechoic lesion was seen within the spleen in a patient who had been febrile for 6 days.

storage in phagocytes are included in the category of reticuloendotheliosis.

Sonographic Findings. On ultrasound, the spleen appears isoechoic.

Letterer-Siwe Disease. In Letterer-Siwe disease, sometimes called *nonlipid reticuloendotheliosis,* proliferation of reticuloendothelial cells occurs in all tissues, but particularly in the splenic lymph nodes and bone marrow. This disease is generally found in children younger than 2 years of age. Clinical features include hepatosplenomegaly, fever, and pulmonary involvement. It is rapidly fatal.

Sonographic Findings. Usually, the spleen is only moderately enlarged, although the change may be more severe in affected older infants.

Hand-Schüller-Christian   Disease. Hand-Schüller-Christian disease is benign and chronic, in spite of many features similar to those of Letterer-Siwe disease. It usually affects children older than 2 years of age. Clinical features include a chronic course, diabetes, and moderate hepatosplenomegaly.

Lymphopoietic Abnormalities

Lymphopoietic abnormalities include lymphocytic leukemias, lymphoma, and **Hodgkin disease** (Figure 15-16).

Sonographic Findings. Ultrasound shows a diffusely hypoechoic splenic pattern with focal lesions. Patients with **non-Hodgkin lymphoma** have been reported to have an isoechoic echo pattern.

Leukemia. Chronic myelogenous leukemia may be responsible for more extreme splenomegaly than any other disease. Chronic lymphocytic leukemia produces less severe splenomegaly.

Focal Disease

Focal disease of the spleen may be single or multiple and may be found in the normal or enlarged spleen. Major nontraumatic causes of focal splenic defects include

tumors (benign and malignant), infarction, abscesses, and cysts. Splenic defects may be discovered incidentally, as in another imaging study, or specifically, as in the case of a splenic infarct or abscess.

Splenic Abscess. Splenic abscesses are uncommon, probably because of the phagocytic activity of the spleen's efficient reticuloendothelial system and leukocytes. The system may be infected by the following: subacute bacterial endocarditis, septicemia, decreased immunologic states, or drug abuse. In the majority of patients, the infection is spread from distant foci in the abdomen, or an inflammatory process extends directly from adjacent organs. Extrinsic processes (i.e., perinephric or subphrenic abscess, perforated gastric or colonic lesions, or pancreatic abscess) may invade the splenic parenchyma.

Clinical findings may be subtle and may include fever, left upper quadrant tenderness, abdominal pain, left shoulder and flank pain, and splenomegaly.

Sonographic Findings. Sonography shows a simple cystic pattern to mixed echo pattern (Figure 15-17). The lesion may be hypoechoic, often with hyperechoic foci that represent debris or gas. Other findings include the following: thick or shaggy walls, anechoic (without

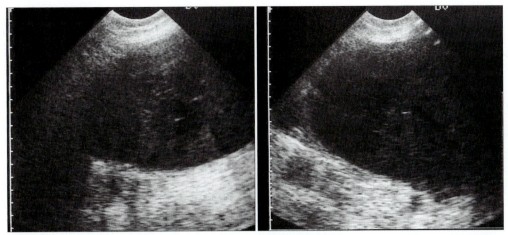

FIGURE 15-18 Patient came to the emergency room with fever and upper abdominal pain after undergoing dental work 2 days earlier. The spleen was enlarged, with areas of inhomogeneity representing a splenic infection.

echoes within a mass) appearance, poor definition of the lesion, and increased to decreased transmission (depending on the presence of gas). An abscess may be difficult to distinguish from an infarct, neoplasm, or hematoma, and clinical correlation is necessary.

Splenic Infection. Many infections can affect the spleen. The most prominent feature is splenomegaly. Many immunocompromised patients also have multiple nodules within the spleen.

Sonographic Findings. Patients with hepatosplenic candidiasis may show irregular masses within the spleen, the "wheels-within-wheels" pattern, with the outer wheel representing the ring of fibrosis surrounding the inner echogenic wheel of inflammatory cells, and a central hypoechoic area (Figure 15-18). Other patterns seen include bull's eye (hypoechoic rim with an echogenic central core), hypoechoic nodule, or hyperechoic nodule. On ultrasound examination, patients with mycobacterial infections show tiny, diffuse echogenic foci throughout the spleen. Active tuberculosis shows echopoor or cystic masses, representing small abscess lesions.

Acquired Immunodeficiency Syndrome. In patients with acquired immunodeficiency syndrome (AIDS), the most common finding is splenomegaly. These patients may have multiorgan involvement (i.e., liver, spleen, and kidneys). Focal lesions include *Candida, Pneumocystis jiroveci* pneumonia, *Mycobacterium*, disseminated *Pneumocystis*, Kaposi's sarcoma, and lymphoma.

Sonographic Findings. The most common finding is moderate splenomegaly. Additional findings may demonstrate focal splenic lesions displaying small round lesions that may be multiple, hypoechoic, and well defined. Many of these lesions were caused by disseminated *Mycobacterium tuberculosis* infection, *Candida, Pneumocystis jiroveci*, or *Mycobacterium avium*. In addition, hepatomegaly with focal lesions, retroperitoneal lymphadenopathy, and ascites may be seen.

Splenic Infarction. Splenic infarction is the most common cause of focal splenic lesions resulting from occlusion of the major splenic artery or any of its branches. They are almost always the result of emboli that arise in the heart, produced from mural thrombi or from vegetation on the valves of the left side of the heart. Other causes include septic emboli and local thrombosis in patients with pancreatitis, leukemia, lymphomatous disorders, sickle cell anemia, sarcoidosis, or polyarteritis nodosa.

Sonographic Findings. Ultrasound may show a localized hypoechoic area, depending on the time of onset (Figure 15-19). Fresh hemorrhage has a hypoechoic appearance; healed infarctions appear as echogenic, peripheral, wedge-shaped lesions with their base toward the subcapsular surface of the spleen. The infarction may become nodular or hyperechoic with time.

Splenic Trauma. The spleen is most commonly injured as a result of blunt abdominal trauma. If the patient has severe left upper quadrant pain secondary to trauma, a splenic hematoma or subcapsular hematoma should be considered. The tear may result in linear or stellate lacerations or capsular tears, puncture wounds from foreign bodies or rib fractures, or subcapsular hematomas.

Blunt trauma has two outcomes. If the capsule is intact, the outcome may be intraparenchymal or subcapsular hematoma; if the capsule ruptures, a focal or free intraperitoneal hematoma may form. In delayed rupture, a subcapsular hematoma may develop with subsequent rupture. Quick assessment of free fluid that may surround the splenic capsule in blunt abdominal trauma can lead to a life-saving diagnosis for the patient.

Sonographic Findings. Sonography is a sensitive and specific test used to examine trauma patients for abdominal injury requiring surgery (Figure 15-20). Routine abdominal ultrasound examination can be performed at the bedside in the trauma center. The use of screening ultrasound can improve clinical decision making for the use of emergency laparotomy.

A study was conducted to evaluate the efficiency of emergency ultrasound scans for blunt abdominal trauma

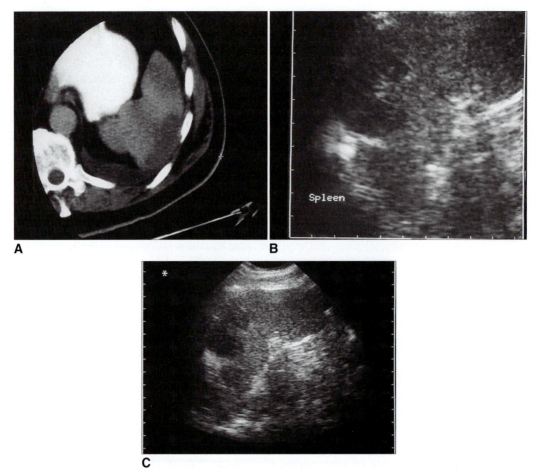

FIGURE 15-19 Splenic infarct. **A,** Computed tomography demonstrates the area of infarct in the spleen. **B** and **C,** Ultrasound shows the hypoechoic area near the peripheral margin of the spleen.

performed by surgeons and radiologists in a trauma center. Two groups of medical personnel were compared; the first consisted of surgeons and residents with minimal training in emergency ultrasound, and the second group consisted of radiologists attending in the emergency department. Overall results revealed an accuracy rate on ultrasound readings of 99% for the surgical team and 99% for the attending radiologists. The conclusion was that surgeons and surgical residents at different levels of training can accurately interpret emergency ultrasound examinations for blunt trauma from real-time images at a level comparable with that of attending radiologists.

The patient typically presents with left upper quadrant pain, left shoulder pain, left flank pain, or dizziness. On clinical evaluation, the patient may have tenderness over the left upper quadrant, hypotension, and decreased hemoglobin, indicating a bleed. A timely response to this emergent situation may save the patient undergoing peritoneal lavage or exploratory surgery. The sonographer should quickly examine the four abdominopelvic quadrants: the area surrounding the kidneys (Morison's pouch), the subdiaphragmatic areas, the liver and splenic capsule, and the bladder and anterior rectal area to determine whether free fluid is present. The patient's bladder may be filled retrograde to help serve as a window in the pelvic cavity. The entire screening examination should take less than 5 minutes and may be recorded on video tape.

If the spleen has been lacerated and blood is contained within the splenic capsule, the most prominent ultrasound finding is splenomegaly, with progressive enlargement as the bleeding continues. In addition, an irregular splenic border, hematoma, contusion (splenic inhomogeneity), subcapsular and pericapsular fluid collections, free intraperitoneal blood, or left pleural effusion may be present.

Focal hematomas may have intrasplenic fluid collections. Perisplenic fluid is seen in patients with subcapsular hematomas. The sonographer should be aware that blood exhibits various echo patterns, depending on the time that has passed since the trauma. Fresh hemorrhage may appear hypoechoic and may be difficult to distinguish from normal splenic tissue. The sonographer should look for a double-contour sign depicting the hematoma as separate from the spleen. As the protein and cells resorb the hematoma, the fluid becomes organized, hyperechoic, and similar to splenic tissue. In focal

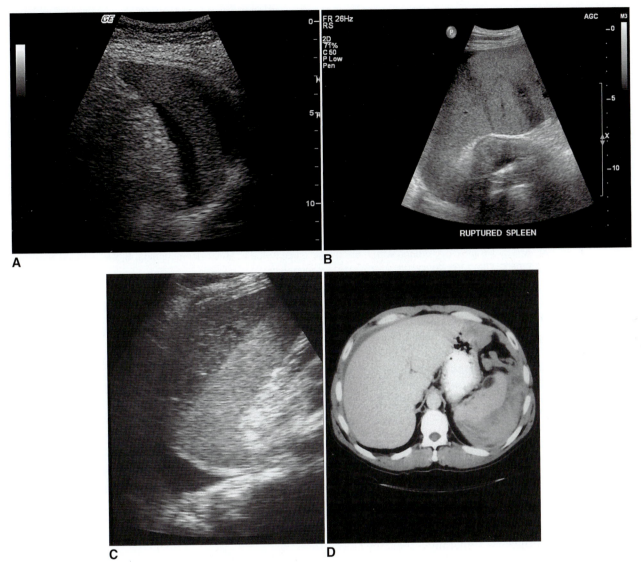

FIGURE 15-20 Splenic hematoma. **A,** Small hypoechoic separation medial to the splenic capsule represents a splenic hematoma. **B,** Inhomogeneity of the splenic texture represents a laceration in the spleen. **C,** Separation of the splenic capsule from the spleen secondary to a large hematoma resulting from an automobile accident. **D,** Computed tomography demonstrates the splenic hematoma along the posterolateral wall of the abdomen.

areas, tiny splenic lacerations give rise to small collections of blood interspersed with disrupted splenic pulp (contusion). Over time, the hematoma becomes more fluid or appears lucent.

The echo-free, intraperitoneal fluid is probably blood mixed with peritoneal transudate. Healing of the lesion often takes months. The free fluid disappears more quickly because the fluid is moved across the pleural and peritoneal membranes rapidly (2 to 4 weeks). Intrasplenic hematomas and contusions take longer because the fluid, protein, and necrotic debris must be resorbed from within a solid organ in which the blood supply has already been focally disrupted. When the spleen returns to normal, small irregular foci may remain, or the parenchyma may be normal.

Splenic Cysts. Splenic cysts may be classified as parasitic or nonparasitic in origin. Most cysts are con-

sidered secondary cysts caused by trauma, infection, or infarction.

Echinococcus is the only parasite that forms splenic cysts; it is uncommon in the United States. Parasitic cysts appear as anechoic lesions with possible daughter cysts and calcification, or as solid masses with fine internal echoes and poor distal enhancement. Nonparasitic cysts of the spleen have been categorized as primary or true.

Primary, or epidermoid, cysts contain an epithelial lining and are considered to be of congenital origin. False or secondary cysts lack a cellular lining, which probably develops as a result of prior trauma to the spleen, and account for 80% of nonparasitic splenic cysts. True cysts are usually solitary and unilocular and rarely contain calcification. The internal surface of the cyst may be smooth or trabeculated. The fluid may be clear or turbid, and may contain protein, iron, bilirubin, fat, and

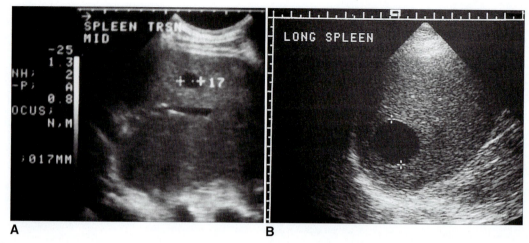

FIGURE 15-21 Splenic cyst. **A**, Tiny anechoic mass found within the splenic parenchyma as an incidental finding. **B**, Well-defined anechoic mass found within an asymptomatic young female.

cholesterol crystals. Primary cysts occur more frequently in females; 50% occur in patients younger than 15 years of age. Clinically, they present with an asymptomatic left upper quadrant mass.

Sonographic Findings. Ultrasound examination shows hypoechoic or anechoic foci with well-defined walls and increased through-transmission (Figure 15-21). The cysts may be small within the splenic parenchyma to very large. Primary cysts can have internal echoes at increased gain. Hemorrhage within the cyst may produce a fluid level. Infectious cysts of *Echinococcus* and hydatid cysts may show calcifications within their walls. Post-traumatic cysts that have no cellular lining are called pseudocysts. These cysts may develop calcifications in their walls.

Benign Primary Neoplasms. Generally speaking, primary tumors of the spleen are rare. The tumors may be divided into two groups: benign and malignant. With benign primary tumors, splenomegaly is the first indication of an abnormality. Most of these tumors appear isoechoic compared with the normal splenic parenchyma. Benign primary tumors include hamartoma, cavernous hemangioma, and cystic lymphangioma.

Hamartoma. The patient with hamartoma is asymptomatic. The tumor may be solitary or multiple and is considered well defined but not encapsulated. The hamartoma consists of lymphoid tissue or a combination of sinuses and structures equivalent to pulp cords of normal splenic tissue. Symptomatic splenic hamartomas are rare in the pediatric age group.

Sonographic Findings. Hamartoma has both solid and cystic components and is generally hyperechoic on sonography (Figure 15-22).

Cavernous Hemangioma. Cavernous hemangioma is usually an isolated inhomogeneous echogenic mass with multiple small hypoechoic areas (Figure 15-23). The patient displays no symptoms and becomes symptomatic only when the size of the spleen increases and it compresses other organs. Complications occur when the

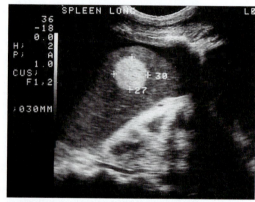

FIGURE 15-22 Hamartoma of the spleen. Small, solitary hyperechoic lesion within the spleen was seen in a young patient with ascites.

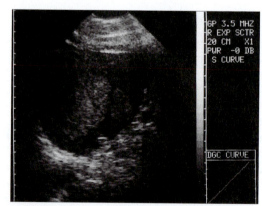

FIGURE 15-23 Cavernous hemangioma. A large inhomogeneous mass nearly fills the entire splenic parenchyma in this middle-aged male.

tumor increases in size to cause a splenic rupture with peritoneal symptoms.

Sonographic Findings. The appearance is variable, from a well-defined echogenic appearance to a complex mixed pattern; infarction with coagulated blood or fibrin

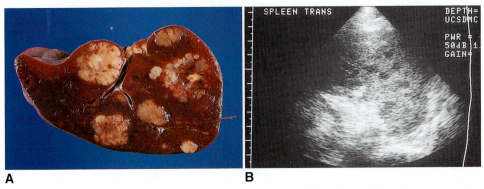

FIGURE 15-24 Metastases. **A,** Gross specimen of splenic metastases. **B,** Multiple diffuse hypoechoic lesions are seen throughout this spleen in a patient with primary breast cancer.

in the cavities may be seen, but is nonspecific. Hydatid cyst, abscess, dermoid cyst, and metastasis should be considered in the differential diagnosis.

Cystic Lymphangioma. Cystic lymphangioma is a benign malformation of lymphatics, consisting of endothelium-lined cystic spaces. Lymphangiomatosis affects predominantly the somatic soft tissue (found in the neck, axilla, mediastinum, retroperitoneum, and soft tissue of the extremities). It may involve multiple organ systems or may be confined to solitary organs, such as the liver, spleen, kidney, or colon.

Sonographic Findings. Cystic lymphangioma appears as a mass with extensive cystic replacement of splenic parenchyma. Splenic involvement is rare, but when it occurs, a multicystic appearance is characteristic.

Malignant Primary Neoplasms

Hemangiosarcoma. Hemangiosarcoma is a rare malignant neoplasm arising from the vascular endothelium of the spleen. Malignant tumors of the spleen are also uncommon. Primary tumors found in the spleen may be lymphoma, Hodgkin tumor, or hemangiosarcoma.

Sonographic Findings. The mixed cystic ultrasound pattern of hemangiosarcoma resembles that of a cavernous hemangioma, but it can also be hyperechoic.

Lymphoma. The spleen is commonly involved in lymphoma.

Sonographic Findings. It may be difficult to detect splenic lymphoma by sonography. When it is seen,

however, it appears to be typically hypoechoic; some focal areas are also seen. Four different sonographic patterns have been reported in patients with malignant lymphoma: (1) diffuse involvement, (2) focal small nodular lesions, (3) focal large nodular lesions, and (4) bulky disease. The diffuse or small nodular pattern was seen predominantly in low-grade lymphomas and in Hodgkin disease.

Metastases. Metastases are the result of a hematogenous spread from another primary site. The spleen is the tenth most common site of metastases, which may originate from the breast, lung, ovary, stomach, colon, kidney, or prostate or from melanoma (Figure 15-24). The metastatic tumors may be microscopic, causing no symptoms.

Sonographic Findings. The splenic parenchyma should be carefully examined by the sonographer to detect abnormalities of the splenic parenchyma. Melanoma deposits appear hypoechoic but are of higher echo amplitude than lymphoma; some are echodense.

Primary tumors and sonographic findings were evaluated in a small number of patients with isolated splenic metastasis to determine when these rare metastases should be suspected. Four of the primary tumors were colonic cancer and one was renal cancer. Care should be taken to image the spleen carefully if focal lesions are identified elsewhere in the body.

The Retroperitoneum

Kerry Weinberg and Shpetim Telegrafi

ANATOMY OF THE RETROPERITONEUM

Normal Anatomy

The retroperitoneal space is the area between the posterior portion of the parietal peritoneum and the posterior abdominal wall muscles (Figure 16-1). It extends from the diaphragm to the pelvis. Laterally, the boundaries extend to the extraperitoneal fat planes within the confines of the transversalis fascia, and medially the space encloses the great vessels. It is subdivided into the following three categories: anterior pararenal space, perirenal space, and posterior pararenal space (Box 16-1).

The perirenal space surrounds the kidney, adrenal, and perirenal fat. The anterior pararenal space includes the duodenum, pancreas, and ascending and transverse colon. The posterior pararenal space includes the iliopsoas muscle, ureter, and branches of the inferior vena cava and aorta and their lymphatics.

The retroperitoneum is protected by the spine, ribs, pelvis, and musculature and has been a difficult area to assess clinically by sonography. Computerized tomography imaging is better to outline the retroperitoneal cavity. Occasionally, however, the sonographer is asked to rule out fluid collection, hematoma, urinoma, or ascitic fluid in the retroperitoneal space.

The retroperitoneum is delineated anteriorly by the posterior peritoneum, posteriorly by the transversalis fascia, and laterally by the lateral borders of the quadratus lumborum muscles and peritoneal leaves of the mesentery. Proceeding from a superior to inferior direction, the retroperitoneum extends from the diaphragm to the pelvic brim. Superior to the pelvic brim the retroperitoneum can be partitioned into the lumbar and iliac fossae. The pararenal and perirenal spaces are included in the lumbar fossa.

Pathologic processes can stretch from the anterior abdominal wall to the subdiaphragmatic space, mediastinum, and subcutaneous tissues of the back and flank.

The retrofascial space, which includes the psoas, quadratus lumborum, and iliacus muscles (muscles posterior to the transversalis fascia), is often the site of extension of retroperitoneal pathologic processes.

Anterior Pararenal Space. The anterior pararenal space is bound anteriorly by the posterior parietal peritoneum and posteriorly by the anterior renal fascia. It is bound laterally by the lateroconal fascia formed by the fusion of the anterior and posterior leaves of the renal fascia. (This space merges with the bare area of the liver by the coronary ligament.) The pancreas, duodenum, and ascending and transverse colon are the structures included in the anterior pararenal space (Figure 16-2).

Perirenal Space. The perirenal space is surrounded by the anterior and posterior layers of the renal fascia (Gerota's fascia), attaching to the diaphragm superiorly. They are united loosely at their inferior margin at the iliac crest level or superior border of the **false pelvis.** Collections in the perinephric space can communicate within the iliac fossa of the retroperitoneum (Figure 16-3).

The lateroconal fascia (the lateral fusion of the renal fascia) proceeds anteriorly as the posterior peritoneum. The posterior renal fasciae fuse medially with the psoas or quadratus lumborum fascia (Figure 16-4). The anterior renal fascia fuses medially with connective tissue surrounding the great vessels. (This space contains the

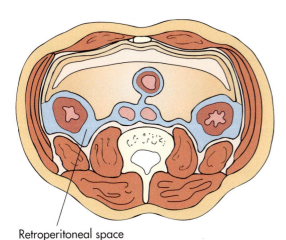

Retroperitoneal space

FIGURE 16-1 Schematic transverse section of the abdominal cavity at the level of the fourth lumbar vertebra. The retroperitoneal space is outlined in blue.

BOX 16-1	Organs in the Retroperitoneal Spaces

Anterior Pararenal Space
- Pancreas
- Duodenal sweep
- Ascending and transverse colon

Perirenal Space
- Adrenal glands
- Kidneys
- Ureter
- Great vessel

Posterior Pararenal Space
- Blood
- Lymph nodes

Iliac Fossa
- Ureter
- Major branches of great vessels
- Lymphatics

Retrofascial Space
Three Compartments
- Psoas
- Lumbar (quadratus lumborum)
- Iliacus

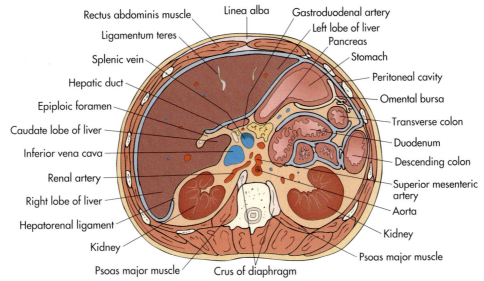

FIGURE 16-2 Transverse drawing of the anterior pararenal space. Cross section of the abdomen at the first lumbar vertebra.

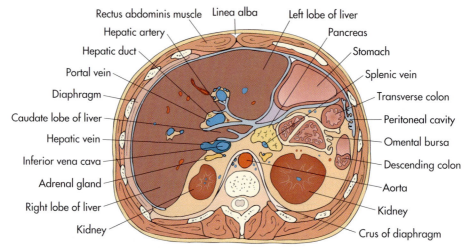

FIGURE 16-3 Transverse drawing of the perirenal space. Cross section of the abdomen at the level of the 12th thoracic vertebra.

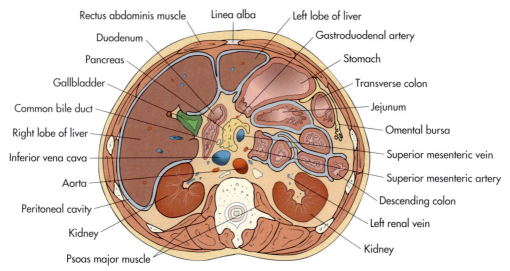

FIGURE 16-4 Transverse drawing of the posterior pararenal space. Cross section of the abdomen at the level of the second lumbar vertebra. This space is located between the posterior renal fascia and the transversalis fascia. It communicates with the peritoneal fat. The space merges inferiorly with the anterior pararenal space and retroperitoneal tissue of the iliac fossa.

adrenal gland, kidney, and ureter; the great vessels, also within this space, are largely isolated within their connective tissue sheaths.) The perirenal space contains the adrenal gland and kidney (in a variable amount of echogenic perinephric fat, the thickest portion of which is posterior and lateral to the kidney's lower pole). The kidney is anterolateral to the psoas muscle, anterior to the quadratus lumborum muscle, and posteromedial to the ascending and descending colon.

The second portion of the duodenum is anterior to the renal hilum on the right. On the left, the kidney is bounded by the stomach anterosuperiorly, the pancreas anteriorly, and the spleen anterolaterally.

Adrenal Glands. In the adult patient the adrenal glands are anterior, medial, and superior to the kidneys (Figure 16-5). The right adrenal is more superior to the kidney, whereas the left adrenal is more medial to the kidney. The medial portion of the right adrenal gland is imme-

diately posterior to the inferior vena cava (above the level of the portal vein and lateral to the crus). The lateral portion of the gland is posterior and medial to the right lobe of the liver and posterior to the duodenum.

The left adrenal gland is lateral or slightly posterolateral to the aorta and lateral to the crus of the diaphragm. The superior portion is posterior to the lesser omental space and posterior to the stomach. The inferior portion is posterior to the pancreas. The splenic vein and artery pass between the pancreas and the left adrenal gland.

The adrenal glands vary in size, shape, and configuration; the right adrenal is triangular and caps the upper pole of the right kidney. The left adrenal is semilunar in shape and extends along the medial border of the left kidney from the upper pole to the hilus. The internal texture is medium in consistency; the cortex and medulla are not distinguished.

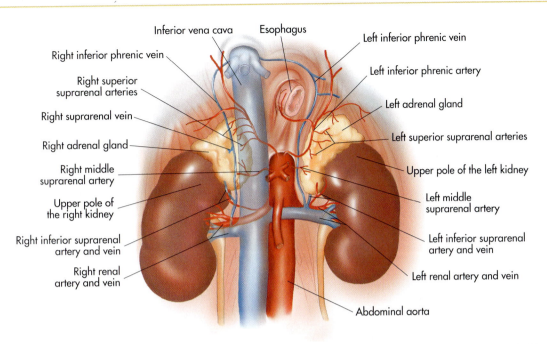

Inferior vena cava — Esophagus — Left inferior phrenic vein
Right inferior phrenic vein — Left inferior phrenic artery
Right superior suprarenal arteries — Left adrenal gland
Right suprarenal vein — Left superior suprarenal arteries
Right adrenal gland — Upper pole of the left kidney
Right middle suprarenal artery — Left middle suprarenal artery
Upper pole of the right kidney — Left inferior suprarenal artery and vein
Right inferior suprarenal artery and vein — Left renal artery and vein
Right renal artery and vein — Abdominal aorta

FIGURE 16-5 The adrenal glands are retroperitoneal organs that lie on the upper pole of each kidney. They are surrounded by perinephric fat. The right adrenal gland is triangular and caps the upper pole of the right kidney. It extends medially behind the inferior vena cava and rests posteriorly on the diaphragm. The left adrenal gland is semilunar and extends along the medial borders of the left kidney. It lies posterior to the pancreas, the lesser sac, and the stomach and rests posteriorly on the diaphragm.

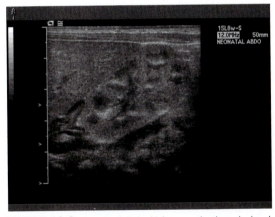

FIGURE 16-6 Neonatal right kidney and adrenal gland.

The adrenal gland is a distinct hypoechoic structure; sometimes highly echogenic fat is seen surrounding the gland. The normal size is usually smaller than 3 cm.

Neonatal Adrenal. The neonatal adrenal glands are characterized by a thin echogenic core surrounded by a thick transonic zone. This thick rim of transonicity represents the hypertrophied adrenal cortex, whereas the echogenic core is the adrenal medulla. An infant adrenal gland is proportionally larger than an adult adrenal gland (one third the size of the kidney; in adults it is one thirteenth the size) (Figure 16-6).

Diaphragmatic Crura. The diaphragmatic crura begins as tendinous fibers from the lumbar vertebral bodies, disks, and transverse processes of L3 on the right and L1 on the left (Figure 16-7). The right crus is longer, larger, and more lobular and is associated with the anterior aspect of the lumbar vertebral ligament. The right renal artery crosses anterior to the crus and posterior to the inferior vena cava at the level of the right kidney. The right crus is bounded by the inferior vena cava anterolaterally and the right adrenal and right lobe of liver posterolaterally.

The left crus courses along the anterior lumbar vertebral bodies in a superior direction and inserts into the central tendon of the diaphragm.

Para-aortic Lymph Nodes. There are two major lymph-node-bearing areas in the retroperitoneal cavity: the iliac and hypogastric nodes within the pelvis and the para-aortic group in the upper retroperitoneum. The lymphatic chain follows the course of the thoracic aorta, abdominal aorta, and iliac arteries (Figure 16-8). Common sites are the para-aortic and paracaval areas near the great vessels, peripancreatic area, renal hilar area, and mesenteric region. Normal nodes are smaller than the tip of a finger, less than 1 cm, and are not imaged on a sonogram. However, if these nodes enlarge because of infection or tumor, they can be seen on a sonogram.

Posterior Pararenal Space. The posterior pararenal space is located between the posterior renal fascia and the transversalis fascia. It communicates with the peritoneal fat, lateral to the lateroconal fascia. The posterior pararenal space merges inferiorly with the anterior pararenal space and retroperitoneal tissues of the iliac fossa (see Figure 16-4).

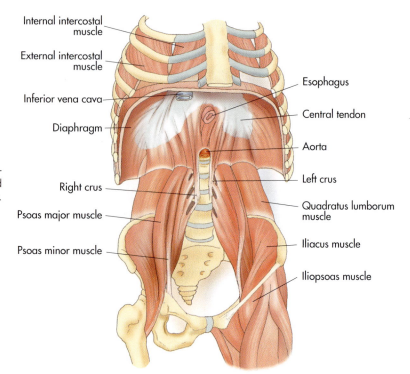

FIGURE 16-7 The crura of the diaphragm begin as tendinous fibers from the lumbar vertebral bodies, disks, and transverse processes of L3 on the right and L1 on the left.

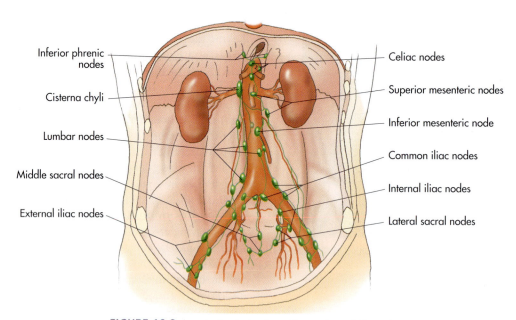

FIGURE 16-8 Lymphatic chain along the aorta and iliac artery.

The psoas muscle, the fascia of which merges with the posterior transversalis fascia, makes up the medial border of this posterior space. This space is open laterally and inferiorly. The blood and lymph nodes embedded in fat may be found in the posterior pararenal space.

Iliac Fossa. The iliac fossa is the region extending between the internal surface of the iliac wings, from the crest to the iliopectineal line. This area is known as the false pelvis and contains the ureter and major branches of the distal great vessels and their lymphatics. The trans-versalis fascia extends into the iliac fossa as the iliac fascia.

Retrofascial Space. The retrofascial space is made up of the posterior abdominal wall, muscles, nerves, lymphatics, and areolar tissue behind the transversalis fascia. It is divided into the following three compartments:

1. The psoas compartment: a muscle that spans from the mediastinum to the thigh (Figure 16-9). The fascia attaches to the pelvic brim.

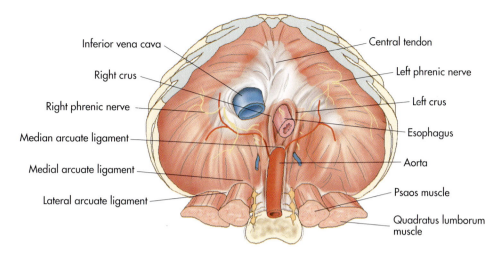

FIGURE 16-9 The psoas muscle extends from the mediastinum to the thigh.

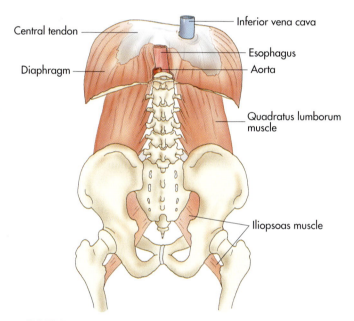

FIGURE 16-10 The quadratus lumborum muscle originates from the iliolumbar ligament, the adjacent iliac crest, and the superior borders of the transverse process of L3 and L4 and inserts into the margins of the 12th rib.

2. The lumbar region consists of the quadratus lumborum, a muscle that originates from the iliolumbar ligament, the adjacent iliac crest, and the superior borders of the transverse process of L3 and L4, and inserts into the margin of the 12th rib (Figure 16-10). It is adjoining and posterior to the colon, kidney, and psoas muscle.

3. The iliac area, which is made up of the iliacus and extends the length of the iliac fossa. The psoas passes through the iliac fossa medial to the iliacus and posterior to the iliac fascia (Figure 16-11). These two muscles merge as they extend into the true pelvis. The iliopsoas takes on a more anterior location caudally to lie along the lateral pelvic side wall.

Pelvic Retroperitoneum. The pelvic retroperitoneum lies between the sacrum and pubis from back to front, between the pelvic peritoneal reflection above and pelvic diaphragm (coccygeus and levator ani muscles) below, and between the obturator internus and piriformis muscles. There are four subdivisions: (1) prevesical, (2) rectovesical, (3) presacral, and (4) bilateral pararectal (and paravesical) spaces.

Prevesical and Rectovesical Spaces. The prevesical space spans from the pubis to the anterior margin of the bladder. It is bordered laterally by the obturator fascia. The connective tissue covering the bladder, seminal vesicles, and prostate is continuous with the fascial lamina within this space. The space is an extension of the retroperitoneal space of the anterior abdominal wall deep to the rectus sheath, which is continuous with the transversalis fascia. The space between the bladder and rectum is the rectovesical space (Figure 16-12).

Presacral Space. The presacral space lies between the rectum and fascia covering the sacrum and posterior pelvic floor musculature.

Bilateral Pararectal Space. The pararectal space is bounded laterally by the piriformis and levator ani fascia and medially by the rectum. It extends anteriorly from the bladder, medially to the obturator internus, and laterally to the external iliac vessels (Figures 16-13 and 16-14).

The paravesical and pararectal spaces are traversed by the two ureters. The pelvic wall muscles, iliac vessels, ureter, bladder, prostate, seminal vesicles, and cervix are retroperitoneal structures within the true pelvis. The obturator internus muscle lines the lateral aspect of the pelvis. Posteriorly the piriformis muscle is seen extending anterolaterally from the region of the sacrum.

Vascular Supply

Aorta. The aorta enters the abdomen posterior to the diaphragm at the level of L1 and passes posterior to the

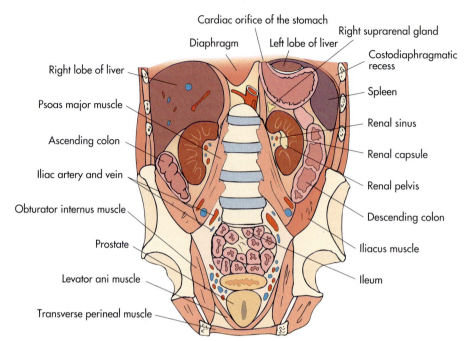

FIGURE 16-11 The iliacus muscle extends the length of the iliac fossa. The psoas muscle passes through the iliac fossa medial to the iliacus. The psoas and iliacus muscles merge as they extend into the true pelvis. The iliopsoas muscle takes on a more anterior location caudally to lie along the lateral pelvic side wall.

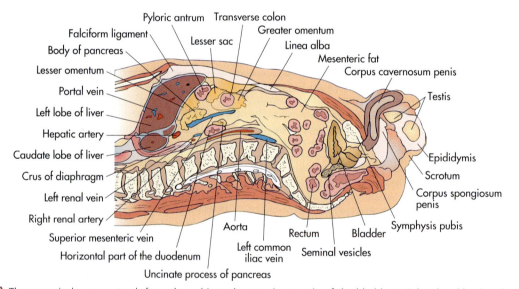

FIGURE 16-12 The prevesical space extends from the pubis to the anterior margin of the bladder. It is bordered by the obturator fascia on its lateral margins. The space between the bladder and rectum is the rectovesical space.

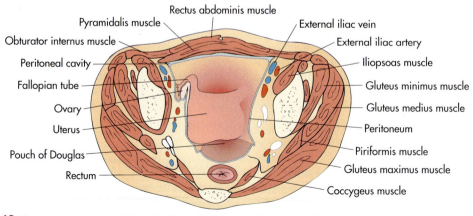

FIGURE 16-13 The pararectal space is bounded laterally by the piriformis and levator ani fascia and medially by the rectum.

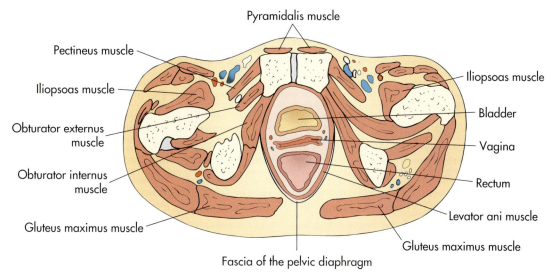

Pyramidalis muscle

Pectineus muscle

Iliopsoas muscle

Obturator externus muscle

Obturator internus muscle

Gluteus maximus muscle

Iliopsoas muscle

Bladder

Vagina

Rectum

Levator ani muscle

Gluteus maximus muscle

Fascia of the pelvic diaphragm

FIGURE 16-14 The pararectal space extends anteriorly from the bladder, medially to the obturator internus, and laterally to the external iliac vessels.

left lobe of the liver. The aorta has a straight horizontal course to the level of L4, where it bifurcates into the common iliac arteries. A slight anterior curve of the aorta is the result of lumbar lordosis.

Inferior Vena Cava. The inferior vena cava extends from the junction of the two common iliac veins to the right of L5 and travels cephalad. Unlike the aorta, it curves anterior toward its termination into the right atrial cavity.

Adrenal Glands. Three arteries supply each adrenal gland: the suprarenal branch of the inferior phrenic, the suprarenal branch of the aorta, and the suprarenal branch of the renal artery (see Figure 15-5). A single vein from the hilum of each gland drains into the inferior vena cava on the right, and on the left, the vein drains into the left renal vein.

PHYSIOLOGY AND LABORATORY DATA OF THE RETROPERITONEUM

Each adrenal gland is made up of two endocrine glands. The **cortex,** or outer part, secretes a range of steroid hormones; the **medulla,** or core, secretes epinephrine and norepinephrine.

Cortex

The steroids secreted by the adrenal cortex fall into the following three main categories: mineralocorticoids, glucocorticoids, and sex hormones (androgen and estrogen).

Mineralocorticoids. Mineralocorticoids regulate electrolyte metabolism. Aldosterone is the principal mineralocorticoid. It has a regulatory effect on the relative concentrations of mineral ions in the body fluids and therefore on the water content of tissue. An insufficiency of this steroid leads to increased excretion of sodium and

chloride ions, and water into the urine. This is accompanied by a fall in sodium, chloride, and bicarbonate concentrations in the blood, resulting in a lowered pH or acidosis.

Glucocorticoids. Glucocorticoids play a principal role in carbohydrate metabolism. They promote deposition of liver glycogen from proteins and inhibit use of glucose by the cells, thus increasing blood sugar level. Cortisone and hydrocortisone are the primary glucocorticoids. They diminish allergic response, especially the more serious inflammatory types (rheumatoid arthritis and rheumatic fever).

Sex Hormones. Androgens are the male sex hormones, and estrogens are the female sex hormones. The adrenal gland secretes both types of hormones regardless of the patient's gender. Normally these are secreted in minute quantities and have almost insignificant effects. With oversecretion, however, a marked effect is seen. Adrenal tumors in women can promote secondary masculine characteristics. Hypersecretion of the hormone in prepubertal boys accelerates adult masculine development and the growth of pubic hair. The adrenal cortex is controlled by **adrenocorticotropic hormone (ACTH)** from the pituitary. A diminished glucocorticoid blood concentration stimulates the secretion of ACTH. Consequent increase in adrenal cortex activity inhibits further ACTH secretion.

Hypofunction of the adrenal cortex in humans is called **Addison's disease.** Symptoms and signs include hypotension, general weakness, fatigue, loss of appetite and weight, and a characteristic bronzing of the skin (hyperpigmentation).

Oversecretion of the adrenal cortex may be caused by an overproduction of ACTH resulting from a pituitary tumor, **hyperplasia,** or a tumor in the cortex itself. Hypersecretion of the cortical hormones produces distinct syndromes. The features of the syndromes often overlap and can be either acquired or congenital. Adrenal hyperfunction can cause Cushing's syndrome, Conn's syndrome, or adrenogenital syndrome (see Adrenal Pathology).

Medulla

The adrenal medulla makes up the core of the gland in which groups of irregular cells are located amid veins that collect blood from the sinusoids. The adrenal medulla produces epinephrine and norepinephrine. Both of these hormones are amines, sometimes referred to as catecholamines. They elevate the blood pressure, the former working as an accelerator of the heart rate and the latter as a vasoconstrictor. The two hormones together promote glycogenolysis, the breakdown of liver glycogen to glucose, which causes an increase in blood sugar concentration.

The adrenal medulla is not essential for life and can be removed surgically without causing untreatable damage. An increase in the production of the medulla hormones may be caused by a **pheochromocytoma**.

SONOGRAPHIC EVALUATION OF THE RETROPERITONEUM

No specific patient preparation is necessary to image the retroperitoneal cavity, although 6 to 8 hours of fasting may help to eliminate bowel gas. To image the retroperitoneum, scans should be made in the longitudinal and transverse planes from the diaphragm to the iliac crest, with the patient in a supine or prone position, and from the crest to the symphysis, with the patient in a supine position and having a full bladder. The upper abdomen may also be scanned with the patient in a decubitus position. All scans should include the kidneys and retroperitoneal muscles.

Adrenal Glands

Although sonography has proven useful in evaluating soft tissue structures within the abdominal cavity, visualization of the adrenal glands has been difficult because of their small size, medial location, and surrounding perirenal fat. Sonography is not the imaging modality of choice for evaluation of an adrenal mass. If the adrenal gland becomes enlarged secondary to disease, it is easier to image and separate from the upper pole of the kidney.

Visualization of the adrenal area depends on several factors: the size of the patient and the amount of perirenal fat surrounding the adrenal area, the presence of bowel gas, and the ability to move the patient into multiple positions.

With the patient in the decubitus position, the sonographer should attempt to align the kidney and ipsilateral paravertebral vessels (inferior vena cava or aorta). The right adrenal gland has a "comma" or triangular shape in the transaxial plane. The best visualization is obtained by a transverse scan with the patient in a left lateral decubitus position. When the patient assumes this position, the inferior vena cava moves forward, and the aorta rolls over the crus of the diaphragm, offering a good window to image the upper pole of the right kidney and adrenal gland. If the patient is obese, it may be difficult to recognize the triangular- or crescent-shaped adrenal gland. The adrenal should not appear rounded; if it does, the finding suggests a pathologic process.

The longitudinal scan is made through the right lobe of the liver, perpendicular to the linear right crus of the diaphragm. The retroperitoneal fat must be recognized as separate from the liver, crus of the diaphragm, adrenal gland, and great vessel (Figure 16-15).

The left adrenal gland is closely related to the left crus of the diaphragm and the anterior-superior-medial aspect of the upper pole of the left kidney. It may be more difficult to image the left adrenal gland because of the stomach gas interference. The patient should be placed in a right lateral decubitus position and transverse scans made in an attempt to align the left kidney and the aorta. The left adrenal gland is seen by scanning along the posterior axillary line (Figure 16-16). The patient should be in deep inspiration in an effort to bring the adrenal and renal area into better view.

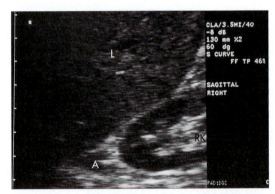

FIGURE 16-15 Longitudinal scan of the right adrenal gland is made through the right lobe of the liver (*L*), adrenal gland (*A*), and upper pole of the right kidney (*RK*).

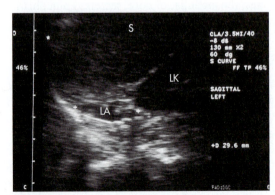

FIGURE 16-16 Longitudinal scan of the left adrenal gland (*LA*) and the anterior superior aspect of the upper pole of the left kidney (*LK*) and spleen (*S*).

Sonography Pitfalls

- Right crus of the diaphragm
- Second portion of the duodenum
- Gastroesophageal junction (cephalad to the left adrenal gland)
- Medial lobulations of the spleen
- Splenic vasculature
- Body-tail region of the pancreas
- Fourth portion of the duodenum

The normal right adrenal gland can be visualized in more than 90% of patients, whereas the left is seen in 80% of patients.

Diaphragmatic Crura

The crus of the diaphragm may be imaged in the transverse or longitudinal coronal plane. The right crus is seen in a plane that passes through the right lobe of the liver, kidney, and adrenal gland (Figure 16-17). The left crus is seen using the spleen and left kidney as a window, with the crus to the left of the aorta.

Para-aortic Lymph Nodes

Sonography patterns associated with nodes include rounded, focal, echo-poor lesions (1 to 3 cm in size and larger), and confluent, echo-poor masses, which often displace the kidney laterally. The sonographer may also detect a "mantle" of nodes in the paraspinal location, a "floating" or anteriorly displaced aorta secondary to the enlarged nodes or the mesenteric "sandwich" sign representing the anterior and posterior node masses surrounding mesenteric vessels (Figures 16-18 to 16-21).

The lymph nodes lie along the lateral and anterior margins of the aorta and inferior vena cava (Figures 16-22 and 16-23); thus, the best scanning is done with the patient in the supine or decubitus position. A left

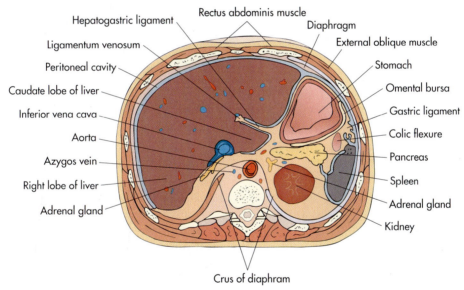

FIGURE 16-17 The right crus of the diaphragm passes posterior to the inferior vena cava, and the left crus passes anterior to the aorta.

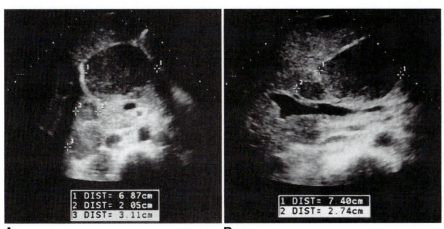

A   B

FIGURE 16-18 A, A 39-year-old female with lymphoma. Three nodes were seen peripancreatic (*crossbars*): *1,* anterior to the pancreas; *2,* lateral to the pancreas head; and *3,* paracaval. **B,** Two nodes paraportal (*crossbars*): *1,* anterior and compressing the main portal vein; and *2,* a smaller, sonolucent homogeneous node.

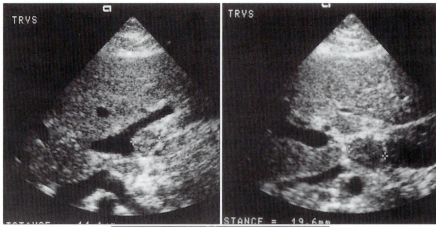

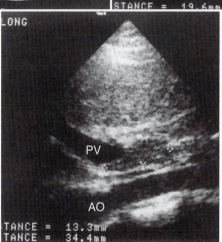

FIGURE 16-19 A 32-year-old female with right upper quadrant pain and fever. Two paracaval nodes were seen anterior to the aorta *(AO)* and inferior to the portal vein *(PV)*.

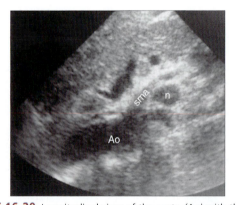

FIGURE 16-20 Longitudinal view of the aorta *(Ao)* with the superior mesenteric artery *(sma)*. If the angle of the SMA exceeds 15 degrees, lymphadenopathy should be considered. *N*, Node.

coronal view using the left kidney as a window may be used to discover para-aortic nodes (Figure 16-24).

It is always important to examine the patient in two planes because in only one plane the enlarged nodes may mimic an aortic aneurysm or tumor.

Longitudinal scans may be made first to outline the aorta and to search for enlarged lymph nodes. The aorta provides an excellent background for the hypoechoic nodes. Scans should begin at the midline, and the transducer should be angled both to the left and right at small angles to image the anterior and lateral borders of the aorta and inferior vena cava.

Transverse scans are made from the level of the xiphoid to the symphysis. Careful identification of the great vessels, organ structures, and muscles is important. Patterns of a fluid-filled duodenum or bowel may make it difficult to outline the great vessels or may cause confusion in diagnosing **lymphadenopathy.**

Scans below the umbilicus are more difficult because of interference from the small bowel. Careful attention should be given to the psoas and iliacus muscles within the pelvis where the iliac arteries run along their medial border. Both muscles serve as a hypoechoic marker along the pelvic side wall. Enlarged lymph nodes can be identified anterior and medial to these margins. A smooth sharp border of the muscle indicates no nodal involvement. The bladder should be filled to help push the small bowel out of the pelvis and to serve as an acoustic window to better image the vascular structures. Color Doppler may be used to help delineate the vascular structures.

Splenomegaly should also be evaluated in patients with lymphadenopathy. As the sonographer moves caudal from the xiphoid, attention should be on the splenic size and great vessel area to detect nodal

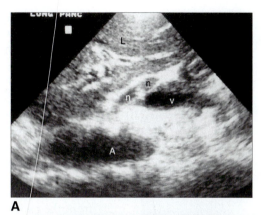

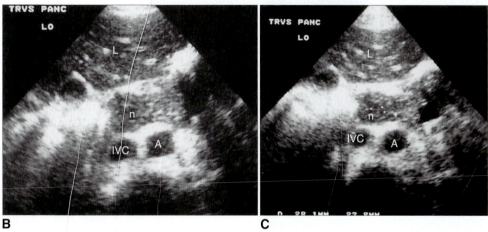

FIGURE 16-21 A 46-year-old male with a history of acquired immune deficiency syndrome (AIDS). Liver function tests were abnormal. Hepatosplenomegaly was present. Adjacent to the pancreas are numerous small nodal masses, the largest measuring 2 cm. **A,** Longitudinal view. *A,* aorta; *L,* liver; *n,* nodes; *v,* superior mesenteric vein. **B** and **C,** Transverse view. *A,* aorta; *IVC,* inferior vena cava; *L,* liver; *n,* nodes.

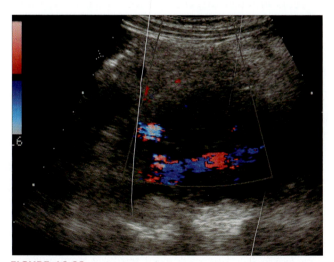

FIGURE 16-22 Sagittal view of lymph nodes anterior and posterior to the aorta, the "sandwich sign." *(Courtesy M. Robert DeJong, RDMS, RVT, FSDMS.)*

involvement near the hilus of the spleen (Figures 16-25 and 16-26).

Lymph nodes remain as consistent patterns, whereas bowel and the duodenum display changing peristaltic patterns when imaged with a sonogram. As gentle pres-sure is applied with the transducer in an effort to displace the bowel, the lymph nodes remain constant in shape. The echo pattern posterior to each structure is different. Lymph nodes are homogeneous and thus transmit sound easily; the bowel presents a more complex pattern with dense central echoes from its mucosal pattern. Often the duodenum has air within its walls, causing a shadow posteriorly. Enlarged lymph nodes should be reproducible on a sonogram in two projections. After the abdomen is completely scanned, repeat sections over the enlarged nodes should demonstrate the same pattern as on the earlier scan.

PATHOLOGY OF THE RETROPERITONEUM

Adrenal Cortical Syndromes

The cortical syndromes that the sonographer may encounter while scanning for an adrenal mass are as follows:

- *Addison's disease (adrenocortical insufficiency).* Affects males and females equally and can be diag-nosed in any age group. It is characterized by atrophy

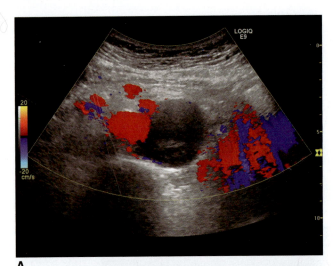

A,

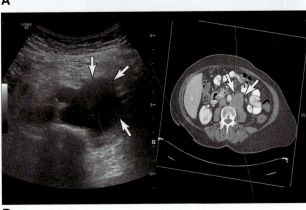

B,

FIGURE 16-23 A, Transverse view of the aorta with a large para-aortic node. **B,** Sonogram and CT of a large para-aortic lymph node (arrows). *(Courtesy Robert DeJong, RDMS, RVT, FSDMS.)*

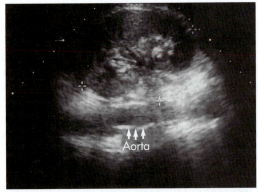

FIGURE 16-24 Decubitus scan using the left kidney as a window to see the aorta.

of the adrenal cortex with decreased production of cortisol and sometimes aldosterone. Usually the majority of the cortical tissue is destroyed before adrenal insufficiency is diagnosed. Primary causes of reduced adrenal cortical tissue include an autoimmune process, tuberculosis (TB), an inflammatory process, a primary neoplasm, or metastases.

Secondary adrenal insufficiencies are caused by pituitary dysfunction and a decrease in production of the pituitary hormone ACTH (adrenocorticotropic hormone). The clinical signs and symptoms usually manifest during metabolic stress or trauma. Symptoms include increased sodium retention, which leads to tissue edema; increased plasma volume; increased potassium excretion; hyperpigmentation; and a mild alkalosis. Fatigue and muscle and bone weakness are common. Prognosis is good with steroid replacement therapy.

- *Adrenogenital syndrome (adrenal virilism).* Results from the excessive secretion of the sex hormones and adrenal androgens. It is caused either by an adrenal tumor or by hyperplasia. The symptoms and clinical signs vary depending on the age and sex of the person. In a newborn there may be ambiguous genitalia with or without adrenal hyperplasia. (Things other than adrenal hyperplasia can also cause ambiguous genitalia.) Adrenal virilism has masculinizing effects on adult women. The clinical signs and symptoms in a female adult include hirsutism, baldness, and acne; deepening of the voice; atrophy of the uterus; decreased breast size; clitoral hypertrophy; and increased muscularity. Prepubescent males will have signs of masculine development, deepening voice, and an increase in body hair. The imaging modality of choice to confirm the presence or absence of an adrenal tumor is computerized tomography (CT) and magnetic resonance imaging (MRI) scan.

- *Conn's syndrome (aldosteronism).* Conn's syndrome occurs in 0.5% of patients with sustained hypertension and is caused by excessive secretion of aldosterone, usually because of a cortical **adenoma** of the glomerulosa cells or less frequent causes, including adrenal hyperplasia or adrenal carcinoma. Hyperplasia is more common in males and adrenal adenomas are more common in females. Adenomas measure 0.5 to 3 cm in diameter and contralateral adrenal atrophy is identified. Clinical signs and symptoms include muscle weakness, hypertension, and abnormal electrocardiogram. If an adenoma is causing the hyperaldosteronism, removal of the adenoma is performed. In rare cases a bilateral adrenalectomy is necessary. In cases of secondary aldosteronism, the hypertension may be caused by renal artery disease.

- *Cushing's syndrome.* **Cushing's syndrome** is caused by excessive secretion of cortisol resulting from adrenal hyperplasia, cortical adenoma, adrenal carcinoma, or elevated ACTH resulting from a pituitary adenoma. Cushing's syndrome symptoms include truncal obesity, pencil thin extremities, "buffalo hump," "moon face," hypertension, renal stones, irregular menses in females, and psychiatric disturbances. If an adrenal tumor is present, the secretion of androgens may increase and cause masculinizing effects in women. Cushing's syndrome can also be caused by an anterior pituitary

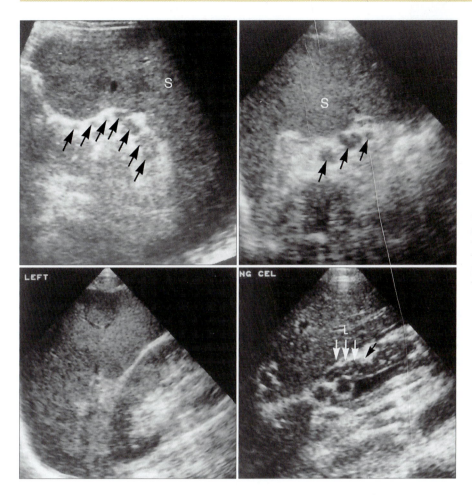

FIGURE 16-25 Splenomegaly should be evaluated in patients with lymphadenopathy. Enlarged nodes are seen in the area of the hilus of the spleen *(S)*. This patient also has a metastatic lesion near the periphery of the spleen. *L,* liver.

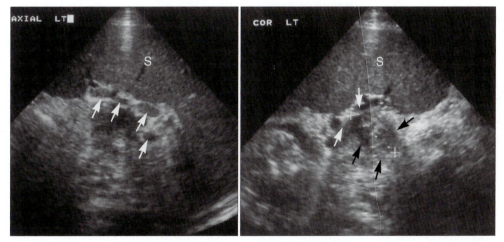

FIGURE 16-26 Axial and coronal scans of a patient with splenomegaly and enlarged nodes in the area of the splenic hilus. Color flow imaging should be used to document that the lesions are nodes and not dilated vascular structures. *Arrows,* nodes; *S,* spleen.

tumor. Treatment to decrease the production of cortisol varies depending on the cause of the hypersecretion. If an adrenalectomy is performed, the patient will require replacement steroids for life. Functioning adrenal adenomas are usually small 2 to 5 cm, and hypoechoic. They typically are associated with contralateral adrenal atrophy.

- *Waterhouse-Friderichsen syndrome.* With Waterhouse-Friderichsen syndrome there is a fulminant bacterial sepsis, shock, and necropsy with evidence of bilateral adrenal hemorrhage that is complicated with acute adrenocortical insufficiency in up to 25% of severely traumatized patients. Adrenal hemorrhage may occur 20% bilateral, which most often is caused by severe

TABLE 16-1	Adrenal Pathology	
Adrenal Diseases	**Hormone Secreted**	**Distinguishing Characteristics**
Addison's disease	Hyposecretion of cortisol, aldosterone	Increases when there is stress or trauma Hypotension, general weakness, loss of appetite, (hyperpigmentation) bronzing of skin, may have renal failure
Adrenogenital syndrome	Excessive secretion of androgens (male) Excessive secretion of estrogen (female)	Prepubertal males accelerate adult masculine development and growth of pubic hair Female: masculine characteristics
Conn's syndrome	Excessive secretion of aldosterone	Cortical adenoma, carcinoma
Cushing's syndrome	Excessive secretion of glucocorticoids	Hyperplasia, benign tumor, carcinoma
Waterhouse-Friderichsen syndrome		Bilateral hemorrhage into adrenal glands
Medulla tumor Pheochromocytoma	Excessive secretion of epinephrine and norepinephrine	Intermittent hypertension; large tumor with varied sonographic pattern (cystic, solid, calcified components)

meningococcal infection. It is characterized by acute adrenal gland insufficiency, which is fatal if not treated immediately. With sonography, depending on the stage of hemorrhage, the echo pattern can range from a hyperechoic to an anechoic suprarenal mass. Subsequently, over a period of time, the mass may shrink, and calcifications may appear as focal hyperechoic areas with acoustic shadowing (Table 16-1).

Adrenal Cysts

Adrenal cysts are uncommon lesions that produce no clinical symptoms when the lesion is small. The cysts affect females more often than males (3:1). Adrenal cysts are usually unilateral and tend to be found incidentally. They may vary in size and can be unilocular or multilocular.

Sonographic Findings. Sonographically, adrenal cysts present a typical cystic pattern, with a strong posterior wall, no internal echoes, and good through-transmission. Adrenal cysts have the tendency to become calcified, which gives them the sonographic appearance of a somewhat sonolucent solid mass appearing with a sharp posterior border and poor through-transmission. (Figures 16-27 and 16-28). Hemorrhage within the cyst would appear as a complex mass with multiple internal echoes and good through-transmission.

Adrenal Hemorrhage

Adrenal hemorrhage in adults is rare and is usually caused by severe trauma or infection. Posttraumatic hemorrhage is usually unilateral and does not cause any major clinical problems. A bilateral hemorrhage may cause adrenal insufficiency. Adrenal hemorrhages are more common in neonates who experienced a traumatic delivery with stress, asphyxia, and septicemia. The adrenal glands in a neonate are very vascular and the

glands are proportionally larger than in an adult. Clinical signs and symptoms include abdominal mass, anemia, and hyperbilirubinemia.

Sonographic Findings. The sonographic appearance of an adrenal hemorrhage will vary depending on the age of the hemorrhage. The adrenal gland will appear as a solid mass initially, and over time the mass will have a more cystic or complex appearance. As the hemorrhage resolves, the mass will decrease in size. The adrenal gland may go back to a normal size with focal areas of calcification (Figure 16-29).

Adrenal Tumors

Sonography can detect 90% of known adrenal masses that were first detected by CT. Sonography is used to characterize a known adrenal mass as cystic or solid, evaluate the position and patency of the IVC and draining veins, evaluate tumor invasion into adjacent structure, and determine the origin of a large retroperitoneal mass. Sonography is also used to follow an adrenal mass that is not surgically removed.

Adrenal Adenoma. Benign nonfunctioning adenoma is the most common primary adrenal tumor. Adrenal nodules are usually less than 2.5 cm. There is a high incidence of adrenal adenomas in older patients with diabetes or hypertension. A significant percentage of the malignant adrenal adenomas may be due to metastases.

Sonographic Findings. In nonfunctioning adenomas, sonographic findings demonstrate a well-defined, round, slightly hypoechoic homogeneous mass. Almost always the mass is detected as an incidental finding. On rare occasions the mass may be so large that it may compress the adjacent structures.

Further pathology of the adrenal glands is related to the tumors arising within them and their hyposecretion or hypersecretion of hormones. Rare nonfunctional adrenal tumors include myelolipomas, hemangiomas,

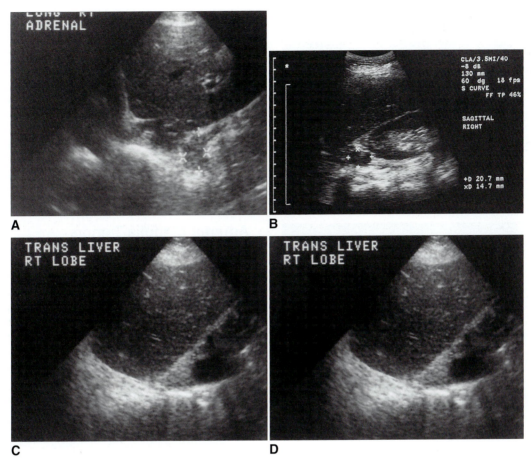

FIGURE 16-27 A, B, Small adrenal cyst is imaged on this longitudinal scan of the right kidney in two asymptomatic females. **C, D,** Transverse images of patient in **(A)** with small adrenal cyst.

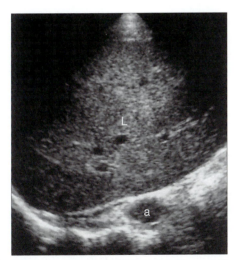

FIGURE 16-28 Adrenal cysts *(a)* may become calcified, which gives them the ultrasound appearance of a "solid" mass with decreased transmission. *L,* liver.

teratomas, lipomas, and fibromas. These tumors are typically not seen on a sonogram and are more frequently imaged with CT or MRI.

Adrenal Malignant Tumors. Primary adrenal carcinomas are rare and may be hyperfunctional or nonfunc-tional. Hyperfunctional malignant tumors are more common in females. Adrenal malignant tumors may be a cause of Cushing's syndrome, Conn's syndrome, or adrenogenital syndrome. The origin of the tumor should be clearly defined. Functional tumors tend to be smaller than nonfunctional tumors because they are typically diagnosed earlier. The tumors are homogeneous with the same echogenicity as the renal cortex (Figure 16-30). The larger neoplasms tend to be nonfunctional and heterogeneous, with a central area of necrosis and hemorrhage.

Sonographic Findings. If the mass is small (2 to 6 cm), it is well defined and homogeneous. If the mass is larger, it tends to have necrosis with central hemor-rhage and often calcifies. In color Doppler, the tumor is hypervascular with a high incidence of invasion of the adrenal or renal vein, IVC, hepatic veins, and lymph nodes. The sonographic appearance of a mass cannot be used to differentiate between a benign or malignant tumor, as this is a histologic diagnosis.

Metastasis. Adrenals glands are the fourth most common site in the body for metastasis, after the lung, liver, and the bones. Primarily there are metastases from lung in 33%, breast carcinomas in 30%, followed by melanoma, gastric carcinoma, colon, kidney, and thyroid.

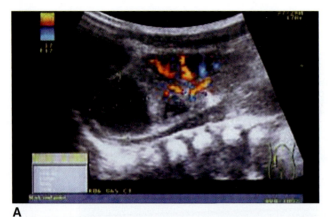

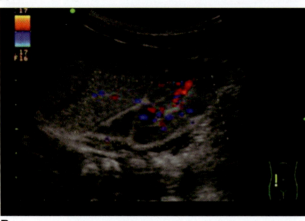

FIGURE 16-29 A, Color Doppler shows a normal kidney displaced inferiorly. **B,** Two months later the hemorrhage is almost reabsorbed and the normal adrenal gland is almost normal.

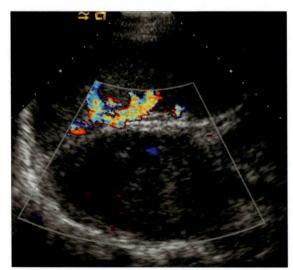

FIGURE 16-30 A coronal scan through the spleen with a large left malignant adrenal mass compressing the splenic hilum. *(Courtesy Robert DeJong, RDMS, RVT, FSDMS.)*

Bilateral involvement is seen in more than half of the patients. Metastases to the adrenal gland typically cause adrenal insufficiency.

Sonographic Findings. Adrenal glands vary in size and echogenicity. Metastatic lesions have a nonspecific appearance. Large masses may contain areas of necrosis and hemorrhage. Sometimes differentiation of a common benign adenoma from a metastatic lesion is difficult when there is no other evidence of metastatic disease and the adrenal mass is unilateral (Figures 16-31 and 16-32). Often central necrosis causes sonolucent areas within the tumor.

Adrenal Medulla Tumors

Pheochromocytoma. The pheochromocytes of the adrenal medulla may produce a tumor called a **pheochromocytoma,** which secretes epinephrine and norepinephrine in excessive quantities. A small percentage of patients will have ectopic adrenal pheochromocytomas rising from the **neuroectodermal tissue;** these tumors tend to be malignant. The clinical symptoms include

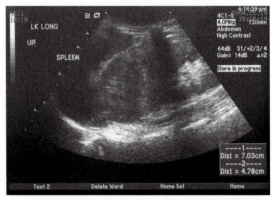

FIGURE 16-31 Sagittal image of a 7.3 × 6.7 × 7.0 cm heterogeneous echogenic left adrenal mass. This mass represents either a metastatic mass or adrenal carcinoma. *(Courtesy Elizabeth Polanno, Beth Israel Center, North, New York.)*

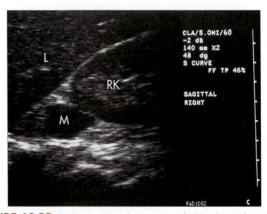

FIGURE 16-32 Patient with a large mass *(M)* in the right adrenal gland representing metastases from a melanoma. *L,* liver; *M,* mass; *RK,* right kidney.

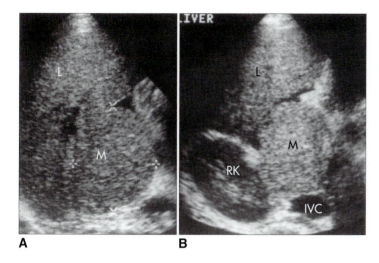

FIGURE 16-33 The pheochromocytoma is a homogeneous tumor that has a weak posterior wall and decreased through-transmission. This tumor can grow quite large. **A,** Longitudinal view. *L,* liver; *M,* mass. **B,** Transverse view. *IVC,* inferior vena cava; *M,* mass; *RK,* right kidney.

intermittent hypertension, severe headaches, heart palpitations, and excess perspiration. Treatment usually is removal of the tumor.

▪ **Sonographic Findings.** The tumor has a homogeneous pattern that can be differentiated from a cyst by its weak posterior wall and poor through-transmission (Figure 16-33). Pheochromocytomas are usually unilateral and may be large, bulky tumors with a variety of sonographic patterns, including cystic, solid, and calcified components.

Adrenal Neuroblastoma. The adrenal **neuroblastoma** is the most common malignancy of the adrenal glands in childhood and the most common tumor of infancy, representing 30% of all neonatal tumors. Neuroblastoma is a well encapsulated tumor that usually displaces the kidney inferiorly and laterally and elevates levels of the vanillylmandelic acid-VMA and homovanillic acid-HVA. More than 90% of fetal neuroblastomas are located in the adrenal glands, and 50% of these have cystic components. Generally, the tumor develops within the adrenal medulla. Although children are usually asymptomatic, some do present with a palpable abdominal mass that must be differentiated from a neonatal hemorrhage and hydronephrosis. It is known to be one of the most common tumors of childhood. Spontaneous regression is common before the age of one. Otherwise it has a poor prognosis and is not responsive to either irradiation or chemotherapy.

▪ **Sonographic Findings.** Lesions generally are heterogeneously echogenic with poorly defined margins. A small percentage of neuroblastomas demonstrate internal calcifications with anechoic "cystic" areas. The "ultrasound lobule" (an area of increased echogenicity in the tumor) seems to be characteristic for neuroblastomas. The use of color Doppler may be helpful in demonstrating capsular flow and low-resistance arterial waveforms (Figure 16-34). Evaluation of the surrounding retroperitoneum and liver should be made to rule out metastases. When a large, solid, upper abdominal mass is identified in an infant or young child, the differential diagnosis should include neuroblastoma, Wilms' tumor (nephroblastoma), and hepatoblastoma.

Retroperitoneal Fat

The anatomic origin of the right upper quadrant mass may be difficult to determine. The reflection produced by the retroperitoneal fat is displaced in a characteristic manner by masses originating from this area. This pattern of displacement helps to localize the origin of the mass. Retroperitoneal lesions cause ventral and often cranial displacement of the lesion.

▪ **Sonographic Findings.** The lesions in the liver or in Morison's pouch displace the echoes posterior and inferior, whereas renal and adrenal lesions cause anterior displacement of structures. An extrahepatic mass may shift the inferior vena cava anteromedially (anterior displacement of right kidney).

Primary Retroperitoneal Tumors

A primary retroperitoneal tumor (PRT) is one that originates independently within the retroperitoneal space. Primary malignancies are more common than benign neoplasms, but both are rare.

Lymphoma is the most common primary retroperitoneal tumor. Sonographic evaluation for abdominal lymphoma is performed to determine the presence or absence of lymphadenopathy and the primary areas to be evaluated include the hepatic and splenic hilum, origin of celiac and SMA (peripancreatic, mesenteric), para-aortic, and renal hilar areas. Accuracy of sonographic detection is close to 90% when the lymph nodes are larger than 2 cm in diameter. The sonographic appearance varies from round, hypoechoic masses to anechoic masses with good posterior enhancement. Color Doppler shows increased intranodal vascularity. The primary criteria for differentiating a malignant from a benign lymph node are size > 2 cm; shape, round; and resistive index (RI) > 0.70 (Figures 16-35 and 16-36).

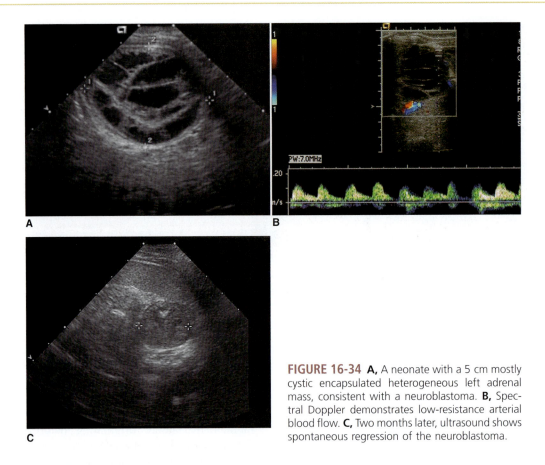

FIGURE 16-34 A, A neonate with a 5 cm mostly cystic encapsulated heterogeneous left adrenal mass, consistent with a neuroblastoma. **B,** Spectral Doppler demonstrates low-resistance arterial blood flow. **C,** Two months later, ultrasound shows spontaneous regression of the neuroblastoma.

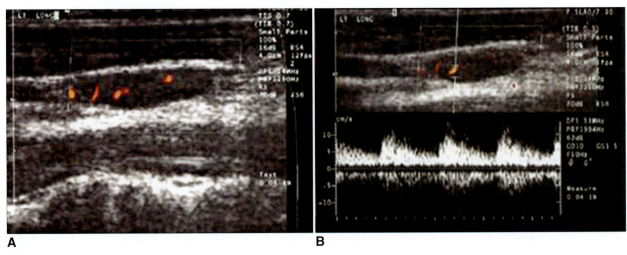

FIGURE 16-35 A, Oval slightly hypoechoic lymph node with normal benign vascularity. **B,** RI 0.63 typical for a benign lymph node.

The other PRT can develop anywhere with most tumors proving to be malignant. The tumor is derived either from mesenchymal or neurogenic tissues. Mesenchymal tumors develop within connective tissues of the retroperitoneum, and most fat-containing tumors are liposarcomas, which is the third most common malignant tumor of soft tissues. More than one third of the tumors originate from perirenal fat including malignant fibrous histiocytomas, fibrosarcomas, and desmoid tumors. All of these tumors are nonspecific by sonography.

Neurogenic tumors are usually encountered in the paravertebral region, where they rise from nerve roots or sympathetic chain ganglia. They extend into the retroperitoneum and may be classified as benign or malignant tumors. The sonographic patterns of neurogenic tumors are quite variable.

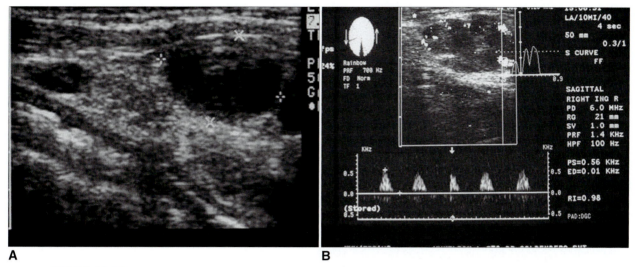

FIGURE 16-36 **A** 1.6 cm round malignant lymph node. **B.** Typical high RI in a malignant lymph node. RI = 0.98.

Tumors of Muscle Origin. Leiomyosarcoma is the second most common PRT. This tumor may originate from smooth muscles of small blood vessels or within GI-tract and extend into the retroperitoneum. On sonography leiomyosarcomas generally present as a large complex mass with areas of necrosis and cystic degeneration.

Fibrosarcomas and rhabdomyosarcomas may be quite invasive and may infiltrate widely into muscles and adjoining soft tissue. They often extend across the midline and appear similar to lymphomas. Sonographically, they are highly reflective tumors.

Germ Cell Tumors. Germ cell tumors can be either benign or malignant and the retroperitoneal space is the fourth most frequent site (ovaries, testes, anterior mediastinum, retroperitoneum, and sacrococcygeal region). Teratomatous tumors may arise within the upper retroperitoneum and the pelvis. They may contain calcified echoes from bones, cartilage, teeth, and soft tissue elements.

Teratomas are seen more commonly in childhood and are usually located in the upper pole of the left kidney. Sonographically they are heterogeneous tumors with solid areas, calcifications, and cystic spaces.

Secondary Retroperitoneal Tumors

Metastatic disease may occur anywhere in the retroperitoneum, secondary to hematogenous, or lymphatic spread, or by direct extension. The most common primary malignancies that spread into the retroperitoneum are from the breast, lung, testis, or the recurrence of previously resected urologic or gynecologic tumor.

Ascitic fluid, along with a retroperitoneal tumor, usually indicates seeding or invasion of the peritoneal surface. Evaluation of the para-aortic region should be made for extension to the lymph nodes. The liver should also be evaluated for metastatic involvement.

Retroperitoneal Fluid Collections

Urinoma. A urinoma is a walled-off collection of extravasated urine that develops spontaneously after trauma, surgery, or a subacute or chronic urinary obstruction. Urinomas usually collect around the kidney or upper ureter in the perinephric space. Occasionally urinomas dissect into the pelvis and compress the bladder.

◣ **Sonographic Findings.** Generally the sonographic pattern of urinomas is sonolucent unless they become infected.

Hemorrhage. A retroperitoneal hemorrhage may occur in a variety of conditions, including trauma, vasculitis, bleeding diathesis, a leaking aortic aneurysm, or a bleeding neoplasm.

◣ **Sonographic Findings.** Sonographically the hemorrhage may be well localized and produce displacement of other organs, or it may present as a poorly defined infiltrative process. Fresh hematomas present as sonolucent areas, whereas an organized thrombus with clot formation shows echo densities within the mass. Calcification may be seen in long-standing hematomas.

Abscess. Abscess formation may result from surgery, trauma, or perforation of the bowel or duodenum.

◣ **Sonographic Findings.** Sonographically the abscess usually has a complex pattern with debris. Gas within the abscess causes a "reflective" pattern on sonography and casts an acoustic shadow. The sonographer should be careful not to mistake a gas-containing abscess for "bowel" patterns. The radiograph should be evaluated in this case. The abscess frequently extends along or within the muscle planes, is of an irregular shape, and

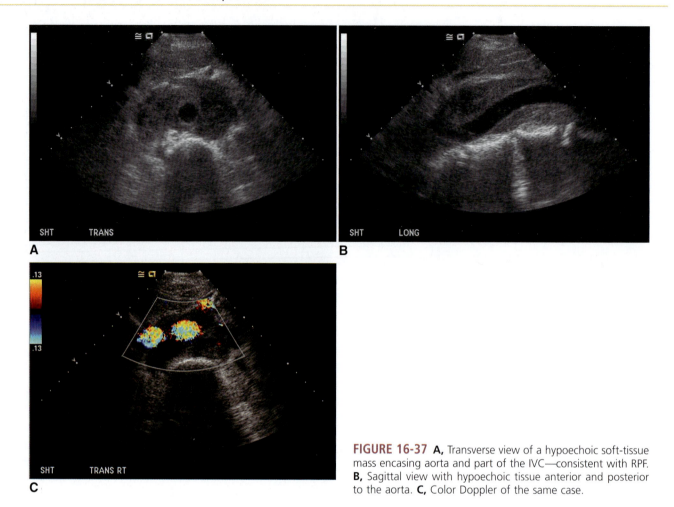

FIGURE 16-37 A, Transverse view of a hypoechoic soft-tissue mass encasing aorta and part of the IVC—consistent with RPF. **B,** Sagittal view with hypoechoic tissue anterior and posterior to the aorta. **C,** Color Doppler of the same case.

lies in the most dependent portion of the retroperitoneal space.

Retroperitoneal Fibrosis (Ormond's Disease)

Retroperitoneal fibrosis (RPF) is an idiopathic condition characterized by thick sheets of fibrous tissue in the retroperitoneal cavity. The fibrosis may encase and obstruct the ureters and vena cava, with resultant hydronephrosis. RPF can be also associated with infiltrating neoplasms, acute immune diseases (Crohn's disease),

ulcerative colitis, sclerosing cholangitis, and so on. Clinically the patient may present with abdominal pain, hypertension, and oligo-anuria. Radiographically an intravenous pyelogram shows medial displacement and bilateral (one third are unilateral) hydronephrosis. Sonography may demonstrate abnormal hypoechoic tissue surrounding the anterolateral aspect of the aorta or IVC. Sonography may also be useful to evaluate the kidneys, as well as fibrosis regression in response to steroids. Further imaging with CT may be necessary to establish whether there is a benign or malignant disease process (Figure 16-37).

The Peritoneal Cavity and Abdominal Wall

Sandra L. Hagen-Ansert

ANATOMY AND SONOGRAPHIC EVALUATION OF THE PERITONEAL CAVITY AND ABDOMINAL WALL

Peritoneal Cavity

The peritoneal cavity is made up of multiple peritoneal ligaments and folds that connect the viscera to each other and to the abdominopelvic walls. Within the cavity are the lesser and greater **omentum**, the mesenteries, the ligaments, and multiple fluid spaces (lesser sac, perihepatic and **subphrenic** spaces). The peritoneum is a smooth membrane that lines the entire abdominal cavity and is reflected over the contained organs. The part that lines the walls of the cavity is the parietal peritoneum, whereas the part covering the abdominal organs to a greater or lesser extent is the visceral peritoneum. In the male, the peritoneum forms a closed cavity; in the female, there is a "communication" outside the peritoneum through the uterine tubes, uterus, and vagina. In reality, however, the complex linings of the uterus and fallopian tubes tend to close off any potential space and prohibit the entrance of air into the peritoneal cavity.

The relationship of the peritoneum to the abdominal structures may be understood with the visualization of an inflated balloon (the peritoneum) within an empty box (the abdominal cavity) (Figure 17-1). If one were to place objects within the box, yet outside the balloon, these objects might impinge on the balloon shape. This is the same condition that the kidneys and the ascending and descending colon have on the peritoneal cavity. Because these structures lie along the posterior surface of the peritoneal cavity, they are considered "retroperitoneal," and they are overlaid by visceral peritoneum. If an object bulges so far into the balloon that it loses contact with the box, the object would become surrounded by a fold of the balloon. This is the situation with the small intestine, transverse colon, and the sigmoid colon; they are suspended from the posterior abdominal wall by a double fold of peritoneum called the **mesentery**, transverse mesocolon, and sigmoid mesocolon. Thus, the peritoneal cavity is really empty of abdominal organs, as they bulge into or are covered by the cavity but are not located within the cavity.

The general peritoneal cavity is known as the greater sac of the peritoneum. With the development of the

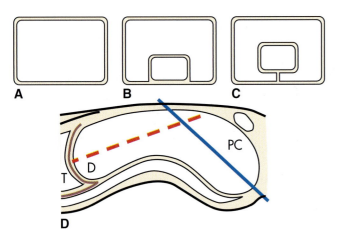

FIGURE 17-1 A, The "abdominal cavity" containing a "balloon" (peritoneum). **B,** An organ inside the abdomen and partly covered by peritoneum, such as the kidney, which is said to be in the retroperitoneal cavity. **C,** An organ suspended from the abdominal wall by a fold of peritoneum, such as the small intestine suspended by its mesentery. **D,** When supine, the backward tilt of the pelvis makes it the lowest part of the peritoneal cavity. Long axis of abdomen *(dotted line)*; long axis of pelvis *(solid line)*; *PC,* pelvic part of peritoneal cavity; *D,* diaphragm; *T,* thorax.

stomach and the spleen, a smaller sac, called the lesser sac (omental bursa), is the peritoneal recess posterior to the stomach (Figure 17-2). This sac communicates with the greater sac through a small vertical opening known as the epiploic foramen. The epiploic foramen is just inferior to the liver and superior to the first part of the duodenum; the inferior vena cava is posterior, and the portal vein is anterior.

The attachments of the peritoneum to the abdominal walls and organs help determine the way abnormal collections of fluid within the peritoneal cavity can collect or move. When the patient is lying supine, the lowest part of the body is the pelvis (Figure 17-3). On a transverse view, the flanks are lower than the midabdomen. Fluid will accumulate in the lowest parts of the body; therefore, the pelvis and lateral flanks (**gutters**) should be carefully examined for pathologic collections of fluid.

The lesser omentum is a double layer of peritoneum, extending from the liver to the lesser curvature of the stomach. This structure acts as a sling for the stomach, suspending it from the liver.

The greater omentum is an apron-like fold of peritoneum that hangs from the greater curvature of the stomach (Figure 17-4). The omentum lies freely over the intestine except for the upper part, which is fused with the transverse colon and mesocolon. The greater omentum is able to adhere to diseased organs, which in turn helps prevent further spread of infected fluid by essentially "walling it off" from the rest of the body. The greater omentum is profusely supplied with blood vessels

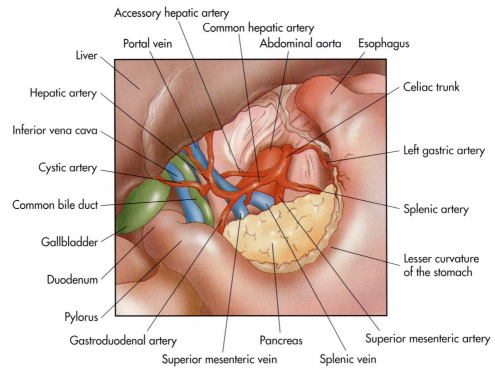

FIGURE 17-2 Upper abdominal dissection, with part of the left lobe of the liver and the lesser omentum removed to show the celiac trunk, portal vein, bile duct, and related structures.

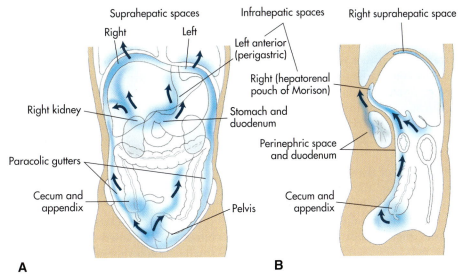

FIGURE 17-3 **A,** Anterior view of the collection of fluid in the abdominal and pelvic cavities. **B,** Sagittal view of the right abdomen shows how the fluid collects in the most dependent areas of the abdomen and pelvis.

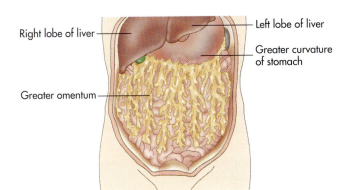

FIGURE 17-4 Anterior view of the greater omentum.

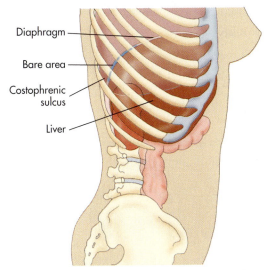

FIGURE 17-5 Sagittal plane of the body shows the diaphragm and liver with the highlighted "bare" area of the liver. The costophrenic sulcus forms the sharp border posterior to the liver and may be identified when fluid is present.

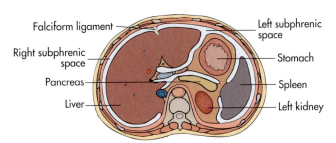

FIGURE 17-6 Transverse view of the subphrenic spaces.

by the epiploic branches of the gastroepiploic vessels and thus can bring masses of blood phagocytes to the areas it adheres to, which helps combat infection.

Determination of Intraperitoneal Location. The determination of intraperitoneal fluid from pleural, subdiaphragmatic, subscapular, or retroperitoneal fluid is necessary to determine a differential diagnosis or to locate a fluid pocket for aspiration or a biopsy.

Pleural versus Subdiaphragmatic. Because of the coronary ligament attachments, collections in the right posterior subphrenic space cannot extend between the bare area of the liver and the diaphragm. On the other hand, because the right pleural space extends medially to the attachment of the right superior coronary ligament, pleural collections may appear apposed to the bare area of the liver (Figure 17-5). Unless it is loculated, the pleural fluid tends to distribute posteromedially in the chest.

Subcapsular versus Intraperitoneal. Subcapsular liver and splenic collections are seen when they are inferior to the diaphragm unilaterally, and they conform to the shape of an organ capsule (Figure 17-6). They may extend medially to the attachment of the superior coronary ligament.

Retroperitoneal versus Intraperitoneal. A mass is confirmed to be within the retroperitoneal cavity when anterior renal displacement or anterior displacement of the dilated ureters can be documented (Figure 17-7). The mass interposed anteriorly or superiorly to kidneys can be located either intraperitoneally or retroperitoneally.

Fatty and collagenous connective tissues in the perirenal or anterior pararenal space produce echoes that are best demonstrated on sagittal scans. Retroperitoneal lesions displace echoes ventrally and cranially; hepatic and **subhepatic** lesions produce inferior and posterior displacement.

The anterior displacement of the superior mesenteric vessels, splenic vein, renal vein, and inferior vena cava excludes an intraperitoneal location. A large, right-sided retroperitoneal mass rotates the intrahepatic portal veins to the left. This causes the left portal vein to show reversed flow.

Right posterior hepatic masses of similar dimensions may produce minor displacement of the intrahepatic portal vein. Primary liver masses should move simultaneously with the liver.

Intraperitoneal Compartments

Perihepatic and Upper Abdominal Compartments.

Ligaments on the right side of the liver form the subphrenic and subhepatic spaces. The falciform ligament divides the subphrenic space into right and left components. The ligamentum teres hepatis ascends from the umbilicus to the umbilical notch of the liver within the free margin of the falciform ligament before coursing within the liver.

The bare area is delineated by the right superior and inferior coronary ligaments, which separate the posterior subphrenic space from the right superior subhepatic space (**Morison's pouch**). Lateral to the bare area and right triangular ligament, the posterior subphrenic and subhepatic spaces are continuous (Figure 17-8).

A single large and irregular perihepatic space surrounds the superior and lateral aspects of the left lobe of the liver, with the left coronary ligaments anatomically separating the subphrenic space into anterior and posterior compartments (see Figure 17-2).

The left subhepatic space is divided into an anterior compartment (the gastrohepatic recess) and a posterior compartment (the lesser sac) by the lesser omentum and stomach (Figure 17-9). The lesser sac lies anterior to the pancreas and posterior to the stomach.

With fluid in the lesser and greater omental cavities, the lesser omentum may be seen as a linear, undulating echodensity extending from the stomach to the porta hepatis.

Gastrosplenic Ligament. The gastrosplenic ligament is the left lateral extension of the greater omentum that connects the gastric greater curvature to the superior splenic hilum and forms a portion of the left lateral border of the lesser sac (see Figure 17-9).

Splenorenal Ligament. The splenorenal ligament is formed by the posterior reflection of the peritoneum of the spleen and passes inferiorly to overlie the left kidney (see Figure 17-9). It forms the posterior portion of the left lateral border of the lesser sac and separates the lesser sac from the renosplenic recess.

The Lesser Omental Bursa. The lesser omental bursa is subdivided into a larger lateroinferior and a smaller mediosuperior recess by the gastropancreatic folds, which are produced by the left gastric and hepatic arteries. The lesser sac extends to the diaphragm. The superior recess of the bursa surrounds the anterior, medial, and posterior surfaces of the caudate lobe, making the caudate a lesser sac structure. The lesser sac collections may extend a considerable distance below the plane of the pancreas by inferiorly displacing the transverse mesocolon or extending into the inferior recess of the greater omentum.

Lower Abdominal and Pelvic Compartments. The supravesical space and the medial and lateral inguinal fossae represent intraperitoneal paravesical spaces formed by indentation of the anterior parietal peritoneum by the bladder, obliterated umbilical arteries, and inferior epigastric vessels.

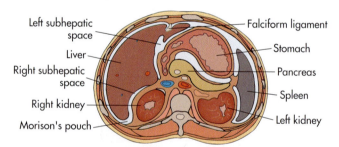

FIGURE 17-8 Transverse view of the subhepatic spaces and Morison's pouch.

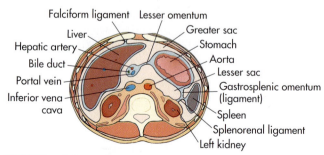

FIGURE 17-9 Transverse view of the abdomen showing the greater and lesser sac, the falciform ligament, the gastrosplenic ligament, and the splenorenal ligament.

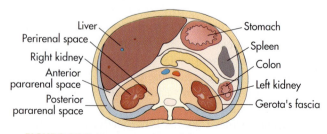

FIGURE 17-7 Transverse view of the retroperitoneal space.

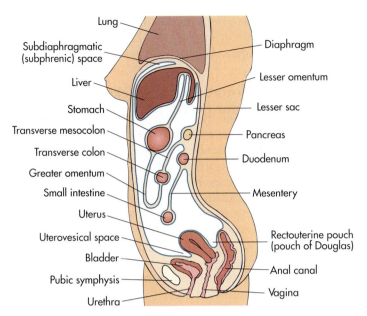

FIGURE 17-10 Sagittal view of the abdomen delineating the peritoneal cavity.

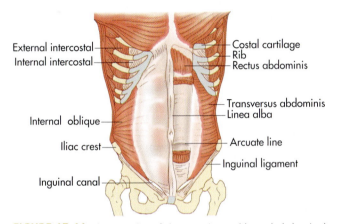

FIGURE 17-11 The muscles of the anterior and lateral abdominal walls include the external oblique, internal oblique, transversus, rectus abdominis, and pyramidalis.

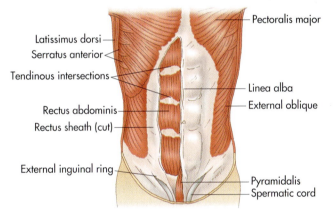

FIGURE 17-12 The rectus abdominis muscle rises from the front of the symphysis pubis and the pubic crest. On contraction, its lateral margin forms a palpable curved surface, termed the *linea semilunaris,* that extends from the ninth costal cartilage to the pubic tubercle. The anterior surface of the rectus muscle is crossed by three tendinous intersections, which are firmly attached to the anterior wall of the rectus sheath. The pyramidalis muscle arises by its base from the anterior surface of the pubis and inserts into the linea alba. It lies anterior to the lower part of the rectus abdominis muscle.

The retrovesical space is divided by the uterus into an anterior vesicouterine recess and a posterior rectouterine sac (pouch of Douglas) (Figure 17-10).

The peritoneal reflection over the dome of the bladder may have an inferior recess extending anterior to the bladder. Ascites displaces the distended urinary bladder inferiorly but not posteriorly. Intraperitoneal fluid compresses the bladder from its lateral aspect in cases of loculation. Fluid in the extraperitoneal prevesical space has a "dumbbell" configuration, displacing the bladder posteriorly and compressing it from the sides along its entire length.

Abdominal Wall

The paired rectus abdominis muscles are delineated medially in the midline of the body by the linea alba (Figure 17-11). Laterally the aponeuroses of external oblique, internal oblique, and transversus abdominis muscles unite to form a bandlike vertical fibrous groove called the linea semilunaris or spigelian fascia. The sheath of the three anterolateral abdominal muscles invests the rectus both anteriorly and posteriorly. Midway between the umbilicus and symphysis pubis, the aponeurotic sheath passes anteriorly to the rectus (Figure 17-12).

Below the peritoneal line, the rectus muscle is separated from the intraabdominal contents only by the transversalis fascia and the peritoneum. The rectus muscles are seen as a biconvex muscle group delineated by the linea alba and linea semilunaris. The peritoneal line is seen as a discrete linear echogenicity in the deepest layer of the abdominal wall.

PATHOLOGY OF THE PERITONEAL CAVITY

Ascites

Ascites is the accumulation of serous fluid in the peritoneal cavity. The amount of intraperitoneal fluid depends on the location, volume, and patient position. Factors other than fluid volume that affect the distribution of intraperitoneal fluid include peritoneal pressure, the area from which fluid originates, rapidity of fluid accumulation, presence or absence of adhesions, density of fluid with respect to other abdominal organs, and degree of bladder fullness.

Sonographic Findings. Serous ascites appears as echo-free fluid regions indented and shaped by the organs and viscera it surrounds or between where it is interposed. The fluid first fills the pouch of Douglas, then the lateral paravesical recesses, before it ascends to both paracolic gutters. The major flow from the pelvis is via the right paracolic gutter. Small volumes of fluid in the supine patient first appear around the inferior tip of the right lobe in the superior portion of the right flank and in the pelvic cul-de-sac, then in the paracolic gutters, before moving lateral and anterior to the liver (Figures 17-13 through 17-15).

The small bowel loops, sinks, or floats in the surrounding ascitic fluid, depending on relative gas content and amount of fat in the mesentery. The middle portion of the transverse colon usually floats on top of fluid because of its gas content, whereas the ascending portions of the colon, which are fixed retroperitoneally, remain in their normal location with or without gas.

Floating loops of small bowel, anchored posteriorly by the mesentery and with fluid between the mesenteric folds, have a characteristic anterior convex fan shape or arcuate appearance. An overdistended bladder may mask small quantities of fluid.

Inflammatory or Malignant Ascites. The sonographer should look for findings within the ascitic fluid that may suggest an inflammatory or malignant process.

Sonographic Findings. In searching for inflammatory or malignant ascites, the sonographer should look for fine or coarse internal echoes; loculation; unusual distribution, matting, or clumping of bowel loops; and thickening of interfaces between the fluid and neighboring structures (Figure 17-16).

Hepatorenal Recess. Generalized ascites, inflammatory fluid from acute cholecystitis, fluid resulting from pancreatic autolysis, or blood from a ruptured hepatic neoplasm or ectopic gestation may contribute to the formation of hepatorenal fluid collections (Figure 17-17). Abdominal fluid collections do not persist 1 week after abdominal surgery as a normal part of the healing process.

Sonographic Findings. Loculated ascites tends to be more irregular in outline, shows less mass effect, and may change shape slightly with positional variation.

Abscess Formation and Pockets in the Abdomen and Pelvis

An **abscess** is a cavity formed by necrosis within a solid tissue or a circumscribed collection of purulent material. The sonographer is frequently asked to evaluate a patient to rule out an abscess formation. The patient may present with a fever of unknown origin or with tenderness and swelling from a postoperative procedure. Other clinical signs include chills, weakness, malaise, and pain at the localized site of infection. Laboratory findings include normal liver function values, increased white blood cell count (**leukocytosis**), generalized **sepsis**, and bacterial cultures (if superficial).

Sonographic Findings. Abscess collections can appear quite varied in their texture depending on the length of time the abscess has been forming and the space available for the abscess to localize. Therefore, many collections appear predominantly fluid filled with irregular borders; they can also be complex, with debris floating within the cystic mass, or they may show a more solid pattern. If the collection is in the pelvis, careful analysis of bowel patterns and peristalsis should be made in an attempt to separate the bowel from the abscess collection.

Classically an abscess appears as an elliptical sonolucent mass with thick and irregular margins (Figure 17-18). The margins tend to be under tension and displace surrounding structures. A septated appearance may result from previous or developing adhesions. Necrotic debris produces low-level internal echoes that may be seen to float within the abscess. Fluid levels are secondary to layering, probably because of the settling of debris.

Gas-Containing Abscess. Scattered air reflectors may be the sonographer's clue in a gas- or air-filled abscess collection.

Sonographic Findings. Gas-containing abscesses have varying echo patterns. Generally, they appear as a densely echogenic mass with or without acoustic shadowing and otherwise increased through-transmission (Figure 17-19). A teratoma may mimic the pattern of a gas-containing abscess, but clinical history and x-rays exclude this tumor from the diagnosis. A gas-containing abscess may be confused with a solid lesion because it can be difficult to determine the presence of through-transmission.

Peritonitis. **Peritonitis** and the resultant abscess formation may be a generalized or localized process. Multiloculated abscesses or multiple collections should be recorded and their size determined as accurately as possible to help plan drainage and improve accuracy in follow-up studies.

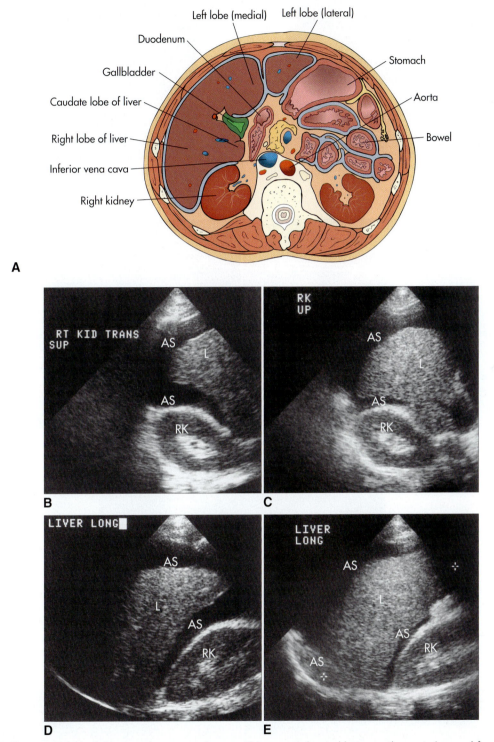

FIGURE 17-13 A, Transverse view of the posterior pararenal space. This space is located between the posterior renal fascia and the transversalis fascia. It communicates with the peritoneal fat, lateral to the lateroconal fascia. The space merges inferiorly with the anterior pararenal space and retroperitoneal tissue of the iliac fossa. Ascites may fill the peritoneal cavity. Small volumes of fluid in the supine position first appear around the inferior tip of the right lobe of the superior portion of the right flank. **B,** Transverse view. *AS,* ascites; *L,* liver; *RK,* right kidney. **C,** Transverse view. **D,** Longitudinal view with fluid in Morison's pouch. **E,** Longitudinal view.

Lesser-Sac Abscess. The small slitlike epiploic foramen usually seals off the lesser sac from inflammatory processes extrinsic to it. If the process begins within the lesser sac, such as with a pancreatic abscess, the sac may be involved along with other secondarily affected peritoneal and retroperitoneal spaces. Differential diagnosis should include pseudocyst, pancreatic abscess, gastric outlet obstruction, and fluid-filled stomach.

Subphrenic Abscess. The left upper quadrant may be difficult to examine because of the air interference. The

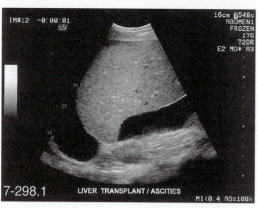

FIGURE 17-14 Ascites secondary to liver transplant is shown in this sagittal image.

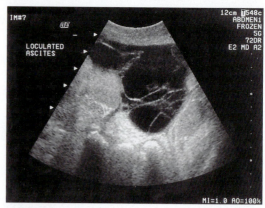

FIGURE 17-15 Loculated ascites with matted bowel.

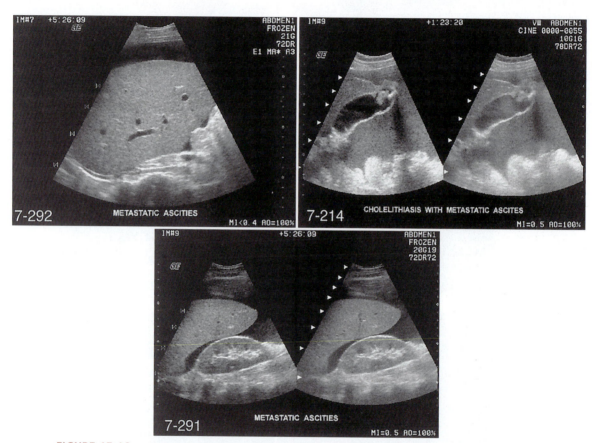

FIGURE 17-16 Malignant ascites. Fine internal echoes are seen in these images of malignant ascites.

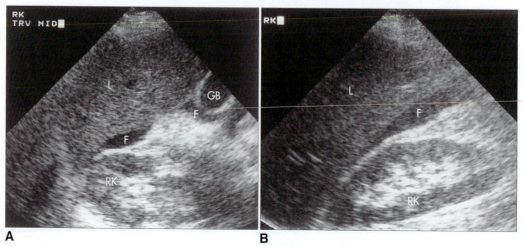

FIGURE 17-17 Fluid in Morison's pouch. Transverse **(A)** and sagittal **(B)** views. *F,* fluid; *GB,* gallbladder; *L,* liver; *RK,* right kidney.

sonographer may alter the patient's position to a right lateral decubitus position to scan along the coronal plane of the body, or prone, to use the spleen as a window.

Sonographic Findings. A sonographer must be careful of pleural effusions that appear above the diaphragm (Figure 17-20). The sonographer may perform the scan with the patient upright to better demonstrate the pleural and subdiaphragmatic areas.

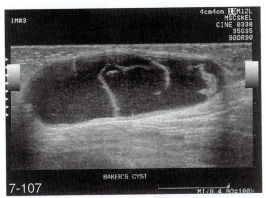

FIGURE 17-18 Collection of fluid was found posterior to the knee in a patient with a Baker's cyst. Multiple septations are seen within the fluid along with low-level debris echoes.

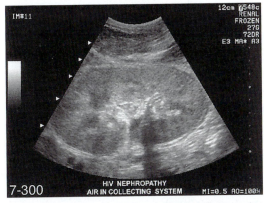

FIGURE 17-19 Patient with human immunodeficiency virus *(HIV)* nephropathy showed air with shadowing in the renal collecting system.

Subcapsular Collections. Subcapsular collections of fluid within the liver can mimic loculated subphrenic fluid.

Sonographic Findings. Intraabdominal fluid may be differentiated by its smooth border and its tendency to conform to the contour of the liver. It displaces the liver medially, rather than indenting the border locally, as subcapsular fluid might. A tense subphrenic abscess can displace the liver.

It may be difficult to distinguish a subphrenic abscess from ascites. To do so, the sonographer can look at the margins of the fluid collection or look for other collections of fluid (in the pelvis) to distinguish ascites from abscess. Preperitoneal fat anterior to the liver may mimic a localized fluid collection.

An abscess collects in the most dependent area of the body; therefore, all the gutters should be examined, including the "pockets" and "pouches" and the spaces above and around the various organs (Box 17-1).

Liver Abscess. There are five major pathways through which bacteria can enter the liver and cause abscess formation:

1. Through the portal system
2. By way of ascending cholangitis of the common bile duct (this is the most common cause in the United States)
3. Via the hepatic artery secondary to bacteremia
4. By direct extension from an infection
5. By implantation of bacteria after trauma to the abdominal wall

Biloma Abscess. Bilomas are extrahepatic loculated collections of bile that may develop because of iatrogenic, traumatic, or spontaneous rupture of the biliary tree.

Sonographic Findings. On ultrasound examination, a biloma abscess may appear cystic with weak internal echoes or a fluid-fluid level if clots or debris are not present. They usually have sharp margins. The extrahepatic bilomas are usually crescentic, surrounding and compressing structures with which they come in contact.

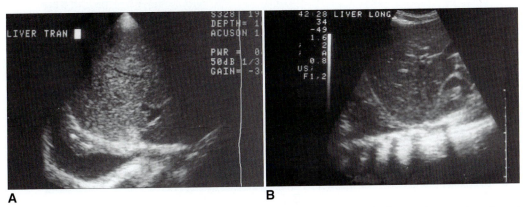

A **B**

FIGURE 17-20 Pleural effusion. **A,** Transverse image shows the pleural effusion posterior to the liver as the transducer is angled in a cephalic direction. **B,** Sagittal images of a patient with a moderate pleural effusion shown superior to the liver.

Kidney Abscess. Renal abscesses are classified according to their locations. A renal carbuncle is an abscess that forms within the renal parenchyma. Clinical symptoms vary from none to fever, leukocytosis, and flank pain. Sonography may show a discrete mass within the kidney, which may be cystic, cystic with debris, or solid.

A perinephric abscess is usually the result of a perforated renal abscess that leaks purulent material into the tissue adjacent to the kidney.

Sonographic Findings. Sonographic findings include a fluid collection around the kidney or an adjacent mass, which can vary from a cystic to a more solid appearance.

General Abdominal Abscess. A high percentage of abdominal and pelvic abscesses appear after surgery or trauma. The hepatic recesses and perihepatic spaces are the most common sites for abscess formation. The pelvis is another common site. (Free fluid below the transverse mesocolon often flows into the pouch of Douglas and perivesical spaces.)

BOX 17-1   Sonography of Abscesses

If an abscess is suspected (e.g., the patient has a fever of unknown origin), the sonographer should evaluate the following areas:

- Subdiaphragmatic area (liver and spleen)
- Splenic recess and borders
- Hepatic recess and borders
- Pericolic gutters
- Lesser omentum
- Transverse mesocolon
- Morison's pouch
- Gastrocolic ligament
- Phrenicosplenic ligament
- Recesses between intestinal loops and colon
- Extrahepatic falciform ligament
- Pouch of Douglas
- Broad ligaments (female)
- The area anterior to the urinary bladder

Sonographic Findings. An abscess may form in the right subhepatic space. The fluid ascends the right pericolic gutter into Morison's pouch. When the fluid fills Morison's pouch, it spreads past the coronary ligament over the dome of the liver. The presence of a right subhepatic abscess generally implies previous contamination of the right subhepatic space.

Appendiceal Abscess. Acute appendicitis is the most common abdominal pathologic process that requires immediate surgery. The cause of obstruction of the appendix is a fecalith at its origin in the cecum. The appendix becomes distended rapidly after obstruction.

Clinical symptoms include fever and severe pain near McBurney point in the right lower quadrant. (To locate this point, draw a straight line between the umbilicus and the anterior superior iliac spine and then move 2 inches along the line from the iliac spine.) Laboratory findings show an increased white blood cell count. The differential diagnosis includes pelvic inflammatory disease, twisted or ruptured ovarian cyst, acute gastroenteritis, and mesenteric lymphadenitis.

Sonographic Findings. On sonography, a complex mass is found in the right lower quadrant (Figure 17-21). The sonographer should also examine other gutters to rule out differentials. For further information on the appendix, see Chapter 13.

PATHOLOGY OF THE MESENTERY, OMENTUM, AND PERITONEUM

A mass or lesion within the mesentery and omentum may have solid or cystic characteristics, whereas a mass within the peritoneum may show an infiltrative pattern (Table 17-1). With an omental mass, at least one third of these lesions are malignant, and secondary neoplasms are more frequent than primary. In the mesentery, a benign primary tumor is more common than a malignant tumor, and secondary neoplasms are more frequent than primary. A cystic mass is more common than a solid

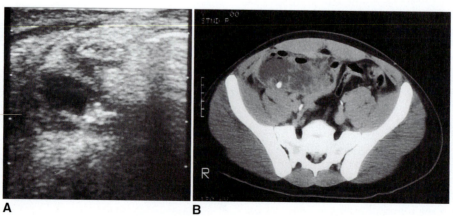

A   **B**

FIGURE 17-21 Appendiceal abscess. **A,** Transverse image of the inflamed appendix with a collection of pus posterior. **B,** Computed tomography scan of the same patient.

TABLE 17-1	Description of Peritoneal, Omental, and Mesenteric Masses	
Solid	**Cystic**	**Infiltrative**
Peritoneal Mass		
• Peritoneal mesothelioma • Peritoneal carcinomatosis	• Cystic mesothelioma • Pseudomyxoma peritonei • Bacterial/mycobacterial infection	• Peritoneal mesothelioma
Solid	**Cystic**	**Infiltrative**
Omental Mass		
• Benign: leiomyoma, lipoma, neurofibroma • Malignant: leiomyosarcoma, liposarcoma, fibrosarcoma, lymphoma, peritoneal mesothelioma, hemangiopericytoma, metastases • Infection: tuberculosis	• Hematoma	
Round	**Loculated Cystic**	**Ill-Defined/Stellate**
Mesenteric Mass		
• Metastases, especially from colon, ovary • Lymphoma • Leiomyosarcoma • Neural tumor • Lipoma, lipomatosis, liposarcoma • Fibrous histiocytoma • Hemangioma • Desmoid tumor (most common primary)	• Cystic lymphangioma • Pseudomyxoma • Peritonei • Cystic mesothelioma • Mesenteric cyst • Mesenteric hematoma • Benign cystic teratoma • Cystic spindle cell tumor	• Metastases (ovary) • Lymphoma • Fibromatosis • Fibrosing mesenteritis • Lipodystrophy • Mesenteric panniculitis • Stellate: peritoneal mesothelioma, retractile mesenteritis, fibrosis reaction of carcinoid, desmoid tumor, tuberculous peritonitis, metastases, diverticulitis, pancreatitis

mass. Malignant solid tumors are more likely found near the root of the mesentery, whereas benign solid tumors are found in the periphery near the bowel.

Cysts

Abdominal cysts may have (1) embryologic, (2) traumatic or acquired, (3) neoplastic, or (4) infective and degenerative origins. It is important to determine the organ of origin of the mass. If the mass is adherent to the mesentery or small intestine, it may be difficult for ultrasound to distinguish the anatomic landmarks necessary to determine the point of origin. Therefore, many patients will have a CT or MRI of the abdomen to better define these borders. **Hemorrhage** into omental or mesenteric cysts may cause rapid distention and clinically mimic ascites. Peritoneal inclusion cysts are considered in the differential diagnosis when large adnexal cystic structures are identified in a young woman. Fungal infections present as peritoneal cystic lesions.

◤ Sonographic Findings. Mesenteric and omental cysts may be uniloculated or multiloculated with smooth walls and thin internal septations. The internal echoes are correlated with fat globules, debris, superimposed hemorrhage, or infection. They may follow the contour of the underlying bowel and conform to the anterior abdominal wall rather than produce distention.

Urachal Cyst. A urachal cyst is an incomplete regression of the urachus during development. The apex of the bladder is continuous with the allantois, which becomes obliterated and forms a fibrous core, the urachus. The urachus persists throughout life as a ligament that runs from the apex of the bladder to the umbilicus and is called the median umbilical ligament.

◤ Sonographic Findings. On ultrasound examination, the sonographer may see a cystic mass between the umbilicus and the bladder. The mass may be small or giant, multiseptated, and extend into the upper abdomen.

Urinoma

A **urinoma,** an encapsulated collection of urine, may result from a closed renal injury or surgical intervention or may develop spontaneously secondary to an obstructing lesion. The extraperitoneal extravasation may be subcapsular or perirenal: the latter collections are sometimes termed uriniferous pseudocysts. The extravasation may leak around the ureter, where the perinephric fascia is weakest, or into adjoining fascial planes and peritoneal cavity.

◤ Sonographic Findings. Cystic masses are most often oriented inferomedially, with upward and lateral displacement of the lower pole of the kidney along with medial displacement of the ureter. They usually present

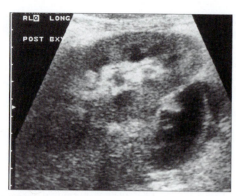

FIGURE 17-22 Right lower quadrant pain in young adult with renal transplant shows a fluid collection posterior to the transplanted kidney indenting its posterior wall. This represented a postoperative urinoma.

on ultrasound as anechoic or contain low-level echoes (Figure 17-22).

Peritoneal Metastases

Peritoneal metastases develop from cellular implantation across the peritoneal cavity. The most common primary sites are the ovaries, stomach, and colon. Other less common sites are the pancreas, biliary tract, kidneys, testicles, and uterus. Metastases may arise from tumors, such as sarcomas, melanomas, teratomas, or embryonic tumors.

Sonographic Findings. The metastases form a nodular, sheetlike, irregular configuration. Multiple small nodules are seen along the peritoneal line. The larger masses obliterate the line and cause adhesion to bowel loops.

Lymphomas of the Omentum and Mesentery

Lymphoma presents as a uniformly thick, hypoechoic, band-shaped structure that follows the convexity of the anterior and lateral abdominal wall, creating the omental band.

Sonographic Findings. On ultrasound examination, omental and mesenteric lymphomas present as a lobulated, confluent, hypoechoic mass surrounding a centrally positioned echogenic area. The **sandwich sign** represents a mass infiltrating the mesenteric leaves and encasing the superior mesenteric artery.

Tumors of the Peritoneum, Omentum, and Mesentery

Secondary tumors and lymphoma are neoplasms that most commonly involve the peritoneum and mesentery. **Peritoneal and Omental Mesothelioma.** Peritoneal and omental mesotheliomas most often occur in middle-aged men as the result of exposure to asbestos. The

common symptoms are abdominal pain, weight loss, and ascites.

Sonographic Findings. The tumor may present as a large mass with discrete smaller nodes scattered over large areas of the visceral and parietal peritoneum, or it may present as diffuse nodes and plaques that coat the abdominal cavity and envelope and mat together in the abdominal viscera.

PATHOLOGY OF THE ABDOMINAL WALL

Abdominal Wall Masses

Lesions found within the superficial abdominal wall include inflammatory lesions, hematomas, neoplasms, hernias, and postsurgical lesions. Symmetry of the rectus sheath muscles is a key factor in determining if an abdominal wall mass is present. The higher-resolution transducers may help the sonographer distinguish between the amount of fat and muscle present and an abnormal lesion.

Lymphoceles. A lymphocele is a collection of fluid that occurs after surgery in the pelvis, retroperitoneum, or recess cavities.

Sonographic Findings. Lymphoceles generally look like loculated, simple fluid collections, although they may have a more complex, usually septated, morphology. Differentiation from loculated ascites is usually possible because the mass effect of a lymphocele that is under tension displaces the surrounding organs. Differentiation from other fluid collections is mainly made by aspiration.

Extraperitoneal Hematoma

Extraperitoneal rectus sheath hematomas are acute or chronic collections of blood lying either within the rectus muscle or between the muscle and its sheath. They occur as the result of direct trauma, pregnancy, cardiovascular and degenerative muscle diseases, surgical injury, anticoagulation therapy, steroids, or extreme exercise. Clinically the patient may present with acute, sharp, persistent nonradiating pain.

Hematomas are caused by surgical injury to tissue or by blunt trauma to the abdomen. Laboratory values may show a decrease in hematocrit and red blood cell count; the patient may go into shock.

Sonographic Findings. On ultrasound examination, the sonographer notices an asymmetry between the rectus sheath muscles. The hematoma may appear as an anechoic mass with scattered internal echoes.

The sonographic appearance depends on the stage of the bleed. Acute bleeds are primarily cystic, with some debris and blood clots; as the blood begins to organize and clot, the mass becomes more solid in appearance. Newly formed clots may be very homogeneous. Hematomas can become infected and at any stage may be sonographically indistinguishable from abscesses. They may mimic subphrenic fluid.

Bladder-Flap Hematoma. A bladder-flap hematoma is a collection of blood between the bladder and lower-uterine segment, resulting from a lower-uterine transverse cesarean section and bleeding from the uterine vessels.

Subfascial Hematoma. A subfascial hematoma is found in the prevesicular space and is caused by a disruption of the inferior epigastric vessels or their branches during a cesarean section.

Inflammatory Lesion (Abscess)

An abscess or inflammation in the abdominal wall may occur after surgery. The sonogram may show cystic, complex, or solid characteristics. Generally the masses are superficial and are easy to locate and needle aspirate with ultrasound guidance if necessary. A high-frequency, linear array transducer should be used to image the superficial area.

The patient may present with leukocytosis, **septicemia**, or a previous history of **pyogenic** infection.

▨ **Sonographic Findings.** On ultrasound examination, an abdominal wall abscess presents as an anechoic or echoic mass with internal echoes from debris. The mass usually has irregular margins and shape. It may have gas bubbles within that show shadowing on the ultrasound image.

Neoplasm or Peritoneal Thickening

Neoplasms of the abdominal wall include lipomas, desmoid tumors, or metastases. The desmoid tumor is a benign fibrous neoplasm of aponeurotic structures. It most commonly occurs in relation to the rectus abdominis and its sheath (Figure 17-23). The tumor may present as hypoechoic to cystic (except lipomas).

▨ **Sonographic Findings.** On ultrasound examination, a desmoid tumor presents as anechoic to hypoechoic, with smooth and sharply defined walls. The peritoneal lining is not seen as a distinct structure during sonography unless it is thickened. This is usually secondary to metastatic implants or to direct extension of the tumor from the viscera or mesentery. Primary mesotheliomas occur rarely.

Hernia

An abdominal hernia is the protrusion of a peritoneal-lined sac through a defect in the weakened abdominal wall (Figure 17-24). The viscera beneath the weakened tissue may protrude, resulting in a hernia. The most common areas of weakness are the umbilical area and the femoral and inguinal rings. (The inguinal hernia is discussed in Chapter 19.) An incarcerated hernia is one that cannot be "reduced" or pushed back into the abdominal cavity. Complications may arise if edema develops or if the opening constricts so much that the protrusion cannot be placed back into position.

Strangulation (interruption of the blood supply) of the bowel can also occur in an incarcerated hernia that is not surgically repaired in a timely manner. This bowel can become necrotic and require resection.

The abdominal wall hernia consists of three parts: the sac, the contents of the sac, and the covering of the sac. Common locations for hernias are umbilical (congenital or acquired), epigastric, inguinal, femoral, and at the separation of the rectus abdominis. The hernia may involve the omentum only or it may mimic other masses. The hernia commonly originates near the junction of the linea semilunaris and arcuate line in the paraumbilical area.

Epigastric hernias are found in the widest part of the linea alba between the xiphoid process and the umbilicus. This hernia is usually filled with fat, which over the years may carry a piece of omentum along with it.

A spigelian hernia is a variant of the ventral hernia, which is found more laterally in the abdominal wall.

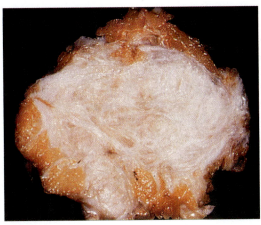

FIGURE 17-23 Gross pathology of a desmoid tumor of the abdominal wall.

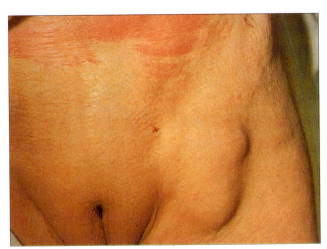

FIGURE 17-24 Femoral hernia causing a bulging enlargement of the femoral canal.

Sonographic Findings. Many hernias are palpable and do not require sonographic evaluation. However, if the mass is not well defined on physical examination, ultrasound evaluation may be helpful. If a hernia is suspected, the sonographer will note an interruption of the peritoneal line separating the muscles and abdominal contents.

Sonography may outline the contents of the mass where it is fluid-filled or contains peristaltic bowel or mesenteric fat. If a hernia is suspected, the sonographer should look for a peristalsing bowel within the mass, although the peristalsis may be absent with incarceration. If the hernia is not readily apparent, the patient may be asked to lift the head or to strain (Valsalva maneuver) to see if the mass moves or changes shape.

The sonographic criteria for a hernia include (1) demonstration of an abdominal wall defect, (2) presence of bowel loops or mesenteric fat within a lesion, (3) exaggeration of the lesion with strain (Valsalva), and (4) reducibility of the lesion by gentle pressure.

Abdominal Applications of Ultrasound Contrast Agents

Daniel A. Merton

OBJECTIVES

On completion of this chapter, you should be able to:
- List the current limitations of ultrasound imaging that may be enhanced with ultrasound contrast agents
- Describe the properties that an ultrasound contrast agent must have to be clinically useful
- Describe the difference between tissue-specific ultrasound contrast agents and vascular agents
- Define harmonic ultrasound imaging
- Describe the clinical applications of contrast agents in the liver

OUTLINE

The use of contrast media has become a routine part of radiography, computed tomography (CT), and magnetic resonance imaging (MRI). The addition of contrast to these modalities has significantly increased their capabilities to the extent that, in many cases, contrast is an essential component of the diagnostic imaging examination. Medical sonography, however, has not benefited to the same degree from the potential of contrast agents. Since the 1980s, a significant amount of research has been conducted toward the development of **ultrasound contrast agents (UCAs)**.[68] Most of the work has centered on developing agents that can be administered intravenously to evaluate blood vessels, blood flow, and solid organs.

The clinical utilization of **contrast-enhanced sonography (CES)** has been shown to reduce or eliminate some of the current limitations of ultrasound (US) imaging and Doppler blood flow detection. These include limitations of spatial and contrast resolution on gray-scale US and the detection of low velocity blood flow and flow in very small vessels using Doppler flow detection modes, including color flow imaging (CFI) and pulsed Doppler with spectral analysis. Advances in US equipment technology following the development of UCAs have resulted in "contrast-specific" imaging modes, including gray-scale US methods that allow detection of blood flow without the limitations of Doppler US. There are now published clinical guidelines that describe the most appropriate use of CES for a variety of abdominal, retroperitoneal, and other applications.[79] Ultrasound contrast agents hold the promise of improving the sensitivity and specificity of current US diagnoses and have the potential of expanding sonography's already broad range of clinical applications.

TYPES OF ULTRASOUND CONTRAST AGENTS

Vascular UCAs

Sonographic detection of blood flow is limited by factors including the depth and size of a vessel, the attenuation properties of intervening tissue, or low-velocity flow. Limitations of US equipment sensitivity and the operator dependence of Doppler US are also factors that may impact the results of a vascular examination. Vascular or blood-pool UCAs enhance Doppler (color and spectral) flow signals by adding more and better acoustic scatterers to the bloodstream (Figures 18-1 and 18-2). The use of these UCAs improves the detection of blood flow from vessels that are often difficult to assess without their use, such as the renal arteries, intracranial vessels, and small capillaries within organs (i.e., tissue perfusion) (Figure 18-3). In addition to enhancing Doppler signals, vascular UCAs also improve gray-scale US visualization of flowing blood and demonstrate changes to the gray-scale echogenicity of tissues with the use of contrast-specific imaging software such as **harmonic imaging (HI)**.

The concept of an UCA was first introduced by Gramiak and Shah in 1968 who, in their initial work, injected agitated saline directly into the ascending aorta and cardiac chambers during echocardiographic examinations.[35] The microbubbles formed by agitation resulted in strong reflections arising from within the normally echo-free lumen of the aorta and chambers of the heart. Eventually other solutions were discovered that could produce similar effects. However, microbubbles produced by simple agitation are nonuniform in size, relatively large, and unstable, which makes them unsuitable for sonographic evaluations of the left heart and systemic circulation, because the microbubbles do not persist through passage of the pulmonary and cardiac circulations. Furthermore, to provide contrast enhancement, agitated saline required direct injection into the vessel under evaluation (e.g., the aorta) and a more clinically practicable administration method, such as **intravenous (IV) injection,** was desired.

Numerous attempts have been made to encapsulate gas and make a more suitable microbubble-based UCA that can be administered intravenously. For a UCA to be clinically useful, it should be nontoxic, have microbubbles or microparticles that are small enough to traverse the pulmonary capillary beds (i.e., less than 8 microns in size), and be stable enough to provide multiple recirculations.

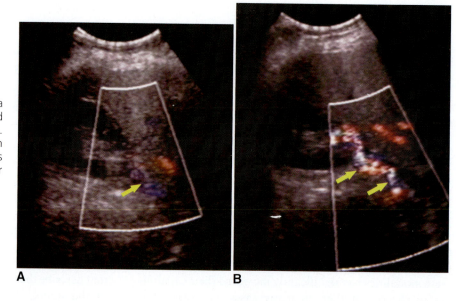

FIGURE 18-1 Color Doppler imaging of a patient's right renal artery before **(A)** and after **(B)** administration of a vascular UCA. Note the increased visualization of flow in the renal artery *(arrows)* after intravenous injection of contrast. In this case no vascular abnormality was detected.

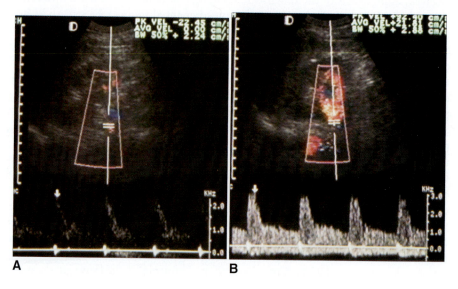

FIGURE 18-2 Color flow imaging and spectral Doppler analysis of renal artery flow. **A,** Before contrast, the spectral waveforms are weak and there is minimal color flow information. **B,** After intravenous administration of a contrast, the spectral wave forms have a higher signal intensity and additional color flow information is provided.

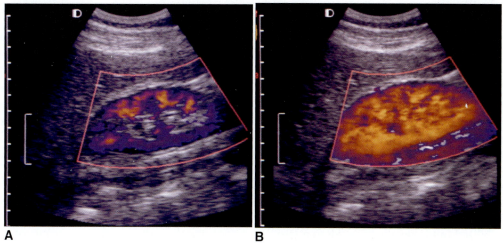

FIGURE 18-3 Power Doppler imaging of a normal right kidney before **(A)** and after **(B)** injection of a vascular UCA. Note the improved demonstration of flow in the renal parenchyma after intravenous injection of contrast.

A number of agents possess these desirable traits, and presently several microbubble-based UCAs are commercially available worldwide. In 1994, Albunex (Mallinckrodt Medical, Inc., St. Louis, Missouri) was the first UCA to receive Food and Drug Administration (FDA) approval in the United States for use in echocardiography applications. However, Albunex was eventually removed from the market primarily because of the commercial availability of agents with increased clinical utility.

Currently in the United States Optison (GE Healthcare, Buckinghamshire, England), Definity (Lantheus Medical Imaging, N. Billerica, Massachusetts), and Imagent (Alliance Pharmaceutical Corp., San Diego, California) are FDA approved for use in echocardiographic applications. (As of February 2011 only Optison and Definity are being marketed.) Several other transpulmonary agents, including Levovist (Schering AG, Berlin, Germany) and SonoVue (Bracco Diagnostics, Milan, Italy), are available in Europe, Asia, and elsewhere. A number of other agents are currently in various stages of clinical trials.[48]

The following sections describe several vascular UCAs that have been approved for clinical applications. These details are provided to demonstrate the diversity of approaches used to produce UCAs. This is not a complete list of agents currently approved for clinical use or in development.

Albunex consists of 5% sonicated human serum albumen (HSA) microspheres containing room air. After IV injection, Albunex reportedly enhanced the detection of blood flow in the heart chambers and improved endocardial border definition (EBD).[17] However, in a large percentage of patients studied, contrast-enhancement was limited, particularly in the apex of the left ventricle and during systole. These limitations combined with the development and availability of more robust UCAs eventually led to the removal of Albunex from the market.

The specific type of gas contained within a UCA microbubble and its shell composition influence the microbubble's acoustic behavior (e.g., reflectivity and elasticity), method of metabolism, and stability within the blood pool.[12,100] In 1998, Optison (FSO 69) became the second commercially available UCA in the United States. Like Albunex, the microbubble shell of Optison is also 5% HSA. However, unlike the low-molecular-weight air-filled microbubbles of Albunex, Optison contains a high-molecular weight gas (perfluoropropane), which improves the stability and plasma longevity of the agent. Agents like Albunex that contain room air are commonly referred to as **first-generation agents,** whereas agents containing heavy gasses are referred to as **second-generation agents.** Optison has shown potential for use with gray-scale HI and Doppler modes for echocardiography as well as systemic vascular, tumor characterization, and abdominal applications.[24,26,50,101]

Levovist (SHU-508A) is another transpulmonary UCA approved for clinical use in several European countries and Australia. The shell of Levovist is composed of 99.9% galactose microparticles with 0.1% palmitic acid. A significant amount of work has been done utilizing Levovist since its European debut in 1996, and there are numerous published reports on its use. Experiments in animals and humans have demonstrated that Levovist can provide contrast-enhancement in excess of 3 minutes duration.[32] Human trials with Levovist have demonstrated its ability to enhance color and spectral Doppler flow signals from both normal and tumor vessels.[6,13,16,76] Temporal measurements of Levovist uptake and washout have been reported in the evaluation of breast masses.[43] This represents a unique quality of CES that may have the potential to help differentiate benign from malignant tumors in a variety of anatomic locations. Contrast kinetics appears to vary between malignant and benign tumors, with a much faster washout seen in malignancies (likely as a result of intratumoral arteriovenous shunts).

More research is being conducted to confirm these findings and to evaluate this application of CES.

In addition to the more common bolus method of administration, Levovist has also been administered via slow infusion. Albrecht and colleagues have shown that the infusion of Levovist results in contrast enhancement lasting as much as 12 minutes or more compared to just over 2 minutes with a bolus injection.[2] The additional enhancement time provided by the infusion of contrast would likely be useful for difficult and time-consuming evaluations of vessels such as the renal arteries. Infusion of Definity has also been approved by the FDA and evaluated in clinical trials.[39]

SonoVue (BR-1) is an aqueous suspension of phospholipid-stabilized sulfur hexafluoride (SF-6) microbubbles having a low solubility in blood.[38] SonoVue enhances the echogenicity of blood and provides opacification of the cardiac chambers resulting in improved left ventricular EBD. In clinical trials it has been shown to increase US's accuracy in detection or exclusion of abnormalities in intracranial, extracranial carotid and peripheral arteries. SonoVue also increases the quality of Doppler flow signals and the duration of clinically useful signal enhancement in portal vein assessments. SonoVue improves the detection of liver and breast lesion vascularity resulting in more specific lesion characterization.[86,87] SonoVue has been approved for use in Europe for echocardiography and macrovascular applications. In the United States at the time of this writing, FDA clinical trials using SonoVue for liver lesion characterization are pending.

Tissue-Specific Ultrasound Contrast Agents

The kinetics of UCA microbubbles following IV injection is complex, and each agent has its own unique characteristics.[7] In general, after IV administration, blood pool UCAs are contained exclusively in the body's vascular spaces. In general, when a vascular agent's microbubbles are ruptured or otherwise destroyed, the microbubble shell products are metabolized or eliminated by the body, and the gas is exhaled.[100]

Tissue-specific ultrasound contrast agents differ from vascular agents in that the microbubbles of these agents are removed from the blood pool and taken up by or have an affinity toward specific tissues, for example, the reticuloendothelial system (RES) in the liver and spleen, or thrombus. Over time the presence of contrast microbubbles within or attached to the tissue changes its sonographic appearance. By changing the signal impedance (or other acoustic characteristics) of normal and abnormal tissues, these agents improve the detectability of abnormalities and permit more specific sonographic diagnoses. Tissue-specific UCAs are typically administered by IV injection. Some tissue-specific UCAs also enhance the sonographic detection of blood flow and

are, therefore, potentially multipurpose. Because tissue-specific UCAs target specific types of tissues and their behavior is predictable, they can be considered in the category of **molecular imaging agents**.[62]

Sonazoid (NC100100; GE Healthcare, Buckinghamshire, England) is a tissue-specific UCA that contains microbubbles of perfluorobutane gas in a stable lipid shell.[48] Sonazoid is currently approved for use in Japan.[92] After being injected intravenously, Sonazoid behaves as a vascular agent (i.e., enhances the detection of flowing blood) and, over time, the microbubbles are phagocytosed by the RES (macrophage Kupffer cells) of the liver and spleen.[7] The intact microbubbles may remain stationary in the tissue for several hours. When insonated after uptake, the stationary contrast microbubbles increase the reflectivity of the contrast-containing tissue. If an appropriate level of acoustic energy is applied to the tissue, the microbubbles first oscillate (emitting harmonic signals that can be detected with gray-scale HI) and then rupture. The rupture of the microbubbles results in random Doppler shifts appearing as a transient mosaic of colors on a color Doppler display (Figure 18-4). This effect has been termed **induced acoustic emission** (IAE), *stimulated acoustic emission* (SAE), or simply **acoustic emission** (AE).[29,36] By exploiting the color Doppler-depicted AE phenomenon, masses that have destroyed or replaced the normal Kupffer cells will be displayed as color-free areas and, thus, become more sonographically conspicuous. These same AE effects can also be demonstrated using gray-scale HI (see the HI discussion that follows) (Figure 18-5).[25,36]

Initial work using VX-2 tumors grown in the livers of rabbits has clearly demonstrated the capability of Sonazoid's AE characteristics to improve detection of small tumors that were not detectable prior to the injection of contrast.[25] The AE effect is not unique to Sonazoid. Other UCAs have been found to demonstrate this effect, including Levovist, but the effect with Levovist is short-lived and it is unclear as to whether there is true RES

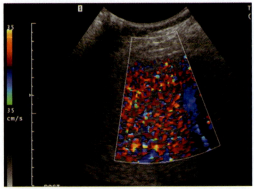

FIGURE 18-4 Color Doppler imaging display of acoustic emission after IV injection of a tissue-specific UCA. The rupture of contrast microbubbles present within the RES cells of the liver results in the characteristic random color display.

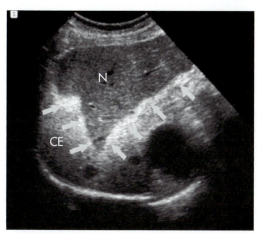

FIGURE 18-5 Gray-scale harmonic imaging display of the acoustic emission effect after IV injection of a tissue-specific UCA. As the acoustic energy traverses through the liver parenchyma, it causes the contrast microbubbles to rupture, resulting in a characteristic wave of intense echoes (*arrows*). The normal echogenicity of the liver parenchyma in the near field (*N*) is restored after the microbubbles have ruptured, whereas deep to the AE wave the contrast enhanced tissue (*CE*) remains echogenic because of the presence of intact microbubbles. This effect is dramatic when visualized in real time.

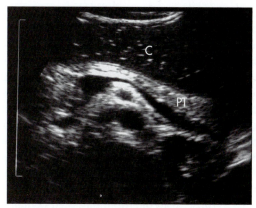

FIGURE 18-6 Transverse view of the pancreas after administration of an oral UCA. The contrast-filled stomach (*C*) provides an acoustic window that enhances visualization of the normal pancreatic tail (*PT*).

uptake of Levovist microparticles or if they are simply trapped within the vascular sinusoids.[36]

It is important to remember that the AE effects are independent of contrast motion. In other words, the AE effect can result from oscillation and eventual rupture of stationary contrast microbubbles, and agents that demonstrate the AE phenomenon also can be utilized for nonvascular applications where there is little or no movement of the microbubbles.

Currently, tissue-specific agents that are taken up by the RES appear to be most useful in the assessment of patients with suspected liver abnormalities, including the ability to both detect as well as characterize liver tumors using CES. However, the properties that cause some UCA's microbubbles to be taken up by the RES (while other UCA microbubbles are not) is not completely understood.[7] Other target- or tissue-specific agents are being developed to enhance the detection of thrombus and tumors.

Oral Ultrasound Contrast Agents

Limitations of the sonographic assessment of the upper abdomen include patient obesity and the presence of gas-filled bowel, which can produce shadowing artifacts. Ingestion of degassed water has been used to improve sonographic examinations of the upper abdominal and retroperitoneal structures such as the pancreas.[58] However, water simply displaces gas and traverses the gastrointestinal tract in an inconsistent and unpredictable manner.

Oral contrast agents have been developed for sonographic applications. SonoRx (Bracco Diagnostics,

Princeton, New Jersey) is an oral UCA that contains simethicone-coated cellulose as its active ingredient.[9,58] Ingestion of SonoRx results in a homogeneous transmission of sound through the contrast-filled stomach (Figure 18-6). Clinical trials have demonstrated that the administration of SonoRx increased the diagnostic capabilities of US and, at times, obviated the need for additional imaging studies, including CT or MRI.[9] Although SonoRx was approved by the U.S. FDA in 1998 and was commercially available, it is no longer being marketed in the United States.

ULTRASOUND EQUIPMENT MODIFICATIONS

Microbubble-based UCAs enhance the detection of blood flow when used with conventional ultrasound imaging techniques, including gray-scale US, and Doppler techniques (i.e., color flow imaging and Doppler spectral analysis). However, research and experience have led to a better understanding of the complex interactions between acoustic energy (i.e., the US beam) and UCA microbubbles, which in turn has led to advances in US instrumentation. The use of "contrast-specific" US imaging modes has been found to greatly improve the clinical utility of CES. Because current US system platforms are digital and software driven, the necessary changes can be implemented relatively quickly.

Harmonic imaging (HI) uses the same broadband transducers used for conventional US, but in HI mode the US system is configured to receive only echoes at the second harmonic frequency, which is twice the transmit frequency (e.g., 7.0 MHz for a 3.5 MHz transducer).[22,51] When using a microbubble-based UCA, the microbubbles oscillate (i.e., they get larger and smaller) when subjected to the acoustic energy present in the US field. The reflected echoes from the oscillating microbubbles contain energy components at the fundamental frequency as well as at the higher and lower harmonics (subharmonics). The majority of the development efforts involving HI have focused on **gray-scale harmonic imaging (GSHI)**, which allows detection of contrast-enhancement of blood flow and organs with gray-scale US. The use of GSHI for CES avoids many of the limitations and artifacts encountered when using Doppler US techniques and UCAs, such as angle dependence and "color blooming" artifacts.[23] In HI mode the echoes from the oscillating microbubbles have a higher signal-to-noise ratio than would be provided by using conventional US, so that regions with microbubbles (e.g., blood vessels and organ parenchyma) are more easily appreciated visually. Although body tissues also generate harmonic signals, compared to those from microbubbles their contribution to the image is negligible. Recent advances in HI technology (e.g., wideband HI, phase-inversion HI, and pulse-inversion HI) employ image processing algorithms to subtract echoes arising from body tissues while echoes arising from contrast microbubbles are preferentially displayed.[51] Thus, wideband GSHI provides a way to better differentiate areas with and without contrast and has the potential to demonstrate real-time gray-scale blood pool imaging (i.e., "perfusion imaging"). In most cases the benefits of using GSHI for CES (e.g., higher frame rates, improved contrast resolution, reduced artifacts) are so great that conventional (non-HI) color flow imaging is neither necessary nor advised.

Harmonic Doppler US modes (e.g., harmonic power Doppler imaging, power modulation imaging) have also been developed. Preliminary investigations with harmonic Doppler modes have identified some potential benefits including enhanced detection of very low-velocity blood flow in organs and suppression of color "flash" artifacts.[18]

When using microbubble-based UCAs, the energy present within the acoustic field can have a detrimental effect on the contrast microbubbles.[12] A significant number of the microbubbles can be destroyed by the acoustic pressure even though the actual pressure contained within the US field is relatively low. Some UCAs are more susceptible to this phenomenon than others. Once the microbubble is destroyed, contrast enhancement is no longer provided, which reduces the clinical utility and duration of contrast enhancement. Several approaches have been used to minimize this problem. One relatively easy technique is to use a low acoustic output power as defined by the **mechanical index (MI)**.[77] Low-MI US is a useful technique for a variety of CES applications including assessment of liver tumors. However, reducing the MI also limits tissue penetration, so this is not always an adequate solution. Furthermore, the MI may be an imprecise predictor of the effect of acoustic energy on contrast microbubbles.[27,36]

Equipment manufacturers have incorporated intermittent imaging capabilities on their systems to provide an additional option to the user seeking to reduce microbubble destruction during contrast-enhanced examinations.[51,77] In this mode the system is gated to only transmit and receive data at predetermined intervals. The gating may be triggered on a specific portion of the ECG (e.g., the r-wave) or a time interval such as once or twice per second. Intermittent imaging reduces the exposure of contrast microbubbles to the acoustic energy and allows additional microbubbles to enter the field between signal transmissions. The additional microbubbles then contribute to an even greater increase in reflectivity of the contrast-containing blood or tissue than would be possible by continuous real-time imaging. A disadvantage to intermittent imaging is its lack of a real-time display of data, but advances in instrumentation such as "flash echocardiography" have begun to address this drawback.[72] This same effect can be obtained by using "frame-one imaging" during CES[61] (Figure 18-7). Intermittent imaging can be combined with wideband HI to further improve the clinical utility of CES.

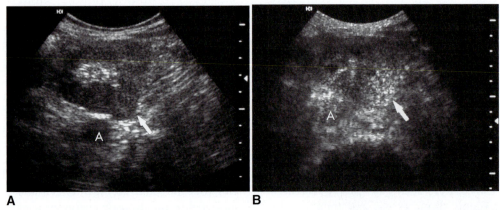

A   **B**

FIGURE 18-7 Enhanced detection of a hypervascular renal tumor using harmonic imaging and interval delay imaging. **A,** A transverse US image obtained precontrast demonstrates the aorta *(A)* and a suspicious contour defect *(arrow)* near the lower pole of the left kidney. **B,** After IV contrast administration using gray-scale harmonic imaging and a manual interval delay, the aorta is filled with contrast and there is increased echogenicity of the suspicious area compared to the normal renal parenchyma. The suspicious area represented a renal cell carcinoma.

Moriyasu used intermittent imaging for CES of hepatic tumors.[64] This study showed that the signal intensity is dependent on an interscan delay time during which the acoustic power is lowered under the threshold for passive cavitation of the microbubbles. Another study by Sirlin demonstrated that intermittent imaging improved image contrast resolution and a one frame-per-second rate had greater contrast resolution than was provided by continuous real-time imaging.[84]

Other system modifications in development include on-board video densitometry, calculation of the integrated backscatter from contrast, and advanced three-dimensional (3D) imaging (Figures 18-8 and 18-9). Furthermore, the administration of contrast provides the capability to measure the transit time of contrast-containing blood through normal and diseased tissue, blood volume estimates, and tissue perfusion.[5,46,98] Systems will likely be developed that will allow on-board

calculation of these unique contrast-specific measurements and calculations provided by the use of UCAs. In the future additional advancements can be expected including modifications to the operator interfaces of US equipment and computer-assisted diagnosis (CAD) software to facilitate the clinical use of contrast.[91]

CLINICAL APPLICATIONS

Hepatic Applications

There are limitations to the sonographic evaluation of hepatic lesions and other hepatic abnormalities. Although US is usually sensitive for the detection of medium to large hepatic lesions, it is limited in its ability to detect small (<10 mm), isoechoic, or peripherally located lesions, particularly in obese patients or patients with diffuse liver disease. Furthermore, sonography is not as effective as CT or MRI for characterization of hepatic tumors.

Hepatic US blood flow studies are limited by low-velocity blood flow (e.g., in cases of portal hypertension) or for the detection of flow in the intrahepatic artery branches. Ultrasound contrast agents have shown the potential to improve the accuracy of hepatic sonography, including enhanced detection and characterization of hepatic masses and improved detection of intra- and extrahepatic blood flow.

Hepatic Blood Flow. Vascular UCAs have been shown to improve the detection of hepatic blood flow in normal subjects as well as in patients with liver disease and **portal hypertension (PHT)**.[1,53,81] Most sonographic examinations for PHT include qualitative assessment of blood flow with color flow imaging to identify the presence and direction of flow in the splenic and superior mesenteric veins, as well as the main portal vein and the intrahepatic portal and hepatic veins. When scanning patients with PHT, slow-moving portal flow can be difficult to detect. In these cases a UCA could potentially be used to increase the reflectivity of portal vein blood, thus enhancing its detectability. The addition of contrast during US evaluations of patients with PHT could potentially also improve the detection of portal-systemic collaterals and evaluations of surgically created porto-systemic shunts as well as improve the confidence of diagnoses in cases of complete or partial portal system thrombosis.

In a study of both normal volunteers and patients with cirrhosis, Sellars et al. found that Doppler flow signals from the portal vein were enhanced in all cases after administration of Levovist.[81] This study compared the duration of enhancement provided by a bolus administration to that of three different infusion rates (slow, medium, and fast). A bolus delivery provided the shortest duration of contrast enhancement, whereas the slow infusion technique provided the longest duration. Contrast enhancement persisted for 113 seconds (mean

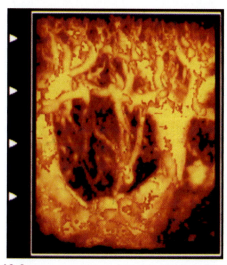

FIGURE 18-8 Contrast-enhanced 3D PDI of a kidney in an animal model. Note the fine detail of the renal vasculature.

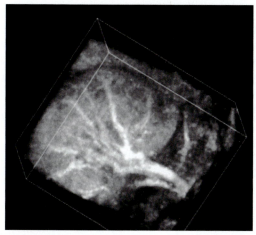

FIGURE 18-9 The combination of 3D gray-scale harmonic imaging and administration of a vascular UCA results in an "ultrasound angiogram."

duration) after a bolus injection compared to as much as 569 seconds (mean duration) following a slow infusion.

Contrast enhanced sonography has also been used effectively in the assessment of flow through transjugular intrahepatic porto-systemic shunts (TIPS).[85,96] Uggowitzer et al. found that Levovist provided Doppler signal enhancement lasting from 30 seconds to 7 minutes, and Levovist-enhanced scans improved the diagnosis of stent stenosis compared to the conventional US examinations.[96]

Published reports have described CES-detectable alterations in blood flow transit time through the livers of patients with diffuse hepatic disease when compared to normal controls.[1,54,81] In cases of cirrhosis there is often reduced portal venous flow and a compensatory increase in hepatic artery flow. Albrecht reported that after IV injection of Levovist in patients with cirrhosis the arrival of contrast in the hepatic veins was 24 seconds compared to 49.8 seconds for normal controls.[1] The authors postulated that the increased hepatic artery flow in the cirrhotic patients resulted in the more rapid appearance of contrast in the hepatic veins. Evaluation of blood flow through the liver has also been investigated as a means to identify hepatic metastases.[37,102] Zhou, et al. examined blood flow in the hepatic arteries and hepatic veins of 52 patients with metastases and 23 normal control subjects after bolus injections of SonoVue.[102] The parameters that were evaluated included contrast arrival time, time to peak enhancement, and peak intensity values in the vessels. Additionally, the difference between the arrival times in the hepatic artery and the hepatic veins was calculated. The arrival times and transit times in the patient group were significantly shorter than those of the control group, and the peak intensity values in the patient group were significantly higher than those of the control group. The results of this study suggest that CES assessment of changes in the hemodynamic parameters of the hepatic artery and vein can be used to improve diagnosis of liver metastases possibly before sonographic detection of focal lesions. Although these preliminary reports on the use of CES to detect changes in hepatic hemodynamics appear promising, additional research in this intriguing application of CES is necessary.

Hepatic Tumors. Many patients who have hepatic tumors first identified sonographically eventually require a CT or MRI examination to better determine the extent of disease as well as to more accurately characterize the lesions. Using CES, it is possible to distinguish the various phases of blood flow to and within the liver. In normal situations after IV administration of an UCA, contrast-enhanced flow in the hepatic artery is identified first (arterial or early vascular phase), followed by enhanced portal venous flow (portal venous phase). Detection of flow in the hepatic capillaries is identified later (late vascular phase) as a parenchymal blush (Figure 18-10). If a RES-specific agent is utilized, identification of the delayed enhancement phase representing the enhancement from the stationary microbubbles that have been phagocytosed by the RES is possible.[92]

Similar diagnostic criteria currently used for contrast-enhanced CT or MRI including evaluation of the phase, degree, and pattern of vascularity in and around hepatic tumors can also be applied to CES.[41,55] In fact, CES, because of its ability to image dynamic events in real time, may prove to be better than CT or MRI in the evaluation of hemodynamics that occur in the various hepatic vascular phases. Numerous published reports suggest that CES can improve the detection and characterization of liver lesions.[6,20,24,25,29,31,37,41,47,49,50,54,55,76,86,87,90,92,93,97,101,102]

Goldberg et al. used NC100100 (Sonazoid), a tissue-specific agent for evaluation of solid liver lesions.[31] Using power Doppler imaging in the vascular phase, enhanced detection of blood flow from vessels in and around hepatic tumors was demonstrated in all patients. In the delayed phase (10 to 30 minutes post UCA injection) there was increased echogenicity of the normal hepatic parenchyma and improved visualization of tumors that were not detected before contrast administration including detection of tumors as small as 3 mm. Some lesions demonstrated an echogenic rim.

Blomley et al. used Levovist to evaluate the detectability of tumors using stimulated AE during US examinations of patients with known liver metastases.[6] They found that all metastases appeared as areas of reduced or absent AE on color Doppler imaging scans of the liver. No AE defects were observed in the livers of three control subjects. The lack of AE from the hepatic metastases improved the conspicuity of lesions and improved the detection of tumors including detection of tumors not visualized using conventional gray-scale US.

Strobel and colleagues evaluated the diagnostic accuracy of CES for diagnosis of liver tumors in 1349 patients who had hepatic tumors that could not be definitively diagnosed with conventional sonography.[89,90] Low-MI, phase inversion HI was utilized to assess contrast enhancement patterns in the focal lesions during the arterial, portal, and late phases, and CES results were compared to histology, CT, or MRI. The diagnostic accuracy of CES was 83% for all benign lesions (82% for hemangiomas and 87% for focal nodular hyperplasia lesions) and 96% for all malignant lesions (91% for metastases and 85% for hepatocellular carcinomas). Late phase hypo-enhancement was seen in 95% of all liver metastases.

Cavernous hemangiomas are common benign solid neoplasms of the liver and are frequently detected during hepatic US examinations. Not all hemangiomas have the classic US appearance of a rounded, homogeneously hyperechoic mass with well-defined margins, nor can they be accurately characterized sonographically (Figure 18-11). Several recent reports have suggested that CES can improve the assessment of hemangiomas.[87,89,91,99]

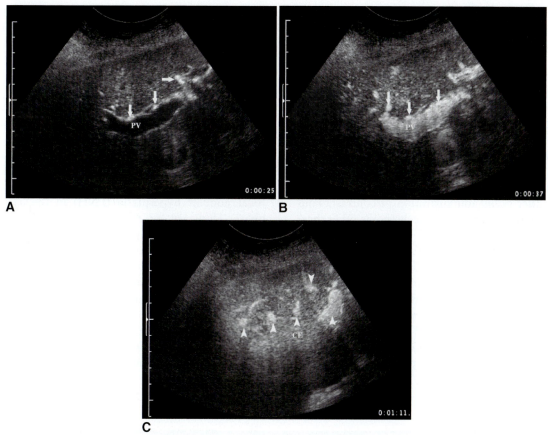

FIGURE 18-10 Contrast-enhanced demonstration of the various phases of hepatic blood flow. **A,** Twenty-five seconds after IV injection of an UCA, the first vessels to demonstrate contrast enhancement in the liver are the hepatic arteries *(arrows),* whereas the portal vein *(PV)* remains anechoic in the arterial phase. **B,** In this patient, the portal venous phase occurred 37 seconds after injection with contrast seen in the portal vein. **C,** In the late vascular phase at 71 seconds after injection, the liver parenchyma is becoming echogenic (i.e., contrast-enhanced; *CE*) and there is persistent enhancement of the major hepatic vessels *(arrowheads).*

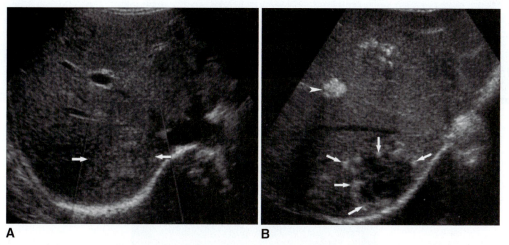

FIGURE 18-11 Improved detection and characterization of a liver hemangioma. **A,** A conventional ultrasound exam identified a poorly demarcated mass *(arrows)* in the right posterior lobe of the liver. **B,** After contrast administration using GSHI there is pooling of contrast-containing blood at the periphery of the lesion and increased echogenicity of the normal liver parenchyma. This pattern is characteristic for hemangiomas.

Weskott reported using US contrast and interval delay gray-scale harmonic imaging (GSHI) in an attempt to identify the hemodynamic patterns most consistent with hemangiomas.[99] Fifteen atypical (i.e., hypoechoic) hemangiomas ranging in size from 8 mm to 45 mm were evaluated before and after bolus administration of Levovist. Correlation was made with CT or MRI. All small hemangiomas demonstrated near complete enhancement with three of the small tumors possessing a central nonenhanced area. The time interval for refill of lesions less than 2 cm in size was under 4 seconds, whereas larger lesions required up to 3 minutes to enhance. A few larger masses demonstrated areas that did not enhance, which the author suggested was because of focal intratumoral thrombosis. Westcott concluded that most atypical hemangiomas show rapid refilling of contrast, suggesting that their blood supply was via arteries. Early and late vascular phase imaging provided a means to accurately characterize hemangiomas sonographically.

SonoVue was used in another study of atypical hemangiomas reported by Solbiati et al.[87] Seven atypical hemangiomas (1.5 to 6.5 cm) were evaluated with GSHI before and after bolus administration of contrast. Four lesions appeared hypoechoic or anechoic; the other three were isoechoic and "almost undistinguishable" on baseline (unenhanced) US. Arterial, portal, and late vascular phase imaging was performed following contrast administration. In the arterial phase, all lesions demonstrated only peripheral enhancement. In the portal phase, and even more so in the late vascular phase, progressive centripetal filling lasting from 5 to 7 minutes was observed in all lesions. The lesions got progressively more echogenic over time, which permitted a confident

diagnosis. The authors concluded that multiphase sonography was necessary for accurate diagnosis of atypical hemangiomas and that CES has the potential to obviate the need for CT scans. They also suggested that contrast-enhanced multiphase imaging may be useful to sonographically characterize other hepatic lesions.

Several reports have described the CES appearance of **hepatocellular carcinoma (HCC)** as having intense enhancement in the early arterial phase and relatively rapid wash-out of contrast in the portal phase.[45,86,101] (Figure 18-12). In our experience (using a RES-specific agent), HCC lesions can have a similar appearance to **focal nodular hyperplasia (FNH)** in the early arterial phase. However, on delayed phase imaging the HCC tumor will be hypoechoic relative to the surrounding normal liver tissue (because of the lack of Kupffer cells within the tumor), whereas FNH tumors, because they contain abundant amounts of Kupffer cells, will be isoechoic to the surrounding normal liver tissue (Figure 18-13). The central feeding artery and spoke-wheel radiating branches that are characteristic of FNH on dynamic CTA can also be depicted by CES, which may help to differentiate HCC from FNH.[45,89,95,97]

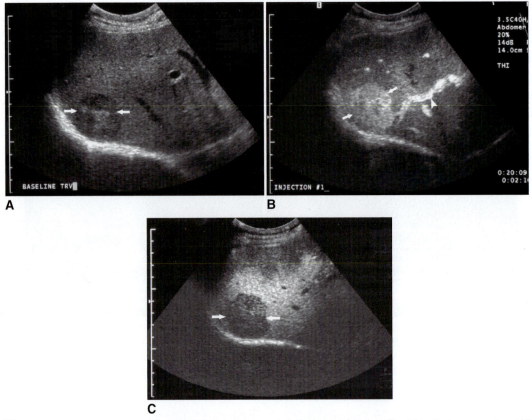

FIGURE 18-12 Improved characterization of hepatocellular carcinoma (HCC) using a RES-specific UCA. **A,** A conventional US exam identified a mass *(arrows)* in the right posterior lobe of the liver having mixed echogenicity. **B,** After contrast administration using GSHI, the hepatic artery and portal veins filled with contrast *(arrowheads)* and the mass became brightly echogenic compared to the surrounding liver tissue in the arterial and portal venous phases. **C,** On delayed imaging the lesion was hypoechoic compared to the surrounding liver tissue. This CES pattern is characteristic for HCC.

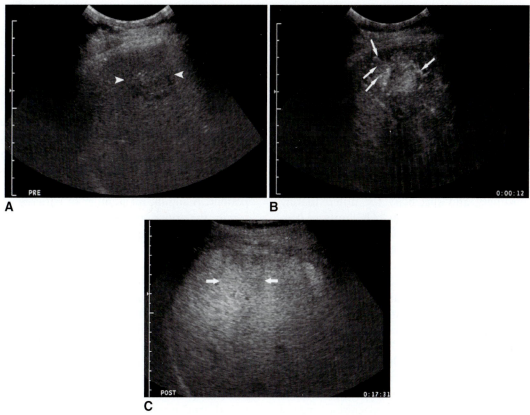

FIGURE 18-13 Improved characterization of focal nodular hyperplasia (FNH) using a RES-specific UCA. **A,** A conventional US exam identified a hypoechoic mass *(arrowheads)* in the right anterior lobe of the liver. **B,** After contrast administration using GSHI, the mass became brightly echogenic and intratumoral vessels having a radiating spoke-like pattern could be identified *(arrows)*. A central hypoechoic area within the mass that did not enhance represents a scar. **C,** On delayed imaging the lesion was isoechoic compared to the surrounding liver tissue. This CES pattern is characteristic for FNH.

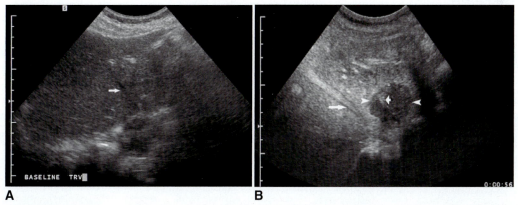

FIGURE 18-14 Improved detection and delineation of a colorectal carcinoma liver metastasis. **A,** A transverse conventional US image at the level of the middle hepatic vein *(arrow)* did not identify the mass, which had been detected on a prior CT examination. **B,** After UCA administration using GSHI in the portal venous phase, there was increased echogenicity of the surrounding liver parenchyma which results in improved delineation of the tumor *(arrowheads)*. Contrast-enhanced blood flow could also be identified in the hepatic vein *(arrow)* and small vessels within the mass *(short arrow)*. In this case the patient was being evaluated for possible US-guided radiofrequency ablation of this nonresectable tumor, and the CES results enhanced the ability to identify the location of the tumor as well as its size and margins.

Contrast-enhanced sonography has been shown to improve the detection and delineation of liver metastases[6,37,92,95,102] (Figure 18-14). However, accurate characterization of metastatic liver tumors with CES can be problematic because the degree of vascularity in these lesions is related to the primary cancer.[101] Therefore, some metastatic liver lesions will be hypervascular, whereas others are hypovascular. One imaging characteristic of liver metastases that has been identified during delayed phase imaging using an RES-specific UCA is an echogenic rim around the tumor.[55] The echogenic rim is thought to reflect the higher concentration of Kupffer cells around metastases or a higher degree of contrast, which results from compression of the normal liver parenchyma around the metastases. [55]

A recent report described the results of a multicenter study that compared CES to CT or MRI for characterization of focal liver lesions.[95] The study included 134 patients with one focal liver lesion detected in baseline ultrasound imaging. The lesions were classified as malignant, benign, or indeterminate based on imaging findings. Compared with unenhanced US, CES markedly improved sensitivity and specificity for differentiating malignant from benign liver lesions. The authors concluded that CES was the most sensitive, most specific, and most accurate imaging modality for the characterization of focal liver lesions.

By providing a means to detect and differentiate the various vascular enhancement patterns (e.g., degree, architecture, and phasicity) in and around hepatic lesions in real time, CES has been proven to improve characterization of liver lesions including HCC, FNH, metastases, and hemangiomas. Numerous published reports have confirmed the clinical utility and diagnostic accuracy of CES for liver lesion characterization. CES for liver lesion characterization is rapidly gaining recognition around the world as one of the most important applications of CES. CES has established itself as an important diagnostic tool for the evaluation of patients with focal liver lesions of unknown origin.

Renal Applications

Published reports have described the use of UCAs in a variety of renal applications including the evaluation of suspected renal masses and renal artery steno-sis.[14,19,52,56,61, 63,66,74,80,98] These reports provide an indication as to what may be expected once vascular UCAs become available for widespread clinical use in the United States.

Renal Artery Stenosis (RAS). The sonographic evaluation of the main and intrarenal renal arteries in patients with suspected **renal artery stenosis (RAS)** is fraught with problems. Because the main renal arteries are retroperitoneal in location, these vessels are typically difficult to evaluate sonographically. Signal attenuation over depth and overlying bowel often limit sonographic visualization of the main renal arteries, particularly in the obese patient. A significant number of patients will have anatomic variations of the renal vasculature, including duplicate or accessory renal arteries, and these variations can be difficult to identify using noncontrast US. Furthermore, there may be limited sonographic windows that can be used to view the renal arteries, and these windows may not be in optimal locations from which to obtain adequate Doppler-to-flow angles. US examinations for RAS are often time consuming and are extremely operator dependent. These factors likely contribute to the wide variability reported in the accuracy of US when used for RAS examinations.[4,71]

By improving the signal intensity of Doppler flow signals and increasing the likelihood of obtaining adequate Doppler flow information, UCAs hold the promise of improving examinations of patients with suspected RAS (Figure 18-15).[67] Vascular contrast agents significantly increase the ability to visualize blood flow using color flow imaging and improve the intensity of spectral Doppler flow signals. Therefore, in cases where the renal arteries are not visualized or the spectral waveforms are of poor quality, the IV administration of contrast can improve the examination process and potentially reduce the number of technically inadequate

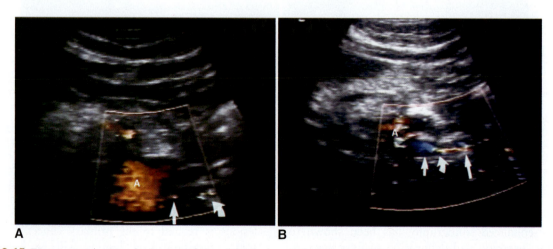

A   **B**

FIGURE 18-15 Transverse color Doppler images of the abdominal aorta and proximal left renal artery in a patient with suspected renal artery stenosis. **A,** Before intravenous administration of contrast, flow in the aorta *(A)* and proximal most renal artery *(arrow)* are visualized and there is aliasing of the color flow display *(curved arrow)*. **B,** After injection of contrast, the stenotic vessel lumen *(arrows)* can be clearly visualized.

or otherwise nondiagnostic examinations (see Figures 18-1 and 18-2).

Needleman reported on the use of contrast in phase III clinical trials including evaluations of RAS.[56] In this series there were 12 kidneys with dual renal arteries identified with magnetic resonance angiography (MRA). Nine of these were correctly identified with CES, whereas only two cases of dual renal arteries were identified before contrast administration. There were 12 confirmed cases of RAS, three (25%) of which were only detected with CES.

Missouris and colleagues reported on the use of Levovist-enhanced sonography compared to angiography in the evaluation of 21 patients with suspected RAS.[63] Sensitivity and specificity for the detection of RAS improved from 85% and 79%, respectively, on noncontrast studies to 94% and 88% with the addition of Levovist. They also reported that the mean examination time was halved by the addition of Levovist. These studies suggest that the use of US contrast agents will improve the sonographic evaluations of patients with suspected RAS, while potentially reducing examination time.

Renal Masses. Diagnostic sonography has been a reliable method of evaluating patients with renal masses, particularly in the differentiation of cystic from solid lesions. Sonography is usually accurate in its ability to identify large (>2 cm) renal cell carcinomas and to identify tumor thrombus in the renal veins or inferior vena cava (IVC). However, in a small percentage of cases sonography cannot identify small neoplasms or differentiate solid hypoechoic renal lesions from hemorrhagic cysts or other benign processes (Figure 18-16). Furthermore, normal anatomic variations such as a prominent column of Bertin or persistent fetal lobulation may mimic renal tumors. In these cases other imaging studies such as CT or MRI or needle biopsy may be indicated for a definitive diagnosis.

By improving the detection of flow in the intrarenal vessels, UCAs may provide a means of identifying and demonstrating the normal renal vasculature and detecting the presence of lesions that distort the vascular architecture[61,74] (see Figure 18-7). Contrast is also likely to improve the detection of abnormal vessels present in renal tumors and to identify flow voids that result from tumor thrombus in cases of renal vein or IVC involvement (Figures 18-17 and 18-18).

Splenic Applications

Several reports have described the clinical value of CES for the evaluation of the spleen.[10,11,59,70,75] Picardi et al. compared CES to CT and fluorodeoxyglucose positron emission tomography (PET) for the detection of nodular infiltration in the spleen of 100 patients with newly diagnosed Hodgkin lymphoma.[75] Malignant nodules were detected with CT in 13 patients, with PET in 13 patients, and with CES in 30 patients. The authors concluded that CES provides a higher sensitivity than does CT or PET in the detection of splenic involvement by Hodgkin lymphoma.

Catalano and colleagues studied 55 patients with a variety of suspected splenic abnormalities including traumatic injuries and tumors.[11] The CES results were compared to baseline (noncontrast) US, CT, or MRI. In this series, parenchymal injuries were detected with a sensitivity of 63% on baseline US, whereas the sensitivity improved to 89% after CES. Parenchymal injuries included posttraumatic infarctions that were not identified on baseline US but were identified with CES. CES also identified 35 of 39 proven focal lesions in patients with Hodgkin disease, whereas baseline US detected only 23 lesions.

In another report, two pediatric patients were evaluated for traumatic splenic injuries.[70] In both cases CES identified splenic hematomas that were not detected on

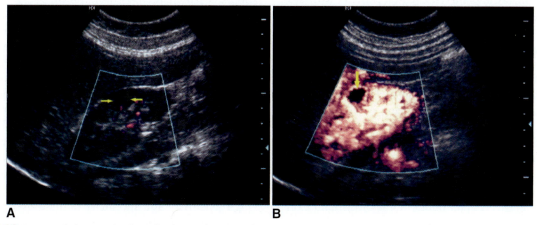

A   **B**

FIGURE 18-16 Improved characterization of a hypoechoic renal mass. **A,** On the precontrast power Doppler image, a hypoechoic mass *(arrows)* is visualized in the midpole of the right kidney. **B,** After injection of a vascular UCA, blood flow is demonstrated with PDI within the normal renal parenchyma but no flow was detected from within the mass *(arrow)*. The mass was later determined to represent a benign hemorrhagic cyst.

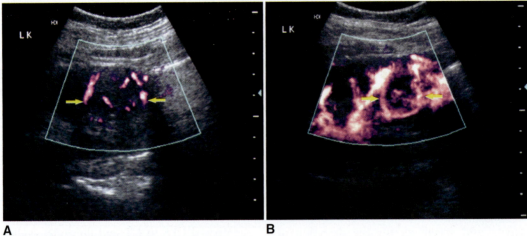

FIGURE 18-17 Power Doppler imaging (PDI) of a suspicious renal mass before and after IV administration of contrast. **A,** On the precontrast image a subtle hypoechoic mass was identified near the lower pole of the left kidney but PDI only demonstrates flow around the mass. **B,** After injection of contrast there are significantly more flow signals detected including intratumoral flow. This was later confirmed to represent a renal cell carcinoma.

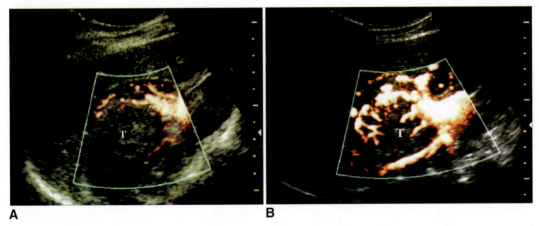

FIGURE 18-18 Power Doppler imaging of a large renal cell carcinoma before and after IV administration of contrast. **A,** On the precontrast image blood flow is only detected around the tumor periphery. **B,** With contrast enhancement there are significantly more flow signals detected including intratumoral flow.

unenhanced US scans. Contrast-enhanced US may prove to be a viable alternative to other diagnostic tests for the initial assessment and surveillance of patients with suspected splenic trauma.

Pancreatic Applications

Sonographic visualization of the pancreas is often hampered by the gland's deep location within the retroperitoneum and the presence of overlying bowel. Although ingestion of water or an oral UCA have been shown to improve the visualization of the pancreas, currently no oral UCAs are available, and, therefore, the potential benefits of oral agents will not be discussed here. Those desiring this information should review the references cited earlier in this chapter under "Oral Ultrasound Contrast Agents."

Advances in US technology (e.g., endoscopic US, HI, etc.) combined with UCAs has led to a significant improvement in the diagnostic potential of US for a

range of pancreatic disorders.[60] Several published reports describe the ability of microbubble-based UCAs to improve pancreatic US evaluations.[8,21,42,44,60,65,67,78] Rickes et al. compared contrast-enhanced power Doppler imaging (PDI) to conventional gray-scale US and PDI in 137 patients suspected of having a pancreatic tumor.[78] Of the 137 patients, a normal pancreas was found in 10; 47 had pancreatic cancer; 41 had lesions associated with pancreatitis; 17 had neuroendocrine tumors; 12 had cystic lesions of the pancreas; and 10 had other pancreatic diseases. The sensitivity of contrast-enhanced PDI for the diagnosis of pancreatic carcinoma was 87% and its specificity 94%. The corresponding values for chronic pancreatitis were 85% and 99%, respectively. The authors concluded that contrast-enhanced PDI had a high sensitivity and specificity in the differential diagnosis of pancreatic tumors.

Kersting et al. evaluated the value of transabdominal CES for differential diagnosis of pancreatic ductal adenocarcinoma (PDAC) and focal inflammatory masses resulting from chronic pancreatitis.[44] Time-intensity curves were obtained in two regions of interest within the lesion and within the normal pancreatic tissue, and CES data were evaluated using quantification software. Of the 60 patients examined, histology revealed 45 PDACs and 15 inflammatory masses. The time-dependent parameters (arrival time and time-to-peak) were significantly longer in PDACs compared to focal masses. The authors concluded that PDAC and focal inflammatory masses exhibit different perfusion patterns that can be visualized with CES. Additionally, the contrast quantification software provided objective criteria that could be used to facilitate pancreatic lesion diagnoses.

In Japan Numata et al. evaluated the vascularity of autoimmune pancreatitis lesions with contrast-enhanced GSHI in six patients and compared their findings to pathology.[67] The vascularity of three of the six lesions studied was also evaluated by CES before and after treatment with corticosteroids. The pancreatic lesions exhibited mild (n = 1), moderate (n = 3), or marked (n = 2) enhancement throughout almost their entirety. The grade of lesion vascularity on the CES images correlated with the pathologic grade of inflammation and inversely correlated with the grade of fibrosis associated with autoimmune pancreatitis. After steroid therapy the vascularity of all treated lesions had decreased. The authors concluded that CES may be useful for evaluating the vascularity of autoimmune pancreatitis lesions and the therapeutic efficacy of steroid therapy.

Organ Transplants

Sonography is routinely used to evaluate kidney, liver, and pancreas transplants. The modality is often employed as a first-line examination tool in the immediate postsurgical period as well as for serial studies to confirm organ viability. After organ transplantation, sonography is used to detect postsurgical fluid collections, to identify urinary or bile obstructions, and to assess blood flow to and from the transplanted organ. Conventional sonography is also useful in the evaluation of blood flow within the organ, but it does not have an adequate level of sensitivity to detect flow at the microvascular level (i.e., tissue perfusion). When a vascular abnormality is suspected, angiography or contrast-enhanced CT can provide a definitive diagnosis. However, angiography is invasive, CT requires ionizing radiation, and administration of contrast media required for these exams may be contraindicated.

The enhanced detection of blood flow provided by CES improves the assessment of blood flow in the arteries and veins that supply the transplanted organ and the vessels to which these vessels are anastomosed. CES has also been found to improve the ability to detect the lack of flow within transplanted organs (i.e., ischemic regions) within renal and pancreatic grafts.[3,8,21,42,49] This is a clinically important application of CES because of the frequent use of sonography to evaluate organ recipients.

Numerous studies suggest that CES is useful for the evaluation of liver transplant recipients.[3,57,82,83] Leutloff et al. reported their findings of 21 patients (31 examinations) who received orthotopic liver transplants.[49] After Levovist was administered, significantly better arterial flow signals were detected in the porta hepatis as well as in the right and left lobes of the liver. The authors concluded that the use of contrast-enhanced CFI significantly improved the detection of hepatic arterial flow in transplant recipients.

For renal transplants, CES can permit better differentiation of regions that have decreased perfusion from true vascular defects resulting from a renal artery branch occlusion or acute rejection.[15] Contrast-enhanced sonography has also been found to be superior to conventional sonography for differentiating parenchymal abnormalities like **acute tubular necrosis (ATN)** from other abnormalities. Benozzi et al. performed serial CES and PDI of 39 kidney recipients within 30 days of transplantation and compared the imaging results with clinical findings and functional assessments.[3] Both CES and PDI identified grafts with early dysfunction, but only some CES-derived parameters distinguished ATN from acute rejection episodes. The authors concluded that the use of CES in the early postoperative period provided important prognostic information about renal transplants.

Other Applications

Other common abdominal/retroperitoneal applications of US include assessment of flow in the mesenteric arteries for mesenteric ischemia; the aorta, and iliac arteries to evaluate suspected aneurysms, stenoses, endovascular leaks, or dissections; and the IVC for evaluation of filters or thromboses. Often these examinations are limited by the presence of overlying bowel and bowel gas, or the effects of signal attenuation resulting from the deep location of the vessels. Vascular UCAs have been used with success to improve the assessment of the abdominal vasculature and blood flow.[28,40,69,73]

In one published study, CES was used for surveillance of aortic stent grafts.[28] Thirty patients were serially evaluated with CES and the results were compared to either computed tomographic angiography (CTA) or magnetic resonance angiography (MRA) as the gold standard. All CTA/MRA-detected endoleaks were also detected by CES (yielding a rate of 100% sensitivity for CES). However, CES also detected endoleaks that were not identified by the comparative studies and, therefore, the authors considered these to represent false positives, even though some of the leaks may have been true positives. They concluded that CES may be a useful stent graft surveillance tool by itself or in conjunction with CTA/MRA but that additional studies were necessary.

At our institution, using animal models, we created bleeding sites in the bowel, spleen, and other organs.[30] After IV injection of contrast, the bleeding sites were visualized as areas with the characteristic mosaic color AE display corresponding to the contrast-containing blood pooling in the region of the lacerations. Similar results were obtained using gray-scale wideband HI of bleeding sites.[10,34] In the future, the use of CES to improve the detection of internal bleeding and for surveillance may prove useful in cases of trauma.

Finally, contrast has been used successfully to diagnose and monitor treatment of patients with focal tumors who are going to have or have had chemotherapy, radiofrequency, ethanol, or other focal tumor ablation techniques[33,88,94] (see Figure 18-14). Ultrasound contrast agents used during the planning stage of a US-guided ablation can provide a means to better define tumor size and delineate tumor margins, which would help ensure that the entire tumor is ablated while normal tissue is preserved. Patients that have had a tumor ablation procedure receive serial imaging examinations to check for residual viable tumor at the ablation site and to screen for tumor recurrence. Currently, CT and MRI are most commonly used for these serial studies. However, in the future CES could be used for the follow-up examinations. If a radiofrequency ablation procedure is being considered, it is conceivable that if additional ablations are indicated by the CES study, they could be performed (under US guidance) at the time of diagnosis, thus reducing the time between diagnosis and treatment, and possibly improving the patient's outcome.

CONCLUSION

Two UCAs are currently being marketed in the United States—Optison and Definity—but they are FDA approved for echocardiographic applications only. In the future, additional agents or clinical applications of existing agents are likely to become available. Many published reports on the efficacy and clinical utility of CES are coming from European and Asian investigators because of the greater availability and utilization of UCAs in those regions of the world. Vascular agents have been shown to improve the detection of blood flow in small and deep vessels throughout the body. Reports have also described the ability of UCAs to improve the sonographic detection and characterization of tumors and other abnormalities within the abdomen as well as in other anatomic areas.

The enhancement capabilities of UCAs have been shown to have the ability to salvage nondiagnostic US examinations and render them diagnostic. The use of UCAs has also resulted in new US evaluations (e.g., the assessment of contrast transit time and phasicity of blood flow in and around liver tumors) that were not possible without their use. Improvements in US technology designed to exploit the acoustic behavior of contrast

microbubbles are complementing the use of UCAs. Advances in both US instrumentation and the development of UCAs will continue to have a positive impact on the future of diagnostic sonography.

REFERENCES

1. Albrecht T, Blomley MJ, Cosgrove DO, et al: Non-invasive diagnosis of hepatic cirrhosis by transit-time analysis of an ultrasound contrast agent, *Lancet* 353:1579-1583, 1999.
2. Albrecht T, Urbank A, Mahler M, et al: Prolongation and optimization of Doppler enhancement with a microbubble US contrast agent by using continuous infusion: preliminary experience, *Radiology* 207:339-347, 1998.
3. Benozzi L, Cappelli G, Granito M, et al: Contrast-enhanced sonography in early kidney graft dysfunction, *Transplant Proc* 41(4):1214-1215, 2009.
4. Berland LL, Koslin DB, Routh WD, Keller FS: Renal artery stenosis: prospective evaluation of diagnosis with color duplex US compared with angiography, *Radiology* 174:421-423, 1990.
5. Blomley MJ, Lim AK, Harvey CJ, et al: Liver microbubble transit time compared with histology and Child-Pugh score in diffuse liver disease: a cross sectional study, *Gut* 52(8):1188-1193, 2003.
6. Blomley MJK, Albrecht T, Cosgrove DO, et al: Improved imaging of liver metastases with stimulated acoustic emission in the late phase of enhancement with the US contrast agent SH U 508A: early experience, *Radiology* 210:409-416, 1999.
7. Blomley MJK, Harvey CJ, Eckersley RJ, Cosgrove DO: Contrast kinetics and Doppler intensitometry. In Goldberg BB, Raichlen JR, Forsberg F, editors: *Ultrasound contrast agents: Basic principles and clinical applications*, ed 2, London, 2001, Martin Dunitz, pp. 81-89.
8. Boggi U, Morelli L, Amorese G, et al: Contribution of contrast-enhanced ultrasonography to nonoperative management of segmental ischemia of the head of a pancreas graft, *Am J Transplant* 9(2):413-418, 2009.
9. Bree LB, Platt J: Clinical applications of an oral ultrasound contrast agent in the upper abdomen: overview of a phase II clinical trial, *Appl Rad* 28(S):28-32, 1999.
10. Catalano O, Aiani L, Barozzi L, et al: CEUS in abdominal trauma: multi-center study, *Abdom Imaging* 34(2):225-234, 2009.
11. Catalano O, Lobianco R, Sandomenico F, et al: Realtime contrast-enhanced ultrasound of the spleen: examination technique and preliminary clinical experience, *Radiol Med* 106(4):338-356, 2003.
12. Chomas JE, Dayton PA, Allen J, Ferrara KW: Optical and acoustical observation of contrast-agent destruction. In Goldberg BB, Raichlen JS, Forsberg F, editors: *Ultrasound contrast agents*, ed 2, London, 2001, Martin Dunitz, pp. 259-266.
13. Claudon M, Rohban T: Levovist in the diagnosis of renal artery stenosis: results of a controlled multicenter study, *Radiology* 205(P):242, 1997.
14. Correas J, Claudon M, Tranquart F, Helenon O: Contrast-enhanced ultrasonography: renal applications, *J Radiol* 84:2041-2054, 2003.
15. Correas J, Helenon O, Moreau JF: Contrast-enhanced ultrasonography of native and transplanted kidney diseases, *Eur Radiol* 9(Suppl 3):S394-S400, 1999.
16. Cosgrove D, Kedar, R, Bamber JC, et al: Color Doppler in the differentiation of breast masses, *Radiology* 189:99-104, 1993.

17. Crouse LJ, Cheirif J, Hanly DE, et al: Opacification and border delineation improvement in patients with suboptimal endocardial border definition in routine echocardiography: results of the phase III Albunex multicenter trial, *J Am Coll Cardiol* 22:1494-1500, 1993.

18. De Jong N, Bouakaz A, Frinking PJA, Ten Cata FJ: Contrast-specific imaging methods. In Goldberg BB, Raichlen JS, Forsberg F, editors: *Ultrasound contrast agents*, ed 2, London, 2001, Martin Dunitz, pp. 25-36.

19. Dowling RJ, House MK, King PM, et al: Contrast-enhanced Doppler ultrasound for renal artery stenosis, *Australas Radiol* 43(2):206-209, 1999.

20. Ernst H, Hahn EG, Balzer T, et al: Color Doppler ultrasound of liver lesions: signal enhancement after intravenous injection of the ultrasound contrast agent Levovist, *J Clin Ultrasound* 24:31-35, 1996.

21. Faccioli N, Crippa S, Bassi C, D'Onofrio M: Contrast-enhanced ultrasonography of the pancreas, *Pancreatology* 9(5):560-566, 2009.

22. Forsberg F, Goldberg BB, Liu JB, et al: On the feasibility of real-time, in vivo harmonic imaging with proteinaceous microspheres, *J Ultrasound Med* 15:853-860, 1996.

23. Forsberg F, Liu JB, Burns PN, Merton DA, Goldberg BB. Artifacts in ultrasound contrast agent studies, *J Ultrasound Med* 13:357-365, 1994.

24. Forsberg F, Liu JB, Merton DA, et al: Tumor detection using an ultrasound contrast agent, *J Ultrasound Med* 4:S8, 1995.

25. Forsberg F, Liu JB, Merton DA, et al: Gray scale second harmonic imaging of acoustic emission signals improves detection of liver tumors in rabbits, *J Ultrasound Med* 19:557-563, 2000.

26. Forsberg F, Liu JB, Rawool NM, et al: Gray-scale and color Doppler flow harmonic imaging with proteinaceous microspheres, *Radiology* 197(P):403, 1995.

27. Forsberg F, Shi WT, Merritt CRB, et al: Does the Mechanical Index predict destruction rates of contrast microbubbles? *J Ultrasound Med* 20:S12, 2001.

28. Giannoni MF, Palombo G, Sbarigia E, et al: Contrast-enhanced ultrasound for aortic stent-graft surveillance, *J Endovasc Ther* 10(2):208-217, 2003.

29. Goldberg BB, Forsberg F, Fitzsch T, et al: Induced acoustic emission as a contrast mechanism for detection of hepatic abnormalities, *J Ultrasound Med* 14:S7, 1995.

30. Goldberg BB, Forsberg F, Merton DA, et al: Sonographic detection of bleeding sites and other structures with use of a contrast agent, *Radiology* 201(P):197, 1996.

31. Goldberg BB, Leen E, Needleman L, et al: Contrast enhanced ultrasound imaging of liver lesions: a phase II study with NC100100, *J Ultrasound Med* 18(S):43, 1999.

32. Goldberg BB, Liu JB, Burns PN, et al: Galactose-based intravenous sonographic contrast agent: experimental studies, *J Ultrasound Med* 12:463-470, 1993.

33. Goldberg BB, Liu JB, Merton DA, et al. The role of contrast-enhanced US for RF ablation of liver tumor, *Radiology* 217(P):607, 2000.

34. Goldberg BB, Merton DA, Forsberg F, Liu, JB. Evaluation of bleeding sites with a tissue-specific sonographic contrast agent: preliminary experiences in an animal model, *J Ultrasound Med* 17:609-616, 1998.

35. Gramiak R, Shah PM: Echocardiography of the aortic root, *Invest Radiol* 3:356-366, 1968.

36. Harvey CJ, Blomley MJK, Cosgrove DO: Acoustic emission imaging. In Goldberg BB, Raichlen JS, Forsberg F, editors: *Ultrasound contrast agents*, ed 2, London, 2001, Martin Dunitz, pp. 71-80.

37. Hohmann J, Müller C, Oldenburg A, et al: Hepatic transit time analysis using contrast-enhanced ultrasound with BR1: a prospective study comparing patients with liver metastases from colorectal cancer with healthy volunteers, *Ultrasound Med Biol* 35(9):1427-1435, 2009.

38. www.astratech.se/Main.aspx/Item/214433/navt/8/navl/46951/nava/46952. Accessed 02/16/04.

39. www.definityimaging.com. Accessed 2/19/04.

40. Iezzi R, Cotroneo AR, Basilico R, et al: Endoleaks after endovascular repair of abdominal aortic aneurysm: value of CEUS, *Abdom Imaging* May 15, 2009.

41. Isozaki T, Numata K, Kiba T, et al: Differential diagnosis of hepatic tumors by using contrast enhancement patters at US, *Radiology* 229(3):798-805, 2003.

42. Karamehic J, Scoutt LM, Tabakovic M, Heljic B: Ultrasonography in organs transplantation, *Med Arh* 58(1 Suppl 2):107-108, 2004.

43. Kedar RP, Cosgrove DO, McCready VR, Bamber JC: Microbubble Doppler angiography of breast masses: dynamic and morphologic features, *Radiology* 189(P):154, 1993.

44. Kersting S, Konopke R, Kersting F, et al: Quantitative perfusion analysis of transabdominal contrast-enhanced ultrasound of pancreatic masses and carcinomas, *Gastroenterology* Aug 25, 2009.

45. Kim EA, Yoon KH, Lee YH, et al: Focal hepatic lesions: contrast-enhancement patterns at pulse-inversion harmonic US using a microbubble contrast agent, *Korean J Radiol* 4:224-233, 2003.

46. Kishimoto N, Mori Y, Nishiue T, et al: Renal blood flow measurement with contrast-enhanced harmonic ultrasonography: evaluation of dopamine-induced changes in renal cortical perfusion in humans, *Clin Nephrol* 59(6):423-428, 2003.

47. Kitamura H, Miyagawa Y, Yokoyama T, et al: Kupffer cell imaging with ultrasound contrast agent for diagnosis of histological grade of hepatocellular carcinoma, *J Ultrasound Med* 20:S10, 2001.

48. Klein HG: Ultrasound contrast agents: A commercial perspective. In Goldberg BB, Raichlen JS, Forsberg F, editors: *Ultrasound contrast agents*, ed 2, London, 2001, Martin Dunitz, pp. 387-405.

49. Koda M, Matsunaga Y, Ueki M, et al: Qualitative assessment of tumor vascularity in hepatocellular carcinoma by contrast-enhanced coded ultrasound: comparison with arterial phase of dynamic CT and conventional color/power Doppler ultrasound, *Eur Radiol* 16, 2003.

50. Kono Y, Mattrey RF, Pinnell SP, et al: Contrast-enhanced B-mode harmonic imaging for the evaluation of HCC viability after therapy in cirrhotic patients, *J Ultrasound Med* 20:S10, 2001.

51. Kono Y, Mattrey RT: Harmonic imaging with contrast microbubbles. In Goldberg BB, Raichlen JS, Forsberg F, editors: *Ultrasound contrast agents*, ed 2, London, 2001, Martin Dunitz, pp. 37-46.

52. Lacourciere Y, Levesque J, Onrot JM, et al: Impact of Levovist ultrasonographic contrast agent on the diagnosis and management of hypertensive patients with suspected renal artery stenosis: a Canadian multicentre pilot study, *Can Assoc Radiol J* 53(4):219-227, 2002.

53. Lee KH, Choi BI, Kim, KW, et al: Contrast-enhanced dynamic ultrasonography of the liver: optimization of hepatic arterial phase in normal volunteers, *Adbom Imaging* 28(5):652-656, 2003.

54. Leen E, Anderson WG, Cooke TG, McArdle CS: Contrast enhanced Doppler perfusion index: detection of colorectal liver metastases, *Radiology* 209(P):292, 1998.

55. Leen E: Radiological applications of contrast agents in the hepatobiliary system. In Goldberg BB, Raichlen JS, Forsberg F, editors: *Ultrasound contrast agents*, ed 2, London, 2001, Martin Dunitz, pp. 278-288.

56. Lencioni R, Pinto S, Cioni D, Bartolozzi C: Contrast-enhanced Doppler ultrasound of renal artery stenosis: pro-

logue to a promising future, *Echocardiography* 16(7, Pt 2):767-773, 1999.

57. Leutoff UC, Scharf J, Richter GM, et al: Use of ultrasound contrast medium Levovist in after-care of liver transplant patients: improved vascular imaging in color Doppler ultrasound, *Radiology* 38:399-404, 1998.

58. Lev-Toaff AS, Goldberg BB: Gastrointestinal ultrasound contrast agents. In Goldberg BB, editor: *Ultrasound contrast agents*, London, 1997, Martin Dunitz, pp. 121-135.

59. Manetta R, Pistoia ML, Bultrini C, et al: Ultrasound enhanced with sulphur-hexafluoride-filled microbubbles agent (SonoVue) in the follow-up of mild liver and spleen trauma, *Radiol Med* 114(5):771-779, 2009.

60. Martínez-Noguera A, Montserrat E, Torrubia S, et al: Ultrasound of the pancreas: update and controversies, *Eur Radiol* 11(9):1594-1606, 2001.

61. Merton DA: An easily implemented method to improve detection of ultrasound contrast in body tissues: frame one imaging, *J Diag Med Sonography* 16(1):14-20, 2000.

62. Postema M, Gilja OH: Contrast-enhanced and targeted ultrasound, *World J Gastroenterol* 7, 17(1):28-41, 2011.

63. Missouris CG, Allen CM, Balen FG, et al: Non-invasive screening for renal artery stenosis with ultrasound contrast enhancement, *J Hypertens* 14(4):519-524, 1996.

64. Moriyasu F, Kono Y, Nada T, et al: Flash echo (passive cavitation) imaging of the liver by using US contrast agents and intermittent scanning sequence, *Radiology* 201(P):196, 1996.

65. Nagase M, Furuse J, Ishii H, Yoshino M: Evaluation of contrast enhancement patters in pancreatic tumors by coded harmonic sonographic imaging with a microbubble contrast agent, *J Ultrasound Med* 22(8):789-795, 2003.

66. Needleman L: Review of a new ultrasound contrast agent—EchoGen emulsion, *Appl Rad* 26 (S):8-12, 1997.

67. Numata K, Yutaka O, Noritoshi K, et al: Contrast-enhanced sonography of autoimmune pancreatitis: comparison with pathologic findings, *J Ultrasound Med* 23(2):199-206, 2004.

68. Ophir J, Gobuty A, McWhirt RE, Maklad NF. Ultrasonic backscatter from contrast producing collagen microspheres, *Ultrasound Imaging* 2:67-77, 1980.

69. Oka MA, Rubens DJ, Strang JG: Ultrasound contrast agent in evaluation of abdominal vessels, *J Ultrasound Med* 20:S84, 2001.

70. Oldenburg A, Hohmann J, Skrok J, Albrecht T: Imaging of paediatric splenic injury with contrast-enhanced ultrasonography, *Pediatr Radiol* 34(4):351-354, 2004.

71. Olin JW, Piedmonte MR, Young JR, et al: The utility of duplex ultrasound scanning of the renal arteries for diagnosing significant renal artery stenosis, *Ann Intern Med* 122:833-838, 1995.

72. Pelberg RA, Wei K, Kamiyama N, et al: Potential advantage of flash echocardiography for digital subtraction of B-mode images acquired during myocardial contrast echocardiography, *J Am Soc Echocardigr* 12:85-93, 1999.

73. Pfister K, Rennert J, Uller W, et al: Contrast harmonic imaging ultrasound and perfusion imaging for surveillance after endovascular abdominal aneurysm repair regarding detection and characterization of suspected endoleaks, *Clin Hemorheol Microcirc* 43(1):119-128, 2009.

74. Peterson CL, Barr RG: Contrast-enhanced sonography in patients with renal pathology, *J Diag Med Sonography* 16(2):53-56, 2000.

75. Picardi M, Soricelli A, Pane F, et al: Contrast-enhanced harmonic compound US of the spleen to increase staging accuracy in patients with Hodgkin lymphoma: a prospective study, *Radiology* 251(2):574-582, 2009.

76. Plew J, Sanki J, Young N, et al: Early experience in the use of Levovist ultrasound contrast in the evaluation of liver masses, *Australas Radiol* 44:28-31, 2000.

77. Porter TR, Xie F: Accelerated intermittent harmonic imaging. In Goldberg BB, Raichlen JS, Forsberg F, editors: *Ultrasound contrast agents*, ed 2, London, 2001, Martin Dunitz, pp. 67-70.

78. Rickes S, Unkrodt K, Neye H, et al: Differentiation of pancreatic tumours by conventional ultrasound, unenhanced and echo-enhanced power Doppler sonography, *Scand J Gastroenterol* 37(11):1313-1320, 2002.

79. Ripollés T, Puig J: Update on the use of contrast agents in ultrasonography: a review of the clinical guidelines of the European Federation of Societies for Ultrasound in Medicine and Biology (EFSUMB), *Radiologia* 51(4):362-375, 2009.

80. Robbin ML, Lockhart ME, Barr RG: Renal imaging with ultrasound contrast: current status, *Radiol Clin North Am* 41(5):963-978, 2003.

81. Sellars ME, Sidhu PS, Heneghan M, et al: Infusions of microbubbles are more cost-effective than bolus injections in Doppler studies of the portal vein: a quantitative comparison of normal volunteers and patients with cirrhosis, *Radiology* 217(P):396, 2000.

82. Sidhu PS, Marshall MM, Ryan SM, et al: Clinical use of Levovist, an ultrasound contrast agent, in the imaging of liver transplantation: assessment of the pre- and post-transplant patient, *Eur Radiol* 10(7):1114-1126, 2000.

83. Sidhu PS, Shaw AS, Ellis SM, et al: Microbubble ultrasound contrast in the assessment of hepatic artery patency following liver transplantation: role in reducing frequency of heaptic artery arteriography, *Eur Radiol* 14(1):21-30, 2004.

84. Sirlin CB, Girard MS, Baker K, et al: Effect of gated US acquisition on liver and portal vein contrast enhancement, *Radiology* 201(P):158, 1996.

85. Skjoldbye B, Weislander S, Struckmann J, et al: Doppler ultrasound assessment of TIPS patency and function-the need for echo enhancers, *Acta Radiol* 39:675-679, 1998.

86. Solbiati L, Cova L, Ierace T, et al: Characterization of focal lesions in patients with liver cirrhosis using second generation contrast-enhanced (CE) wideband harmonic sonography (WBHS) in different enhancement phases, *J Ultrasound Med* 20:S10, 2001.

87. Solbiati L, Cova L, Ierace T, et al: Diagnosis of atypical hemangioma using contrast-enhanced wideband harmonic sonography (CE-WBHS), *J Ultrasound Med* 20:S9, 2001.

88. Solbiati L, Goldberg SN, Ierace T, et al: Radio-frequency ablation of hepatic metastases: post procedural assessment with a US microbubble contrast agent: early experience, *Radiology* 211:643-649, 1999.

89. Strobel D, Seitz K, Blank W, et al: Tumor-specific vascularization pattern of liver metastasis, hepatocellular carcinoma, hemangioma and focal nodular hyperplasia in the differential diagnosis of 1,349 liver lesions in contrast-enhanced ultrasound (CEUS), *Ultraschall Med* 30(4):376-382, 2009.

90. Strobel D, Krodel U, Martus P, et al: Clinical evaluation of contrast-enhanced color Doppler sonography in the differential diagnosis of liver tumors, *J Clin Ultrasound* 28:1-13, 2000.

91. Sugimoto K, Shiraishi J, Moriyasu F, Doi K: Computer-aided diagnosis of focal liver lesions by use of physicians' subjective classification of echogenic patterns in baseline and contrast-enhanced ultrasonography, *Acad Radiol* 16(4):401-411, 2009.

92. Sugimoto K, Shiraishi J, Moriyasu F, et al: Improved detection of hepatic metastases with contrast-enhanced low mechanical-index pulse inversion ultrasonography during the liver-specific phase of Sonazoid: observer performance study with JAFROC analysis, *Acad Radiol* 16(7):798-809, 2009.

93. Tanaka S, Kitamra T, Yoshioka F, et al: Effectiveness of galactose-based intravenous contrast medium on color Doppler sonography of deeply located hepatocellular carcinoma, *Ultrasound in Med Biol* 21:157-160, 1995.

94. Tawada K, Yamaguchi T, Kobayashi A, et al: Changes in tumor vascularity depicted by contrast-enhanced ultrasonography as a predictor of chemotherapeutic effect in patients with unresectable pancreatic cancer, *Pancreas* 38(1):30-35, 2009.

95. Trillaud H, Bruel JM, Valette PJ, et al: Characterization of focal liver lesions with SonoVue® enhanced sonography: International multicenter-study in comparison to CT and MRI, *World J Gastroenterol* 15(30):3748-3756, 2009.

96. Uggowitzer MM, Hausegger KA, Machan L, et al: Echo-enhanced Doppler sonography in the evaluation of transjugular intraheptic portosystemic shunts: Clinical applications of a new transpulmonary US contrast agent, *Radiology* 201(P):266, 748, 1996.

97. von Herbay A, Vogt C, Haussinger D: Pulse inversion sonography in the early phase of the sonographic contrast agent Levovist: differentiation between benign and malignant focal liver lesions, *J Ultrasound Med* 21:1191-1200, 2002.

98. Wei K, Le E, Bin JP, et al: Quantification of renal blood flow with contrast-enhanced ultrasound, *J Am Coll Cardiol* 15;37(4):1135-1140, 2001.

99. Weskott HP: Contrast-enhanced Reperfusion imaging in atypical hepatic hemangiomas, *J Ultrasound Med* 20:S9, 2001.

100. Wheatley MA: Composition of contrast microbubbles: Basic chemistry of encapsulated and surfactant-coated bubbles. In Goldberg BB, Raichlen JS, Forsberg F, editors: *Ultrasound contrast agents*, ed 2, London, 2001, Martin Dunitz, pp. 3-13.

101. Wilson SR, Burns PN, Muradali D, et al: Harmonic hepatic US with microbubble contrast agent: initial experience showing improved characterization of hemangioma, hepatocellular carcinoma, and metastasis, *Radiology* 215:153-161, 2000.

102. Zhou JH, Li AH, Cao LH, et al: Haemodynamic parameters of the hepatic artery and vein can detect liver metastases: assessment using contrast-enhanced ultrasound, *Br J Radiol* 81(962):113-119, 2008.

Ultrasound-Guided Interventional Techniques

M. Robert De Jong

Ultrasound has been used to assist in interventional procedures since the 1970s by means of specially designed A-mode and B-mode transducers. The use of ultrasound as a primary imaging modality to guide interventional examinations continues to grow. Multiple factors contribute to this growth: increased system resolution, new developments in transducer designs, new technology developments like compound imaging and fusion technologies, as well as the development of more versatile transducer needle guide attachments, which offer multiple angles. Another important factor is economics, as ultrasound-guided procedures are less costly than other imaging modalities. The other economic benefit is that performing the biopsy under ultrasound allows patients throughout to continue through the computed tomography (CT) scanner. Performing a biopsy under CT would mean a decrease of four to five patients per hour in the CT scanner as opposed to one less patient in the ultrasound room. Ultrasound is now being used to perform a variety of invasive procedures on various organs and masses located in the neck, chest, abdomen, retroperitoneum, musculoskeletal, and pelvis, as well as to drain various fluid and abscess collections. There has been an increase in the number of nonimaging physicians who use ultrasound for the placement of peripherally inserted central catheters, PICC lines, subclavian and jugular lines, and even to assist in starting IVs.

ULTRASOUND-GUIDED PROCEDURES

In recent years, there has been a movement to perform more and more procedures under ultrasound guidance. Retroperitoneal masses, pleural based masses, deep masses in the liver, and musculoskeletal masses that were once typically biopsied under CT guidance or in open surgical biopsies are now being successfully performed using ultrasound guidance (Figure 19-1).

Ultrasound can be used to do the following:

- Biopsy malignant or benign masses.
- Biopsy organs for parenchymal disease or transplant rejection.
- Drain fluid collections, such as cysts, ascites, or pleural fluid.
- Drain or obtain samples of abscesses to determine the type of organism, especially on patients who are not responding to antibiotic therapy.
- Assist in placement of drainage tubes or catheters.
- Assist in placement of catheters in arteries and veins.
- Mark spots for fluid taps to be performed without direct sonographic guidance.

The main advantage of using ultrasound for guidance is to have continuous real-time visualization of the biopsy needle, which allows adjustment of the needle as

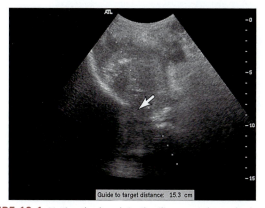

FIGURE 19-1 Notice the break in the iliac crest (arrow) where the tumor has broken through the cortex. The biopsy was positive for Ewing's sarcoma.

needed during the procedure. As the biopsy specimen is being obtained, the needle tip can be watched in real time to ensure that it does not slip outside the mass. This is especially important for small masses or if patients have trouble holding their breath. Ultrasound also has the advantage of allowing different patient positions and approaches to be considered. The patient may be turned into a decubitus or oblique position to allow safe access to the mass (Figure 19-2). Subcostal approaches can allow the use of steep angles with the needle directed cephalic in liver masses. This can reduce the risk of a pneumothorax or bleeding from an injury to an intercostal artery when using intercostal techniques. Using ultrasound the patient can be placed in a comfortable position and not be made to lie supine or prone. For example, the patient's head may be slightly elevated or the patient can move slightly between passes to relieve back or joint pain. Another benefit is the ability to comfort and reassure the patient as the sonologist, sonographer, and nurse are all with the patient during the procedure. Even the most anxious patients can be coached to cooperate when the team is by their side and not constantly in and out of the room. Other advantages include the ability to perform the biopsy in a single breath hold, portability, lack of radiation, and shorter procedure times.

Despite all its benefits, ultrasound guidance does have some limitations. Not all masses can be visualized with ultrasound, as the mass may be isoechoic to the normal tissue. The sonographer should look for indirect signs of the presence of a mass, such as displaced vessels, capsule bulges, or the presence of tumor vessels (Figure 19-3). Abdominal masses may also be obscured by bowel gas. Sometimes the sonographer can press the gas out of the way with the transducer, allowing for a successful biopsy. Gas may move during the procedure causing difficulty in seeing the mass, which can delay the biopsy until the

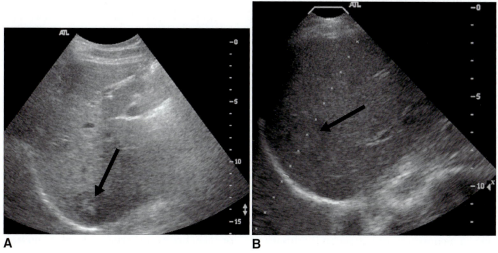

A **B**

FIGURE 19-2 A, With the patient supine, the liver mass (arrow) is 15 cm deep. **B,** The patient is now in the left lateral decubitus position, the liver has fallen forward, and the same mass (arrow) is now only 7 cm deep. An easy, successful biopsy showed metastatic disease from a pancreas primary.

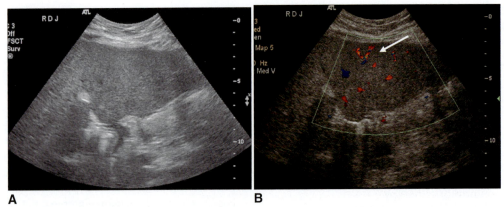

FIGURE 19-3 A, Although a definite mass was seen on a contrast MRI, it was not appreciated by ultrasound. **B,** Using the MRI as a guide and color Doppler to assess for areas of abnormal flow, a successful biopsy was performed on this patient with infiltrative hepatocellular carcinoma *(arrow).*

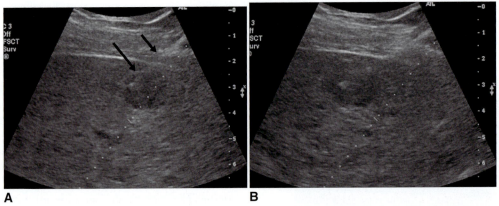

FIGURE 19-4 A, The needle *(arrows)* deviated from the projected path of the guide *(dotted line).* **B,** Because of the constant deviation of the needle from the projected path, the sonographer had to compensate by moving the transducer laterally so that the needle would pass through the center of the mass. Note that the projected path does not even go through the mass. A diagnosis of hepatocellular carcinoma was obtained.

gas moves or even in some cases canceling the biopsy under ultrasound and finishing it under CT. The needle tip may be difficult to see if it deviates from the projected path because of bending or deflection of the needle. This can call upon the sonographer's scanning skills to maneuver the transducer to find the needle tip or to correct for needle deviation (Figure 19-4). Other disadvantages may include sonographer inexperience, the comfort level of the radiologist with performing biopsies with CT, and having to use fixed angles when using needle guides.

INDICATIONS FOR A BIOPSY

The most common indication for a biopsy is to confirm malignancy in a mass. The mass may be the primary tumor in a patient with an undiagnosed malignancy or a metastatic mass in a patient with a known primary malignancy. Other indications include the need to differentiate between a metastatic and a second primary mass, to determine the cause of metastases in a patient with multiple primaries, to differentiate recurrent tumor from postoperative or therapy scarring, to differentiate

malignancy from inflammatory or infectious disease, to determine metastatic lymph adenopathy from lymphoma, and to characterize a benign mass. Other common reasons for a biopsy are to obtain a sample of the parenchyma in an organ to determine the severity or progression of a disease process such as hepatitis or renal failure or to determine the cause of rejection in a transplanted organ (Figure 19-5).

CONTRAINDICATIONS FOR A BIOPSY

Contraindications of ultrasound-guided procedures are few because of the procedure's minimally invasive nature. However, contraindications do include an uncorrectable bleeding disorder, the lack of a safe needle path (Figure 19-6), or an uncooperative patient. Patient cooperation is needed so that the mass may be biopsied safely. If the patient will not hold still, is jumpy, or cannot control his or her breathing, the risk of a complication for the patient increases significantly, as does the risk to the sonographer or sonologist of being stuck by a contaminated needle.

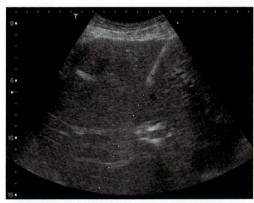

FIGURE 19-5 Liver core biopsy in a patient with hepatitis C.

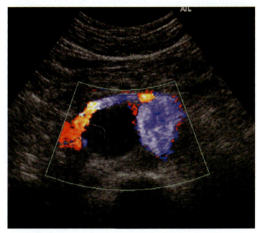

FIGURE 19-6 This retroperitoneal lymph node could not be biopsied under ultrasound because of the vessels that surrounded it.

LABORATORY TESTS

With the exception of bleeding times, blood or urine tests typically are not requested before an ultrasound-guided procedure. Usually, an abnormal lab value will be part of the patient's work-up that led to the biopsy. Some abnormal examples that may trigger a request for a procedure include an elevated alpha-fetoprotein (AFP) when there is a liver lesion, elevated prostate-specific antigen (PSA) to evaluate for prostate cancer, changes in thyroglobulin levels in a patient with a history of thyroid cancer, increased white blood cell count (leukocytosis) when an abscess is suspected, and hematuria along with a renal mass.

Laboratory tests that should be reviewed before most procedures are the patient's bleeding times. These tests measure the time it takes the blood to form a clot. This is especially true for patients who are on blood thinners such as Coumadin, heparin, or aspirin therapy. Because vitamin K is essential in the blood clotting process, patients with liver disease are at risk for prolonged bleeding and the formation of hematomas. To eliminate patient rescheduling or cancellation, test results should be obtained as close to the date of the procedure as possible, although results may be acceptable up to 3 to 4 weeks

before the scheduled procedure. These simple blood tests can also be performed the morning of the procedure as results can usually be obtained in 2 to 3 hours.

At least a dozen factors are needed to form a blood clot to stop bleeding; they all interact through a complex series of reactions called the coagulation cascade. There are three pathways in the blood clotting process: intrinsic, extrinsic, and common. To evaluate all three pathways, both prothrombin time (PT) and partial thromboplastin time (PTT) are evaluated. PTT can be used to evaluate the effects of heparin, aspirin, and antihistamines on the blood-clotting process. PTT evaluates factors found in the intrinsic and common pathways. PTT values may vary depending on the method and activators used, with normal values typically between 60 and 70 seconds. PT is used to evaluate factors found in the extrinsic pathway, which may be affected by patients on Coumadin. Normal values are typically between 10 and 13 seconds.

Because of the variability of PT results between laboratories, a method of standardization was developed called the **international normalized ratio (INR)**. The INR was created in 1983 by the World Health Organization to account for the various thromboplastin reagents used to determine PT, which caused fluctuations in normal values. The INR is a calculation that adjusts for the variations in PT processing and values so that test results from different laboratories can be compared. The INR is expressed as a number. Values of less than 1.4 are needed to ensure a safe procedure. The INR/PT is not used on patients with liver disease or on heparin. It is evaluated on patients taking anticoagulants, especially Coumadin.

PT, PTT, and platelet count are required before most procedures. Some departments may not require a hemostatic evaluation for fluid aspirations and superficial or low-risk biopsies such as of the thyroid, neck nodes, or the prostate. Anticoagulants should be discontinued before the biopsy to reduce the risk of postprocedural bleeding. Patients should be off their blood thinners before the procedure as follows: 4 to 6 hours for heparin, 3 to 4 days for Coumadin, and 5 to 7 days for aspirin, although these values can be different for different hospitals or imaging centers. Patients should also be informed to stop taking supplements that can prolong bleeding times such as omega-3, fish oils, and flaxseed oil. Patients with a defect in their blood-clotting mechanism (coagulopathy) will need to have a platelet transfusion just before and during the procedure to ensure that they do not have excessive bleeding.

TYPES OF PROCEDURES

Biopsies are used to confirm if a mass is benign, malignant, or infectious. Most biopsies are easily and safely performed as an outpatient procedure. Biopsy success rates have been reported to have sensitivities of greater than 85% and specificities of greater than 95%. Cell type is often needed to determine treatment type and options, as specific tumors respond better to certain types of chemotherapy or to radiation therapy.

Fine needle aspiration (FNA), or cytologic aspiration, uses thin-gauge needles to obtain cells from within the mass. FNAs are performed using a 20- to 25-gauge needle with a cutting tip, such as a Franseen, Chiba, or spinal needle (Figure 19-7). These types of needles have the least risk associated with their use, allowing multiple passes as needed. The number of the gauge corresponds to the diameter of the needle: the higher the number, the smaller the diameter. Needles are described by their length and gauge. For example, if the physician asks for a 20, 15, or 20 × 15, he or she wants a 20-gauge needle that is 15 cm in length. If different types of needles are available, the physician might ask for a Franseen 20, 15. A word of caution: Seeing the length of the needle may cause a patient to become quite apprehensive. The sonographer should explain to the patient that the thickness of the needle is what is important, not the length, as part of the needle will be in the needle guide. The specimen is obtained by using a capillary action technique. This involves a steady, quick up-and-down motion of the needle (after the stylet is removed), which obtains the needed cells through a scraping or cutting action. As the needle is removed from the body, the physician will place his thumb over the open hub so that the cells are not sucked back into the body. An FNA technique reduces the trauma to the cells and decreases the amount of background blood. If the sample is scant, suction techniques can be used. Suction technique involves using a syringe and tubing attached to the needle. As the needle is being moved up and down, suction is applied to draw up the cells into the needle. Once the needle is removed, the physician will place the tip of the needle over the slide to deposit the cells so that they can be smeared for staining and evaluation. The physician may also express the cells into a container holding special fluid to preserve the cells. Because of its thin size, the needle can safely go through the large or small bowel and near vascular

structures. FNA in conjunction with onsite cytopathology can help ensure that the procedure is diagnostic and minimize the number of passes.

A core biopsy utilizes an automated, spring-loaded device, termed a biopsy gun, to obtain a core of tissue for histologic analysis. The biopsy device is cocked and the needle tip is placed just inside the mass, on the outside edge of the mass or inside the organ itself. The button is then pushed and the cutting needle is thrown obtaining a core of tissue, which is deposited into a slot on the inner needle (Figure 19-8). Various throw lengths are available, ranging from 10 to 23 mm, which will also correspond to the length of specimen that is obtained. The throw length is the distance that the needle will advance when fired. The proper throw distance needs to be determined so that the needle does not go through the back wall of the mass and damage underlying structures or vessels (Figure 19-9). The snapping sound that the device makes can be startling to the patient, and it is advised to let the patient hear the sound before obtaining the specimen. This also ensures that the device is not defective. Core biopsy needles are larger in diameter and range in size from 14 to 20 gauge. A core biopsy can be used in conjunction with FNA techniques, especially if a definitive diagnosis could not be determined from just the FNA or if the cytopathologist requires more tissue for a more accurate diagnosis or special stains. Core biopsies are used to diagnose diffuse parenchymal disease of the liver or kidney, in transplanted organs, masses in the breast and in prostate biopsies.

Ultrasound is routinely used to guide needle placement to drain or obtain samples from ascites or pleural effusions. Usually, these procedures are performed without the use of a needle guide unless the fluid is multiloculated, is only a small amount, or is unsafe to drain by free hand techniques. If a small amount of fluid is needed, a 22- or 20-gauge needle may be used. If the fluid is viscous, an 18- or 16-gauge needle may be required. If the goal is to drain as much fluid as possible, a special needle called a centesis catheter is used (Figure

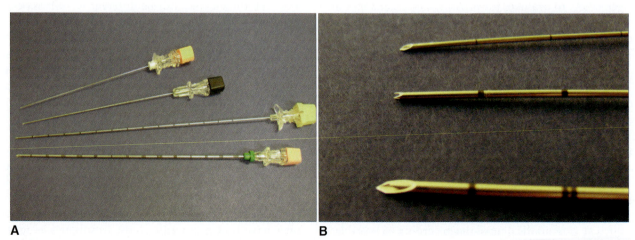

A   **B**

FIGURE 19-7 **A,** Different types of needles and gauges used for FNA biopsies. From top: 25g, 22g, 20g, 18g. **B,** Example of different types of needle tips. From top: Chiba, Franseen, Spinal.

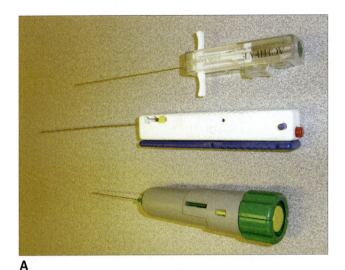

A

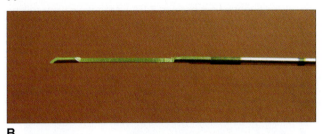

B

FIGURE 19-8 Different types of biopsy devices used for core biopsies. **B,** Close-up of a core needle where the specimen is deposited.

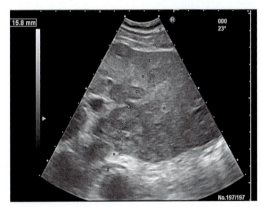

FIGURE 19-9 The sonographer measured the lesion (calipers) to determine the size of the core needle to be used. The diameter of the lesion along the needle path is 15.8 mm, so a 15-mm throw is needed to stay within the lesion.

19-10). After the needle is properly placed, the stylet is removed, leaving a catheter with side holes to safely drain the fluid. For large volume drainage, one-liter vacuum bottles are used to remove the fluid. Ultrasound can be used to periodically check the amount of fluid remaining or to help reposition the catheter to free it from bowel that may be sucked against the wall of the catheter (Figure 19-11). The sonographer can usually scan outside the sterile field. In a patient with massive ascites, a large volume of fluid may be drained for patient comfort. It is usually recommended that no more than 5 liters be drained because more than that can place the

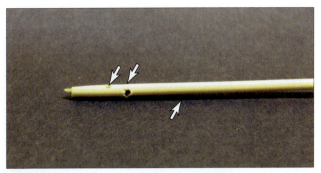

FIGURE 19-10 A centesis catheter. The arrows are pointing to the side holes.

patient at risk for electrolyte imbalance, **hypovolemia, hypotension,** and **hepatorenal syndrome.** If more than 5 liters are to be removed, the patient is usually given intravenous albumin to decrease the chance of these complications.

Fluid or abscess collections are usually performed using a needle guide. Abscess or fluid collections may be located in or around the liver, peripancreatic, perinephric, intraabdominal, pelvic, intramuscular, or in the prostate gland. Ultrasound can also be used to provide guidance to drain the gallbladder in patients who have cholecystitis, especially acalculous cholecystitis, or in patients too sick for surgery. The needle gauge used to drain the abscess depends on the thickness of the fluid. For pelvic collections, depending on their location, an endovaginal approach should be considered in women, and endorectal approaches in both men and women. For prostatic abscess drainage, an endorectal technique is used. Fluid is obtained to determine the type of organism present, so that the correct antibiotics can be administered to the patient. For a larger abscess, catheters may be left in place to drain the collection. Patients may have follow-ups to monitor that the cavity is getting smaller and to check that the catheter is still in the correct position. These follow-up examinations are usually performed under fluoroscopy in a procedure called a sinogram, although ultrasound can also be used.

Ultrasound is currently being used to guide placements of catheters and lines in various vessels including the subclavian, jugular, brachial, and femoral vessels; to assist in transjugular intrahepatic porto-systemic shunt (TIPSS) procedures; and to place nephrostomy tubes in obstructed kidneys. There are even dedicated ultrasound units available to help with image-guided peripheral IV insertion.

ULTRASOUND GUIDANCE METHODS

There are two methods in performing ultrasound-guided procedures: free hand techniques and the use of needle guides. The **free hand technique** is performed without the use of a needle guide on the transducer. The transducer is placed in a sterile cover, and the radiologist or physician that performs the biopsy will hold the transducer in one hand and the needle in the other hand. Care

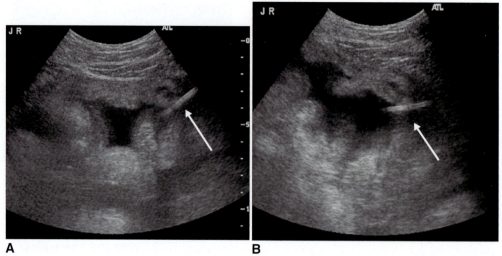

FIGURE 19-11 A, Bowel has been sucked up against the catheter *(arrow),* obstructing the flow of fluid. **B,** By having the patient roll into an oblique position, the fluid collected to the dependent portion and the bowel loop floated away from the catheter *(arrow),* allowing drainage to continue.

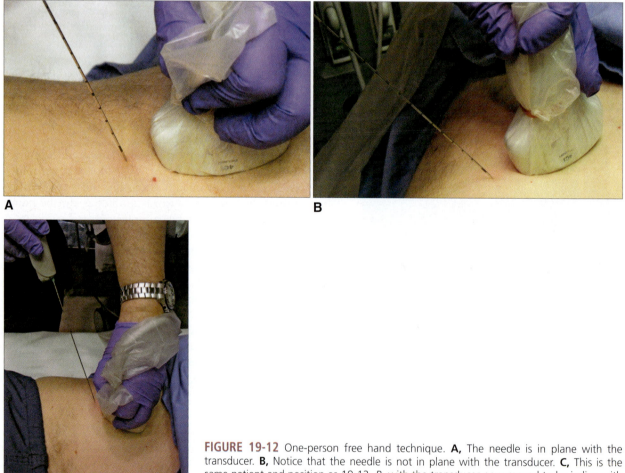

FIGURE 19-12 One-person free hand technique. **A,** The needle is in plane with the transducer. **B,** Notice that the needle is not in plane with the transducer. **C,** This is the same patient and position as 19-12, *B,* with the transducer now moved to be in line with the needle.

must be taken to align the needle with the transducer and the sound beam or else the needle tip will not be seen. If the needle tip disappears while advancing the needle on the image, the transducer should be repositioned in alignment with the needle path to bring the needle tip back into view. The free hand technique allows more flexibility in choosing the needle path, but it is more technically challenging, especially on deep lesions (Figure 19-12). A variation of this technique allows the sonographer to scan outside the sterile field while the physician performs the biopsy (Figure 19-13). Again, it is important to remember that to see the needle tip, the transducer must be aligned to the needle path. If the needle is not going to the area of interest, then either the transducer must be realigned to the needle path to find the needle or the needle must be removed and reinserted toward the transducer. If there is a light or color mark on the transducer, the sonographer can tell the physician to go toward the light. Free hand techniques are typically used to drain ascites (Figure 19-14), pleural fluid, and in superficial lesions. Some physicians prefer using free hand techniques for thyroid, native renal, and renal transplant biopsies.

The second method involves using a needle guide that is attached to the transducer (Figure 19-15). The predicted needle path is displayed on the screen either as a

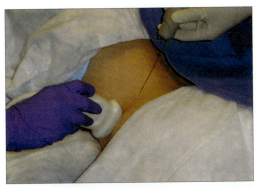

FIGURE 19-13 Two-person free hand technique with the sonographer scanning outside the sterile field.

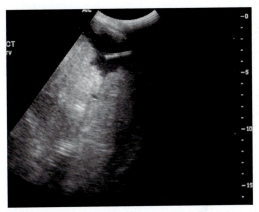

FIGURE 19-14 This paracentesis was performed without the use of a guide, as the fluid was superficial.

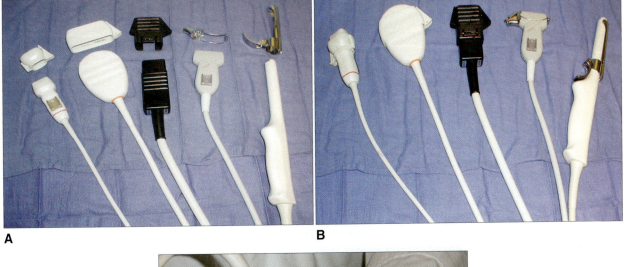

A   **B**

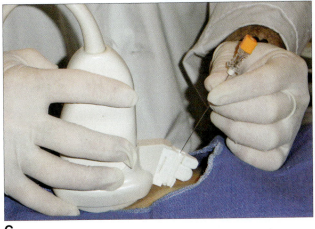

C

FIGURE 19-15 **A,** Various types of transducers and their guides. **B,** Same transducers with their guides attached. **C,** Biopsy using a needle guide.

single line or as two parallel lines. The mass is then lined up along the path, either on the single line or between the two lines. Some transducers offer a choice of angles, usually a steep angle and a shallow angle (Figure 19-16). This gives some flexibility around vessels or other structures. There are many benefits to using a needle guide, including a faster learning curve, faster placement of the needle, and the ability to keep the needle going through

the anesthetized area when multiple passes are required (Figure 19-17). The use of needle guides has expanded the role of ultrasound-guided procedures by allowing biopsies of pleural-based lung lesions, deep retroperitoneal lesions, small masses, and musculoskeletal masses. When the sonographer attaches the needle guide to the transducer, it is important to attach it correctly and set the angle on the guide the same as the angle on the

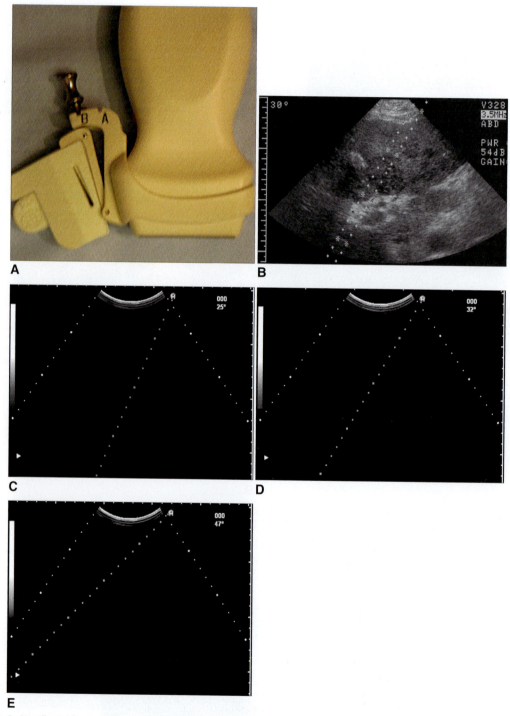

FIGURE 19-16 A, Needle guide attachment that offers a choice of two angles. The guide is in position for angle B. **B,** Needle guide attachment that offers a choice of a 15- or 30-degree angle. The transducer is set up for the 30-degree angle. This patient was determined to have metastatic liver disease from a lung primary. **C,** A transducer that offers three angles set at 25 degrees. **D,** A transducer that offers three angles set at 32 degrees. **E,** A transducer that offers three angles set at 47 degrees.

screen. The needle guides are precision-made devices and need to be handled with care and attached properly. If another angle is set on the transducer, the needle will appear to deviate, as it is not following the projected path on the screen; if the guide is put on backward, the needle will come in from the opposite side of the guide (Figure 19-18).

Both methods have their pros and cons, and the physician performing the biopsy or procedure will decide which technique—free hand or needle-guided—to use.

CYTOPATHOLOGY

Some ultrasound departments collaborate with the cytopathology department by having the cytopathology team present during the procedure. Usually, one to three passes are made, placed on the sterile slides, and stained in the ultrasound room. The cytopathologist looks at the slides to determine if the material is diagnostic. This can ensure that enough diagnostic material is obtained and help to minimize the number of passes. The cytopathologist may

request additional material for special stains and flow cytometry. (Flow cytometry may be needed when lymphoma is suspected.) The cytopathologist may also request that a core sample be obtained to enhance the chances of obtaining a diagnosis for the patient. It typically takes 3 to 5 minutes to stain and evaluate the slides per pass or group of passes. The benefit of having cytopathology onsite is that it does increase the percentage of successful biopsies, helps to minimize the number of passes, and possibly reduces overall procedure time.

Inconclusive Specimens

Unfortunately, not all biopsies yield sufficient material to provide a diagnosis. There are multiple reasons that lead to an inconclusive result, including insufficient material, necrotic lesion, and not biopsying the area of malignancy. If this occurs, a repeat biopsy may be required. This possibility should have been explained to the patient during the consent process. To increase the success of the repeat biopsy, a cytopathologist should be present.

BIOPSY COMPLICATIONS

Complications from an ultrasound-guided biopsy are usually minor and may include post-procedural pain or discomfort, vasovagal reactions, and hematomas. Serious complications, although rare, include bleeding, hemorrhage, pneumothorax, pancreatitis, biliary leakage, peritonitis, infection, and possibly death. Seeding of the needle track by malignant cells is rare, with an estimated occurrence in 1/20,000 patients. These potential complications must be explained to the patient during the consent process. It is important for the sonographer to look for signs of a complication both by observing the patient and with ultrasound. The sonographer should scan after every pass to look for any sonographic sign of a complication using both gray scale and color Doppler

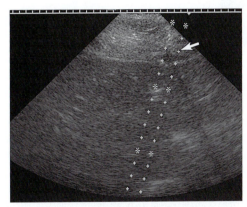

FIGURE 19-17 The arrow is pointing to a hypoechoic area, which is the lidocaine that was injected adjacent to the liver capsule. It is important for the sonographer to keep the transducer in this position so that the biopsy needle goes through the anesthetized area.

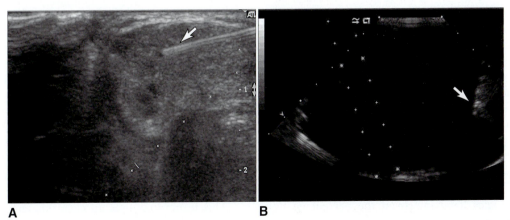

A   **B**

FIGURE 19-18 A, The arrow is pointing to the needle, which appears to be deviating. What is actually happening is that the guide on the transducer is set for angle A, but the biopsy line displayed on the screen is set for angle B. **B,** The transducer was attached backward. When the needle is inserted (*arrow*), it appears from the opposite side of the screen.

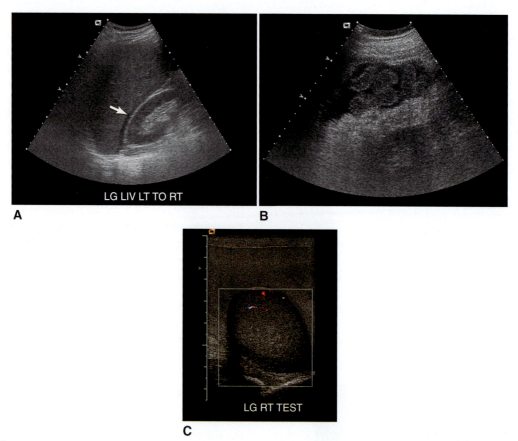

FIGURE 19-19 A, Hematoma *(arrow)* in Morison's pouch after a core biopsy. **B,** Same patient with free fluid along the left flank. **C,** The hematoma extended into the scrotal sac. Color Doppler verified that flow was present in the testicle.

(Figure 19-19). The sonographer should also help in observing the patient for any indications of a vasovagal reaction, pain, or bleeding from the biopsy site. Any visual or sonographic signs of a complication should be reported to the physician immediately. Applying pressure with the transducer over the area of bleeding can treat both internal and external bleeding. For bleeding from the skin at the biopsy site, cover the puncture site with a sterile 4 × 4 or other sterile material and press with the transducer. The sterile 4 × 4 will absorb the blood so that it does not drip down the patient's side and lend stability to the transducer so that it is not slippery. Vasovagal symptoms include the patient's profuse sweating, complaining of feeling faint or lightheaded, and nausea. Patients who experience any or all of these symptoms should be placed in a Trendelenburg position or have their feet elevated with a stack of sheets. A cold cloth or compress should also be placed on the forehead. After these feelings pass, the biopsy can continue.

FUSION TECHNOLOGY

Newer technologies have improved the percentage of procedures that can be performed using ultrasound guidance. Harmonic imaging and compound imaging have improved resolution by improving visualization of subtler lesions as well as of the needle tip. However, there are still a small percentage of lesions that cannot be seen by ultrasound. These are typically isoechoic lesions, especially in the liver. These lesions may also only be seen on a contrast-enhanced CT, thus making it difficult to perform the biopsy under CT guidance. Recently, some ultrasound companies have developed ultrasound equipment that has the capabilities to import the patient's CT or MRI scan directly into the ultrasound unit. This allows the sonographer to compare the MRI or CT scan directly with the ultrasound image in side-by-side images. As the ultrasound scan is being performed, the MRI or CT images move to the corresponding area, following the sonographer as they scan. Thus, the same anatomy is seen in real time on both the ultrasound image and the corresponding imported images (Figure 19-20). Another option allows fusing or superimposing of the two image sets on top of one another. Controls allow the ultrasound image or CT/MRI image to be given preference. For example, while locating the mass, the CT/MRI image may be emphasized, whereas the ultrasound image will be emphasized during the actual biopsy (Figure 19-21).

This technology uses an electromagnetic transmitter, which is placed near the area of scanning, and electromagnetic sensors that are connected to the transducer. Both the electromagnetic transmitter and the transducer sensors are connected to a position-sensing unit inside the ultrasound machine. The position-sensing equipment allows the ultrasound unit to track the transducer's position as the sonographer scans, and with it the image position, within the electromagnetic field (Figure 19-22).

To begin, the MRI or CT data set must be imported into the ultrasound unit. This can either be done via the network or uploaded from a DVD (Figure 19-23). Next, the sonographer needs to register the ultrasound image with the CT or MRI data set. This is accomplished by choosing a common anatomic point that can be identified easily on both the ultrasound image and the MRI or CT data set. Some common reference points may be the

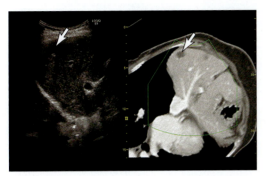

FIGURE 19-20 Fused studies of an ultrasound and CT demonstrating a simple liver cyst in the dome of the liver *(arrows).*

bifurcation of a vessel, the border of an organ, or even an area inside the mass. After locking in these points, the machine builds a transformation matrix based on this information. This transformation matrix is then used to display the multiplanar reconstructed image from the 3D MRI or CT data set that corresponds to the current live ultrasound image. As the ultrasound image is moved, the MPR, MRI, or CT image tracks in real time. The images can then be displayed either side by side or in a blended, overlapping format. The ultrasound image can also be removed, allowing the sonographer to scan and see only the CT or MRI image. This can be helpful in allowing the sonographer to scan and locate the area using the other imaging modality. Once the area of concern is located, the ultrasound image can be activated, and the sonographer can either remove the image from the other modality, scan in a fused method, or scan in a side-by-side format.

Once the two imaging modalities have been registered, the sonographer can use the CT or MRI scan to locate the area in question with ultrasound. If the area is not well seen by ultrasound, a marker can be placed on the MRI or CT image so that the radiologist knows where to obtain the specimen. Once this marker is placed on the MRI or CT image, a corresponding marker will appear on the ultrasound image (Figure 19-24). Another use for marking or targeting the mass is to quickly locate

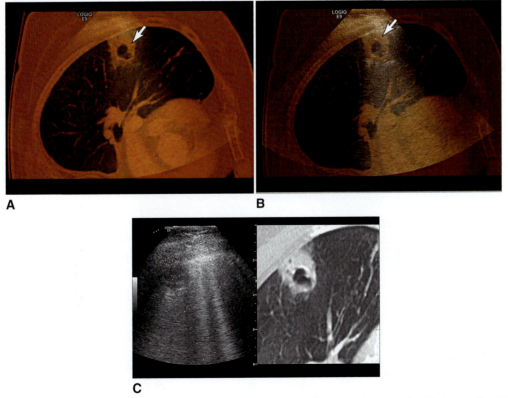

FIGURE 19-21 A, Fused imaged of a chest CT and ultrasound. The arrow is pointing to the mass. In this image, the CT has preference over the ultrasound image. **B,** Same two images, but this time the ultrasound has preference over the CT image. **C,** Side-by-side images used to guide the biopsy. This patient had adenocarcinoma of the lung.

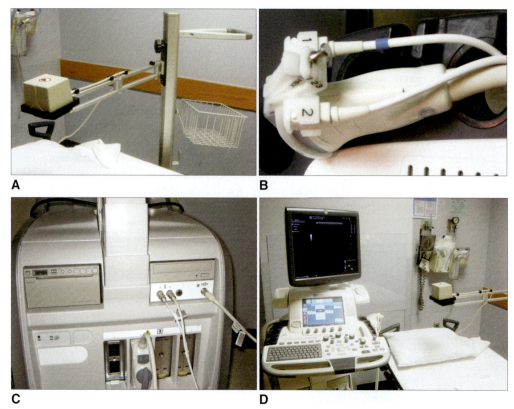

A **B**

C **D**

FIGURE 19-22 A, An electromagnetic transmitter unit. **B,** An example of sensors attached to the transducer. **C,** The cord from the transmitter unit and the paired cords from the transducer are plugged into the position sensing unit. **D,** The ultrasound unit and accessories needed to perform fusion imaging.

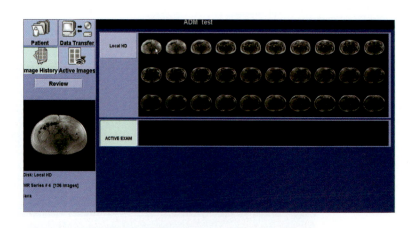

FIGURE 19-23 An MRI series that has been imported into the ultrasound unit.

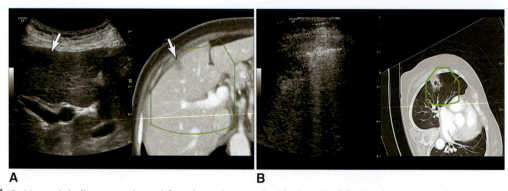

A **B**

FIGURE 19-24 A, Very subtle liver mass *(arrow)* found on ultrasound with the aid of fusing the ultrasound with the imported CT scan. **B,** The biopsy was performed in a fused mode. The green box marks the liver mass. The biopsy specimen came back positive for metastatic colon cancer.

it when the transducer needs to be removed from the patient's skin. When the area that has been marked is on the screen, the marker will appear as a small square. As the sonographer scans away from the area, the marker grows larger. For difficult lesions, marking the area on the scans allows the sonographer to rest his or her arm between passes or before the procedure begins, thus helping to prevent MSK injuries from prolonged holding of the transducer in one place. The sonographer can place the transducer back on the patient when the biopsy is ready to proceed, look for the marker, and adjust the scanning plane until the marker is small and the area of interest is displayed (Figure 19-25). This can be a time-saver when the transducer is removed from the patient's skin, especially for difficult-to-see lesions, as the tracking boxes will help the sonographer quickly return to the lesion with confidence. Fusion techniques are also helpful if multiple lesions are visible on the MRI or CT and there is a specific lesion that the clinician wants biopsied.

At the time of this writing, companies were starting to show needles with electromagnetic sensors embedded in them. By using a system consisting of a reusable sensor and a disposable needle, the radiologist will know exactly where the needle tip is at all times. This will help the radiologist to find the needle tip quickly if the needle is deflected or bends, as well as ensure that the needle is in the proper place for small or difficult to access masses.

This technology will help the radiologist always know where the needle tip is during the insertion stage. Once the needle tip is in the proper location, the sensor is removed and the biopsy performed.

ULTRASOUND BIOPSY TECHNIQUES

1. Before beginning the procedure, the patient's medical history, lab values, and imaging studies should be reviewed and blood work checked. If the patient's PT, PTT, and INR are normal, the procedure can safely begin.
2. The next step is to explain the procedure to the patient. A well-informed patient is usually more relaxed and cooperative. The patient must be informed of the potential risks, alternate methods of obtaining the same information, and what would be the course of the disease if the biopsy is not performed and the correct treatment cannot be planned. The benefits of the procedure and what to expect during the procedure, especially the need for multiple passes, should be discussed, as well as any potential complications, including the possibility of a nondiagnostic procedure. The patient's role in the procedure should be explained: how the patient needs to keep still and to follow breathing instructions. A summary of all personnel in the room and

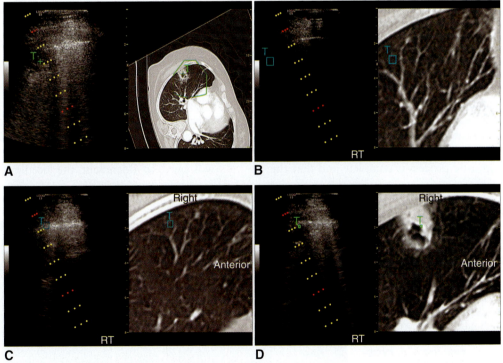

FIGURE 19-25 A, This lung lesion is found, the biopsy path determined, and a target marker placed on the CT image. The marker is duplicated on the ultrasound image (*small green T and +*). **B,** The sonographer removed the transducer while waiting for the procedure to begin to rest the arm. Upon placing the transducer back on the patient, the blue box and T appeared on both the CT and ultrasound image. This denotes that the lesion is close. **C,** As the sonographer scans closer to the lesion, the blue box gets smaller. **D,** The box is small and has turned green as the site marked on image A is now in view.

their roles is given; the room can become crowded with the following people: sonographer, attending, fellow or resident, nurse, and, possibly, a cytopathology team. At this time the psychological needs of the patient should be determined and sedatives ordered as needed. Patients need to be awake for the procedure so that they can stay in the needed position and control their breathing. Time should also be allowed for the patient to ask questions. The consent form is then signed and witnessed. The sonographer may serve as the witness. If the sonographer did not see the patient sign the form, he or she should show the signature to the patient and verify that it is the patient's signature.

3. After obtaining the patient's consent for the procedure, the next step in the process is to review any diagnostic imaging studies, such as an ultrasound, CT, MRI, or PET scan. If possible, the film demonstrating the mass should be hung in the room. This is one of the positive aspects of fusion technology, as the images will be imported directly into the machine for review. You can review the images without fusing the studies together. In areas with PACS, if there are no viewing monitors in the room, a film with the necessary images should be printed, especially for chest, retroperitoneal masses, and other challenging masses. With new fusion technologies, the sonographer should start the importing of the needed images. While the sonographer is reviewing or importing the images, the patient can be brought into the scanning/procedure room, changed into a gown, and have their vital signs taken. The nurse will also complete the preprocedural checklist at this time. An electrocardiogram and pulse oximeter machine will be connected to the patient if there is a chance of a pneumothorax.

4. Next, a limited ultrasound is performed to localize the mass and choose the optimal approach as well as the best transducer type and frequency (Figure 19-26). It is important to realize that for a biopsy that the diagnostic process is complete and that the transducer type and frequency needed for the biopsy might not be the same used for a clinical examination. For example, it may be necessary to use a high-frequency linear array for a superficial liver or abdominal mass, and a mid- to low-frequency phased array transducer or even an endocavitary transducer for a subclavicular mass (Figure 19-27). Again, it's important to think "approach to the mass or lesion" and not penetration and resolution. When appropriate, older units may be used for biopsies, freeing up newer machines for diagnostic studies. This is especially true for lower-resolution procedures such as paracentesis, thoracentesis, renal cores, and liver cores. The sonographer should determine multiple approaches, if needed, and review them with the radiologist. An X or a dot is marked on the skin with a marker, at the site where the needle will pierce the skin. To determine the needle length required to reach the mass, measure the distance to the mass by placing a caliper at the bottom of the mass. This should be performed with the needle guidelines on the screen, as the machine will now take into account the length of the needle that is inside the needle guide, which is typically 2 to 4 centimeters (Figure 19-28). Common needle lengths are 6, 9, 15, and 20 centimeters. Usually it is best to have the sonographer on one side of the patient, preferably next to the ultrasound machine, and the physician on the other side of the patient. Sometimes the best path requires the sonographer and physician to be on the same side of the patient. If this is the situation, then the two of them will need to determine the best position so that they both can see the ultrasound monitor. One solution is for the sonographer to sit on a stool so that he or she is shorter than the radiologist. This allows the sonographer to still have access to the controls and see the monitor. Good ergonomics should be maintained. If the sonographer must scan from the opposite side of the stretcher, someone else will need to document the needle tip and adjust

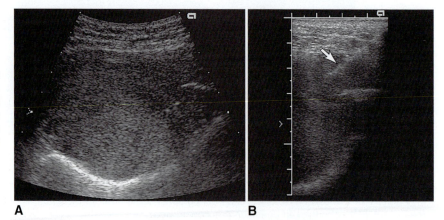

FIGURE 19-26 A, A large mediastinal mass is seen with a 5-MHz curved array transducer. **B,** This same patient is biopsied *(arrow)* using a 7-MHz linear array, as a hypoechoic area in the mass was better appreciated. This is the area from which positive cells were found. A primary mediastinal tumor was diagnosed.

A   B

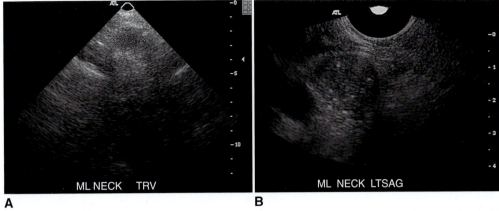

A **B**

FIGURE 19-27 A, It proved difficult to image around the clavicle using a linear array transducer. To angle under the clavicle, a phased array transducer was first used. **B,** The same patient is now being evaluated with an endocavity transducer. This proved to be the best transducer, allowing an easy and safe path to the lymph node as well as the resolution to see the small calcifications. Metastatic thyroid cancer was diagnosed.

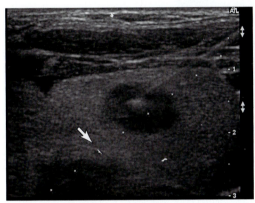

FIGURE 19-28 The arrow is pointing to the cursor along the biopsy line that determined the length of the needle needed to reach this point. As each mark represents 5 mm, the distance to the back wall of this thyroid lesion is 6.5 mm. A 9-cm needle length was used to perform the biopsy on this patient who was determined to have a benign thyroid nodule compatible with an adenoma. Notice the slight needle deviation.

controls as needed, such as another sonographer or even a sonography student. The sonographer can also consider rearranging the relationship of the stretcher and machine to accommodate both the sonographer and the physician on the same side of the patient.

5. The national patient safety standards (found at www.jcaho.org) mandate that a "time-out" be performed before beginning any procedure. A member of the biopsy team should ask the patient to recite his or her full name. The patient's ID or history number is confirmed as is the type and location of the procedure. The time-out needs to be documented. This documentation may be part of the consent form. The words "time-out" can also be typed on the screen and an image documented as part of the ultrasound examination. This is helpful, as there will be preprocedural image, the "time-out"

image, which documents date and time, and then the needle tip documentation images (Figure 19-29).

6. The radiologist/sonologist may start prepping the skin, usually after the time-out, while the sonographer preps and bags the transducer. Prepping the transducer often requires the assistance of another person, such as a nurse, a sonography student, a radiologist, or even another sonographer, to help maintain sterility of the transducer. Transducer preparation consists of attaching the needle guide to the transducer and covering the transducer with a sterile cover (Figure 19-30). Depending on the transducer, the needle guide may be covered by the sterile bag or it may also be sterile and placed over the sterile bag. Please note that the use of sterile bags and sterile guides varies among institutions. For example, one institution may bag the transducer and guide, keeping it sterile for a thyroid biopsy, whereas another may use the transducer and guide in a clean but not sterile fashion. After the transducer guide is attached, the correct size needle gauge insert is attached to the transducer guide. These guides are based on the gauge of the needle or catheter being used. These may need to be changed during the procedure. For example, a 22-gauge guide may be used during the FNA, but it may be changed to an 18-gauge guide for the core. Also, on a deep lesion, the radiologist may start with a 22-gauge needle but, because it keeps deviating, switch to a sturdier 20-gauge needle.

7. After the patient and transducer are prepped, sterile gel is used to rescan and check the mark. Once the area of the biopsy has been rechecked, local skin anesthesia is given, usually with a 25-gauge needle.

8. Next, deeper numbing is given along the needle path using the needle guide. This is important for patient comfort, especially on deep masses and liver masses, as the liver capsule is very sensitive. The transducer

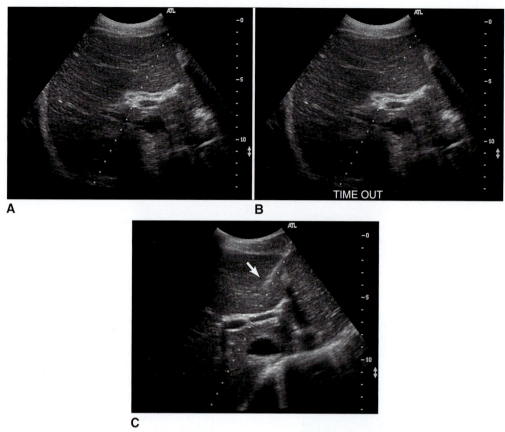

FIGURE 19-29 A, Preprocedural image for a liver core in a patient with hepatitis C demonstrating the needle path. **B,** Time-out verifying patient's name, ID number, and type of procedure. **C,** The procedure has begun. The arrow is pointing to the needle tip.

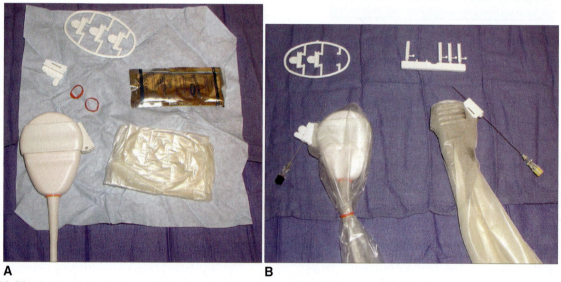

FIGURE 19-30 A, Transducer and sterile kit, which includes the bag, guide attachment, needle gauge inserts, rubber bands, and sterile gel. **B,** Prepped transducers.

should stay on the anesthetized area to ensure that the needle is always passing through the numbed tissue (see Figure 19-17). Typically, a 9-centimeter, 22-gauge spinal needle is used for the deeper numbing. It is important that the physician squirt the lidocaine or numbing agent through the needle

to push out the air inside the needle before inserting the needle into the patient. Otherwise, air will be introduced into the patient's tissue, obscuring the mass and the needle path. Patients should be reminded that they should not feel any sharp pain but that they may feel pressure. Some patients will complain of "pain" during the procedure when what they are really feeling is the pressure of the needle passing through their tissue. A good analogy is having a tooth filled. The patient feels the sensation of the drilling but not the sharp pain. Also, it is a good idea to let patients know that they may feel some pressure from the transducer as it is held steadily in place.

9. The sonographer holds the transducer as the radiologist performs the biopsy. In some institutions, the radiologist may be the person who holds the transducer while performing the biopsy. When a free hand technique is used, the radiologist will usually hold the transducer. When a sonographer assists with the procedure, he or she will have one sterile hand, which is holding the transducer, while the other hand will be dirty, as it will be optimizing the controls, taking images to document the needle tip and procedure, and maybe even holding the patient's hand or patting the patient on the shoulder. The needle should be advanced in a swift motion while it is being tracked. Echogenic tip needles should be used, as the tip of the needle has been scored to produce an increase of scattered echoes, causing it to be echogenic. The shaft of the needle is echogenic, as it is a specular reflector, whereas the tip of the needle is more echogenic because it has been scored. Some needles have the stylet scored to enhance visualization of the needle (Figure 19-31).

10. For neck, chest, abdominal, and retroperitoneal biopsies, the patient is asked to stop breathing while the needle is inserted. A typical FNA pass lasts between 20 to 40 seconds. Patients who cannot hold their breath for this long should be instructed to breathe shallowly until the needle is removed, as deep breaths may cause the needle to bend. The sonographer can be helpful by coaching and encouraging patients with their breathing and breath holding. When locating the mass, try to let patients breathe normally as much as possible, having them hold their breath to verify the selected path. This will allow the patient to be "fresh" for the biopsy and not out of breath already from the prescans. For masses that move a lot with breathing, it can be helpful to show patients the mass and biopsy line and how their breathing affects the location of the mass.

11. After the procedure is finished, the patient's skin is cleaned and a bandage placed over the biopsy site. A cold compress should also be placed over the biopsy site to reduce swelling and pain. The bag should be placed over the patient's gown or it can be wrapped in a towel or a few paper towels, as direct skin contact may be uncomfortable for the patient. The sterile bag and guide is removed from the transducer. Care should be taken not to accidentally throw the reusable guide in the garbage, as these guides are expensive. The sonographer should scan the area to look for any postprocedural complications such as a hematoma. Color or power Doppler can be used to ensure that there is no active bleeding. This is especially useful in renal biopsies. If an active bleed is discovered, the sonographer can use the transducer to apply pressure over the area to stop the bleeding. Usually the bleeding can be stopped within 5 to 10 minutes. If the bleeding cannot be stopped, interventional radiology should be contacted immediately (Figure 19-32).

12. Before the patient leaves the room, the nurse will assess the patient's pain level and take vital signs. The sonographer should take the transducer and guide, clean the gel and any blood or other body fluids off of them, and soak them in a disinfectant solution, according to the hospital's infection control

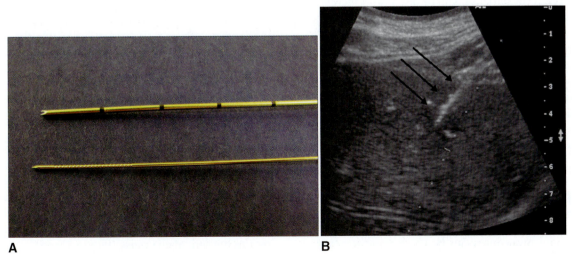

A   **B**

FIGURE 19-31 **A,** A biopsy needle with a scored stylet. **B,** Needle with an echogenic stylet *(arrows)* allowing easy visualization of the needle. This hypoechoic mass was a metastatic lesion from a colon primary.

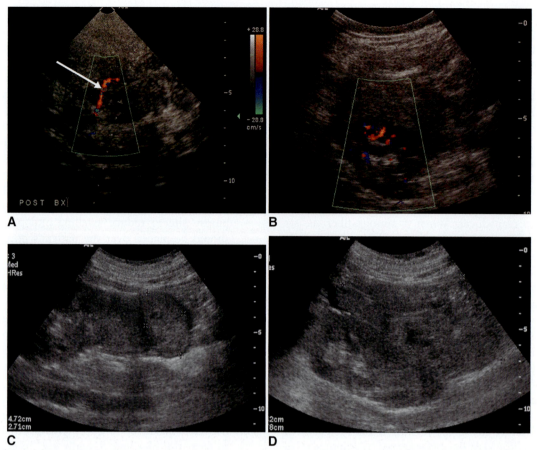

FIGURE 19-32 A, Perinephric bleed *(arrow)* and hematoma postnative renal biopsy in a patient with proteinuria. **B,** Same patient as after pressing over the area of the bleed with the curved linear array transducer. After 5 minutes, the bleeding has stopped. **C,** Patient with a 5-cm bleed after a native renal biopsy. **D,** Same patient as in image C after 35 minutes of applied transducer pressure. The hematoma keeps increasing in size and is now 11.4 cm in size. The patient was sent to interventional radiology because the bleeding could not be stopped with outside pressure.

policies and the recommendations of the transducer manufacturer.

13. The patient is then taken to a holding or observation area. Depending on the type of procedure, the patient may remain in this area between 15 to 120 minutes. If the patient's pain or discomfort increases, the sonographer should rescan to look for a hematoma (Figure 19-33). Stable patients can be discharged with appropriate instructions. Patients who have had chest procedures or procedures near the lungs will be sent to radiology for a chest x-ray to evaluate for a pneumothorax (Figure 19-34).

14. Typically, the nurse makes a follow-up phone call within the next 24 to 72 hours to ensure that the patient did not experience any complications.

THE SONOGRAPHER'S ROLE IN INTERVENTIONAL PROCEDURES

Interventional procedures can be challenging for everyone involved. A sonographer that has an interest in interventional ultrasound can be a valuable asset to the biopsy team. Sonographers may work closely with a radiologist, sonologist, or with other physicians such as a nephrologist in native kidney biopsies, surgeons in kidney transplant or liver biopsies, or other clinicians for ascites taps or during thoracentesis.

Sonographer involvement has many benefits. Sonographers can locate the pathology and determine various approaches, offering recommendation for the best and safest needle path to the mass. Using their scanning skills, sonographers can optimize the image to locate subtle masses and use Doppler to ensure that there are no vessels in the needle path. The sonographer can place the patient in a variety of positions to determine the best approach. For example, by placing the patient in a left posterior oblique or left lateral decubitus position, the liver may drop into a more subcostal position or a mass may roll away from a vessel. Placing the patient in a prone position may give better access to a renal mass. Knowledge of new technologies such as harmonic and compound imaging may facilitate finding or better defining the borders of the mass (Figure 19-35).

It is also important to use the proper transducer. This means choosing not only the right frequency but also the

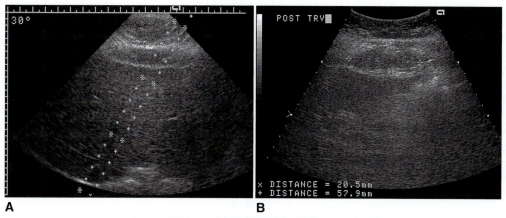

FIGURE 19-33 A, Prelive scan to determine the needle path in this patient with hepatitis C. Notice the prominent rectus abdominis muscle anterior to the liver. **B,** The patient developed a hematoma postbiopsy. Notice the similar appearance to the rectus abdominis muscle, which can be mistaken for a hematoma. It is recommended that a pre-biopsy image be taken for a comparison.

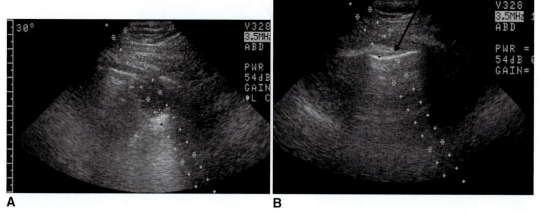

FIGURE 19-34 A, Pleural based lung lesion. **B,** The needle nicked the lung, causing a small pneumothrox *(arrow)*. Fortunately, an adequate specimen was obtained, which proved to be adenocarcinoma of the lung.

correct transducer type. Sometimes it may be better to use a transducer not normally associated in a routine examination for that area—for example, using an endocavitary transducer for a mediastinal or subclavicular mass or a phased array transducer to get to masses that require an intercostal approach in the chest (Figure 19-36). Because of the angle provided, a linear array may provide a safer choice in a pelvic node than a curved array. In the abdomen and pelvis, both a curved array and a phased array transducer should be evaluated. Different transducer types offer different angles and approaches to the mass.

Another aspect of preparing for the procedure is determining the effects of the patient's breathing on the mass. It is important to determine how much the mass moves with respiration and also how well and how long the patient can hold his or her breath. Determining this gives both sonographer and patient a chance to practice breathing so that the patient knows what is expected of him or her during the actual biopsy. The sonographer can also point out the mass on the screen and show the patient how breathing affects the location of the mass. They can

then work together so that the patient can watch the screen and know how much of a breath to take so that the mass lines up on or between the dotted lines on the screen. Besides abdominal and chest masses, neck and thyroid masses can also move with respiration.

The sonographer should not be afraid to speak to the physician performing the procedure. For example, if the sonographer realizes that the needle is approaching a major vessel, he or she should calmly and professionally tell the physician to stop (Figure 19-37). Sonographers may also need to discuss and determine solutions to problems like needle deviation. If a hematoma is forming, the sonographer may want to alert the physician so that he or she can decide whether to proceed or stop the procedure. Patients tend to talk to the sonographer more, and their questions or fears can then be relayed to the physician. The sonographer can also gently remind the physician that the patient is holding his or her breath if the physician is taking a longer time than usual to obtain the specimen. Similarly, the sonographer can catch the signal that the patient needs to breathe and can let the physician know.

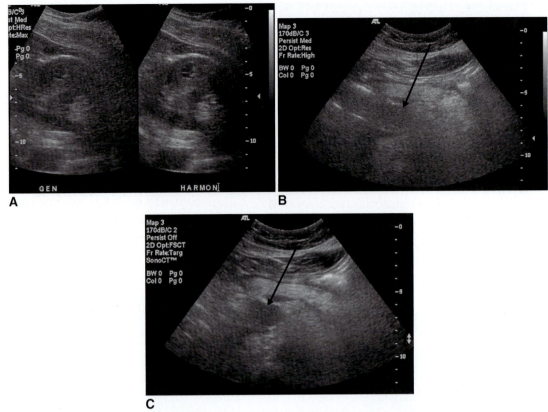

FIGURE 19-35 A, Cystic renal cell carcinoma *(arrow),* which was better visualized using harmonic imaging (Gen = normal image, Harmon = harmonic image). **B,** Image of a pancreas head mass *(arrow)* using normal imaging parameters. **C,** With compound imaging activated, the borders of the mass were better defined, leading to a successful biopsy and a diagnosis of adenocarcinoma of the pancreas.

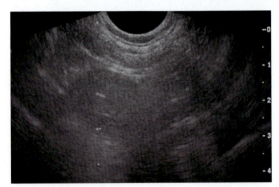

FIGURE 19-36 Using an endocavitary transducer gave better access and resolution on this metastatic supraclavicular node in a patient with a history of thyroid cancer.

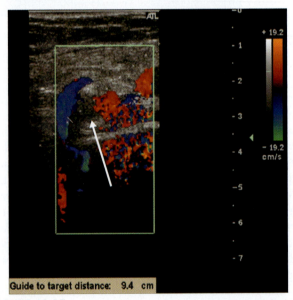

FIGURE 19-37 The sonographer must communicate to the physician if the needle deviates to any of the iliac vessels around this 1-cm node *(arrow)* in the pelvis. This node was positive in this HIV patient.

Importantly, a sonographer can be a second set of hands as needed to adjust imaging controls, freeze and unfreeze the image, and document the needle tip. When using biopsy guides, the sonographer can hold the transducer, freeing the physician's hands. This can be especially helpful when aspiration techniques are used. The sonographer can use the transducer to press bowel out of the way, allowing the mass to be seen. This increased transducer pressure needs to be maintained during the procedure and requires another set of hands. This technique can also be used to minimize the distance between the skin and the mass on deep lesions (Figure 19-38).

The sonographer can assist and encourage the patient during the procedure. This can be valuable in helping the patient control breathing and giving the patient someone to talk to as needed. The sonographer can coach and support the patient emotionally, allowing the physician

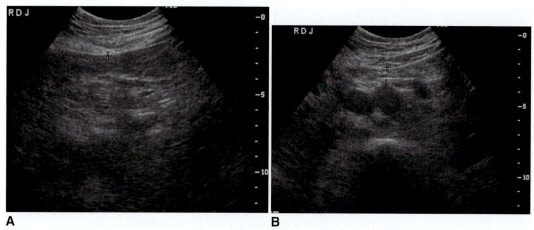

FIGURE 19-38 These deep retroperitoneal lymph nodes are difficult to see with normal scanning techniques. There is 5.4 cm of tissue between the abdominal wall and the anterior surface of the nodes. **B,** By applying pressure with the transducer, the distance from the abdominal wall and the nodes has decreased to 1.2 cm, allowing visualization of the nodes. This amount of pressure was applied during the biopsy, allowing a successful biopsy and a diagnosis of lymphoma.

to concentrate on the procedure or discuss the specimen with the cytopathologist, if present. While the radiologist and nurse are busy with the specimen, the sonographer can talk to the patient to make sure that the patient is doing okay, look for signs of a complication, assure the patient that he or she is doing a great job, and, importantly, communicate to the patient what the next step will be.

Using their Doppler skills, the sonographer can locate vessels that may potentially traverse the needle path or be in close proximity to the mass. The sonographer can help guide the needle safely to deep retroperitoneal masses that may be near major vessels. Also, by using color or power Doppler, the sonographer can locate vessels in a mass, as this may represent areas of viable tumor tissue. This can be beneficial in masses that have necrotic areas (Figure 19-39).

Finally, the sonographer can be a time-saver for the busy physician. The sonographer can assist with probe preparation as well as with cleaning up. Sonographers can be scanning the next patient while the physician signs up the following patient or checks and dictates other studies. With a sonographer involved, a second physician may not be required for some procedures, thus allowing patient flow to continue in the department.

Experienced sonographers may find being involved with procedures a welcome change from routine scanning. It allows them to interact with the patient in a different way, be part of an important team, and bring into play all their scanning skills and knowledge.

FINDING THE NEEDLE TIP

The needle tip should appear as an echogenic dot on the ultrasound image. Visualizing the needle tip depends on several factors, including the type of needle (specially designed echogenic needles are better seen than normal needles), the gauge of the needle (larger-gauge needles

cause brighter reflections), the transducer frequency (using the highest frequency possible), placement of the focal zone (which should be at or just below the level of the needle tip), using only one focal zone (multiple focal zones may decrease the frame rate), and the echogenicity of the mass (hypoechoic masses allow easier visualization of the needle than more echogenic masses) (Figure 19-40). The needle should be inserted quickly and steadily and the tip followed as it advances toward the mass. The needle may deviate out of the projected path and away from the ultrasound beam, causing loss of visualization of the needle tip. This deviation of the needle can be caused by the physician bending or tilting the needle as it is being advanced or by the tissue and muscle planes it is traversing (Figure 19-41). Echogenic needle tips or scored stylets improve needle and needle tip visualization.

Tricks to try to see the needle tip include the following:

1. Moving the needle up and down in a bobbing motion.
2. Bobbing or jiggling the stylet inside the needle.
3. Scanning and angling the transducer in a superior and inferior motion. This is helpful when the needle is bent out of the plane of the sound beam.
4. Using harmonics or compound imaging.
5. A last resort is to remove the needle and start again, closely watching the displacement of the tissue as the needle advances.

At times the patient may move or breathe at the time that the biopsy core is fired, preventing the needle path from being visible for documentation. In these instances, the sonographer can scan the area and look for the needle track. This will be seen as an echogenic line caused by the air that is introduced into the tissue during the firing/cutting process (Figure 19-42).

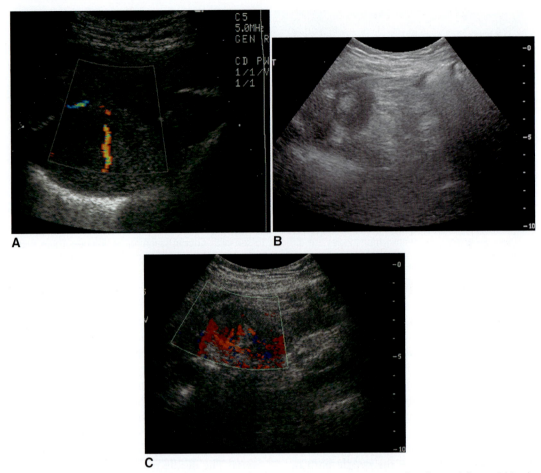

FIGURE 19-39 A, After several specimens showed only necrotic tissue, color Doppler was used to located flow within the mass. Viable tissue was found in this location, and a diagnosis of a mediastinal adenocarcinoma was made. **B,** Transverse image of the upper abdomen in a patient with a suspected hepatic flexure tumor. **C,** Using color Doppler, the colon mass was defined and an ultrasound-guided biopsy was performed confirming the suspicion of colon cancer.

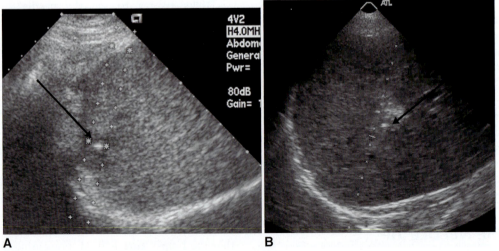

FIGURE 19-40 A, The needle tip is easily seen *(arrow)* in this patient with a hypoechoic metastatic lesion. **B,** The needle tip is hard to see *(arrow)* in this patient with a hyperechoic metastatic lesion.

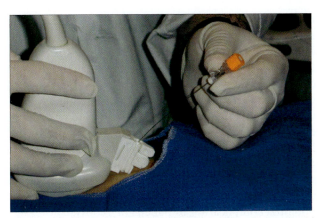

FIGURE 19-41 Notice that the needle is being inserted with bending, which causes the needle to bend out of plane and lose visualization of the needle tip.

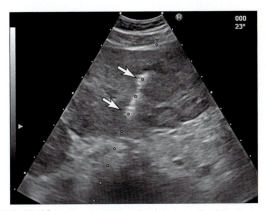

FIGURE 19-42 The patient breathed just as the biopsy gun was fired. The needle was not seen to document the location of the biopsy. By scanning the echogenic line from the needle track was found *(arrows)*, allowing documentation of the biopsy area.

WHAT TO DO WHEN THE NEEDLE DEVIATES

Deviation of the needle from the projected path can be an issue and a challenge for the sonographer. The tissue and organs between the skin and the mass are usually the cause of this problem. For example, in pancreatic biopsies, the needle is often deflected as it passes through the posterior wall of the stomach. If it is a constant problem, the sonographer can overcorrect—that is, move the transducer more lateral or medial so that the path that the needle is following will intersect the mass. It is important that the sonographer verify that the correct size needle guide insert was used, because if the guide is too large, there will be some play within the needle guide that can cause this problem. As previously discussed, the sonographer should ensure that the guide on the transducer is set to the correct angle. Also, the sonographer should make sure that the transducer is perpendicular and that the needle guide touches the patient's skin. It is vital that the sonographer become familiar with the various transducers and guides, how they should be placed on the body, and how to correct or adjust their

scanning as needed. If the problem persists, sometimes using a 20-gauge as opposed to a 22-gauge needle may correct the situation, as the larger gauge needle is sturdier and does not bend as easily. In extreme cases, another pathway may need to be determined. The sonographer can also watch how the physician is inserting the needle to make sure that the needle is not bending as it is being inserted into the skin. Finally, the position of the tip of the needle can influence deviation on certain types of needles (see Figure 19-8, *B*). When the needle is inserted with the tip of the needle at the bottom (sometimes called bevel-up), the needle will encounter less resistance as it passes through the tissues; when bevel down, the needle may deviate as it passes through the same tissues.

Another problem is when a mass is pushed out of the way by the needle. This can be a problem with small nodes and masses. Again, the sonographer needs to understand how to counter these situations. Applying firm pressure with the transducer against the mass or trying to get the needle to approach the center of the mass so that it doesn't push the mass to the left or to the right can stabilize the mass and allow the needle to enter it. Sometimes another approach may be needed, which would require breaking down the sterile field and starting again. When any of these situations arise, the sonographer should be thinking of possible solutions to suggest. The physician can also try to quickly insert the needle or try to rotate the bevel of the needle into a different position.

BIOPSIES AND PROCEDURES BY ORGAN

Liver

The liver is one of the most common organs of which a biopsy is requested, either of a specific area or mass in the liver or for diffuse parenchyma abnormalities, such as hepatitis. Liver masses are amenable to ultrasound-guided biopsy in the majority of cases and can include metastatic masses, suspected hepato-cellular carcinoma (HCC) or other primary cancer, atypical benign lesions, and small abscesses (Figure 19-43). A biopsy of a hypoechoic area in a cirrhotic liver may be requested, especially in a patient with elevated AFP, to differentiate it from a regenerating liver nodule. The inability to biopsy a liver mass can be caused by either the failure to visualize the mass or a lack of a safe approach to the mass. Whenever possible, a subcostal approach should be used to avoid the possibility of a pneumothorax or damage to the intercostal arteries. Intercostal biopsies also tend to be painful to the patient (Figure 19-44). Masses at the dome of the liver are easier to biopsy under ultrasound than CT, although a steep angle approach is often required. In some cases, scanning and biopsying in a sagittal plane is helpful. Core biopsies may be obtained on patients with hepatitis, cirrhosis, or increased liver function tests. Usually the left lobe of the liver is biopsied using a subcostal approach, as there are fewer major structures in the way, such as the gallbladder and porta hepatis. A biopsy of the left lobe in this group of patients is easier to perform and more comfortable for the patient than the traditional blind approach through the ribs of the right lobe. Specific complications of liver biopsies include pneumothorax for masses near the dome of the liver, bile leak, and hematomas. Use zoom techniques for easier visualization of a small mass (Figure 19-45). Consider multiple patient positions to try to decrease the distance to the mass and to avoid intercostal approaches.

Pancreas

Most pancreatic mass biopsies are performed to confirm the diagnosis of adenocarcinoma, unresectable adenocarcinoma, or to confirm pancreatitis in patients with unusual imaging studies. Although the needle has to traverse the stomach or colon, complications are rare. Color

Doppler is useful to map out vessels, especially if they are encased by the mass. Good specimens can usually be obtained near the biliary drainage tube, if the patient has one. A curved linear array transducer is preferred, as it can help display bowel gas with its large footprint. Pancreatic biopsies can be challenging because gas can move into the field and interfere with visualization of the mass, even after the biopsy has started. Other challenges include finding a safe path around the various vessels, deflection or bending of the needle as it goes through the stomach, and patient breathing, which can cause the pancreas to move with respirations (Figure 19-46). Pancreatitis is a potential complication of pancreatic biopsy.

Kidney

Most solid renal tumors are surgically resected without obtaining a biopsy, as the majority of them will be malignant or premalignant. However, a biopsy of a renal mass may be requested to differentiate an incidental renal cell carcinoma from a renal metastasis in a patient with a known primary cancer or if the patient has a prior history of renal cell carcinoma. Atypical cysts, especially those with thick septations, need to be biopsied to differentiate between a cystic renal cell carcinoma and a benign complex cyst. Renal parenchymal biopsies are requested on patients with proteinuria, nephrotic syndrome, or in renal failure. Because the disease process affects both kidneys, either kidney can be biopsied. The left kidney is preferred, as it offers a safer approach than the right, as the spleen is well above the left kidney, while the liver may be potentially in the way. These biopsies are performed with the patient prone, biopsying the lower pole of the left kidney, usually with an 18-gauge core needle. The sonographer should guide the needle through the parenchymal tissue, as the cortical tissue is

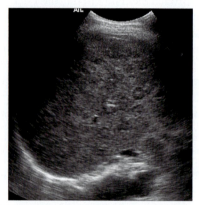

FIGURE 19-43 Patient with AIDS and multiple liver lesions. Biopsy was requested to determine the nature of the lesions. They were found to be amebic liver abscesses.

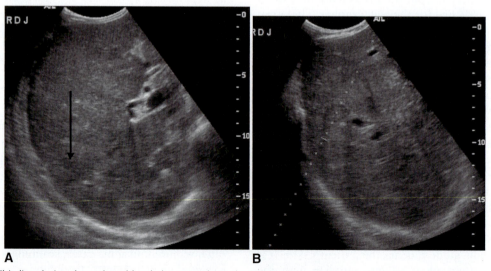

FIGURE 19-44 This liver lesion (arrow) could only be seen along the intercostal margin with the patient supine. **B,** With the patient in a right posterior oblique, the liver rolled out from under the ribs, allowing better visualization of the mass, and a subcostal approach could be used on this metastatic mass.

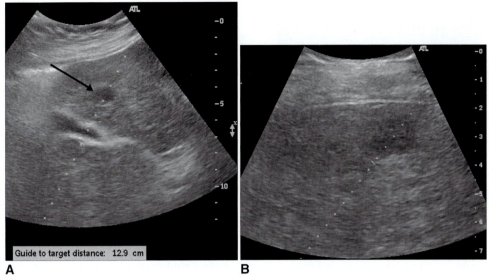

FIGURE 19-45 A, A small 1-cm hypoechoic metastatic lesion *(arrow)* at normal scale size. **B,** Visualizing the same small 1-cm metastatic lesion using a write zoom to magnify the lesion made the mass and needle tip easier to see.

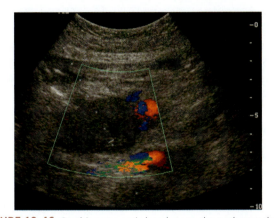

FIGURE 19-46 On this pancreatic head mass, the path was chosen to avoid the mesenteric vessels.

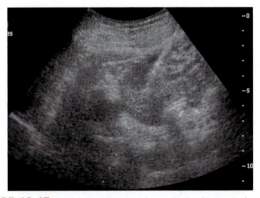

FIGURE 19-47 Renal core biopsy through the lower pole of the left kidney in this patient with proteinuria.

needed to make the diagnosis (Figure 19-47). Specific complications of renal biopsies include perinephric hematoma and hematuria. The sonographer should evaluate the needle track area with color Doppler immediately post biopsy to ensure that there is no active bleeding. If the patient develops hematuria, the bladder should be scanned for the presence of a clot. If a clot is discovered, the patient should be rolled into a steep oblique position to determine if the clot is mobile or attached to the bladder wall. This is important, as the clot may be positioned over the urethral opening, causing an outlet obstruction. For biopsies of renal masses, various patient positions should be evaluated including supine, decubitus, oblique, and prone (Figure 19-48).

Renal Transplants

Ultrasound is used to guide biopsies when there is elevation of the creatinine or when the cause of rejection needs to be determined for treatment. Locate the main renal vessels using color Doppler. Typically, the upper

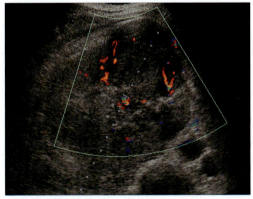

FIGURE 19-48 Biopsy of a right renal mass with the patient in a left lateral decubitus position. The diagnosis was metastatic disease from melanoma.

pole of the kidney is biopsied to avoid possible lacerations of the main renal vessels and ureter. It is also recommended that a color Doppler image of the entire kidney be obtained to use as a baseline in case there are complications such as an arteriovenous fistula (AVF) or

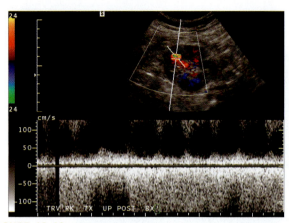

FIGURE 19-49 A postbiopsy image of this renal transplant demonstrates an arteriovenous fistula. Notice the mosaic color and turbulent Doppler flow.

pseudoaneurysm formation of intrarenal vessels. Ultrasound can also be used to direct drainage of perinephric fluid collections such as lymphoceles. Specific complications include hematomas, hematuria, and AVF (Figure 19-49).

Adrenal Glands

The most common indication for an adrenal biopsy is to differentiate an adenoma from a metastatic mass, particularly in patients with a known malignancy, especially melanoma. The right adrenal gland is usually more accessible and can be reached via a transhepatic approach. Left adrenal mass biopsies can be more difficult, and the patient may need to be biopsied in an oblique, decubitus, or even a prone position. A solid, homogenous adrenal mass that is discovered incidentally probably represents an adenoma and a biopsy is not required. This is especially true if the mass is less than 3 centimeters, if there is no primary cancer, and if there is no evidence of an endocrine abnormality. Also, it is important to exclude a pheochromocytoma with clinical and laboratory data, because biopsying one can cause a hypertensive crisis. Specific complications can include a pneumothorax and hematomas.

Spleen

Masses in the spleen are rare. Most lesions are metastatic in origin or are from lymphoma involvement. Because the spleen is highly vascular, there is an increased risk for bleeding or hemorrhage. Multiple patient positions should be evaluated to determine the best approach to the mass, including supine, anterior oblique, posterior oblique, decubitus, and prone positions.

Retroperitoneal Lymph Nodes

Most retroperitoneal masses, including paraaortic and pericaval lymph nodes, are amenable to ultrasound guid-

ance. These can be technically challenging, especially with small masses and in larger patients, so the use of a needle guide is essential. Usually an anterior approach is preferred, and by applying a firm and steady pressure with the curved linear array transducer, overlying bowel loops and intraabdominal fat can be displaced. This technique also reduces the depth at which the needle needs to be placed. To avoid major vessels and other structures, multiple biopsy transducers and guides may need to be evaluated to determine the safest path (Figure 19-50). Real-time monitoring of the needle tip ensures that the needle excursions during the biopsy stay within the node. In patients with suspected lymphoma, tissue needs to be obtained not only to diagnose lymphoma but also to determine the subtype, as this is critical for treatment. Usually part of the sample is sent for flow cytometric studies and a core may also be required. Specific complications include retroperitoneal hematomas. Because the sonographer may have to apply transducer pressure, the patient may feel more discomfort than usual from the increased pressure. The sonographer should explain this to the patient. Also, this increased pressure can add fatigue to the sonographer's wrist, hand joints, and shoulder. Therefore, sonographers should relax the pressure and their grip on the transducer to reduce MSK injuries between passes.

Lung

Ultrasound guidance has been shown to be a safe alternative to CT for biopsy of pleural, parenchymal, or mediastinal masses abutting the chest wall. This technique is associated with a high success rate and lower complications than CT and is particularly valuable for small peripheral masses in close proximity to a rib and diaphragmatic masses where slight respiratory excursion can affect the position of the mass. The transducer is placed parallel to the intercostal space, and the needle is advanced in a single breath hold to minimize trauma to the pleura. The tip is monitored to ensure it does not slip out of the mass into normal aerated lung. Intraparenchymal tumors are generally not amenable to ultrasound guidance, unless they are within an area of consolidation or if the patient has a large pleural effusion that can be used as an acoustic window. Lung lesions can be challenging by ultrasound, and it is always helpful to have the CT films present for guidance. New fusion technology can assist in finding these masses quickly and accurately. These lesions are usually small and mobile with respiration. Creative positioning may be needed to get between ribs and around the scapula. The patient may need to be placed in an oblique, decubitus, or prone position. A pillow or sponges may be placed under the patient to spread the ribs apart. The patient's arm may also need to be adjusted to get the scapula out of the way in apical lesions. Transducer type also needs to be evaluated, as sometimes a phased array transducer

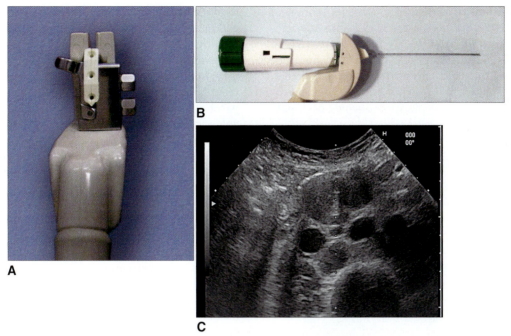

FIGURE 19-50 **A,** This specially designed transducer has the biopsy slots in the middle of the transducer, allowing zero angle or straight down biopsies. **B,** The same transducer with the biopsy gun in the zero degree biopsy hole. **C,** The patient with massive abdominal lymphadenopathy being biopsied by the transducer shown in part B.

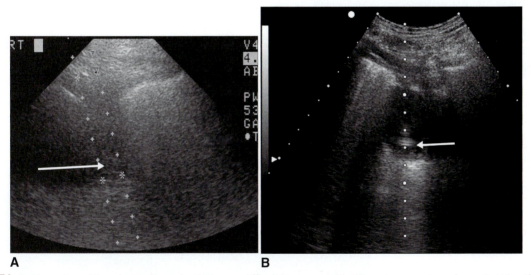

FIGURE 19-51 **A,** Pleura-based lung lesion *(arrow)*, which was difficult to access with this sector array transducer. **B,** Using this transducer with the biopsy guide, this lung mass was better defined and offered a safe approach. The arrow is pointing to the needle tip.

provides better access than a linear array transducer (Figure 19-51). Remember that resolution is not as much an issue as is accessibility. Start with a small footprint phased array transducer, as it helps to image between the ribs and allows the sonographer to angle through the rib space. Once the lesion is located, the linear array transducer can be evaluated for path access. In lung biopsies, patient breathing is crucial because the lesion will move with respirations. The sonographer will need to evaluate the patient in various degrees of inspiration and expiration. These lesions can be challenging for the sonographer to find, as there are few landmarks to use. Specific complications include pneumothorax. If the patient starts to cough up blood (hemoptysis), the biopsy needs to stop immediately for patient safety.

Thyroid Gland

Thyroid biopsies can be helpful in distinguishing malignant masses from goiters or adenomas. Biopsies should be taken in various portions of the mass to confirm colloid or abnormal cells. The sonographer should look for small calcifications, as there is a higher percentage of positive cells in these areas (Figure 19-52). The sonographer should remember to evaluate if the thyroid gland moves with respiration. If it does, the patient should be told to hold his or her breath as the needle is inserted. Usually the patient can breathe shallowly during the biopsy process. Specific complications include neck pain and hematomas.

Neck Nodes and Masses

Biopsies of neck masses can easily be performed with ultrasound guidance. In a patient with a history of

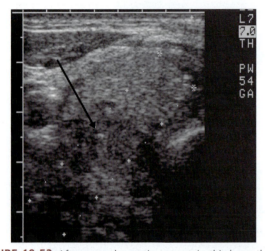

FIGURE 19-52 After several negative passes in this large thyroid nodule, positive cells were obtained in the area of the small calcifications (arrow).

thyroid cancer, it is important to differentiate between malignant and benign lymph nodes. Round, homogenous lymph nodes are usually suspicious for cancer as opposed to oval nodes with echogenic centers from a fatty hilum. Other causes of neck masses include lymphoma and submandibular gland tumors. Masses of the parotid gland can also be biopsied under ultrasound guidance. Large masses seen in a supraclavicular location may be difficult to access using a linear array transducer. High-frequency curved arrays, phased arrays, or even an endocavitary transducer may give more access to these masses.

Musculoskeletal Biopsies

Ultrasound has also proven successful in biopsying masses in the extremities. These may be muscular in origin, such as a leiomyosarcoma or rhabdomyosarcoma, or from nerves, such as a schwannoma or neurofibroma. If a bony lesion has broken through the cortex, ultrasound can be used to guide the biopsy. Ewing's sarcoma, osteosarcoma, and metastatic disease from prostate cancer are some examples of bone cancers.

Pelvis

A variety of pelvic masses can be biopsied using ultrasound guidance. Pelvic lymph nodes can be seen and color Doppler used to identify the location of the iliac vessels. Perisacral masses may be seen with the patient supine, using a curved linear array transducer (Figure 19-53). If unable to see the mass with the patient supine, the radiologist should evaluate a prone approach. In

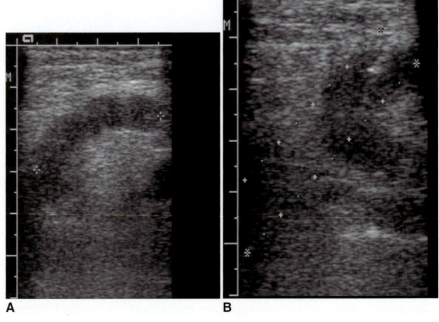

FIGURE 19-53 A, This lymph node exhibits the characteristic of a benign lymph node: oval in shape with a fatty hilum. **B,** The specimen came back positive for metastatic disease.

A   B

females, pelvic masses or fluid collections should be evaluated with both a transabdominal approach and a transvaginal approach. Transvaginal biopsies are usually performed with the patient in stirrups.

Prostate Gland

Men with elevated PSA levels or palpable nodules found on a rectal digital examination may be referred for a prostate biopsy. If a full scan is needed before the biopsy, the biopsy guide should be placed on the transducer so that the probe does not need to be removed and reinserted. The patient is biopsied in the left lateral decubitus position. Because the biopsy is through the rectal wall, the patient should be placed on a broad-spectrum antibiotic the day before and usually 2 days after the biopsy to reduce the chance of infection. Transrectal prostate biopsies are considered clean procedures, not sterile procedures. Random samples are taken from the prostate gland as follows: one each from the apex, mid, and base of the peripheral zone and one through the central gland on both the right and left sides of the gland. Extra passes should also be obtained through any suspicious hypoechoic area seen in the peripheral zone. For the peripheral zone area, the needle tip is placed on the edge of the prostate gland and fired. For central gland passes, the needle tip is placed inside the prostate gland, just inside the central gland (Figure 19-54). The number of passes obtained will vary among departments, with 8 to 10 total passes being a common number. On the patient where a rectal approach is not feasible because of rectal surgery, a transperineal biopsy can be performed. The best transducer is typically a phased array transducer, as a small footprint is required. The patient is placed in stirrups with the perineum exposed. The penis and scrotum need to be positioned out of the biopsy field and held in place with towels and tape. The patient is usually given intravenous sedation in addition to plenty of local numbing. Because of the lack of resolution, two to three random specimens are obtained from both the right and left sides of the prostate gland. In the patient with a prostatic abscess, ultrasound is used to obtain a specimen from the abscess if the patient is not responding to antibiotic therapy. These patients are very tender, and care and gentleness need to be used when inserting the transducer.

FLUID COLLECTIONS AND ABSCESSES

Pleural Fluid

Patients who have pleural effusions may be marked for a thoracentesis and returned to the unit for the actual procedure, or they may have it performed under sonographic guidance. The patient should be scanned in the same position that the procedure will be performed, which is usually an upright position, through the back. In cases of loculated fluid, the procedure may be performed with the use of a needle guide (Figure 19-55). Care should be taken to identify the diaphragm and examine above the diaphragm so that the spleen or liver is not accidentally mistaken for a collection because of poor technical settings. Misidentification may happen because of air artifact and using reduced overall gain. A guide may not be necessary if the fluid is not complicated and the pocket large enough. When just marking the patient who is having the tap performed blindly, it is important not to press too hard on the skin, as this will change the depth to the fluid and may cause the clinician not to advance the needle far enough to reach the fluid. The distance to the fluid and the distance to midpocket are usually measured. To scan between the ribs, a phased array or curved linear transducer is used (Figure 19-56). The clinician who is unable to see any fluid may scan the patient supine to see if there are any fluid layers above the diaphragm. While the fluid is being drained, the patient may start to cough as the lung reexpands with air.

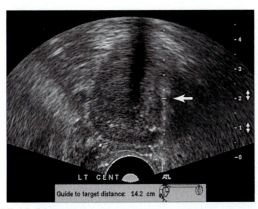

FIGURE 19-54 Prostate biopsy of a patient with an elevated PSA. Although no discrete mass was seen, adenocarcinoma of the prostate was found in one of the biopsy specimens. The arrow points to the needle.

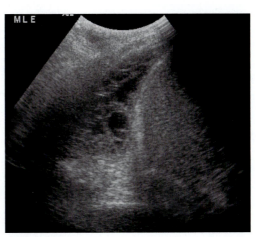

FIGURE 19-55 Because of the loculations in this pleural fluid, an ultrasound-guided thoracentesis was performed to remove fluid for cytology.

After the procedure the patient may be sent for a chest x-ray to make sure that there is no pneumothorax.

Ascites

Ascites drainage is a common sonography request. Patients with intraabdominal fluid may be marked for an ascites tap (paracentesis) to have the procedure performed in their room or have the procedure performed under sonographic guidance. The entire abdomen and pelvis should be evaluated for the extent of fluid and to locate the largest area or "pocket" of fluid. To pool the fluid in the pelvis, the patient may be scanned in a reverse Trendelenburg position of 30 to 45 degrees. If the fluid is septated, the pocket is small, or if there are organs or bowel loops in the way, a guide may be used. During the procedure, the patient may be rolled into an oblique position so that the fluid drains to the dependent portion where the needle or centesis catheter is located. When marking the fluid, care should be taken to apply just enough pressure with the transducer to make contact with the skin, as pressure will influence the measure-ments to the fluid (Figure 19-57). If the procedure is to be performed on the floor blindly, the distance to the fluid and the distance to midpocket should be measured and reported (Figure 19-58). A postprocedural image should be taken to document the remaining amount of fluid (Figure 19-59).

Abscess Drainage

As mentioned before, ultrasound can be used to drain abscesses and fluid collections from different locations in the body, including abdominal, pelvic, hepatic, perirenal, prostate, and peripancreatic. In some instances, only a small amount of fluid is removed to determine the organism that is causing the infection or to determine the proper type of antibiotics for treatment. Infected fluid is typically complex and may contain low-level echoes. Larger bore needles from 16 to 18 gauge may be needed to remove the viscous fluid. Drains may be left in place and ultrasound or radiology used for follow-up as needed.

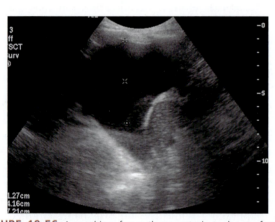

FIGURE 19-56 A marking for a thoracentesis to be performed without ultrasound guidance. The distance to the fluid is 1.27 cm and to midpocket it is between 4.16 to 7.21 cm.

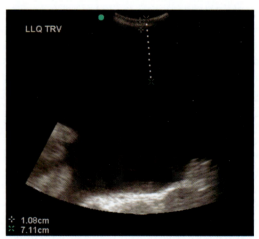

FIGURE 19-58 An example of marking for a paracentesis. The distance to the fluid is 1.08 cm, and it is 7.11 cm to about the middle of the fluid.

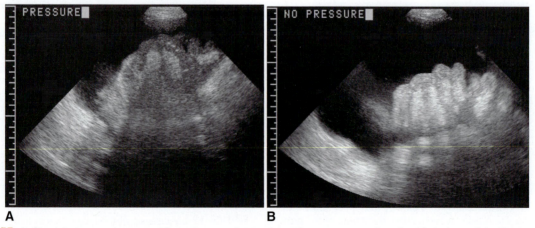

FIGURE 19-57 A, There is too much pressure from the transducer, giving the appearance that there is only a minimal amount of fluid in this area. **B,** The same patient with minimal transducer pressure demonstrates the true amount of fluid.

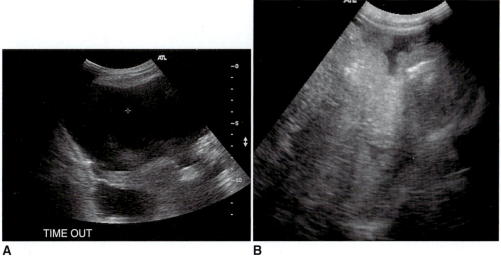

FIGURE 19-59 A, The predrainage image in this patient with a pelvic ascites. **B,** The postdrainage image demonstrating the residual fluid after the paracentesis.

NEW APPLICATIONS

With the introduction of small, portable ultrasound units, sonography is being used outside the traditional areas of radiology, obstetrics, vascular medicine, and cardiology. These low-cost units are designed for ease of use and can be designed for specific applications including guidance for placing lines into various arteries and veins in the body. Physicians and nonphysicians such as internists, surgeons, emergency room personnel, residents, IV therapists, nurses, and interventional physicians are using these units for brachial IV guidance, performing the ascites tap in the patient's room, guiding superficial biopsies, and other applications. These procedures are performed by a nonsonologist without the assistance of either a sonologist or sonographer.

Ultrasound guidance is also used in the operating room to verify the number and location of tumors, locate vessels, and determine resection approaches as well as in guidance of biopsies on sedated patients, especially pediatric patients. The sonographer may be involved in setting up the equipment with the operating room personnel, documenting images, and assisting the surgeon with the identification of structures, because if more lesions are found on intraoperative ultrasound than are documented by MR or CT, the surgery may be canceled. Some dedicated operating room ultrasound units have ultrasound laparoscopic capabilities. The sonographer is a valuable member of the operating team and can assist the surgeon by offering ultrasound knowledge and skills. The problem is that operating room (OR) cases can involve the sonographer for many hours or involve multiple trips to the OR as needed.

Ultrasound can be used for guidance for the various types of ablation procedures, which include radio frequency (RF), cryoablation, laser, microwave, and high-intensity focused ultrasound (HIFU). The goal of ablation is to destroy the cancerous tissue while limiting the damage done to the normal tissue. Ablation procedures can be performed either in the OR or percutaneously through small incisions. These ablation therapies typically have fewer complications, as well as a shorter recovery, time than surgical resections. Ablation is used when the patient is not a candidate for surgery or on masses that are not resectable, and it can be used on various organs in the body including but not limited to the liver, kidney, breast, and prostate. Unfortunately, not all patients will be able to be treated with ablation and not all diseases or masses are amenable to this technique. On some patients, the procedure may be difficult to perform in a minimally invasive or safe manner.

Ablation utilizes cold or hot temperatures to kill cells. The extreme heating or cooling of the tissue results in death of the tissue. Most ablation techniques use heat to kill the cells. As the tissue is heated, dissolved gases, primarily nitrogen, are released from the cells forming microbubbles within the tissue. These microbubbles are visible by ultrasound and are seen as hyperechoic echoes. Seeing this streaming effect of the microbubbles assists in confirming the area that is being treated (Figure 19-60). The ablation area is roughly the diameter of the prongs, with different configurations available to create the proper size of ablation zone. Although ultrasound can be used for guidance, CT or MR will be the imaging modality of choice for documenting the postablation area for residual tumor and for follow-up.

In radiofrequency ablation, the patient is grounded for the procedure by placing grounding pads on the appropriate place on the body like, for example, the upper legs. When introduced, the expandable electrodes are collapsed within a 14- to 15-gauge needle. Once correctly positioned, the prongs or tines are deployed, resulting in a final configuration that resembles an

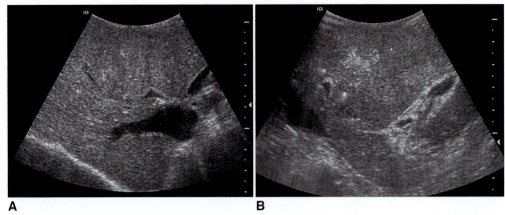

A   **B**

FIGURE 19-60 A, Liver lesion being measured pre-RFA. **B,** Same patient undergoing RFA. Notice the 60-cycle noise that is seen during the ablation. The bright echoes seen represent the microbubbles produced.

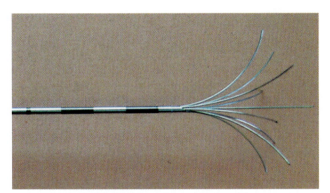

FIGURE 19-61 Deployed RF needle.

umbrella (Figure 19-61). The needle is connected to a radiofrequency generator to create an electrical circuit. The tip of the probe releases a high-frequency current that heats and destroys the cancer cells. Tissue that is farther away from the prongs is heated by thermal conduction, with the temperature decreasing as the distance from the prongs increases. The temperature of the tissue will be the highest directly adjacent to the prongs and can reach about 100° C or 212° F. Irreversible damage and cell death occur at temperatures over 60° C or 140° F. The amount of tissue reaching these lethal temperatures depends on the type of tumor and the surrounding tissue. The body reabsorbs the destroyed cells. The procedure is performed under conscious sedation, although general anesthesia may be used. Each session of treatment lasts between 10 and 30 minutes, depending on the size of the lesion. Tumors smaller than 7 cm have a greater success rate of being totally ablated than larger tumors. At the end of the procedure, the needle is withdrawn at a lower power output to prevent bleeding and seeding of the needle track. RF ablation is used in conjunction with other types of therapy such as chemotherapy. The advantages of RF ablation include low complication rate, reduced cost, and increased patient compliance. The hospital stay is short and most patients can resume normal activities within a few days. Complications are rare and are related to thermal injury to either the skin or nearby organs.

Unlike the other forms of ablation, which use heat to destroy the tissue, cryoablation uses extremely cold temperatures. Cryoablation uses repetitive freezing and thawing of tissue to produce cellular death and necrosis. Irreversible tissue destruction will occur at temperatures below −20 to −30° C or −4° to −22° F. Temperatures as low as −160° C or −256° F can be achieved with cryoablation using liquid nitrogen and argon for the gases to freeze the tissue. As the tissues are frozen, crystals will form within, which causes the cells to expand. Both the formation of crystals and expansion of the cell wall cause cellular damage. Thawing the cell also results in cellular disruption and death. Just as in RF ablation, the body absorbs the destroyed cells. Different size and shape cryoprobes are available to map out the area to be treated.

Cryoablation is performed either in the OR with the patient open, or percutaneously using smaller diameter cryoprobes. Ultrasound is often used to guide the cryoprobe into position and to monitor the size of the ice ball. Once the cryoprobe is in place, the gases are released to freeze the tissue, followed by periods of tissue thawing. The development of the ice ball can be monitored using ultrasound with an accuracy of 1 to 5 mm (Figure 19-62). It is important that the ultrasound transducer does not touch the cryoprobe, as it will freeze the ultrasound transducer, causing it temporarily not to work.

There are several potential advantages of cryoablation over the various thermal ablation techniques. One main advantage is that the ice ball formed during the ablation process is highly visible with ultrasound, which allows precise control of the ablation area and limits injury to adjacent structures. A second advantage is that larger masses of up to 12 cm in size can be ablated with cryoablation. Some of the risks of cryoablation include freezing of nontarget tissues and internal bleeding.

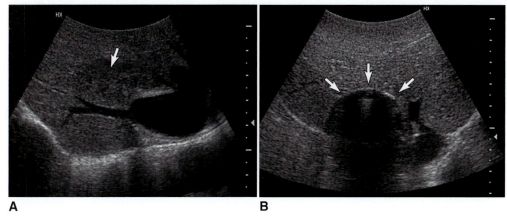

FIGURE 19-62 A, Precryoablation image. The arrow is pointing to the liver mass. **B,** The arrows are pointing to the ice ball that formed during the cryoablation.

Emergent Abdominal Ultrasound Procedures

Sandra L. Hagen-Ansert

OBJECTIVES

On completion of this chapter, you should be able to:

- Discuss the advantages and disadvantages of sonography for the trauma patient
- Define the goal of sonography in the assessment of blunt trauma
- Describe the protocol for focused assessment with sonography for trauma (FAST)

- Describe the sonographic findings for aortic dissection, three types of hernia, free fluid in the abdominopelvic region, acute pelvic pain, and scrotal trauma and torsion
- Identify the modalities commonly used to evaluate flank pain

OUTLINE

Sonography is well recognized as a powerful and efficient tool for the diagnosis and evaluation of the patient in the emergency room. The development of smaller, inexpensive, portable units has brought the ultrasound system into controversy as to who may be qualified to perform the studies on an emergent basis.

The most common reasons people go to the emergency room include problems in the following areas: lower gastrointestinal system, genitourinary system, cardiac system, orthopedics, respiratory system, nervous system, locations of lacerations, limbs and joints, skin, and upper gastrointestinal system.

The primary focus of this chapter is to cover the more common emergent abdominal procedures that the

sonographer is likely to encounter in a "call back" situation from the emergency department. Potential life-threatening emergencies such as abdominal emergencies, internal hemorrhage following blunt trauma, ectopic pregnancy, pericardial tamponade, and ruptured aortic aneurysm are rapidly assessed with sonography.

ASSESSMENT OF ABDOMINAL TRAUMA

The assessment of the abdomen for possible sustained abdominal injury caused by blunt abdominal trauma is a common clinical challenge for surgeons and emergency medicine physicians. The physical findings may be unreliable because of the state of patient consciousness, neurologic deficit, medication, or other associated injuries. The health care staffs in emergency departments in the United States have used ultrasound with great success since the late 1990s.

Peritoneal Lavage

Peritoneal lavage is used to sample the intraperitoneal space for evidence of damage to the viscera and blood vessels. It is usually used as a diagnostic technique in certain cases of blunt abdominal trauma, and this technique has been used as a surgical tool for the diagnosis of **hemoperitoneum** since 1965. A sensitivity of 95% has been found with this tool in the evaluation of intraperitoneal hemorrhage.

For this procedure the patient is placed in the supine position and the urinary bladder is emptied by catheterization. The patient's stomach is emptied by a nasogastric tube because a distended stomach may extend to the anterior abdominal wall. The skin is anesthetized, and a small vertical incision is made. The incision is made either in the midline or at the paraumbilical site with multiple layers of tissue penetrated before the parietal peritoneum is located (Figure 20-1).

Although peritoneal lavage has been used successfully to assess abdominal injuries, it is an invasive procedure that carries a risk of bowel perforation, bladder penetration,

vascular laceration, and wound complications. It also is limited to injuries of the retroperitoneum and pancreas or contained injuries to solid intraperitoneal organs. Moreover, this procedure is inappropriate for alert patients in stable condition, who represent the majority of patients with blunt abdominal trauma. Finally, peritoneal lavage decreases the specificity of subsequent ultrasonography or computed tomography (CT) because of the introduction of intraperitoneal fluid and air.

Computed Tomography

CT remains the radiology standard for investigating the injured abdomen but requires patient transfer and inevitable delay (bowel preparation). CT is usually performed in patients in whom intraabdominal injury is strongly suspected. Other indications for CT include equivocal findings of abdominal examination in stable patients, persistent abdominal pain, and decreasing hematocrit. CT is unsuitable for patients who are clinically unstable.

Ultrasound

The clinical utilization of sonography in the evaluation of blunt trauma has existed in Europe and Asia since the 1980s. Using sonography as a screening procedure involves many factors. The clinicians are looking for a

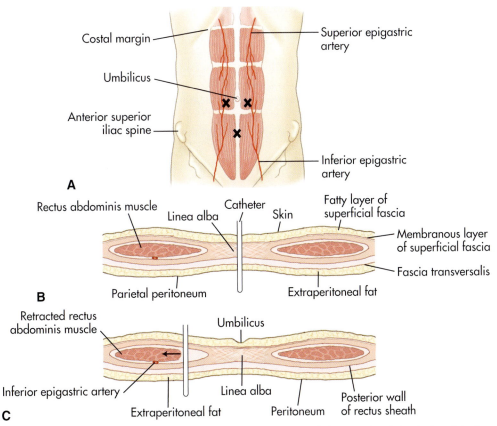

FIGURE 20-1 A, The two common sites for peritoneal lavage. **B,** Cross section of the anterior abdominal wall in the middle. Note the structures pierced by the catheter. **C,** Cross section of the anterior abdominal wall just lateral to the umbilicus.

screening tool that will be fast, accurate, portable, and easy to perform. Sonography is now well established as a noninvasive and easily repeatable tool to image many areas of the body.

FOCUSED ASSESSMENT WITH SONOGRAPHY FOR TRAUMA

Focused assessment with sonography for trauma is also known as the **FAST** scan in the emergency department. This is a limited examination of the abdomen or pelvis to evaluate free fluid or pericardial fluid. In the context of traumatic injury, free fluid is usually the result of

hemorrhage and contributes to the assessment of the circulation.

The FAST scan area of evaluation is widespread, extending from the pericardial sac to the urinary bladder and includes the perihepatic area (including Morison's pouch), perisplenic region (including splenorenal recess), paracolic gutters, and cul-de-sac (Figure 20-2). The visceral organs are assessed for heterogeneity and evaluated with color Doppler if necessary.

Accessibility and speed of performance are critical in the trauma setting. Onsite personnel who are educated in performing the ultrasound examination provide the highest success rate. Limitations of ultrasound include

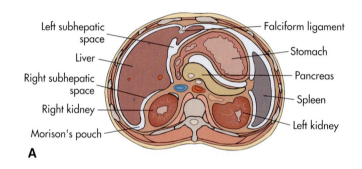

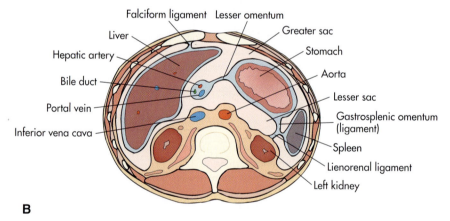

FIGURE 20-2 **A,** Transverse view of the perihepatic space and Morison's pouch. **B,** Transverse view of the perisplenic area and the splenorenal ligament. **C,** Anterior view of the collection of fluid in the abdomen and pelvic cavities. **D,** Sagittal view of the right abdomen shows how the fluid collects in the most dependent areas of the abdomen and pelvis.

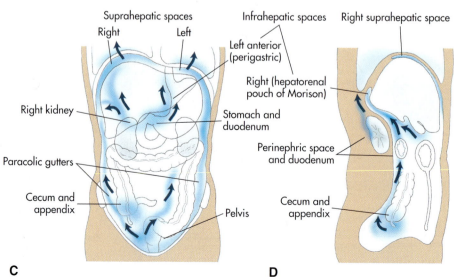

its dependence on operator skill, which becomes particularly important if surgeons or emergency physicians with limited training perform the studies. Although CT remains the standard of reference for intraperitoneal and retroperitoneal assessment, this application is not readily available at the bedside.

Assessment of Blunt Trauma with Ultrasound

Ultrasound of the abdomen and pelvis is performed simultaneously with the physical assessment, resuscitation, and stabilization of the trauma patient. The examination usually takes about 5 minutes. The goal is to scan the four quadrants, pericardial sac, and cul-de-sac for the presence of free fluid or hemoperitoneum. Ultrasound has been found to be highly sensitive for the detection of free intraperitoneal fluid, but it is not sensitive for the identification of organ injuries. If the patient is hemodynamically stable, the value of ultrasound is limited by the large percentage of organ injuries that are not associated with free fluid.

Protocol for Focused Assessment with Sonography for Trauma. The ultrasound examination is performed with the proper transducer according to the patient size. The patient is usually in the supine position. The right and left upper quadrants of the abdomen, epigastrium, paracolic gutters, retroperitoneal space, and pelvis are evaluated with ultrasound (Box 20-1). If there is no contraindication to catheterization, the empty bladder is filled with 200 to 300 ml of sterile saline through a Foley catheter to ensure bladder distention to allow adequate visualization of the pelvic cavity. The examination is focused to look for the presence of free fluid, the texture of the visceral organs, and the pericardial sac around the heart.

The initial survey is directed in the subcostal plane with the transducer angled in a cephalic direction toward the four-chamber view of the heart to image the pericardial sac (Figure 20-3). The right upper quadrant is then evaluated, including the diaphragm, dome of the liver, subhepatic space (Morison's pouch), right kidney, and right flank (Figure 20-4). The liver is quickly scanned to look for texture abnormalities (Figure 20-5).

BOX 20-1	Fast Scan Protocol

- Fill urinary bladder
- Scan subxiphoid to look for pericardial effusion
- Evaluate RUQ: diaphragm, subhepatic space/Morison's pouch, right kidney, right flank
- Evaluate liver for texture abnormalities
- Evaluate epigastrium
- Evaluate LUQ: diaphragm, spleen, left kidney, left flank
- Evaluate RLQ
- Evaluate LLQ

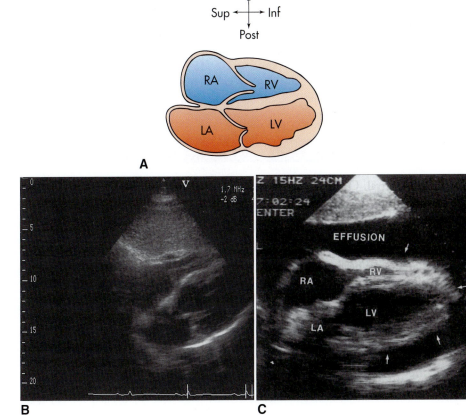

FIGURE 20-3 **A,** Subcostal view of the four chambers of the heart. The transducer is angled sharply in a cephalic direction in the subcostal area. Cardiac pulsations are noted and the four chambers of the heart should be seen. **B,** Normally, there is no significant fluid that separates the outer layer of the heart (epicardium) within the pericardial sac. **C,** Subcostal four-chamber view shows a tip of the left lobe of the liver anterior to the large pericardial effusion that fills the pericardial cavity.

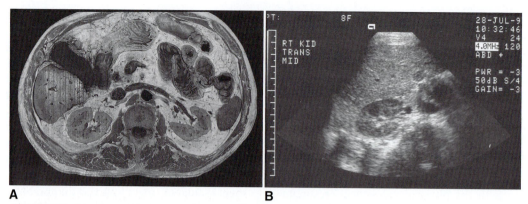

FIGURE 20-4 Gross anatomy **(A)** and transverse **(B)** images of the right upper quadrant and normal liver.

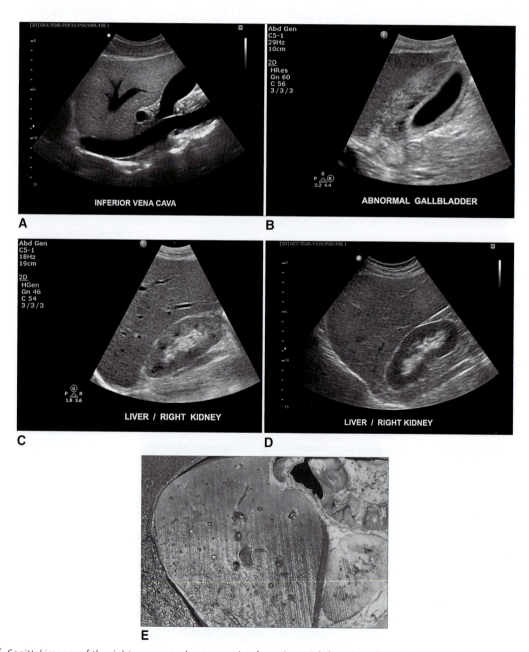

FIGURE 20-5 Sagittal images of the right upper quadrant sweeping from the IVC **(A)** to the inflamed gallbladder **(B)** to the lateral abdominal wall **(C** and **D)** demonstrate a good border between the liver and right kidney with no fluid in Morison's pouch. Gross anatomy **(E)** of the liver and right kidney.

The epigastrium is briefly examined (Figure 20-6). The transducer is then moved to the left upper quadrant to observe the diaphragm, spleen, left kidney, and left flank and to search for the presence of fluid (Figure 20-7). The pelvic cavity (with the bladder distended) is evaluated for the presence of free fluid in the cul-de-sac (Figure 20-8).

Sonographic Findings. In the trauma setting, free fluid usually represents hemoperitoneum, although it may also represent bowel, urine, bile, or ascitic fluid. Hemorrhage in the peritoneal cavity collects in the most dependent area of the abdomen (Figure 20-9). The fluid is usually hypoechoic or hyperechoic, with a few internal echoes, and conforms to the anatomic site it occupies. The most common site of fluid accumulation is the subhepatic space (Morison's pouch), regardless of the site of the injury (Figure 20-10). The next most common space is the pelvis. The blood in the pelvis may collect centrally

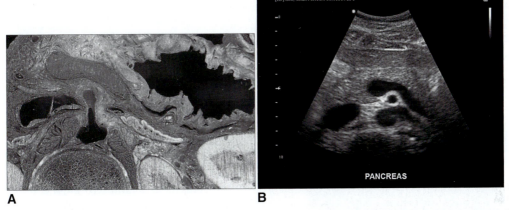

FIGURE 20-6 Gross anatomy **(A)** and transverse image **(B)** of the epigastric area of the abdomen. The horseshoe shape of the spine is the most posterior reflection with the aorta and inferior vena cava directly anterior. The celiac axis arises from the anterior wall of the aorta. The left lobe of the liver is identified anterior to the pancreas, which lies directly anterior to the prevertebral vessels (aorta, inferior vena cava, celiac axis, and splenic vein).

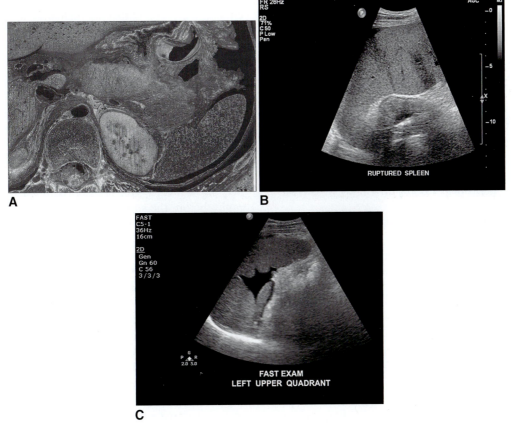

FIGURE 20-7 **A,** Gross anatomy of the left upper quadrant. **B,** Sagittal image of the diaphragm, enlarged ruptured spleen, and upper pole of the left kidney. **C,** Sagittal image of the left upper quadrant with fluid in the splenic hilum.

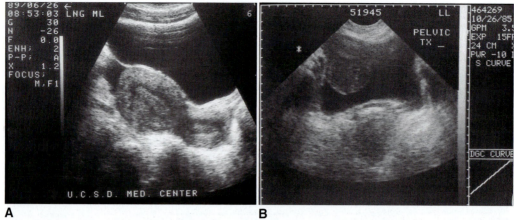

A **B**

FIGURE 20-8 A, Normal sagittal pelvic image with a distended urinary bladder and uterus posterior. It is not uncommon to see a small amount of fluid in a female of menstrual age. **B,** Transverse image of the distended urinary bladder as it provides a window for the uterus and adnexal area.

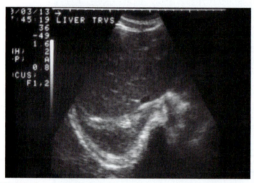

FIGURE 20-9 Transverse image of a patient with pleural effusion as seen posterior to the right lobe of the liver. Fluid will collect in the most dependent area of the abdomen and should not be confused with ascitic fluid.

in the pouch of Douglas or laterally in the paravesical space (Figure 20-11). When fluid is present, the poorly visualized loops of bowel are separated by triangular collections of fluid. If there is a massive hemoperitoneum, the intraperitoneal organs will float in the surrounding fluid.

If the collection of fluid is small, the surgeon may not want to do an immediate laparotomy. Close monitoring of the patient with either ultrasound or CT imaging may help to define the further extent of the injury after the patient stabilizes.

Parenchymal Injury

The ultrasound appearance of hepatic and splenic injury will vary with both the type and time of injury. Liver lacerations or contusions are more easily detected with ultrasound than any other visceral abdominal injury. Such injuries appear as heterogeneous or hyperechoic. Hematomas and localized lacerations will appear initially hypoechoic with low-level echoes from the red

blood cells or echogenic as the blood begins to coagulate, which over time will become more anechoic with the onset of hemolysis (Figure 20-12). Pitfalls of abdominal ultrasound include failure to show contained solid-organ injuries; injuries to the diaphragm, pancreas, and adrenal gland; and some bowel injuries. Therefore, a negative ultrasound does not exclude an intraperitoneal injury, and close clinical observation or CT is warranted.

A brisk intraparenchymal hemorrhage may be identified as an anechoic region within the abnormal parenchyma, whereas a global parenchymal injury may project in the liver as a widespread architectural disruption with absence of the normal vascular pattern. An extensive splenic injury presents as a diffusely heterogeneous parenchymal pattern with both hyperechoic and hypoechoic regions.

The early diagnosis of parenchymal injury can affect patient treatment. The clinically stable patient with a hemoperitoneum and an obvious splenic injury seen on ultrasound can be taken directly to surgery. However, if extensive hepatic disruption is demonstrated, the surgeon may want further investigation with CT or even angiography before the surgery is performed.

Free Pelvic Fluid in Women. In female patients of reproductive age with trauma, free fluid isolated to the cul-de-sac is likely physiologic and clinical follow-up should suffice. Female patients with fluid elsewhere usually have a clinically important injury and require further evaluation.

Pitfalls and Limitations. As in other ultrasound procedures, obesity may prevent adequate visualization of the anatomic structures. In some cases the presence of subcutaneous emphysema precludes adequate ultrasound views. The presence of subcutaneous air from a pneumothorax that dissects into the abdominal cavity may collect over the liver or spleen.

An intraperitoneal clot is usually hyperechoic relative to the neighboring structures; occasionally, though, it is

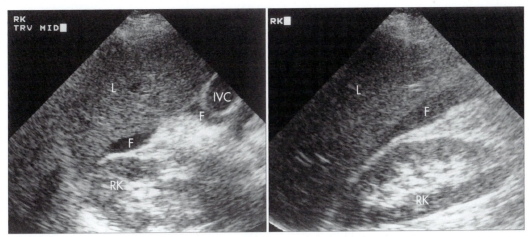

FIGURE 20-10 RUQ fluid is present in a patient after trauma. There is a small amount of fluid seen in Morison's pouch anterior to the kidney. *F,* fluid; *IVC,* inferior vena cava; *L,* liver; *RK,* right kidney.

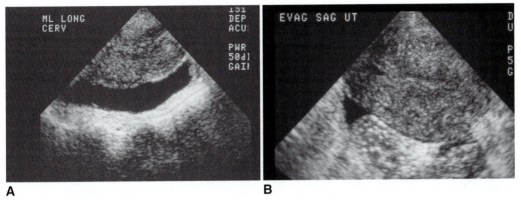

FIGURE 20-11 **A** and **B,** Transvaginal images of fluid in the pouch of Douglas.

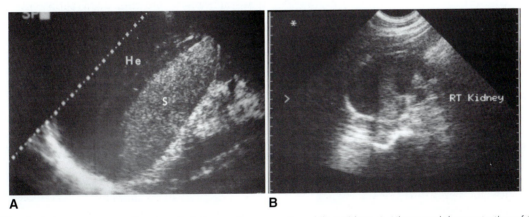

FIGURE 20-12 Splenic hematoma secondary to splenic trauma from an automobile accident. **A,** Ultrasound demonstration of the somewhat hypoechoic mass with low-lying echoes adjacent to the spleen. **B,** Perinephric hematoma in a patient after a renal biopsy procedure.

isoechoic, and intraperitoneal bleeding or parenchymal injury may go unrecognized.

Contained parenchymal injuries of the liver and spleen, as well as bowel injuries, may not be accompanied by hemoperitoneum and may therefore be missed if screening ultrasound alone is used to evaluate for blunt trauma. Ultrasound may not depict injuries to the diaphragm, the pancreas, the adrenal gland, and bone.

RIGHT UPPER QUADRANT PAIN

Acute Cholecystitis versus Cholelithiasis

One of the most frequent complaints in the emergency department is the onset of severe right upper quadrant pain. The patient may have other medical conditions, such as diabetes or peptic ulcer disease, which may contribute to the pain. A myocardial infarction may also present with right upper quadrant pain. Thus, a clinically focused physical examination in conjunction with historical and laboratory information should provide the information necessary for decision making.

If the patient is female with symptoms of right upper quadrant pain with point tenderness, fever, and leukocytosis, acute cholecystitis should be ruled out. The most common cause of acute cholecystitis is cholelithiasis with a cystic duct obstruction.

Sonographic Findings. Sonographic findings of acute cholecystitis include an irregular, thickened gallbladder wall, a positive sonographic Murphy's sign, sludge, pericholecystic fluid, and a dilated gallbladder greater than 5 cm in transverse diameter (Figure 20-13). The presence of biliary stones within the inflamed gallbladder is recognized as tiny echogenic foci collected along the posterior wall with a well-demarcated acoustic shadowing in at least two planes (Figure 20-14). The sonographer must be careful to make sure the shadowing is secondary to gallstones and not to surrounding bowel gas. By holding the transducer carefully over the area of interest, the presence of peristalsis in the bowel may cause shifting

of the dirty shadow. Alterations in the patient position will cause movement of the gallstones, with resultant movement of the acoustical shadow. If the stones are very small, they have a chance of becoming lodged within the neck of the gallbladder and may be too small to render an acoustical shadow. The gallbladder will show signs of inflammation. Cholesterol stones are usually smaller than the biliary stones and on sonography are less echogenic. They may be seen to "float" within the thick bile and demonstrate a "comet tail" artifact on sonography.

Biliary Dilatation

The common bile duct (CBD) is demonstrated on sonography by identifying the portal vein. The duct is seen anterior and to the right of the portal vein on a transverse image and does not fill in with color Doppler (Figure 20-15). Recall the hepatic artery is anterior and medial of the portal vein. The normal upper limit of the CBD is 6 mm, although with age this diameter may extend up to 10 mm in size. The presence of stones within the duct should be carefully assessed.

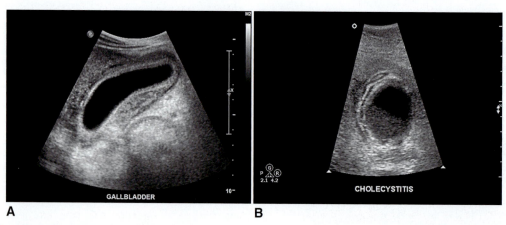

FIGURE 20-13 Sagittal **(A)** and transverse **(B)** images of the distended gallbladder with edema and wall thickening secondary to acute cholecystitis and sludge.

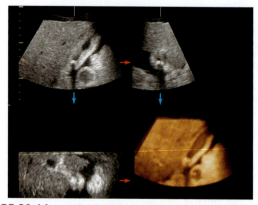

FIGURE 20-14 Multiple images of the chronic cholelithiasis show an edematous thick-walled gallbladder with a large gallstone within the gallbladder bed. This stone may obstruct the bile in the area of Hartmann's pouch, causing extreme right upper quadrant pain.

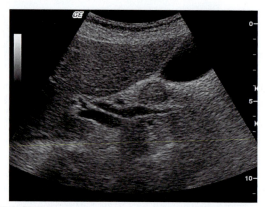

FIGURE 20-15 Prominent common bile duct is seen anterior to the portal vein in this sagittal image. Careful sweep of the transducer should demonstrate echo density with shadowing if stones are present and large enough to be detected with sonography.

The sonographer should look for echogenic foci with acoustical shadowing beyond the foci. Adjustment of gains should be made to delineate the CBD, and alterations in patient position may allow the visualization of the duct to be separated from bowel gas interference.

EPIGASTRIC PAIN

Pancreatitis

Midepigastric pain that radiates to the back is characteristic of acute pancreatitis. Pancreatitis occurs when the toxic enzymes escape into the parenchymal tissue of the gland, causing obstruction of the acini, ducts, small blood vessels, and fat with extension into the peripancreatic tissue. Clinical findings of fever and leukocytosis are found along with elevated enzymes. The serum amylase levels increase within the first 24 hours of onset but fall rather quickly, whereas the lipase levels take longer to elevate (as much as 72 hours) and remain elevated for a longer period of time. Sonographic findings in acute pancreatitis show a normal to edematous gland that is somewhat hypoechoic to normal texture (Figure 20-16). The borders are irregular secondary to

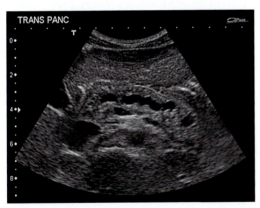

FIGURE 20-16 Acute epigastric pain may be secondary to pancreatitis. This image also demonstrates the enlarged pancreatic duct.

the inflammation. Increased vascular flow may be apparent because of the inflammatory nature of the disease.

Abdominal Aortic Aneurysm

The patient who presents with classic abdominal pain radiating to the back, with hypotension and a pulsatile abdominal mass, is not a diagnostic dilemma in the emergency department (Figure 20-17). Sonography can rapidly separate the emergent patient with a possible aortic dissection from the elderly patient with vague abdominal complaints or the middle-aged patient with symptoms that mimic nephrolithiasis (Figure 20-18). If a dissection is suspected, CT with contrast is generally more specific than sonography, as the full length of the aorta may be clearly imaged in a matter of minutes without bowel gas interference. Sonography may identify the abdominal aortic aneurysm in relation to the renal vessels, which is important because in the event a dissection occurs, extension may extend into the renal arteries. Recall that the aorta and iliac arteries are measured from the outside margin of the wall on one wall to the outside margin on the other wall. This measurement should be performed in two planes, transverse and longitudinal. Most aneurysms occur at the level of the umbilicus, at the junction of the bifurcation into the iliac vessels. Aneurysms may expand in the transverse diameter as well as in the AP diameter. The sonographic examination may be inhibited by obesity, bowel gas interference, or extreme abdominal tenderness.

The sonographer should be aware of several pitfalls when scanning the abdominal aorta. If bowel gas precludes adequate visualization of the aorta from the anterior wall, the transducer may be directed from the lateral abdominal wall, using the liver or spleen as an acoustic window to image both the aorta and inferior vena cava. Alternately, the patient could be rolled into a decubitus position and imaged from the lateral wall. The true diameter of the aorta should be measured with the transducer perpendicular to the vessel; an oblique or angled

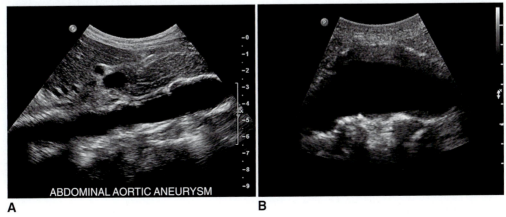

A   **B**

FIGURE 20-17 Abdominal aortic aneurysm. **A,** This sagittal image of the abdominal aorta demonstrates a small aneurysm just superior to the bifurcation of the vessel. **B,** Prominent dilation of the abdominal aorta extending from the umbilicus to the proximal aorta.

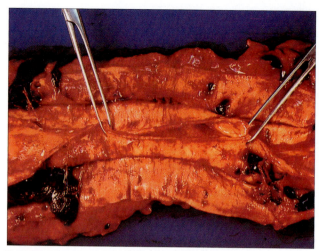

FIGURE 20-18 Gross pathology of a dissecting aortic aneurysm demonstrates the layers of the aortic wall separated by the blood.

image would exaggerate the true aortic diameter. A small aneurysm does not preclude rupture. The sonographer should also assess for free intraperitoneal fluid when a patient with an acute abdominal aortic aneurysm is examined. Paraaortic nodes may be confused with the aorta, mimicking an aneurysm. These nodes often are anterior to the aorta, but they can be found posterior as well, encasing the aorta and displacing it from the vertebral body. The nodes are irregular in shape without luminal flow.

EXTREME SHORTNESS OF BREATH

Pericardial Effusion

The primary application of cardiac ultrasound in an emergent situation is to rule out the presence of pericardial effusion or to evaluate cardiac function in patients with sudden cardiac arrest. Body habitus and underlying

pathologic conditions will affect the accessibility of the heart to sonographic evaluation. Patients with pulmonary hyperinflation have poor parasternal windows but generally have adequate apical and subcostal windows.

Other emergent situations such as cardiac tamponade involve a more complex evaluation of the cardiac structures that require high-end ultrasound equipment that is not commonly found in the emergency department. The diastolic collapse of any chamber in the presence of a moderate to large effusion may be indicative of tamponade. This is usually seen in the right atrial collapse or right ventricular collapse. Further Doppler evaluation of both the tricuspid and mitral valve inflow patterns with a respirator monitor is made to look for alterations of flow secondary to cardiac tamponade. Clinically, the presence of the pulsus tardus may be present in the setting of tamponade.

The evaluation of acute right ventricular dysfunction or acute pulmonary hypertension in the clinical setting of acute and unexplained chest pain, dyspnea, or hemodynamic instability is best evaluated by the high-end ultrasound equipment. In this case, patients with suspected pulmonary embolism are usually referred for a rapid CT scan to demonstrate the presence of clot or thrombus lodged within the pulmonary arteries.

The sonographer should be aware that when a pericardial effusion is demonstrated, several observations should be made. The pericardial effusion usually images as an anechoic or hypoechoic fluid collection within the pericardial space (Figure 20-19). With inflammatory, malignant, or hemorrhagic etiologies, this fluid may have a more complex echogenic texture. Fluid usually initially collects dependently. The size of the effusion is important to document. In the parasternal long axis view, the fluid is demonstrated within the pericardial sac beyond the epicardial border of the left ventricle. If the fluid collection is small (< 1 cm between the epicardium and posterior border of the fluid in diastole), it may only be seen

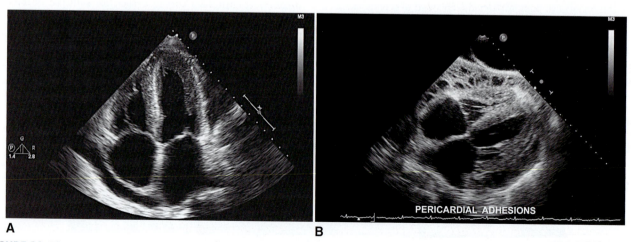

A   **B**

FIGURE 20-19 A, Apical four-chamber view shows a small separation between the right atrium and the diaphragm. This pericardial effusion is not large enough to cause compromise of the right heart. **B,** Subcostal window shows a complex moderate size pericardial effusion representing adhesions from previous interventions.

in the posterior of the heart. As the fluid increases, it becomes circumferential, reflecting off the great vessels and not extending beyond the atrial appendage. A moderate size effusion measures between 1 to 2 cm in diastole, usually circumferential. Beyond 2 cm in diastole the fluid is considered large. The fluid should be assessed in multiple planes, short axis, apical four chamber, and subcostal views.

In the acute hemopericardium trauma patient with clotted blood, the fluid may have a soft echogenic to isoechoic to the myocardium texture representing blood within the pericardial space. Hypoechoic fatty tissue found in the epicardial layer surrounding the heart may sometimes mimic pericardial effusion. It is important to note that a small rapidly forming effusion may lead to tamponade, whereas extremely large, slowly forming effusions may be tolerated with minimal symptoms.

Care should also be taken not to confuse pleural effusions with a pericardial effusion. Patients with congestive heart failure who present with acute failure may have both pericardial and pleural effusion. Again in a long axis view of the heart, the pericardial effusion will be seen posterior to the epicardial border of the left ventricular and anterior to the descending aorta. The pleural effusion will also be found in that similar area, but will be seen posterior to the descending aorta.

AORTIC DISSECTION

A dissecting aortic aneurysm is a condition in which a propagating intramural hematoma actually dissects along the length of the vessel, stripping away the intima and, in some cases, part of the media (Figure 20-20). The resultant aortic dissection is a defect or tear in the aortic intima with concomitant weakness of the aortic media.

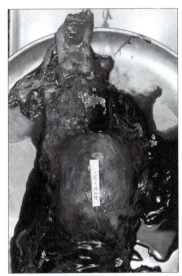

FIGURE 20-20 Surgical revelation of a large abdominal aortic aneurysm that has dissected and ruptured into the abdominal cavity.

At this point, blood surges into the media, separating the intima from the adventitia. This channel is called the "false lumen." This blood in the false lumen can reenter the true lumen anywhere along the course of the dissection. Most aortic dissections will occur at one of three sites: (1) at the root of the aorta with possible extension into the arch, descending aorta, and abdominal aorta; (2) at the level of the left subclavian artery, with extension into the descending aorta or abdominal aorta; and (3) only at the level of the ascending aorta.

Approximately 70% of dissections are located in the ascending aorta, 10% to 20% in the aortic arch, and 20% in the abdominal aorta. Most often, the dissection will propagate distally in the aorta into the iliac vessels, although proximal extension can occur.

Causes of Aortic Dissection

Systemic hypertension is nearly always associated with aortic dissection (Box 20-2). The age of most patients affected ranges from 50 to 70 years, with a higher prevalence in males than females. In the under-age-40 group, the incidence is equal. In women, 50% of dissections occur during pregnancy. (Hormonal imbalance, associated hypertension, and sclerosis and necrosis of both the medial layer and the vasa vasorum all play a contributory role.) Without treatment, a dissecting aorta may result in death if the dissection obstructs the blood flow to the brain or the tear is so great that volumes of blood loss occur.

Clinical Findings for Aortic Dissection

The most typical presentation is that of a sudden onset of severe, tearing chest pain radiating to the arms, neck, or back. Syncope occurs in a small percentage of patients. The complexity of the symptoms will depend on the extension of the dissection, the specific branches of the aorta involved, and the location of external rupture if present (Table 20-1). If the carotid artery is affected, hemiplegia may result. Involvement of the subclavian or iliac vessels will appear with decreased or absent pulses in the arms or legs.

The location of the pain may be a clue to the site of the dissection. If the pain centers in the anterior thorax,

BOX 20-2	Causes of Aortic Dissection

- Hypertension (70% to 90%)
- Marfan's syndrome (16%)
- Pregnancy
- Acquired or congenital aortic stenosis
- Coarctation of the aorta
- Trauma
- Iatrogenic (cardiac catheterization, aortic valve replacement)

TABLE 20-1	Common Emergency Conditions
Clinical Findings	**Sonographic Findings**
RUQ Pain: Cholecystitis	
RUQ pain	Thickened GB wall
Fever	+ Murphy's sign
Nausea, vomiting	Pericholecystic fluid
Leukocytosis	Dilated GB
Epigastric Pain: Pancreatitis	
Midepigastric pain radiating to back	Normal to edematous gland
	Hypoechoic texture
Fever	Irregular borders
Leukocytosis	Increased vascular flow
↑ Amylase	
↑ Lipase	
Flank Pain: Urolithiasis	
Spasmodic flank pain	Echogenic foci with shadowing
Pain may radiate into pelvis	Hydronephrosis may be present
Hematuria	Look for ureteral jets in bladder
Fever	
Leukocytosis	
Thoracic or Abdominal Pain: Aortic Dissection	
Sudden onset of severe chest pain with radiation to arms, neck, or back	Aneurysm
	Look for flap at site of dissection
Syncope may be present	Look for false lumen
RLQ Pain: Appendicitis	
Intense RLQ pain	Distended, noncompressible appendix
Nausea, vomiting	
Fever	↑ Color flow
Leukocytosis	McBurney sign
Lower Abdominal Pain: Paraumbilical Hernia	
Asymptomatic to mild discomfort	Lower abdominal mass; look for peristalsis of bowel in hernia
Palpable mass	
Valsalva: shows exaggeration of mass	
Reduce sac with gentle pressure	

On sonography, the classic finding is the visualization of the flap at the site of the dissection. An echogenic intimal membrane within the aorta or the iliac arteries may be seen to move freely with arterial pulsations on sonography if both the true and false lumen are patent (Figure 20-21). However, if the membrane is thick and the lumen is thrombosed, the membrane may not move. Color Doppler may demonstrate slow flow in both the true and false lumen. The flow is decreased or reversed in the false lumen. The sonographer should look for the presence of the intimal membrane with concomitant clotting in the iliac, celiac, and superior mesenteric arteries.

A **pseudodissection** on color flow demonstrates a turbulent blood flow pattern, indicating a hypoechoic thrombus near the outer margin of the aorta with an echogenic laminated clot. No intimal flap is seen with a pseudodissection.

FLANK PAIN: UROLITHIASIS

Flank pain caused by urolithiasis is a common problem in patients coming to the emergency department. Radiology plays a vital role in the evaluation of these patients through the use of **intravenous urography (IVU)**, ultrasonography, and limited noncontrast helical CT studies. The most sensitive and specific for the presence of stones are the IVU and helical CT. Traditional evaluation of the patient with flank pain consisted of conventional radiography followed by IVU with noniodinated contrast. In those patients unable to undergo IVU safely (i.e., patients with dye allergies, renal insufficiency, congestive heart failure, or suspected pregnancy), ultrasound was used to evaluate for secondary signs of obstruction, namely hydronephrosis. Computerized tomography has largely replaced these other modalities with its ability to identify calculi and their location, determine the size, and guide the management.

Clinical Findings for Urolithiasis

Acute ureteral obstruction usually manifests as renal colic, a severe pain that is often spasmodic, that increases to a peak level of intensity, and then decreases before increasing again. The pain can also manifest as steady and continuous. The pain usually begins abruptly in the flank and increases rapidly to a level of discomfort that often requires narcotics for adequate pain control. Over time, the pain may radiate to the lower abdomen and into the scrotum or labia as the stone moves into the more distal portion of the ureter.

Urinalysis is the initial laboratory examination. Hematuria is the common finding in 85% of the patients. However, if the stone completely obstructs the ureter, no hematuria will be present. Clinical symptoms such as fever, leukocytosis, and urine gram staining can help identify a superimposed urinary tract infection.

a proximal dissection may be present; severe pain in the interscapular area is more common with distal involvement. However, the majority of patients with distal dissection of the aorta have back pain. Occlusion of the visceral arteries may appear with abdominal pain.

Sonographic Findings. In the acute aortic dissection, time is of the essence and therefore magnetic resonance imaging (MRI) or contrast-enhanced CT are the imaging modalities of choice for evaluating aortic dissections. In the stabilized patient with a suspected dissection, sonography may be performed. Because most dissections are seen in the ascending aorta, a transesophageal echocardiogram will be performed in the cardiology division. If the dissection is suspected in the abdomen, an abdominal ultrasound may be requested. The size of the aorta may be somewhat enlarged but not necessarily aneurysmal.

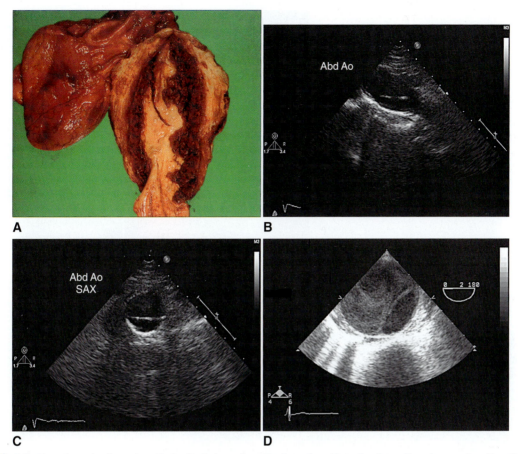

FIGURE 20-21 A-D, Type 1 aortic dissection. **B,** Sagittal view of aortic dissection. Note the linear line demarcating the site of dissection. **C,** Short axis (*SAX*) or transverse image. **D,** Transesophageal image of the dissection is shown as clear with homogeneous blood swirling in the thoracic aorta.

Radiographic Examination for Urolithiasis

Intravenous urography (IVU) is the least expensive initial examination for the patient suspected of having urolithiasis, because the majority of urinary calculi are radiopaque. The IVU has been the traditional modality of choice for evaluation of patients suspected of having urolithiasis. After the IV administration of contrast material, the classic signs of ureteral obstruction include delayed opacification of the collecting system and a persistent delayed nephrogram that increases in intensity with time.

Sonographic Findings. The calculi imaged with sonography are highly echogenic foci with distinct acoustic shadowing. Stones as small as 0.5 mm may be seen. When obstruction occurs, ultrasound is effective in demonstrating the secondary sign of hydronephrosis (Figure 20-22). Overlying bowel gas in the pelvis may obscure the evaluation of the distal ureters. With the bladder distended, color Doppler is an excellent tool to image the presence of ureteral jets in the bladder. The transducer should be angled in a cephalic presentation through the distended urinary bladder. Color Doppler is turned on and the probe is held stationary to watch for the appearance of ureteral jets. The pulse repetition frequency (PRF) should be decreased to assess the low velocity of the ureteral jet flow. The color gain should be turned up just enough to barely see color in the background. Usually within 2 to 3 minutes the jet will light up with color as the urine drains into the bladder (Figure 20-23). Be sure to look for the presence of both the right and left ureteral jet with this technique. Power Doppler may also be used to image the ureteral jets and is very effective.

The presence of hydronephrosis in a pregnant patient may be more problematic because it is not uncommon for the kidneys to become slightly hydronephrotic during the latter stage of pregnancy because the uterus enlarges and causes pressure on the ureter. This is seen especially in the right kidney because it lies lower than the left and is more likely to show minimal hydronephrosis. Therefore, the appearance of ureteral jets may help to rule out the presence of obstruction secondary to calculi.

RIGHT LOWER QUADRANT PAIN: APPENDICITIS

Acute appendicitis is one of the most common diseases that necessitates emergency surgery and is the most common atraumatic surgical abdominal disorder in children 2 years of age and older. Appendicitis is the result

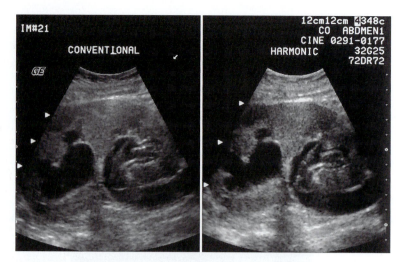

FIGURE 20-22 Ultrasound demonstration of hydrone-phrosis secondary to a stone in the urinary system.

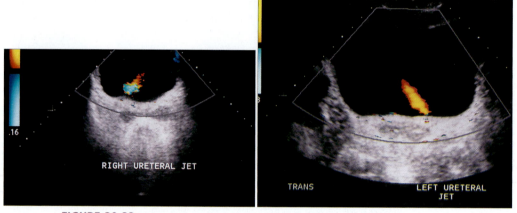

FIGURE 20-23 Normal ureteral jets in bladder as imaged with color flow Doppler.

of luminal obstruction and inflammation, leading to ischemia of the vermiform appendix. The early diagnosis of acute appendicitis is essential in the prevention of perforation, abscess formation, and postoperative complications. The classic clinical symptoms include exquisite lower abdominal pain, nausea, vomiting, fever, and leukocytosis. The quick release maneuver is performed by applying pressure with the fingertips directly over the area of the appendix and then quickly letting go. With appendicitis, the patient will usually have rebound tenderness, "McBurney sign," associated with peritoneal irritation.

The sonographer should utilize a high-frequency linear transducer to image the right lower quadrant. Careful explanation of the technique to the patient with care over the tender abdomen is essential in performing an adequate examination. The inflamed appendix will demonstrate a thickened edematous wall > 2 mm thick (Figure 20-24). If the wall is asymmetric, perforation may have occurred and the search for fluid collections around the appendiceal area should be made. The inflamed appendix may also demonstrate a "target" lesion on transverse images demonstrating a hypoechoic, fluid-distended lumen, with a hyperechoic inner ring,

and an outer hypoechoic ring representing the muscularis externa. There is a lack of peristalsis and compressibility of the inflamed appendix. Gradual pressure with the transducer is placed over the point of tenderness in an effort to displace the bowel to image the area of inflammation (see Table 20-1).

PARAUMBILICAL HERNIA

A common cause of abdominal pain and intestinal obstruction is the presence of an abdominal wall hernia. The hernia may be classified into one of three types: (1) **reducible hernia** is one in which the visceral contents can be returned to the normal intraabdominal location; (2) **incarcerated hernia** means the visceral contents cannot be reduced; and (3) **strangulated hernia** is an incarcerated hernia with vascular compromise.

A hernia forms when the abdominal wall muscles are weakened, which allows the viscera to protrude into the weakened abdominal wall. The weakest area of the abdomen is the site of the umbilicus, and this paraumbilical hernia occurs more often in females, whereas the inguinal hernia is more common in males (Figure 20-25, *A*).

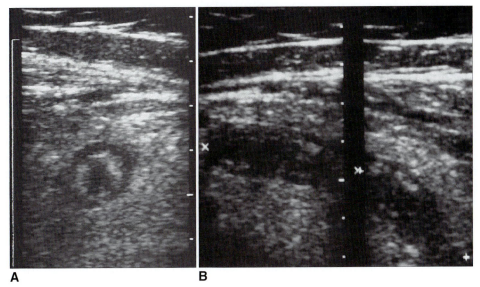

FIGURE 20-24 Appendicitis. Transverse **(A)** and sagittal **(B)** images of the inflamed appendix that was not compressed with the linear array transducer.

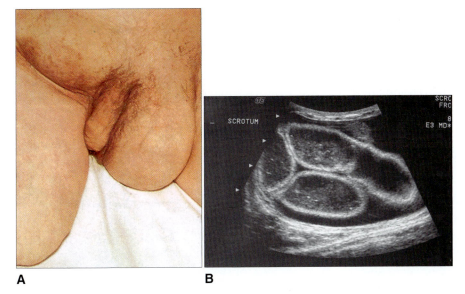

FIGURE 20-25 A, Right inguinal hernia that causes a bulging enlargement of the inguinal canal. **B,** Ultrasound evaluation in real time shows the peristalsis of the multiple bowel loops in the swollen scrotal sac.

Causes of Herniation

Common causes of herniation include congenital defect or weakening of the abdominal wall, increased abdominal pressure secondary to ascites, abdominal mass, bowel obstruction, obesity, and repeated pregnancy. Strangulation of the colon and omentum is a complication of the hernia. Another complication of a hernia is rupture of the abdominal wall in severe chronic ascites.

Sonographic Findings. The real-time visualization of the bowel within the hernia provides critical information for the clinician. Sonography allows visualization of the peristaltic movement of the bowel during Valsalva maneuvers and determines the presence or absence of vascular flow within the defect.

The sonographic criteria for a paraumbilical hernia include (1) demonstration of an anterior wall defect, (2) presence of bowel loops within the sac, (3) exaggeration of the sac during the Valsalva maneuver, and (4) reducibility of the sac with gentle pressure (Figure 20-25, *B*). Most paraumbilical hernias contain colon, omentum, and fat. The large intestine will display a complex pattern of fluid, gas, and peristalsis. Of course, the mesenteric fat is very echogenic.

The high-frequency linear array transducer allows the sonographer to demonstrate a wide area of the abdominal wall. Reduced gain to demonstrate the layers of the abdominal wall will be useful to see the distinction between the hernia, bowel, and muscular layers of tissue. Color flow will be necessary to determine the vascular flow within the hernia sac. The patient should be instructed to perform a Valsalva maneuver to determine the site of wall defect and confirm the presence of the protruding hernia. It is important to visualize the peristalsis of the bowel loops within the hernia to confirm the diagnosis (see Table 20-1).

ACUTE PELVIC PAIN

The evaluation of the patient in acute pelvic pain can be challenging for the sonographer in the middle of the night. These patients usually appear in the emergency department when the pain is so intense that they cannot bear it any longer. The sonographer must rule out acute pathology such as tubo-ovarian abscess, ruptured ovarian cyst, or ectopic pregnancy. Ovarian torsion is likewise an emergent situation for the patient with severe pelvic pain.

Sonography of Pelvic Structures

Sonography of the pelvic structures should include evaluation in at least two planes of the uterus, cul-de-sac, ovaries, fallopian tubes, and adnexal area. Transabdominal imaging will provide an overview of the entire pelvic area, whereas transvaginal imaging allows exquisite detail of the uterus, ovaries, and fallopian tubes. A full bladder technique is required with transabdominal sonography to serve as a window to image the pelvic structures.

Uterus. On sonography the uterus should appear as a homogeneous structure with an echogenic line in the center representing the endometrial canal (Figure 20-26). The long axis plane should demonstrate the uterus from fundus to cervix with the endometrial cavity well demonstrated. The entire uterus should be evaluated to look for inhomogeneity in texture that may represent degenerating fibroids or an interstitial pregnancy. Fibroids may cause significant pain and bleeding. A pregnancy that is within 5 to 7 mm from the edge of the myometrium is at risk for becoming an interstitial ectopic pregnancy. The presence of a normal gestational sac implanted high in the uterine cavity is the sign of an intrauterine pregnancy. Viability may be assessed with transvaginal ultrasound with demonstration of the fetal heart rate.

Cul-de-Sac. This area may normally contain a small amount of fluid in the healthy female that is dependent on her point in the menstrual cycle. However, large amounts of fluid are abnormal. An ectopic pregnancy that has ruptured may lead to increased amounts of fluid in the cul-de-sac. A pelvic inflammatory disease may also expand with pus into the cul-de-sac. Ascites or other free fluid secondary to trauma will accumulate in this dependent area of the pelvis.

Ovaries. The ovaries are best imaged with transvaginal sonography. Careful evaluation of the texture of the ovary should separate an enlarged ovarian cyst, ectopic pregnancy, or other ovarian masses that may lead to pelvic pain. Torsion of the ovary shows an enlarged

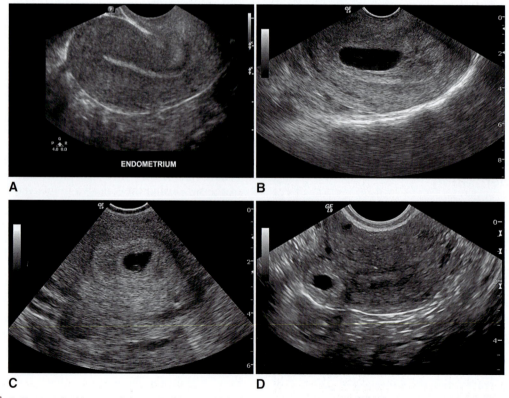

FIGURE 20-26 **A,** Transvaginal image of the normal uterus with the endometrial stripe. **B,** Blighted ovum shows dilatation of the endometrium without products of conception, **C,** Tiny yolk sac is seen within the endometrial cavity in this very early pregnancy, **D,** The uterine cavity is normal; however, the gestational sac is lying outside the uterine cavity in the adnexal cavity.

edematous with severe reduction of flow on color Doppler.

Fallopian Tubes. Again, the fallopian tubes are best imaged with transvaginal ultrasound, as they originate from the cornua of the uterus. The presence of enlarged anechoic to slightly heterogeneous tubes may signify hydrosalpinx or the presence of a tubo-ovarian abscess.

SCROTAL TRAUMA AND TORSION

Scrotal trauma presents a challenge to the sonographer because the scrotum is often painful and swollen. The trauma may be the result of a motor vehicle accident, athletic injury, direct blow to the scrotum, or a straddle injury. The most important goal of the sonographic examination is to determine if a rupture has occurred. Rupture of the testis is a surgical emergency requiring a prompt diagnosis. If surgery is performed within 72 hours following injury, at least 90% of testes can be saved; this number decreases to 45% after 72 hours. Hydrocele and hematocele are both complications of trauma. Hematoceles contain blood and are also found in advanced cases of epididymitis or orchitis (Figure 20-27).

On sonography, findings associated with scrotal rupture include a focal alteration of the testicular parenchymal pattern, interruption of the tunica albuginea, irregular testicular contour, scrotal wall thickening, and hematocele. These findings may also be associated with abscess, tumor, or other clinical conditions; but when combined with a history of trauma, they suggest rupture.

Torsion of the spermatic cord occurs as a result of abnormal mobility of the testis within the scrotum. Torsion is a surgical emergency, and it is important to obtain diagnostic images as soon as possible. The abnormality is seen more frequently in the adolescent and young adult. The patient presents with a sudden onset of pain and swelling on the affected side. On sonography, the early stages of torsion may show the testis to have a normal homogeneous pattern. After 4 to 6 hours, the testis becomes swollen and hypoechoic. The lobes within the testis are well identified during this time secondary to interstitial and septal edema. After 24 hours, the testis becomes heterogeneous as a result of hemorrhage, infarction, necrosis, and vascular congestion. The epididymal head appears enlarged and may have decreased echogenicity or become heterogeneous. Color Doppler is useful to differentiate torsion from epididymo-orchitis. An absence of perfusion in the symptomatic testis with normal perfusion demonstrated in the asymptomatic side is considered to be diagnostic of torsion.

EXTREMITY SWELLING

The evaluation of deep venous thrombosis in the patient with swelling of the proximal lower extremities may be made in the emergency department. There are essentially two types of evaluation: one is a superficial "compression" of the venous structures to see if there is an obstruction in the venous system, and the other is the thorough examination of the entire lower venous structures with gray scale, color, and spectral Doppler evaluation. The thrombosis may be acute, chronic, distal, or superficial in the venous system. Other causes of extremity pain and swelling include Baker's cyst (posterior swelling of the knee with extension into the lower calf), cellulitis, abscess, muscle hematoma, and fasciitis (Figure 20-28). Often the patient with extremity swelling presents with a swollen, tender extremity that is painful to the touch. Care must be taken to adequately evaluate the leg with gentle compression. The use of color and spectral Doppler allows the sonographer to determine the arterial from venous flow patterns to avoid the false negative or false positive result (Figure 20-29). In the obese patient, the large superficial veins may be mistaken for the deep veins and may prevent adequate compression of the venous structures. The unclotted thrombus may be isoechoic to slightly hypoechoic and thus not well seen in the lower-level equipment.

The proximal deep veins of the lower extremity are those in which thrombus poses a significant risk of pulmonary embolization. These veins include the common femoral, superficial femoral, and popliteal veins. (Note the superficial femoral vein is part of the deep system, not the superficial system.) The deep femoral vein is not considered to be a source of embolizing thrombi and is not included in the evaluation for deep venous thrombosis.

The sonographic evaluation is performed with a high-frequency linear array transducer using both real-time imaging and compression of the venous structures. The compression should be made with the vein directly under the transducer while watching for complete apposition

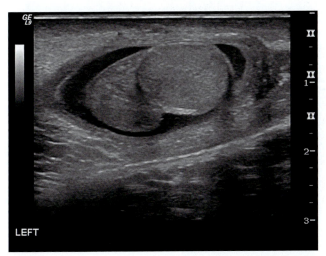

FIGURE 20-27 Acute scrotal pain with hydrocele and epididymitis.

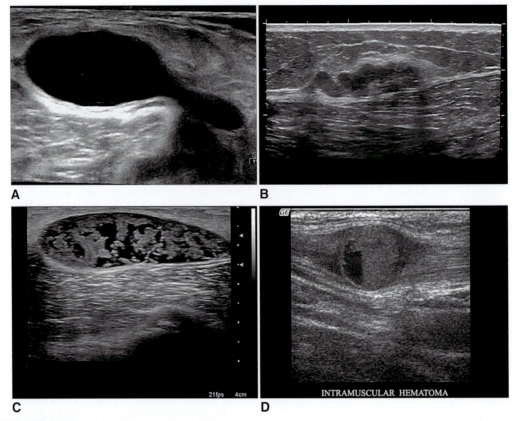

FIGURE 20-28 **A**, Baker's cyst. **B**, Musculo-fascitis. **C**, Large Baker's cyst with complex fluid. **D**, Intramuscular hematoma.

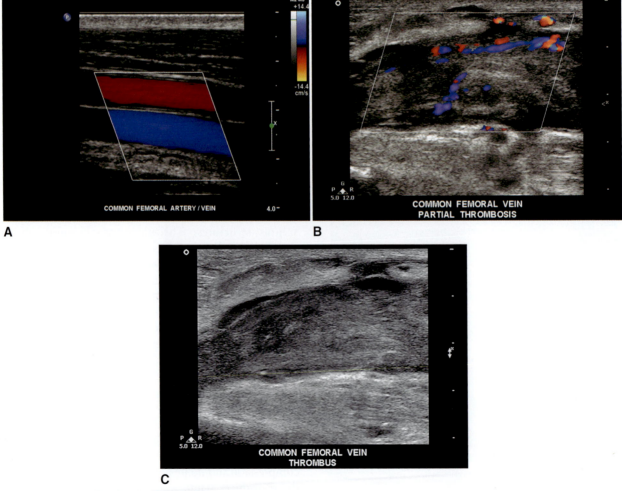

FIGURE 20-29 **A,** Sagittal color image of the normal femoral artery and vein. **B** and **C**, Large thrombosis of the common femoral vein.

of the anterior and posterior walls. If thrombus is present, complete compression will not be possible.

Other structures may be inflamed next to the venous structures as in cases of lymphadenopathy. The enlarged lymph nodes are hypoechoic with a small echogenic center and will not compress; these may be mistaken for thrombus within the venous structures.

The inferior vena cava and iliac veins should also be assessed for a possible source of emboli or thrombi, causing lower extremity pain and swelling.

PART III

Superficial Structures

The Breast

Sandra L. Hagen-Ansert, Tamara L. Salsgiver, and M. Elizabeth Glenn

OBJECTIVES

On completion of this chapter, you should be able to:
- Describe breast anatomy and sonographic layers.
- Discuss breast physiology.
- Know the difference between breast screening and breast imaging.
- Summarize the indications for the use of ultrasound in breast imaging.
- Describe the correct technique for imaging the breast using ultrasound.

- Know how to use methods of identifying and labeling breast anatomy and masses.
- Identify the sonographic characteristics associated with benign and malignant breast masses.
- Identify the mammographic characteristics associated with malignant breast masses.
- Discuss ultrasound-guided interventional procedures.

OUTLINE

One out of eight American women will develop **breast cancer.** It is the most common type of cancer among women in the United States and is the second leading cause of cancer death among women between the ages of 40 and 59. Early detection of breast cancer is vital, because cancer can be difficult to eradicate once it has spread. Delays in early detection and treatment can be particularly tragic because the survival rate for localized breast cancer adequately treated is 98% after 5 years and 95% after 10 years, whereas metastatic cancer shows survival rates of only 30% to 50% after 10 years. Ultrasound evaluation of the breast plays a vital role in the early detection and characterization of breast masses and provides real-time guidance during interventional breast procedures.

This chapter presents an overview of breast anatomy, physiology, sonographic evaluation techniques, and breast pathology with emphasis on breast cancer diagnosis and staging.

HISTORICAL OVERVIEW

John Wild published the first paper on breast ultrasound in 1951. This early paper described the A-mode technique of ultrasound imaging. Advancements in ultrasound equipment design allowed increased tissue characterization, and by 1970, gray-scale ultrasound technique had significantly improved diagnostic accuracy. Dedicated whole breast ultrasound units were tested as a potential screening method for the detection of breast cancer. This effort, unfortunately, failed. Whole breast ultrasound imaging units gave way to smaller units with hand-held transducers for breast evaluation. Although ultrasound was not an effective primary tool in **breast cancer screening,** its usefulness as an adjunctive tool to mammography for breast lesion characterization has become increasingly evident. Screening mammograms have long been considered the gold standard for breast cancer screening, although accumulating evidence suggests that ultrasound screening in conjunction with mammography may be beneficial in patients with very dense tissue, complicated mammograms, or very high risk factors for breast cancer.

Most clinical laboratories today use high-resolution, real-time sonography as an adjunct to mammographic screening. Although screening the entire breast with ultrasound is not routinely done, most ultrasound laboratories currently perform the breast examination within a localized area to characterize palpable lesions or suspicious areas seen on a mammogram. High-frequency 10- to 15-MHz transducers have the optimum resolution and the short-to-medium focus necessary for obtaining high-quality images of the breast parenchyma. The high frame-rates available with real-time ultrasound systems in use today facilitate ultrasound guidance during interventional procedures of the breast to include **cyst aspirations,** core biopsies, preoperative localization techniques, and vacuum-assisted biopsies for small lesion diagnosis and removal.

ANATOMY OF THE BREAST

Normal Anatomy

The **breast** is a modified sweat gland located in the superficial fascia of the anterior chest wall. The major portion of the breast tissue is situated between the second and third rib superiorly, the sixth and seventh costal cartilage inferiorly, the anterior axillary line laterally, and the sternal border medially. In many women, the breast extends deep toward the lateral upper margin of the chest and into the **axilla.** This extension is referred to as the axillary tail of the breast, or the **tail of Spence** (Figure 21-1).

The surface of the breast is dominated by the nipple and the surrounding **areola.** A few women may have ectopic breast tissue or accessory (supernumerary) nipples. Ectopic breast tissue and accessory nipples are usually located along the mammary milk line, which extends superiorly from the axilla downward and medially in an oblique line to the symphysis pubis of the pelvis.

Sonographically, the breast is divided into three layers located between the skin and the pectoralis major muscle on the anterior of the chest wall. These layers include the **subcutaneous layer,** the **mammary** (glandular) **layer,** and the **retromammary layer** (Figure 21-2, Box 21-1). The subcutaneous and retromammary layers are usually quite thin and consist of fat surrounded by connective tissue septa. Although fat is often highly echogenic in other parts of the body, it is the least echogenic tissue within the breast. The fatty tissue appears **hypoechoic,** and the ducts, glands, and supporting ligaments appear echogenic (Figure 21-3).

The mammary/glandular layer includes the functional portion of the breast and the surrounding supportive

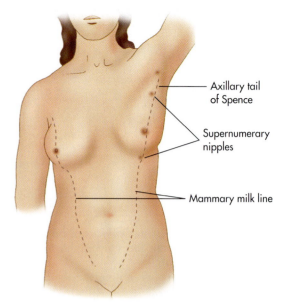

FIGURE 21-1 The mammary milk line is the anatomic line along which breast tissue can be found in some women. The axillary tail of Spence is an extension of breast tissue into the axilla that is present in some women.

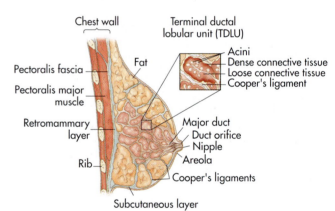

FIGURE 21-2 Breast anatomy. Fifteen major ductal systems are present within the breast. Each gives rise to many separate terminal ductal lobular units (TDLUs) containing the terminal ducts, at least one lobule, and the separate acinar units (milk-producing glands) within each lobule. Each TDLU is surrounded by varying amounts of loose and dense connective tissue. The TDLU represents the site of origin of nearly all pathologic processes of the breast. Cooper's ligaments surround and suspend each of the TDLUs within the surrounding fatty tissue. The ligaments extend to the subcutaneous layer of the skin and the deep retromammary layer next to the pectoralis fascia overlying the chest wall.

(stromal) tissue. The functional portion of the breast is made up of 15 to 20 lobes, which contain the milk-producing glands, and the ductal system, which carries the milk to the nipple. The lobes emanate from the nipple in a pattern resembling the spokes of a wheel. The upper, outer quadrant of the breast contains the highest concentration of lobes. This concentration of lobes in the upper outer quadrant of the breast is the reason why most tumors are found here, as most tumors originate from within the ducts. The lobes of the breast resemble

Subcutaneous layer: thin layer
- Fatty tissue
- Cooper's ligaments

Mammary layer: functional portion of the breast
- 15 to 20 lobes radiate from the nipple.
- Lactiferous ducts carry milk from acini to the nipple.
- Terminal ductal lobular unit (TDLU) is made up of acini and terminal ducts.
- Fatty tissue is interspersed between lobes.
- Cooper's ligaments extend from the retromammary fascia to the skin and provide support.

Retromammary layer: thin layer
- Fatty tissue
- Cooper's ligaments

Pectoralis major muscle

Pectoralis minor muscle

Ribs

Chest wall

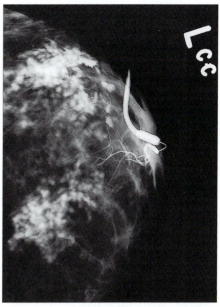

FIGURE 21-4 Galactogram (contrast injected retrograde into a single ductal system) showing opacification of individual glands (terminal ductal lobular units, or TDLUs). Normally, TDLUs are 2 mm or less in diameter. The TDLU is the site of origin of most pathologic processes within the breast.

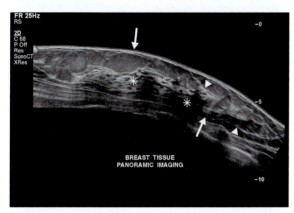

FIGURE 21-3 Sonographic layers of breast tissue. The three layers of breast tissue are bordered by the skin and chest wall muscles (*arrows*). The subcutaneous fat layer and the retromammary fat layer are usually very thin (*arrowheads*). The mammary layer (*asterisks*) varies remarkably in thickness and in echogenicity, depending on location within the breast (most glandular tissue is located in the upper outer quadrant) and the patient's age, hormonal status (e.g., pubertal, mature, gravid, lactating, postmenopausal), and inherited breast parenchymal pattern.

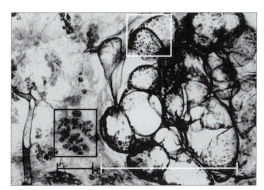

FIGURE 21-5 Three-dimensional histology showing normal terminal ductal lobular units (TDLUs) and dilated TDLUs. Normal TDLUs are usually no larger than 2 mm. Fibrocystic condition and other pathologic processes can cause marked enlargement of the TDLU. Note the difference between the normal TDLU within the black box and the dilated TDLU filling the right half of the image. The white box shows a single dilated acinus within the enlarged TDLU, showing cellular changes of apocrine metaplasia (one of the tissue changes of fibrocystic condition recognized by pathologists), and causing the lining cells to enlarge and overproduce fluid.

a grapevine branch; the major duct branches into smaller branches called lobules. Each lobule contains **acini** (milk-producing glands), which are clustered on the terminal ends of the ducts like grapes on a vine. Literally hundreds of acini (*sing.* **acinus**) are present within each breast (Figures 21-4 and 21-5). The terminal ends of the duct and the acini form small lobular units referred to as **terminal ductal lobular units (TDLUs),** each of which is surrounded by both loose and dense connective tissue. The TDLUs are invested within the connective tissue skeleton of the breast (see Figures 21-2, 21-4, and 21-5). Normal TDLUs measure 1 to 2 mm and usually are not differentiated sonographically. The TDLU is significant in that nearly all pathologic processes that occur within

the breast originate here. The space between the lobes is filled with connective and fatty tissue known as stroma. These stromal elements are located both between and within the lobes and consist of dense connective tissue, loose connective tissue, and fat. The connective tissue septa within the breasts form a fibrous "skeleton," which is responsible for maintaining the shape and structure of the breast. These connective tissue septa are collectively called **Cooper's ligaments;** they connect to the fascia around the ducts and glands and extend out to the skin.

The pectoralis major muscle lies posterior to the retromammary layer. It originates at the anterior surface of the medial half of the clavicle and anterolateral surface of the sternum and inserts into the intertubercular groove on the anteromedial surface of the humerus (see Figure 21-2). The lower border of the pectoralis major muscle forms the anterior margin of the axilla. The pectoralis minor muscle lies superolateral and posterior to the pectoralis major. The pectoralis minor courses from its origin near the costal cartilages of the third, fourth, and fifth ribs to where it inserts into the medial and superior surface of the coracoid process of the scapula. These muscles sonographically appear as a hypoechoic interface between the retromammary layer of the breast and the ribs (Figure 21-6). Although most lesions are found within the glandular tissue of the breast, it is important to evaluate tissue all the way to the chest wall.

Sonographic Appearance

The boundaries of the breast are the skin line, nipple, and retromammary layer. These generally give strong, bright echo reflections. The areolar area may be recognized by its slightly lower echo reflection as compared with the nipple and the skin. The internal nipple may show low to bright reflections with posterior shadowing, and it has a variable appearance (Figure 21-7).

Subcutaneous fat generally appears hypoechoic, whereas Cooper's ligaments and other connective tissue appear echogenic and are dispersed in a linear pattern (Figure 21-8). Cooper's ligaments are best identified when the beam strikes them at a perpendicular angle; compression of the breast often enhances the ability to visualize them.

The mammary/glandular layer lies between the subcutaneous fatty layer anteriorly and the retromammary layer posteriorly (Figure 21-9). The fatty tissue interspersed throughout the mammary/glandular layer dictates the amount of intensity reflected from the breast parenchyma. If little fat is present, a uniform architecture

with a strong echogenic pattern (because of collagen and fibrotic tissue) is seen throughout the mammary/glandular layer. When fatty tissue is present, areas of low-level echoes become intertwined with areas of strong echoes from the active breast tissue. Analysis of this pattern becomes critical to the final diagnosis, and one must be able to separate lobules of fat from a marginated lesion.

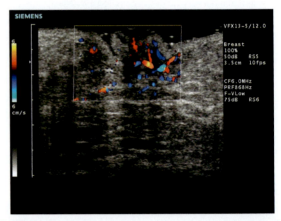

FIGURE 21-7 Shadow from the areolar area prevents imaging directly posterior to the nipple. The transducer should be moved away from the nipple area to image the mammary and retromammary layers.

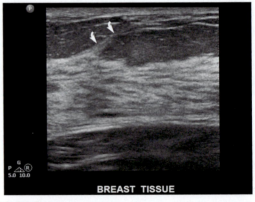

FIGURE 21-8 Subcutaneous fat is hypoechoic, whereas Cooper's ligaments appear echogenic within the subcutaneous layer (arrows).

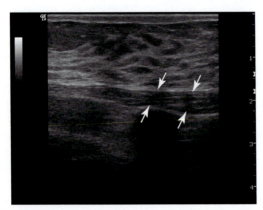

FIGURE 21-6 The hypoechoic pectoralis muscle (arrows) is seen between the retromammary layer and the ribs.

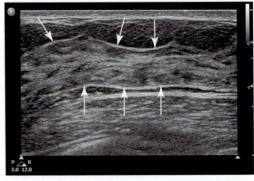

FIGURE 21-9 Mammary-glandular layer lies between the subcutaneous fatty layer anteriorly and the retromammary layer posteriorly (arrows).

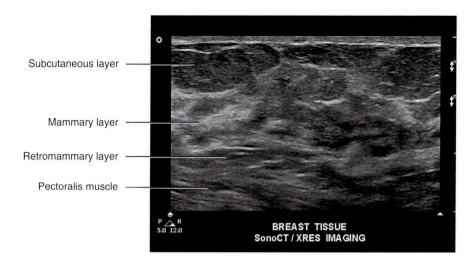

Subcutaneous layer

Mammary layer

Retromammary layer

Pectoralis muscle

BREAST TISSUE
SonoCT / XRES IMAGING

FIGURE 21-10 The retromammary layer is similar in echogenicity and echo texture to the subcutaneous layer.

The retromammary layer is similar in echogenicity and echotexture to the subcutaneous layer, although the boundary echoes resemble skin reflections (Figure 21-10). The pectoral muscles appear as low-level echo areas posterior to the retromammary layer. The ribs appear sonographically as hyperechoic rounded structures with dense posterior shadowing. They are easily identified by their occurrence at regular intervals along the chest wall.

Several normal structures within the breast can appear abnormal, unless care is taken to prevent this during the sonographic examination. The ducts immediately behind the nipple frequently cause acoustic shadowing and can be mistaken for a suspicious breast mass. Angling of the transducer in the retroareolar tissue will usually improve visualization and eliminate doubt. The distinction of a subtle **isoechoic** or hypoechoic sonographic mass from normal fibroglandular tissue in the breast can sometimes be troublesome. The adipose or fatty tissue can situate itself in and among the areas of glandular tissue and, in some scanning planes, can mimic isoechoic or hypoechoic masses. It is helpful to turn on the structures to see if they are consistent or lengthen out within the scanning plane. To see whether a structure will lengthen out geometrically, one should rotate the transducer 90 degrees during real-time. In the case of a true sonographic mass, a mass will maintain its shape in both dimensions, confirming its three-dimensional character, whereas glandular tissue elements will elongate and appear less like a mass.

Parenchymal Pattern

The size and shape of the breasts vary remarkably from woman to woman. Some women have more glandular tissue, some have less. Some have more fatty tissue than others, and some have more connective tissue, so their breasts are firmer. Some women have very little breast tissue. The size and shape of the breasts also vary over time because of changes that occur during the menstrual cycle, with pregnancy and breast-feeding, and during menopause. Most differences in breast size between women are due to the amount of fatty tissue within the breasts.

The involutional changes that occur in the breast throughout life affect the appearance and pattern of the breast parenchyma. Involution is hallmarked in breast imaging by the remodeling process that causes glandular tissue to be slowly replaced by fatty tissue. This accounts for differences in the size, shape, and architecture of breast tissue.

Generally, in a young woman, fibrous tissue elements predominate, and the resulting appearance on mammography and ultrasound is a dense echogenic pattern of tissue (Figure 21-11). In a pregnant or lactating woman, the glandular portions of the breast proliferate remarkably in both density and volume, creating interfaces that are less echogenic. As a woman ages, the glandular breast tissue undergoes cell death and is remodeled by the infiltration of fatty tissue. The tissue is progressively replaced by fat and, with the onset of menopause, the ducts atrophy, resulting in a mammographic and sonographic pattern with less fibrous tissue elements (Figure 21-12). This fatty breast is most difficult to image by sonography, as all three layers of the breast appear hypoechoic, with less distinction between the layers. Sonographically, cancers can be difficult to differentiate in the fatty breast because most cancers appear hypoechoic and can be difficult to differentiate from normal breast tissue. Although sonography of the fatty breast is difficult, mammography images this type of breast very well.

Vascular Supply

The main arterial supply to the breast comes from the internal mammary and the lateral thoracic arteries. More than half of the breast—mainly the central and medial portions—is supplied by the anterior perforating

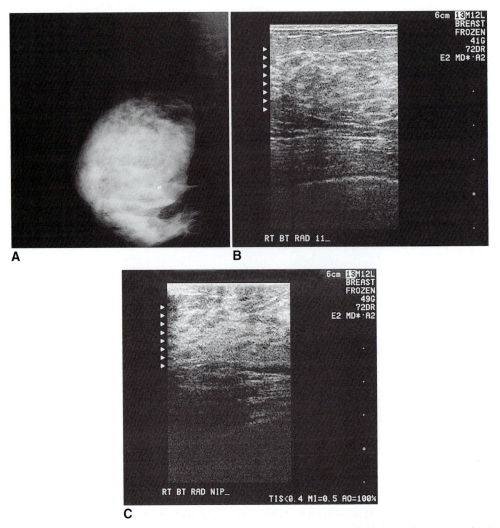

FIGURE 21-11 Dense breast. **A,** Example of dense breast tissue on mammogram. Mammographic technique emphasizes tissue contrast. As a result, the skin often is not visible on routine images. The skin is separated in this case by nearly 2 cm from the outer margins of the dense mammary layer. **B,** Example of ultrasound appearance of dense breast tissue. **C,** Example of variation in breast tissue pattern at different locations even within the same breast.

branches of the internal mammary artery. The remaining portion—the upper outer quadrant—is supplied by the lateral thoracic artery; intercostals and subcapsular and thoracodorsal arteries contribute in lesser ways to the blood supply.

Venous drainage is mainly provided by superficial veins that can be seen sonographically just under the skin. These surface veins are often enlarged with superior vena cava syndrome or chronic venous thrombosis of the subclavian vein, as well as when arteriovenous shunts are placed in patients with chronic renal insufficiency. Figure 21-13 shows an example of a grossly dilated surface vein in the breast. When there is doubt concerning the vascular nature of a long, tubular, **anechoic** structure on breast ultrasound, such as the distinction between a dilated duct and a vessel, color flow vascular imaging or Doppler ultrasound techniques can easily resolve this situation.

Lymphatic System

Lymphatic drainage from all parts of the breast generally flows to the axillary lymph nodes. The flow of lymph is promoted by valveless lymphatic vessels that allow the fluid to mingle and proceed unidirectionally from superficial to deep nodes of the breast. The flow of lymph moves from the intramammary nodes and deep nodes centrifugally toward the axillary and internal lymph node chains. It has been estimated that only about 3% of lymph is eliminated by the internal chain, whereas 97% of lymph is removed by the axillary chain.

Part of the standard surgical therapy of invasive breast cancer involves axillary lymph node dissection. This is vital in the staging and management of breast cancer because nodal status affects the patient's prognosis and is important in guiding adjunctive therapy. Although most tumors can infiltrate and spread via the axillary

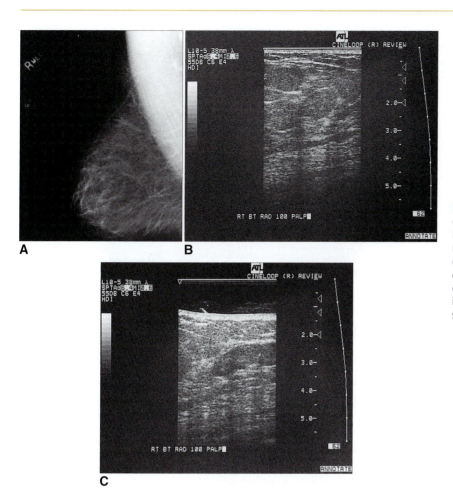

FIGURE 21-12 Fatty breast. **A,** Example of predominantly fatty tissue on mammogram. **B,** Example of ultrasound appearance of predominantly fatty tissue. Note the loss of sonographic detail in the deeper layers of the breast and chest wall. Fat deflects the ultrasound beam and degrades detail. **C,** Example of improved visualization of skin and subcutaneous tissues with a stand-off pad.

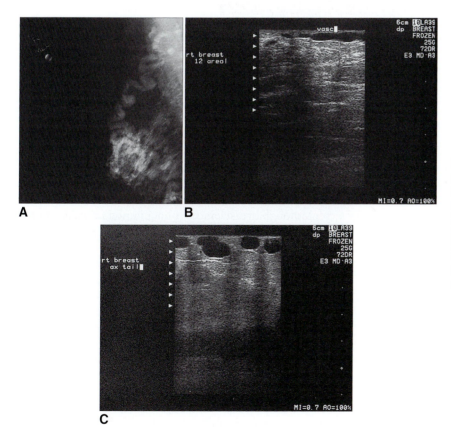

FIGURE 21-13 Dilated veins in the breast. **A,** Mammographic image of a breast showing markedly dilated surface veins in an elderly woman. **B** and **C,** Ultrasound images of veins just under the skin of the breast in the same patient. In cases in which there is doubt, color flow mapping or Doppler techniques will easily confirm the vascular nature of these dilated tubular structures and will distinguish them from dilated ducts.

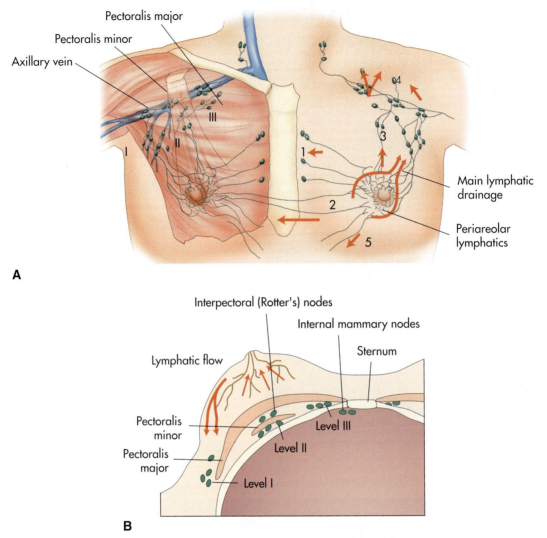

FIGURE 21-14 Lymphatic drainage of the breast. **A,** General position of the major axillary lymphatic groups I, II, and III in relation to the pectoralis major and minor muscles of the chest wall. On the right side of the figure, the major lymphatic flow from the periareolar plexus toward the axilla is shown. Alternative routes of lymphatic flow include (1) retromammary nodes, (2) contralateral flow to the opposite breast, (3) interpectoral (Rotter's) nodes located between the pectoralis major and minor muscles, (4) supraclavicular nodes, and (5) diaphragmatic nodes. **B,** Same information in cross section.

lymph nodes, they may begin their infiltration by using alternative lymph channels, such as the internal mammary chain within the chest, across the midline to the contralateral breast, deep into the interpectoral (Rotter's) nodes, or into the supraclavicular nodes (Figures 21-14, 21-15, and 21-16).

The Male Breast

In males, the nipple and the areola remain relatively small. The male breast normally retains some ductal elements beneath the nipple, but it does not develop the milk-producing lobular and acinar tissue. The ductal elements usually remain small but can hypertrophy during puberty and later in life under the influence of hormonal fluctuations, disease processes, or medications. This condition, in which the ductal elements

hypertrophy, is called benign **gynecomastia** (Figure 21-17). Imaging with mammography and ultrasound is often requested to exclude breast cancer as a cause.

Although breast cancer is uncommon in males, it does occur. Approximately 1300 new cases are diagnosed each year within the United Sates. The occurrence approximates 1% of the incidence in women. Box 21-2 lists male patients who have an increased risk for breast cancer.

PHYSIOLOGY OF THE BREAST

The primary function of the breast is fluid transport. The breast includes fat, ligaments, glandular tissue, and a ductal system that work together to provide fluid transport. The ductal system is critical in the transport of

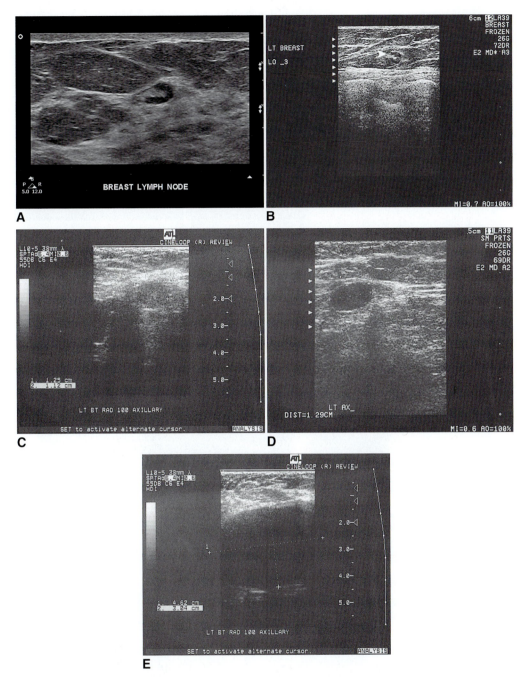

FIGURE 21-15 Normal and abnormal lymph nodes. **A** and **B,** Sonographic images of a normal lymph node showing a smooth homogeneously hypoechoic cortex and an echogenic fatty internal hilum. **C** through **E,** Images of abnormal lymph nodes. Signs of suspicion for metastatic involvement of lymph nodes include an irregular, inhomogeneous cortex and loss of the fatty hilum. **C,** Lymph node that has nearly lost the fatty hilum and has a poorly defined but relatively homogeneous cortex. This may be a reactive lymph node or one with early metastatic involvement. **D,** Similar lymph node that has completely lost its fatty hilum but has a smooth homogeneous cortex. **E,** Large hypoechoic mass that has no sonographic characteristics of a normal lymph node. This mass was sampled by ultrasound-guided core biopsy, confirming a low axillary lymph node nearly completely replaced with metastatic cancer.

fluids within the breast. The ductal system is also where many pathologic conditions originate.

An important function of the breast during the reproductive years is to make milk from nutrients and water taken from the bloodstream. Milk is produced within the acini and is carried to the nipple by the ducts. During lactation, the transport of milk depends on the action of the two epithelial cells that make up the ductal network:

luminal cells, which secrete the milk components into the ductal lumen, and myoepithelial cells, which contract to aid in the ejection of milk.

The female breast is remarkably affected by changing hormonal levels during each menstrual cycle and is further affected by both pregnancy and lactation (breast-feeding). Breast development begins before menarche and continues until the female is approximately 16 years old.

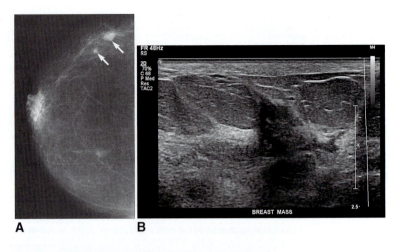

FIGURE 21-16 Metastatic spread of breast cancer to the opposite breast. **A,** Mammogram showing several moderate-to-low density, relatively benign appearing masses *(arrows)* in a patient with a history of mastectomy for cancer in the opposite breast. **B,** Image of one of the masses shows a solid mass with an irregular, poorly defined margin and heterogeneous echogenicity. These lesions were all metastatic lesions from the opposite breast, likely from an alternative route of lymphatic spread across the midline.

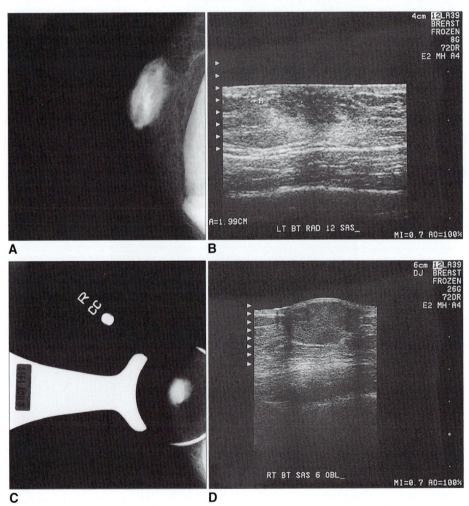

FIGURE 21-17 Two male patients with palpable breast masses. **A,** Mammographic appearance of benign gynecomastia. This condition is nearly as often unilateral as bilateral. **B,** Ultrasound example of the frequently masslike appearance of gynecomastia. **C,** Mammography example of male breast cancer. **D,** Sonographic image with stand-off pad of palpable suspicious breast mass in elderly male. Note the heterogeneous echogenicity and the elevation of skin over the mass.

During this time, the ductal system proliferates under the influence of estrogen. During pregnancy, acinar development is accelerated to enable milk production by estrogen, progesterone, and prolactin. Prolactin is a hormone produced by the pituitary gland that stimulates the acini

to produce and excrete milk. Prolactin levels usually rise during the latter part of pregnancy, but milk production is suppressed by high levels of progesterone. Expulsion of the placenta after the birth of a baby causes a drop in circulating progesterone, initiating milk production

BOX 21-2	Male Patients at Increased Risk for Breast Cancer

Klinefelter's syndrome
Male-to-female transsexual
History of prior chest wall irradiation (especially for Hodgkin lymphoma)
History of orchitis or testicular tumor
Liver disease
Genetic predisposition (BRCA2 gene mutation, breast cancer in female relatives, p53 mutation)

BOX 21-3	Breast Cancer Screening

Breast self-examination (BSE)
- Monthly beginning at age 20
Clinical breast examination (CBE) by a health care provider
- Ages 20 to 39: every 3 years
- Ages 40 on: yearly
Screening mammography
- Yearly starting at age 40

Exceptions: Personal history of breast cancer, first-degree relative (mother or sister) with premenopausal breast cancer, atypical hyperplasia or lobular carcinoma in situ (LCIS) on prior breast biopsy, and known breast cancer gene mutation (BRCA1 or BRCA2)

within the breasts. The physical stimulation of suckling by the baby initiates the release of oxytocin (produced by the hypothalamus and released by the pituitary gland), which further incites prolactin secretion, stimulating additional milk production. Full maturation of the acini occurs during lactation and is thought to be mildly protective against the development of breast cancer. At the end of lactation, the breast tissue parenchyma involutes. Breast evaluation by mammography can be difficult in a dense, lactating breast; therefore, mammographic screening of the breast usually is not performed until at least 6 months after cessation of lactation.

BREAST EVALUATION OVERVIEW

Breast Screening

The primary purpose of breast screening is the detection and diagnosis of breast cancer in its earliest and most curable stage. Accurate identification of benign breast lesions during cancer screening is also important for good care because it can save the patient from unnecessary surgical procedures and resultant tissue scarring.

Three general categories of **diagnostic breast imaging** are available, two of which involve breast ultrasound. These three categories include breast cancer screening (generally performed by physical breast evaluation with mammography), diagnostic interrogation (consultation, problem solving, workup), and interventional breast procedures (histologic diagnosis and/or localization).

Breast cancer screening is recommended in women without clinical signs of breast cancer (Box 21-3). According to the American Cancer Society, breast cancer screening involves monthly **breast self-examination (BSE)**, regular **clinical breast examination (CBE)** by a physician or other health care provider, and annual screening mammography. Monthly BSE is best performed at the end of menses and should begin at age 20. CBE should be performed once every 3 years from ages 20 to 39 and at least yearly from age 40 on. Screening mammography should be performed yearly starting at age 40. BSE and CBE are important steps in breast cancer screening because 70% of cancers are found as lumps felt during BSE and CBE. BSE and CBE may also identify other signs or symptoms of possible breast

BOX 21-4	Clinical Signs and Symptoms of Possible Breast Cancer

New or growing dominant, discrete breast lump
- Hard, gritty, or irregular surface
- Usually (not always) painless
- Does not fluctuate with hormonal cycle
- Different from "lumpy" breast texture
Unilateral single-duct nipple discharge
- Spontaneous, persistent; serous or bloody
Surface nipple lesions
- Nonhealing ulcer
- Focal irritation
New nipple retraction
New focal skin dimpling or retraction
Unilateral new or growing axillary lump
Hot, red breast

Note: Although these clinical signs and symptoms may indicate the presence of breast cancer, it is important to understand that in most cases, the cause is not cancer, but rather a benign condition.

cancer that require further evaluation by diagnostic breast imaging (Box 21-4).

Mammography, sonography, and magnetic resonance imaging (MRI) are the primary imaging tools used for diagnostic breast evaluation. Mammography provides a sensitive method of screening for breast cancer, whereas ultrasound and MRI are used to provide additional characterization and further interrogation of breast lesions that are not well visualized by mammography. The mammographic signs of breast cancer are listed in Box 21-5. Because ultrasound examination is performed by scanning in cross-sectional planes, it is difficult to adequately screen the entire breast in most patients. Ultrasound may be used for screening purposes in young, dense breasts, which are difficult to penetrate by mammography, to evaluate palpable masses that are not visible on a mammogram, and to image the deep **juxtathoracic** tissue not normally visible by mammography. Ultrasound is also useful in differentiating structures within uniformly dense breast tissue in which mammography is limited (e.g., in differentiating solid, round masses from fluid-filled **cysts** and in visualizing tissue adjacent to implants

BOX 21-5	Signs of Breast Cancer on Mammography

Primary Signs

Common	Irregular (spiculated), high-density mass
	Clustered pleomorphic microcalcifications
	Focal distortion (with no history of prior biopsy, infection, or trauma)
Less common	Focal asymmetric density (with associated palpable lump or solid sonographic mass)
	Developing density

Secondary Signs

Common	Nipple or skin retraction
	Skin thickening
	Lymphedema pattern
	Increased vascularity

BOX 21-6	Risk Factors for Breast Cancer

Female gender
Increasing age
Family history of breast cancer
Personal history of breast cancer
- First-degree relative (mother, sister, daughter)
- Premenopausal breast cancer
- Multiple affected first- and second-degree relatives
- Associated cancers (ovarian, colon, prostate)
Biopsy-proven atypical proliferative lesions
- Lobular neoplasia (lobular carcinoma in situ)
- Atypical epithelial hyperplasia
Prolonged estrogen effect
- Early menarche
Late menopause
Nulliparity
Late first pregnancy

or other structures that limit visualization by mammography). MRI is also a useful tool in breast imaging but is prohibitively expensive for screening purposes. Because a strong magnetic field is used to create images, not all patients are good candidates for MRI (e.g., patients with pacemakers or artificial joints). Patients who suffer from uncontrolled claustrophobia are also not good candidates for MRI.

Breast Evaluation

The overall goal of breast evaluation is the proper classification of a breast lesion according to the level of suspicion for breast cancer. Thorough evaluation takes into account the results of both the breast imaging assessment and the clinical assessment. The appropriate next step in patient management is dictated by the level of suspicion for cancer in any breast lesion and takes into account the age and individual risk factors for each particular patient. Risk factors for breast cancer are listed in Box 21-6.

Clinical Assessment. It is important to recognize clinical signs or symptoms of possible breast cancer (see Box 21-4). Patients with clinical indications of breast cancer generally undergo diagnostic breast interrogation. Diagnostic imaging of the breast is tailored to the patient's age and specific clinical problem. Clinical history and examination of the patient with a breast problem (Box 21-7) help determine the next diagnostic step. In the patient with no signs or symptoms of possible breast cancer, screening mammography is typically the first diagnostic test performed.

Screening Mammography. In women aged 40 and over who are **asymptomatic** (without clinical signs of possible breast cancer), annual screening by mammography is recommended. Usually less than 10% of these women will have abnormalities detected on the screening examination that require further workup. When a breast lesion is identified by mammography, it is normally

TABLE 21-1	ACR BI-RADS® Assessment Categories for Mammographic Masses

BI-RADS® Category/ Recommended Action	Description
1. Negative	Nothing to comment on. Breasts are symmetric; no masses, architectural distortion, or suspicious calcifications.
2. Benign finding(s)	Involuting, calcified fibroadenomas, multiple secretory calcifications, fat-containing lesions.
3. Probable benign finding(s)/initial short-term follow-up	Noncalcified circumscribed solid mass; focal asymmetry; cluster of round (punctate) calcifications. Less than 2% chance of malignancy.
4. Suspicious abnormality/ consider biopsy	Findings do not have classic appearance of malignancy but have wide range of probability of malignancy greater than those in Category 3.
5. Highly suggestive of malignancy/appropriate action needed	Classic breast cancers with a 95% or greater likelihood for malignancy.

Used with permission of the American College of Radiology (ACR).

described using guidelines contained within the **breast imaging reporting and data system (BI-RADS)**. The BI-RAD system was developed by the American College of Radiology (ACR). A key component of this system is an overall outcome assessment category that indicates the suspicion of malignancy (Table 21-1). Figures 21-18, 21-19, 21-20, and 21-21 present mammographic and

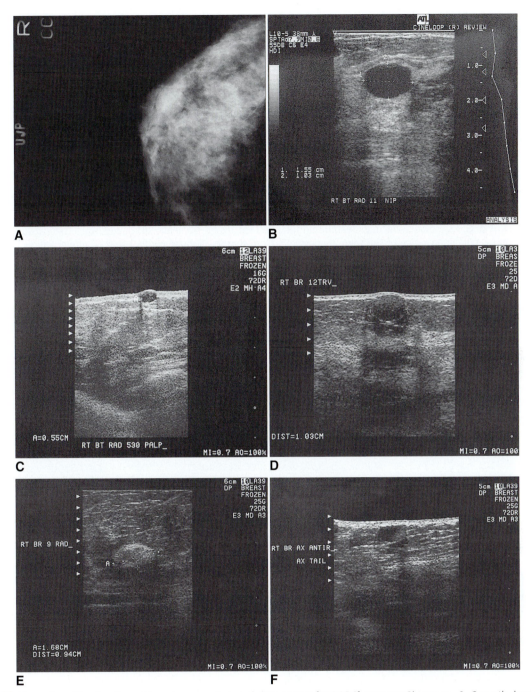

FIGURE 21-18 Examples of benign (breast imaging reporting and data system [BI-RADS] category 2) masses. **A,** Smooth, benign appearing mammographic mass. **B,** Same mass on ultrasound showing classic features of a simple cyst. **C,** Example of a sebaceous cyst. Note the smooth, hypoechoic appearance and classic location within the skin. **D,** Example of an isoechoic mass abutting the dermis. This is an epidermal inclusion cyst, often indistinguishable from a sebaceous cyst. These lesions appear within the skin or at the junction of the dermis and the subcutaneous fatty layer. **E,** Vague, low-density mammographic mass correlated with this echogenic mass on ultrasound. Echogenic masses are nearly always benign, but the level of suspicion should be determined by the mammographic appearance. **F,** Small mass on mammogram in this hospitalized patient on warfarin appears as a small, superficial complex cyst with a "fluid-fluid" level consistent with a small, resolving hematoma (a galactocele in a lactating patient has a similar appearance, but is located within the mammary layer). This superficial hematoma may resolve completely or may evolve into an oil cyst. *Continued*

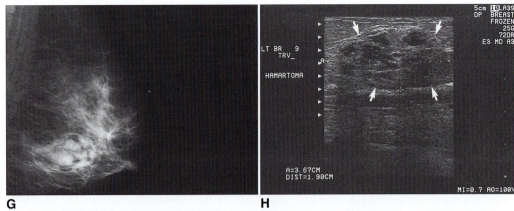

FIGURE 21-18, cont'd **G,** Mammographic mass with mixed fatty and soft tissue elements, surrounded by a thin capsule. This is a breast hamartoma. **H,** Sonographic appearance of the same hamartoma. Note that its high fat content makes differentiation from surrounding fatty tissue difficult.

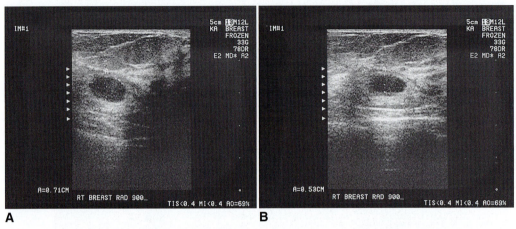

FIGURE 21-19 Example of probably benign (breast imaging reporting and data system [BI-RADS] category 3) mass. **A,** Sonographic appearance of a smooth, benign appearing mass with homogeneous echogenicity, wider than tall, showing low-level posterior acoustic enhancement. This image is taken without applied compression. **B,** Same mass with applied compression, showing the decreased anteroposterior dimension. Most benign masses are soft and compressible.

BOX 21-7	Clinical Evaluation of the Patient with a Breast Problem

History
- Patient age
- Risk factors for breast cancer
- Onset and duration of mass
- Relation to menstrual cycle

Breast examination (for palpable mass)

Location of mass
- Clock face or quadrant

Characteristics of mass:
- Size
- Shape (round, oval, lobular, irregular)
- Surface contour (smooth, irregular)
- Consistency (soft, rubbery, firm, hard, gritty)
- Mobility (movable, fixed)

sonographic examples of various BI-RADS category masses.

Diagnostic Breast Interrogation. Diagnostic breast interrogation (consultation, workup, problem solving) is performed on all patients who present with any clinical signs of possible breast cancer found on CBE or BSE, and on patients who are recalled for additional evaluation because of an abnormal screening mammogram. Diagnostic mammography involves specialized detailed views to analyze specific areas of the breast in question. In at least one third of cases, adjunctive ultrasound of the breast is used to further evaluate questionable mammographic or clinical findings (see discussion below).

Interventional Breast Procedures. In some breast lesions, interventional procedures are necessary for definitive diagnosis. A common example is a smooth, benign appearing mass identified by mammography that correlates with a hypoechoic sonographic lesion but does not meet the criteria for interpretation as a simple cyst. Cyst aspiration can be performed to determine whether the lesion is a complex cyst or truly a solid mass. Under real-time sonographic guidance, a needle is guided into

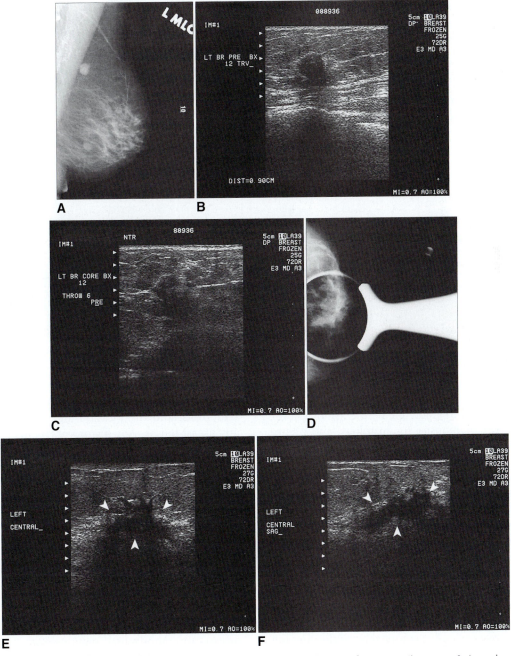

FIGURE 21-20 Examples of suspicious (breast imaging reporting and data system [BI-RADS] category 4) masses. **A,** Irregular mammographic mass that had shown interval growth. **B,** Sonographic appearance of the same mass, with a heterogeneous echogenicity but only a slightly irregular margin. Weak posterior acoustic shadowing can be seen. **C,** Fourteen-gauge core-biopsy needle traversing the mass. Pathologic condition confirmed an infiltrating ductal carcinoma. **D,** Mammographic area of focal distortion that persisted with detail imaging. Transverse **(E)** and sagittal **(F)** ultrasound images confirm a three-dimensional area of focal distortion. The patient had no history of previous surgery, injury, or infection in this breast to explain the distortion.

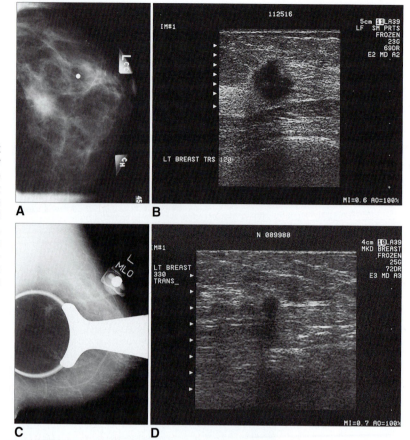

FIGURE 21-21 Example of highly suspicious (breast imaging reporting and data system [BI-RADS] category 5) mass. **A,** Magnification view of a palpable lump showing a spiculated, highly suspicious mammographic mass. **B,** Sonographic image of the same mass. Note the heterogeneous echogenicity, poorly defined and irregular margin, and "higher than wide" appearance, which does not change with most cancers even with applied compression. **C,** Spot compression mammogram of a small spiculated mass. **D,** Ultrasound image showing a small mass with features similar to those in **B.**

the lesion in an attempt to aspirate fluid. Successful fluid aspiration is diagnostic of a complex cyst. The same approach can be used to guide fine-needle aspiration for cytology, core-needle biopsies for histology, and preoperative needle wire localization of masses for surgery, and for the injection of radioactive tracers for **sentinel node** identification and mapping.

In some cases, a patient has a clinical sign or symptom of possible breast cancer, and yet diagnostic breast imaging shows no abnormality. The most common clinical scenario is the patient with a breast lump and negative breast imaging. If no imaging correlation can be identified to explain the patient's breast lump, the patient must be managed clinically, which means that she is examined sequentially through at least one menstrual cycle. In the overwhelming majority of cases, the breast lump will improve or resolve completely, confirming the diagnosis of clinical fibrocystic condition. If the breast lump does not improve or continues to grow, surgical biopsy is performed.

SONOGRAPHIC EVALUATION OF THE BREAST

Indications for Sonographic Evaluation

The sonographer must have basic clinical information regarding any patient who is referred for breast ultra-

sound. Pertinent clinical information includes the patient's age, risk factors for breast cancer (see Box 21-6), and symptoms, and the location and clinical impression of any breast lumps. Any history of trauma to the breast or previous breast surgery is also helpful. Inspection of the breast during the ultrasound examination often reveals pertinent findings. For example, the examiner should make note of any surface nipple erosion (possible **Paget's disease**), nipple or skin retraction, skin thickening (edema, scarring, or **peau d'orange**), scars, signs of inflammation (induration and erythema), or contusion. Sonography is normally used as an adjunct to mammography but may be the initial method of imaging when a breast lump is palpable; it may also be used in a young patient with dense breasts, in a pregnant or lactating patient, in a patient with breast augmentation, or in a patient with a difficult or compromised mammogram.

Palpable Breast Lump. Patients are often referred for breast ultrasound because of a **palpable** breast lump. Pertinent clinical information that should be provided by the referring physician includes size and location of the lump, when it was noticed, and its relation to the menstrual cycle. The physician's clinical impression (e.g., suspicion of cancer, probable fibrocystic condition, possible abscess) can help focus the sonographer's examination. The sonographer can often feel the mass of concern while scanning the breast. This can help guide the examination and over time will lead to improved expertise on the part of the sonographer in differentiating lesions. For example, a dominant cyst is frequently round or oval (long axis toward nipple), smooth, soft (some cysts under tension can be firm and are usually very tender), and easily movable. Fibroadenomas are usually similar in shape, but are often firm and rubbery in consistency and homogeneously solid on ultrasound. Breast cancer, by contrast, will generally be painless (although some cancers are associated with focal pain), lobular or irregular in shape, uneven in surface contour (sometimes gritty in texture), and fixed or poorly movable (Box 21-8).

Young Patient With Dense Breasts. Ultrasound is the primary tool in breast imaging for all women younger than age 30, according to most authors. Mammography is added as necessary on a limited basis between ages 20 and 30, mainly to rule out microcalcifications (a sign of possible breast cancer that may not be visible by ultrasound). Mammography is rarely indicated for patients younger than age 20 and, in some centers, younger than age 25. The three main reasons for this are that breast cancer is rare in women younger than 25 years, that breast tissue at this age is generally denser and more difficult to analyze by mammography, and that young breast tissue is more sensitive to damage from radiation.

Most breast masses that arise during the teen years are fibroadenomas (Figure 21-22). Other common causes of breast lumps include the developing breast bud immediately behind the nipple (which must never be mistaken for an abnormal mass and surgically removed) or a dominant cyst. Less commonly, a hyperplastic lymph node, abscess, hematoma, or giant fibroadenoma can present before age 20. Malignant breast lesions in patients younger than 20 years are extremely rare. When they do occur, they generally are not of breast origin, but rather are metastatic or of soft tissue origin (such as soft tissue sarcomas). If a young patient has a rapidly enlarging or painful mass, surgical excision should be considered.

Pregnant or Lactating Patient. Sonography is the primary tool for breast imaging in a pregnant patient. Mammography is added (with abdominal shielding) to allow accurate characterization of a breast mass as necessary. Diagnostic evaluation of a breast mass (including biopsy if indicated) should not be delayed because of the pregnancy.

Most masses that present in a pregnant or lactating patient are benign fibroadenomas. These can often enlarge rapidly because of the marked increase in circulating hormone levels during pregnancy and lactation. The increase in circulating hormones, however, can have a similar effect on breast cancers. In patients who develop breast cancer during pregnancy, cancers are often diagnosed at a later stage than in the nonpregnant patient.

Other breast problems that may arise during pregnancy or lactation include mastitis, abscesses, cysts, or galactoceles (cysts containing milk). In the case of a galactocele, a fat-fluid level may be visible both by mammography and by ultrasound, but more commonly, this lesion appears as a complex cyst. Galactoceles or cysts can be aspirated easily under ultrasound guidance.

Patient With Breast Augmentation. Sonographic evaluation of the breast in a patient who has had breast augmentation or reconstruction with silicone implants has been shown to be of benefit. Mammography is often limited in its ability to image beyond the implant, whereas ultrasound has the ability to evaluate the tissue surrounding the implant, search for the presence of defects in the membrane, and look for leakage into the breast parenchyma. An intracapsular implant rupture occurs when there is a breach of the membrane surrounding an implant, but the silicone that leaks out is still confined within the fibrous scar tissue, which forms a "capsule" around the implant. As the implant collapses and the membrane folds inward, a series of discontinuous echogenic lines parallel to the face of the transducer may be seen and are referred to as the "stepladder sign" or "linguine sign" (Figure 21-23). Caution must be used when evaluating internal echoes within an implant because the internal architecture of an implant may appear heterogeneous as a result of reverberation artifacts and/or a mixture of the gel with other fluids that may have been injected into the implant during surgery, giving a false-positive stepladder sign. An implant rupture allowing

BOX 21-8	Differential Diagnoses

Smooth Mass

Common	Simple cyst
	Complex cyst
	Fibroadenoma
	Lymph node
	Oil cyst
Less common	Galactocele
	Seroma
	Hematoma
	Phyllodes tumor
	Cancer

Focal Distortion

Common	Postsurgical scar
	Fibrocystic condition
	Cancer
Less common	Prior infection
	Old hematoma
	Degenerating fibroadenoma
Uncommon	Fibrocystic condition

Palpable Breast Lump With Negative Breast Imaging

Common	Fibrocystic condition
Less common	Resolving trauma
Uncommon	Cancer

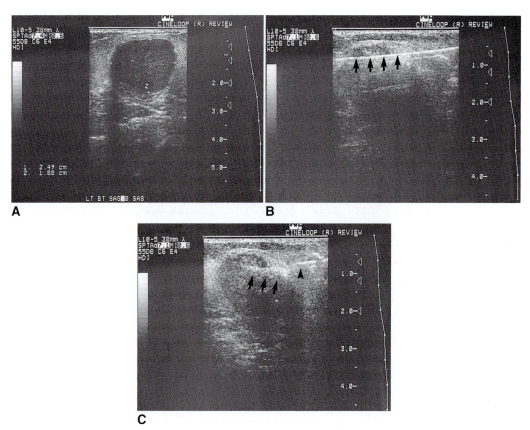

FIGURE 21-22 Smooth, solid mass (fibroadenoma). **A,** Ultrasound image of a growing palpable mass in a teenage female. This was one of several similar masses. Fibroadenomas are frequently multiple and often run in families. Please note the hypoechoic, homogeneous echogenicity of the mass, and the low-level posterior acoustic enhancement and the edge refraction. **B,** The patient was referred for large core-needle biopsy for diagnosis. This ultrasound image shows the 14-gauge core-biopsy needle in postfire position traversing the superficial portion of the mass. The approximate area of the sample notch from which tissue is obtained is indicated by the arrows. Multiple passes are made to ensure adequate sampling and a reliable tissue diagnosis. **C,** Note the echogenic core biopsy tract within the mass *(arrows).* Fresh hemorrhage along the needle tract caused the echogenic appearance. The prefire position of the needle adjacent to the mass, in preparation for the next tissue sampling, is also visible *(arrowhead).*

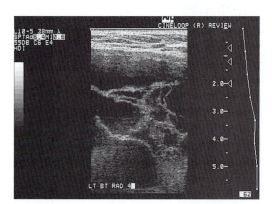

FIGURE 21-23 Seroma. This chronic seroma (noninfected fluid collection) has been repeatedly aspirated in this patient with previous silicone implants that ruptured. Note the thick septations (synechiae) within the seroma.

extracapsular leakage of silicone into the tissue sonographically appears as an indistinctly marginated area of increased echogenicity along the margin of the implant, with dirty posterior acoustic shadowing and the presence of noise. The depiction of an extracapsular rupture has

been described as having a "snowstorm" appearance. Ultrasound is often the first choice among imaging procedures to examine the implant. If the image is unclear, MRI may be used to further define the area in question.

Patient With a Difficult or Compromised Mammogram. For some patients, breast imaging by mammography is limited in its sensitivity (as in the case of very dense breast tissue) or in its ability to visualize the breast tissue (as in the case of retroglandular breast implants) (Figure 21-24). Distinguishing between scar tissue and breast cancer is difficult with mammography. With more women having breast reduction surgeries, these reduction scars, along with previous open biopsy scars, form tissue that is distorted and is difficult to distinguish from breast cancer distortion of normal tissue.

For other patients, examination of breast tissue is compromised because of postsurgical or postradiation changes (Figures 21-25 and 21-26). This is a common situation in the patient who has had breast-conserving therapy for early-stage breast cancer located close to the chest wall or in the axillary tail near the armpit. As

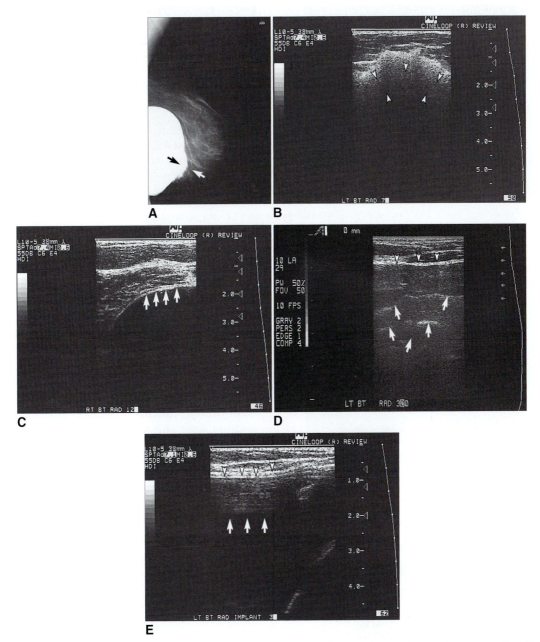

FIGURE 21-24 Ruptured silicone breast implants. **A,** Mammogram showing retroglandular implant with extracapsular silicone *(arrows)*. **B,** Ultrasound image of the same case showing typical "snowstorm" appearance of free extracapsular silicone *(arrowheads)*. **C,** Ultrasound image of normal intact silicone implant. Note the anechoic appearance of the silicone and the double echogenic margin of the implant perpendicular to the incident sound waves *(arrows)*. **D** and **E,** Two ultrasound images of the same silicone breast implant taken at separate times showing intracapsular rupture. **D,** Note the echogenic fibrous capsule *(arrowheads)* that is no longer a double line, but only a single line. Note the nonparallel echogenic interfaces *(arrows)* within the silicone. These interfaces represent portions of the collapsed and ruptured envelope surrounded by silicone still contained within the fibrous capsule. Compare this appearance with **(E),** the same patient at an earlier time, showing the double echogenic interface *(arrowheads)*. Note the faint parallel lines under the echogenic capsule *(arrows)* representing reverberation artifact.

technologic advances in ultrasound continue to improve its sensitivity and specificity, the routine use of adjunctive breast ultrasound and mammography in certain high-risk or complicated patients is being advocated (Box 21-9). Although sonography is an invaluable aid to breast imaging, it should not be used as a substitute for mammography because microcalcifications and focal distortion, two of the three principal signs of breast cancer seen by mammography, are often difficult to visualize with ultrasound.

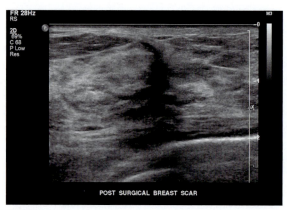

FIGURE 21-25 Postsurgical breast scar causes interruption in the ultrasound beam at the site of the scar (area of shadowing).

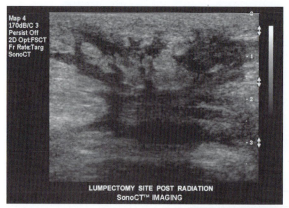

FIGURE 21-26 Lumpectomy site after radiation demonstrates an irregular area that appears to be "masslike" without defined borders in the breast.

BOX 21-9 | **Breast Ultrasound Applications**

Further characterization of mammographic masses
Evaluation of a palpable breast lump
Young patient with dense breasts
Pregnant or lactating patient
Patient with breast augmentation
Difficult or compromised mammogram
Image-guided procedures

Technique

Scanning is performed using the real-time technique. In most laboratories and clinics, hard copy images are produced to document the examination. The image first must be optimized using electronic focusing, overall gain, and time gain compensation (TGC) adjustment. The goal is to balance the image from the low-level echoes of the subcutaneous fat to the low-level echoes of the retromammary fat. This should result in an image that clearly shows all levels of the breast from the skin level through the echogenic breast core and the deeper echogenic chest wall layers. Moderate compression

---

BOX 21-10 | **Breast Scanning Points to Remember**

Image optimization (image tissue from skin through chest wall equally)
Lesion location and annotation methods
- Clock face
- Quadrant
- Distance from nipple
- "1,2,3 ... A,B,C" method
Three-dimensional measurement methods
- Sagittal/transverse
- Radial/antiradial
Ultrasound pitfalls
- Pseudomass
- Infiltrative pattern
- Large, fatty breast

---

applied with the transducer during scanning will improve detail and decrease the depth of tissue that the ultrasound beam must traverse. In the case of a negative breast ultrasound examination, the usual practice is to record representative images of each quadrant, the subareolar ducts, or specific radial images of the breast, depending on the protocol of the imaging center.

Positioning. Patients are usually scanned in the supine position with the use of a hand-held, high-resolution transducer. The patient is positioned with her arm behind her head on the side of the breast to be examined. This spreads the breast tissue more evenly over the surface of the chest and provides a more stable scanning surface and easier access to the axilla. When the medial portion of the breast is scanned, a supine position works well. For the lateral margin of the breast, the patient can be rolled slightly toward the opposite side (approximately 30 to 45 degrees) and stabilized with a cushion under her shoulder and hips.

If a lesion identified on a mammogram cannot be located sonographically, it may be helpful to sit the patient upright and position the breast in the same positions used to obtain the mammogram. This allows easier localization and a similar frame of reference.

Scanning Technique. When examining for a palpable mass or for correlation with an abnormal mammogram, some centers scan only the area of interest. For example, if a mass in the upper inner quadrant of the right breast is seen on the mammogram, then only the upper inner quadrant of the right breast will be scanned by ultrasound. This is a more specific approach to lesion evaluation, results in fewer cases of false-positive sonographic findings, and is more cost effective than scanning the entire breast. Other centers, however, routinely scan the entire breast. Breast scanning points to remember are listed in Box 21-10.

When a patient is evaluated for a palpable breast mass or for a specific abnormality seen on a mammogram, the abnormality is first located with a preliminary scan. It is helpful to mark the external skin over the mass. The transducer orientation should remain the same as with conventional ultrasound examination (i.e., the patient's right side is oriented to the left of the screen on transverse images, and the notch of the transducer is directed cephalad on longitudinal images). The mass is then thoroughly scanned in orthogonal planes (90 degrees apart) for evaluation of the lesion in three dimensions. This can be recorded using sagittal and transverse images or using radial/antiradial transducer positions (Figure 21-27). Use of radial/antiradial positions is unique to the breast and can often pick up subtle abnormalities extending toward the nipple along the ductal system from the mass. All dominant solid masses are generally recorded with three-dimensional measurements (length, width, and height) to facilitate management decisions and future follow-up.

Annotation. Labeling sonographic images of the breast is extremely important in the identification and correlation of breast images with images from other modalities. Most imaging centers have traditionally used the quasi-grid pattern. This views the breast as a clock face. Directly above the nipple on either breast is 12 o'clock. Right medial breast and left lateral breast are 3 o'clock. Directly below the nipple bilaterally is 6 o'clock, and right lateral breast and left medial breast are 9 o'clock, respectively (Figure 21-28).

Many imaging centers will further subdivide the breast with three concentric circles, with the center being the nipple (Figure 21-29, *A*). The first ring circles one third of the breast tissue, encompassing the area just outside the nipple, or zone 1. The second ring is about two thirds of the breast surface from the nipple, or zone

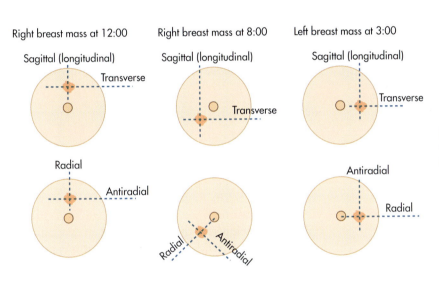

FIGURE 21-27 Examples of sagittal and transverse, plus radial and antiradial, transducer positions.

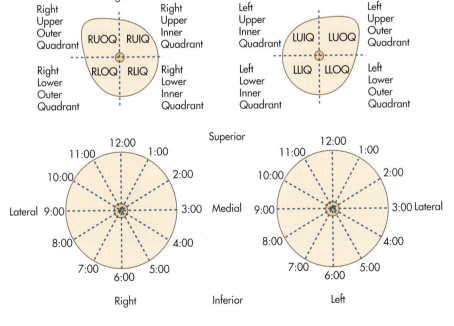

FIGURE 21-28 Breast anatomy is described by two methods: the quadrant method (right/left, upper/lower, and inner/outer quadrants) and the clock face method.

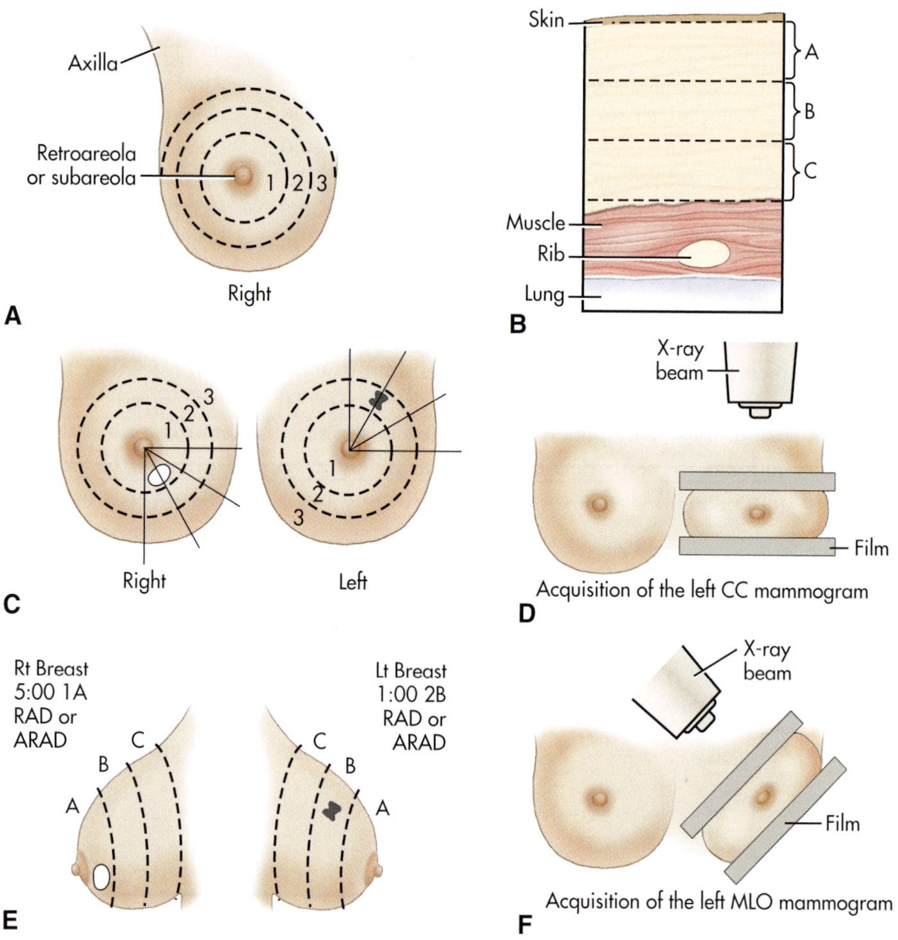

FIGURE 21-29 **A**, Zones of the breast are shown. **B**, Documentation of depth of tissue. **C**, Localization of mass in the right breast. **D**, Anterior and posterior mammogram of the breast. **E**, Longitudinal view of the breast mass. **F**, Medial to lateral mammogram acquisition.

2. The final ring is to the breast periphery, or zone 3. Lesions located close to the nipple are labeled "A," lesions in the middle of the breast are labeled "B," and lesions located at the outer margin of the breast are labeled "C" (Figure 21-29, *B* and *E*).

Finally, the depth of any pathologic condition is documented. The breast again is divided into thirds from the skin to the pectoralis major. Depth A is the most superficial third of the breast, depth B is the middle layer, and depth C is the deepest third of the breast. Superficial lesions located close to the skin surface are labeled "1," lesions in the middle of the breast are labeled "2," and deeper lesions located toward the chest wall are labeled "3."

With solid lesions, it is important to document the orientation of the mass, in addition to its location. The orientation of a lesion is determined by aligning the transducer with the longest axis of a lesion and identifying whether the long axis is oriented in a **radial** or **antiradial** plane. This is important because malignancies tend to grow within the ducts and often follow the ductal system in a radial plane toward the convergence at the nipple. The various methods of annotation described earlier can be combined to relay a specific location and orientation of a lesion. For example, a lesion labeled "RT BREAST 2:00 B3 RAD" can be relocated easily for follow-up; this lesion in the right breast is deeply situated toward the chest wall in the 2 o'clock position approximately midway between the nipple and the outer margin of the breast, and its long axis is oriented radially toward the nipple.

Sonographic Characteristics of Breast Masses

Sonographic evaluation of a breast lesion normally begins with determination of whether a lesion is cystic or solid (Box 21-11). The distinction between a cyst and a solid mass is extremely important for management purposes; a cyst that meets the criteria of a simple cyst on ultrasound is universally considered benign. Solid masses, however, have a malignant potential. Although a vast majority of solid masses are benign, further characterization of a solid lesion is necessary.

To be considered a simple cyst, a lesion must meet several criteria on ultrasound: It must be devoid of internal echoes (anechoic), show smooth inner margins with an imperceptible capsule, and demonstrate posterior acoustic enhancement (Table 21-2). Cysts within the breast can be multilocular with thin internal septations. In the case of simple cysts, no further workup is usually necessary. In some cases, however, these cysts will be

BOX 21-11   Sonographic Characteristics of Breast Lesions

Simple cyst
- Smooth walls
- Anechoic
- Posterior enhancement

Complicated cyst
- Wall thickening or irregularities
- Septations
- Internal echoes

Solid mass
- Margins
  Benign: smooth, rounded
  Malignant: indistinct, fuzzy, spiculated
- Disruption of breast architecture
  Benign: grow within tissue, causing compression of the tissue adjacent to the mass
  Malignant: grow through tissue without compressing adjacent tissue and may cause retraction of the nipple or dimpling of the skin
- Shape
  Benign: rounded or oval, large lobulations (<3)
  Malignant: sharp, angular microlobulations (≥3)
- Orientation
  Malignant: taller-than-wide highly suspicious; radial growth suspicious for intraductal lesions
- Internal echo pattern
  Benign: isoechoic, hyperechoic
  Malignant: hypoechoic, weak internal echoes, clustered microcalcifications
- Attenuation effects
  Benign: posterior enhancement
  Malignant: strongly attenuating
- Mobility
  Benign: some mobility
  Malignant: firmly fixed
- Compressibility
  Benign: fatty tumors are usually compressible
  Malignant: rigid, noncompressible
- Vascularity
  Malignant: hypervascular; feeder vessel may be identified

TABLE 21-2   Sonographic Characteristics of Common Lesions

Mass	Characteristics
Simple cyst	Oval or round, anechoic, imperceptible capsule, posterior acoustic enhancement, edge refraction shadowing, often compressible
Fibrocystic changes	Multiple cysts, well circumscribed, thin walls, increased fibrous stroma
Complex cyst	Irregular or thickened wall, mural nodule, fluid levels, debris, particulate echoes, variable degrees of shadowing
Benign fibroadenoma	Oval or gently lobular, hypoechoic, uniform echogenicity, smooth, distinct margins, wider-than-tall, posterior acoustic enhancement, edge refraction shadow
Lipoma	May be large, smooth walls, hypoechoic (isoechoic with fat), posterior acoustic enhancement, easily compressible
Fat necrosis	Irregular, complex mass with low-level echoes; may have posterior acoustic shadow, separate from breast parenchyma
Abscess	Hypoechoic, complex lesion, posterior enhancement, thick walls, fluid levels
Cystosarcoma phyllodes	Large, hypoechoic tumor, well-defined margins, decreased through-transmission, fine or coarse internal echoes, variable amounts of shadowing
Intraductal papilloma	Intracystic lesion with fibrovascular stalk
Malignant	Irregular, spiculated, indistinct, or angular margins, hypoechoic, heterogeneous echogenicity, taller-than-wide, posterior acoustic shadowing, noncompressible, hypervascular with feeder vessel
Ductal carcinoma	Calcifications and ductal enlargement with extension within the ducts in situ (DCIS)
Invasive ductal	Begins in the ducts, invades the fatty tissue of the breast carcinoma (IDC)
Lobular carcinoma in situ (LCIS)	Confined to the gland, difficult to distinguish sonographically
Invasive lobular carcinoma (ILC)	Begins in the lobule, extends into the fatty tissue; often bilateral, multicentric, or multifocal

painful or disturbing to the patient (Figure 21-30). Aspiration can be performed quickly and easily under ultrasound guidance.

If the cyst has internal echoes, wall irregularity, mural nodularity or septation, shadowing, nonuniform internal echoes, or any other feature not associated with a simple cyst, it is by definition a complex cyst, and aspiration and/or biopsy should be considered. Complex cysts are often indistinguishable from homogeneous solid sonographic masses because of their thick proteinaceous fluid content. Other complex cysts have thick or irregular capsules, a possible intracystic mass, or dependent debris. Cysts with layering calcifications or floating crystals (these can be seen moving on real-time scanning) are benign, although careful ultrasound technique is required

to distinguish these cysts from those requiring further evaluation.

The usual approach to a small, smooth, round or oval, benign appearing solid mass in low-risk patients favors close-interval follow-up breast imaging. Color Doppler has been successfully used to interrogate solid masses to check for increased vascular flow. The demonstration of increased vascular flow could accelerate the need for biopsy of these masses.

Tissue diagnosis is suggested in high-risk patients or patients with larger masses. The size cutoff for tissue diagnosis versus follow-up varies. In a low-risk patient with a single, dominant, smooth, solid mass, follow-up is offered for masses with a diameter of up to 1 cm. Some physicians recommend following lesions up to 1.2 or even 1.5 cm in size, especially in the case of multiple bilateral masses. In a high-risk patient or in a patient who is not comfortable waiting on follow-up for an answer, tissue diagnosis can be pursued more aggressively. Options include fine-needle aspiration cytology, large-core needle biopsy, vacuum-assisted biopsy, and surgical excisional biopsy (Figure 21-31). High-quality sonographic imaging of a solid breast mass is accurate in characterizing a lesion as probably benign or probably

malignant in a majority of cases (see Table 21-2). It is important, however, to realize that there is significant overlap in the appearance of benign and malignant lesions; ultrasound cannot be used as a substitute for tissue diagnosis when sonographic findings are indeterminate or when a biopsy is indicated by clinical examination or patient history.

Margins. The margins of a mass should be investigated carefully. A technique called **fremitus** can be used to identify and confirm the margins of a mass. Fremitus is a palpable tremor or vibration of the chest wall. Using power Doppler, have the patient hum. The vibrations of the chest wall will carry through to the breast tissue, creating a power Doppler signal. The lesion is normally void of signal, making it easier to identify its margins. This technique can be useful in confirming the presence of a mass when in doubt, identifying multifocal masses, differentiating diffuse masses, and locating palpable masses that are isoechoic with the breast parenchyma.

Benign lesions usually have smooth, rounded margins (Figure 21-32, *A* through *C*). Malignant tumors are aggressive and tend to grow through tissue via finger-like extensions called **spiculation** (Figure 21-32, *D*). Spiculated margins are the ultrasound finding with the highest positive predictive value of malignancy and correlate with mammographic spiculation. Sonographic spiculations appear as small lines that radiate outward from the surface of a mass. They are typically alternating hypoechoic and hyperechoic lines. Ductal extensions project radially from the tumor and are oriented toward the nipple. Small extensions may not be visible sonographically, but may make the margins of a lesion appear indistinct or fuzzy.

Disruption of Breast Architecture. Benign tumors are usually slow growing and do not invade surrounding tissue. They tend to grow horizontally within the tissue planes, parallel to the chest wall. Larger benign lesions often cause compression of tissue adjacent to the mass,

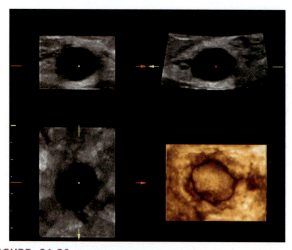

FIGURE 21-30 Symptomatic cyst. Simple cyst on ultrasound (notice the lack of internal echoes and the smooth internal margin, imperceptible capsule, strong posterior acoustic enhancement, and edge refraction) is large enough to create a painful lump in the patient's breast.

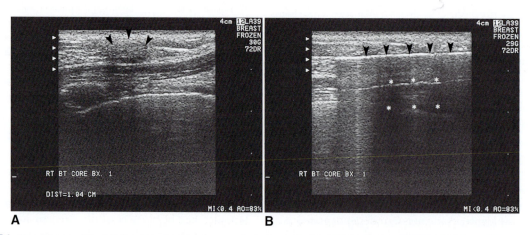

FIGURE 21-31 Core biopsy of isoechoic mass close to chest wall. **A,** Sonographic image of an isoechoic mass *(arrowheads)* located immediately adjacent to the pectoralis muscle *(arrows)*. **B,** Core-biopsy needle *(arrowheads)* is directed parallel to the chest wall. Note the loss of information posterior to the needle caused by acoustic shadowing and reverberation echoes *(asterisks)*.

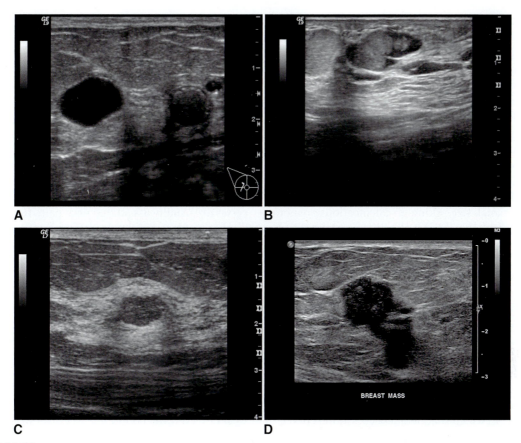

FIGURE 21-32 Benign lesions of the breast. **A,** Cyst. **B,** Complex. **C,** Fibroadenoma. **D,** Malignant solid mass with spiculation.

implying that the mass is pushing against adjacent breast tissue, as opposed to infiltrating it.

Malignant lesions, on the other hand, tend to grow right through the normal breast tissue. As malignant masses enlarge, they may cause retraction of the nipple or dimpling of the skin as the spiculations pull on Cooper's ligaments (Figure 21-33).

Shape. A rounded or oval shape is usually associated with benign lesions; sharp, angular margins are associated with malignancy. Mild undulations in contour can be seen in benign masses such as fibroadenomas; however, microlobulations (very small 1- to 2-mm lobulations) are more often associated with malignancy. Lobulations associated with benign fibroadenomas are usually large, rounded lobulations and do not exceed three in number. Microlobulations associated with malignancy are usually smaller, sharper, and more numerous.

Orientation. The normal tissue planes of the breast are horizontally oriented. Benign lesions tend to grow within the normal tissue planes, and their long axis lies parallel to the chest wall. Malignant lesions are able to grow through the connective tissue and may have a vertical orientation when the breast is imaged from anterior to posterior. If a mass measures longer in the anteroposterior dimension (height) than in the transverse or sagittal plane (width), it has a vertical orientation, is usually

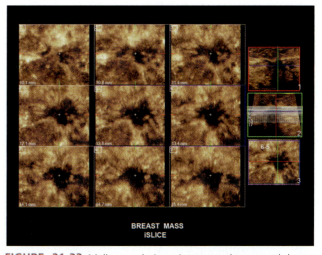

FIGURE 21-33 Malignant lesions interrupt the normal breast architecture as they spread throughout the tissue, as shown on this tomographic presentation.

described as "taller-than-wide," and is suspicious for malignancy.

Internal Echo Pattern. Lesions that appear isoechoic with the breast parenchyma or have echoes equivalent to or brighter than that of fat are most often benign. A solid lesion that is hypoechoic relative to the normal breast parenchyma is more suspicious for malignancy. Malignant lesions tend to be highly hypoechoic relative to fat and usually have weak internal echoes. They are often associated with dense posterior shadowing, making the lesion difficult to penetrate.

Microcalcifications within a solid mass are associated with a breast malignancy. Ultrasound is less sensitive than mammography in the detection of microcalcifications due to the heterogeneous appearance of normal breast tissue. Microcalcifications seen with ultrasound are typically very small echogenic foci that do not create shadows because of their small size. Although calcifications are not visualized frequently by sonography, their detection in a hypoechoic mass is suspicious for malignancy.

Attenuation Effects. Enhancement behind a lesion is normally caused by a weakly attenuating structure; it usually indicates that the lesion is made up of fluid and is a characteristic associated with benign lesions. Most solid lesions, with the exception of a fibroadenoma, will not enhance.

Shadowing behind a solid breast mass is another suspicious sonographic sign for malignancy because malignant tumors tend to be highly attenuating. Posterior shadowing should not be confused with edge or refraction shadowing, in which shadowing occurs at the curved edge of a smooth, benign mass.

Mobility. Benign lesions normally demonstrate a limited degree of mobility or may roll away as they are palpated. Because of the spiculations associated with malignancy, malignant lesions are normally very fixed or rigid in their position.

Compressibility. If pressure applied by the transducer causes the lesion to compress or change shape, the lesion is probably benign and most likely represents a fat lobule. Malignant lesions normally are very hard and noncompressible.

Vascularity. Doppler interrogation of a breast lesion is an essential element of the study. Although breast lesions are not associated with consistent resistance patterns on Doppler ultrasound, malignant masses often demonstrate increased vascularity within the lesion and often have a feeder vessel, which can be identified upon careful evaluation. Vessels that penetrate a mass are highly suspect for malignancy and should be checked using color or power Doppler to ascertain the number and to look for intratumoral vessels.

PATHOLOGY

The most common pathologic lesions of the female breast are, in order of decreasing frequency, fibrocystic disease, carcinoma, fibroadenoma, intraductal papilloma, and duct ectasia. Benign lesions are the most common breast lesions, representing 70% of proved lesions in biopsies after they are removed. Several parameters, including the patient's age, physical characteristics

of the mass, and previous medical history, must be considered when a dominant mass has been palpated. Lesions common to younger women are fibrocystic disease and fibroadenomas. Older or postmenopausal women are more likely to have intraductal papilloma, duct ectasia, and cancer.

Differential Diagnosis of Breast Masses

Symptoms of breast masses include pain, a palpable mass, spontaneous or induced nipple discharge, skin dimpling, ulceration, and nipple retraction. Benign processes are usually associated with pain, tumor, and nipple discharge. Skin dimpling or ulceration and nipple retraction nearly always result from cancer. Benign tumors are rubbery, mobile, and well defined (as seen in a fibroadenoma), whereas malignant tumors are often stone hard and irregular with a gritty feel. Soft tumors usually represent a lipoma (fat tissue). Cystic masses are like a balloon of water, well delineated but not as mobile as fibroadenomas because they form part of the breast parenchyma, whereas a fibroadenoma has a capsule.

Benign Conditions

Cysts. Cysts are commonly seen in women 35 to 55 years of age. Symptoms include history of changing with the menstrual cycle, pain (especially when the cyst is growing rapidly), recent lump, and tenderness. Small cysts may not regress completely and may persist from one cycle to the next.

Fibrocystic Condition. Fibrocystic changes produce histologic alterations in the terminal ducts and lobules of the breast in both epithelial and connective tissue. Fibrocystic changes are usually accompanied by pain or tenderness in the breast and represent normal physiologic processes of breast tissue that fluctuate under the influence of normal female hormonal cycles. These processes become magnified in some patients to the point of causing symptoms that are upsetting to the patient (mainly pain and tenderness or recurrent cysts). In some cases, fibrocystic condition (FCC) causes changes that are frankly worrisome for breast cancer. In all age groups, the most common diagnosis at breast biopsy is FCC. These biopsies are prompted by a growing or dominant clinically suspicious breast lump.

The terms *fibrocystic condition* and *fibrocystic change* (use of the term *fibrocystic disease* is discouraged) actually encompass many different processes under a single term. An abundance of inaccuracy and confusion results from using the term *fibrocystic condition*. In some cases, FCC may refer to the normal hormonal fluctuations in breast texture. At the other end of the spectrum, a surgical biopsy may be undertaken because of a growing suspicious breast lump. In a few cases, a biopsy reveals tissue changes that mean the patient is at increased risk for subsequent development of breast cancer.

Clinical signs and symptoms of FCC include the lumps and pain that the patient feels that fluctuate with every monthly cycle. In most cases, both breasts are equally involved. In some cases, FCC may affect just one area of one breast. This can be frightening for the patient and is a frequent cause of referral for diagnostic breast imaging.

Imaging signs of FCC may be visible on the mammogram or breast ultrasound. On mammogram, FCC may cause diffuse benign microcalcifications, **adenosis,** and multiple round masses. Ultrasound of the breast shows the round masses as multiple cysts (Figure 21-34).

Many separate tissue processes of FCC are recognized by the pathologist in reviewing breast tissue under a microscope, including **apocrine metaplasia,** fibrosis, **epithelial** ductal **hyperplasia,** and sclerosing adenosis. In correlating the pathologic results of a breast biopsy with the indication for biopsy (i.e., palpable breast lump, suspicious mammographic or sonographic mass, or clustered microcalcifications), it is very important for the physician to document that the pathologic results are concordant with the targeted lesion. If a breast biopsy was performed because of suspicious microcalcifications, for example, the pathology report should state that microcalcifications were seen. If no microcalcifications were seen on pathology slides, then this is a discordant result, and further investigation will be required.

In an attempt to create a more clinically relevant classification of tissue processes under the enormous and confusing heading of fibrocystic condition, these processes have been separated into three categories: (1) nonproliferative lesions (no increased risk of subsequent development of breast cancer); (2) proliferative lesions without atypical cells (mildly elevated risk of subsequent breast cancer); and (3) proliferative lesions with atypical cellular changes (moderately increased risk of subsequent breast cancer). Any woman with an atypical proliferative breast lesion (especially lobular neoplasia) who also has a family history of a first-degree relative with breast cancer will have double the risk of subsequent breast cancer compared with the patient with an atypical proliferative lesion alone (Table 21-3).

Fibroadenoma. The most common benign breast tumors are **fibroadenomas,** and they occur primarily in young women. They may be found in one breast or in both breasts. The growth of a fibroadenoma is stimulated by estrogen. Under normal circumstances, hormonal influences on the breast (estrogen) result in the proliferation of epithelial cells in lactiferous ducts and in stromal tissue during the first half of the menstrual cycle. During the second half of the cycle, this condition regresses, allowing breast tissue to return to its normal resting state. In certain disturbances of this hormonal mechanism, regression fails to occur, resulting in the development of fibrous and epithelial nodules that become fibroadenomas, fibromas, or adenomas, depending on the predominant cell type. They may also be related to pregnancy and lactation.

Clinically, a fibroadenoma is firm, rubbery, freely mobile, and clearly delineated from the surrounding breast tissue (Figure 21-35). It is round or ovoid and smooth or lobulated, and usually does not cause loss of contour of the breast unless it develops to a large size. It rarely causes mastodynia, and it does not change size during the menstrual cycle. Fibroadenomas tend to grow very slowly. A sudden increase in size with acute pain may be the result of hemorrhage within the tumor. Calcification may follow hemorrhage or infarction; thus the tumor may have calcifications and may mimic the appearance of a carcinoma on mammography. Sonographically, fibroadenomas have benign characteristics with smooth, rounded margins and low-level homogeneous internal echoes and may demonstrate intermediate

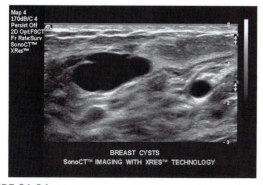

FIGURE 21-34 Fibrocystic condition shows two sonolucent structures within the breast.

TABLE 21-3	**Fibrocystic Condition: Common Breast Lesions—Risk of Subsequent Breast Cancer**
Classification	**Description**
Nonproliferative lesions: no increased risk	Cyst Apocrine metaplasia Fibroadenoma Ductal ectasia Mild epithelial ductal hyperplasia Benign microcalcifications
Proliferative lesions without atypical features: mildly increased risk (1.5 to 2×)	Moderate or florid epithelial ductal hyperplasia Sclerosing adenosis Radial scar (complex sclerosing lesion) Intraductal papilloma
Proliferative lesions with atypical features: moderately increased risk (4 to 6×)	Atypical ductal hyperplasia Atypical lobular hyperplasia Lobular neoplasia (alternative term for lobular carcinoma in situ [LCIS])

Note: Patients with an atypical proliferative lesion and a first-degree relative with breast cancer are at even greater risk for subsequent breast cancer.

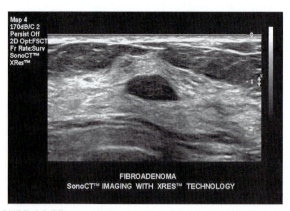

FIGURE 21-35 Fibroadenoma. Smooth, ovoid, solid mass with a low-level internal echo pattern.

posterior enhancement. Fibroadenomas are normally hypoechoic, but occasionally are **hyperechoic** to the fat within the breast.

Lipoma. A pure lipoma consists entirely of fatty tissue. Other forms of lipoma consist of fat with fibrous and glandular elements interspersed (fibroadenolipoma). A lipoma may grow to a large size before it is clinically detected. It is usually found in middle-aged or menopausal women. Clinically, on palpation, a large, soft, poorly demarcated mass is felt that cannot be clearly separated from the surrounding parenchyma. No thinning or fixation of the overlying skin is noted. Sonographically, it may be difficult or impossible to detect a lipoma in a fatty breast. Lipomas typically have smooth walls, are hypoechoic, and appear similar to fat. They often demonstrate posterior enhancement and are easily compressible.

Fat Necrosis. Fat necrosis may be caused by trauma to the breast, surgery, radiation treatments, or plasma cell mastitis or may be related to an involutional process or other disease present in the breast, such as cancer. It is more frequently found in older women. Clinical palpation reveals a spherical nodule that is generally superficial under a layer of calcified necrosis. A deep-lying focus of necrosis may cause scarring with skin retraction and thus may mimic carcinoma. Sonographically, fat necrosis appears as an irregular, complex mass with low-level echoes; it may mimic a malignant lesion and may appear as fat, but it is separate and distinct from the rest of the breast parenchyma. Acoustic shadowing may or may not be present.

Acute Mastitis. Acute mastitis may result from infection, trauma, mechanical obstruction in the breast ducts, or other conditions. It often occurs during lactation, beginning in the lactiferous ducts and spreading via the lymphatics or blood. Acute mastitis causes an enlarged, reddened, tender breast, and is often confined to one area of the breast. Diffuse mastitis results when infection is carried via the blood or breast lymphatics and thus affects the entire breast. Patients are treated initially with antibiotics and are referred for breast imaging

when acute inflammatory symptoms are sufficiently reduced to allow good quality mammography and breast ultrasound to rule out inflammatory breast cancer as a cause.

Chronic Mastitis. An inflammation of the glandular tissue is considered to be chronic mastitis. This is very difficult to differentiate by ultrasound; the echo pattern is mixed and diffuse with sound absorption. The condition is usually found in elderly women. Thickening of the connective tissue results in narrowing of the lumina of the milk ducts. The cause is inspissated intraductal secretions, which are forced into the periductal connective tissue. Clinically, the patient usually has a nipple discharge; frequently, the nipple has retracted over a period of years. Palpation reveals some subareolar thickening, but no dominant mass.

Abscess. Abscesses may be single or multiple. Acute abscesses have a poorly defined border, whereas mature abscesses are well encapsulated with sharp borders. A definite diagnosis cannot be made from a mammogram alone. Aspiration is necessary. Clinical findings include pain, swelling, and reddening of the overlying skin. The patient may be febrile, and swollen painful axillary nodes may be present. Sonographic findings may show a diffuse, mottled appearance of the breast, irregular margins, posterior enhancement, and low-level internal echoes (Figure 21-36). If associated with mastitis, skin thickening is almost always present, and edema leads to diffusely increased echogenicity of the breast tissue. Color or power Doppler of the breast may be helpful to document hyperemia associated with increased vascularity, which may tip the scales toward abscess rather than hematoma.

Cystosarcoma Phyllodes. Cystosarcoma phyllodes is a rare, predominantly benign breast neoplasm. It accounts for less than 1% of all breast neoplasms, yet it is the most frequent sarcoma of the breast. It is more commonly found in women in their 50s and usually is unilateral. It may arise from a fibroadenoma. Many patients may notice that a small breast mass that has been present for a long time suddenly begins to grow rapidly. Although it is considered a benign lesion, 27% of these tumors are malignant, and 12% metastasize.

When the tumor is small, it is well delineated, firm, and mobile, much like a fibroadenoma. As it enlarges, the surface may become irregular and lobulated. Skin changes can develop from increasing pressure. Edema may produce a skin change. Increasing pressure causes trophic changes and eventual skin ulcerations. Infection and abscess formation may be a secondary complication. The tumor never adheres to adjacent soft tissue or underlying pectoral muscle; therefore, dimpling of the skin or fixation of the tumor is not observed. Sonographic findings include a large, hypoechoic tumor with well-defined margins and decreased through-transmission. Internal echoes may be fine or coarse with variable amounts of shadowing.

Intraductal Papilloma. An intraductal papilloma is a small, benign tumor that grows within the acini of the breast. It occurs most frequently in women 35 to 55 years of age. The predominant symptom is spontaneous nipple discharge arising from a single duct. When the discharge is copious, it is usually preceded by a sensation of fullness or pain in the areola or nipple area that is relieved as the fluid is expelled. It has a "raspberry-like" configuration on the mammogram and in this way helps to promote correlation between the mammogram and the sonogram.

Papillomas are usually small, multiple, and multicentric. They consist of simple proliferations of duct epithelium projecting outward into a dilated lumen from one or more focal points (Figure 21-37), each supported by a vascular stalk from which it receives the blood supply. Trauma may rupture the stalk, filling the duct with blood or serum. Papillomas may grow to a large size and thus become palpable lesions. They are some-

what linear, resembling the terminal duct, and are usually benign.

Malignant Conditions

Malignancies generally develop over a long time. It is not unusual for several years to pass from the first appearance of **atypical hyperplasia** to the final diagnosis of in situ cancer. Malignant cells grow along a line of least resistance, such as in fatty tissue. In fibrotic tissue, most cancer growth occurs along the borders. Lymphatics and blood vessels are frequently used as pathways for new tumor development. If the tumor is encapsulated, it continues to grow in one area, compressing and distorting the surrounding architecture. When the carcinoma is contained and has not invaded the basal membrane structure, it is considered in situ. Most cancer originates in the terminal ductal lobular units, whereas a smaller percentage originates in the glandular tissue. The breast lobules are concentrated in the upper outer quadrant of the breast, and so it is not surprising that a majority of breast cancers (50%) are found there, followed by lesser incidence in the retroareolar area (17%), upper inner quadrant (15%), lower outer quadrant (10%), and lower inner quadrant (5%). Multifocal masses are least common and occur in approximately 3% of cases.

Cancer of the breast is of two types: sarcoma and carcinoma. Sarcoma refers to breast tumors that arise from supportive or connective tissues. Sarcomas tend to grow rapidly and invade fibrous tissue. Carcinoma refers to breast tumors that arise from the epithelium, in the ductal and glandular tissue, and usually has tentacles. Other malignant diseases affecting the breast result from systemic neoplasms, such as leukemia or lymphoma.

Breast carcinomas are generally categorized by two factors: where the cancer cells originate (ductal or lobular), and whether the cancer is prone to spreading

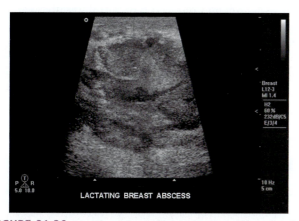

FIGURE 21-36 Lactating breast abscess shows a diffuse mottled appearance of the breast with irregular margins and posterior enhancement.

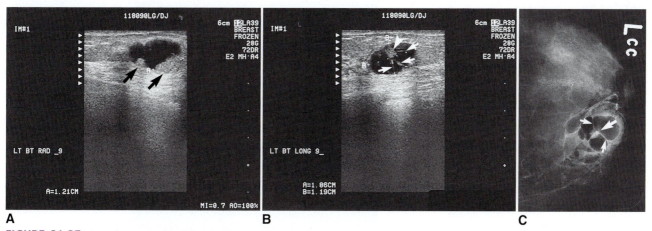

FIGURE 21-37 Complex cyst with debris and intracystic mass. **A,** Ultrasound image of a complex cyst with irregular dependent debris *(arrows).* **B,** Another image of the same complex cyst showing an intracystic mass *(arrowhead)* and thickened septations *(arrows).* **C,** Postaspiration pneumocystogram (air in cyst cavity) showing the intracystic mass *(arrow)* and the septations *(small arrows).* Intracystic masses are usually benign papillomas, but sometimes may be papillary carcinomas.

(noninvasive or invasive). Most breast carcinomas begin within the ducts of the breast and are called ductal or intraductal carcinomas. Breast cancers that form in the lobules are called lobular carcinomas. Carcinomas that do not normally spread outside of the duct or lobule are called noninvasive, noninfiltrating, or in situ cancer, whereas cancers that spread into nearby tissue are said to be invasive or infiltrating.

Ductal Carcinoma In Situ (DCIS). DCIS is also known as intraductal carcinoma. DCIS is characterized by cancer cells that are present inside the ducts but have not yet spread through the walls of the ducts into the fatty tissue of the breast (Figure 21-38). Because these are confined to the duct and have not spread, they usually have a 100% cure rate. Calcifications and ductal enlargement with extension within the ducts are common (Figure 21-39).

Invasive Ductal Carcinoma (IDC). IDC accounts for nearly 80% of breast cancers. Similar to DCIS, these cancers begin in the ducts, but in contrast to DCIS, they invade the fatty tissue of the breast and have the potential to metastasize via the bloodstream or the lymphatic system. It is important to get a definitive diagnosis and begin treatment before cancer spreads to other organs.

Lobular Carcinoma In Situ (LCIS). Lobular carcinoma in situ (LCIS) is not considered a "cancer" because it has a low malignant potential. LCIS is often referred to as *lobular neoplasia* and is classified as a precancerous

growth that begins in the lobule. LCIS is confined to the gland and does not penetrate through the wall of the lobule. LCIS does not usually form a distinct mass and therefore can be difficult to pick up with the use of only mammography and ultrasound screening. Women with LCIS are at higher risk of developing invasive breast cancer later on.

Invasive Lobular Carcinoma (ILC). ILC begins in the lobule, where it extends into the fatty tissue of the breast. Similar to IDC, invasive lobular carcinoma has the potential to metastasize and spread to other parts of the body. ILC is the second most common type of invasive tumor, accounting for 10% to 15% of all breast cancers. ILC is often bilateral, **multicentric,** or **multifocal** (Figure 21-40).

Breast cancers are considered multifocal when more than one tumor is identified and when they are located within the same quadrant or ductal system and are within 5 cm of each other. Breast cancers are considered multicentric when they are located in different quadrants and are located at least 5 cm apart. Multifocal lesions tend to be of the same cell type histologically, whereas multicentric lesions are more likely to be of two different cell types.

The more favorable cancers remain localized to the breast longer, and treated patients have a 75% survival rate after 10 years. They represent only 10% to 12% of all breast cancers. This group includes medullary,

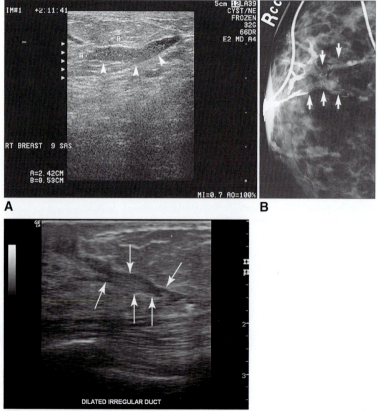

FIGURE 21-38 Intraductal masses. **A,** Sonographic image shows a large intraductal mass in a patient with a unilateral single-duct discharge *(arrowheads)*. **B,** Magnification view from a galactogram, in which contrast was injected retrograde into the duct orifice from which the discharge was expressed. Note the large filling defect *(arrows)*. **C,** Sonographic image from another patient showing a small intraductal mass *(arrows)*. Most intraductal masses are benign papillomas. It is generally difficult, however, to distinguish an intraductal papilloma from an early intraductal cancer.

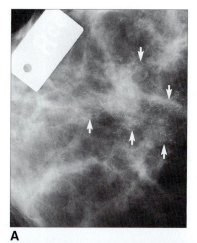

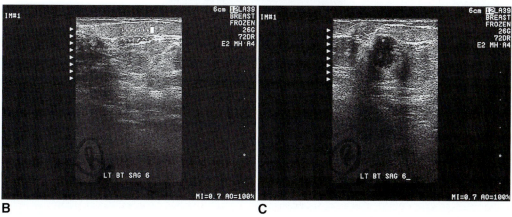

FIGURE 21-39 Suspicious microcalcifications (ductal carcinoma in situ [DCIS]) and occult infiltrating ductal carcinoma. **A,** Magnification mammogram image of pleomorphic (irregular shapes) suspicious microcalcifications identified on screening mammogram in this asymptomatic young woman. No mass was visible on the mammogram. **B,** Sonographic demonstration of echogenic microcalcification within a dilated duct *(arrows)*. **C,** Image of the same breast showing an unsuspected sonographic mass with suspicious features (note that the mass is taller than wide, shows an irregular indistinct margin, and shows asymmetric posterior shadowing and heterogeneous echogenicity). Ultrasound-guided large-needle core biopsy proved infiltrating malignancy. This altered the patient's management, requiring a mastectomy and axillary node dissection for staging.

intracystic papillary, papillary, colloid, adenoid cystic, and tubular carcinomas. Other malignant tumors that have a better than average prognosis after treatment include malignant cystosarcoma phyllodes and stromal sarcomas, because they rarely metastasize to regional nodes.

Definitive identification of a tumor type can be made only by histologic (tissue) examination. Although many solid lesions have definite malignant characteristics, crossover of benign and malignant characteristics is often seen on ultrasound, and the nature of the lesion is indeterminate by sonographic evaluation alone. It is not uncommon for malignant lesions to have a benign appearance on ultrasound, thus making it extremely important to consider the patient's risk factors and clinical history when considering the differential diagnosis. The following is a brief description of the more common malignancies affecting the breast.

Comedocarcinoma. Intraductal solid carcinoma in which the lactiferous ducts are filled with a yellow paste-like material that looks like small plugs (comedones) when sectioned is called comedocarcinoma. Histologically, the ducts are filled with plugs of an epithelial tumor that have a central necrosis, giving rise to the pastelike material. Both invasive and noninvasive forms exist.

Noninvasive forms may lack any clinical or palpatory findings. If a nipple discharge occurs, it is more frequently clear than bloody (unlike papillary carcinoma, in which bloody discharge is typical). The patient may complain of pain or the sensation of insects crawling on the breast. With early invasion, minimal thickening of the surrounding breast tissue may be palpated. In the advanced stage, clinical signs include nipple retraction, dominant mass, and fixation.

Microcalcifications are commonly seen on mammography and may be picked up sonographically. Intraductal carcinomas have malignant characteristics, including irregular margins, a diffuse internal echo pattern, and attenuation with shadowing.

Juvenile Breast Cancer. Juvenile breast cancer is similar to ductal carcinoma in situ and invasive ductal

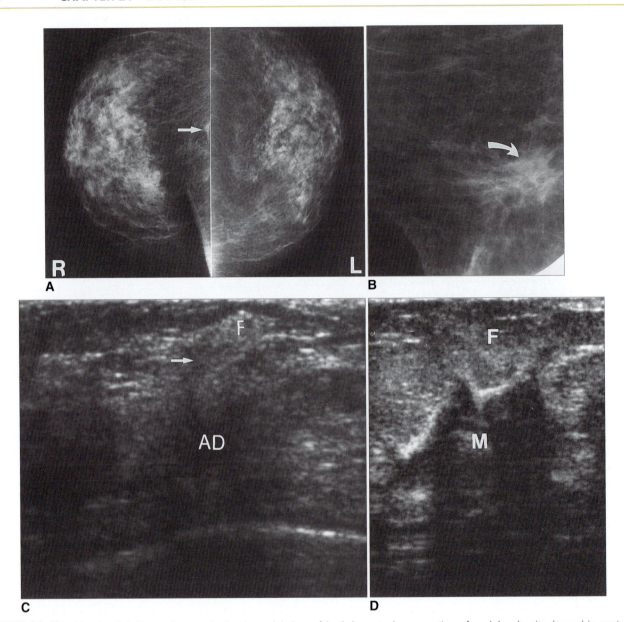

FIGURE 21-40 Infiltrating lobular carcinoma. **A,** Craniocaudal view of both breasts shows portion of nodular density *(arrow)* in posterior central right breast. **B,** Spot compression magnification view shows wispy area *(arrow)* of parenchymal density in the inframammary fold corresponding to the nodule on the craniocaudal view. **C,** Sonogram of area of mammographic abnormality shows hypoechoic, ill-defined area of architectural distortion *(AD)* with infiltration *(arrow)* into the adjacent fibroglandular parenchyma *(F)*; ultrasound-guided biopsy confirmed the diagnosis of infiltrating lobular carcinoma. **D,** In another patient with vague thickening on self-examination, a mammogram showed dense glandular tissue but no focal mass. Ultrasound demonstrates an extensive hypoechoic angular mass *(M)* occupying nearly two thirds of the breast. Fibroglandular tissue *(F)*.

carcinoma as found in adults. Generally, it occurs in young females, between 8 and 15 years of age, and has a good prognosis when treated early.

Papillary Carcinoma. Papillary carcinoma is a tumor that initially arises as an intraductal mass. It may also take the form of an intracystic tumor, which is rare. The early stage of papillary carcinoma is noninvasive. The tumor occasionally arises from a benign ductal papilloma. It is associated with little fibrotic reaction.

Both intraductal and intracystic forms exist, and these represent 1% to 2% of all breast carcinomas. The earliest clinical sign of intraductal papillary carcinoma is bloody nipple discharge. Occasionally, a mass can be palpated as a small, firm, well-circumscribed area and may be mistaken for a fibroadenoma (Figure 21-41). Nodules of blue or red discoloration may be found under the skin with central ulceration. A diffusely nodular appearance overlying the skin is a special variant of multiple intraductal papillary carcinoma. Intracystic papillary carcinoma is clinically indistinguishable in its early stages from a cyst or fibroadenoma. When the tumor has invaded through the cyst wall, it is palpable as a poorly circumscribed mass. Papillary carcinoma typically has a more favorable prognosis than other types of carcinoma.

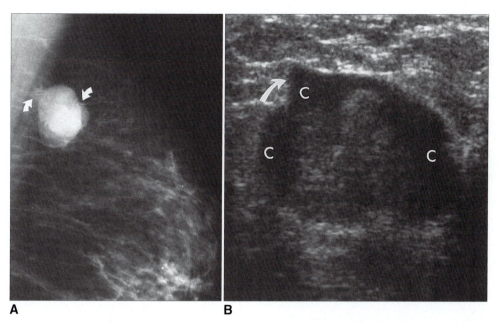

FIGURE 21-41 Papillary carcinoma. **A,** Mediolateral oblique view of the left breast shows well-circumscribed mass containing area of increased density. Slight marginal irregularity is seen *(arrows)*. **B,** Circumscribed complex mass with anterior protuberance *(curved arrow)*. Central area of echogenicity is surrounded circumferentially by what most likely represents the cystic component *(C)* of this in situ papillary carcinoma with stromal invasion.

Paget's Disease. Paget's disease arises in the retroareolar ducts and grows in the direction of the nipple, spreading into the intraepidermal region of the nipple and areola, and has a rashlike appearance that may be confused with a melanoma. Any ulceration, enlargement, or deformity of the nipple and areola should suggest Paget's disease. This is a relatively rare tumor, accounting for 2.5% of all breast cancers. It typically occurs in women over 50 years of age. Differential diagnosis includes benign inflammatory eczematous condition of the nipple, because palpatory findings frequently are not present. The primary ductal cancer may be quite deep or embedded in fibrotic tissue. Sonographically, Paget's disease will present as a retroareolar mass with irregular margins, heterogeneous internal echoes, and attenuation with posterior shadowing.

Scirrhous Carcinoma. Scirrhous carcinoma is a type of intraductal tumor with extensive fibrous tissue proliferation (very dense fibrosis). Focal calcification may also be present. Histologically, the cells are found in narrow files or strands, clusters, or columns and may form lumina with varying frequency.

Scirrhous carcinoma is the most common form of breast cancer and often has no specific histologic findings or patterns; therefore it is often classified as ductal carcinoma that is not otherwise specified (NOS). The classic clinical signs include a very firm nodular, frequently nonmovable mass, often with fixation and flattening of overlying skin and nipple retraction. The retraction is a result of an infiltrative shortening of Cooper's ligaments caused by productive fibrosis (see Figure 21-22). Fixation and retraction of the nipple may be the result of a subareolar

carcinoma, but may also be caused by benign fibrosis of the breast. It is important to note that some patients normally have inverted nipples. The size of the cancer may vary from a few millimeters to involvement of nearly the entire breast. The deep-lying scirrhous carcinoma may grow into and become fixed to the thoracic wall. A bloody discharge is rare with this tumor.

Medullary Carcinoma. Medullary carcinoma is a densely cellular tumor that contains large, round, or oval tumor cells. It usually is a well-circumscribed mass, with the center frequently necrotic, hemorrhagic, and cystic (Figure 21-42). Medullary carcinomas are relatively rare, accounting for less than 5% of breast cancers. The age of occurrence is slightly lower than for the average breast cancer, with a majority of cases occurring in women younger than 50. Medullary carcinomas are usually well circumscribed, often large, and resemble fibroadenoma with a fairly benign appearance. Discoloration of the overlying skin is often seen as a clinical finding, and bilateral occurrence is more frequent with medullary carcinoma than with other cancers.

Colloid Carcinoma. Colloid carcinoma (mucinous) is a relatively rare type of ductal carcinoma that accounts for approximately 3% of breast carcinomas. The cells of the tumor produce secretions that fill lactiferous ducts or stromal tissues in which the tumor cells are invading. Clinically, the tumor presents in older women as a slow-growing, smooth, and not particularly firm mass upon palpation. The sonographic appearance is often similar to a fibroadenoma with smooth margins and posterior enhancement. The echotexture has been described as having a "salt and pepper" appearance (Figure 21-43).

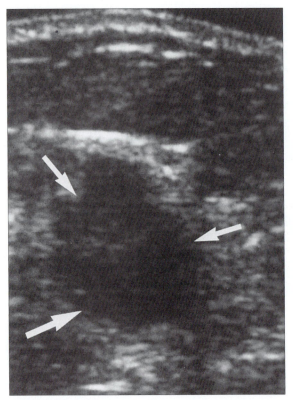

FIGURE 21-42 Medullary carcinoma. Sonogram depicts lobulated mass *(arrows)* with ill-defined margins, low-level internal echoes, and a small amount of posterior acoustic enlargement.

Tubular Carcinoma. Tubular carcinoma represents an extremely well-differentiated form of **infiltrating (invasive) ductal carcinoma** usually less than 2 cm in dimension. Tubular carcinoma occurs in women with an average age of 50 and has a favorable prognosis with a low rate of recurrence or metastasis. Death is rare. Tubular carcinoma typically has poorly circumscribed margins and a hard consistency (Figure 21-44).

Ultrasound-Guided Interventional Procedures

Ultrasound is an important guide for many diagnostic and interventional procedures in the breast. These include cyst aspiration, fine-needle aspiration cytology (FNAC), abscess or seroma drainage, large-core needle biopsy, vacuum-assisted needle biopsy, ultrasound-guided preoperative needle wire localization for surgical excision, and injection of a radiopharmaceutical agent for sentinel node identification and biopsy (Box 21-12). Sterile coupling gel is available commercially, as are sterile plastic transducer sleeves. It is possible and more cost effective to use isopropyl alcohol as a coupling agent during procedures.

When ultrasound is used to guide any diagnostic or interventional procedure in the breast, the high-frequency, narrow-beam linear array transducer is a valuable tool. Even narrow-gauge needles (22 or 25 gauge) can be seen and accurately guided into cysts or masses. The key to

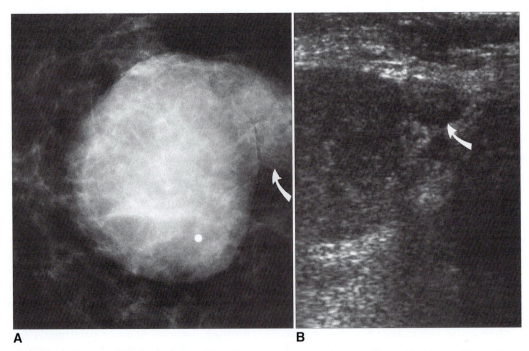

A   **B**

FIGURE 21-43 Mucinous (colloid) carcinoma. **A,** Spot compression mammographic view of palpable (denoted by radiopaque marker) circumscribed mass. A satellite nodule suggestive of diverticulum is seen laterally *(curved arrow)*. **B,** Sonography of a portion of the mass shows that the sonographic margins are well defined and the diverticulum-like satellite *(curved arrow)* is easily seen. This homogeneous mass shows posterior acoustic enhancement.

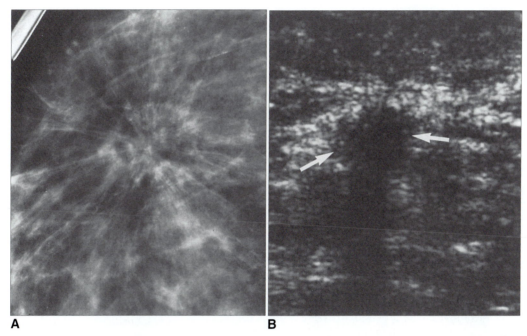

A   **B**

FIGURE 21-44 Tubular carcinoma. **A,** Magnified mammographic view shows mass with central radiolucent areas and very long radiating spiculation, suggesting radial scar. **B,** Sonogram depicts 0.7-cm, solid, hypoechoic mass with irregular, poorly defined margins *(arrows)* and posterior acoustic attenuation—common features of carcinoma.

BOX 21-12	**Ultrasound-Guided Interventional Procedures**

Cyst aspiration
Fine-needle aspiration cytology (FNAC)
Drainage procedures
Preoperative needle (wire) localization
Large-core needle biopsy
Vacuum-assisted needle biopsy
Sentinel node biopsy

---

visualizing the needle is to keep it oriented as nearly parallel to the transducer face as possible. Accuracy in placing the needle tip within the target lesion is also aided when the lesion is kept in the field of vision along with the needle (Figure 21-45). This protects the patient, because the main hazard for the patient is inadvertent piercing of the chest wall. Puncture of the lung resulting in a pneumothorax can occur in some cases with asthenic patients (especially those with emphysema, in which case the lung may protrude between ribs). If care is taken to maintain the needle parallel to the transducer face, the needle tip will remain parallel to the chest wall, and this will help prevent potential complications.

Another important consideration in planning needle procedures in the breast is the approach. When dealing with any breast lesion that has the potential for malignancy, selection of the needle approach can have consequences in future therapeutic and reconstructive surgical procedures. Although the shortest approach from skin

to target lesion has been advocated in the past for preoperative needle wire localizations and is often the favored route for ultrasound-guided core biopsy, a more horizontal approach will often facilitate a better cosmetic outcome for the patient if a mastectomy is necessary. Preprocedure consultation with the referring surgeon concerning the approach for needle wire localizations and core biopsies will ensure the best final outcome for the patient.

Cyst Aspiration. Cyst aspiration is a common interventional technique used in the breast. The cystic fluid is usually "straw-colored" when it is withdrawn, unless it is tinged with blood. The two main indications are a symptomatic cyst (one large enough to create a palpable lump or to cause a patient pain) and a hypoechoic lesion on ultrasound that does not meet criteria for a simple cyst (Figure 21-46). In the latter situation, aspiration determines whether the lesion is simply a complex cyst or a solid mass. This distinction is important for patient management. Occasionally, cyst aspiration will be undertaken because cysts are so large or so numerous that visualization of breast tissue by mammogram is significantly compromised.

Fine-Needle Aspiration Cytology (FNAC). The FNAC procedure uses a fine needle (usually 25 gauge) and an aspiration technique intended to harvest individual cells for diagnosis. The technique is used in the United States and many other countries. It is fast, easy for the patient, and generally very cost effective. The single greatest problem in FNAC is obtaining an adequate specimen. Another limitation in FNAC is the requirement for a

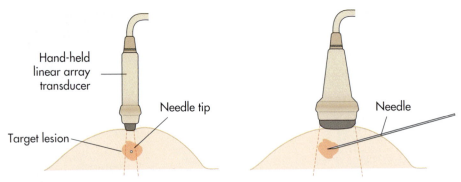

FIGURE 21-45 Placement of the needle tip is facilitated by keeping it in the field of vision and as parallel as possible to the transducer surface.

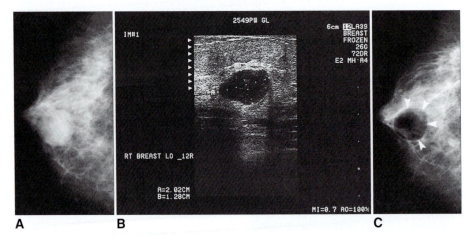

FIGURE 21-46 Complex cyst. **A,** Mammogram shows a smooth, benign appearing dominant mass. **B,** Ultrasound shows a lobular, smooth, hypoechoic lesion with weak posterior acoustic enhancement. Cyst aspiration attempt under ultrasound guidance was done to assess this lesion as cystic or solid. Benign cyst fluid was obtained, and a pneumocystogram (air injected through the aspiration needle into the cyst cavity with a postaspiration mammogram) was performed. **C,** Postaspiration view of a normal pneumocystogram *(arrowheads)* after successful aspiration of a complex cyst. Pneumocystography can be used to exclude the possibility of an intracystic mass and may prevent or retard cyst recurrence.

specially trained and experienced pathologist (cytopathologist)—not available in many centers. This technique has not been as popular in the United States in part because of the somewhat greater inaccuracy of FNAC diagnosis (especially in fibrous malignant lesions and in proliferative benign lesions), and because of the greater availability of the more accurate (although more invasive) large-core needle biopsy.

Drainage Procedures. When clinically indicated, most cases of breast abscess, seroma, or hematoma will be easily palpated and drained in a simple office procedure by a breast surgeon or other physician. In some cases, the physician or surgeon may request ultrasound guidance. These lesions differ from simple cysts in that they typically require a larger needle (at least 18 gauge); have thicker, more fibrous capsules; have thicker fluid, often with abundant cellular debris; and frequently have numerous fibrous synechiae within the lesion that can interfere with complete evacuation of contents. The goal in therapy of a breast abscess is complete eradication of the abscess, usually accomplished through a combina-

tion of drainage and antibiotic therapy. Seromas and hematomas are fluid accumulations within the breast that are not infected. These lesions have similar imaging characteristics (smooth mammographic mass, complex cyst on ultrasound). They differ in the quantity of blood and blood by-products within the fluid. They usually are encountered during healing from surgical procedures and are not infrequently seen after lumpectomy or following a large-core needle biopsy. In some cases, blunt trauma may lead to a hematoma, and occasionally, foreign body reaction or implant rupture may cause a seroma.

Preoperative Needle Wire Localization. Ultrasound offers a quick method for placement of a percutaneous needle wire assembly for preoperative localization of a **nonpalpable** breast lesion for surgical excision (Figure 21-47). Ultrasound guidance offers a significant advantage in complicated cases, such as localization of a lesion adjacent to a breast implant (Figure 21-48), a lesion close to the chest wall, or a lesion in other areas not easily approached under mammographic guidance.

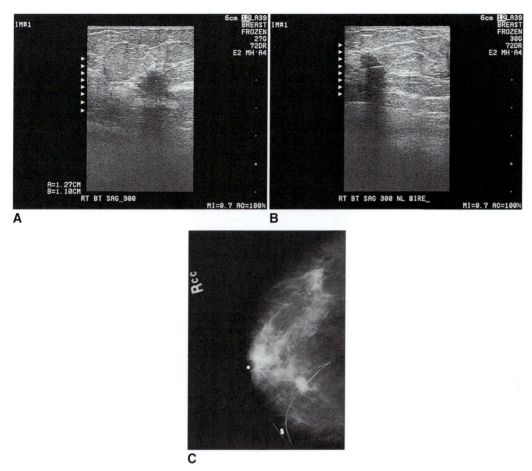

FIGURE 21-47 Preoperative needle wire localization of spiculated cancerous mass. **A,** Ultrasound image shows a sonographic mass with suspicious features. **B,** Ultrasound image shows the echogenic wire through the center of the mass. **C,** Mammogram taken after wire placement shows the hook wire through the center of the cancerous mass. This wire placement aids the surgeon in identifying and removing tissue around the target mass.

Large-Core Needle Biopsy. Ultrasound offers a fast and easy method for guiding large-core needle biopsy of solid masses. Patient comfort is enhanced, procedure time is often shorter, and ultrasound guidance is more cost effective in general than prone stereotactic procedures. It should be noted, however, that stereotactic guidance is still the preferred method for evaluation of clustered pleomorphic microcalcifications, which are difficult to see by ultrasound. An exception to this rule is illustrated in Figure 21-49, in which ultrasound scanning of a patient with multiple suspicious microcalcifications noted on a screening mammogram revealed an unsuspected solid mass. Ultrasound-guided core biopsy of the solid mass revealed infiltrating malignancy, which altered the patient's management.

Vacuum-Assisted Needle Biopsy. A relatively new breast biopsy technique is vacuum-assisted breast biopsy. This type of biopsy is a percutaneous procedure that relies on stereotactic mammography or ultrasound imaging for guidance. Stereotactic mammography is performed using computers to pinpoint the exact location of a breast mass taken from two different angles. The computer coordinates help the physician guide the needle

to a position posterior to the mass. Ultrasound may also be used to guide the needle and allows the physician to observe the biopsy procedure in "real-time." Vacuum-assisted biopsy is a minimally invasive procedure that allows the removal of multiple larger tissue samples with a single insertion of the needle. A special biopsy probe and needle are used. The needle used in a vacuum-assisted biopsy is generally of a larger gauge than needles used for core biopsies and has a special cutting blade at its tip to make the needle easier to insert. The opening of the needle (aperture) is located along the side of the needle on the distal end. Under ultrasound guidance, the needle is inserted immediately posterior to the tumor. Once sampling is initiated, a vacuum pulls the tumor into the opening on the needle, and a rotating cutting blade slices the tissue. The tissue sample is sent to a special chamber in the biopsy probe, where it can be retrieved without removal of the needle. This technique allows multiple tissue samples to be taken with minor rotations of the needle. It is also possible to completely remove smaller masses by taking multiple samples.

Sentinel Node Biopsy. Standard surgical therapy for breast cancer has, for many years, involved a full level I

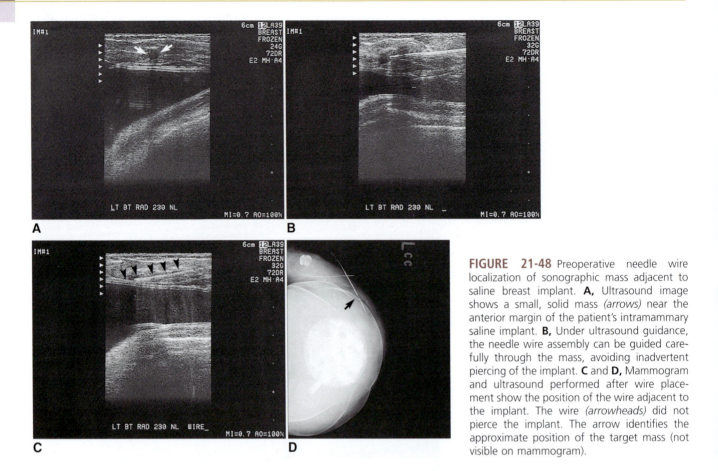

FIGURE 21-48 Preoperative needle wire localization of sonographic mass adjacent to saline breast implant. **A,** Ultrasound image shows a small, solid mass *(arrows)* near the anterior margin of the patient's intramammary saline implant. **B,** Under ultrasound guidance, the needle wire assembly can be guided carefully through the mass, avoiding inadvertent piercing of the implant. **C** and **D,** Mammogram and ultrasound performed after wire placement show the position of the wire adjacent to the implant. The wire *(arrowheads)* did not pierce the implant. The arrow identifies the approximate position of the target mass (not visible on mammogram).

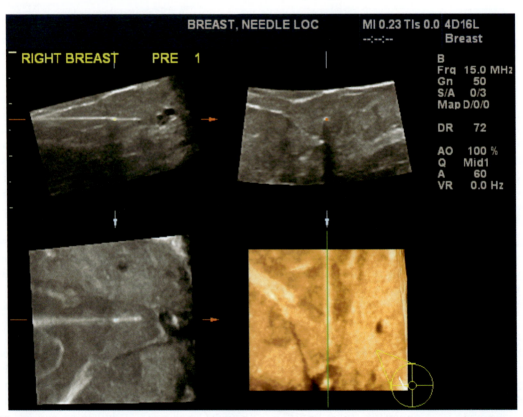

FIGURE 21-49 Ultrasonic guidance for a needle biopsy may aid the clinician in accurate needle placement when the suspected mass is large enough to be imaged with sonography. The needle is shown as the linear bright straight line as it approaches the solid mass. Three-dimensional imaging assures the clinician that the needle is correctly placed within the lesion for biopsy.

and at least a partial level II axillary lymph node dissection. This results in a small but significant rate of morbidity from lymphedema or nerve damage, or, in severe cases, loss of arm and shoulder function. An important step forward in surgical therapy for breast cancer involves sentinel node biopsy (SNB). In this procedure, the superficial subcutaneous tissues around the tumor bed and/or the areola are injected with methylene blue dye and/or radioactive-labeled solution (usually technetium-labeled filtered sulfur colloid). Both of these substances are taken up by the lymphatics and transported to the first, or "sentinel," lymph node along the axillary node chain. This lymph node is then identified in surgery and is carefully analyzed for evidence of metastasis. This is generally followed by a limited axillary node dissection. Early experience with this procedure shows an excellent accuracy rate for detecting lymph node metastases, which results in a reduced rate of morbidity and a faster recovery for the patient (Figure 21-50).

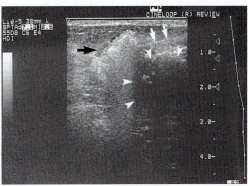

FIGURE 21-50 Injection of radiopharmaceutic agent around tumor for sentinel lymph node identification. Ultrasound image showing echogenic fluid *(arrow)* being injected into the superficial tissue around a mass *(arrowhead)*. The needle is visible *(small arrow)*. Injection of radioactive tracer in a saline solution can be done around the tumor, in the subcutaneous tissue over the tumor, and/or in the periareolar tissue. Over several hours, the radioactive tracer will move through the breast lymphatic system and into the first or "sentinel" lymph node, usually the lowest node in the level I axillary lymph node chain.

The Thyroid and Parathyroid Glands

Sandra L. Hagen-Ansert

The thyroid gland is the part of the endocrine system that maintains body metabolism, growth, and development through the synthesis, storage, and secretion of thyroid hormones. These hormones include triiodothyronine (T_3), thyroxine (T_4), and calcitonin. Disorders of the thyroid may result from pituitary or thyroid gland dysfunction.

Unless the thyroid gland is enlarged, it is not easily palpated by physical examination. A general enlargement of the gland is called a **goiter** with obvious swelling in the neck area. A localized enlargement is a nodular goiter. Both deficient and excessive secretion may cause enlargement.

High-resolution sonography is used to evaluate the thyroid gland as it lies superficially within the neck. The examination is easy to perform and is well tolerated by patients. Sonography of the thyroid is used to define the texture of a palpable lesion (i.e., solid or cystic, complex or calcified) and to determine whether the lesion is single or multiple. The size and location of the nodule and the evaluation of the adjacent lymph node adenopathy may be imaged. Sonography and color Doppler are utilized to define the anatomic structures within and surrounding the thyroid gland rather than to determine the physiology of the gland. The functional state is better determined by nuclear scintigraphy and laboratory measurements of the thyroid hormone present in the blood. Interventional procedures under ultrasound guidance, including **fine-needle aspiration** and alcohol ablation of parathyroid adenomas, are an important application of sonography. Evaluation of the parathyroid gland and other lesions of the neck will also be presented in this chapter.

ANATOMY OF THE THYROID GLAND

The thyroid gland is located in the anteroinferior neck at the level of the thyroid cartilage. The gland consists of a right and a left lobe located along either side of the

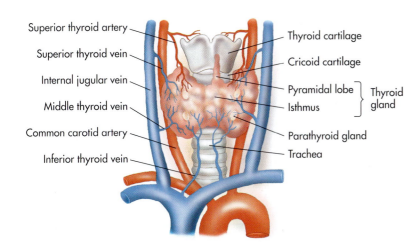

Superior thyroid artery
Superior thyroid vein
Internal jugular vein
Middle thyroid vein
Common carotid artery
Inferior thyroid vein

Thyroid cartilage
Cricoid cartilage
Pyramidal lobe
Isthmus
Parathyroid gland
Trachea

} Thyroid gland

FIGURE 22-1 Anterior view of the thyroid and parathyroid glands.

TABLE 22-1	Size of the Thyroid	
Dimension	**Adults**	**Children**
Length	40–60 mm	20–30 mm
Anteroposterior	20–30 mm	12–15 mm
Width	15–20 mm	10–15 mm

trachea and connected across the midline by the thin bridge of thyroid tissue called the **isthmus.** The thyroid straddles the trachea anteriorly, whereas the paired lobes extend on either side of the trachea, bounded laterally by the carotid arteries and jugular veins (Figure 22-1). When present, the **pyramidal lobe** arises from the isthmus and tapers superiorly just anterior to the thyroid cartilage. This segment may be seen in the pediatric population but usually atrophies in the adult.

Size

The size and shape of the thyroid gland vary with gender, age, and body surface area, with females having a slightly larger gland than males (Table 22-1). In tall individuals, the lateral lobes of the thyroid have a longitudinally elongated shape on sagittal scans, whereas in shorter individuals, the gland is more oval. As a result, the normal dimensions of the gland have a wide range of variability. The lobes are normally equal in size. In the newborn, the gland measures 18 to 20 mm long, with an anteroposterior (AP) diameter of 8 to 9 mm. By age 1, the mean length is 25 mm and the AP diameter is 12 to 15 mm. The normal adult thyroid measures 40 to 60 mm in length, 20 to 30 mm in AP diameter, and 13 to 18 mm in width. The gland is considered enlarged when the AP diameter measures greater than 20 mm. The isthmus is the smallest part of the gland with an AP diameter of 4 to 6 mm. A pyramidal lobe that extends superiorly from the isthmus is present in 15% to 30% of patients.

The thyroid volume may be useful to determine the size of the goiter to assess the need for surgery, to calculate the dose of iodine-131 for thyrotoxicosis, or to evaluate the response to suppression treatments. The method commonly used to calculate thyroid volume is based on the ellipsoid formula with a correction factor (length × width × thickness × 0.52 for each lobe). The normal mean thyroid volume is 18.6 ± 4.5 ml. The volume in males is slightly greater than in females.

Relational Anatomy

Anterior. Along the anterior surface of the thyroid gland lie the **strap muscles,** including the sternothyroid, omohyoid, sternohyoid, and **sternocleidomastoid muscles** (Figure 22-2). The sternohyoid and omohyoid muscles are seen on ultrasound as thin, hypoechoic bands anterior to the gland. The sternocleidomastoid muscle is seen as a larger oval band that lies anterior and lateral to the gland.

Posterior. Posterolateral anatomy includes the carotid sheath with the common carotid artery, internal jugular vein, and vagus nerve. The **longus colli muscle** is posterior and lateral to each thyroid lobe and appears as a hypoechoic triangular structure adjacent to the cervical vertebrae (see Figure 22-2).

Medial. Medial anatomy consists of the larynx, trachea, inferior constrictor of the pharynx, and esophagus. The esophagus, primarily a midline structure, may be found to the left of the trachea (see Figure 22-2). It is identified by the target appearance in the transverse plane and by its peristaltic movements when the patient swallows. The posterior border of each thyroid lobe is related to the superior and inferior parathyroid glands and the anastomosis between the superior and inferior thyroid arteries.

Blood Supply

Blood is supplied to the thyroid by four arteries. Two superior thyroid arteries arise from the external carotids and descend to the upper poles. Two inferior thyroid arteries arise from the thyrocervical trunk of the subclavian artery and ascend to the lower poles. Doppler peak systolic velocities reach 20 to 40 cm/sec in the major thyroid arteries and 15 to 30 cm/sec in the

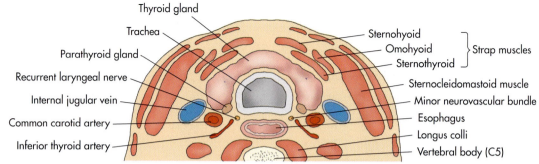

FIGURE 22-2 Cross section of the thyroid region showing the thyroid gland and vascular and muscular relationships to one another.

intraparenchymal arteries. Corresponding veins drain into the internal jugular veins (see Figure 22-1).

THYROID PHYSIOLOGY AND LABORATORY DATA

As part of the endocrine system, the role of the thyroid is to maintain normal body metabolism, growth, and development by the synthesis, storage, and secretion of thyroid hormones. The mechanism for producing thyroid hormones is iodine metabolism. The thyroid gland traps iodine from the blood and, through a series of chemical reactions, produces the thyroid hormones triiodothyronine (T_3) and thyroxine (T_4). These are stored in the colloid of the gland. When thyroid hormone is needed by the body, it is released into the bloodstream by the action of thyrotropin, or **thyroid-stimulating hormone (TSH)**, which is produced by the pituitary gland.

The secretion of TSH is regulated by thyrotropin-releasing factor, which is produced by the hypothalamus (located in the brain). The level of thyrotropin-releasing factor is controlled by the basal metabolic rate. A decrease in the basal metabolic rate—a result of a low concentration of thyroid hormones—causes an increase in thyrotropin-releasing factor. This causes increased secretion of TSH and a subsequent increase in the release of thyroid hormones. When the blood level of hormones is returned to normal, the basal metabolic rate returns to normal and TSH secretion stops.

Calcitonin decreases the concentration of calcium in the blood by first acting on bone to inhibit its breakdown. With less bone being resorbed, less calcium moves out of bone into blood, decreasing the concentration of calcium in the blood. Calcitonin secretion increases after any concentration of blood calcium increases. Thus calcitonin helps to maintain homeostasis of blood calcium and helps prevent an excess of calcium in the blood (hypercalcemia).

Euthyroid, Hypothyroidism, and Hyperthyroidism

Euthyroid. When the thyroid is producing the correct amount of thyroid hormone, it is considered to be

BOX 22-1	Disorders Associated With Hyperthyroidism

Common (account for 99% of cases)
Diffuse toxic hyperplasia (Graves' disease)
Toxic multinodular goiter
Toxic adenoma

Uncommon
Acute or subacute thyroiditis
Hyperfunctioning thyroid cancer
Choriocarcinoma or hydatidiform mole
Thyroid-stimulating hormone (TSH)-secreting pituitary adenoma
Neonatal thyrotoxicosis associated with maternal Graves' disease

normal, or **euthyroid.** Abnormal secretions of the thyroid hormone may result in hypothyroidism (undersecretion) or hyperthyroidism (oversecretion).

Hypothyroidism. The undersecretion of thyroid hormones is **hypothyroidism.** This condition may be caused by low intake of iodine (goiter) in the body, inability of the thyroid to produce the proper amount of thyroid hormone, or a problem in the pituitary gland that does not control thyroid production.

Clinical signs and symptoms of hypothyroidism include myxedema, weight gain, hair loss, increased subcutaneous tissue around the eyes, lethargy, intellectual and motor slowing, cold intolerance, constipation, and a deep husky voice. Treatment with thyroid hormone can reverse the condition.

Hyperthyroidism. The oversecretion of thyroid hormones is **hyperthyroidism.** This occurs when the entire gland is out of control, or when a localized neoplasm (such as an adenoma) causes overproduction of the thyroid hormone.

Hyperthyroidism dramatically increases the metabolic rate; clinical signs include weight loss, increased appetite, high degree of nervous energy, tremor, excessive sweating, heat intolerance, and palpitations, and many patients show signs of exophthalmos (protruding eyes). Box 22-1 lists the common disorders associated with hyperthyroidism, which account for 99% of cases of hyperthyroidism.

Tests of Thyroid Function

Nuclear medicine is used to determine the function of the thyroid. A small amount of radioactive iodine is injected into the bloodstream. In normal individuals, a certain percentage of the amount injected will be taken into the thyroid gland within 24 hours. In patients with hyperthyroidism, a greater percentage is taken up; in patients with hypothyroidism, a smaller percentage is taken up. The amount taken up by the thyroid is determined by measuring the radioactivity accumulated in the gland with a gamma camera.

The laboratory tests for thyroid measure the amount of T_3 or T_4 in the blood. This amount is elevated in patients with hyperthyroidism and is decreased in patients with hypothyroidism.

SONOGRAPHIC EVALUATION OF THE THYROID

The sonographer should obtain a patient history before the ultrasound examination. Pertinent information regarding the patient's general health, thyroid medications, previous imaging studies (i.e., scintigraphy), family history of hyperparathyroidism or thyroid cancer, or prior history of radiation or surgery to the neck should be noted in the examination record.

The patient is placed in the supine position with a pillow under both shoulders to provide a moderate hyperextension of the neck. This position allows the lower lobes of the gland to be more readily visualized with ultrasound.

A high-frequency (7.5- to 15-MHz) linear-array transducer should be used. Each lobe requires careful scanning in longitudinal and transverse planes. The lateral, mid, and medial parts of each lobe are examined in the longitudinal plane (Figure 22-3) and are so labeled. The superior, mid, and inferior portions of each gland are examined individually and labeled in the transverse plane (Figure 22-4). If possible, the patient's head should be turned to the opposite side to enable better visualization of each lobe. Having the patient swallow allows visualization of the lower pole of the thyroid gland. Swallowing raises the entire gland and brings the lower pole into the field of view.

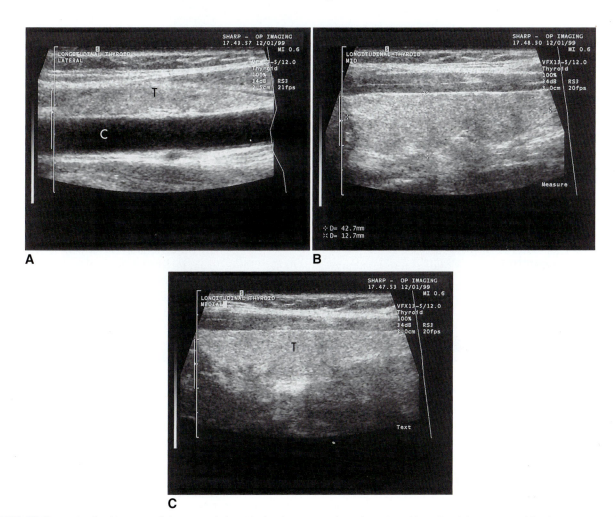

FIGURE 22-3 Longitudinal images of the normal thyroid gland. **A,** Long, lateral. *C,* Carotid; *T,* thyroid. **B,** Long, mid. Measurement of the length and anteroposterior (AP) dimension of the gland. **C,** Long, medial. *T,* Thyroid.

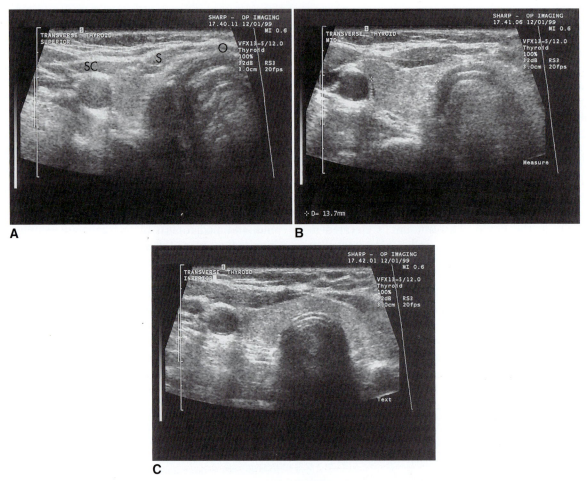

FIGURE 22-4 Transverse images of the normal thyroid gland. **A,** Trans, superior. *O,* Omohyoid muscle; *S,* sternohyoid muscle; *SC,* sterno-cleidomastoid. **B,** Trans, mid. Measurement of the width of the gland. **C,** Trans, inferior.

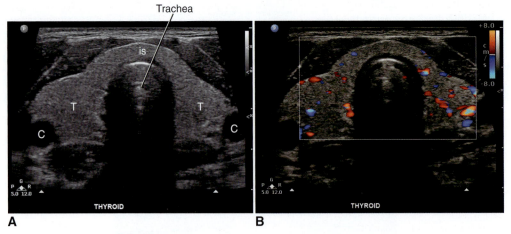

FIGURE 22-5 Normal image **(A)** and color Doppler **(B)** of both lobes of the thyroid show the comparable homogeneity of each lobe. *C,* Carotid; *T,* thyroid; *is,* isthmus.

Landmarks for the transverse image include the common carotid artery, the trachea, and the jugular vein (Figure 22-5). The common carotid artery is a circular, pulsatile structure directly adjacent to the gland. The oval-shaped jugular vein is lateral to the carotid artery. The trachea is noted in the middle of the neck with posterior shadowing.

Transverse and longitudinal images of the isthmus must also be obtained (Figure 22-6). The examination should extend laterally to include the region of the carotid artery and jugular vein to identify enlarged cervical lymph nodes.

The normal thyroid gland has a fine homogeneous echotexture that is slightly more echogenic than the

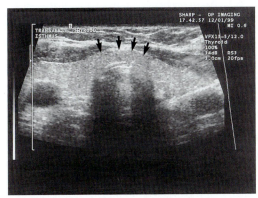

FIGURE 22-6 The isthmus (arrows) is shown in the transverse view at the inferior border of the thyroid gland.

surrounding muscle structure. The thyroid capsule is imaged as a thin hyperechoic line that clearly outlines the gland from the other anatomy. The tiny vascular structures may be seen as tubular anechoic structures within the gland. Color Doppler with low pulse repetition frequency (PRF) will distinguish these structures as blood-filled. The superior thyroid artery and vein may be found in the upper pole of the lobes, and the inferior thyroid artery and vein are found in the lower part of the lobes. Flow velocities in peak systole are 20 to 40 cm/sec in the major arteries and 15 to 30 cm/sec in intraparenchymal arteries.

The muscles surrounding the gland are hypoechoic compared with the thyroid tissue. The sternohyoid and omohyoid muscles are anterior to the gland, and the sternocleidomastoid muscle is lateral to the gland. The longus colli muscle is found posterior to either lobe of the thyroid. The recurrent laryngeal nerve and the inferior thyroid artery pass in the angle between the trachea, esophagus, and thyroid lobe. On longitudinal scans, the recurrent laryngeal nerve and inferior thyroid artery may be seen between the thyroid lobe and esophagus on the left and between the thyroid lobe and longus colli muscle on the right. The esophagus may be seen midline or slightly to the left of the midline, next to the trachea, with a hypoechoic rim surrounding an echogenic center.

If an abnormality is encountered, all sonographic characteristics (i.e., cystic areas, calcifications, or a halo) should be demonstrated. It is not uncommon for sonography to demonstrate multiple nodules in a gland previously suspected of having only a solitary lesion.

PATHOLOGY OF THE THYROID GLAND

Congenital abnormalities of the thyroid gland include agenesis, hypoplasia, and ectopia. Agenesis may occur in one lobe or in the entire gland. Hypoplasia refers to underdevelopment of part of the gland.

Nodular Thyroid Disease

Hyperplasia and Goiter. Nodular hyperplasia, multinodular goiter, and adenomatous hyperplasia are some of the terms used to describe goiter, which is the most common thyroid abnormality. Approximately 80% of nodular thyroid disease is due to hyperplasia of the gland. This condition occurs in up to 5% of the population. The most common cause of thyroid disorders worldwide is iodine deficiency, which leads to goiter formation and hypothyroidism. In areas not deficient in iodine, autoimmune processes are believed to be the basis for most cases of thyroid disease, which ranges from hyperthyroidism to hypothyroidism. When hyperplasia leads to overall enlargement of the thyroid gland, the term *goiter* is used. Women are more likely to have this disease, which peaks at between 30 and 50 years. Table 22-2 lists the clinical findings, sonographic findings, and differential considerations for nodular thyroid disease.

Hyperplasia develops at the cellular level of the thyroid acini, leading to micronodule and macronodule formation. These nodules then undergo liquefactive degeneration with resultant accumulation of blood, serous fluid, and colloid substance. At this point pathologically they are known as hyperplastic, adenomatous, and colloid nodules. Many of the cystic thyroid lesions are hyperplastic nodules that have undergone extensive liquefactive degeneration. The function of these hyperplastic nodules may be decreased, normal, or increased (toxic nodules).

Goiter is an enlargement of the thyroid gland that is often visible as an anterior protrusion on the neck. The enlargement is due to compensatory hypertrophy and hyperplasia of the follicular epithelium caused by a derangement that hampers hormone secretion. A goiter may become very large, compressing the esophagus and interfering with swallowing, or it can cause pressure on the trachea. Other causes of goiter include Graves' disease, thyroiditis, neoplasm, or a cyst. Goiters may be diffuse and symmetrical or irregular and nodular. They may result from hyperplasia, neoplasia, or an inflammatory process.

Endemic goiter may affect large groups of people in a specific geographic area. This usually occurs in areas where iodine levels in the soil and food are low (e.g., mountainous areas, areas around the Great Lakes). Normally, iodine is trapped by the thyroid gland and is used to synthesize the T_3 and T_4 hormones. This dietary deficiency leads to low T_3 and T_4 production and a compensatory increase in TSH from the pituitary, producing hyperplasia and hypertrophy in the thyroid gland. For the most part, the use of iodized salt has solved this problem.

Certain types of foods may block the synthesis of T_3 and T_4 but increase TSH secretion. Thus TSH causes hyperplasia of the gland and can promote goiter

TABLE 22-2	Thyroid Findings: Nodular Thyroid Disease	
Clinical Findings	**Sonographic Findings**	**Differential Considerations**
Nontoxic Simple Goiter		
Thyroid enlargement	Sometimes smooth, sometimes nodular; possible compression of surrounding structures	Thyroiditis Hypothyroidism Neoplasm
Toxic Multinodular Goiter		
Thyroid enlargement	Enlarged inhomogeneous gland; can have focal scarring, focal ischemia, necrosis, and cyst formation	Neoplasm Cyst
Graves' Disease		
Diffuse toxic goiter	Diffusely homogeneous and enlarged	Neoplasm Ophthalmopathy Cutaneous manifestations Hyperthyroidism
Thyroiditis		
Swelling and tenderness of the thyroid; later, hypothyroidism	Homogeneous enlargement with nodularity; later, inhomogeneous	Neoplasm
Benign Lesions		
Cysts		
Solitary nodules or multiple nodules	Anechoic areas, echogenic fluid, or moving fluid levels	Toxic multinodular goiter
Adenoma		
Usually euthyroid or hyperthyroid	Compression of adjacent structures; fibrous encapsulation; ranges from anechoic to hyperechoic; may have halo	Graves' disease

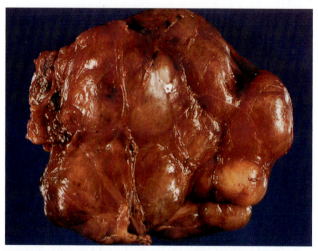

FIGURE 22-7 Gross pathology of a nodular goiter. The thyroid is enlarged with nodules that vary in size and shape.

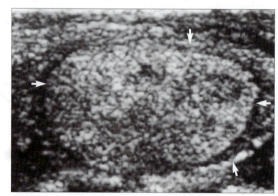

FIGURE 22-8 The heterogeneous appearance is well seen within the adenoma with well-defined, discrete borders. The hypoechoic halo is shown surrounding the lesion *(arrows).*

formation when such food (i.e., cabbage, turnips, and other related vegetables) is ingested in large quantities.

A toxic goiter is a hyperthyroid condition resulting from hyperactivity of the thyroid gland, perhaps caused by excessive stimulation from TSH, which produces a large nodular gland.

Nontoxic (simple) goiter occurs as a diffuse thyroid enlargement not resulting from a neoplasm or inflammation. It is not initially associated with hypothyroidism or hyperthyroidism. The goiter is formed when the gland is unable to provide an adequate supply of thyroid hormone. This deficiency may be the result of iodine shortage (dietary) or malfunction of the gland itself. The gland becomes diffusely and uniformly enlarged in an attempt to trap and use every atom of iodine. Often the gland is able to keep up with the demand and provides normal release of hormones. However, in some cases, the gland lags behind the demand and the patient develops hypothyroidism. In the first stage, hyperplasia occurs; in the second stage, colloid involution occurs (Figure 22-7). Progression of this process leads to an asymmetrical and multinodular gland with hemorrhage and calcification (Figure 22-8). Laboratory data reveal evidence of hypothyroidism.

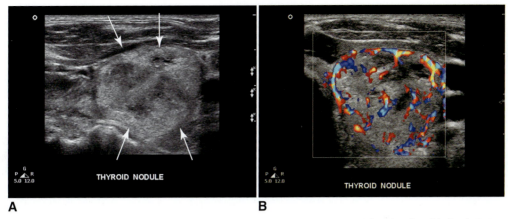

FIGURE 22-9 A, Multinodular goiter is seen as an inhomogeneous enlarged tissue mass within the thyroid gland. **B,** Increased vascularity is shown in a patient with a multinodular goiter.

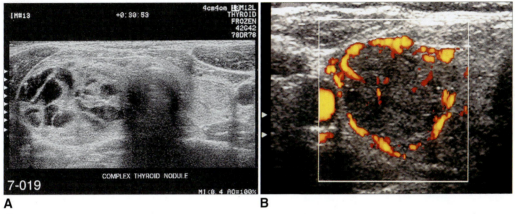

FIGURE 22-10 A, A patient with an asymmetrical, multinodular goiter on the right shows a complex sonographic pattern. The left lobe is normal. **B,** Increased vascularity is seen surrounding the heterogeneous lesion.

◆ Sonographic Findings. Most hyperplastic or adenomatous nodules are isoechoic compared with normal thyroid tissue. As the gland enlarges, it may become hyperechoic as a result of numerous interfaces between cells and colloid substance. As the disease progresses, areas of focal scarring and ischemia, as well as necrosis and cyst formation, may appear within the gland (Figure 22-9). Fibrosis or calcifications may also manifest. Some of the nodules are poorly circumscribed; others appear to be encapsulated (Figure 22-10). Enlargement can involve one lobe to a greater extent than the other and sometimes causes difficulty in breathing and swallowing (Figure 22-11).

When the nodule is isoechoic or hyperechoic, a thin peripheral hypoechoic halo is commonly seen as a result of perinodular blood vessels and mild edema. Hyperfunctioning nodules usually demonstrate increased perinodular and intranodular vascularity on color Doppler.

Benign Lesions

A discrete nodule of the thyroid gland is the most common reason for an ultrasound examination. Nodular thyroid disease is frequently encountered in the adult

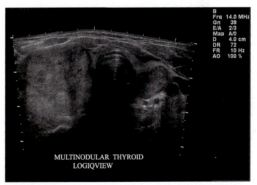

FIGURE 22-11 Multinodular goiter shows an inhomogeneous pattern. Right lobe is more than twice the size of the left lobe.

population, with up to 7% found to have a benign nodule, with women affected more frequently than men. Nodules can be imaged with ultrasound and described to help determine whether the nodule is benign or malignant. Confirmation of the complex or solid lesion may be made through fine-needle biopsy.

Cyst. A cyst in the thyroid gland is thought to be representative of cystic degeneration of a follicular adenoma.

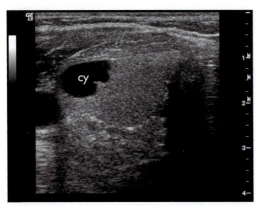

FIGURE 22-12 A large, anechoic cyst *(cy)* is seen within the normal thyroid gland.

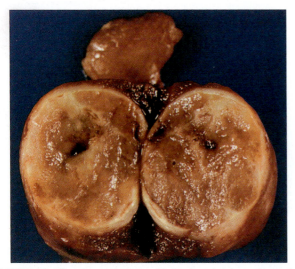

FIGURE 22-13 Gross pathology of follicular adenoma. The nodule is well circumscribed with a fibrous capsule separating it from the normal parenchyma.

🔖 **Sonographic Findings.** The degenerative changes of nodules correspond to their sonographic appearance. Purely anechoic areas result from serous or colloid fluid, echogenic fluid, or moving fluid; fluid levels correspond to hemorrhage. Approximately 20% of solitary nodules are cystic. Blood or debris may be present within the nodule (Figure 22-12). As with all simple cysts, the sonographic appearance of a simple thyroid cyst must be anechoic and must reveal sharp, well-defined walls and distal acoustic enhancement.

Adenoma. A follicular **adenoma** is a benign thyroid neoplasm characterized by complete fibrous encapsulation. Adenomas represent only 5% to 10% of all nodular diseases of the thyroid and are seven times more common in females than in males. The benign follicular adenoma is a true thyroid neoplasm that is characterized by compression of adjacent tissue and fibrous encapsulation (Figure 22-13).

Adenomas are homogeneous with variable size. Usually the lesion is solitary with areas of hemorrhage or necrosis. The adenoma is slow growing

unless hemorrhage occurs, causing sudden and painful enlargement. Most patients are euthyroid or hyperthyroid. Some nodules produce a thyroid hormone; if they do, they may or may not be controlled by the usual hormonal controls.

🔖 **Sonographic Findings.** Adenomas have a broad spectrum of ultrasound appearances. They range from anechoic to completely hyperechoic and commonly have a peripheral halo. The halo, or thin echolucent rim surrounding the lesion, may represent edema of the compressed normal thyroid tissue or the capsule of the adenoma (Figure 22-14). In a few instances, blood may surround the lesion. Although the halo is a relatively consistent finding in adenomas, additional statistical information is necessary to establish its specificity. Hyperfunction of the adenoma can exhibit enhanced blood flow patterns as seen on Doppler along the peripheral borders or within the lesion.

Adenomas that contain anechoic areas are a result of cystic degeneration (probably from hemorrhage) and usually lack a well-rounded margin. This lack of a discrete cystic margin is helpful in differentiation from a simple cyst. Calcification along the rim can also be associated with adenoma. Its acoustic shadow may preclude visualization posteriorly. Color Doppler has not been found to add specific information to the examination performed in an effort to separate a benign from a malignant process.

Malignant Lesions

Carcinoma of the thyroid is rare. A solitary nodule may be malignant in a small percentage of cases, but the risk of malignancy decreases with the presence of multiple nodules. A solitary thyroid nodule in the presence of cervical adenopathy on the same side suggests malignancy.

🔖 **Sonographic Findings.** The ultrasound appearance of thyroid cancer is highly variable. The neoplasm can be of any size, single or multiple, and can appear as a solid, partially cystic, or largely cystic mass. Occasionally, thyroid cancer presents as a small, solid nodule. Thyroid cancer is usually hypoechoic relative to normal thyroid, but thyroid carcinomas with the same echo texture as normal thyroid have been reported. Calcifications are present in 50% to 80% of all types of thyroid carcinoma. Increased vascularity may be noted.

Papillary Carcinoma. The most common of the thyroid malignancies is called **papillary carcinoma**. Females are affected more often than males. Round, laminated calcifications are seen in 25% of cases (Figure 22-15). The major route of spread of papillary carcinoma is through the lymphatics to the nearby cervical lymph nodes. Approximately 20% of patients with papillary thyroid cancer have metastatic cervical adenopathy.

🔖 **Sonographic Findings.** Sonographic characteristics of papillary carcinoma include hypoechogenicity (90% of

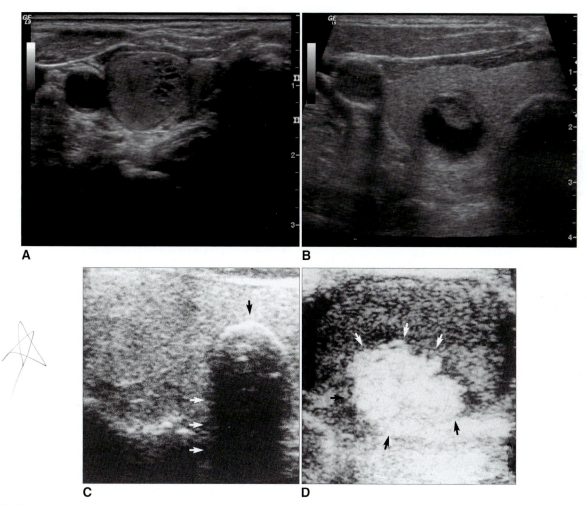

FIGURE 22-14 Sonographic variations of adenomas. **A,** A well-defined adenoma with a hypoechoic halo is seen on the right lobe. **B,** Thyroid adenoma demonstrating a halo. **C,** Large calcification within a thyroid adenoma *(black arrow)*. Shadowing from the calcification *(white arrows)*. **D,** Large, echogenic mass within the hemorrhagic adenoma *(arrows)*.

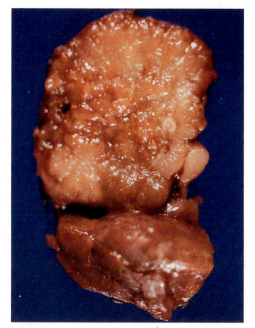

FIGURE 22-15 Gross pathology of papillary carcinoma. Large solid tumor mass nearly replaced one lobe of the thyroid gland.

cases), **microcalcifications** that appear as tiny, punctate hyperechoic foci (with or without acoustic shadowing), hypervascularity (90% of cases), and cervical lymph node metastasis (in approximately 20% of cases) (Figure 22-16).

Follicular Carcinoma. Follicular carcinoma is the second subtype of well-differentiated thyroid cancer. Two types of follicular carcinoma are known: minimally invasive and widely invasive. The minimally invasive type is well encapsulated; histologically, the demonstration of focal invasion of capsular blood vessels of the fibrous capsule permits differentiation from follicular adenoma. The widely invasive type is not encapsulated; however, invasion of the blood vessels and adjacent thyroid tissue occurs. This type of cancer spreads through the bloodstream rather than by the lymphatics, with mestastases to bone, lung, brain, and liver. Follicular carcinoma of the thyroid is usually a solitary mass of the thyroid and is more aggressive than papillary cancer (Figure 22-17).

Sonographic Findings. An irregular margin with a thick irregular halo, nodular enlargement, and tortuous

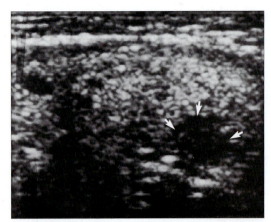

FIGURE 22-16 Solitary lesion representing a papillary carcinoma upon biopsy *(arrows).*

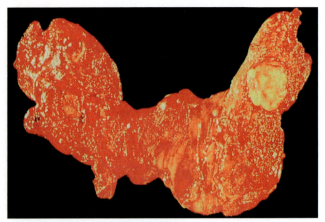

FIGURE 22-18 Gross pathology of medullary carcinoma shows a well-defined mass in the thyroid gland.

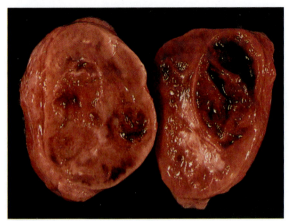

FIGURE 22-17 Gross pathology of follicular carcinoma shows a well-circumscribed tumor.

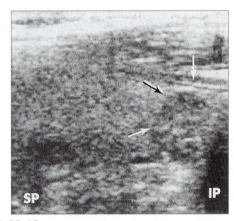

FIGURE 22-19 Arrows indicate a medullary carcinoma causing enlargement of the inferior pole of the right thyroid gland. *IP,* Inferior pole; *SP,* superior pole.

internal blood vessels is characteristic, but not specific, for follicular carcinoma.

Medullary Carcinoma. **Medullary carcinoma** accounts for 5% of thyroid cancers. This cancer is often familial (20%) and is an essential component of the multiple endocrine neoplasia (MEN) type II syndromes. The disease may be multicentered and/or bilateral in familial cases. A high incidence of metastatic involvement of the lymph nodes has been reported (Figure 22-18).

Sonographic Findings. In patients with medullary thyroid carcinoma, thyroid lesions appear similar to those of papillary carcinoma as a hypoechoic mass (Figure 22-19). Calcium deposits are often noted. Sonography is highly sensitive in detecting metastatic lymphadenopathy in these patients; thus careful evaluation of the entire neck area and liver is important to rule out metastases.

Anaplastic Carcinoma. **Anaplastic carcinoma** (*anaplastic* means undifferentiated) is rare and accounts for less than 2% of thyroid cancers. It usually occurs after age 50. This lesion presents as a hard, fixed mass with rapid growth. Its growth is locally invasive in surrounding neck structures, and it usually causes death by compression and asphyxiation due to invasion of the trachea.

Sonographic Findings. The sonographic appearance of this type of thyroid cancer is as a hypoechoic mass, with invasion of surrounding muscles and vessels of the neck.

Lymphoma. Lymphoma in the thyroid is primarily the non-Hodgkin type. The tumor affects older females and accounts for 4% of all thyroid malignancies. Clinically, the patient has a rapidly growing mass in the neck area. In many cases of lymphoma, the patient has a preexisting chronic lymphocytic thyroiditis (Hashimoto's disease) with subclinical or overt hypothyroidism.

Sonographic Findings. The sonographic appearance of lymphoma is characterized by a nonvascular hypoechoic and lobulated mass. Large areas of cystic necrosis may be noted within the tumor or encasement of adjacent neck vessels. The adjacent thyroid parenchyma may be heterogeneous secondary to associated chronic thyroiditis.

Diffuse Thyroid Disease

Several diseases of the thyroid are characterized by diffuse involvement of the gland. This generally causes diffuse enlargement of the gland (goiter) without palpable nodules. Conditions that produce diffuse enlargement of the gland include Graves' disease, thyroiditis, and colloid or adenomatous goiter. Specific diagnosis is made on the basis of clinical and laboratory findings. Sonography is usually not indicated in this condition as the gland is diffusely enlarged; however, it may be indicated if a suspected thyroid mass may be present. In diffuse enlargement, the isthmus of the gland may measure 1 cm or greater.

Thyroiditis. Types of thyroiditis include acute suppurative thyroiditis, subacute granulomatous thyroiditis (de Quervain's disease), and chronic lymphocytic thyroiditis (Hashimoto's disease). Swelling and tenderness of the thyroid is called **thyroiditis,** which is caused by infection or can be related to autoimmune abnormalities. Sonography can be utilized to locate an abscess within the thyroid gland, which appears as an irregular, ill-defined, hypoechoic, heterogeneous mass with internal debris with or without septa and/or gas. Adjacent inflammatory nodes may also be present.

Subacute (de Quervain's) thyroiditis is probably caused by a viral infection of the thyroid, which results in diffuse inflammation of the thyroid with enlargement and tenderness. The disease has a gradual or fairly abrupt onset, and the pain may be severe. de Quervain's thyroiditis may cause transient hyperthyroidism, but, in a period of weeks or months, the swelling and pain subside and the gland functions normally. With sonography the gland may appear enlarged and hypoechoic with normal or decreased vascularity secondary to diffuse edema of the gland, or the process may appear as focal hypoechoic regions.

Hashimoto's thyroiditis, the most common form of thyroiditis, is characterized by a destructive autoimmune disorder, which leads to chronic inflammation of the thyroid. The outstanding feature is a painless, diffusely enlarged gland in a young or middle-aged female. The entire gland is involved with an inflammatory reaction; enlargement is not necessarily symmetrical (Figure 22-20). On sonography, the gland shows a diffuse coarsened parenchymal texture that is slightly more hypoechoic than a normal thyroid (Figure 22-21). Homogeneous enlargement initially occurs with nodularity; as the disease progresses, the gland shows inhomogeneous enlargement (micronodulation). Mild to moderate tenderness is present. Color Doppler shows normal to decreased flow velocity, although occasionally, the "thyroid inferno" pattern is seen when hypothyroidism develops. Eventually, the gland becomes severely damaged with resultant hypothyroidism. Cervical lymphadenopathy may also develop.

Graves' Disease. Graves' disease occurs more frequently in women over 30 years of age and is related to an autoimmune disorder. It is characterized by thyrotoxicosis and is the most frequent cause of hyperthyroidism. Graves' disease is characterized by a triad of the

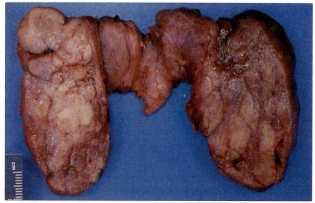

FIGURE 22-20 Gross pathology of a patient with Hashimoto's thyroiditis. The enlarged gland is multinodular with multiple lymphoid infiltrates.

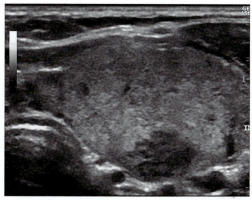

FIGURE 22-21 Sonographic image of a patient with Hashimoto's thyroiditis demonstrates the inhomogeneous enlarged thyroid gland.

following findings: hypermetabolism, diffuse toxic goiter, exophthalmos (inflammatory infiltration of the orbital tissue resulting in proptosis, or bulging of the eyes), and cutaneous manifestations (thickening of the dermis of the pretibial areas and the dorsum of the feet). Hyperthyroidism associated with a diffuse hyperplastic goiter is present (Figure 22-22). Clinically, the thyroid gland is diffusely homogeneous and enlarged.

Exophthalmos is characterized by the presence of protruding, staring eyes with decreased movement. This results from increased tissue mass in the orbit that pushes the eyeball forward, and from increased sympathetic stimulation that affects the eyelids.

Thyrotoxic crisis, or thyroid storm, is an acute situation in a patient with uncontrolled hyperthyroidism, usually precipitated by infection or surgery. It may be life threatening because of resulting hyperthermia, tachycardia, heart failure, and delirium.

❯ Sonographic Findings. The gland appears more inhomogeneous than it is in diffuse goiter primarily because of the presence of multiple large intraparenchymal vessels. In younger patients, the gland may be hypoechoic secondary to extensive lymphocytic infiltration or

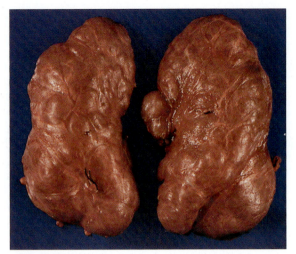

FIGURE 22-22 Gross pathology of a patient with Graves' disease shows symmetrical enlargement of the thyroid gland.

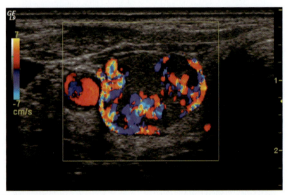

FIGURE 22-23 Increased color Doppler indicates increased vascularity in the thyroid gland in a patient with Graves' disease.

predominant cellular content of the parenchyma that is devoid of colloid substance. The overactivity of Graves' disease is manifested sonographically by increased vascularity on color Doppler imaging, leading to the term "thyroid inferno" (Figure 22-23). Spectral Doppler may show velocities greater than 70 cm/sec.

ANATOMY OF THE PARATHYROID GLAND

The parathyroid glands are normally located on the posterior medial surface of the thyroid gland. Most people have four parathyroid glands, but some have three or five parathyroid glands. Parathyroid glands have been found in ectopic places, such as the neck and mediastinum. The four parathyroid glands are paired; two lie posterior to each superior pole of the thyroid, and the other two lie posterior to the inferior pole (see Figure 22-1).

Each gland is flat and disk-shaped. The echo texture is similar to that of the overlying thyroid gland. For this reason, normal-size glands (less than 4 mm) are usually not seen with sonography, but occasionally a single

gland may be imaged and appear as a flat hypoechoic structure posterior and adjacent to the thyroid. Enlarged glands (greater than 5 mm) have a decreased echo texture and appear sonographically as elongated masses between the posterior longus colli and the anterior thyroid lobe.

PARATHYROID PHYSIOLOGY AND LABORATORY DATA

The parathyroid glands are the calcium-sensing organs in the body. They produce **parathyroid hormone (PTH)** and monitor the **serum calcium** feedback mechanism. The stimulus to PTH secretion is a decrease in the level of blood calcium. When the serum calcium level decreases, the parathyroid glands are stimulated to release PTH. When the serum calcium level increases, parathyroid activity decreases. PTH acts on bone, kidney, and intestine to enhance calcium absorption. Patients with unexplained hypercalcemia detected on routine blood chemistry screening are the most common referrals for parathyroid sonography. Symptomatic renal stones, ulcers, and bone pain are other indications.

SONOGRAPHIC EVALUATION OF THE PARATHYROID GLAND

For successful sonographic detection of parathyroid abnormalities, a high-resolution (7.5- to 15-MHz) transducer must be used. The patient is placed supine with the neck slightly hyperextended. From the upper neck, just under the jaw, to the sternal notch, transverse and longitudinal planes of the thyroid/parathyroid area must be examined and observations recorded. To detect the inferiorly located parathyroid glands, the patient is asked to swallow to elevate the thyroid gland during real-time scanning. Under usual circumstances, it is not common to be able to visualize the normal parathyroid glands because they are closely attached to or embedded in the thyroid glands and therefore lack acoustic differences. This anatomic relationship, coupled with the small size of the parathyroid glands, makes visualization a challenge. However, with high-resolution technology and three-dimensional (3D) and harmonic imaging, visualization of the parathyroid glands is not as difficult as it once was.

The parathyroid gland measures about 5 mm × 3 mm × 1 mm. The glands are oval or bean-shaped, but have also been reported as spherical, elongated, or lobulated.

In some cases, a prominent **longus colli muscle** appears as a discrete area posterior to the thyroid; it is important not to confuse this normal anatomy with a mass. Longitudinal sections can usually solve the problem, and the linear appearance of the muscle is evident in this plane. The minor neurovascular bundle, consisting of the inferior thyroid artery and recurrent laryngeal nerve, may also be a source of confusion. Longitudinal scans can often eliminate this confusion by identifying the bundle's tubular appearance.

PATHOLOGY OF THE PARATHYROID GLAND

Primary Hyperparathyroidism

Primary hyperparathyroidism is a state of increased function of the parathyroid glands. Women have primary hyperparathyroidism two to three times more frequently than men; it is particularly common after menopause. Primary hyperparathyroidism is characterized by hypercalcemia, hypercalciuria, and low serum levels of phosphate (**hypophosphatasia**).

Most patients are asymptomatic at the time of diagnosis and have no manifestations of **hyperparathyroidism,** such as nephrolithiasis and osteopenia. Primary hyperparathyroidism occurs when increased amounts of PTH are produced by an adenoma, primary hyperplasia, or, rarely, carcinoma located in the parathyroid gland.

Primary Hyperplasia. Of patients with hyperparathyroidism, approximately 10% have **parathyroid hyperplasia.** Primary hyperplasia is defined as hyperfunction of all parathyroid glands with no apparent cause. Only one gland may significantly enlarge, with the remaining glands only mildly affected, or all glands may be enlarged (Figure 22-24). In any case, glands rarely reach more than 1 cm in size. Hyperplasia usually involves all the glands; however, multiple adenomas may involve two or three of the glands. As the glands become inconsistently enlarged, it becomes more difficult to separate the lesions with sonography.

Pitfalls to be aware of in diagnosing parathyroid enlargement include recognition of normal cervical structures (veins, arteries, esophagus, muscles), which can simulate adenomas and produce false-positive results.

Adenoma. Adenoma is the most common cause of primary hyperparathyroidism (80% of cases). A solitary adenoma may involve any of the four glands with equal frequency. The most common shape of a parathyroid adenoma is oval (Figure 22-25). As the adenoma enlarges, it dissects between the longitudinal tissue planes of the neck to assume an oblong, tubelike, or bilobar shape. The texture of the adenoma is homogeneously solid. Occasionally, calcifications are seen in the adenoma.

Sonographic Findings. Parathyroid adenomas are hypoechoic (Figure 22-26), and a vast majority are solid. Benign adenomas are usually less than 3 cm in size, with larger adenomas measuring 5 cm or greater in length. Superior parathyroid adenomas are located adjacent to the posterior aspect of the mid portion of the thyroid. The location of inferior thyroid adenomas is more variable, but they may be found close to the caudal tip of the lower pole of the thyroid. The parathyroid gland may also be ectopic, making it difficult to locate with ultrasound or for the surgeon to treat. Common ectopic locations are mediastinal, retrotracheal, intrathyroid, and carotid sheath/undescended.

Adenomas are encapsulated and have a discrete border. Differentiation of adenomas and hyperplasia is difficult on histologic and morphologic grounds. Color Doppler may show a hypervascular pattern or a peripheral vascular arc that may aid in differentiation from hyperplastic regional lymph nodes, which have hilar flow.

Parathyroid Carcinoma. The histologic differentiation of adenoma and carcinoma is very difficult. Metastases to regional nodes or distant organs, capsular invasion,

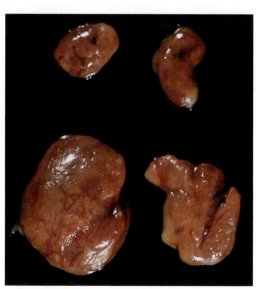

FIGURE 22-24 Parathyroid hyperplasia shows enlargement of all four parathyroid glands.

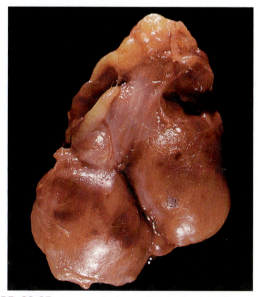

FIGURE 22-25 Gross pathology of parathyroid adenoma. The gland is enlarged and nodular.

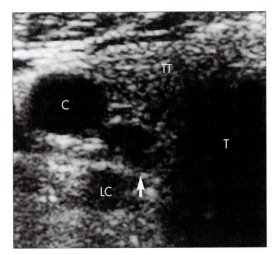

FIGURE 22-26 Transverse image of an enlarged parathyroid gland. Parathyroid *(arrow)*. *C,* Carotid; *LC,* longus colli; *T,* trachea; *TT,* thyroid tissue.

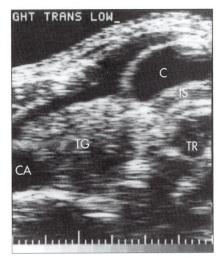

FIGURE 22-27 Transverse image at the level of the thyroid gland *(TG)*, demonstrating a thyroglossal duct cyst *(C)* in the midline anterior to the trachea *(TR)*. *CA,* Carotid artery; *IS,* isthmus of thyroid gland.

or local recurrence must be present for cancer to be diagnosed. Most cancers of the parathyroid glands are small, irregular, rather firm masses. The mass may adhere to surrounding structures. On sonography, the carcinoma is usually larger than the adenoma. The malignant tumor has a lobular contour, heterogeneous internal architecture, and internal cystic components. A large adenoma may also exhibit these features.

Secondary Hyperparathyroidism

Secondary hyperparathyroidism is a chronic hypocalcemia caused by renal failure, vitamin D deficiency (rickets), or malabsorption syndromes. These abnormalities induce PTH secretion, which leads to secondary hyperparathyroidism. Hyperfunction of the parathyroids is apparently a compensatory reaction; renal insufficiency and intestinal malabsorption cause hypocalcemia, which leads to stimulation of PTH. All four glands are usually enlarged.

MISCELLANEOUS NECK MASSES

The role of ultrasound in evaluating palpable neck masses is to determine the site of origin and assess lesion texture.

Developmental Cysts

Thyroglossal Duct Cysts. Congenital anomalies that appear in the midline of the neck anterior to the trachea are called **thyroglossal duct cysts** (Figure 22-27). They are oval or spherical masses rarely larger than 2 or 3 cm. A remnant of the tubular development of the thyroid gland may persist between the base of the tongue and the hyoid bone. This narrow, hollow tract, which connects the thyroid lobes to the floor of the pharynx,

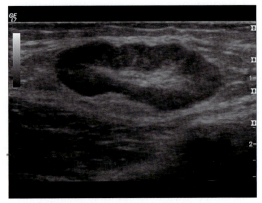

FIGURE 22-28 Enlarged lymph node.

normally atrophies in the adult. Failure to atrophy creates the potential for cystic masses to form anywhere along it.

Branchial Cleft Cysts. **Branchial cleft cysts** are cystic formations usually located lateral to the thyroid gland. During embryonic development, the branchial cleft is a slender tract extending from the pharyngeal cavity to an opening near the auricle or into the neck. A diverticulum may extend laterally from the pharynx or medially from the neck. Although primarily cystic in appearance, these lesions may present with solid components, usually of low-level echogenicity, particularly if they have become infected.

Abscess

Abscesses can arise in any location in the neck.

◢ **Sonographic Findings.** The sonographic appearance of an abscess ranges from primarily fluid-filled to completely echogenic. Most commonly, it appears as a mass of low-level echogenicity with rather irregular walls. Chronic abscess may be particularly difficult to demonstrate because the indistinct margins blend with surrounding tissue. The role of ultrasound in evaluating abscess consists of localization for percutaneous needle aspiration and follow-up examination during and after treatment.

Lymphadenopathy

Lymphadenopathy is the term for any disorder characterized by localized or generalized enlargement of the lymph nodes or lymph vessels.

Sonographic Findings. In the neck, the shape of the node is important. A normal lymph node is oval in shape and has a homogeneous texture with a central core echo complex. The more rounded the node, the more likely the node is malignant. Low-level echogenicity of well-circumscribed masses is the classic sonographic appearance of enlarged lymph nodes (Figure 22-28). In some cases, however, the node appears echo-free. Inflammatory processes may also exhibit a cystic nature. Differentiation of inflammation from neoplastic processes is not always possible by sonographic criteria alone. To confirm a neoplastic process, a fine-needle biopsy is performed.

The Scrotum

Cindy A. Owen

Ultrasound is the imaging modality of choice for evaluating the scrotum. High-frequency ultrasound imaging, combined with color and spectral Doppler, quickly and reliably provides valuable information in the assessment of scrotal pain or mass. In particular, color Doppler has a central role in the evaluation of suspected testicular torsion because it can demonstrate absence of flow in the affected testis. Color Doppler also plays a key role in the evaluation of testicular infection by demonstrating hyperemic flow on the affected side. Ultrasound imaging accurately differentiates intratesticular from extratesticular masses and cystic from solid masses. Advances in the development of ultrasound equipment have provided improved spatial and contrast resolution, reduced speckle artifact, and increased sensitivity to the display of scrotal perfusion. The steady progress in ultrasound image quality has enhanced our ability to clearly define the scrotal anatomy and to more accurately depict and differentiate abnormalities. This chapter covers the pertinent anatomy of the scrotum and its contents, including the vascular supply. The ultrasound scanning protocol is discussed along with tips on scanning techniques and potential pitfalls. A review of the disease processes affecting the scrotum is provided, including a description of sonographic findings.

ANATOMY OF THE SCROTUM

The testes are symmetrical, oval-shaped glands residing in the **scrotum**. In adults, the testis measures approximately 3 to 5 cm in length, 2 to 4 cm in width, and approximately 3 cm in height. Each testis is divided into more than 250 to 400 conical lobules containing the seminiferous tubules. These tubules converge at the apex of each lobule and anastomose to form the rete testis in the mediastinum. The rete testis drains into the head of the epididymis through the efferent ductules (Figure 23-1). Sonographically, the testes appear as smooth, medium gray structures with a fine echo texture.

The epididymis is a 6- to 7-cm tubular structure beginning superiorly and then coursing posterolateral to the testis. It is divided into head, body, and tail. The head is the largest part of the epididymis, measuring 6 to 15 mm in width. It is located superior to the upper pole of the testis (Figure 23-2). It contains 10 to 15 efferent ductules from the rete testis, which converge to form a single duct in the body and tail. This duct is known as the ductus epididymis. It becomes the vas deferens and continues in the spermatic cord. The body of the epididymis is much smaller than the head. It is difficult to see with ultrasound on normal individuals. It follows the

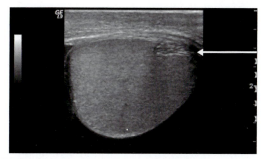

FIGURE 23-1 Transverse ultrasound scan of the normal rete testis. With the use of high-resolution imaging and transducer frequencies of 10 MHz or greater, the normal rete testis can sometimes be depicted with ultrasound. It appears as tiny tubules adjacent to the epididymal head and the testis mediastinum *(arrow)*.

posterolateral aspect of the testis from the upper to the lower pole. The tail of the epididymis is slightly larger and is positioned posterior to the lower pole of the testis. The appendix of the epididymis is a small protuberance from the head of the epididymis. Postmortem studies have shown the appendix epididymis in 34% of testes unilaterally and 12% of testes bilaterally. The normal epididymis usually appears as isoechoic or hypoechoic compared with the testis, although the echo texture is coarser.

At the upper pole of the testis, the appendix testis is attached. It is located between the testis and the epididymis. Postmortem studies have shown the appendix testis to be present in 92% of testes unilaterally and 69% bilaterally (Figure 23-3).

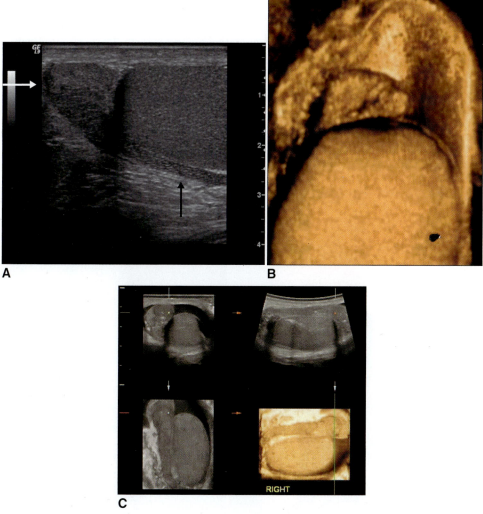

FIGURE 23-2 A, Sagittal ultrasound scan of a normal epididymis and testis. The head of the epididymis is seen superior to the upper pole of the testis *(white arrow)*. The body of the epididymis is seen posterior to the testis *(black arrow)*. Note the coarse echo texture of the epididymis compared with the fine texture of the testis. **B,** Three-dimensional (3D) view rendered in the coronal plane demonstrates the relationship of the normal epididymal head to the superior pole of the testis. **C,** 3D view shows orthogonal planes of enlarged epididymis in patient with epididymitis. An axis point *(small white dot)* is placed on the epididymal head to demonstrate the same point in three orthogonal views. The 3D dataset allows manipulation of the volume in an infinite number of imaging planes. This allows the sonographer to adjust the display, so that the entire length of the epididymis can be demonstrated.

The testis is completely covered by a dense, fibrous tissue termed the **tunica albuginea.** The posterior aspect of the tunica albuginea reflects into the testis to form a vertical septum known as the **mediastinum testis.** Multiple septa (**septa testis**) are formed from the tunica albuginea at the mediastinum. They course through the testis and separate it into lobules. The mediastinum supports the vessels and ducts coursing within the testis. The mediastinum is often seen on ultrasound as a bright hyperechoic line coursing craniocaudad within the testis (Figure 23-4, A, B). The **tunica vaginalis** lines the inner walls of the scrotum, covering each testis and epididymis. It consists of two layers: parietal and visceral. The parietal layer is the inner lining of the scrotal wall. The visceral layer surrounds the testis and epididymis. A small bare area is posterior. At this site, the testicle is against the scrotal wall, preventing torsion. Blood vessels, lymphatics, nerves, and spermatic ducts travel through the area (see Figure 23-1). The space between the layers of the tunica vaginalis is where hydroceles form. It is normal to see a small amount of fluid in this space.

The **vas deferens** is a continuation of the ductus epididymis. It is thicker and less convoluted. The vas deferens dilates at the terminal portion near the **seminal vesicles.** This portion is termed the ampulla of the deferens. The vas deferens joins the duct of the seminal vesicles to form the **ejaculatory duct,** which, in turn, empties into the **urethra.** The junction of the ejaculatory ducts with the urethra is termed the **verumontanum.** The urethra courses from the bladder to the end of the penis. In men, the urethra transports both urine and semen outside the body.

The vas deferens, testicular arteries, venous pampiniform plexus, lymphatics, autonomic nerves, and fiber of the cremaster form the **spermatic cord.** The cord extends from the scrotum through the inguinal canal and internal inguinal rings to the pelvis. The spermatic cord suspends the testis in the scrotum.

VASCULAR SUPPLY

Right and left **testicular arteries** arise from the abdominal aorta just below the level of the renal arteries. They are the primary source of blood flow to the testis. The testicular arteries descend in the retroperitoneum and

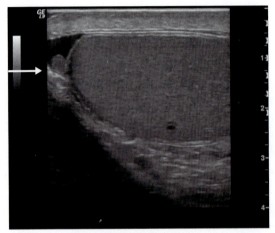

FIGURE 23-3 Sagittal ultrasound scan of the normal testis demonstrates the appendix testis as a small structure superior to the testis *(arrow)*. The appendix testis is isoechoic to the testis. A small hydrocele improves the visibility of the appendix testis.

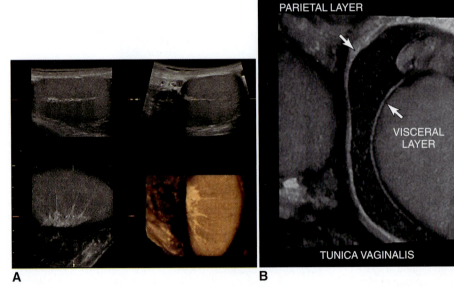

FIGURE 23-4 **A,** Three-dimensional (3D) view showing the mediastinum testis in orthogonal planes with the septa. This image was obtained with a 3D transducer sweeping in the sagittal plane *(upper left)*. The transverse image is derived from the 3D volume and is displayed upper right. 3D allows visualization of the coronal plane *(lower left)*. The coronal plane is rarely imaged with traditional 2D imaging. A rendered view of the testis is seen in the lower right. **B,** 3D coronal view demonstrating the layers of the tunica vaginalis *(arrows)*. This is well demonstrated because of the presence of a hydrocele. Hydroceles form between the parietal and visceral layers of the tunica vaginalis.

enter the spermatic cord in the deep inguinal ring. Then they course along the posterior surface of each testis and pierce the tunica albuginea, forming the capsular arteries, which branch over the surface of the testis. With high-frequency ultrasound imaging, the capsular artery is sometimes seen as a hypoechoic linear structure on the surface of the testis. Color Doppler can be used to confirm its identity (Figure 23-5). The capsular arteries give rise to **centripetal arteries,** which course from the testicular surface toward the mediastinum along the septa. Before reaching the mediastinum, they curve backward, forming the **recurrent rami** (centrifugal arteries) (Figure 23-6). These centrifugal arteries branch farther into arterioles and capillaries. With sensitive color Doppler settings, the recurrent rami may be seen giving a candy cane appearance (Figure 23-7).

In approximately one half of normal testes, a transmediastinal (or transtesticular) artery is visualized coursing through the mediastinum toward the testicular capsule. A large vein is often identified adjacent to the artery (Figure 23-8). On color Doppler, the

transmediastinal artery will have a different color than the centripetal arteries because its flow is directed away from the mediastinum and toward the capsule. Upon reaching the testicular surface opposite the mediastinum, the transmediastinal artery courses along the capsule as capsular arteries. Spectral Doppler waveforms obtained from the capsular, centripetal, or transmediastinal arteries show a low-resistance waveform pattern in normal individuals (Figure 23-9). Box 23-1 diagrams arterial branching in the testicles.

BOX 23-1	**Testicular Arterial Branching**

Testicular artery
↓
Capsular artery
↓
Centripetal artery
↓
Recurrent rami

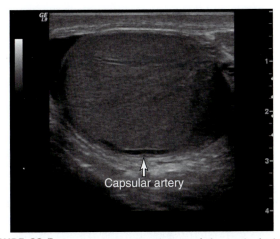

FIGURE 23-5 Transverse ultrasound view of the testis depicting the capsular artery in a patient with orchitis. The capsular artery is seen as an anechoic structure coursing along the surface of the testis *(arrow).*

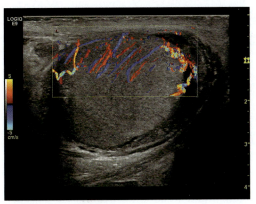

FIGURE 23-7 Color Doppler image of the testis depicting the recurrent rami. A centripetal artery is seen coursing from the testicular capsule. Before reaching the mediastinum, it turns backward in a candy cane pattern, forming the recurrent rami.

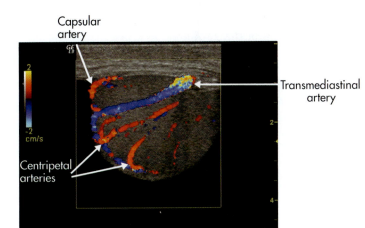

FIGURE 23-6 Color Doppler image of the testis depicting the capsular artery giving rise to centripetal arteries. A transmediastinal artery is seen coursing from the mediastinum to the testicular surface. It then branches across the top of the testis as capsular arteries. The flow direction in the transmediastinal artery *(blue)* is opposite that in the centripetal arteries *(red).* The centripetal arteries rise from the capsular arteries with a flow direction through the testis toward the mediastinum, whereas the blood flow in the transmediastinal artery courses from the mediastinum to the testicular capsule.

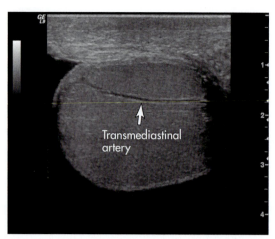

FIGURE 23-8 Transverse ultrasound (US) image shows a normal transmediastinal artery coursing from the mediastinum to the testicular capsule. It appears as an anechoic or hypoechoic tube. Transmediastinal arteries are seen in approximately 50% of testes.

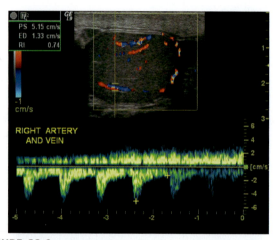

FIGURE 23-9 Spectral Doppler image showing the normal low-resistance waveform pattern of the intratesticular arteries. A low-resistance waveform demonstrates forward flow during both systole and diastole. In this image, the Doppler sample volume includes both a transmediastinal artery and its accompanying vein. The venous and arterial flow signals are on opposite sides of the Doppler baseline, as their flow is in opposite directions.

The **cremasteric** and **deferential arteries** accompany the testicular artery within the spermatic cord to supply the extratesticular structures. They also have anastomoses with the testicular artery and may provide some flow to the testis. The cremasteric artery branches from the inferior epigastric artery (a branch of the external iliac artery). It provides flow to the **cremasteric muscle** and peritesticular tissue. The deferential artery arises from the vesicle artery (a branch of the internal iliac artery). It mainly supplies the epididymis and vas deferens. The scrotal wall is also supplied by branches of the **pudendal artery.**

Venous drainage of the scrotum occurs through the veins of the **pampiniform plexus.** The pampiniform plexus exits from the mediastinum testis and courses in the spermatic cord. It converges into three sets of anastomotic veins: testicular, deferential, and cremasteric. The right **testicular vein** drains into the inferior vena cava, and the left testicular vein joins the left renal vein. The deferential vein drains into the pelvic veins, and the cremasteric vein drains into tributaries of the epigastric and deep pudendal veins.

PATIENT POSITIONING AND SCANNING PROTOCOL

Ultrasound examination of the scrotum is performed with the patient in the supine position. The penis is positioned on the abdomen and covered with a towel. The patient is asked to place his legs close together to provide support for the scrotum. Alternatively, a rolled towel placed between the thighs can support the scrotum. It is often unnecessary to place a towel for support if the legs are positioned close together. This may be more comfortable for the patient in pain.

A generous amount of warmed gel is applied to the scrotum to ensure adequate probe contact and eliminate air between the probe and the skin surface. Rarely, a stand-off pad may be necessary to improve imaging of very superficial structures such as a tunica albuginea cyst. However, with the use of high-frequency probes (10 to 14 MHz), this is usually not necessary. Instead of a stand-off pad, an extra thick mound of gel may be adequate to improve near-field imaging.

Before beginning the scrotal ultrasound, it is necessary to determine clinical findings. Was this patient referred because of a palpable mass, scrotal pain, swollen scrotum, or other reason? It is important to ask the patient to describe his symptoms, including history, location, and duration of pain. Can he feel a mass? If so, ask the patient to find the lump. Then place the probe exactly over this location to examine the site. Did the patient experience trauma? When did the trauma occur? Ask him to describe what happened. Has he had a vasectomy? When? Not only is this information helpful in guiding the examination, but it is important to the interpreting physician and gives confidence to the patient regarding the quality of the ultrasound study. Box 23-2 lists important tips when performing an ultrasound examination of the scrotum.

BOX 23-2 | Sonographer Tips

- Explain procedure and preparation to patient, and then allow the patient to get ready in private.
- Be sure to take an image of right and left testicles together for comparison in both gray-scale and color Doppler.
- Perform Valsalva maneuver when a varicocele is suspected.
- Sensitize color Doppler for slow flow when evaluating torsion.
- Torsion is a surgical emergency; perform the examination in a timely manner.

Scrotal ultrasound is always a bilateral examination, with the asymptomatic side used as a comparison for the symptomatic side. To begin, it is best to perform a brief survey scan to determine what abnormalities, if any, are present. Each testis is scanned from superior to inferior and is carefully examined to determine whether abnormal findings are present. The size, echogenicity, and structure of each testis are evaluated. The testicular parenchyma should be uniform with equal echogenicity between sides. Think of these questions as you scan: Is the parenchyma homogeneous or heterogeneous? Is there a mass? If so, is it cystic or solid? Is it intratesticular or extratesticular? Is one testis much larger than the other? Which side is swollen, or is one side shrunken? All testes should appear similar in size and shape. Is the epididymis normal? Is the skin thickened? Turn on color Doppler to assess the flow. Is there an absence of flow in the testis, or is it hyperemic? How does the color Doppler compare between sides? Testes should show about the same amount of flow when the same color Doppler setup is used. Check the flow in each epididymis. Again, compare between sides. They should be similar. After the survey scan, images are obtained that demonstrate the findings.

Representative images are obtained in at least two planes—transverse and sagittal—with additional imaging planes scanned as needed to demonstrate the findings. In transverse, images are taken that show the superior, mid, and inferior portions of each testis. The width of the testis is measured in the mid-transverse view. A transverse view of the head of the epididymis is included. Superior to the epididymal head, an image is obtained to demonstrate the area of the spermatic cord. In the sagittal plane, images are taken to show the medial, mid, and lateral portions. A long axis measurement of testicular length is obtained in the midsagittal image. Again, additional images may be taken to demonstrate abnormal areas. An image is obtained of the epididymal head superior to the **testicle**. The body and tail of the epididymis can be demonstrated coursing posteriorly on each side. Scrotal skin thickness is evaluated and compared from side to side. At least one image is taken to show both testes at the same time, so the interpreting physician can compare size and echogenicity (Figure 23-10). Additional views may be taken in patients with suspected varicocele. These include upright positioning and the Valsalva maneuver. Color and spectral Doppler are used in all examinations, with representative images taken to demonstrate both arterial and venous flow in each testis. Table 23-1 lists the scanning protocols for scrotal ultrasound.

TECHNICAL CONSIDERATIONS

High-frequency linear-array transducers are preferred for scrotal imaging because they provide the best spatial resolution. However, the field of view is limited with

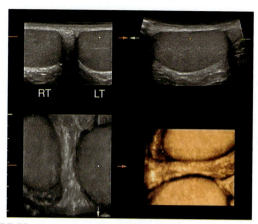

FIGURE 23-10 Transverse three-dimensional (3D) sweep obtained at the midline in a normal patient demonstrating both testes. The size, echogenicity, and texture are similar between sides. It is advisable to obtain an image like this in all cases to allow comparison between the testes.

TABLE 23-1	Ultrasound Scrotal Scan Protocol
Transverse Image	**Sagittal Image**
Spermatic cord area	Spermatic cord area
Epididymal head	Epididymal head with superior testis
Superior testis	Long axis mid-testis with
Mid testis with	measurement
measurement	Medial long axis
Inferior testis	Lateral long axis
Transverse view showing	Color Doppler of epididymal head
both testes	Color Doppler of mid testis
	Spectral Doppler of artery
	Spectral Doppler of vein

Note: In patients with suspected varicocele, additional views include upright view of spermatic cord with and without Valsalva maneuver.

linear arrays. Occasionally, a larger field of view is required to measure anatomy or display anatomic relationships. Ultrasound systems provide numerous methods to meet this need, including virtual convex imaging, panoramic imaging, stitching images together, and using a curved-array transducer.

Real-time imaging of the scrotum is performed with a high-frequency linear-array probe of at least 7.5 MHz. Because high-frequency transducers have better spatial and contrast resolution compared with lower-frequency transducers, they are preferred for scrotal imaging. Probes with frequencies of 10 to 15 MHz are usually best. Because there is a tradeoff between frequency and penetration, the highest frequency providing adequate penetration should be used. In patients with considerable wall edema and thickening, frequencies as low as 5 to 7.5 MHz may be necessary to adequately penetrate the testis.

Many ultrasound systems have a trapezoid or virtual convex feature that can be selected with the linear-array probe. This is very helpful for measuring the long axis of the testis, or when an abnormal area cannot be entirely imaged with the standard linear format (Figure 23-11, *A*). It is best to use this feature selectively instead of routinely, because steering the beam to create the wider format has a negative impact on image quality; steering widens the distance between scan lines and degrades lateral resolution.

In cases of large hydroceles, hematomas, or swelling, an even larger field of view may be required. In these cases, a panoramic tool may be useful. This tool allows the image to build as the probe is moved over the skin surface. A very long image can be obtained that shows anatomic relationships (Figure 23-11, *B*). Images may also be stitched together in a combined mode. The first

image is obtained in one window; then the probe is moved, and another image is obtained by attempting to match the boundaries of the first image (Figure 23-11, *C*). Another way to obtain a larger field of view is to use a 5- to 7.5-MHz curved-array transducer for a portion of the examination to demonstrate the entire scrotal contents. Again, this should be done selectively to obtain the necessary images and should be followed by a return to the high-frequency linear-array probe for further evaluation of each testis (Figure 23-11, *D*).

Most modern ultrasound scanners offer additional features that enhance the quality of the ultrasound image. These features include, but are not limited to, compound imaging, harmonics, extended field-of-view imaging, virtual convex, speckle reduction algorithms,

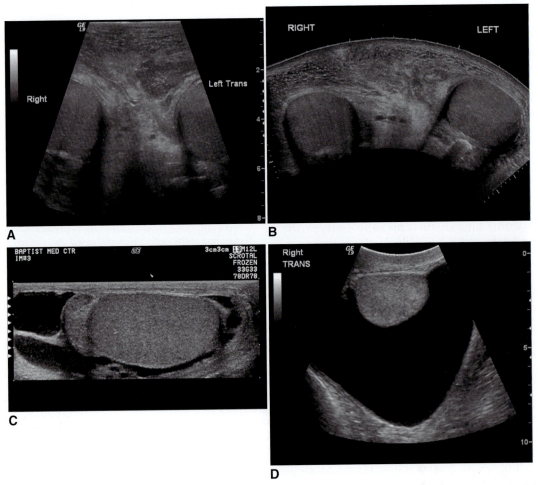

FIGURE 23-11 A, Transverse ultrasound scan of a scrotal hematoma using a virtual convex to create a sector or trapezoidal format using a linear-array probe. The field of view is enlarged to allow better depiction of the size and location of the hematoma compared with the testes. This feature is useful for measuring testicular length and showing abnormal areas that are too large to view with the standard linear format. However, because the scan lines are steered to create this image, lateral resolution is decreased compared with the standard format. **B,** Transverse ultrasound view of the same scrotal hematoma using a panoramic setting. This feature allows the image to build as the transducer is moved across the anatomy. It is very useful for showing large masses and anatomic relationships. **C,** Sagittal ultrasound image in a patient with epididymitis and hydrocele. The image was obtained by stitching together two images in a combined mode. This is another useful tool when a larger field of view is necessary to demonstrate anatomy. **D,** Sagittal ultrasound image of the testis surrounded posteriorly by a large hydrocele. The linear-array format could not display the entire hydrocele, so a 7-MHz curved-array transducer was used to better demonstrate a pathologic condition.

and use of multiple focal zones (Table 23-2). All of these controls may be adjusted to improve image quality.

Color and spectral Doppler play an important role in scrotal ultrasound. The typical color/spectral Doppler frequencies used for scrotal ultrasound are between 4 and 8 MHz. The upper frequency range is used to improve sensitivity to slow flow. This is important in evaluation of testicular torsion or tumor vascularity. Penetration is decreased with higher frequencies, so it is important to make sure that the color penetrates to the depth of interest. Color and spectral Doppler findings on the symptomatic side are always compared with the asymptomatic side.

Power Doppler is often used as a way to quickly get to a sensitive setting that will demonstrate slow flow. Power Doppler shows the amplitude or power of the moving signal, whereas color Doppler shows the frequency shift. Power Doppler does not demonstrate flow direction or aliasing, and to some offers a more straightforward display of blood flow. Presets for power Doppler are often set at a lower pulse repetition frequency (PRF) than color Doppler because aliasing is not an issue, so pushing the power Doppler button may show more flow with fewer adjustments to the controls. This often provides a quick way to get to a more sensitive flow setting. Persistence is usually much greater with power Doppler, requiring a steady hand and slower movement of the probe. To further enhance power Doppler, the same parameters are adjusted as for color Doppler.

Familiarity with color Doppler controls is very important when performing scrotal ultrasound. The sonographer may need to adjust some of the following color Doppler parameters throughout the study to enhance the visibility of scrotal perfusion (Table 23-3):

- **Gain**—The color gain control is used to amplify the reflected color Doppler signal. Whenever the expected amount of color is not visible in the image, the color gain should be increased until noise is present. Once color noise is visible, the gain can be decreased until it just disappears. At this point, the color gain setting is optimized.
- **Scale/pulse repetition frequency (PRF)**—The PRF is the number of pulses transmitted in one second. This important color parameter affects the sensitivity of the system in displaying slow flow. It also sets the point at which color aliasing occurs (Nyquist limit). The control has different names depending on the ultrasound equipment being used. It is variably named scale, PRF, or flow rate. The PRF is reduced to improve sensitivity to slow flow. This is critical when ruling out testicular torsion. If the PRF is set too high, slow flow may not be visible. When the PRF is set too low, excessive color aliasing occurs, which makes it impossible to determine flow direction or to assess flow quality. Neither of these factors is significant in scrotal ultrasound, so it is common to use low PRF settings. However, flash artifact from patient motion is more apparent with very low PRFs and may make scanning difficult. It is recommended to adjust the PRF so that the asymptomatic testicular flow is well demonstrated without excessive flash artifact. Then compare the same settings on the contralateral side (Figure 23-12).
- **Wall filter**—The wall filter acts as an electronic eraser. Color echoes that lie below the filter cutoff do not appear on the image display. The wall filter is adjusted downward to enhance flow sensitivity. It is turned up to reduce flash artifact. On most ultrasound systems, the wall filter is automatically adjusted with the PRF.

TABLE 23-2	Scanning Features		
Feature	**What Is It?**	**Advantage**	**Disadvantage**
Harmonics	Selective reception of penetration (uses frequencies generated within tissue)	Improved contrast resolution Improved visibility of low-level echoes Reduction of artifacts	Less harmonic penetration (uses higher frequency)
Compound imaging	Uses multiple-angled firings to create one image	Improved border definition Reduced speckle Less angle dependence	Slowed frame rate Loss of some beneficial artifacts (i.e., shadowing, refraction, and enhancement)
Speckle reduction algorithms	Sophisticated algorithms applied to the image to reduce speckle (salt and pepper appearance of ultrasound image)	Improved contrast resolution Improved conspicuity of masses	None
Extended field of view imaging	Image builds up as probe is moved across anatomy	Improved ability to show anatomic relationships of structures too large to fit in linear-array format	May be difficult to perform on uncooperative patient or over sharply curving interface
Trapezoid or virtual convex imaging	Steering of linear-array probe to create sector format	Larger field of view with linear-array probes	Reduced lateral resolution
Multizone focus	Use of multiple focal zones to create an extended area of focus on one image	Improved lateral resolution	Slowed frame rate

TABLE 23-3	Color/Power Doppler Parameters	
Parameter	**What Is It?**	**How to Adjust**
Gain	Amplification of selected frequency shift signal	Turn up until noise is present and then decrease until noise goes away
PRF (pulse repetition frequency)	PRF is the number of pulses transmitted per second; sets the Nyquist limit; main control affecting sensitivity to flow	Adjust on the asymptomatic side so that flow is visible without too much flash or motion artifact; decrease to improve sensitivity to slow flow; increase to reduce aliasing
Wall filter	Color signals received below the wall filter setting do not appear on the image	Decrease to improve sensitivity and to reduce flash/motion artifact
Line density	Density of scan lines contained within the color box	Turn up to improve lateral resolution of vessels; turn down to increase frame rate
Threshold	Level of gray-scale brightness that is allowable to be overwritten by color when both gray-scale and color information are obtained for the same pixel location within the image	Turn up so that color information is prioritized compared with gray-scale information; if the threshold (also known as color/write priority) is set too low, small intratesticular vessels will not be filled with color
Packet size	Number of pulses on each color scan line sensitivity	Turn up to improve signal-to-noise ratio and turn down to improve frame rate
Color box size	Region of interest that is color encoded within the image	Set just over the area of interest; increasing color box size or depth will slow frame rate

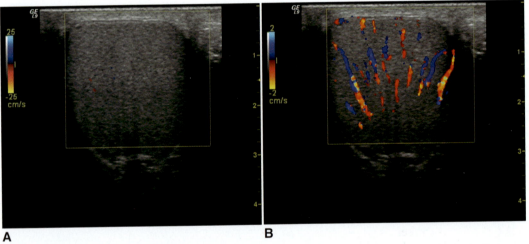

FIGURE 23-12 A, Transverse color Doppler image of a normal testis. Almost no color signal is apparent in the testis because of the high pulse repetition frequency (PRF) setting. The velocity scale values adjacent to the color bar show a velocity sensitivity of 25 cm/sec. **B,** Image of the same testis, using a much lower PRF setting. The velocity scale shows a flow sensitivity of 2 cm/sec. Many intratesticular vessels can now be seen with color Doppler.

But in some instances, it may be beneficial to make further adjustments.

- **Line density**—The line density is the number or density of scan lines contained within the color box. It affects the lateral resolution of the color display. As line density is increased, lateral resolution is improved. The size of the intratesticular arteries is displayed more accurately when line density is high. Frame rate becomes slower as line density is increased, because more transmitted pulses are required to create each image frame. If the frame rate becomes too slow, the line density can be decreased. The user must choose the tradeoff between resolution and frame rate (Figure 23-13).

- **Threshold**—The B/Color threshold is used to determine whether a gray scale or a color pixel is displayed in any given location on the image. Color and power Doppler images are color overlays on top of an existing gray-scale image. A problem arises when gray-scale and color information is received for the same pixel location. The threshold control allows the user to prioritize gray scale or color. For ultrasound of most small parts, including scrotal imaging, it is best to set the threshold so that color is prioritized. Based on the setting, when color and gray-scale information is received for the same pixel location, the one displayed is based on the brightness (amplitude) of the gray-scale dot and the frequency shift and/or power

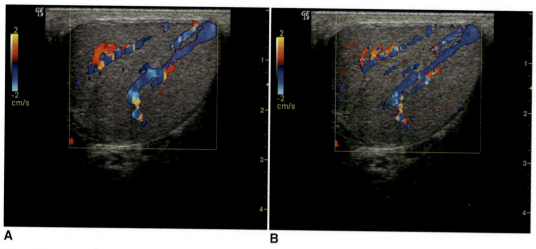

FIGURE 23-13 A, This image was obtained at a low line density setting. The vessels appear wider than expected (poor lateral resolution). **B,** When the line density is increased, the vessel size is more accurately displayed. Frame rate is slower because more scan lines are present within the same-sized color box.

level of the color signal. This feature is not as important when looking at large vessels, such as the common carotid artery, because the vessel lumen typically does not contain gray-scale information, and color can be freely displayed in those pixels. However, in small parts imaging, most vessels are so small that the lumen may not be seen or may be filled with gray-scale echoes caused by volume averaging. In these instances, color will not be displayed unless the threshold control is set to a level that prioritizes color.

- **Packet size**—The packet size is the number of sound pulses transmitted on each scan line within the color box. The packet size is usually set at between 8 and 16 pulses on each scan line. The packet size affects the signal-to-noise ratio, improving color sensitivity when more pulses are used. The frame rate gets slower as the number of packets (pulses) is increased on each scan line. The packet size can be reduced to raise the frame rate when necessary, or increased to improve color sensitivity. The key factor affecting color sensitivity, however, is the PRF.
- **Color box/region of interest**—The color box or region of interest is the area within the gray-scale image where flow is color encoded. The width of the color box affects the frame rate. If the color box is very wide, more scan lines are required to complete each image frame. This means that a greater number of pulses must be transmitted. This takes more time, so the frame rate is reduced. Color box depth also affects frame rate. When the color box is placed deep in the image, the round-trip time for the sound is increased. This slows down the frame rate.

An understanding of the factors affecting color frame rate, sensitivity, and resolution allows the sonographer to optimize the color parameters for each clinical situation. Most systems have specific presets for each

ultrasound application. Selection of the scrotal preset will set the color parameters near an optimal setting for a typical normal examination. However, the user must further adjust the controls to enhance the visibility of scrotal perfusion in abnormal states.

SCROTAL PATHOLOGY

Table 23-4 lists the pathology and sonographic appearance associated with scrotal trauma, infection, and fluid collection. Although the sonographer is not responsible for the interpretation of ultrasound images, an understanding of the various differential considerations is useful to fully evaluate the lesion. Table 23-5 lists many of the common and uncommon masses or fluid collections found within or surrounding the testes.

Acute Scrotum

Scrotal Trauma. Scrotal trauma presents a challenge to the sonographer because the scrotum is often painful and swollen. Trauma may be the result of motor vehicle accident, athletic injury, direct blow to the scrotum, or straddle injury. The most important goal of the ultrasound examination in testicular trauma is to determine whether a rupture has occurred. Rupture of the testis is a surgical emergency that requires prompt diagnosis. If surgery is performed within 72 hours following injury, up to 90% of testes can be saved, but only 45% can be saved after 72 hours. Hydrocele and hematocele are both complications of trauma. However, neither is specific to trauma. Hematoceles contain blood and are also found in advanced cases of epididymitis or orchitis.

Sonographic Findings. The sonographic findings associated with scrotal rupture include focal alteration of the testicular parenchymal pattern, interruption of the tunica albuginea, irregular testicular contour, scrotal

TABLE 23-4	Scrotal Infection, Trauma, and Fluid Collections
Pathology	**Sonographic Appearance**
Infection	
Epididymitis	Enlarged epididymis
	Heterogeneous texture
	Hypoechoic, may contain hyperechoic areas
	Blood flow in the epididymis
Focal orchitis	Hypoechoic area within testis
	Blood flow in the testis
Diffuse orchitis	Enlarged, hypoechoic testis
	Echogenicity of the whole testis
Trauma	
Rupture	Irregular contour
	Focal alteration in echogenicity
Hematoma	Heterogeneous area
	Becomes hyperechoic as the blood clot ages
	Avascular
Torsion	Gray-scale image of testis normal when duration <4 hours
	Testis enlarged and hypoechoic 4 to 12 hours
	Testis heterogeneous after 24 hours
	Absence of testicular flow
Fluid Collections	
Hydrocele	May be anechoic, but often contains low-level echoes
	Surrounds anterolateral aspect of testis
Spermatocele	Located in head of epididymis
	May contain internal echoes and/or septations
	Smooth walls
	Posterior acoustic enhancement
Epididymal cyst	May be located anywhere in epididymis
	Usually small, anechoic
	Ultrasound cannot differentiate between spermatocele and epididymal cyst
	Posterior acoustic enhancement
Varicocele	Tortuous, dilated veins
	Increased size with Valsalva maneuver or patient standing
	Dilated veins fill with color on Valsalva maneuver
	Spectral Doppler confirms venous flow
Hematocele	Contains low-level echoes
	May contain septations and loculations

TABLE 23-5	Differential Considerations: Extratesticular Fluid Collections or Masses
Scrotal Masses	
Common:	Hydrocele
	Varicocele
	Ascites
	Hematocele
	Spermatocele
	Epididymitis
Uncommon:	Cysts
	Pyoceles
	Herniated bowel
	Metastasis
	Polyorchidism
	Extratesticular
	Seminoma
Extratesticular Cystic Mass	
Common:	Hematocele
	Spermatocele
Uncommon:	Pyocele
	Epididymal cyst
	Herniated bowel
Hypoechoic Lesion	
Common:	Seminoma
	Embryonal cell carcinoma
	Choriocarcinoma
	Mixed cell tumor
	Lymphoma
	Leukemia
Uncommon:	Teratoma
	Torsion
	Metastasis
	Epididymal tumor
	Abscess
Enlarged Testicle	
Common:	Tumor
	Edematous testis caused by trauma
	Torsion
Uncommon:	Myeloma of testicle
	Idiopathic macro-orchidism
Enlarged Epididymis	
Common:	Epididymitis
	Sperm granuloma
Uncommon:	Polyorchidism
	Lipoma
Hypoechoic Band in Testis	
Common:	Normal mediastinum testis
	Normal vessels

wall thickening, and **hematocele**. These findings may also be associated with abscess, tumor, or other clinical conditions. When combined with a history of trauma, they suggest rupture.

The sonographic appearance of hematoceles varies with age. An acute hematocele is echogenic with numerous, highly visible echoes that can be seen to float or move in real-time. Over time, hematoceles show low-level echoes and develop fluid-fluid levels or septations. The presence of a hematocele does not confirm rupture. Hematoceles result from bleeding of the pampiniform plexus or other extratesticular structures.

Hematomas associated with trauma may be large and may cause displacement of the associated testis. Hematomas appear as heterogeneous areas within the scrotum. They tend to become more complex over time, developing cystic components. Hematomas may involve the testis or epididymis, or they can be contained within the scrotal wall. Because hematomas are avascular, color Doppler is helpful in identifying them as areas with no flow (Figure 23-14).

Other uses of color Doppler in testicular trauma include identification of blood flow disruption across the surface of the testis. This is an indication of rupture. Color Doppler can aid in separating a normally vascularized testis from one that is disrupted by hematoma. Epididymitis may result from trauma, and color Doppler imaging can be used to identify the associated increased vascularity in the **epididymis**. Torsion may also be associated with trauma. Color Doppler is used to confirm absence of flow in the testis with torsion.

Epididymo-orchitis. Epididymo-orchitis is infection of the epididymis and testis. It most commonly results from the spread of a lower urinary tract infection via the spermatic cord. Less common causes include mumps, syphilis, tuberculosis, viruses, trauma, and chemical causes. Epididymo-orchitis represents the most common cause of acute scrotal pain in adults. The epididymis is the organ primarily involved with infection, which spreads to the testis in about 20% to 40% of cases. Orchitis almost always occurs secondary to epididymitis. Patients typically have increasing scrotal pain over 1 or 2 days. The pain may be mild or severe. Symptoms may also include fever and urethral discharge.

Sonographic Findings. Epididymitis appears as an enlarged, hypoechoic gland. If secondary hemorrhage has occurred, the epididymis may contain focal hyperechoic areas. Hyperemic flow is confirmed with color Doppler (Figure 23-15). The normal epididymis shows little flow with color Doppler. The amount of color flow signal should be compared between sides. The affected side shows significantly more flow than the asymptomatic epididymis. It is important to use the same color Doppler settings when comparing the amount of flow between sides.

With epididymitis, Doppler waveforms demonstrate increased velocities in both systole and diastole. A low-resistance waveform pattern is present (see Figure 23-15). If the infection is isolated to the epididymis, the testis will appear normal. When orchitis has developed, ultrasound imaging will show an enlarged testis. The infection may be focal or diffuse, and affected areas may appear hypoechoic compared with surrounding tissue. Focal areas of infection within the testis will result in a heterogeneous appearance on ultrasound. A diffusely infected testis will appear enlarged and homogeneous with a hypoechoic echogenicity (Figure 23-16). Up to 20% of cases will have a normal appearing epididymis and testis on ultrasound. Ultrasound gray-scale findings associated with epididymo-orchitis are not specific and may also be seen with torsion or tumor. Color and spectral Doppler are key tools in differentiating between epididymo-orchitis and torsion in the patient with acute scrotal pain.

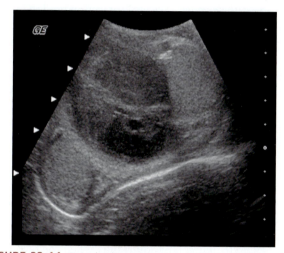

FIGURE 23-14 Complex hematoma in a patient with hemophilia following scrotal trauma. Transverse ultrasound scan of both testes shows a large heterogeneous mass adjacent to the left testis. Color Doppler *(not shown)* demonstrated the mass to be avascular.

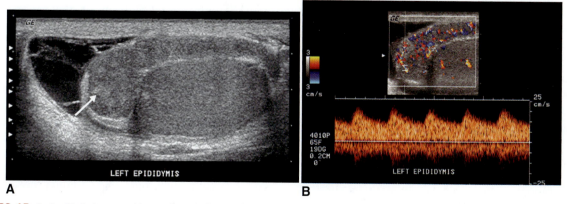

FIGURE 23-15 A, Sagittal ultrasound image in a patient with severe epididymitis shows an enlarged epididymis with a heterogeneous echo texture. Focal hyperechoic areas *(arrow)* within the epididymis may represent hemorrhage. A complex hydrocele with numerous septations is shown near the epididymal head. **B,** Color Doppler shows hyperemic flow within the epididymis. A Doppler waveform obtained from the epididymal head shows increased diastolic flow associated with inflammation.

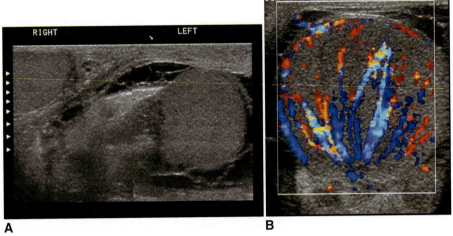

FIGURE 23-16 A, Orchitis in a patient presenting with severe scrotal pain and swelling. Transverse stitched ultrasound scan shows an enlarged left testis and a normal right testis. A complex hydrocele surrounds the left testis. Marked skin thickening is present on the left side compared with the normal right side. **B,** Color Doppler shows hyperemic flow.

Epididymo-orchitis causes hyperemic flow with a significantly greater number of visible vessels on color Doppler compared with the asymptomatic side. Hyperemic flow is seen in the epididymis and testis when both are involved but is isolated to the epididymis when the testis is normal. Documentation of findings on ultrasound must include an image showing both testes, so the size and echogenicity can be compared. It is also recommended to obtain an image with the color box opened wide enough to show portions of both testes, so that the amount of flow between sides can be easily compared.

Other findings associated with epididymitis and epididymo-orchitis include scrotal wall thickening and **hydrocele.** Hydroceles are found around the anterolateral aspect of the testis. They may appear anechoic or may contain low-level echoes. Complex hydroceles may be associated with severe epididymitis and orchitis. These have thick septations and contain low-level echoes. In severe cases, a pyocele may be present. A **pyocele** occurs when pus fills the space between the layers of the tunica vaginalis. It usually contains internal septations, loculations, and debris. This same appearance may be noted following trauma or surgery.

In severe cases of orchitis, testicular infarction may occur. The swollen testis is confined within a rigid tunica albuginea. Excessive swelling can cause obstruction to the testicular blood supply. Color Doppler will show decreased or absent flow compared with the contralateral testis. With decreased flow, spectral Doppler waveforms will have high resistance with little or no diastolic flow. A Doppler waveform demonstrating reversed diastolic flow is a serious finding, indicating threatened testicular infarction (Figure 23-17). Infarction can affect the entire testis or may be confined to a focal area. With focal infarction, color will show perfusion only in portions of the testis that have an absence of color signals in the affected areas. Gray-scale imaging will depict a

heterogeneous pattern. Areas of infarction tend to appear hypoechoic compared with the surrounding testicular parenchyma. If the entire testis becomes infarcted, findings cannot be differentiated from testicular torsion.

Torsion. Torsion of the spermatic cord occurs as a result of abnormal mobility of the testis within the scrotum. An anomaly termed the *bell clapper deformity* is the most common cause of this condition. Normally, the testis and epididymis are surrounded by the tunica vaginalis, except at the bare area where they are attached to the posterior scrotal wall. The bell clapper anomaly occurs when the tunica vaginalis completely surrounds the testis, epididymis, and distal spermatic cord, allowing them to move and rotate freely within the scrotum. This movement is similar to that of a clapper inside a bell, hence the name. Torsion results when the testis and epididymis twist within the scrotum, cutting off the vascular supply within the spermatic cord. Up to 60% of patients with torsion will have an anatomic anomaly on both sides. Undescended testes are 10 times more likely to be affected by torsion than normal testes. Torsion compromises blood flow to the testis, the epididymis, and the intrascrotal portion of the spermatic cord. Venous flow is affected first, with occluded veins causing swelling of the scrotal structures on the affected side. If torsion continues, the arterial flow is obstructed, and testicular ischemia follows.

Torsion of the spermatic cord is a surgical emergency. It is important to obtain diagnostic images as quickly as possible because the salvage rate of the testis depends on the elapsed time since torsion. If surgery is performed within 5 to 6 hours of the onset of pain, 80% to 100% of testes can be salvaged. Between 6 and 12 hours, the salvage rate is 70%, but after 12 hours, only 20% will be saved. The degree of torsion (or number of twists) also affects testicular salvage.

Torsion is the most common cause of acute scrotal pain in adolescents. Although it is more common in

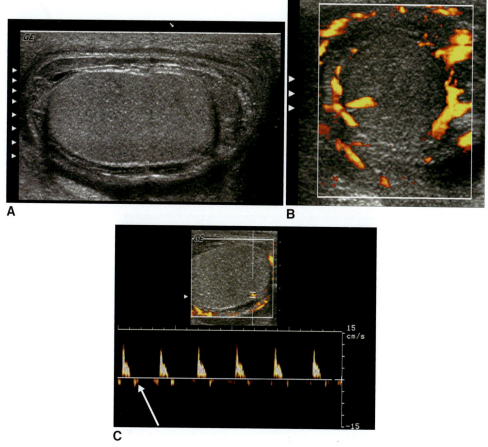

FIGURE 23-17 A, Severe epididymo-orchitis in patient with scrotal pain, swelling, and edema. The testis is swollen against a rigid tunica albuginea. Scrotal skin thickening is evident. **B,** Power Doppler shows hyperemic perfusion surrounding the testis but little intratesticular flow, despite the use of sensitive Doppler settings. **C,** Spectral Doppler waveform of an intratesticular artery demonstrates a high-resistance waveform. Reversed flow is seen in diastole *(arrow).* This is a serious finding, indicating threatened infarction.

young adults and adolescents, torsion can occur at any age, with peak incidence at age 14. Patients with torsion most often present with sudden onset of scrotal pain accompanied by swelling on the affected side. The severe pain causes nausea and vomiting in many patients. Patients with torsion frequently report previous episodes of scrotal pain. The clinical differentiation between torsion and epididymo-orchitis is difficult in that patients have similar symptoms. Ultrasound plays a key role in helping to differentiate these entities.

Sonographic Findings. Gray-scale findings on ultrasound depend on how much time has passed since the torsion occurred. In early stages, scrotal contents may have a normal sonographic appearance. After 4 to 6 hours, the testis becomes swollen and hypoechoic (Figure 23-18). The lobes within the testis are usually well identified during this time as a result of interstitial and septal edema. After 24 hours, the testis becomes heterogeneous as a result of hemorrhage, infarction, necrosis, and vascular congestion (Figure 23-19).

The epididymal head appears enlarged and may have decreased echogenicity or may become heterogeneous. In some cases, the twisted spermatic cord knot may be seen

as a round or oval extratesticular mass that can be traced back to normal spermatic cord. Other findings may include scrotal skin thickening and reactive hydrocele.

Because ultrasound gray-scale findings are similar to those noted with epididymo-orchitis, Doppler evaluation in testicular torsion is very important. Color Doppler imaging is used to make diagnostic images of torsion. Absence of perfusion in the symptomatic testis with normal perfusion on the asymptomatic side is considered to be diagnostic of torsion. Color or power Doppler parameters must be adjusted for optimal detection of slow flow. The PRF and wall filter should be set at a low level. Flow around the ischemic testis will appear normal or decreased.

Spontaneous detorsion can produce a very confusing picture both clinically and by ultrasound. Depending on how long the testis was torsed and how long it has been since relief was attained, the intratesticular flow may be minimal or hyperemic. Extratesticular flow is usually increased. This is very difficult to differentiate from epididymo-orchitis.

Torsion of the appendix epididymis and the appendix testis also occurs and further complicates the clinical

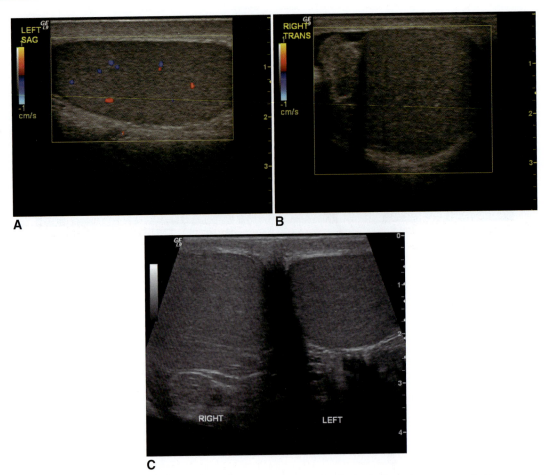

FIGURE 23-18 Testicular torsion in an adolescent patient with sudden onset of right testicular pain, accompanied by nausea and vomiting. **A,** Color Doppler shows normal flow within the parenchyma of the left testis. **B,** The right testis and epididymis are avascular with color Doppler imaging, with the same settings used to show flow on the asymptomatic side. **C,** Transverse ultrasound image showing both testes in right testicular torsion. The right testis is swollen and hyperechoic compared with the normal left testis.

picture. The clinical presentation is similar to that of testicular torsion and epididymo-orchitis. Ultrasound may show a small, hypoechoic mass located between the head of the epididymis and the superior testis. Color Doppler shows increased flow around the mass. Hemorrhage may cause the mass to appear hyperechoic.

Extratesticular Masses

Epididymal Cysts, Spermatoceles, and Tunica Albuginea Cysts. Cysts are benign fluid collections that may be located within the testis or in the extratesticular structures. Most scrotal cysts are extratesticular. Extratesticular cysts are found in the tunica albuginea or epididymis. These include spermatoceles, epididymal cysts, and tunica albuginea cysts. **Spermatoceles** are cystic dilatations of the efferent ductules of the epididymis. They are always located in the epididymal head. Spermatoceles contain proteinaceous fluid and spermatozoa. They may be seen more often following vasectomy.

Epididymal cysts are small, clear cysts that contain serous fluid (Figure 23-20). They can be found anywhere within the epididymis. Small cysts are sometimes found between the layers of the tunica vaginalis or between the tunica vaginalis and the tunica albuginea. All three entities are generally asymptomatic, although they may be palpable and may cause the patient to be concerned.

▶ **Sonographic Findings.** Spermatoceles may be seen as simple cysts or multilocular cystic collections that contain internal echoes. Epididymal cysts appear as simple fluid-filled structures with thin walls and posterior acoustic enhancement. Ultrasound imaging cannot reliably differentiate epididymal cysts from spermatoceles. Tunica albuginea cysts are usually small and appear as anechoic, thin-walled structures on ultrasound. They can become large and cause displacement and distortion of the testis. This helps to differentiate them from hydroceles, which do not distort the testis.

Varicocele

A **varicocele** is an abnormal dilatation of the veins of the pampiniform plexus (located within the spermatic cord). Varicoceles are usually caused by incompetent venous valves within the spermatic vein. These are called primary varicoceles. They are more common on the left. This is

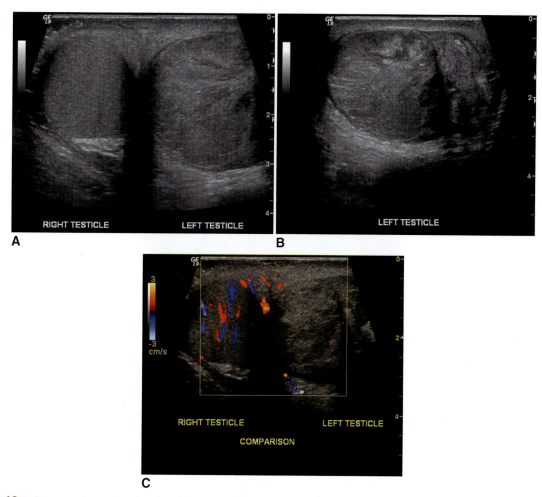

FIGURE 23-19 Left spermatic cord torsion in adolescent with a history of scrotal pain of duration greater than 24 hours. **A,** Transverse ultrasound image showing both testes. The left testis is enlarged and heterogeneous. **B,** Sagittal ultrasound image of the left testis. The infarcted testis has a mixed echo pattern caused by the hemorrhage, necrosis, and vascular congestion associated with spermatic cord torsion exceeding 24 hours. **C,** Transverse color Doppler image showing normal perfusion to the right testis with absence of detectable signal on the left side. Paratesticular blood flow is increased around the abnormal testis.

probably due to the mechanics pertaining to the left spermatic vein and the left renal vein. The spermatic vein empties into the left renal vein at a steep angle, which may inhibit blood flow return. The left renal vein can become compressed between the aorta and the superior mesenteric artery. Secondary varicoceles are caused by increased pressure on the spermatic vein. This may be the result of renal hydronephrosis, an abdominal mass, or liver cirrhosis. An abdominal malignancy invading the left renal vein may cause a varicocele with noncompressible veins. Any noncompressible varicocele in a man older than 40 years of age should prompt a search for a retroperitoneal mass.

Varicoceles have a relationship with impaired fertility. They are more common in infertile men. Treatment of the varicocele has been shown to improve sperm count in up to 53% of cases, but controversy surrounds the treatment of varicoceles for infertility. Uncommonly, varicoceles may extend within the testis. These will be located near the mediastinum. Intratesticular varicoceles have unknown clinical significance, but it is possible that

they will affect male fertility by the same mechanism as extratesticular varicoceles.

Sonographic Findings. Ultrasound imaging of a varicocele shows numerous tortuous tubes of varying sizes within the spermatic cord near the epididymal head. The tubes may contain echoes that move with real-time imaging. This represents slow venous flow (Figure 23-21, *A*, *B*). Varicoceles measure more than 2 mm in diameter. They tend to increase diameter in response to the Valsalva maneuver. Scanning with the patient in an upright position will enhance the visibility of a varicocele because the veins will become more distended. Some authors advocate using a standing position routinely; others believe that supine scanning with the Valsalva maneuver and color Doppler imaging is adequate. With either protocol, color and spectral Doppler are used to confirm the presence of venous flow and to demonstrate retrograde filling with the Valsalva maneuver (Figure 23-21, *C*). Color Doppler settings must be sensitized for slow flow to detect the venous signal in varicoceles. Flash artifact may be a problem with color Doppler imaging during a

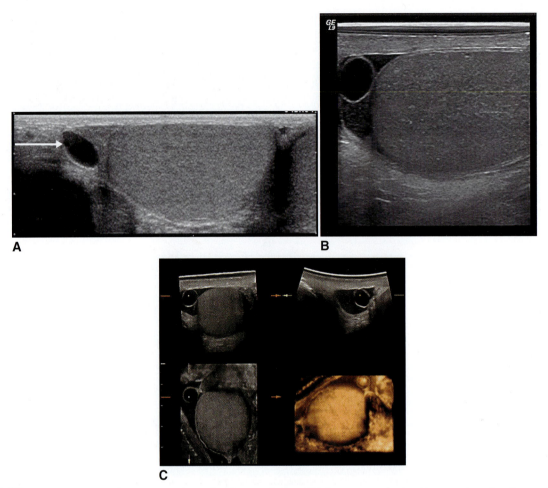

FIGURE 23-20 A, Sagittal image of a patient with a palpable scrotal mass. This image was obtained by scanning directly over the palpable area. It shows a fluid-filled mass with posterior acoustic enhancement located in the head of the epididymis *(arrow)*. This finding is consistent with both spermatocele and epididymal cyst. **B,** Conventional two-dimensional (2D) sagittal image demonstrated a cystic mass slightly superior and lateral to the right testis. **C,** 3D volume from the same patient showing orthogonal planes and surface rendering *(lower right)* demonstrated smooth walls and confirmed the extratesticular location of the cyst near the epididymal head. The coronal plane image *(lower left image)* demonstrated a stalk connecting the cyst to the epididymal head, confirming the diagnosis of a pedunculated cystic appendix epididymis.

Valsalva maneuver. It is helpful to instruct the patient to hold as still as possible during the maneuver, and to carefully adjust the color settings so that the PRF and wall filter are sensitized, but not so low that flash artifact fills the screen with a small movement.

Intratesticular varicocele has the sonographic appearance of straight or serpiginous channels coursing from the mediastinum into the testicular tissue. Color and spectral Doppler are used to identify these channels as dilated veins. On gray-scale imaging, the appearance can mimic that of tubular ectasia of the rete testis. Color Doppler will differentiate between intratesticular varicocele and tubular ectasia of the rete testis, as the latter shows no flow (Figure 23-22).

Scrotal Hernia

Hernias occur when bowel, omentum, or other structures herniate into the scrotum. Clinical diagnosis is usually sufficient, but ultrasound imaging is helpful when findings are equivocal. The bowel is the most commonly herniated structure, followed by the omentum.

Sonographic Findings. Peristalsis of the bowel, seen on real-time imaging, confirms the diagnosis of a scrotal hernia (Figure 23-23). This can be captured on videotape or as a cine clip for the interpreting physician to review. Unfortunately, peristalsis may not always be visible. Fluid-filled bowel loops are easily recognizable by ultrasound. Air-filled loops and loops that contain solid stool are more difficult to recognize. On ultrasound, air appears as bright echoes with a dirty acoustic shadow or ring artifact. Omental hernias appear brightly echogenic because of the omental fat (Figure 23-24).

Hydrocele, Pyocele, and Hematocele

A potential space exists between the visceral and parietal layers of the tunica vaginalis. This space is the place

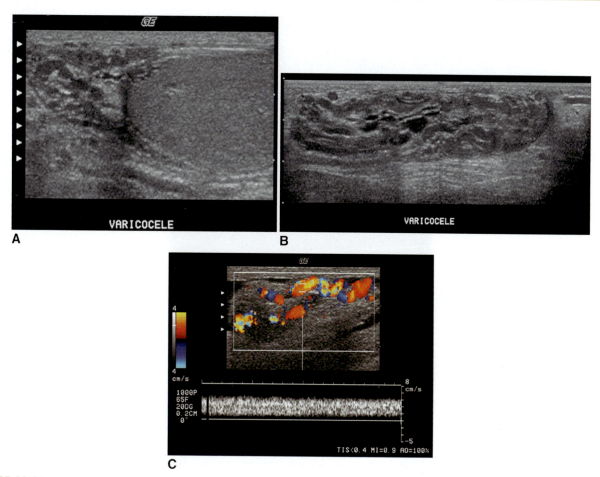

FIGURE 23-21 Varicocele in patient being evaluated for infertility. **A,** Sagittal view of the testis shows dilated tubular structures superiorly. **B,** Stitched ultrasound image shows prominent serpiginous venous channels forming a large varicocele on·the left. **C,** Doppler ultrasound with Valsalva maneuver shows venous flow within the dilated vascular channels, confirming the diagnosis of varicocele.

where a hydrocele, pyocele, or hematocele will develop. Normally, a small amount of fluid is present in this cavity, and this should not be confused with the presence of a hydrocele. A hydrocele contains serous fluid and is the most common cause of painless scrotal swelling. Hydroceles may have an unknown cause (idiopathic), but are commonly associated with epididymo-orchitis and torsion. They may also be found in patients following trauma or development of a neoplasm. Hydroceles associated with neoplasms tend to be smaller than those associated with other causes. Pyoceles and hematoceles are much less common than hydroceles.

A pyocele is a collection of pus. Pyoceles occur with untreated infection or when an abscess ruptures into the space between the layers of the tunica vaginalis. Hematoceles are associated with trauma, surgery, neoplasms, or torsion. They are collections of blood.

▶ **Sonographic Findings.** A hydrocele displays a fluid-filled collection located outside the anterolateral aspect of the testis. Hydroceles may be anechoic but most often contain some low-level echoes as a result of cellular debris (Figure 23-25). The display of low-level echoes is enhanced by high-frequency transducers and harmonic imaging. Hydroceles are more likely to appear anechoic with transducer frequencies below 7 MHz, or when low dynamic range settings are used. Hydroceles associated with infection show more internal echoes and septations. Sonographically, pyoceles and hematoceles are indistinguishable. They both contain internal echoes, thickened septations, and loculations (Figures 23-26 and 23-27). Ultrasound depiction of air within the space indicates an abscess, although an abscess may occur without the presence of air.

Sperm Granuloma

Sperm granulomas occur as a chronic inflammatory reaction to extravasation of spermatozoa. They are most frequently seen in patients with a history of vasectomy. A sperm granuloma may be located anywhere within the epididymis or the vas deferens. The main role of ultrasound imaging is to determine whether the mass is intratesticular or extratesticular. Extratesticular masses have a much lower rate of malignancy compared with intratesticular masses. Sperm granulomas cannot be reliably differentiated from epididymal tumors by ultrasound

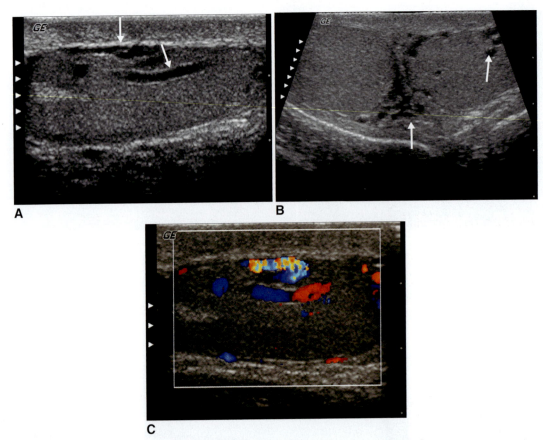

FIGURE 23-22 Intratesticular varicocele. **A,** Sagittal ultrasound image shows prominent connecting tubes with the testis *(arrows)*. **B,** Transverse ultrasound image of both testes shows an intratesticular and extratesticular varicocele on the left side *(arrows)*. **C,** Color Doppler is used to detect flow within the dilated intratesticular veins during Valsalva maneuver.

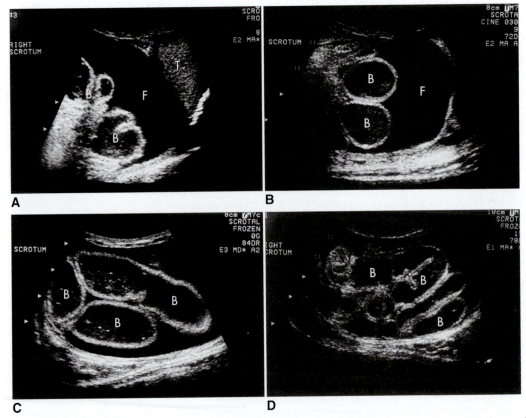

FIGURE 23-23 **A** through **D,** Small bowel herniated into the scrotum, representing scrotal hernia. Peristalsis was noted on real-time imaging. *B,* Bowel; *F,* fluid; *T,* testicle.

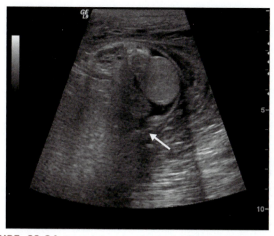

FIGURE 23-24 Scrotal hernia. Sagittal ultrasound image in a patient with chronic heart failure and scrotal edema. A large amount of edema is seen in the tissue surrounding the normal testis. A small hydrocele is present. A large hernia is seen protruding into the scrotum and displacing the testis inferiorly *(arrow)*. The hyperechoic appearance of the hernia suggests omental fat content.

imaging. However, a clinical history of vasectomy will help to target the differential diagnosis. Additionally, sperm granulomas are often painful. This aids in their differentiation from epididymal tumors, which are usually painless.

Sonographic Findings. Sonographic imaging shows a well-defined solid mass that may appear hypoechoic or isoechoic to the epididymis. These masses are often heterogeneous (Figure 23-28). Calcifications are not commonly present. Increased flow may be seen with color Doppler when inflammation is present.

Benign Testicular Masses

Tubular Ectasia of the Rete Testis. The **rete testis** is located at the hilum of the testis where the mediastinum resides. Tubular ectasia of the rete testis is an uncommon, benign condition. It is associated with the presence of a spermatocele, an epididymal or testicular cyst, or

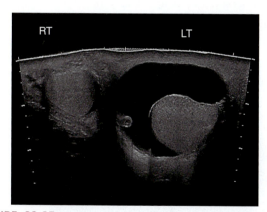

FIGURE 23-25 Idiopathic hydrocele formation in patient with scrotal swelling and tenderness. Panoramic view shows the normal right testis. The left testis is compressed because of the large hydrocele.

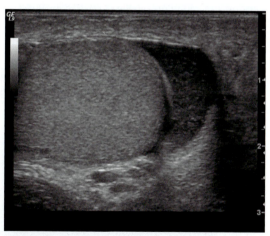

FIGURE 23-27 Hematocele in patient from the emergency room with scrotal trauma. Sagittal ultrasound image shows a small fluid collection with numerous bright echoes.

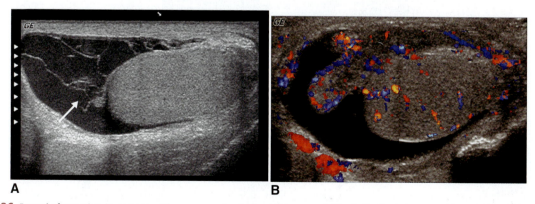

A   **B**

FIGURE 23-26 Pyocele formation in patient with severe, untreated epididymo-orchitis. **A,** Sagittal ultrasound image shows the multiseptated fluid collection containing internal debris *(arrow)*. **B,** Color Doppler image shows increased perfusion in the epididymis, testis, and surrounding tissue.

other epididymal obstruction on the same side as the dilated tubules. It is more commonly seen in patients 45 years of age or older.

Sonographic Findings. The normal rete testis may not be clearly depicted with ultrasound imaging. High-resolution imaging sometimes allows visualization of the normal rete testis as very tiny tubular structures near the mediastinum. Tubular ectasia appears as prominent hypoechoic channels near the echogenic **mediastinum testis** (Figure 23-29). Color Doppler can confirm the avascular nature of the tubules. Tubular ectasia has a similar sonographic appearance to intratesticular varicocele. These conditions can be differentiated using Doppler interrogation because the varicocele will demonstrate slow venous flow. To demonstrate slow flow, the color Doppler must be sensitized by using a low PRF and wall filter setting. The Valsalva maneuver should be used to enhance flow if a varicocele is present. If these and other adjustments are not made to the color controls, flow within a varicocele may not be detected, and results may be misinterpreted.

Cyst. Intratesticular cysts were once thought to be uncommon but are seen more often with more frequent use of ultrasound imaging. Cysts are common in men older than 40 years of age and have an association with extratesticular spermatoceles. They are located near the mediastinum. They may be single or multiple and of variable size. Cysts are incidental findings on sonography and do not require treatment.

Sonographic Findings. The sonographic appearance of cysts is the same throughout the body. Simple cysts

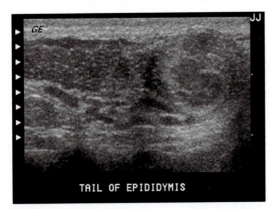

FIGURE 23-28 Painful epididymal mass in patient with history of vasectomy. Sagittal ultrasound image of epididymis shows a small, heterogeneous mass in the tail of the epididymis, possibly representing a sperm granuloma.

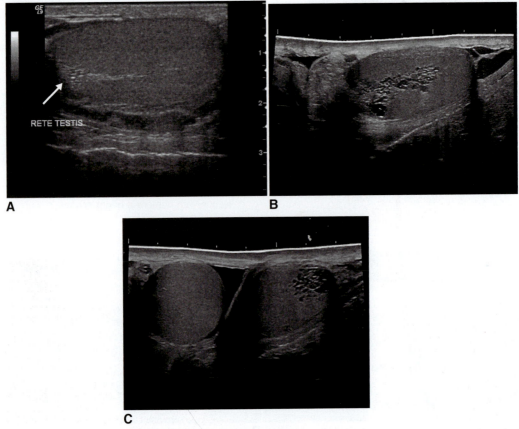

FIGURE 23-29 A, Mild dilatation of the rete testis in patient with spermatocele. Sagittal ultrasound image shows enlarged tubular structures located near the mediastinum testis. **B,** Sagittal panoramic view on the same patient demonstrates the dilated tubules of the rete testis in the area of the testicular mediastinum. **C,** Panoramic transverse image through the right and left testis shows dilatation of the rete testis on the left in a patient with a large spermatocele *(not shown)*.

are anechoic with posterior acoustic enhancement and a smooth border (Figure 23-30).

Microlithiasis. This is an uncommon condition characterized by tiny calcifications within the testis. These microcalcifications are smaller than 3 mm. Microlithiasis is usually a bilateral condition. It has been reported to have an association with testicular malignancy, but the exact nature of this is unknown. Annual follow-up of patients with testicular microlithiasis is recommended by some to exclude the development of neoplasm. Microlithiasis has also been associated with cryptorchidism, Klinefelter's syndrome, infertility, varicoceles, testicular atrophy, and male pseudohermaphroditism.

▶ **Sonographic Findings.** The sonographic appearance of testicular microlithiasis is of multiple bright, nonshadowing foci scattered throughout the testis (Figure 23-31).

The microliths may be numerous or few but are not considered to be abnormal unless more than five appear on any single image (Figure 23-32).

Malignant Testicular Masses

Table 23-6 lists the sonographic findings for solid malignant masses.

Germ Cell Tumors. Testicular cancer is not common, accounting for only 1% of cancers in men, but it is the most common malignancy in men between the ages of 15 and 35 years. Fortunately, testicular cancer is one of the most curable forms of cancer. It is more common in white men than black men. Testicular cancer occurs most frequently between the ages of 20 and 34. Undescended testes are 2.5 to 8 times more likely to develop cancer.

Most patients have no other symptoms except a painless lump, testicular enlargement, or vague discomfort in the scrotum. The primary goal of the ultrasound examination in testicular tumors is to determine mass location and differentiate between cystic and solid composition. Extratesticular masses are usually benign, whereas intratesticular masses are more likely to be malignant. Intratesticular cysts are benign masses, but care must be taken to ensure that a cyst is simple because some testicular cancers contain cystic components. Some benign conditions may mimic malignancy. These include hematoma, orchitis (especially when focal), abscess, infarction, and sperm granuloma. Obtaining a thorough patient history is very important because it will help to differentiate between these conditions.

In general, testicular tumors are divided into germ cell and non–germ cell tumors. Germ cell tumors are associated with elevated levels of human chorionic gonadotropin and alpha-fetoprotein. Approximately 95% of all testicular tumors are of germ cell type and are highly malignant. Non–germ cell tumors are generally benign. The most common type of germ cell tumor is seminoma,

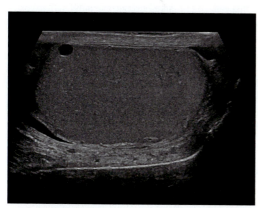

FIGURE 23-30 Simple testicular cyst. Sagittal ultrasound image was obtained using virtual convex to obtain a wide field of view. A small, simple cyst is shown in the superior pole of the testis. Note the smooth borders and the posterior acoustic enhancement.

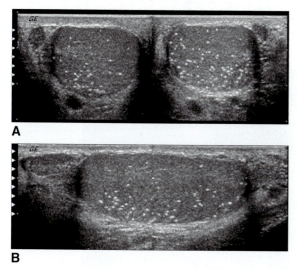

FIGURE 23-31 Testicular microlithiasis. **A,** Stitched transverse ultrasound image showing both testes with numerous brightly echogenic foci throughout. **B,** Sagittal ultrasound image showing testis with fewer microliths.

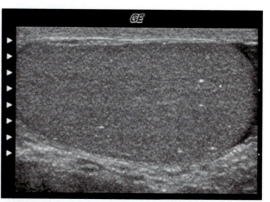

FIGURE 23-32 Sagittal ultrasound image showing testis with fewer microliths. More than five microcalcifications per image is considered abnormal. Note the absence of shadowing.

followed by mixed embryonal cell tumors and teratocarcinomas. Other less common germ cell tumors include yolk sacs, choriocarcinomas, teratomas, and other combinations of these cell types. The sonographer must remember that although testicular masses can be clearly described and differentiated using ultrasound, the examination cannot confirm the histology of the neoplasm. However, the sonographic features of a mass may suggest a certain type of tumor.

▶ **Sonographic Findings.** Ultrasound is nearly 100% sensitive for detecting tumors. Sonographically, most tumors appear as focal, hypoechoic masses (see Table 23-6). Seminomas tend to be homogeneous, hypoechoic masses with a smooth border (see Figure 23-27) (Figures 23-33 and 23-34). They often do not contain calcification or cystic components. In comparison, embryonal cell carcinoma is heterogeneous and is less well circumscribed. It may contain areas of increased echogenicity resulting from calcification, hemorrhage, or fibrosis (see Figure 23-28). Cystic components are found in up to one third of embryonal cell carcinomas (Figure 23-35). Embryonal cell tumors are more aggressive than seminomas, often invading the tunica albuginea and distorting the testicular contour. Teratomas may show dense foci that produce acoustic shadowing. They are normally heterogeneous but have well-defined borders. Teratomas are usually benign in children but malignant in adults. Choriocarcinoma has a varied sonographic appearance because of mixed cell types. Its appearance is determined by the dominant cell type, but it typically has irregular borders (see Figure 23-29). Ultrasound imaging cannot differentiate malignant from benign masses. Neither color Doppler nor Doppler waveforms can reliably distinguish between flow patterns of benign and malignant tumors.

Metastasis. Metastasis to the testicle is rare, normally occurring later in life. The primary tumor may originate from the prostate or kidneys; less common sites include lung, pancreas, bladder, colon, thyroid, and melanoma. Metastasis to the testicle is bilateral, with multiple lesions found.

▶ **Sonographic Findings.** Sonographically, metastasis appears as a solid hypoechoic mass, although it has been reported as hyperechoic or a mixture of both (see Table 23-6).

TABLE 23-6	Solid Malignant Masses
Tumor	**Sonographic Findings**
Seminoma	Hypoechoic lesion Smooth, well-defined borders
Embryonal cell carcinoma	Small hypoechoic mass Areas of increased echogenicity due to calcification Irregular borders May contain cystic areas
Teratoma	Complex mass, usually cystic and/or solid Well-defined borders Acoustic shadowing
Choriocarcinoma	Irregular borders Complex lesion Metastasis usually seen
Metastasis	Solid hypoechoic lesion (uncommonly may appear as hyperechoic or mixed echogenicity)
Lymphoma and leukemia	Enlarged testis Diffuse or focal areas of decreased echogenicity
Chronic lymphocytic leukemia	Well-circumscribed Anechoic Through-transmission

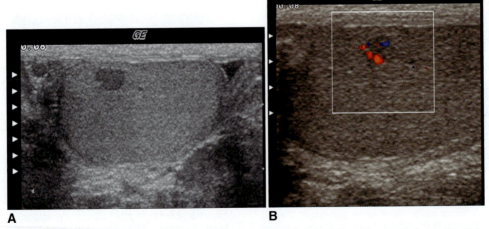

FIGURE 23-33 Small seminoma. **A,** Sagittal ultrasound image shows a small, hypoechoic mass within the testis. Note the presence of a small hydrocele. **B,** Color Doppler shows increased vascularity to the mass.

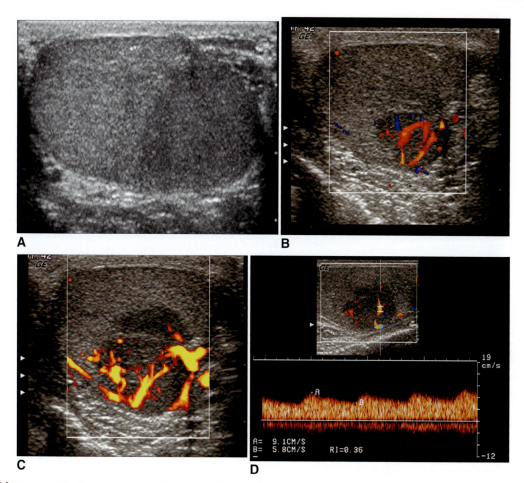

A, **B,** **C,** **D,**

FIGURE 23-34 Germ cell testicular tumor. **A,** Transverse ultrasound image shows heterogeneous echo texture throughout the testis. The tumor is primarily hypoechoic. **B,** Color Doppler shows distortion of the normal vessel architecture within the testis. Increased flow is seen within the mass. **C,** Power Doppler clearly shows the distorted vasculature of the testis within the mass. **D,** Spectral Doppler waveforms obtained within the mass show low resistance with prominent end-diastolic velocities characteristic of tumor flow. Doppler waveforms have not been shown to reliably differentiate between benign and malignant flow patterns.

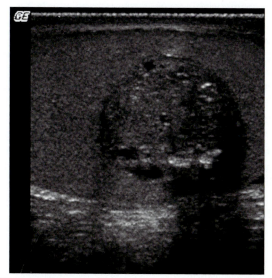

FIGURE 23-35 Heterogeneous testicular tumor. Sagittal ultrasound image of a testicular tumor containing calcium and cystic components. Although this pattern is not specific, it is typical of embryonal cell tumor.

Lymphoma and Leukemia

Malignant lymphoma makes up 1% to 7% of all testicular tumors and is the most common bilateral secondary testicular neoplasm affecting men older than 60 years.

Leukemic involvement of the testicle is the next most common secondary testicular neoplasm, most often found in children. Of children with leukemia, 8% have been reported to have testicular involvement.

Clinically, patients may experience weight loss, anorexia, and weakness. The testicle may become enlarged, and the tumor may be bilateral or unilateral.

◆ **Sonographic Findings.** Sonographically, lymphoma and leukemia appear similar. The testes may appear homogeneously hypoechoic or may contain multiple focal areas of decreased echogenicity (see Table 23-6). Chronic lymphocytic leukemia may appear as a focal, well-circumscribed, anechoic mass with through-transmission. Increased vascularity is seen with color Doppler imaging.

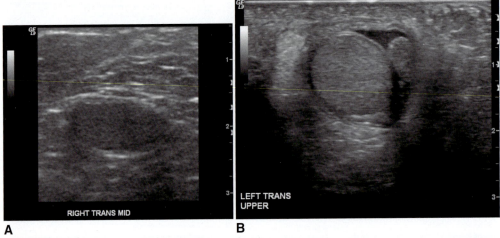

FIGURE 23-36 Undescended right testicle **(A)** with normal left testicle **(B)**. The undescended testis is smaller and hypoechoic compared with the normal left testis. The right testicle was located within the right inguinal canal.

Congenital Anomalies

Cryptorchidism (Undescended Testicle). During fetal growth, the testes first appear in the retroperitoneum near the kidneys. They descend into the scrotum from the inguinal canal shortly before birth or early in the neonatal period. The terms *undescended testis* and *cryptorchidism* describe a condition in which the testis has not descended into the scrotum and cannot be brought into the scrotum with external manipulation. The undescended testis may be located in the abdomen, inguinal canal, or other ectopic location. In most cases (up to 80%), the testis is found in the inguinal canal and is usually palpable. Because the testes do not descend until late in pregnancy, this condition is more common in premature babies. Cryptorchidism is bilateral in 10% to 25% of cases.

Surgical treatment of an undescended testicle by freeing it from the structures and implanting it into the scrotum is known as *orchiopexy*. If orchiopexy is not performed at an early age, multiple complications can occur. Exposure of the testis to higher temperatures than that found in the scrotum can prohibit spermatogenesis and result in infertility. Undescended testes are much more likely to develop testicular cancer. The risk of cancer is not reduced by orchiopexy, but it does allow the testis to be more easily palpated, so that a lump may be detected and treated earlier. Testicular torsion is also more common with undescended testes.

Sonographic Findings. On ultrasound, the undescended testis is smaller and less echogenic than the normal testis. It is usually oval with a homogeneous texture (Figure 23-36). Rarely, the mediastinum is seen.

Testicular Ectopia. Testicular ectopia is a very rare condition. Unlike an undescended testicle, an ectopic testicle cannot be manipulated into the correct path of descent. The most common site for the ectopic testicle to rest is the superficial inguinal pouch. Other sites include perineum, femoral canal, suprapubic area, penis, diaphragm, and the other scrotal compartment.

Anorchia. Anorchia is also rare. Unilateral anorchia, or monorchidism, is found in 4% of patients with a nonpalpable testis. It is more common on the left side, and definitive diagnosis depends on surgical diagnosis. Causes include intrauterine testicular torsion and other forms of decreased vascular supply to the testicle in utero. Bilateral anorchia is found in only 0.6% to 1.0% of patients with a nonpalpable testis. Patients have a male XY genotype. On physical examination, the **scrotum** is an empty, hypoplastic sac with a micropenis. These patients also have delayed onset of puberty, usually caused by an imbalance of hormones.

Polyorchidism (Testicular Duplication). Polyorchidism is a very rare disorder, with only 80 cases reported. It is more common on the left side (75%) and is bilateral in 5% of cases. Testicular duplication is usually found in the scrotum, but has also been found in the inguinal canal or retroperitoneum. The incidence of malignancy, cryptorchidism, inguinal hernia, and torsion is increased with polyorchidism. The duplicated testis is usually small, and its efferent spermatic system is completely absent.

The Musculoskeletal System

Susan Raatz Stephenson

OBJECTIVES

On completion of this chapter, you should be able to:
- Identify the normal anatomic location and function of the tendon, ligament, muscle, nerve, and bursa
- Know the advantages and disadvantages of sonographic artifacts in musculoskeletal imaging
- Summarize the basic sonographic examinations of the shoulder, wrist, knee, ankle, and foot
- Distinguish normal anatomy from common pathologic conditions

OUTLINE

In the early 1990s, a radiologist asked me to try to image a torn suprapatellar tendon. It was difficult to image the torn tendon because of technologic limitations and our inexperience in musculoskeletal (MS) ultrasound imaging. Musculoskeletal imaging is now gaining in popularity in the United States, following in the wake of magnetic resonance imaging (MRI). However, ultrasound of the musculoskeletal system has been widely used outside of the United States.

Many things have changed since then, both in the delivery of medical care and in the production of sonographic images. The decrease in medical reimbursements has forced the development of less expensive modalities to complement or replace computed tomography (CT) or MRI. Ultrasound equipment manufacturers have also continued to improve and refine technology, and this has resulted in improved soft tissue imaging. The 5- or 7-MHz transducer commonly used in the nineties is hardly acceptable for scanning superficial structures today. Current transducers create images with frequencies as high as 17 MHz.

This chapter is intended to provide a solid foundation for basic musculoskeletal ultrasound (MSUS). Imaging of the muscular system is not limited to the muscles themselves, but also includes the tendons, nerves, liga-ments, and bursa. Other areas of MS imaging include the joints, pediatric imaging, bone, skin, many disease processes, foreign bodies, and postoperative scanning. Add the joint-specific scanning of shoulder, knee, ankle, elbow, and wrist, and you begin to understand that MSUS imaging is a significant area that we have just begun to explore.

ANATOMY OF THE MUSCULOSKELETAL SYSTEM

Normal Anatomy

Skeletal muscle contains long organized units called muscle fibers. The characteristic long fibers are under voluntary control, allowing us to contract a **muscle** and move a joint. The blood vessels, lymphatics, and nerves follow the fibrous partitions between the bundles of muscle.

Several different types of muscles are present in the human body. Muscles have fibers that run parallel to the bone, have a fan shape, or form a **pennate** pattern. These feather-like muscle patterns run oblique to the long axis of the muscle and are unipennate, bipennate, multipen-nate, or circumpennate. Think of a feather and how the fibers grow from a central section. Half of this feather is unipennate, whereas the whole feather is bipennate. A multipennate muscle is a division of several feather-like sections in one muscle, whereas the circumpennate is the convergence of fibers to a central tendon (Figure 24-1, *A*). The deltoid muscle is an example of a unipennate muscle; it has feather-like fascicles with a unipennate, bipennate, or multipennate attachment (Figure 24-1, *B*). The gastrocnemius muscle in the calf is a bipennate muscle in which the fibers have a central origin (Figure 24-1, *C*). The large, flat muscles of the external oblique or the trapezius attach with a large, flat aponeurosis (Figure 24-1, *D*).

Attachment of the muscle occurs at the proximal and distal portions of the bundle. This attachment, a collection of tough collagenous fibers, is a **tendon.** These attachments may be cordlike or flat sheets called **aponeuroses.** This type of attachment occurs in flat muscles, such as the rectus abdominis in the abdomen. The elastic tendon consists of collagen fibers that enable it to stretch and flex around structures. This avascular structure heals slowly and has a whitish appearance. Because of the lack of vascularity, tendons heal slowly; this is why an injury can incapacitate a patient.

Tendons occur with or without a **synovial sheath.** This tubular sac surrounding a tendon has two layers. Fluid separates the two layers of the sheath and is found in the shoulder, hand, wrist, and ankle. This sheath plays an important role in imaging these structures with sonography. The biceps tendon of the shoulder is one example of a tendon with a synovial sheath. Other tendons, such as the Achilles' and patellar, lack this sheath and have a surrounding fat layer or loose connective tissue, which makes this type of tendon more difficult to image with sonography.

The support and strength of a joint are due in part to the **ligaments.** These short bands of tough fibers connect bones to other bones. This type of connective tissue is especially important in the knees, ankles, and shoulders.

The saclike structure surrounding joints and tendons that contains a viscous fluid is the **bursa.** This potential space provides an area for synovial fluid to aid in the reduction of friction between two musculoskeletal structures, such as tendon and bone or ligament and bone. For example, two of the knee joints that have such a bursa are the patellofemoral and femorotibial joints. The suprapatellar pouch has a continuous connection with the joint cavity but is often referred to as a bursa. The knee joint itself has nine bursae—three located anterior and six on the popliteal side of the joint.

Nerves are the conduits for impulses to and from the muscles and the central nervous system (CNS). Muscle action is under the control of the muscle system with the

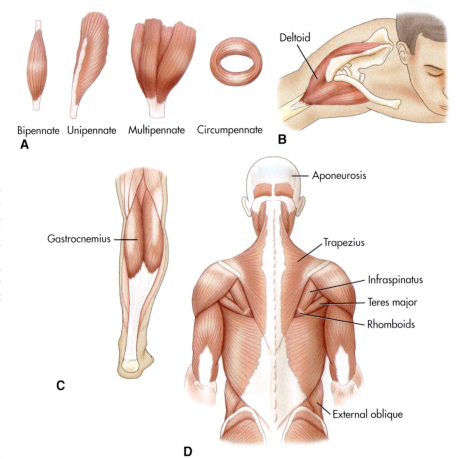

FIGURE 24-1 Different types of muscle. **A,** Unipennate, bipennate, multipennate, and circumpennate muscle patterns. **B,** The deltoid muscle is an example of a unipennate muscle and has feather-like fascicles with a unipennate, bipennate, or multipennate attachment. **C,** The gastrocnemius muscle in the calf is a bipennate muscle, whose fibers have a central origin. **D,** The large, flat muscles of the external oblique or the trapezius attach with a large, flat aponeurosis.

nerves in contact with the muscle through motor end plates. Elements of the nerves include the nerve fibers, arranged into bundles (**fasciculi**) and surrounded by dense insulating sheaths of **myelin** (forms the sheath of Schwann cells), and connective tissue.

Normal Sonographic Appearance

Imaging of the musculoskeletal system can be overwhelming because so many different muscles, attachments, ligaments, and tendons can be seen. All joints contains similar anatomic structures, and tendons and ligaments have the same sonographic imaging characteristics whether they are part of an ankle or a shoulder. Muscle attachments also have a similar sonographic appearance. The first step in sonographic imaging of any MS structure is knowledge of the normal appearance.

Tendons. Magnetic resonance imaging (MRI) has been the modality of choice for physicians in the United States when diagnosing MS problems. The advent of high-resolution ultrasound has challenged the superiority of

MRI for imaging tendons, especially when the examination is performed by a skilled sonographer using high-quality equipment. The evolution of real-time ultrasound allows demonstration of the full range of motion of the tendon. High resolution of modern transducers also allows imaging of the fine tendon fibers and comparison of normal versus abnormal using dual imaging techniques.

The tendon occurs in two forms: with and without a synovial sheath (Figure 24-2). Wrapped around the tendon, the smooth inner layer of this tubular sac lies in close contact with the tendon. Between this inner layer and an outer layer, a small amount of thick mucinoid material helps facilitate movement. The biceps tendon is one example of a sheath-covered tendon that images well (Figure 24-3). The thickness of this sheath measures only a couple of millimeters and is sonographically imaged as a hypoechoic halo surrounding the tendon. Inflammation of this sheath and tendon often aids in imaging and diagnosing problems with this tendon. Acute disease may reveal a sheath that is thicker than the contained tendon. Areas of high stress in the hand, wrist, and ankle also contain tendons with sheaths.

Paratenon, a loose areolar connective tissue, fills the fascial compartment of the tendon lacking a synovial sheath. The dense epitendineum, another layer of connective tissue, closely adjoins the tendon. The epitendineum images as an echogenic layer adjacent to the tendon. The lack of density differences in these interfaces makes the tendon somewhat difficult to image. Fortunately, many of the tendons without a synovial sheath are large and image relatively well. The accompanying bursa may also be abnormal, thus enhancing the tendon. Examples of this type of tendon include Achilles', patellar, proximal gastrocnemius, and semimembranosus tendons (Figure 24-4).

Interwoven and interconnected collagen fibers found in the tendon run in a parallel path. The numerous interfaces of the collagen fascicles provide a strong linear

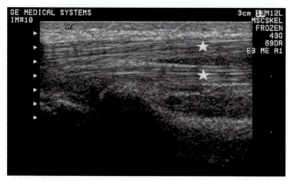

FIGURE 24-2 Superficial and deep flexor tendons *(stars)* have a surrounding synovial sheath that allows smooth motion of the pulley system of the hand. Tendon movement can be seen in real-time with movement of the fingers.

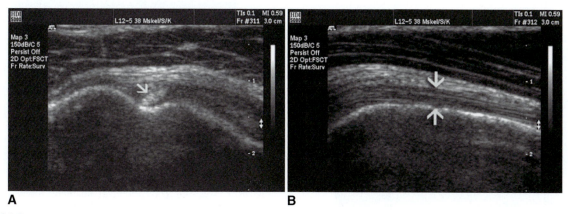

A   B

FIGURE 24-3 This transverse view of the rounded biceps tendon **(A)** images the tendon as a hyperechoic structure sitting within the bicipital groove of the humerus *(arrow)*. The longitudinal view **(B)** has the characteristic pattern seen with tendons encased within a synovial sheath *(arrows)*.

reflector that images well with ultrasound. The higher the frequency of the imaging transducer, the better these fibers image—a fact that underscores the need for a transducer of 7 MHz or greater. This normal fibrillar hypoechoic pattern and imaging detail become very important when diagnosing abnormalities.

Care must be taken when imaging the tendon because even a slight rotation off axis may produce an image that incorrectly suggests tendinitis. Both transverse and longitudinal planes help image the tendon, along with a side-by-side (dual) comparison of the contralateral side.

The tendon insertion site has its own sonographic characteristics. The joining of the tendon to the bone (enthesis) occurs with a narrow band of fibrocartilage. This avascular structure is approximately 1 cm long and images longitudinally as a triangular hypoechoic area in the distal tendon. Familiarity with the normal sonographic appearance is important because injury to this area of the tendon results in thickening of the insertion site (Figure 24-5).

Ligaments. Ligaments are thin, superficial structures, which makes them difficult to image. This superficial location requires the use of a higher-frequency transducer—10 MHz or greater—and possibly a stand-off pad to aid in imaging ligaments outside the joint. Critical to ligament identification is the equipment parameter adjustment. Adding too much gain to the image using overall gain or time gain compensation (TGC) results in loss of detail due to the strong bone reflections. Unlike imaging in other areas of the body, longitudinal imaging of the ligament is the only method used to image injuries. Transverse planes are of little help when imaging the ligament because they blend with the surrounding fat. The difficulty of imaging the ligament is helped by using a dual or side-by-side technique to compare normal and abnormal anatomy.

Many ligaments in the large joints of the body image well as hyperechoic straplike structures (Figure 24-6). One exception is the cruciate ligament within the knee joint, which appears hypoechoic. The large joints include

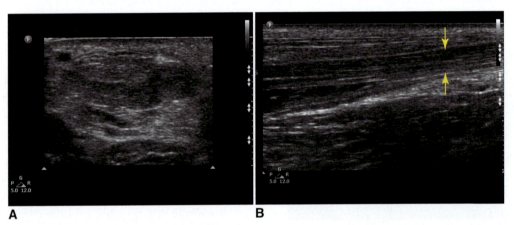

A **B**

FIGURE 24-4 A cross section or transverse view of the distal Achilles tendon **(A)** demonstrates the characteristic oval appearance. The tendon changes shape with decreased use, becoming round in the sedentary individual. The lack of synovial sheath is evident on the longitudinal image of the tendon **(B)**. The slight increase in echogenicity *(arrows)* on each side of the tendon is the epitendineum.

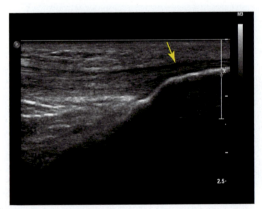

FIGURE 24-5 The normal Achilles tendon insertion *(arrow)* images at that insertion on the calcaneus and mimics cartilage found in other parts of the body.

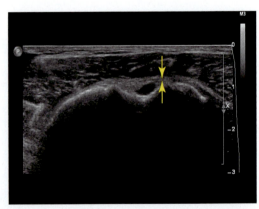

FIGURE 24-6 The coracohumeral ligament *(between arrows)* helps maintain the proper location of the long biceps tendon within the bicipital groove. This biceps tendon demonstrates tenosynovitis and inflammation of the tendon and sheath, which results in a hypoechoic appearance.

the hip, shoulder, ankle, wrist, and knee. Part of the difficulty associated with imaging the ligament is the lack of a contiguous structure, such as muscle, to aid in location. The dense fibers have a slightly less regular appearance and may help hold a tendon in place. Usually the ligament measures 2 to 3 mm thick and images as a hypoechoic band with a homogeneous appearance. These ligament structures are found close to both ends attaching to the bony cortex.

One ligament—the medial collateral ligament (MCL) or tibial collateral ligament, which connects the medial femoral condyle to the medial proximal tibia—deviates from the usual ligament appearance. This wide, smooth ligament is about 9 cm long and has deep and superficial portions. The external superficial portion consists of connective tissue appearing as a dense band that connects the medial femoral condyle to the proximal tibia. The deep layer connects the medial meniscus to the femur and tibia.

Sonographic imaging of the MCL reveals a three-layer structure. The superficial and deep layers have a hypoechoic-separating layer. Loose connective tissue forms the middle layer, which provides a potential space for bursas in some individuals (Figure 24-7).

Muscle. Discussions of muscle often include references to the origin and insertion of the muscle. The proximal portion of the muscle is considered the origin, whereas the insertion is the distal end. A muscle with two or more heads has an origin in more than one place on the bone. Most of us do not think in terms of origins and insertions, so for the purpose of this discussion, we will talk in terms of the location or attachment of the muscle.

To begin to learn the normal appearance of a muscle, it is easy to use the large quadriceps muscle located in the anterior thigh or the posterior calf muscles. Skeletal muscle imaged on a longitudinal plane appears homogeneous with multiple, fine parallel echoes (Figure 24-8). Connective tissue surrounding the fiber bundles produces these echogenic bands. The main portions of the muscle fibers are hypoechoic and radiate toward a central tendon or aponeurosis (Figure 24-9). The transverse plane discloses a less organized pattern of fine punctate echoes scattered through the muscle bundle. Encasing the muscle is a connective tissue fascia that has a bright echogenic appearance (Figures 24-10 and 24-11). This fascia layer, although brighter than the sheathed muscle fibers, has less echogenicity than subcutaneous fat or tendons.

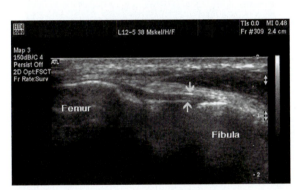

FIGURE 24-7 The fibular collateral ligament connects the fibula to the lateral side of the femur. This hypoechoic linear structure *(arrows)* passes over the lateral meniscus and has a slightly oblique course.

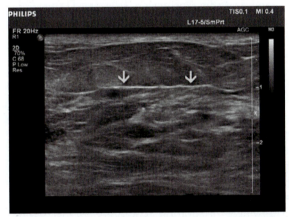

FIGURE 24-9 The dense aponeurosis tissue that connects the muscle to bone images is an echogenic linear structure *(arrows)*.

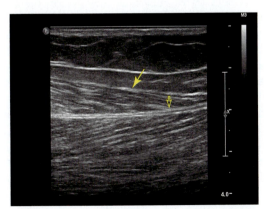

FIGURE 24-8 The bipennate gastrocnemius muscle has echogenic obliquely oriented connective tissue *(solid arrow)* between the muscle bundles. A small central tendon *(open arrow)* serves as the anchor for these bundles.

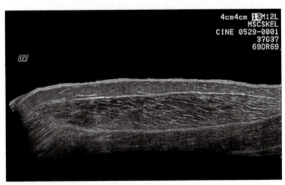

FIGURE 24-10 Panoramic imaging allows global study of this normal gastrocnemius muscle.

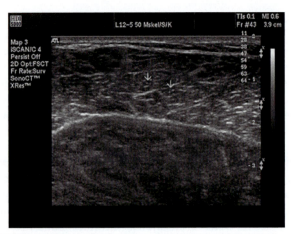

FIGURE 24-11 Small punctate echogenicities *(arrows)* image on the transverse muscle.

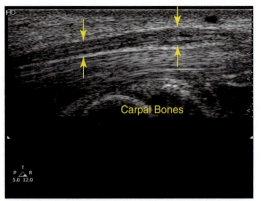

FIGURE 24-12 The median nerve runs on the ventral side of the forearm and wrist, supplying the muscles of the superficial layers of the forearm and hand. The hypoechoic nerve *(right arrows)* sits just anterior to the echogenic deep flexor tendon of the index finger *(left arrows)*.

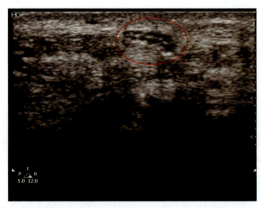

FIGURE 24-13 This transverse scan of the median nerve reveals the hyperechoic nerves with hypoechoic nerve fiber fascicles.

The muscle bundle contains nerves, fascia, tendons, fat, and fibrous connective tissue surrounding the muscle. The epimysium continues into the muscle, developing into the perimysium, which separates the bundles into muscle fibers. These hypoechoic structures, when compared with the muscle fibers, help differentiate muscles. The sonographic appearance of muscle can be deceiving in some areas, such as the hand, because of the similarity of echo texture to a mass or tenosynovitis. Careful scanning and transducer rotation help image the pennate structure of the muscle, aiding in identification of a possible normal muscle variant.

Normal dynamics of the muscle images easily in real-time because contraction of the muscle increases muscle thickness and hypoechogenicity. In addition, echogenic connective tissue bands increase in obliquity. Sustained contraction of the muscle has the same sonographic appearance as muscle bundles found in the athletic patient. This decreased echogenic muscle, as a result of hypertrophy, is normal for this patient population. Compression of the muscle with the transducer condenses the tissue, resulting in an increase in muscle echogenicity.

Transducer orientation is another factor that influences muscle echogenicity. Ensuring a longitudinal and transverse plane with good contact helps negate the possibility of introducing artifactual information. It is helpful to scan the contralateral normal side to ensure technique or to ensure that normal variants do not result in a misdiagnosis.

Nerves. The normal nerve has a hyperechoic appearance when compared with muscle but is hypoechoic when compared with tendons. The echogenicity depends on the surrounding structures and is not constant within the body. The longitudinal plane reveals a fibrillar pattern with parallel inner linear echoes similar to the tendon. In transverse imaging, the nerve fibers appear hypoechoic, with a hyperechoic **perineurium** surrounding each fiber. The collagenous **epineurium**—the outer layer of the nerve—appears as a hyperechoic layer (Figures 24-12 and 24-13).

Differentiating nerves from tendons is a simple task when you contrast the two structures. Real-time imaging shows tendons that move when the corresponding joint or muscle contracts. The nerve will remain stable within the muscle tissue. Sonographic artifacts (anisotropy) are not as evident on the nerve as they are on the tendon, and nerves are imaged best with a transducer of 10 MHz or higher. Power Doppler is especially helpful because vessels accompany the nerves. Table 24-1 lists the nerves that are identifiable with sonography.

Bursa. The small sac between two moving surfaces, usually tendon and bone, is the bursa. These fluid-filled cavities facilitate the movement of tendons or muscles over bony projections. The minute amount of viscous fluid contained within the bursa helps reduce friction between moving parts of the joint (Figures 24-14 and 24-15). The major bursa of the body is the subacromial-subdeltoid bursa, found in the shoulder, covering the deep surface of the deltoid muscle.

Two types of bursas are found in the body: communicating and noncommunicating. This categorization helps explain the relationship of the bursa to the joint

TABLE 24-1	Nerves Identifiable With Sonography
Lower Limb	**Location**
Sciatic	Posterior thigh lateral to the hamstring muscle
Popliteal	Popliteal fossa superficial to the popliteal artery and vein
Upper Limb	**Location**
Suprascapular	Deep to the trapezius to the infraspinatus fossa
Median	Medial to the biceps tendon and brachial artery, elbow, right side of the carpal tunnel
Radial	Between the brachioradialis and brachialis muscles
Ulnar	Median epicondyle of the elbow, medial to the ulnar artery in Guyon's canal

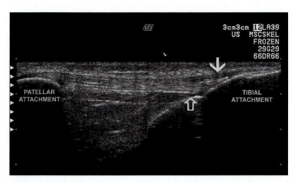

FIGURE 24-14 This normal infrapatellar tendon has multiple bursae, which usually blend in with surrounding tissue. One lies between the skin and fascia anterior to the tibial tuberosity *(arrow)*, and a deep bursa lies between the patellar ligament and the tibial tuberosity *(open arrow)*. The knee itself has a total of nine bursae located in and around the joint.

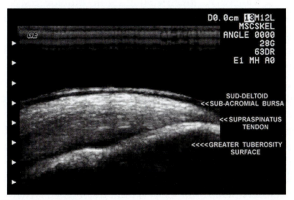

FIGURE 24-15 New technologies, such as three-dimensional (3D) imaging, have the ability to remove surrounding tissue signals from the dataset. This capability makes this modality ideal for imaging of the bursa. This subdeltoid-subacromial bursa image clearly demonstrates the external synovial layer with hypoechoic lubricating fluid.

space. One communicating bursa sonographers often see is **Baker's cyst**, which is located in the medial popliteal fossa. This bursa, located between the semimembranosus and medial gastrocnemius tendons, has a connecting neck to the bursa contained within the knee joint. Usually, sonographers image bursas that do not communicate with the joint space. An example of a superficial noncommunicating type of bursa is the prepatellar bursa.

In the normal patient, the bursae are difficult to image because they often blend in with surrounding tissue and fat. The thin film of viscous fluid found within the bursa contributes to the hypoechoic appearance of the structure because the walls are too thin to image. These potential spaces will appear on ultrasound in the presence of an inflammatory process caused by fluid accumulation. Any bursa larger than 2 mm is enlarged and needs to be compared with the normal contralateral side.

Table 24-2 summarizes the normal sonographic appearance of tendons, ligaments, nerves, muscle, and bursae.

ARTIFACTS

Sonographers and sonologists have the daily challenge of separating artifacts from useful image information. All equipment manufacturers program in some basic assumptions about the interaction between tissue and sound: that the speed of sound is 1540 m/sec, that the area imaged is within the central beam, and that sound travels out and back in a straight line. Artifacts occur when these basic assumptions are not met, and something is created that is not real, is erroneously positioned, has improper brightness, or is absent from the image. Many manufacturers have developed technology to reduce and often eliminate some types of artifacts caused by compound and harmonic imaging.

Musculoskeletal imaging displays the same gamut of artifacts seen in other areas of the body. The superficial nature of MS structures, often anterior to the highly reflective bone, causes artifacts to become more of a problem. Some artifacts aid in identifying pathologic conditions and structures; however, others hinder and even mimic disease.

Several artifact types—anisotropy, reverberation, time of flight artifact, and refractile shadowing—are important in MSUS. Understanding how artifacts occur and how to correct images increases both diagnostic confidence and image accuracy.

Anisotropy

The anisotropic phenomenon is one that occurs not only in sonography but also in other professions, such as astronomy, geology, and chemistry. **Anisotropy** occurs when the sound beam misses the transducer on the return because of the curve of the structure (Figure 24-16). The

TABLE 24-2 | **Normal Sonographic Appearance**

Anatomy	General Sonographic Appearance	Longitudinal Appearance	Transverse Appearance
Tendon	Hyperechoic linear structure Dynamic with movement of corresponding joint/muscle	Cordlike	Oval, round, or cuboid
Ligament	Isoechoic, weakly hyperechoic	Striated structures connecting bone to bone	Difficult to image on the transverse plane
Nerve	Hypoechoic to tendons Hyperechoic to muscle Cannot be mobilized with movement Posterior enhancement lacking	Cordlike tubular structure	Hypoechoic with fascicles
Muscle	Muscular bundles—hypoechoic Perimysium, epimysium, fascia, fat plane—hyperechoic	Parallel echogenic linear appearance within hypoechoic muscle tissue; may appear featherlike depending on the type of muscle imaged	Punctate echogenic areas within the hypoechoic muscle
Bursa	Thin, hypoechoic structure that merges with the surrounding fat	Thin linear hypoechoic structure adjacent to a tendon	Normal bursa are difficult to image on the transverse plane

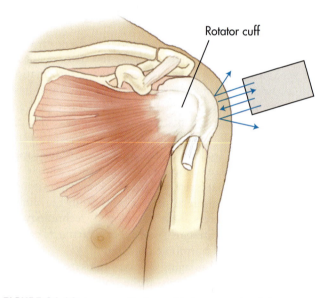

Rotator cuff

FIGURE 24-16 A perpendicular or 90-degree angle of the sound beam to the reflecting tissue surface results in the greatest amount of reflection and optimal images. At nonperpendicular incidence, part of the incident sound beam misses the transducer, resulting in the display of decreased brightness of returning echoes.

angle and direction of the reflected beam depend upon the angle of incidence.

The reflection coefficient is a function of the angle and becomes a problem when the reflected beam misses the receiver. The nonperpendicular tissue interfaces return echoes at an angle that does not return to the transmitting transducer, creating an imaging challenge. This results in differing image properties depending on the angle of incidence.

The loss of definition of the curved upper pole of the right kidney is one example of this artifact. The muscle,

ligaments, and nerves also image as an anisotropic reflector because of the plane they occupy, with tendons having the most pronounced anisotropy in MS imaging. This loss of image requires a heel-to-toe rocking of the transducer to create the optimal 90-degree angle (Figures 24-17 and 24-18).

Reverberation

A reflective surface reverberates sound and may be beneficial or detrimental. We often experience this phenomenon without realizing its impact. Our senses use reverberation as a clue to the location of structures in a room through reflection of sound back to our ears. Any acoustic environment, such as an auditorium, relies on reverberation to transmit sound.

The same is true of sound transmitted into the body. The initial sound beam transmits and returns. Multiple delayed reflections from strong tissue boundaries, such as bone, result in a linear artifact that *decreases* in intensity with depth. This collection of reflected sound is superimposed over the primary signal, often adding distracting information to the image (Figure 24-19).

Reverberation is not always a detrimental process. One type of artifact, comet tail, results from reverberation from metal, such as clips, sutures, staples, or a foreign object like a BB. This type varies slightly from the traditional reverberation, which bounces between the transducer face and the strong reflector. The **comet tail artifact** is a function of the sound bouncing between two closely placed reflectors within the imaged structure. In the case of a pin surgically placed within a bone, the reflecting surfaces are the anterior and posterior borders of the hardware. The ringing occurs within the metal object, and each time the sound returns to the anterior border, some of the sound escapes. The resultant

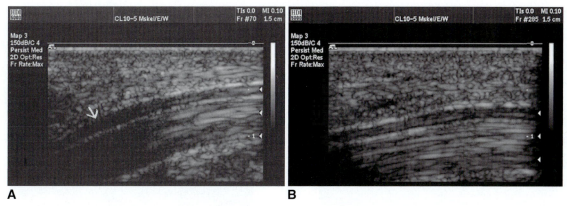

FIGURE 24-17 These images of the median nerve and the deep flexor tendon illustrate the effects of anisotropy. **A,** A large artifact occurred because the angle of incidence is not 90 degrees, resulting in a hypoechoic appearance of the tendon and nerve *(arrow).* **B,** Rocking the transducer or repositioning the structure allows the angle of incidence to be closer to 90 degrees, thus reducing or eliminating the artifact.

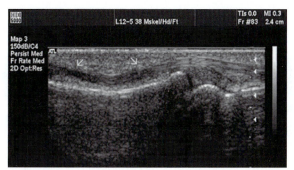

FIGURE 24-18 Change in direction of the imaged structure (digital flexor tendon) causes multiple areas of anisotropy *(arrows)* due to changes in the angle of incidence.

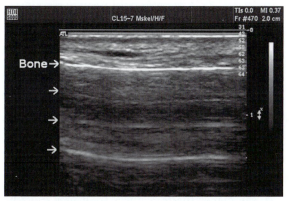

FIGURE 24-19 Reverberation artifact resulting from sound bouncing between the strongly reflecting bone and the transducer face.

artifact resembles a comet tail, hence its name (Figure 24-20).

Refractile Shadowing

The bending of the transmitted sound beam to an oblique path occurs often and is seen as an edge artifact (**refractile shadowing**) on the sonographic image. This change in direction of the sound beam results in a hypoechoic band

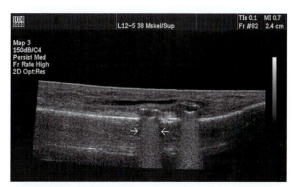

FIGURE 24-20 Comet tail artifact *(arrows)* seen posterior to tibial pins placed to stabilize a tibial fracture. Note the widening of the posterior reverberation, which is due to reverberation within the metal pins. This widening is common with metal placed within musculoskeletal (MS) structures and is still a comet tail artifact even though it does not narrow in the distal area.

posterior to the structure. Another cause of refractile shadowing is a tissue impedance mismatch different than the average speed of sound within soft tissue (1540 m/sec). This is seen at the edge of a round or oval ligament or as the result of a traumatic tear of an MS structure (Figures 24-21 and 24-22). Most commonly seen with a complete tendon tear, the angles formed from the retracted tendon cause refractile shadowing. This shadowing is often used to determine the distance between ligaments by measuring from one artifact edge to the other.

Time of Flight Artifact

Time of flight, or speed of sound, artifacts occur when the returning sound wave has passed between two tissues with markedly different speeds. This misrepresentation of the return time results from the assumption that the speed of sound is a constant 1540 m/sec. If the speed of sound is less than the average in tissue, the artifact appears to be farther away from the transducer. Faster speed results in the artifact being closer to the transducer on the image. Creation of this type of false information

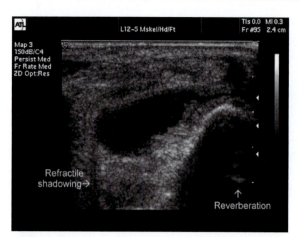

FIGURE 24-21 This ganglion located in the ankle demonstrates refractile shadowing.

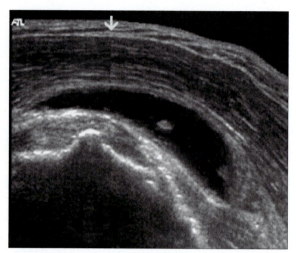

FIGURE 24-23 This panoramic image of a rotator cuff tear demonstrates the very subtle time of flight artifact.

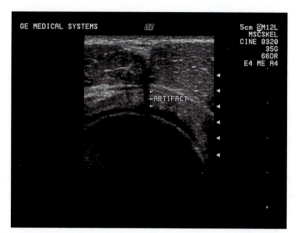

FIGURE 24-22 Refractile shadowing from a normal structure anterior to the area of interest (supraspinatus tendon) makes it difficult to diagnose abnormalities.

TABLE 24-3	Correction Techniques for Artifacts
Artifact	**Correction Technique**
Anisotropy	Heel-to-toe rocking of the transducer creates a perpendicular angle of incidence, removing the anisotropy.
Reverberation	Anterior reverberation can be minimized with the use of a stand-off pad or by changing the angle of incidence.
Refractile	Use of newer technologies, such as compound shadowing imaging or tissue harmonics, helps reduce or eliminate this artifact. Changing the angle of incidence may move the artifact out of the region of interest.
Time of flight	May not be able to eliminate as a result of tissue artifact sound properties. Change the angle of incidence to demonstrate surrounding tissue.

occurs most commonly with MSUS when imaging obese patients at a muscle-fat interface (Figure 24-23).

The speed of sound artifact displaces the image in the anteroposterior (axial) plane. When this speed artifact is coupled with refraction, a structure displays with an incorrect shape. For example, think of a wall of bricks. If one section fails and drops down, the result is that one section is asymmetrical from the surrounding areas. Do not mistake this very subtle artifact with a transducer crystal malfunction. A mechanical failure produces a decrease in image information that begins at the transducer face, but the time of flight artifact affects only the image.

Table 24-3 lists the techniques for correcting the artifacts discussed previously.

SONOGRAPHIC EVALUATION OF THE MUSCULOSKELETAL SYSTEM

Sonographic imaging of the joints begins with the proper choice of transducers. Superficially located joints and structures image well with high-frequency transducers of 5 MHz or higher. The more superficial the imaged structure is, the higher the transducer frequency must be to ensure maximal detail; however, larger joints, such as the shoulder, may require a lower frequency to penetrate the MS structures.

Positioning of the joint of interest is an important part of the examination. The patient should be placed in a comfortable position that allows the sonographer to maintain correct scanning ergonomics to prevent development of MS problems. A final consideration is the dynamic portion of the examination. It is often helpful to be able to move the joint to confirm the imaged structure. Space must be allowed for a full range of motion for the imaged joint.

Rotator Cuff

The American Institute for Ultrasound Medicine (AIUM) recommends middle frequencies of 7 and 10 MHz for imaging shoulder structures; however, deeper rotator cuff structures may require a frequency of 5 MHz. Shoulder anatomy is complex, with numerous bursae, muscles, and tendons surrounding the joint. A basic sonographic examination of the structures found in the rotator cuff includes 11 images. Comparison with the contralateral normal shoulder is always helpful in determining the absence or presence of a pathologic condition.

The biceps tendon is one of the easiest structures to image in the adult shoulder. Similar to any examination, documentation includes both longitudinal and transverse views. Begin by having the patient sit erect on a rotating chair with a back. The rotation of the chair allows quick and easy readjustments to the shoulder. To begin the examination of the biceps tendon, place the patient with a slight internal rotation of the shoulder. To obtain this position, have the patient place the arm on the lap with the fingers of the hand facing the opposite shoulder (Figure 24-24).

Begin the examination by facing the patient and checking the transducer orientation to prevent confusion during scanning. The structures will change with the particular shoulder being imaged. When facing the patient and imaging the right shoulder, the lateral anatomy displays on the left side of the image and the medial anatomy on the right side of the screen. When scanning posterior shoulder structures, the image corresponds to the patient position.

Begin the examination with the 3- to 5-mm-thick biceps tendon. This tendon is easily located in the transverse plane and images as an echogenic oval structure within the bicipital groove of the humerus. This groove, located between the greater and lesser tuberosities, coupled with the overlying transverse ligament, maintains the biceps tendon location. Once identified, images at several different levels help determine normalcy. A small amount of fluid—less than 1.5 mm—is a normal finding. Care must be taken to use minimal transducer pressure because small amounts of fluid may be compressed out of the imaging plane (Figure 24-25). A longitudinal image of the tendon requires some rocking of the transducer to obtain images with minimal anisotropic artifacts. When scanning the biceps tendon, take note of the fibrillar pattern of the normal tendon because disruptions indicate a possible pathologic condition (Figure 24-26).

Finding the subscapularis tendon begins by imaging the biceps tendon on the transverse plane at the level of

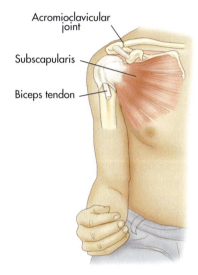

FIGURE 24-24 The subscapularis, the biceps tendon, and the acromioclavicular joint image easily from the anterior approach. This is considered a neutral position for the shoulder.

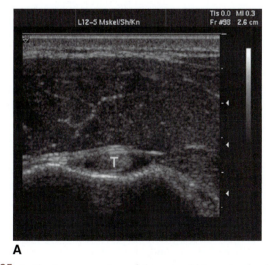

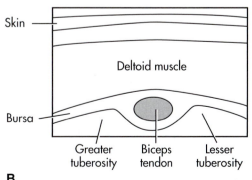

A   **B**

FIGURE 24-25 A, The transverse view of the normal biceps tendon has the echogenic tendon *(T)* within the bicipital groove. The anechoic effusion of tenosynovitis surrounding the tendon aids in visualization. **B,** Diagram of the anatomy.

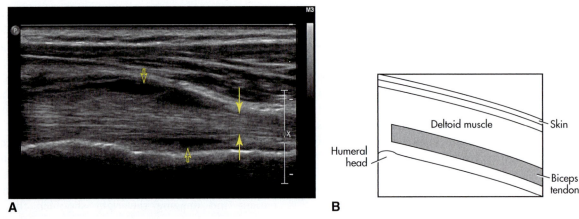

FIGURE 24-26 A, The longitudinal image of the biceps tendon *(arrows)* images the fibrillar pattern seen with tendons. The small amount of effusion *(open arrows)* seen posterior to the tendon indicates mild tenosynovitis. **B,** Diagram of the anatomy.

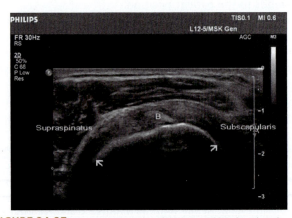

FIGURE 24-27 The biceps tendon *(B)* is a good landmark to locate the subscapularis and supraspinatus tendons. This image shows the transverse tendon between the anteromedially located subscapularis tendon and the posterolateral supraspinatus. Note the anisotropy artifact *(arrows)* seen as the tendons curve with the humeral head.

the humeral head. Using the biceps tendon as a landmark, angle the transducer anteromedially, while locating the subscapularis. The transverse view images the tendon as an oval soft tissue structure. Note that the transverse view of the tendon requires a longitudinal transducer orientation (Figure 24-27). Externally rotating the arm while scanning aids in visualization of the tendon and determination of normal movement. This tendon inserts into the lesser tuberosity at an angle requiring slight rotation to obtain the longitudinal view (transverse transducer position).

The next structure to be located is the 3- to 7-mm supraspinatus tendon located laterally and posteriorly from the biceps tendon. This bandlike tendon has a medium-level echo texture and originates from the greater tuberosity of the humerus. The acromion limits the field of view, necessitating careful transducer and patient positioning. A portion of the tendon, called the critical zone and located 1 cm posterolateral to the biceps tendon, is the most likely location for injury. Care

must be taken here because improper scanning results in a false-positive or false-negative finding. The dual- or split-screen function allows for normal versus injured shoulder comparisons, which help to pinpoint tears.

Initial transverse and longitudinal views begin with the patient's arm in a neutral position; however, after localization of the tendon, the arm is repositioned into the Bouffard or Crass position (Figure 24-28). Whether the shoulder can be externally rotated into these positions depends on the patient's ability to place the arm behind the back or on the hip. This stresses the tendons of the rotator cuff, helping to emphasize any abnormalities. Another benefit is that the supraspinatus moves anterior and out from under the acromion, allowing better visualization of the tendon (Figures 24-29 through 24-32).

The infraspinatus tendon is the next structure to be imaged; two methods are available to localize the tendon. The first involves rotating the patient to gain access to the posterior shoulder and positioning the hand on the patient's opposite shoulder. The posterior glenoid labrum is a good landmark to help find the anteriorly located infraspinatus tendon (Figure 24-33). A second method has the patient's arm in the same position used in imaging the biceps tendon, locating the supraspinatus tendon, moving posterior and parallel to the scapular spine, and locating the infraspinatus tendon at its attachment to the posterior greater tuberosity of the humerus. Fluid imaged superficial to the infraspinatus tendon indicates bursal fluid, whereas posterior fluid indicates joint effusion. Take note of the humeral head contours because irregularities indicate a pathologic condition.

Although injury to the teres minor tendons is uncommon, imaging ensures complete visualization of the infraspinatus tendon because of their close proximity. This tendon lies parallel to the scapular spine and inferior to the infraspinatus tendon. To differentiate the infraspinatus tendon from the teres minor, pay close attention to the plane of the tendon fibers. Horizontal fibers indicate the infraspinatus, whereas the teres minor

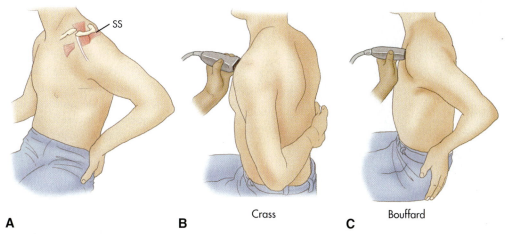

A   **B**   Crass   **C**   Bouffard

FIGURE 24-28 Once the supraspinatus *(SS)* has been located in the neutral position **(A),** move the hand to position the patient in the Crass **(B)** or Bouffard **(C)** position.

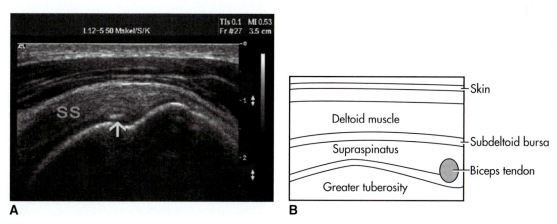

A   **B**

FIGURE 24-29 A, The medially located biceps tendon *(arrow)* helps locate the supraspinatus *(SS).* Scan this tendon from the acromion to the greater tuberosity to locate any echogenicity changes or the presence of fluid. **B,** Diagram of the anatomy.

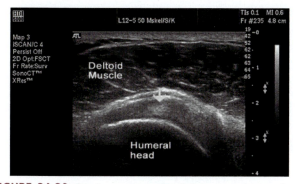

FIGURE 24-30 This transverse scan of the supraspinatus shows the tendon *(arrow)* to be mildly hyperechoic.

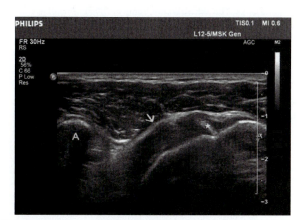

FIGURE 24-31 This image has the arm in a neutral position. To locate the supraspinatus, use the biceps tendon *(star)* as a landmark, and then rotate the transducer until the acromion *(A)* comes into view. The supraspinatus tendon *(arrow)* appears between these two structures. Note the anisotropy artifact that hinders visualization of part of the tendon.

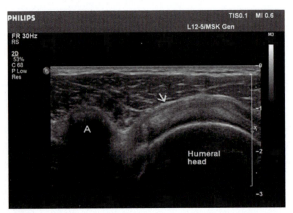

FIGURE 24-32 This image shows the supraspinatus tendon *(arrow)* seen extending to the acromion *(A)* with the shoulder internally rotated into the Bouffard position. Most of the anisotropic artifact disappears because the tendon is closer to parallel to the transducer.

is on an oblique plane. The teres minor appears as a trapezoidal structure inferior to the infraspinatus tendon.

During examination of rotator cuff structures, it is important to note any bursal thickening, tendon calcifications, bony irregularities, loose bodies, or fluid collections. Many other non–rotator cuff structures can also be imaged, such as the **acromioclavicular joint (AC)**. Because of the superficial location of the AC, joint separations are easily imaged, especially when compared with a normal contralateral joint. As with any other portion of the body, soft tissue masses and injury, foreign body localization, and fluid collections are easily identified (Figures 24-34 and 24-35).

Box 24-1 lists the main indications for shoulder sonography. Box 24-2 lists the minimum shoulder views of the rotator cuff.

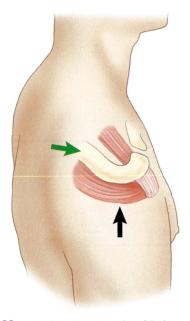

FIGURE 24-33 The infraspinatus tendon *(black arrow)* lies lateral and inferior to the scapular spine *(green arrow)*.

BOX 24-1	Indications for Shoulder Sonography

- Shoulder pain or swelling
- Pain with joint rotation
- Weakness with arm elevation
- Trauma
- Decreased range of motion
- Evaluation of soft tissue masses

BOX 24-2	Minimum Shoulder Views of the Rotator Cuff

View: 1/2: Biceps longitudinal and transverse
View: 3/4: Subscapularis longitudinal and transverse
View: 5/6/7/8: Supraspinatus in neutral and internal rotation
View: 9/10: Infraspinatus/posterior glenoid labrum
View: 11: Teres minor

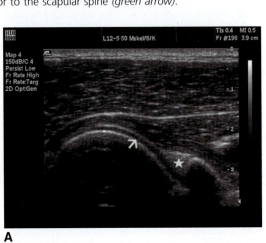

A

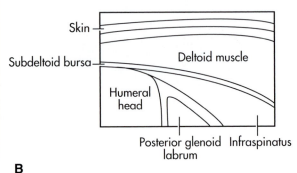

B

FIGURE 24-34 A, The posterior glenoid labrum *(star)* is a triangular hyperechoic structure deep to the infraspinatus tendon. The humeral head cartilage *(arrow)* images as a thin, hypoechoic layer superficial to the bony surface. **B,** Diagram of the anatomy.

Carpal Tunnel

The wrist joint is easily examined because of its accessibility, size, and lack of overlying bony structures. This ease of imaging implies that the wrist is an uncomplicated joint to image; however, familiarity with wrist anatomy reveals a very complex set of structures. The complexity of the wrist is underscored by the fact that some orthopedic surgeons specialize in just this one joint.

Positioning of the wrist entails placing the arm at a 90-degree angle with the palm pronated or supinated on the lap of the patient (Figure 24-36). Placing a small rolled-up towel under the wrist when examining the palmar (**volar**) portion of the wrist places the joint in a neutral position. The towel also helps dorsal imaging of the wrist when the hand is palm down. These positions allow imaging of carpal tunnel structures, ganglion and synovial cysts, tears of the triangular fibrocartilage, tenosynovitis, and any other tumors. Another benefit of sonographic imaging of the wrist is the ability to demonstrate the dynamics of the wrist and associated masses

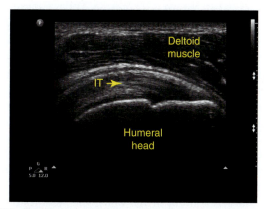

FIGURE 24-35 The infraspinatus tendon *(IT)* has a triangular appearance at the attachment to the posterior greater tuberosity. This image helps determine the echogenic consistency of the tendon when coupled with external and internal rotation maneuvers.

with finger movement. The smaller wrist joint requires a higher-frequency transducer in the 10- to 20-MHz range. Manufacturers also offer transducers with smaller footprints, which allow easier scanning than some of the larger linear transducers.

The carpal tunnel is located between the carpal bones and the flexor retinaculum on the palmar side of the wrist. This fibro-osseous space contains the median nerve, the flexor pollicis longus, and the eight tendons that connect the digital muscles to the wrist (flexor digitorum tendons). The ulnar artery and veins indicate the medial border of the carpal tunnel, whereas the most lateral structures are the radial artery and veins. The flexor retinaculum forms the anterior border by attaching to the scaphoid tubercle, trapezium ridge, pisiform bone, and hook of the hamate. The median nerve, which is of particular interest when diagnosing carpal tunnel syndrome, lies superficial and toward the radial side of the tunnel. **Guyon's canal** is a tunnel on the ulnar side of the wrist formed by the hook of the hamate and pisiform bones. The ulnar nerve may be compressed at this site in long-distance cyclists, by falling on the wrist, or by repetitive wrist actions.

The transverse imaging plane is the easiest approach to use to begin an examination of the carpal tunnel. Locating the ulnar artery at the wrist crease helps orientation and subsequent identification of wrist structures. Care must be taken to maintain a perpendicular scan plane to reduce anisotropic effects. Use of large amounts of gel or a stand-off pad may help in imaging the anterior structures of the wrist. The flexor digitorum tendons are a hypoechoic structure just posterior to the median nerve. Fibrillary hyperechoic tendon patterns help differentiate the median nerve because the nerve is hypoechoic with a hyperechoic border. The rounded or oval median nerve flattens as it continues through the carpal tunnel (Figure 24-37).

The longitudinal nerve images as a parallel structure superficial to the flexor digitorum tendons. The nerve

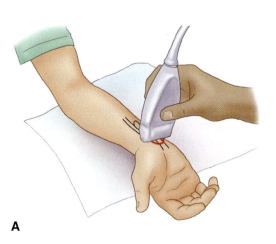

A

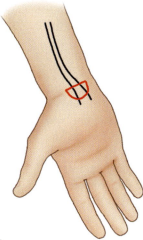

B

FIGURE 24-36 A, The wrist can be positioned on a pillow on the patient's lap to aid in imaging the volar structures. **B,** The retinaculum *(red),* a strong fibrous structure, attaches to the pisiform on the lateral side and the hook of the hamate.

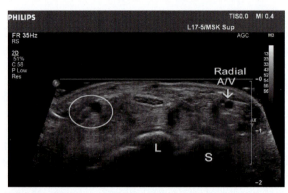

FIGURE 24-37 This image taken from the volar side of the wrist at the crease demonstrates the complicated anatomy from this view. Large amounts of gel allow for imaging with minimal artifact on the lateral curved edges. Guyon's canal *(circle)* contains the ulnar vein and vessels demarcating the medial carpal tunnel border. The lunate *(L)* and scaphoid bone *(S)* mark the posterior boundaries of the carpal tunnel. Laterally, the radial artery and vein mark this border. The median nerve is slightly flattened at this level, which is a normal finding.

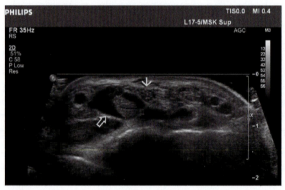

FIGURE 24-38 This image taken proximal to Figure 24-37 demonstrates a rounder median nerve *(solid arrow)*. The flexor pollicis longus tendon and the beginning of the muscle *(open arrow)* appear as a hypoechoic structure.

sheath appears as a continuous hyperechoic structure on the anterior and posterior borders of the nerve. Tendons located posterior to the median nerve have the characteristic hyperechoic fibrillar pattern seen with tendons in other areas of the body (Figure 24-38).

Box 24-3 lists the main indications for wrist sonography.

Achilles Tendon

The Achilles tendon is named after a figure in Greek mythology. Achilles' mother wished to have her son invulnerable to all weapons, so she dipped him in the waters of the river Styx. The only portion that was not bathed in the water was his heel, resulting in a vulnerable spot. A poison arrow would later pierce the unprotected heel during the Trojan wars, resulting in Achilles' death.

This large, strong fibrous tendon connects the gastrocnemius and soleus muscles to the calcaneus. Although this tendon (as with any tendon) has many variations,

---

BOX 24-3 | **Indications for Wrist Sonography**

- Masses
- Loss or decrease of digital mobility
- Pain and swelling
- Trauma
- Foreign body location
- Numbness of the middle and index fingers
- Weakness or clumsiness of the hand
- Tingling with nerve percussion (Tinel's sign)
- Pain with wrist flexion when sustained for a minute or longer (Phalen's sign)

approximately two thirds of the tendon originates from the gastrocnemius muscle and one third from the soleus muscle. This tendon helps move your foot downward, push off when walking, and rise up on your toes. Injury to this tendon can make it impossible to walk without pain.

A limited blood supply increases risk of injury to the Achilles tendon and slows the healing process. The longitudinal arteries that run the length of the gastrocnemius and soleus muscles provide the blood supply. The poorest blood supply is above the insertion of the tendon into the calcaneus, which is also the most frequent site of tendon tears. Chances of rupture and inflammation increase with age as the result of a diminishing blood supply.

A connective tissue sheath called the paratenon surrounds the Achilles tendon. This allows a gliding action of 2 to 3 cm with movement, and the tendon may thicken with increased activity. The lack of a true synovial sheath results in a less echogenic border between the tendon and the surrounding tissue.

The largest tendon of the body, the Achilles tendon, may develop tendinitis in the athletic patient. Any activity that involves jumping and sudden stops and starts will stress the tendon. Female athletes who wear high-heeled shoes and then change into sneakers to exercise also increase their risk of tendinitis. Overstretching the tendon can result in a partial or complete tear, with the most common site being the distal tendon at the area of decreased blood flow (2 to 6 cm from the calcaneus).

Fortunately, the Achilles tendon is relatively easy to scan because of its echo characteristics and location. To begin the examination, position the patient prone with the foot hanging over the edge of the cart or bed. The foot may also be supported on a pillow or sponge for easier scanning and patient comfort. Patients who are unable to lie prone may be scanned while on their side if the injured Achilles tendon is on the upside.

The size of this tendon allows imaging with a 5-MHz linear transducer. Scan the tendon from the origin at the gastrocnemius and soleus muscles to the insertion on the calcaneus. A complete scan includes transverse and sagittal views and measurements of the transverse tendon. The AP diameter of the normal tendon is approximately

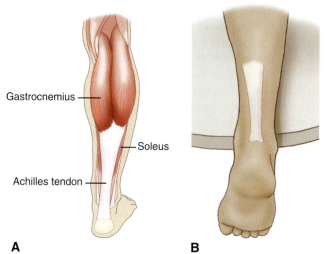

A   **B**

FIGURE 24-39 A, Achilles tendon imaging extends from the origin at the gastrocnemius and soleus muscles to the insertion on the calcaneus. **B,** Placing the patient prone with the foot over the cart edge allows easy access to the tendon and dorsal and plantar flexion of the foot.

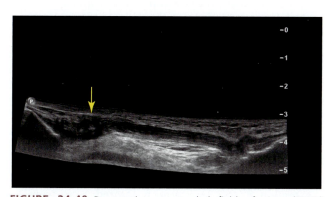

FIGURE 24-40 Panoramic or extended field of view (EFOV) imaging allows imaging of a greater length of the Achilles tendon. This ensures comparison of the echo texture in different areas of the tendon. Kager's fat pad *(arrow)* images as a hypoechoic structure.

5 to 6 mm, varying with patient gender and body habitus. Measurement of the AP tendon diameter on the longitudinal plane tends to overestimate the distance because of the oblique course of the tendon. **Dorsiflexion** and **plantar flexion** of the foot, best imaged on the sagittal plane, increase the chances of imaging an Achilles tendon tear. The **Thompson's test** (plantar flexion with squeezing of the calf) may be used to evaluate the integrity of the Achilles tendon. The patient kneels on the examination table with the feet hanging off; the examiner then squeezes the calf while observing for plantar flexion. The result is positive if no movement of the foot is noted; this indicates an Achilles tendon rupture.

When scanning the patient in the prone position, special attention must be given to the hypoechoic Kager's fat pad or pre-Achilles fat pad located deep in the Achilles tendon. Displacement of this triangular fat pad is one

radiographic marker for the Achilles tendon and can serve as a landmark during the sonographic examination. Scanning the contralateral side also aids in determining normalcy of the tendon (Figures 24-39 and 24-40).

Box 24-4 lists the indications for Achilles tendon sonography.

PATHOLOGY OF THE MUSCULOSKELETAL SYSTEM

Familiarity with the sonographic appearance of injury, inflammation, and chronic problems allows a confident diagnosis of MS problems. Some pathology occurs with increased frequency in a specific joint, but the same problem images similarly in the tendons, ligaments, and muscles, regardless of location.

Shoulder Biceps Tendon Subluxation/Dislocation

The dislocation (also called *subluxation*) of the biceps tendon from the bicipital groove may be due to a problem with the transverse humeral ligament, abnormal development of the bicipital groove or supraspinatus, and/or subscapularis tears. The most common dislocation is deep to the subscapularis anterior to the glenohumeral joint capsule. This medial dislocation results in an empty groove that may fill with granulation and fibrous tissue. Rotating the arm from a neutral to external position allows real-time imaging of the tendon dislocation or subluxation (Figures 24-41 and 24-42).

Rotator Cuff Tears

Tears of the rotator cuff may be classified as partial-thickness or full-thickness tears (Figure 24-43). The two types are differentiated through determination of abnormal communication between the glenohumeral joint and the subacromial bursa. The full-thickness tear has this communication, although the partial-thickness tear does not.

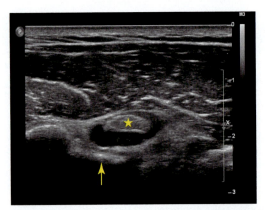

FIGURE 24-41 Subluxation and complete or incomplete dislocation of the biceps tendon *(star)* out of the bicipital groove *(arrow)* of the humerus.

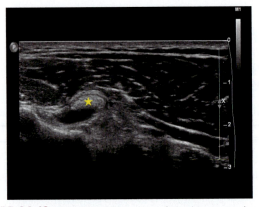

FIGURE 24-42 Complete dislocation of the biceps tendon *(star)* outside of the biceps groove of the humerus.

Rotator cuff problems may occur as an acute or chronic process. Biceps tendon ruptures, falls, and shoulder dislocations are a few causes of an acute rotator cuff tear. A chronic process occurs as a cumulative progression of injury from activities involving placing the arms over the head. This may be due to actions such as placing items on high shelves, playing tennis, swimming, or rock climbing. This microtrauma, due to impingement of the tendon between the humeral head and the acromion, results in cuff degeneration and an eventual tear. Rotator cuff tears are divided into three stages—Stage I: swelling and mild pain; Stage II: inflammation and scarring; and Stage III: partial or complete tears of the rotator cuff.

The supraspinatus, similar to all tendons of the shoulder, is a straplike tendon with three dimensions. Tears in width, length, and thickness occur in tendons, and a complete examination includes a description of the tear in all planes. A tear located on the sagittal plane of the tendon images as a disruption on the thickness or AP dimension of the tendon. This is only part of the picture, and an orthogonal image will identify the location and extent of the tear on the width of the tendon.

Another consideration is that the curved tendons will have an increased chance of producing an anisotropic artifact, which will appear similar to a tear. Moving the patient's arm to an internal rotation or an extended position changes the imaging plane and helps not only to reduce the artifact, but to accentuate the defect.

Partial-Thickness Tear. The partial-thickness tear may involve the bursal or articular cuff surface or the intrasubstance material. An intrasubstance tear is very rare. Tears begin in the critical zone of the anterolateral supraspinatus tendon and image as focal disruptions of the tendon fibers. This zone is located 1 cm from its

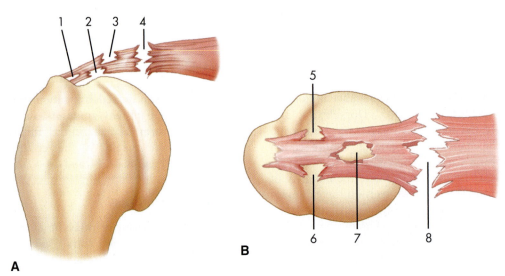

FIGURE 24-43 Coronal view **(A)** and view from above **(B)** showing tears of the supraspinatus tendon. These tears can occur anywhere along the tendon and range from an intrasubstance tear (1) to a complete full-thickness, full-width tear (8). The range includes partial-thickness humeral surface tear (2), partial-thickness bursal surface tear (3), full-thickness tear (4), full-thickness tear posteriorly (partial width) (5), full-thickness tear posteriorly (partial width) (6), and full-thickness tear centrally (partial width) (7).

insertion into the greater tuberosity. When injured, the acute tendon tear images as an anechoic defect in the rotator cuff. A chronic tear may image as an area of hyperechogenicity caused by mixing of blood and bursal granulation tissue in the frayed tendon area. Diffuse thinning of the tendon is another indication of a chronic partial-thickness tear.

The most common type of tear is the articular cuff surface defect. The following criteria help in establishing the presence of a partial-thickness tear:

1. A critical zone focus of mixed hyperechoic and hypoechoic echo texture (focal discontinuity)
2. Bursal or articular extension of any hypoechoic areas imaged in two orthogonal planes
3. An irregularity of the anterior greater tuberosity is seen in up to three fourths of partial-thickness tears. These may appear as bone cortex defects, fragmentation, and/or spurring.
4. Decreased thickness of the tendon with chronic partial-thickness tears

Fluid seen within the biceps tendon indicates the possibility of an articular surface tear. The presence of large amounts of fluid in the subacromial-subdeltoid bursa raises the chance of a nonvisualized full-thickness tear.

Hypoechoic concave bursal surface tears are the next most common type of partial rotator cuff tears (Figure 24-44). These defects, close to the joints and bursa, are tender to palpation.

Box 24-5 lists the sonographic criteria for partial-thickness tears.

Full-Thickness Tear. A tear of the rotator cuff that involves the full thickness and full width of the tendons is considered a full-thickness tear. Retraction of multiple tendons occurs with a separation of 2 to 4 cm between the torn tendon ends. The frequency of tendon tearing in descending order occurs in the supraspinatus, infraspinatus, and subscapularis, and, very rarely, the teres minor.

Images of the tear on sagittal and transverse planes not only confirm the full-thickness tear, but also provide for measurement between the torn tendon edges (Figures 24-45 through 24-47). The largest distance measurement is used to classify the tear. The **cartilage interface sign** is the echogenic line on the anterior surface of the cartilage surrounding the humeral head. The four classifications of rotator cuff vary with the author, but the criteria listed are a composite of published categorizations:

1. Partial-thickness tear
2. Small full-thickness tear 1 to 2 cm in AP dimension over the greater tuberosity
3. Large full-thickness tear of 2 to 4 cm
4. Complete tears of greater than 4 cm

BOX 24-5	**Sonographic Criteria for Partial-Thickness Tears**

- Critical zone of the supraspinatus imaging with a hypoechoic or hyperechoic focus
- Articular or bursal extension of a hypoechoic lesion on two orthogonal planes
- Hypoechoic or echogenic line within the cuff substance
- Anterior greater tuberosity regional irregularities
- Effusions of the biceps tendon sheath
- Concave subdeltoid bursal surface

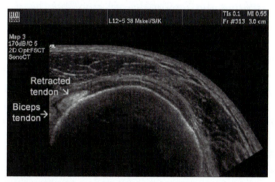

FIGURE 24-45 This complete full-thickness tear (complete rupture) panoramic image shows the biceps tendon retraction in the far left of the image. The deltoid muscle is located anterior to the greater tuberosity.

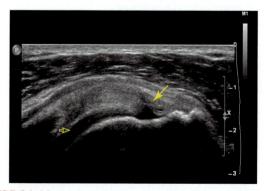

FIGURE 24-44 This bursal side partial-thickness tear *(solid arrow)* has a hypoechoic appearance when compared with the surrounding rotator cuff. Fluid, blood, and debris collect in the bursa, producing an anechoic structure *(open arrow)*.

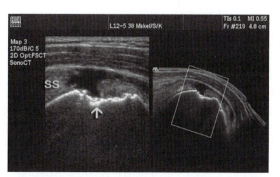

FIGURE 24-46 This magnification and panoramic image shows a complex subdeltoid bursa representing hemorrhage after a rotator cuff tear. The retracted supraspinatus *(SS)* leaves a space for fluid and blood to collect. Note the irregularity of the biceps groove *(arrow)*.

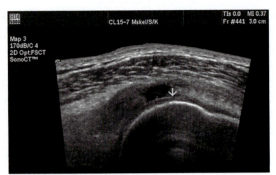

FIGURE 24-47 The cartilage interface sign (arrow) is the echogenic anterior linelike border of the cartilage surrounding the humeral head. This is seen through the anechoic or hypoechoic complete rotator cuff tear.

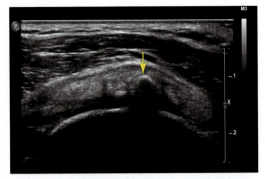

FIGURE 24-48 Intratendinous calcifications (arrow), as seen in this rotator cuff, are a common finding with chronic tendinitis.

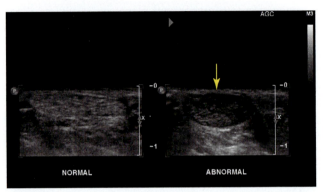

FIGURE 24-49 Comparison of the normal with the injured tendon reveals a focal area of inflammation (arrow).

During the real-time examination, perform a simple compression test over the area of concern. The normal tendon cannot be compressed; however, the injured tendon flattens as the torn edges move apart. Longstanding cuff injury may also result in atrophy or nonvisualization of a muscle. Rupture of the subscapularis tendon results in retraction of muscle between the scapula and the chest wall. Fatty infiltration of the supraspinatus and infraspinatus fossae changes the echo appearance of this area, giving a false appearance of normalcy and underscoring the importance of scanning the normal contralateral side. The **naked tuberosity sign** is defined as the deltoid muscle on the humeral head; it is seen with a full-thickness tear of the rotator cuff.

Joint effusion around the biceps tendon combined with subacromial-subdeltoid (SASD) bursitis results in the double effusion sign. This is a specific sign of a rotator cuff tear and has been quoted as having a positive predictive value as high as 95%. Arm extension and internal rotation help image lateral greater tuberosity bursal fluid. Light transducer pressure is important because a heavy scan technique may compress the fluid into other nonimaged areas of the joint. This indirect sign is important enough to warrant complementary imaging of arthroscopy or MRI.

Box 24-6 lists the primary and secondary sonographic signs of a full-thickness tear.

Tendinitis

One of the most common tendon abnormalities is inflammation due to age-related elasticity loss, disease such as rheumatoid arthritis, overuse, or acute trauma. **Tendinitis** occurs in any tendon, but is seen more often in the shoulder, wrist, heel, and elbow. This inflammatory condition has a characteristic clinical symptom of pain at the tendinous insertion into the bone, a palpable mass in the area of pain, and a decreased range of movement. Treatment is important because chronic tendinitis may lead to weakening of the tendon, resulting in rupture (Figure 24-48).

BOX 24-6	Primary and Secondary Sonographic Signs of a Full-Thickness Tear

Primary Signs
- Naked tuberosity sign
- Tendon edge atrophy in a chronic tear
- Retracted tendons
- Fiber discontinuity with interposed fluid
- A cleft in the cuff of hypoechoic or anechoic echo texture
- Distended SASD bursa in direct communication with the joint
- Compressed tendon
- Absence of the rotator cuff
- Deltoid muscle or SASD bursa herniation into the rotator cuff

Secondary Signs
- Long head biceps tendon effusion
- Double effusion sign
- Erosion of the greater tuberosity of the humerus
- Cartilage interface sign
- Double effusion sign
- Glenohumeral joint effusion

SASD, Subacromial subdeltoid.

Sonography images tendinitis well because of changes in the inflamed area in surrounding tissue (Figure 24-49). Acute tendinitis (also called *tenosynovitis*) involves not only the tendon but also the surrounding synovial sheath. Imaging demonstrates an increase in fluid within the synovial sheath, appearing as a halo effect on the transverse image (Figure 24-50). The normal synovial sheath

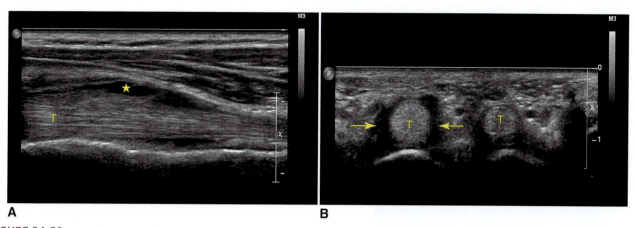

FIGURE 24-50 A, Tenosynovitis of the extensor tendons of the hand displays the characteristic anechoic fluid *(star)* surrounding the tendon *(T).* **B,** The fluid within the tendon sheath creates a halo effect *(arrows)* around the tendon on the transverse image.

appears as a hypoechoic halo around the tendon. Fluid surrounding the tendon may be anechoic or complex because of debris. To differentiate complex fluid from edema, tap the area or increase the output power to encourage movement of the debris.

A focal or diffuse decrease in echogenicity within the tendon fibers is one sonographic sign of tendinitis. This hypoechoic area also demonstrates increased Doppler flow in the periphery, caused by hyperemia. These areas of injury may be very subtle; comparing the normal side versus the abnormal side helps confirm the diagnosis (see Figure 24-49). Any discrepancy in thickness measurements greater than 1.5 mm is highly suspicious of a focal lesion.

de Quervain's tendinitis is one form of tendinitis with which many sonographers and sonologists may be inherently familiar. This type of tendon inflammation results in symptoms of pain over the thumb side of the wrist and may even result in an audible creaking called *crepitus.* Continuous use of the hand and thumb in a twisting, pinching, or grasping fashion increases the chances of developing swelling on the thumb side of the wrist. During the acute phase of this disease, sonographic imaging of the large abductor pollicis longus and small extensor pollicis brevis tendon reveals hypoechoic tendons and synovium. As the process becomes chronic, fibrosis forms, increasing echogenicity. Fibrosis results in restriction of the tendons through the dorsal compartment of the hand, leading to an inability to move the thumb away from the rest of the hand or to straighten the thumb after grasping.

Box 24-7 lists the sonographic features of tendinitis.

Muscle Tears

Ultrasound demonstrates traumatic muscle injury through its ability to reveal subtle changes in the internal structure of the muscle. A tear is the most common pathologic condition of the muscles of the limbs, although other sites are also affected. A muscle strain related to

BOX 24-7	Sonographic Features of Tendinitis

- Focal or diffuse hypoechogenicity
- Enlargement of the tendon in a focal or diffuse pattern
- Echogenic tendon fibrils within the area of inflammation
- Calcifications with chronic tendinitis
- Increased color or power Doppler signal in the periphery
- Coexisting bursitis
- Synovial sheath fluid

exertion does not image with ultrasound because of the lack of a lesion; however, imaging of this type of pain-related problem helps differentiate a tear from a strain. Two types of tears occur in the muscle: distraction (indirect) and compression (direct) tears. Abrupt stretching of the muscle beyond the maximum length results in distraction tears. These are usually due to sudden interruption of a movement, such as kicking, or improper body alignment. External force resulting in a crush injury is considered a compression tear. This type of trauma, which results from muscle crushing against the underlying bone, ranges from a bruise to a large hematoma. Hematomas also occur with muscle injury and have a variable sonographic appearance. This characteristic of a muscle injury helps determine the extent of the underlying damage. The new hematoma is a hyperechoic mass structure that pushes the muscle fibers apart. Often diffuse and ill defined, the acute hematoma images as an area of enlargement with increased echogenicity within the muscle fibers. Within a few days, the hematoma becomes organized; this often increases detection (Figure 24-51). As the hematoma ages, it liquefies into a hypoechoic to anechoic mass, and a **seroma,** an accumulation of serous fluid within tissue, forms within the defect in a few weeks. Healing of this type of injury results in a hyperechoic fibrous scar or calcifications within the muscle after reabsorption of the serous material. The hematoma that conforms to the fibrous layers

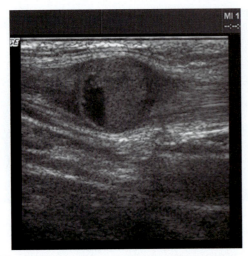

FIGURE 24-51 This intramuscular hematoma images an organized clot with a heterogeneous appearance.

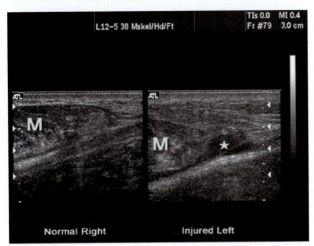

FIGURE 24-52 A tear of the gastrocnemius muscle (*M*) results in a hematoma (*star*) at the area of the injury. Comparison of the normal and injured sides confirms the muscle tear, which may be seen in athletes participating in jumping activities.

TABLE 24-4	Sonographic Appearance of Muscle Tear Grades
Muscle Tear Grade	**Sonographic Appearance**
I (elongation injury)	Normal, flame-shaped focal fiber discontinuity, small hematoma (<1 cm)
II (partial rupture)	<⅓ of muscle fibers disrupted, hematoma <3 cm, interfascial hematoma, hypoechoic gap within the muscle that changes position with transducer pressure
III (complete rupture)	>⅓ rupture of muscle resembling a soft tissue mass, hematoma >3 cm, large interfascial hematoma

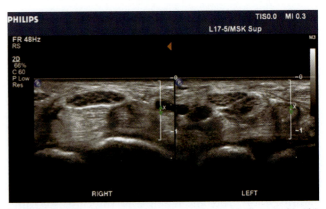

FIGURE 24-53 The right median nerve is notably flattened in this symptomatic patient. The left median nerve is also mildly flattened.

may also mimic deep vein thrombosis (DVT) within the calf or arm muscles.

The sonographic appearance of a muscle tear varies with the type of injury. A tear of the full thickness of the muscle images with the torn muscle end outlined by fluid. The muscle belly will appear thicker with a whorled circular pattern when compared with the contralateral side (Figure 24-52). As the hematoma resolves, it becomes smaller, and echogenicity is increased.

A complete tear of a muscle has a straightforward appearance of a retracted hyperechoic muscle surrounded by a hematoma (**clapper-in-the-bell sign**). The partial tear may be as subtle as a discontinuity of the muscle fibers and septa or as obvious as a hematoma with echoic debris. This type of tear may be difficult to separate from the earlier mentioned edge artifact because of the similar appearance. The true torn muscle with irregular margins will maintain the same sonographic appearance at different angles of incidence, whereas the edge artifact will

appear only with the 90-degree angle. Examination of the injured muscle includes images with the muscle contracted and at rest in both longitudinal and transverse planes. An area of rupture may also image with a hyperechoic halo surrounding the jagged rupture margins. As the muscle heals, the edges of the tear increase in echogenicity and thickness. The normal muscle architecture becomes evident with healing. The hyperechoic linear, stellate, or nodular scar or an intramuscular cyst provides evidence of an abnormal healing process.

Table 24-4 lists the sonographic appearance of muscle tears by grade.

Carpal Tunnel Syndrome

Carpal tunnel syndrome (CTS) is primarily entrapment or compression neuropathy of the median nerve. Occupations that require repetitive motion produce repetitive stress on the nerve, resulting in the pain and paresthesias characteristic of this syndrome. Continued use of the same muscle group results in hypertrophied muscles, and repeated trauma to the tendon sheath may cause enlargement (traumatic synovitis). This increase in size of the muscle and tendon sheath results in tunnel narrowing (Figure 24-53). We are most familiar with the repetitive causes of CTS, but this group of problems can have other causes, including pregnancy, chronic renal failure, diabetes mellitus, rheumatoid arthritis, amyloidosis, and tenosynovitis. Extrinsic causes include accessory muscles, soft tissue masses, and ganglions.

The patient suffering from CTS typically presents with numbness of the middle and index fingers, weakness or clumsiness of the hand, and pain. The clinical examination is positive for **Tinel's sign** or **Phalen's sign,** and weakness is seen in the affected hand.

Normal median nerves are elliptical and flatten with distal progression. The transverse scan on a patient with CTS reveals a nerve that flattens in the distal tunnel and nerve swelling in the distal tunnels; at the level of the distal radius and palmar, bowing is seen in the flexor retinaculum. Because of the varied cross-sectional area, calculation of the area is helpful in determining the presence of an increase in the median nerve. This area esti-

---

BOX 24-8	**Sonographic Appearance of Median Nerve Compression**

- Focal or diffuse proximal enlargement
- Increased cross-sectional area (>15 mm^2)
- Three flattening ratios of the median nerve in distal carpal tunnel
- Tenosynovitis with >4 mm dorsal bowing of the flexor retinaculum

---

mate uses the formula for the ellipse (area = $\pi(D1 \times D2)/4$). Any cross-sectional area greater than 15 mm^2 at the level of the proximal tunnel is considered diagnostic for an increased median nerve.

Box 24-8 describes the sonographic appearance of median nerve compression.

PART IV

Neonatal and Pediatrics

Neonatal Echoencephalography

Sandra L. Hagen-Ansert

Advances in sonography, computed tomography, and magnetic resonance imaging since the early 1980s have brought increased understanding of the intracranial lesions of premature babies. Sonography has been the primary imaging modality for high-risk and unstable premature infants because it is portable, nonionizing, and noninvasive; can be tolerated by even the sickest infants; and does not require sedation. Sonography of the neonatal brain may be performed if there are abnormal findings in the prenatal ultrasound examination or in the premature infant (to evaluate for intracranial bleeds) or if the postnatal examination is abnormal. **Neonates** who suffered a difficult delivery associated with **hypoxia** or **asphyxia** may be examined with ultrasound. Brain damage is one of the primary concerns about the health of premature infants. Intraventricular and subependymal hemorrhages of the **subependyma** occur in 40% to 70% of premature neonates under 34 weeks' gestation. Multifocal necrosis of the white matter

or periventricular leukomalacia may develop in 12% to 20% of infants weighing less than 2000 g. These lesions are associated with increased mortality and an abnormal neurologic outcome.

This chapter discusses the embryology, normal cranial anatomy, sonographic protocols for the neonatal head examination, common developmental problems of the brain, and ultrasound evaluation of neonatal brain lesions. The primary focus of this chapter is neural tube defects, hydrocephalus, infections, and hemorrhagic pathologic conditions of the premature infant. For further detail on lesions of the brain, the reader is referred to Chapter 59.

EMBRYOLOGY OF THE BRAIN

The central nervous system develops from the neural plate. Before the neural tube forms, the neural plate is expanded rostrally where the brain will develop

(Figure 25-1). The neural plate develops at 18 to 20 days after conception. The neural plate forms the neural tube and the neural crest. The neural tube differentiates into the central nervous system, consisting of both the brain and the spinal cord. The neural crest gives rise to most of the structures in the peripheral nervous system.

Temporarily the neural tube is open at both the cranial and the caudal ends (Figure 25-2). The cranial opening closes first at around 24 days after conception. The caudal opening closes two days later. The walls of the tube thicken to form the various portions of the brain and the spinal cord. The lumen of the neural tube becomes the ventricular system of the brain cranially and the central canal of the spinal cord caudally.

The greatest growth and differentiation of the neural tube are at the cranial end. At the end of the fourth week after conception, the cranial end of the neural tube differentiates into three primary brain vesicles. These vesicles consist of the prosencephalon (forebrain), mesencephalon (midbrain), and rhombencephalon (hindbrain) (Figure 25-3). The following week, the forebrain differentiates into the telencephalon (end brain), which is the rostral portion of the brain, and the diencephalon (immediate brain). The hindbrain divides into the metencephalon and the myelencephalon (Table 25-1).

The Forebrain

As the brain flexures form, the forebrain develops rapidly. During the fifth week it develops diverticula called optic vesicles (Figure 25-3, *B*) that will develop into the eyes and cerebral vesicles that will become cerebral hemispheres (Figure 25-3, *C*). The diencephalon is positioned centrally, whereas the telencephalon consists of lateral expansions. The diencephalon (Figure 25-3, *D*) develops from the tissues of the walls of the third ventricle that form three discrete swellings: the epithalamus, the **thalamus**, and the hypothalamus.

The cerebral vesicles enlarge rapidly, expanding in all directions until they cover the diencephalon and part of the brain stem (Figure 25-3, *E*). In the floor and lateral wall of each vesicle, a thickening of nerve cells develops that will become the corpus striatum (see Figure 25-3, *D*) from which the basal ganglia will develop. Fibers from the developing cerebral hemispheres pass through the corpus striatum on their way to the brain stem and spinal cord, dividing the corpus striatum into two parts, the **caudate nucleus** and the lentiform nucleus. These fibers form the internal capsule.

Thickenings appear in the lateral walls of the diencephalon, which will become the thalamus. The thalamus is the dominant portion of the diencephalon and

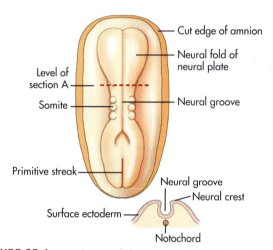

FIGURE 25-1 Dorsal view of the nervous system at 22 days. The neural folds have fused near the middle of the embryo to form the neural tube.

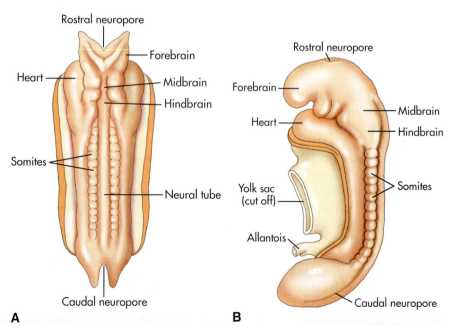

FIGURE 25-2 A, Dorsal view of an embryo at 23 days. Note that the hindbrain and midbrain vesicles have formed and that the neural tube is much longer. **B,** Lateral view. The rostral and caudal neuropores are still open. The rostral neuropore closes on day 25 or 26, and the caudal neuropore closes about 2 days later. Failure of these openings to close results in severe neural tube defects.

A

B

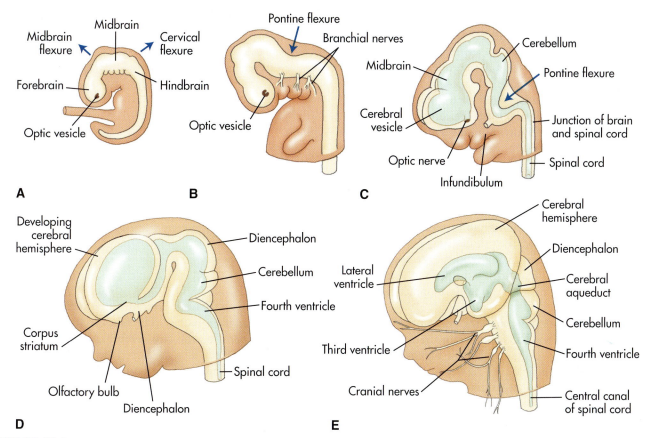

FIGURE 25-3 Development of the brain and the ventricular system. Note how the brain flexures affect the shape of the brain, enabling it to be accommodated in the head. The cerebral hemispheres expand and gradually cover the diencephalon and midbrain. The nerves of the branchial arches become the cranial nerves. **A,** 28 days. **B,** 35 days. **C,** 56 days. **D,** 10 weeks. **E,** 14 weeks.

TABLE 25-1	Progression of Developing Regions of the Brain	
Primary Brain Vesicles	**Secondary Brain Vesicles**	**Regions of the Mature Brain**
Forebrain (Prosencephalon)	Diencephalon	Thalamus, epithalamus, hypothalamus, subthalamus
	Telencephalon	Cerebral hemispheres (consisting of the cortex and medullary center, the corpus striatum, and the olfactory system)
Midbrain (Mesencephalon)	Mesencephalon	Midbrain
Hindbrain (Rhombencephalon)	Myelencephalon	Medulla
	Metencephalon	Pons and cerebellum

enlarges rapidly. At the same time, the thalami bulge into the third ventricle to reduce the ventricular lumen to a narrow cleft. The thalami fuse in the midline and form a fusion called the *massa intermedia.*

The diencephalon also participates in the formation of the pituitary gland. The posterior lobe of the pituitary gland develops from a down growth from the diencephalons known as the infundibulum (see Figure 25-3, *C*). The anterior lobe of the pituitary gland develops from an evagination of the primitive mouth cavity.

The telencephalic or cerebral vesicles communicate with the cavity of the third ventricle. Along the choroidal fissure, the medial wall of the developing cerebral hemisphere becomes thin. Invaginations of vascular pia form

the choroid plexus of the lateral ventricles at this site. The hemispheres cover the surfaces of the diencephalon, the midbrain, and, eventually, the hindbrain. The falx cerebri, or interhemispheric fissure, is formed as the mesenchyme is trapped in the midline with the growth of the hemispheres. This development separates the lateral ventricles from the third ventricle. At this point in development, only the frontal horns, bodies, and atria of the lateral ventricles are developed.

The Midbrain

The midbrain does not change as much as the other parts of the brain, except for considerable thickening of its walls. It is the growth of large nerve fiber tracts through it that thickens its walls and reduces its lumen, which become the cerebral aqueduct (see Figure 25-3, *E*). Four large groups of neurons form in the roof of the midbrain known as the superior and inferior colliculi (quadrigeminal body). In the basal portion of the midbrain, fibers passing from the cerebrum form the cerebral peduncles. A broad layer of gray matter adjacent to these large fiber tracts is known as the substantia nigra.

The Hindbrain

The hindbrain undergoes flexion, which divides the hindbrain into the metencephalon and myelencephalon. The pontine flexure demarcates the division between these two parts (see Figure 25-3, *B*). The myelencephalon becomes the closed part of the medulla oblongata. It resembles the spinal cord both developmentally and structurally.

The metencephalon becomes the pons and the cerebellum. The fourth ventricle forms from the cavity of the hindbrain and also contains choroid plexus, as do the lateral and third ventricles. At 12 weeks, the vermis and cerebellar hemispheres are recognizable.

ANATOMY OF THE NEONATAL BRAIN

The sonographer must be familiar with specific anatomic structures within the brain to perform a complete sonographic examination of the neonatal head. The anatomy presented in this chapter focuses on the cranial anatomy the sonographer needs to understand in order to perform a neonatal cranial ultrasound. The cranial cavity contains the brain and its surrounding meninges and portions of the cranial nerves, arteries, veins, and venous sinuses.

Fontanelle

Fontanelles are the spaces between the bones of the skull (Figure 25-4). In the neonate, the fontanelles have not closed completely. The anterior fontanelle is located at the top of the neonatal head and may be easily felt as the "soft spot." If hydrocephalus is present, this fontanelle is felt to be bulging. If there is overlapping of the cranial bones, the fontanelle may be difficult to palpate and provides a limited window for the transducer to image the cranial structures. The transducer is placed carefully on the anterior fontanelle to record multiple images of the brain in the coronal, axial, and sagittal planes.

Meninges

There are three membranes called **meninges** that surround and form a protective covering for the brain: the dura mater, arachnoid, and pia mater membranes. The

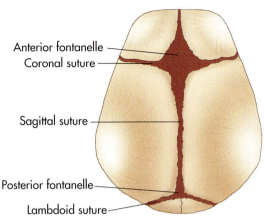

FIGURE 25-4 Neonatal skull showing the sutures and open anterior fontanelle.

dura mater is a double layered outer membrane that forms the toughest barrier. The **falx cerebri** is a fibrous structure separating the two cerebral hemispheres. The **tentorium cerebelli** is a V-shaped echogenic structure separating the cerebrum and the cerebellum; it is an extension of the falx cerebri.

Ventricular System

The lateral ventricles are the largest of the cerebral spinal fluid cavities located within the cerebral hemispheres. They communicate with the third ventricle through the interventricular foramen. There are two lateral ventricles located on either side of the brain. The lateral ventricles are divided into the following four segments: frontal horn, body, and occipital and temporal horns (Figures 25-5 and 25-6). The **atrium** (or **trigone**) **of the lateral ventricle** is the site where the anterior, occipital, and temporal horns join together.

The body of the lateral ventricle extends from the foramen of Monro to the trigone. The **corpus callosum** forms the roof, and the **cavum septum pellucidum** forms the medial wall. The thalamus touches the inferior lateral ventricular wall, and the body of the caudate nucleus borders the superior wall.

The temporal horn extends anteriorly from the trigone through the temporal lobe. The roof is formed by the white matter of the temporal lobe and by the tail of the caudate nucleus. The hippocampus forms the medial wall.

The occipital horn extends posteriorly from the trigone. The occipital cortex and white matter form the medial wall. The corpus callosum forms the proximal roof and lateral wall.

The frontal horn is divided posteriorly by the foramen of Monro near the body of the ventricle. The roof is formed by the corpus callosum. The septum pellucidum forms the medial wall and the head of the caudate nucleus forms the lateral wall.

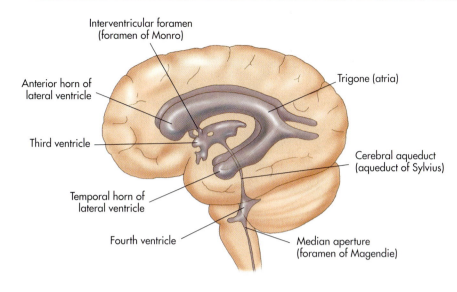

FIGURE 25-5 Sagittal view of the ventricular system.

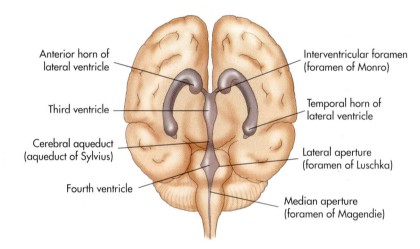

FIGURE 25-6 Anterior view of the ventricles.

The third ventricle is connected by the foramen of Monro to the lateral ventricles. The aqueduct of Sylvius connects the third and fourth ventricles. The medulla oblongata forms the floor of the fourth ventricle. The roof is formed by the cerebellar vermis and posterior medullary vellum. The lateral angles of the fourth ventricle form the foramen of Luschka. The inferior angle, the foramen of Magendie, is continuous with the central canal of the spinal cord.

Cerebrospinal Fluid. The cerebrospinal fluid (CSF) surrounds and protects the brain and spinal cord from physical impact. Approximately 40% of the CSF is formed by the choroid plexuses of the lateral, third, and fourth ventricles. The remainder is produced by the extracellular fluid movement from blood through the brain and into the ventricles. The fluid from the lateral ventricles passes through the foramen of Monro to the third ventricle. The fluid then passes through the aqueduct of Sylvius to the fourth ventricle. From that point, the fluid may leave through the central foramen of Magendie or the lateral foramen of Luschka into the cisterna magna and the basal subarachnoid cisterns. The anterior flow continues upward through the chiasmatic cisterns, sylvian fissure, and the pericallosal cisterns up over the hemispheres, where it is reabsorbed by the arachnoid granulations in the sagittal sinus. Posteriorly the cerebrospinal fluid flow moves around the cerebelli, through the tentorial incisure, the quadrigeminal cistern, the posterior callosal cistern, and up over the hemispheres. A small amount flows down the spinal subarachnoid space.

The cerebrospinal fluid results from the production of fluid by the choroid plexus and from the respiratory and vascular pulsations, ciliary action in the ependyma, and a downhill pressure gradient between the subarachnoid spaces and the venous sinuses. The CSF fluid production does not change appreciably with increased intracranial pressure; however, when the pressure is significantly increased, there will be a change in intracranial pressure.

Cavum Septum Pellucidum. The cavum septum pellucidum is a thin triangular space filled with

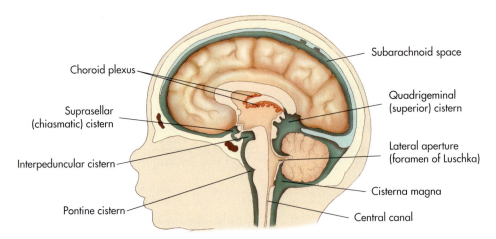

FIGURE 25-7 Sagittal view of choroid plexus and cisterns of the ventricular system.

cerebrospinal fluid, which lies between the anterior horn of the lateral ventricles and forms the floor of the corpus callosum. Thus, the cavum septum pellucidum is anterior to the corpus callosum. The cavum vergae is found at the posterior extension of the cavum septum pellucidum. The cavum septum pellucidum is present at birth and closes within 3 to 6 months of life.

Choroid Plexus. The **choroid plexus** is a mass of special cells located in the atrium of the lateral ventricles. These cells regulate the intraventricular pressure by secretion or absorption of cerebrospinal fluid. The glomus is the tail of the choroid plexus and is a major site for bleeding (Figure 25-7).

Cisterns

The narrow subarachnoid space surrounding the brain and spinal cord contains a small amount of fluid. The subarachnoidal cisterns are the spaces at the base of the brain where the arachnoid becomes widely separated from the pia, giving rise to large cavities. The cisterna magna is one of the largest of these subarachnoidal **cisterns**; it is located in the posterior fossa between the medulla oblongata, cerebellar hemispheres, and occipital bone (Figure 25-8).

Cerebrum

Cerebral Hemispheres. There are two cerebral hemispheres connected by the corpus callosum. They extend from the frontal to the occipital bones above the anterior and middle cranial fossae. Posteriorly, they extend above the tentorium cerebelli. They are separated by a longitudinal fissure into which projects the falx cerebri. The **cerebrum** consists of the gray and white matter. The outermost portion of the cerebrum is the cerebral cortex (composed of gray matter). The white matter is located within the cerebrum. The largest and densest bundle of white matter is the corpus callosum.

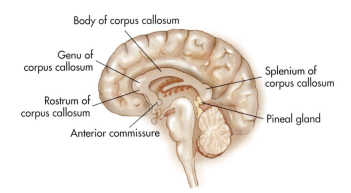

FIGURE 25-8 Sagittal view of cerebral cortex.

Lobes of the Brain. The cortex is divided into four lobes: frontal, parietal, occipital, and temporal, which correspond to the cranial bones with the same names (Figure 25-9).

Gyrus and Sulcus. The gyri are convolutions on the surface of the brain caused by infolding of the cortex. The **sulcus** is a groove or depression on the surface of the brain separating the gyri. The sulci further divide the hemispheres into frontal, parietal, occipital, and temporal lobes.

Fissures. The interhemispheric fissure is the area in which the falx cerebri sits and separates the two cerebral hemispheres. The sylvian fissure is located along the lateralmost aspect of the brain and is the area where the middle cerebral artery is located (Figure 25-10). The quadrigeminal fissure is located posterior and inferior from the cavum vergae. The vein of Galen is posterior, so the sonographer must be aware that Doppler should be performed to make sure it is a fissure and not an enlarged vein of Galen.

Corpus Callosum. The corpus callosum forms broad bands of connecting fibers between the cerebral hemispheres. This structure forms the roof of the lateral ventricles. The corpus callosum sits superior to the cavum

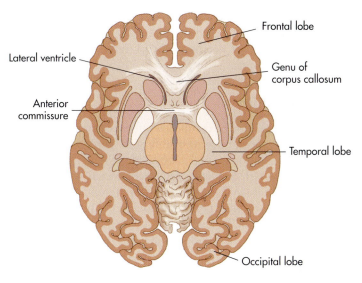

FIGURE 25-9 Axial view of cerebral cortex and corpus callosum.

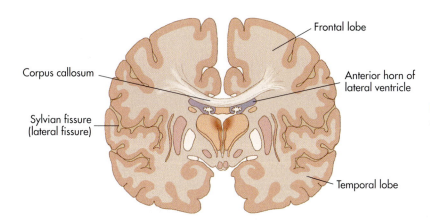

FIGURE 25-10 Coronal view of cerebral lobes, corpus callosum, and sylvian fissure.

septum pellucidum (see Figure 25-7). The development of the corpus callosum occurs between the 8th and 18th week of gestation, beginning ventrally and extending dorsal. The anterior body of the corpus callosum develops earlier than the *genu* (the dorsal element). If a uterine insult occurs, development may be partially arrested or complete agenesis may occur. If partial, then the genu, the splenium (posterior element), and the rostrum are absent. This is known as agenesis of the corpus callosum.

Basal Ganglia

The basal ganglia are a collection of gray matter that includes the caudate nucleus, lentiform nucleus, claustrum, and thalamus. The caudate nucleus is the portion of the brain that forms the lateral borders of the frontal horns of the lateral ventricles and lies anterior to the thalamus (Figure 25-11). It is further divided into the head, body, and tail. The head of the caudate nucleus is a common site for hemorrhage. The caudate nucleus and lentiform nucleus are the largest basal ganglia. They serve as relay stations between the thalamus and the

cerebral cortex. The claustrum is a thin layer between the insula and the lentiform nucleus.

The thalamus consists of two ovoid, egg-shaped brain structures situated on either side of the third ventricle superior to the brain stem. The thalamus borders the third ventricle and connects through the middle of the third ventricle by the massa intermedia.

The hypothalamus forms the floor of the third ventricle. The pituitary gland is connected to the hypothalamus by the infundibulum.

The **germinal matrix** includes periventricular tissue and the caudate nucleus. It is located 1 cm above the caudate nucleus in the floor of the lateral ventricle. It sweeps from the frontal horn posteriorly into the temporal horn.

Brain Stem

The **brain stem** is the part of the brain connecting the forebrain and the spinal cord. It consists of the midbrain, pons, and medulla oblongata.

Midbrain. The midbrain portion of the brain is narrow and connects the forebrain to the hindbrain. It consists of two halves called the cerebral peduncles (Figure 25-12). The cerebral aqueduct is a narrow cavity of the midbrain that connects the third and fourth ventricles. The tectum is part of the tegmentum located behind the cerebral aqueduct. It has four small surface swellings called the superior and inferior colliculi.

Pons. The pons is found on the anterior surface of the cerebellum below the midbrain and above the medulla oblongata.

Medulla Oblongata. The medulla oblongata extends from the pons to the foramen magnum where it continues as the spinal cord (see Figure 25-9). This structure contains the fiber tracts between the brain and the spinal cord, and the vital centers that regulate important internal activities of the body (heart rate, respiration, and blood pressure).

Cerebellum

The **cerebellum** is composed of two hemispheres that have the appearance of cauliflower. The cerebellum lies in the posterior cranial fossa under the tentorium cerebelli. The two hemispheres are connected by the vermis (Figure 25-13). Three pairs of nerve tracts, the cerebellar peduncles, connect the cerebellum to the brain stem. The superior cerebellar peduncles connect the cerebellum to the midbrain. The middle cerebellar peduncles connect the cerebellum to the pons, and the inferior cerebellar

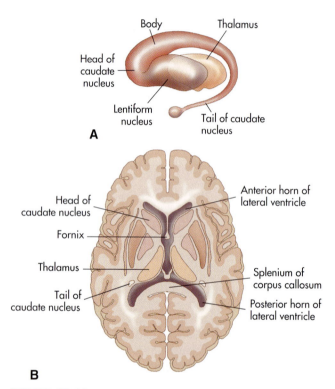

A

B

FIGURE 25-11 **A,** Lateral view of the basal ganglia with the caudate nucleus. **B,** Axial view of the basal ganglia with the thalamus, corpus callosum, and caudate nucleus.

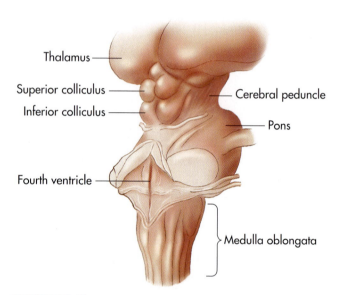

FIGURE 25-12 Oblique view of brain stem showing relationship of thalamus to cerebral peduncles, fourth ventricle, and medulla oblongata.

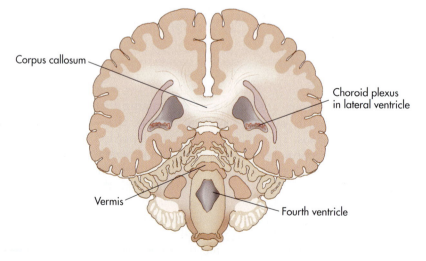

FIGURE 25-13 Coronal view of the medulla oblongata with the vermis and fourth ventricle.

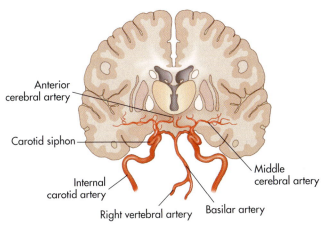

FIGURE 25-14 Coronal view of the cerebral arterial system.

peduncles connect the cerebellum to the medulla oblongata.

Cerebrovascular System

The cerebrovascular system consists of the internal cerebral arteries, vertebral arteries, and circle of Willis (Figure 25-14). The middle cerebral artery (branch of the internal carotid artery) and the circle of Willis are often evaluated with Doppler ultrasound in determining cerebral blood flow patterns. The cerebrovascular system will be discussed in more detail in Chapters 36 and 59.

SONOGRAPHIC EVALUATION OF THE NEONATAL BRAIN

Most neonatal sonographic examinations are performed in the nursery at the bedside. The sonographer must be aware of the infant's condition before the examination. Contact the infant's neonatal nurse to find out the status of the neonate before the examination. A small amount of warm gel should be used; keep in mind that the infant's temperature may be reduced if the isolette is open for extended time during the examination or if a large amount of cold gel is applied to the fontanelle.

If the patient is stable enough to travel to the ultrasound department, the sonographer should take the following considerations into account: First, even though the neonate may be well enough to come to the laboratory, she or he is still fragile and susceptible to any environmental changes. Consequently, blankets, radiant heaters, oxygen hookups, and heating pads are all essential to making the environment in the laboratory suitable. Second, if there are any problems with the neonate, a crash cart and life support systems must be immediately available. A neonatal nurse specialist will accompany the neonate to the laboratory. After all these considerations, you may decide to transport the ultrasound equipment to the neonatal intensive care unit for initial evaluation and follow-up.

NEONATAL HEAD EXAMINATION PROTOCOL

The small sector transducer with a 120-degree sector angle and multifocal capabilities is used to image through the anterior fontanelle. The small diameter transducer makes it possible to obtain excellent contact with the skull through the fontanelles and sutures and to avoid the curvature of the calvarium. Consequently, the brain is visualized well, even in infants with small fontanelles. The small footprint linear array, high-frequency transducers (12 MHz), may also be utilized to image the near field pathology from the anterior fontanelle. This transducer is utilized for subdural hematomas, meningitis, thrombosis in the superior sagittal sinus, and cerebral edema. The broadband width transducer frequencies ranging from 7.5 MHz or higher are most commonly used with the premature infant. In larger babies the studies can be obtained with the higher-frequency transducer for structures located close to the fontanelles and a slightly lower frequency (5 MHz) transducer for visualization of the anatomy in areas situated farther away from the transducer (Box 25-1). The use of multiple focal zones throughout the depth of the image is used for the best lateral resolution.

Sonography of the neonatal brain is evaluated through the anterior fontanelle in multiple planes to study the supratentorial and infratentorial compartments. Supratentorial studies show the cerebral hemispheres, the basal ganglia, the lateral and third ventricles, the interhemispheric fissure, and the subarachnoid space surrounding the hemispheres. Infratentorial studies visualize the cerebellum, the brain stem, the fourth ventricle, and the basal cisterns. In addition, images can be obtained through the posterior and mastoid fontanelles.

Both compartments are studied in the coronal, modified coronal, sagittal, and parasagittal planes. The sagittal, parasagittal, and modified coronal planes are imaged from the anterior fontanelle. Because the structures in the infratentorial compartment are located relatively far from the transducer, the alteration of a deep focal placement or lowering the transducer frequency is recommended, particularly in older infants. The coronal views for the infratentorial compartment are obtained from the mastoid fontanelle and the occipitotemporal area.

A standoff pad may be useful in evaluating a superficial abnormality such as a subdural hemorrhage; however, the higher-resolution transducer is easier to manipulate and should adequately image the near field structures. Color Doppler should be used to demonstrate the normal vascular structures within the neonatal head.

BOX 25-1	Transducer Selection

5.0 MHz for over 34 weeks or macrocephaly
7.5 MHz or higher for under 34 weeks

If pathology is demonstrated, color Doppler is used to demonstrate the presence or absence of flow within the particular structure. Color Doppler is also useful to evaluate the circle of Willis through the posterior fossa. A clot in the occipital horns is best evaluated from the posterior approach. The foramen magnum is useful to evaluate the proximal end of the spinal canal. Scanning may be limited if the anterior fontanelle is not "wide" enough. If the fontanelle is compressed or overlapping because of oligohydramnios or a difficult delivery, it may be difficult to adequately image the structures of the brain. The anterior fontanelle remains open until about 2 years of age, but is wide enough to scan until about 12 to 14 months.

Coronal and Modified Coronal Planes

Technically a view of the **coronal plane** is 90 degrees to Reid's baseline, but a number of different angles to Reid's baseline are actually used in performing the examination. Reid's baseline is the line extending from the lower edge of the orbit to the center of the aperture of the external auditory canal and backward to the center of the occipital bone. When looking at the coronal sections, the vertex of the skull is at the top and the left side of the brain is to the right of the image.

To perform these studies, the transducer is placed on the anterior fontanelle with the scanning plane following the coronal suture (Figure 25-15). The middle of the transducer must be centered in the coronal suture to reduce bone interference and to procure the most extensive image of the brain. It is critical that symmetrical images be obtained; this is accomplished by using the skull bones and the middle cerebral arteries at the sylvian fissure as landmarks (Figure 25-16). The skull bones and the arteries should be the same size bilaterally. In the coronal plane, the transducer is angled from the anterior to the posterior of the skull to completely visualize the lateral and third ventricles, the deep subcortical white matter, and the basal ganglia (Box 25-2).

When the transducer is angled anteriorly, the frontal horns of the lateral ventricles appear as slitlike hypoechoic to cystic formations. As the transducer is angled posteriorly, the ventricles acquire a comma-like shape; the ventricular width increases from 2 mm at the frontal lobes to a maximum of 3 to 6 mm at the region of the choroid plexus (bodies of the lateral ventricles) (Figure 25-17).

The sonographer should be aware that ventricular size varies with gestational age and that the premature infant will normally have larger ventricles than will the term infant. The term infant has small ventricles, which are slitlike in shape. It is important to note the approximate "gestational age" of the premature infant when performing a neonatal sonogram of the head.

The choroid plexus is an intraventricular structure lying along the floor of the lateral ventricles, extending from the temporal horn into the atrium and body of the lateral ventricles (see Figure 25-17). At the foramen of Monro, the choroid plexus enters into the third ventricle. Consequently the frontal (anterior) and the occipital (posterior) horns are devoid of choroid plexus. The choroid plexus becomes enlarged at the level of the atria

---

BOX 25-2 | Coronal Protocol

- Anterior: orbits
- Anterior: anterior horns and lateral ventricles
- Middle: lateral ventricles, cavum septum pellucidum, third ventricle, and corpus callosum
- Posterior: ambient wings and cisterna magnum
- Posterior: tentorium and cisterna magnum
- Posterior: choroid
- Posterior: glomus of choroids
- Posterior: far posterior brain (occipital)

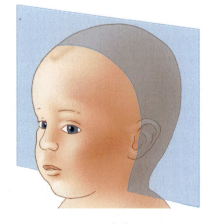
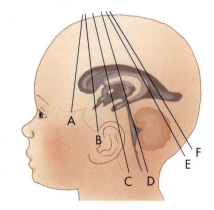

FIGURE 25-15 A, The transducer is placed on the anterior fontanelle, perpendicular to the neonatal head. **B,** Coronal scan planes as the transducer is angled from the anterior to posterior skull as described in the text. *A* through *F* indicate the different scanning planes. *A* is the most anterior, and *F* is the most posterior.

Coronal plane

A   **B**

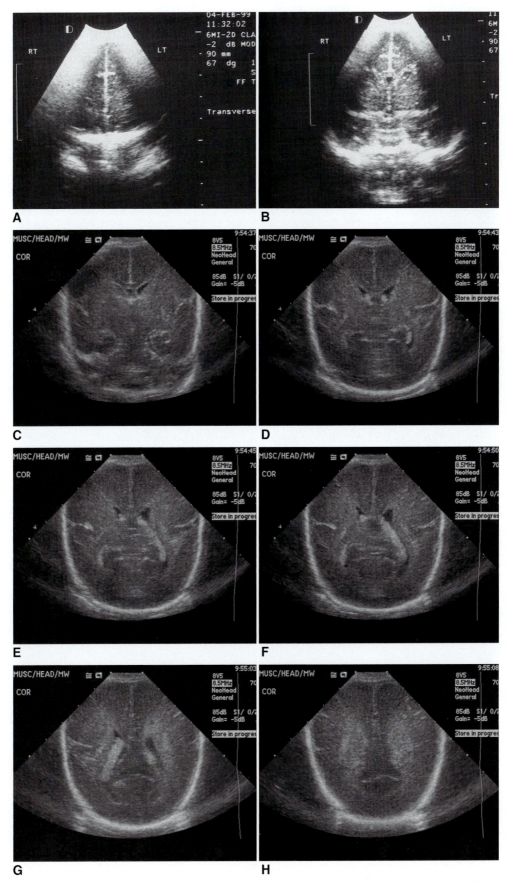

FIGURE 25-16 Normal protocol for coronal images beginning with the transducer angled toward the anterior skull (**A** and **B**), then angled to the midcoronal section (**C, D, E,** and **F**), and finally angled toward the posterior occipital area of the skull (**G** and **H**).

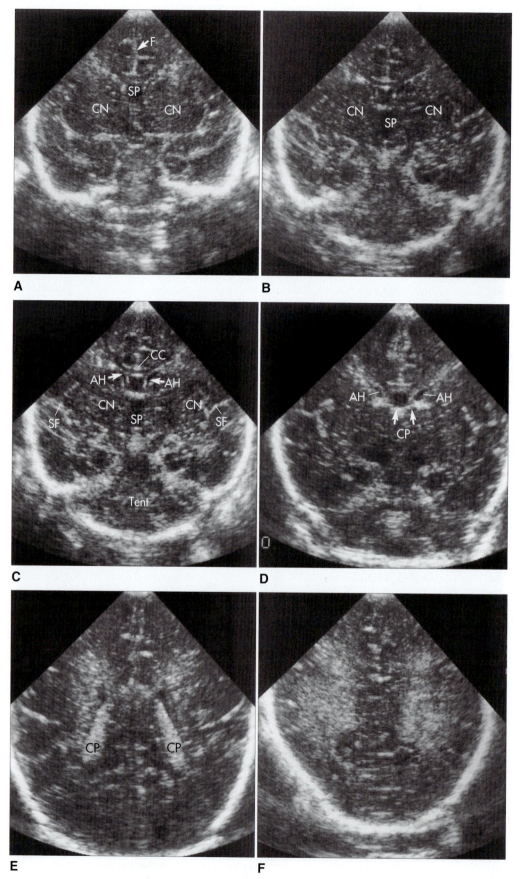

FIGURE 25-17 A, First anterior coronal image. *CN,* Caudate nucleus; *F,* falx; *SP,* septum pellucidum. **B,** Second anterior coronal image. *CN,* Caudate nucleus; *SP,* septum pellucidum. **C,** Midcoronal image. *AH,* Anterior horn; *CC,* corpus callosum; *CN,* caudate nucleus; *SF,* sylvian fissure; *SP,* septum pellucidum; *Tent,* tentorium. **D,** Midcoronal image. *AH,* Anterior horn; *CP,* choroid plexus. **E,** Posterior coronal image. *CP,* Choroid plexus. **F,** Posterior coronal image beyond the level of the ventricles.

(glomus of the choroid plexus). At the atria, the plexus can almost entirely fill the ventricular cavity.

On sonography, the choroid plexus is an echogenic structure inside the ventricular cavities surrounding the thalamic nuclei. The size of the choroid plexus depends on the gestational age of the infants. The plexus is very large in very immature infants (less than 25 weeks), and it should not be mistaken for intraventricular hemorrhages. The plexus becomes smaller with increasing gestational age. Between 30 weeks of gestation and term, the size is approximately 2 to 3 mm at the body of the lateral ventricles and 4 to 5 mm at the atria (glomus of the choroid plexus).

The third ventricle is not visualized in normal conditions in the coronal or modified coronal studies in the full-term fetus. Occasionally a thin and very echogenic formation can be seen in the midline immediately below the septum pellucidum. This echogenic image corresponds to the choroid plexus extending into the third ventricle. The septum pellucidum appears as a midline hypoechoic to cystic structure separating the bodies and frontal horns of the lateral ventricles. The septum constitutes the internal wall of the bodies and posterior part of the frontal horns. The cavum septum pellucidum is anterior to the corpus callosum. In the premature fetus, less than 32 weeks, the third ventricle is prominent and easily seen on sonography.

Coronal and modified coronal views also visualize the basal ganglia and the white matter. The caudate nuclei constitute the inferior and lateral walls of the ventricles at the bodies and posterior part of the frontal horns (see Figure 25-17). In premature infants, the caudate nuclei may have higher echogenicity than the rest of the brain parenchyma. In these infants, the nuclei should not be mistaken for subependymal hemorrhages. The thalamic ganglia are located laterally to the third ventricle, and they are visualized as areas of low echogenicity. The white matter is situated between the lateral ventricles and the cortex. The white matter has low echogenicity, with thin echogenic streaks that correspond to small vessels. This area is known as "watershed zones," which are the terminal ends of the vessel bed and may be used to describe the periventricular white matter.

Modified Coronal Studies of the Ventricles and Posterior Fossa

The modified coronal plane demonstrates the body of the lateral ventricles, the third ventricle, and the posterior fossa. To obtain this view, the transducer is positioned over the anterior fontanelle with an angle of approximately 30 to 40 degrees between the scanning plane and the surface of the fontanelle. In this view the tentorium, the cerebellar vermis, the fourth ventricle, the cerebellar hemispheres, and the cisterna magna can be seen in the infratentorial compartment.

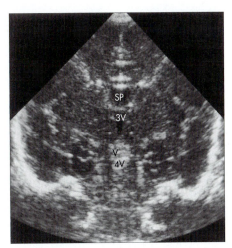

FIGURE 25-18 Midcoronal image of the septum pellucidum (*SP*), third ventricle (*3V*), vermis (*V*), and fourth ventricle (*4V*).

The vermis is a very echogenic structure in the midline (Figure 25-18). The fourth ventricle appears in the midline as a small anechoic space approximately 2 to 3 mm wide, located anteriorly to the vermis. The cerebellar hemispheres have low echogenicity and are contiguous with the echogenic vermis. The cisterna magna corresponds to a nonechogenic space between the vermis, the cerebellar hemispheres, and the occipital bone.

Coronal Studies through the Posterior Fontanelle

If the anatomic structures are difficult to image because of overlapping bones in the area of the fontanelle, the posterior fontanelle is used as an alternative window to image the choroid plexus and lateral ventricles. The transducer is placed 1 cm behind the helix of the ear and 1 cm above the tragus. The fontanelle is located at the junction of the squamosal, lambdoidal, and occipital sutures. The posterior fossa axial images, with the anterior portion of the transducer angled slightly cephalad, will demonstrate the fourth ventricle, posterior cerebellar vermis, cerebellar hemispheres, and the cisterna magna.

Sagittal Plane

Sagittal plane sections are made by rotating the coronal plane approximately 90 degrees. These sections are viewed with the anterior brain to the left and the occipital portion of the brain to the right. To obtain these studies, the transducer is positioned over the anterior fontanelle with the scanning plane following the sagittal suture (Figures 25-19 and 25-20). Sagittal studies provide the most extensive visualization of the brain (Box 25-3).

The straight sagittal study (the only view strictly in the sagittal plane) shows the midline structures in the supratentorial and infratentorial compartments. The

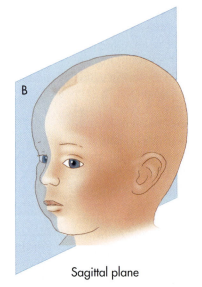
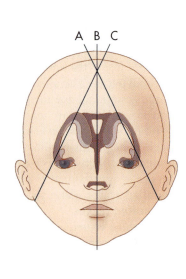

FIGURE 25-19 The transducer is placed in the anterior fontanelle, perpendicular to the skull, and rotated 90 degrees from the coronal plane to the sagittal plane. The transducer uses the midsagittal plane as the primary landmark; slight angulation of the transducer away from the midline will show the parasagittal and midsagittal planes. **A** and **C** indicate the lateral sagittal planes through the ventricles. **B** indicates the midline sagittal plane.

Sagittal plane

BOX 25-3 | **Sagittal Protocol**

These items should be assessed separately for each side of the brain:
- Midline: cavum septum pellucidum, corpus callosum, third ventricle, and foramen of Monro, aqueduct of Sylvius, fourth ventricle, cerebellum (tentorium), cisterna magna
- Thalamus
- Caudothalamic groove (notch)
- Lateral ventricle: anterior, body, and occipital (temporal if hydrocephalic)
- Angle slightly lateral from the lateral ventricle to show the white matter
- Very lateral—sylvian fissure (middle cerebral artery)

---

straight midline view should be obtained before performing the right and left parasagittal studies. This view is a guide to determine if a parasagittal study corresponds to the right or left side (Figure 25-21).

The supratentorial structures shown by the sagittal studies are the corpus callosum, septum pellucidum, and third ventricle (Figure 25-22). The corpus callosum appears as two thin parallel lines separated by a thin echogenic space. The genu and splenium of the corpus callosum may be identified as the anterior-dorsal and posterior portions, respectively. The cingulate sulcus is found anterior and parallel to the corpus callosum. This is a helpful landmark to identify; as with agenesis of the corpus callosum, it is randomized or spiraled because of the midline defect. The septum pellucidum appears as an anechoic (cystic) structure immediately below the corpus callosum. The third ventricle is normally anechoic and is located inferiorly to the septum. The echogenic choroid plexus appears to enter the top of the third ventricle through the foramen of Monro. The supraoptic recess of the third ventricle is shown as a triangular nonechogenic structure extending inferiorly and anteriorly toward the suprasellar region.

In the straight sagittal plane, the infratentorial structures visualized are the cerebellar vermis, the fourth ventricle, the cisterna magna, the supracerebellar and quadrigeminal cisterns, and the brain stem. The vermis of the cerebellum appears as a very echo-dense formation, separated from the occipital bone by an anechoic space that corresponds to the cisterna magna.

The other cisterns also are anechoic spaces located above and behind the cerebellar vermis. The fourth ventricle appears as a small "V" with the vertex oriented posteriorly inside the echogenic vermis. The fourth ventricle is limited anteriorly by the brain stem. The brain stem has low echogenicity, with an echo-dense anterior border demarcated by the basilar artery.

Parasagittal Studies

After having studied the midline, the transducer is moved/angled slightly to the left and right sides to visualize the cerebellar hemispheres in the parasagittal plane (see Box 25-3). The cerebellar hemispheres appear as round, low echogenic formations with moderately hyperechoic surfaces.

The parasagittal views are obtained by angling the transducer to the right or left side of the skull. Three parasagittal studies should be performed. The first parasagittal image should be close to the midline to visualize the caudate nuclei in detail, because subependymal hemorrhages begin in the germinal matrix that is located at the level of these ganglia. These views image the frontal horn and body of the lateral ventricles, the thalamus, the head of the caudate nucleus, and the choroid plexus.

The frontal horns and bodies of the lateral ventricles appear as narrow sonolucent cavities (Figure 25-23). The height of the bodies of the ventricles normally is less than 7 mm at the level of the midthalamus. The floor of the lateral ventricles is determined by the boundary between

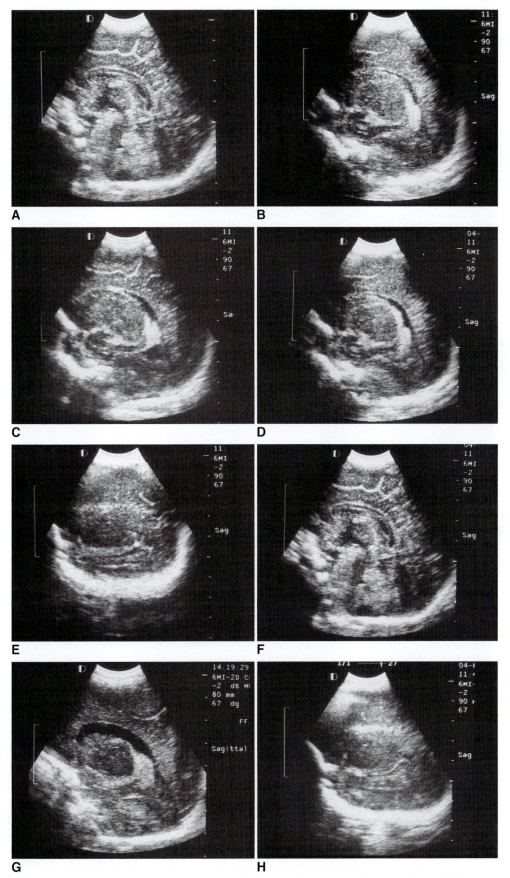

FIGURE 25-20 Normal protocol for sagittal images beginning with the transducer perpendicular to the skull **(A)**, then to the right **(B, C, D,** and **E)**, back to the midline **(F)**, and then to the left **(G** and **H)**.

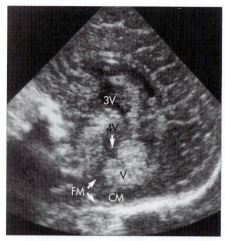

FIGURE 25-21 Slight parasagittal view of the third ventricle *(3V)*, fourth ventricle *(4V)*, vermis *(V)*, foramen magnum *(FM)*, and cisterna magna *(CM)*.

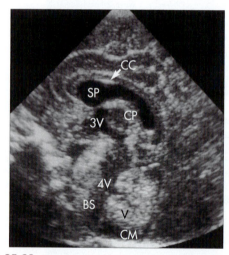

FIGURE 25-22 "Straight" sagittal view of the midline structures. Supratentorial structures: choroid plexus *(CP)*, corpus callosum *(CC)*, septum pellucidum *(SP)*, and third ventricle *(3V)*. Infratentorial structures: brain stem *(BS)*, cerebellar vermis *(V)*, cisterna magna *(CM)*, and fourth ventricle *(4V)*.

the very echogenic choroid plexus and the less echogenic thalamus. The choroid plexus appears as a small (2 to 3 mm height), very echogenic structure lying against the thalamus. The plexus appears to end at the **thalamic-caudate groove,** which is the most common location of subependymal hemorrhages. The floor of the ventricles ventral to the groove is formed by the head of the caudate nucleus, which in small infants has higher echogenicity than the surrounding tissue.

The second parasagittal image is made slightly lateral to the first image and includes the entire ventricular cavity. Because the ventricular cavity is not entirely parallel to the midline (i.e., the posterior horns are more lateral or external than the anterior horns), the transducer must be rotated slightly counterclockwise to form an acute angle with the sagittal suture anteriorly. These views show the entire ventricular horns; the choroid plexus, including the glomus; the thalami; the caudate nuclei; and the white matter superior and anterior to the lateral ventricles.

The third parasagittal view images the white matter located lateral (externally) to the lateral ventricles (Figure 25-24). This view is useful for studying intraparenchymal hemorrhages, porencephaly, and periventricular leukomalacia.

A fourth parasagittal view should demonstrate the lateralmost aspect, the sylvian figure, middle cerebral artery, and insula.

DEVELOPMENTAL PROBLEMS OF THE BRAIN

Neural Tube Defects

A number of different anomalies may occur in fetal brain development. These anomalies, such as anencephaly, meningomyelocele, meningocele, and encephalocele, are discussed in more detail in Chapter 59.

Arnold-Chiari Malformations. A Chiari malformation is a congenital anomaly associated with spina bifida in

FIGURE 25-23 Parasagittal images of the right **(A)** and left **(B)** ventricles *(LV)* with choroid plexus (CP).

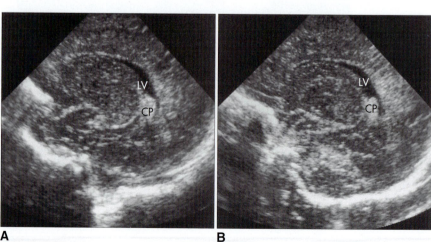

A   B

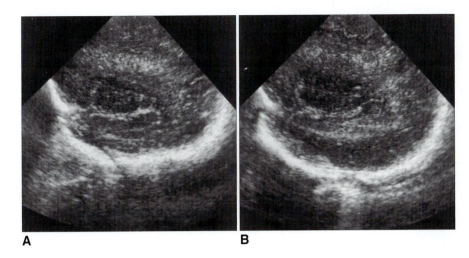

A   **B**

FIGURE 25-24 Parasagittal images of the brain are made as the transducer is angled toward the sylvian fissure to show the white matter of the brain. **A,** Right brain. **B,** Left brain.

which the cerebellum and brain stem are pulled toward the spinal cord and secondary hydrocephalus develops. Chiari malformations have been characterized by variations of the following findings: (1) displacement of the fourth ventricle and upper medulla into the cervical canal, (2) displacement of the inferior part of the cerebellum through the foramen magnum, and (3) defects in the calvarium and spinal column.

Chiari malformations have been classified into three classic groups:

Chiari I. Downward displacement of the cerebellar tonsils, without displacement of the fourth ventricle or medulla.
Chiari II. Most common (and of greatest clinical importance) because of its association with meningomyelocele.
Chiari III. High cervical encephalomeningocele in which the medulla, fourth ventricle, and cerebellum reside.

The failure in neural tube closure during development results in a small posterior fossa. Recall that in early development of the brain, abnormal neural tube closure may result in a spinal defect, such as a myelomeningocele. This decompresses the ventricles and leads to underdevelopment of the posterior fossa bony structures with a resulting small posterior fossa. Chiari malformation is frequently associated with myelomeningocele, hydrocephalus, dilation of the third ventricle, and absence of the septum pellucidum. About 80% to 90% of infants with myelomeningocele have Chiari malformations. Hydrocephalus is usually caused by an obstruction of the CSF pathway at the fourth ventricle or in the posterior fossa, or secondary to aqueductal stenosis, which is present in 40% to 75% of infants with Chiari malformations.

Sonographic Findings. Chiari malformations can be diagnosed with sonography. A failure in the neural tube closure results in a small posterior fossa. In addition, the formation of a myelomeningocele may develop as a result of the open neural tube defect. The

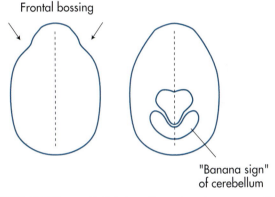

Frontal bossing

"Banana sign" of cerebellum

FIGURE 25-25 Arnold-Chiari malformation shows a small, displaced cerebellum, absence of the cisterna magna, malposition of the fourth ventricle, absence of the septum pellucidum, and widening of the third ventricle.

myelomeningocele in turn decompresses the ventricles, causing underdevelopment of the posterior fossa.

Sagittal studies from the anterior fontanelle show a small cerebellum, absence of the cisterna magna, low position of the fourth ventricle, and displacement of the cerebellum through the foramen magnum associated with hydrocephalus, absence of the septum pellucidum, and widening of the third ventricle (Figures 25-25 and 25-26). With compression of the cerebellum, the cerebellar tonsils and vermis are herniated into the spinal canal through an enlarged foramen magnum. The pons and medulla are inferiorly displaced and the fourth ventricle becomes elongated (Figure 25-27). In addition, enlargement of the massa intermedia may be noted on the coronal and midline sagittal images. This enlargement of the massa intermedia may cause the third ventricle to appear slightly larger than normal. The frontal horns are often small ("bat wing" sign of the anterior and inferior pointing of the frontal horns), whereas the posterior horns of the ventricles are quite enlarged. The septum pellucidum may be partially or completely absent. The interhemispheric fissure may appear widened on the

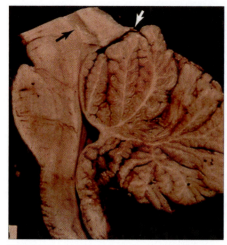

FIGURE 25-26 Gross pathology of Arnold-Chiari malformation shows breaking of the tectum *(black arrow)* and dilatation of the aqueduct *(white arrow)* caused by compression of the fourth ventricle.

coronal scans. The posterior fossa is small and the tentorium is low and hypoplastic. Hydrocephalus is usually present.

Agenesis of the Corpus Callosum. The corpus callosum is a white matter structure that connects both cerebral hemispheres. The presence of the corpus callosum is important in coordinating information and exchanging sensorial stimuli between the two hemispheres. Development of the corpus callosum occurs between the 8th and 12th week of gestation, beginning ventrally and extending dorsally. Depending on the timing of the intrauterine insult, the development of the corpus callosum can be partially arrested or complete agenesis can occur. The corpus callosum is the great commissure connecting the brain hemispheres. Hypoplasia or agenesis of the corpus callosum may occur during the processes of ventral induction or cellular migration. Agenesis of the

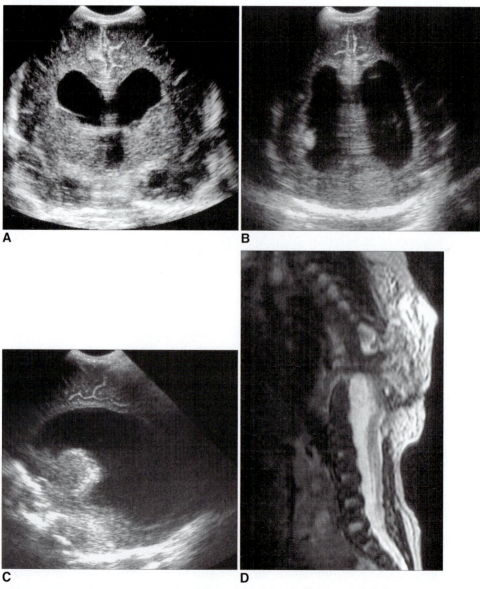

FIGURE 25-27 Infant was delivered by cesarean section at 39 weeks' gestation for thoracic spina bifida. Chiari's malformation, type II, was identified. Enlarged ventricles can be seen in **(A)** anterior and **(B)** posterior coronal views. **C,** Lateral sagittal view of head. **D,** Magnetic resonance imaging shows spinal defect.

corpus callosum is often combined with migrational disorders, such as heterotopias and polymicrogyria. Absence of the corpus callosum may also be induced by ischemic lesions in the midline or by intrauterine encephalomalacia. Other defects associated with this defect are porencephaly, hydrocephalus, microgyria, and fusion of the hemispheres.

The corpus callosum is absent in severe holoprosencephaly. Agenesis of the corpus callosum may be associated with Arnold-Chiari malformation and hydrocephalus. In neonates with this anomaly, the cerebral hemispheres have ventricles with pointed upper corners (bat-wing appearance).

◤ **Sonographic Findings.** Complete absence of the corpus callosum is distinguished by narrow frontal horns and marked separation of the anterior horns and bodies of the lateral ventricles associated with widening of the occipital horns and the third ventricle (Figure 25-28). The ventricular cavities acquire the distinctive appearance of "vampire wings." These characteristics are easily identified by ultrasound (Figure 25-29). Partial agenesis of the corpus callosum occurs when the genu, the splenium, and the rostrum are absent.

Dandy-Walker Malformation. Dandy-Walker syndrome is a congenital anomaly in which a huge fourth

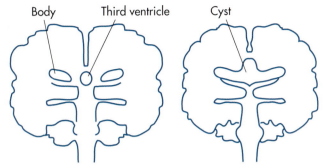

FIGURE 25-28 Complete agenesis of the corpus callosum is characterized by narrow frontal horns with marked separation of the anterior horns and bodies of the lateral ventricles.

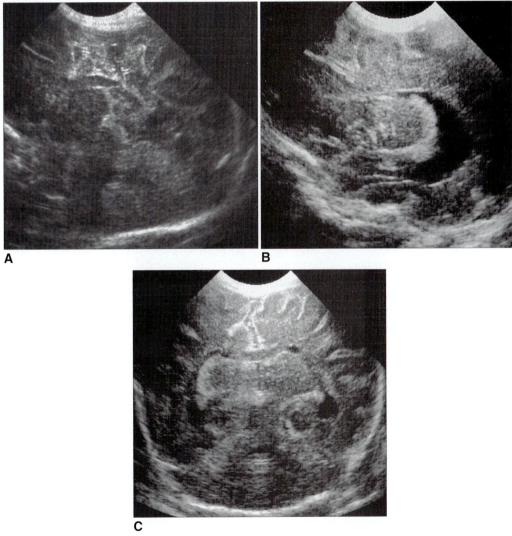

FIGURE 25-29 A, Agenesis of the corpus callosum (ACC) is noted in midline sagittal image of preterm infant. Cingulated gyri also display abnormal configuration. **B,** Rounded occipital horns are also evidence of ACC. **C,** Coronal view shows monoventricle present. Infant was diagnosed with semilobar holoprosencephaly. Bilateral cleft lip was also present. Infant died shortly after birth.

ventricle cyst occupies the area where the cerebellum usually lies, with secondary dilation of the third and lateral ventricles. The **Dandy-Walker malformation** of the cerebellum is the result of a disturbance of the growth of the roof of the fourth ventricle. The vermis is absent in 25% of the population. The fourth ventricle is enlarged. The posterior fossa is enlarged with the elevation of the tentorium cerebelli, straight sinus, and torcular Herophili at the venous sinus confluence. The brain stem may be compressed anteriorly or become hypoplastic. Obstructive hydrocephalus occurs in a high percentage of patients.

Dandy-Walker malformation may be associated with other central nervous system (CNS) anomalies, which include hydrocephalus, partial or complete agenesis of the corpus callosum, encephalocele, holoprosencephaly, microcephaly, infundibular hamartomas, or brain stem lipomas.

▶ **Sonographic Findings.** The typical Dandy-Walker malformation is characterized by hypoplasia or absence of the cerebellar vermis, enlarged fourth ventricle with the development of a large cyst in the posterior fossa (Dandy-Walker cyst), hypoplastic cerebellar hemispheres displaced laterally by the fourth ventricle, small brain stem, and hydrocephalus (Figure 25-30), obstruction above and below the fourth ventricle, and absent corpus callosum. The hydrocephalus is caused by the atresia of the foramina of Luschka and Magendie (congenital obstructive hydrocephalus) (Figure 25-31). When the vermis is absent, the fourth ventricle communicates directly with the cyst. A Dandy-Walker variant is present when there is an enlarged cisterna magna communicating with the fourth ventricle in the presence of a normal or hypoplastic cerebellar vermis (Figure 25-32).

There are two differential diagnoses of posterior fossa cystic lesions that mimic Dandy-Walker syndrome. A mega cisterna magna is a normal variant with no mass effect that is not associated with the development of hydrocephalus and has a normal cerebellar vermis, fourth ventricle, and cerebellar hemisphere. A posterior fossa subarachnoid cyst can be differentiated from Dandy-Walker malformation or variant by the lack of communication of the cyst with the fourth ventricle. The arachnoid cyst displaces the normal fourth ventricle, vermis, and cerebellum.

Disorders of Diverticulation and Cleavage

Holoprosencephaly. Holoprosencephaly is a complex development abnormality of the brain arising from failure of cleavage of the prosencephalon. This failure results early in gestation. It is characterized by a grossly abnormal brain in which there is a common large central ventricle (Figure 25-33). The abnormalities found in holoprosencephaly include cyclopia, cebocephaly, ethmocephaly, median cleft, and holotelencephaly.

Holoprosencephaly represents a spectrum of malformations that form a continuum from most severe, with

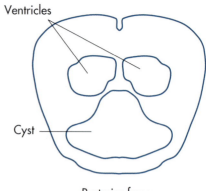

FIGURE 25-30 Dandy-Walker malformation is characterized by the absence of the cerebellar vermis and cystic changes in the fourth ventricle. Hydrocephalus may also be present.

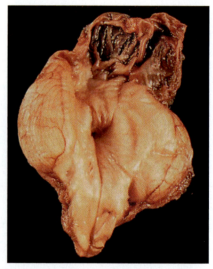

FIGURE 25-31 Dandy-Walker malformation. Hypoplastic vermis and cyst are reflected to expose a dilated fourth ventricle.

no separation of the telencephalon (alobar), to least severe, with partial separation of the dorsal aspects of the brain (lobar). A third classification of intermediate severity between alobar and lobar is semilobar holoprosencephaly. The mildest form of lobar prosencephaly is septoptic dysplasia, in which there is absence of the septum pellucidum and optic nerve hypoplasia.

The neuropathologic features include a single cerebrum with a single ventricular cavity, absence of the corpus callosum and frontal horns, and a thin membrane arising from the roof of the third ventricle, which may extend posteriorly forming a supratentorial cyst (Figure 25-34). In addition, anomalies of the face also accompany this condition.

Alobar Holoprosencephaly. This is the most severe form of holoprosencephaly. Multiple facial anomalies (i.e., cebocephaly, cyclopia, and ethmocephaly) are present. The brain surrounds a single midline crescent-shaped ventricle with a thin, primitive cerebral cortex surrounding the large ventricle. The thalami and

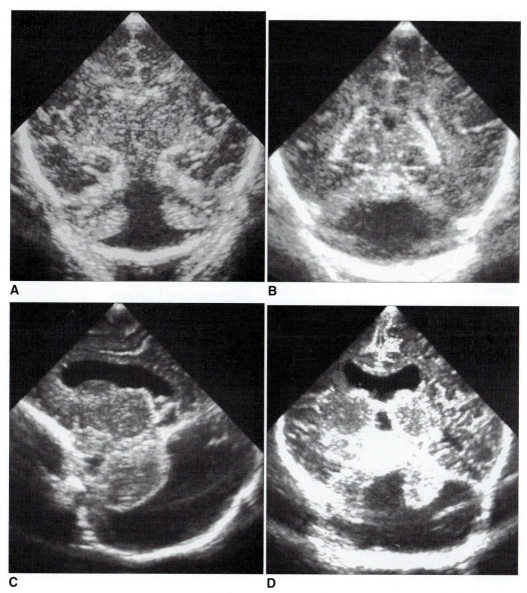

FIGURE 25-32 Dandy-Walker malformation. **A** and **B,** Female infant was born at 37 weeks' gestation, and neonatal head ultrasound was ordered. Mother of the infant had no prenatal care. Sonographic evaluation showed posterior fossa cyst and splaying in cerebellar hemispheres as noted in the coronal images. No hydrocephalus was identified. **C** and **D,** Hydrocephalus was identified in infant with DWM. Lateral sagittal **(C)** and coronal **(D)** views show large posterior fossa cyst and accompanying ventricular enlargement.

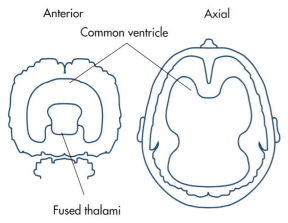

FIGURE 25-33 Holoprosencephaly features a single ventricular cavity with abnormalities of the cerebrum.

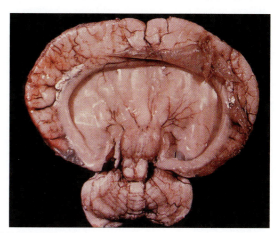

FIGURE 25-34 This posterior view shows the reflected cyst wall communicating with a univentricle.

hemispheres are fused; therefore, the falx, corpus callosum, and interhemispheric fissure are not present. The fused thalami are seen anterior to the fused hyperechogenic choroid plexus (Figure 25-35). The third ventricle is absent, causing the dilated single ventricle to communicate directly with the aqueduct of Sylvius. A large dorsal cyst may also be present.

Semilobar Holoprosencephaly. A single ventricle is evident; however, more brain parenchyma is present. A small portion of the falx and interhemispheric fissure develops in the occipital cortex posteriorly. There may be separate occipital and temporal horns. The splenium and genu of the corpus callosum is often formed and may be seen on midline sagittal images. The thalami are partially separated and the third ventricle is rudimentary. Mild facial anomalies (i.e., hypotelorism and cleft lip) may be present.

Lobar Holoprosencephaly. This is the least severe form of holoprosencephaly. There is nearly complete separation of hemispheres with development of a falx and interhemispheric fissure. There may be fusion of the frontal lobes. The septum pellucidum is absent. The anterior horns of the lateral ventricles are fused; however,

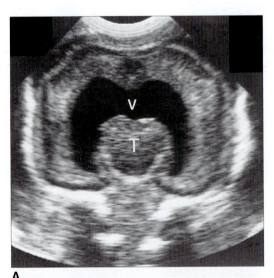

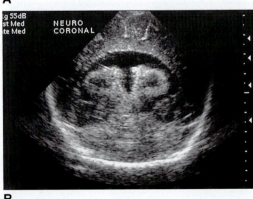

FIGURE 25-35 A, Alobar holoprosencephaly is identified in image demonstrating single ventricle. **B,** Variable fusion identified in semilobar holoprosencephaly is seen in image.

the occipital horns are separated. The third ventricle is present and separates the thalami. The splenium and body of the corpus callosum are present with the absence of the genu and rostrum. Facial anomalies are mild.

Ischemic Lesions. After the ventral induction has occurred, ischemic lesions in the midline may induce malformations of the telencephalon similar to holoprosencephaly. As in holoprosencephaly, there is a single ventricular cavity and absence of the corpus callosum. However, the presence of two frontal horns helps differentiate these malformations caused by ischemic lesions from true holoprosencephaly.

Sonographic Findings. When holoprosencephaly is suspected, it is important to obtain modified coronal studies of the whole frontal lobes to determine whether two frontal horns are present.

Destructive Lesions

Porencephalic Cyst. A porencephalic cyst, also known as porencephaly, is a cyst filled with cerebrospinal fluid that communicates with the ventricular system or subarachnoid space. These cysts may result from hemorrhage, infarction, delivery trauma, or inflammatory changes in the nervous system. The affected brain parenchyma undergoes necrosis, brain tissue is resorbed, and a cystic lesion remains.

Sonographic Findings. A cyst is seen within the brain parenchyma without a mass effect. There may be communication of the cyst with the ventricle or subarachnoid space. A reduction in the size of the affected hemisphere may cause a midline shift and contralateral ventricular enlargement.

Hydraencephaly. Hydranencephaly is believed to be the result of bilateral occlusion of the internal carotid arteries during fetal development, but it may result from any number of intracranial destructive processes. Brain development is destroyed and replaced by cerebrospinal fluid. Because the posterior communicating arteries are preserved, the midbrain and cerebellum are present. The basal ganglia, choroid plexus, and thalamus may also be spared.

Sonographic Findings. There is absence of normal brain tissue with almost complete replacement by cerebrospinal fluid (Figure 25-36). The falx is either absent or partially absent. The midbrain, basal ganglia, and cerebellum are seen. Macrocephaly may be present. Doppler flow in the carotid arteries is absent.

Hydrocephalus

Hydrocephalus results when there is an imbalance between the production of cerebrospinal fluid (CSF) and its drainage by the arachnoid villi. Three mechanisms account for the development of hydrocephalus: obstruction to outflow, decreased absorption, or overproduction.

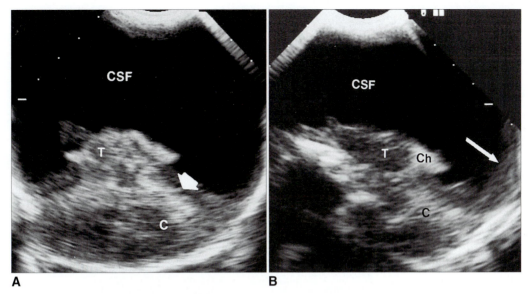

FIGURE 25-36 Hydranencephaly. Coronal **(A)** and sagittal **(B)** midline views. Tentorium cerebelli (*thick arrow*); thin remnant of cerebral cortex (*thin arrow*), *T,* Thalamus, *C,* cerebellum, *Ch,* choroid plexus.

The CSF provides a chemically controlled protective environment that continually bathes and circulates around the CNS. Although the choroid plexus produces the majority of fluid, the ventricular ependyma, the intracranial subarachnoid lining, and the spinal subarachnoid lining also produce it. The CSF fluid flows from the lateral ventricles, through the foramina of Monro, the third ventricle, the aqueduct of Sylvius, the fourth ventricle, the lateral foramina of Luschka or medial foramen of Magendie, and into the basal cisterns. From this point, a small amount circulates down into the spinal subarachnoid space. CSF flows upward around the brain to reach the vertex, where it is reabsorbed by the arachnoid granulations into the superior sagittal sinus.

Congenital Hydrocephalus. Hydrocephalus refers to any condition in which enlargement of the ventricular system is caused by an imbalance between production and reabsorption of CSF. Hydrocephalus is caused by a variety of conditions that cause the ventricles to dilate when there is obstruction of cerebrospinal fluid. Congenital structural malformations, such as myelomeningocele, agenesis of the corpus callosum, and aqueductal stenosis, are all associated with ventricular dilatation. Acquired hydrocephalus occurs after the loss of deep white matter in periventricular leukomalacia (PVL) and after intraventricular hemorrhage caused by either acquired aqueductal stenosis or occlusion of resorptive arachnoid granulations. Posthemorrhagic hydrocephalus (PHH) should not be confused with grade III intraventricular hemorrhage.

Hydrocephalus is divided into communicating and noncommunicating forms; the former is produced by occluded granulations and the latter by some anatomic obstruction to CSF flow. The earlier the hydrocephalus occurs, the greater the enlargement of the neonatal head.

This dilation results in widely separated sutures and huge, bulging fontanelles.

Sonographic Findings. The sonographer should look for the blunting of the lateral angles of the lateral ventricles (Figure 25-37). When this instability of hydrocephalus ensues in the fetus, the widening of the ventricular system is present at birth. Infants born with ventricular enlargement are considered to have congenital hydrocephalus. Hydrocephalus is infrequently caused by overproduction of fluid. Excessive fluid production may occur in infants with papilloma of the choroid plexus, a tumor that actively secretes CSF. Two anatomic types of hydrocephalus are distinguished: obstructive and communicating.

Obstructive Hydrocephalus. Obstructive hydrocephalus is characterized by interference in the circulation of CSF within the ventricular system itself, causing subsequent enlargement of the ventricular cavities proximal to the obstruction.

Communicating Hydrocephalus. In communicating hydrocephalus, the CSF pathways are open within the ventricular system, but there is decreased absorption of CSF. Absorption of CSF can be impeded by occlusion of the subarachnoid cisterns in the posterior fossa or the obliteration of the subarachnoid spaces over the convexities of the brain. The entire ventricular system becomes uniformly distended.

The most common cause of congenital hydrocephalus is **aqueductal stenosis.** The aqueduct of Sylvius is narrowed or replaced by multiple small channels with blind ends. Occasionally, aqueductal stenosis may be caused by extrinsic lesions posterior to the brain stem, such as congenital aneurysm of the vein of Galen.

Sonographic Findings. Aqueductal stenosis can be diagnosed with ultrasound when an infant is born with

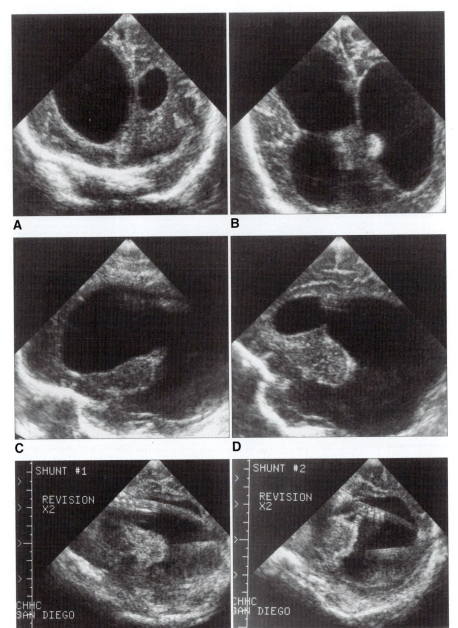

FIGURE 25-37 A through **D,** A 4-month-old infant with hydrocephalus shows dilation of the lateral ventricles. **E** and **F,** Follow-up study of the infant shows the shunt tubing in place for drainage of the hydrocephalus. Ultrasound is very useful in following the shunt placement and monitoring the drainage of the dilated ventricle.

widening of the lateral and third ventricles and a normal-size fourth ventricle. If the hydrocephalus is very large, the posterior fossa is smaller than usual, and the cerebellum is displaced toward the occipital bone with the disappearance of the cisterna magna. However, the cerebellum is not dislodged into the foramen magnum, thus differentiating aqueductal stenosis from the Arnold-Chiari malformation. Arnold-Chiari and Dandy-Walker malformations, other important causes of congenital hydrocephalus, already have been described.

Cystic Lesions

Subarachnoid Cysts. Subarachnoid cysts are lined by arachnoid tissue and contain cerebrospinal fluid. There are three major causes postulated to explain the formation of these cysts: (1) localized entrapment of fluid during embryogenesis, (2) residual subdural hematoma, and (3) fluid extravasation secondary to leptomeningeal tear or ventricular rupture.

The cysts may be located in the infratentorial or supratentorial compartments. Subarachnoid cysts in the posterior fossa are associated with a normal vermis and a normal fourth ventricle, which differentiates subarachnoid cysts from the Dandy-Walker malformation. In a supratentorial compartment, these cysts usually arise from the suprasellar or quadrigeminal plate cisterns. The most frequent locations are the interhemispheric fissure, the suprasellar region, and the cerebral convexities. These cysts may be symptomatic secondary to cerebral

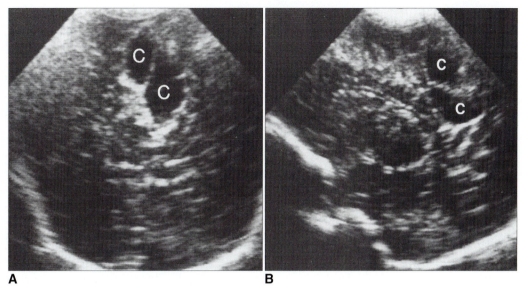

FIGURE 25-38 Midline arachnoid cyst. **A,** Coronal and **B,** sagittal scans show two arachnoid cysts (*C*) in interhemispheric fissure, just above lateral ventricle.

compression or hydrocephalus, or they may be totally asymptomatic.

Sonographic Findings. Subarachnoid cysts usually appear on sonography as a sonolucent structure arising from the quadrigeminal plate cistern or the suprasellar region (Figure 25-38). Sagittal studies are useful to determine the location and size of these cysts. Sequential studies should be obtained in infants with this complication, as the cysts may have progressive growth and may need to be drained by ventriculoperitoneal shunts. Color Doppler may be used to verify that these are not venous malformations, especially when the cysts occur within the quadrigeminal plate cistern or the suprasellar region.

Choroid Plexus Cysts versus Subependymal Cysts. The choroid plexus cysts are common and may be seen in early development as well as after delivery. The cysts tend to be singular and present as an isolated finding, not associated with other CNS or chromosomal abnormalities. However, when the cysts are greater than 10 mm and multiple, these can be associated with chromosomal abnormalities, particularly trisomy 18.

Subependymal cysts present as discrete cysts in the lining of the ventricles. They are most commonly the result of the sequela of germinal matrix hemorrhage in premature infants. These cysts are seen as a smooth-walled spherical cyst in the lateral ventricle.

Sonographic Findings. On sonography, the choroid plexus cyst appears as a well-defined anechoic mass within the dorsal choroid plexus (Figure 25-39). They range in size from 4 to 7 mm and are usually unilateral with the left larger than the right.

Galenic Venous Malformations. The galenic venous malformations represent dilation of the vein of Galen caused by a vascular malformation that is fed by large arteries off the anterior or posterior cerebral artery circulation. Infants with this condition usually present with congestive heart failure.

Sonographic Findings. This malformation appears as an anechoic, cystic mass between the lateral ventricles. It lies posterior to the foramen of Monro, superior to the third ventricle, and primarily in the midline. The large feeding vessels help to differentiate this lesion from other cystic masses. Hydrocephalus may or may not be present and calcification may occur, especially if there is thrombosis in the malformation.

SONOGRAPHIC EVALUATION OF NEONATAL BRAIN LESIONS

Sonography is ideal for timing the onset and sequentially following the evolution of brain lesions that may develop in the premature infant.

Hemorrhagic Pathology

Subependymal-Intraventricular Hemorrhages. Subependymal-intraventricular hemorrhages (SEHs-IVHs) are the most common hemorrhagic lesions in preterm newborn infants. There is an increased risk of subependymal-intraventricular hemorrhage in infants less than 32 weeks' gestational age or less than 1500 grams birth weight. These lesions affect 30% to 50% of infants less than 34 weeks of gestation. SEHs-IVHs are a developmental disease, as they originate in the subependymal germinal matrix (Figure 25-40).

The germinal matrix is the tissue where neurons and glial cells develop before migrating from the subventricular (subependymal) region to the cortex. The germinal matrix is highly cellular, has poor connective supporting tissue, and is richly vascularized with very thin

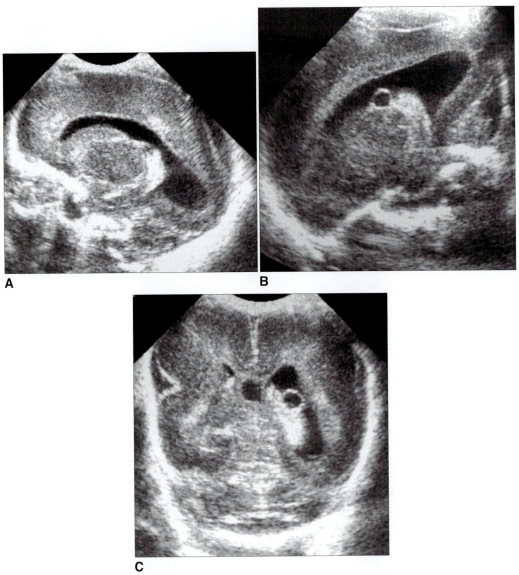

FIGURE 25-39 Choroid plexus cyst. **A,** Subacute choroid plexus hemorrhage. **B** and **C,** Choroid plexus cyst developed after the hemorrhage.

capillaries. This increased capillary fragility may explain the high frequency of these hemorrhages in tiny infants. Furthermore, the germinal matrix has a high fibrinolytic activity that may be important for the extension of the capillary hemorrhages that originate in this tissue. By 24 weeks of gestation, most of the neuronal and glial migration has occurred. However, pockets of germinal matrix remain until 40 weeks of gestation in the subependymal area at the head of the caudate nuclei. This may explain why subependymal hemorrhages occur less frequently in term infants and why the majority of the intraventricular hemorrhages in these infants originate in the choroid plexus.

Subependymal hemorrhages (SEHs) are caused by capillary bleeding in the germinal matrix. The most frequent location is at the thalamic-caudate groove (Figure 25-41). If bleeding continues, the hemorrhage enlarges,

pushing the ependyma into the ventricular cavity, which can then become completely occluded by the subependymal hemorrhage. Eventually, large SEHs rupture through the ependyma into the ventricular cavity, forming an intraventricular hemorrhage (IVH).

◆ **Sonographic Findings.** IVHs and SEHs are easily detected with ultrasound as echogenic structures because fluid and clotted blood have higher acoustic impedance than the brain parenchyma and the CSF. The degree of echogenicity will depend on the acute-chronic process of the hemorrhage. The acute hemorrhage will appear more echogenic than the chronic hemorrhage. SEHs-IVHs can be studied in the coronal, modified coronal, sagittal, parasagittal, and **axial planes.** A subependymal hemorrhage is usually seen at the thalamic-caudate notch as a very echogenic lesion pushing up the floor and external wall of the lateral ventricle with partial obliteration of the ventricular cavity. The SEH can extend by continuous bleeding and perforate the ventricular wall with partial or total flooding of the ventricular system (intraventricular hemorrhage, IVH) (Figure 25-42).

IVHs appear as echogenic structures inside the anechoic ventricular cavities. Depending on the amount of blood, the ventricle can become full and dilated. Subsequently the SEH may obstruct the circulation and absorption of the cerebrospinal fluid, causing the

ventricles to dilate further with CSF and ultimately resulting in posthemorrhagic hydrocephalus.

Studies from the anterior fontanelle may not detect small IVHs, because intraventricular blood tends to "settle out" in the posterior horns. These small IVHs can be diagnosed when the occipital horns are visualized in the axial plane from the mastoid or from the posterior

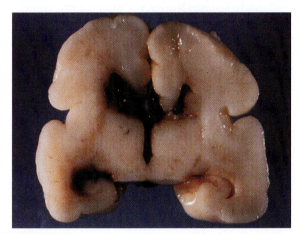

FIGURE 25-40 Subependymal hemorrhage extending into the ventricles. The ventricles contain coagulated blood.

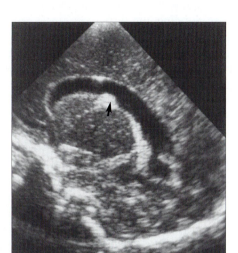

FIGURE 25-41 Sagittal image of a premature neonate with a small subependymal bleed *(arrow)*.

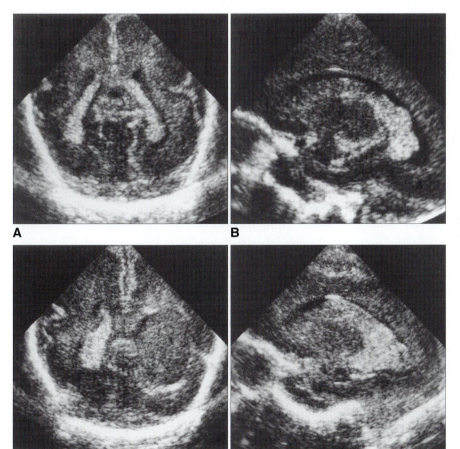

A

B

C

D

FIGURE 25-42 **A** and **B,** Coronal and sagittal images of a premature twin with a grade II bleed shortly after birth that progressed to a grade III bleed in 1 day (**C** and **D**).

fontanelles. Because these fontanelles are closer to the occipital horns than the anterior fontanelle, the occipital horns are within the focal range of the transducer, and a greater amount of ultrasonic energy can reach the sedimented red blood cells.

IVHs-SEHs are not a sudden event; they usually expand slowly. This phenomenon is probably secondary to the high fibrinolytic activity of the germinal matrix. However, in some infants the IVHs-SEHs extend very fast; sudden flooding and distention of the ventricles by hemorrhage is associated with the clinical symptoms of shock, seizures, hypoxemia, and a sudden decrease in the hematocrit. Typically, when a small IVH-SEH progresses to a large IVH-SEH (usually during the first 4 postpartum days), the IVHs-SEHs are asymptomatic. Because approximately 70% of hemorrhages are asymptomatic, it is necessary to have a technique, such as ultrasound, to routinely scan all the infants at risk for these lesions.

Classification of subependymal intraventricular hemorrhages (SEH-IVH) is based on the extension of the hemorrhage and the resultant changes in the ventricular size (Box 25-4). Only ventricular enlargement produced by the intraventricular hemorrhage should be considered. Small SEHs-IVHs may occlude the foramen of Monro or the aqueduct of Sylvius and thereby produce moderate to large dilation of the lateral ventricles by CSF.

The ventricular size is measured in the sagittal plane (height of the body of the ventricles at the midthalamus) and in the axial plane (width of the atrium at the level of the choroid plexus). Based on these measurements, ventricular dilation may be classified as follows:

- *Mild dilation.* Ventricular size measuring 8 to 10 mm.
- *Moderate dilation.* Ventricular size measuring 11 to 14 mm.
- *Large dilation.* Ventricular size greater than 14 mm.

After the hemorrhage has occurred, the blood spreads following the CSF pathways, reaching the fourth ventricle and eventually the cisterns in the posterior fossa, with the development of subarachnoid hemorrhages (SAH) (Figure 25-43). Subsequently, obstruction of the CSF pathways and obliterans arachnoiditis occurs, causing imbalance between production and reabsorption of CSF. Posthemorrhagic ventricular dilation develops as a consequence of this imbalance. If the ventricular dilation is progressive, the patient is considered to have posthemorrhagic hydrocephalus. This complication

occurs in approximately 35% of infants with large hemorrhages. Usually mild to moderate ventricular dilation resolves spontaneously. However, placement of a ventriculoperitoneal shunt may be necessary for severely dilated ventricles.

Posthemorrhagic hydrocephalus may be silent because the white matter of newborn infants is very compliant and easily compressed as the ventricles widen. This factor explains why initial ventricular dilation occurs without changes in the head circumference. The head circumference starts to enlarge only after significant compression of the white matter has developed. Sequential studies are required in infants with SEHs-IVHs to diagnose posthemorrhagic ventricular dilation in the silent phase.

Sonography is the most reliable technique to diagnose and follow changes in the ventricular size and in the intraventricular clots. IVHs-SEHs resolve in several days or weeks, depending on the size of the bleed and on the individual patient. Although CT easily detects intraventricular clots, they resolve as the concentration of hemoglobin decreases, and they are not seen after 10 to 14 days in computed tomography (CT) studies.

Intraventricular clots undergo characteristic changes with time. Initially, they are very echogenic, but then low echogenic areas appear. Eventually they become completely cystic with visualization of the choroid plexus inside the cystic ventricular cast. Large cystic intraventricular clots may cause persistent ventricular dilation despite drainage of the CSF by a ventriculoperitoneal shunt. If the bleed completely fills the ventricular cavity, the ventricle becomes isoechoic with the other structures in the brain and it is more difficult to define the borders of the ventricular wall.

Intraparenchymal Hemorrhages. Intraparenchymal hemorrhages (IPHs) complicate SEHs-IVHs in approximately 15% to 25% of infants. IPHs are a severe complication because they indicate that the brain parenchyma has been destroyed. Although IPHs originally were considered an extension of SEHs-IVHs, evidence suggests that this lesion may actually be a primary infarction of the periventricular and subcortical white matter with destruction of the lateral wall of the ventricle. When the necrotic tissue liquefies, the IVH extends into the necrotic areas.

▶ **Sonographic Findings.** Intraparenchymal hemorrhages appear as very echogenic zones in the white matter adjacent to the lateral ventricles. Echogenic areas in the white matter may correspond to IPHs or to hemorrhagic infarctions or extensive periventricular leukomalacia. In the classic grade IV IPH, there is a clot extending from the white matter into the ventricular cavity (Figure 25-44).

Intraparenchymal clots follow the same evolution as intraventricular clots. A few days after the acute bleeding, the clots become cystic and are reabsorbed completely in 3 or 4 weeks, leaving a cavity communicating with the lateral ventricle (porencephalic cyst).

BOX 25-4	**Classification of Subependymal Intraventricular Hemorrhages**

Grade I: SEH or IVH without ventricular enlargement
Grade II: SEH or IVH with minimal ventricular enlargement
Grade III: SEH or IVH with moderate or large ventricular enlargement
Grade IV: SEH or IVH with intraparenchymal hemorrhage

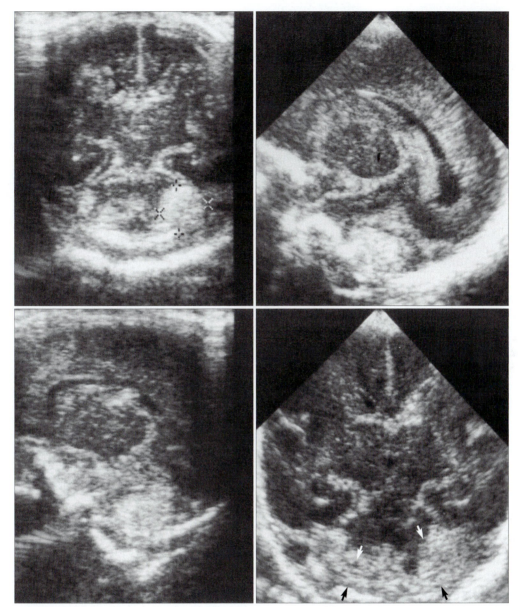

FIGURE 25-43 Multiple coronal and sagittal images in a premature infant born after 27 weeks of gestation with a large cerebellar bleed (*arrows*). In 5 days the bleed had progressed throughout the cerebellar compartment.

When SEHs-IVHs associated with IPH evolve to post-hemorrhagic hydrocephalus, the increased intraventricular pressure is transmitted to the porencephalic cyst. Hydrocephalus after hemorrhage associated with porencephaly is an indication for early ventriculoperitoneal shunt placement to minimize the deleterious effects of progressive compression and ischemia of the brain parenchyma.

Intracerebellar Hemorrhages. Four categories of intracerebellar hemorrhage are described as follows:

1. Primary intracerebellar hemorrhage
2. Venous infarction
3. Traumatic laceration resulting from occipital diastasis
4. Extension to the cerebellum of a large SEH-IVH

In premature neonates, there are areas of germinal matrix located around the fourth ventricle in the cerebellar hemispheres. The cerebellar germinal matrix has the same vulnerability to hemorrhage as the telencephalic germinal matrix. Intracerebellar hemorrhages have been reported in approximately 5% to 10% of postmortem studies of neonatal populations. The incidence in live infants is significantly lower. This discrepancy is probably a result of the difficulties in diagnosing these hemorrhages.

Sonographic Findings. Using modified coronal, sagittal, and parasagittal views of the posterior fossa (infratentorial compartment), it is possible to diagnose unequivocally intracerebellar hemorrhages. These hemorrhages appear as very echogenic structures inside the less echogenic cerebellar parenchyma. Coronal views through the

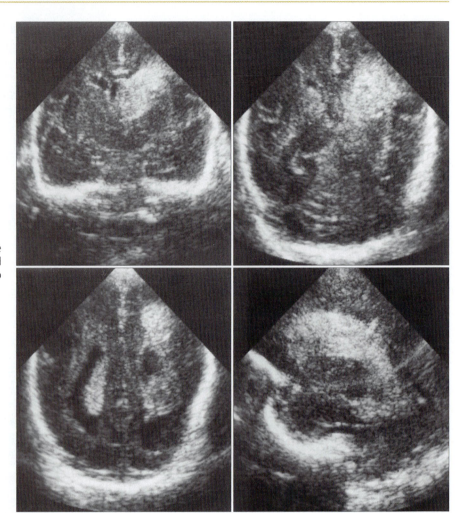

FIGURE 25-44 A 3-day-old premature infant has a grade III bleed on the right and grade IV bleed on the left with extension into the brain parenchyma.

mastoid fontanelle may be essential to differentiate intracerebellar hemorrhages from large SAHs in the cisterna magna, the supracerebellar cistern, or both. Intracerebellar hemorrhages become cystic with time, leaving cavitary lesions in the cerebellar hemispheres. These characteristic sequential changes are useful in making a positive diagnosis of intracerebellar hemorrhages.

Epidural Hemorrhages and Subdural Collections. Epidural hemorrhages and subdural fluid collections are better diagnosed by CT. Because these lesions are located peripherally along the surface of the brain, they are often not adequately visualized by ultrasound.

Sonographic Findings. Subdural collections appear as nonechogenic spaces between the echogenic calvarium and the cortex. Epidural hemorrhages are seen as echogenic formations located immediately underneath the calvarium.

Ischemic-Hypoxic Lesions

Ischemic-hypoxic cerebral injury is a frequent complication of sick newborn infants. The premature neonate is physiologically delicate at birth and as a result is subject to many stresses that in turn can cause hemorrhage and brain injury. Hypoxia is the lack of adequate oxygen to the brain, whereas ischemia is the lack of adequate blood flow to the brain. These occurrences can result from a variety of insults, including respiratory failure, congenital heart disease, and sepsis.

In the term neonate, hypoxic-ischemic injury tends to occur in watershed regions between the vascular territories of the major cerebral vessels. With severe insults, the basal ganglia and thalami may also be involved. The cortex is usually preserved in the preterm infant as a result of anastomotic communicating vessels from the meningeal circulation that serve to preserve cortical blood flow. The preterm infant suffers injury primarily to the periventricular white matter, occurring most commonly near the atria of the lateral ventricles posteriorly and near the foramen of Monro, but can occur anywhere within the corona radiata and even the corpus callosum. White matter ischemia leads to white matter volume loss or periventricular leukomalacia (PVL). These lesions in the brain are usually associated with abnormal neurologic outcome. Five major types of neonatal hypoxic-ischemic brain injury have been described:

1. Selective neuronal necrosis
2. Status marmoratus
3. Parasagittal cerebral injury
4. Periventricular leukomalacia or white-matter necrosis
5. Focal brain necrosis

◢ Sonographic Findings. Sonography is not a precise technique to diagnose necrotic ischemic lesions. In ischemic-hypoxic encephalopathy, sonography may show areas of increased echogenicity in the subcortical and deep white matter and in the basal ganglia (Figure 25-45). The increased echogenicity is caused by congestion and

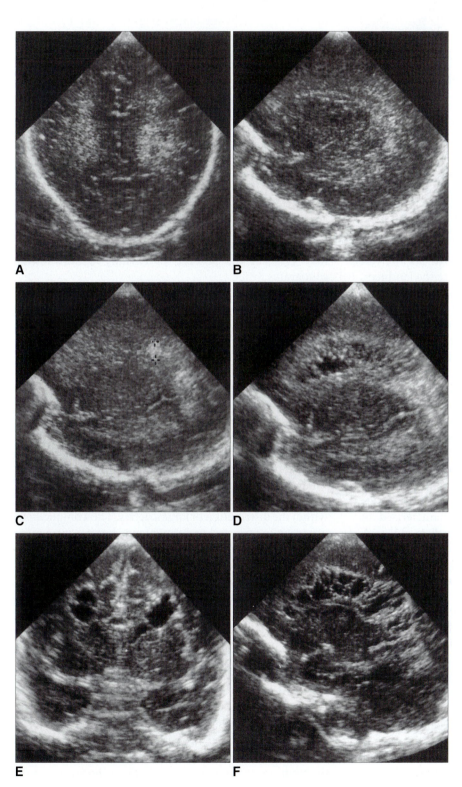

A

B

C

D

E

F

FIGURE 25-45 Progression of periventricular leukomalacia (PVL) in a premature infant. **A,** Posterior coronal image. **B,** Left sagittal image shows white matter congestion and cavitation on day 1. **C,** Day 3 shows progression of the PVL. **D,** Day 14 shows further progression of white matter congestion and cavitation on this sagittal image. **E,** Day 42 demonstrates extensive cavitation throughout both right and left cerebral areas. **F,** Sagittal image shows multiple cavities.

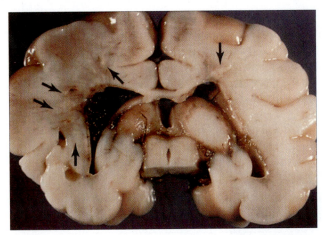

FIGURE 25-46 Periventricular leukomalacia. Chalky white lesions are indicated by arrows.

microhemorrhages, which are characteristically present in the acute stage of ischemic injuries (Figure 25-46). However, echodensities are not pathognomonic of ischemic necrosis, inasmuch as they have been observed in infants having only congestion and microhemorrhages without necrosis. If necrosis is present in the echogenic areas, cavitary lesions appear 2 or more weeks after the ischemic insult. Echolucencies or cysts are the landmark for the diagnosis of ischemic brain injury in newborn infants. Sonography is useful in diagnosing multifocal white matter necrosis (periventricular leukomalacia) and focal ischemic lesions.

Periventricular Leukomalacia or Multifocal White Matter Necrosis. Multifocal white matter necrosis (WMN) or **periventricular leukomalacia (PVL)** is the most frequent ischemic lesion in the immature brain. This lesion is associated with anomalous myelination of the immature brain and abnormal neurologic development, including cerebral palsy. WMN is probably the most important cause of abnormal neurodevelopmental sequelae in preterm infants.

WMN is found in 20% to 80% of neonatal autopsies. Pathologists describe an acute phase characterized by multiple foci or coagulation necrosis in deep and periventricular white matter, and a chronic phase depicted by cavitation and scarring appearing 1 or more weeks after the cerebral insult. Early in the chronic stage, multiple cavities develop in the necrotic white matter adjacent to the lateral walls of the frontal horns, body, atria, and occipital horns of the lateral ventricles. These lesions are frequently located in the lateral wall of the atria and occipital horns, causing damage to the optic radiations. Eventually the cavities resolve, leaving gliotic scars and diffuse cerebral atrophy. Necrotic lesions with only microscopic cavities may also lead to cerebral atrophy.

Currently, WMN may be diagnosed in infants with echoencephalography. The acute stage of WMN is characterized by highly echogenic areas in the cerebral white matter superior and lateral to the frontal horns, bodies,

atria, and occipital horns of the lateral ventricles (Figure 25-47). Echogenic areas are present during the first week after delivery and usually resolve in the following weeks. Microscopically, the echogenicity consists of congestion, microhemorrhages, and foci of necrosis. However, echogenicities may be associated only with congestion and microhemorrhages without necrosis.

◤ **Sonographic Findings.** The chronic stage of WMN is identified with sonography when echolucencies develop in the echogenic white matter (Figure 25-48). Pathologic studies have confirmed that echolucent lesions correspond to cavitary lesions in the white matter. The presence of echolucencies is prima facie evidence that necrotic injury exists in the cerebral white matter. Echogenicity alone suggests, but does not prove, that the echogenic white matter is necrotic. The absence of cystic lesions in the echoencephalogram precludes definitive diagnosis of WMN. Because very echogenic white matter can be simply congestion without coagulation, and in fact not necessarily white matter necrosis at all, careful sequential observations must be made to identify cavitary lesions developing in the echodense white matter. Cystic lesions in WMN may be microscopic or smaller than the resolution of the ultrasound scanners. Consequently, WMN may exist in the absence of cavitary lesions in the sonograms.

Both neuropathologic and echoencephalographic studies have shown that a period of 1 to 6 weeks ensues between the acute stage of WMN and the development of cystic lesions. Echogenic areas and cysts decrease in size and eventually disappear 2 to 5 months after the diagnosis of acute necrosis. If the necrosis was extensive, brain atrophy may be the only indication that WMN occurred during the perinatal period. Sonography is also useful to diagnose the atrophic phase of the chronic stage. This phase is identified by an enlarged subarachnoid space, widened interhemispheric fissure, and persistent ventricular dilation in an infant with a normal or small head circumference.

Focal Brain Necrosis. These necrotic lesions occur within the distribution of large arteries. This complication is present in term and preterm infants, but it is infrequent under 30 weeks' gestational age. Vascular maldevelopment, asphyxia or hypoxia, embolism from the placenta, infectious diseases, thromboembolism secondary to disseminated intravascular coagulation, and polycythemia have been implicated as causal factors in this condition. These insults may occur prenatally or early in postnatal life, leading subsequently to the dissolution of the cerebral tissues and formation of cavitary lesions. The term *porencephaly* is used to describe a single cavity, *multicystic encephalomalacia* for multiple cavities, and *hydranencephaly* for a large single cavity with the entire disappearance of the cerebral hemispheres.

◤ **Sonographic Findings.** Ultrasound images of these injuries show very echogenic localized lesions within the distribution of the major vessel. The echodense lesions

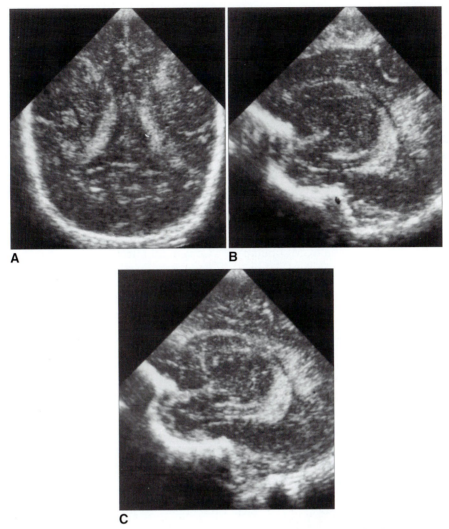

FIGURE 25-47 **A,** Coronal posterior. **B** and **C,** Sagittal scans of a 33-week premature infant with white matter necrosis along the lateral ventricular borders. Follow-up studies will show if this congestion develops into a hemorrhage or clears up completely.

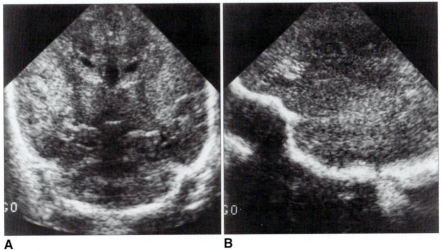

FIGURE 25-48 **A** and **B,** Follow-up study of the patient in Figure 21-47 shows a septal vein in the cavum septum pellucidum and increased ventricular size.

are considered to correspond to cerebral infarctions. After several days, sonolucencies appear within the echogenic areas. Subsequently the infarcted regions are replaced by cavities that may or may not communicate with the ventricle.

Extracorporeal Membrane Oxygenation. Extracorporeal membrane oxygenation (ECMO) is used for pulmonary and circulatory support in many neonatal conditions to allow additional time for the lungs to develop. Infants born with diaphragmatic hernia, persistent pulmonary hypertension, meconium aspiration, and congenital heart disease may be recommended for ECMO to give the infant's lungs a chance to mature. The ECMO cannula is inserted into the right internal jugular vein and carotid artery (the vessels are ligated above their insertion site). Therefore, the ECMO pump procedure can cause a notable change in cerebral circulation, and neonatal ultrasound is used to monitor hemorrhage in the brain tissue.

After the vessel ligation, there is a 50% abrupt decrease in intracranial blood flow with a return of peak systolic velocities to nearly pre-ECMO levels within 3 to 5 minutes. The end-diastolic velocity is increased, and the Doppler is used to monitor for hypoxic-ischemic encephalopathy.

Hemorrhage and ischemia are common in children on ECMO, both from the effects of ECMO itself and from the conditions leading to the use of ECMO. Preexisting hypoxic-ischemic encephalopathy with an abnormal resistive index has been shown to lead to intracranial hemorrhage in a high percentage of infants. Bleeding may occur in the parenchyma, ventricle, or posterior fossa, but the cerebellum also is a common site. Increased extraaxial fluid is a common finding in children on ECMO, usually in the subarachnoid space, and is of little consequence.

BRAIN INFECTIONS

Congenital infections of the brain can have serious consequences for the neonate including mortality, mental retardation, or developmental delay. The most frequent congenital infections are commonly referred to by the acronym TORCH. This refers to the infections *Toxoplasma gondii,* rubella virus, cytomegalovirus (CMV), and herpes simplex type 2. The "O" stands for *other,* such as syphilis, which may cause acute meningitis.

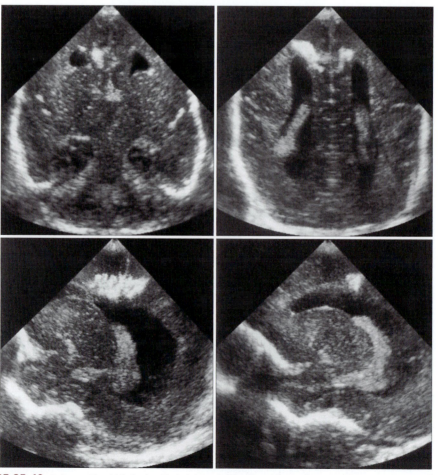

FIGURE 25-49 A 1-month-old infant with bright calcifications bilaterally secondary to cytomegalovirus.

Ventriculitis

Ventriculitis is a common complication of purulent meningitis in newborn infants. Ventriculitis probably is caused by hematogenous spread of the infection to the choroid plexus. The presence of a foreign body in the ventricular cavity, such as a catheter from a ventriculoperitoneal shunt, may provide a nidus for persistent infection of the ventricular cavities.

Sonographic Findings. Ventriculitis leads to compartmentalization of the ventricular cavities by inflammatory adhesions extending from wall to wall. The first stage of ventriculitis is seen in ultrasound as thin septations extending from the walls of the lateral ventricles (Figure 25-49). The septa become thicker and lead to multilocular hydrocephalus and extensive disorganization of the brain anatomy. Sequential studies in patients with meningitis or with ventriculoperitoneal shunts can provide early diagnosis of this severe complication.

Ependymitis

Ependymitis occurs when the ependyma become thickened and hyperechoic as a result of irritation from hemorrhage within the ventricle. This is more common and occurs earlier than ventriculitis developing from interventricular hemorrhage.

The Pediatric Abdomen: Jaundice and Common Surgical Conditions

Sandra L. Hagen-Ansert

In many medical centers, sonography is the first imaging procedure used to evaluate infants and children with acute abdominal problems. This chapter focuses on the cause and sonographic appearance of jaundice in the neonate and pediatric patient. The chapter also focuses on sonographic examination techniques for detecting the more common surgical conditions that may cause pain or vomiting and the ultrasound appearance of these conditions. Specific conditions that affect the **neonate** and pediatric patient will be presented. The reader is referred to the Chapters 10 and 62 for further discussion of liver disease.

EXAMINATION PREPARATION

Gaining the trust of the patient and the patient's family can do much to facilitate the examination. Therefore, the sonographer should first allow sufficient time to explain the examination to the parents and to the child who is old enough to comprehend the proceedings. Sedation and immobilization techniques are generally not required. Toys, books, keys, mobiles, and a variety of other distracting devices can help to quiet the frightened young child. A pacifier may likewise serve well when examining infants. Formula feeding is not recommended if the child

is a surgical candidate. Some laboratories offer glucose water or Pedialyte feedings when examining a neonate for pyloric stenosis. Parents are encouraged to be present during the examination and can help reassure and quiet the patient. Box 26-1 outlines scanning considerations for the pediatric patient.

Virtually no routine patient preparation is required. However, to image the biliary system completely, it is recommended that feeding be withheld for a short time according to the age of the patient (Box 26-2). Adequate distention of the urinary bladder is desirable in many situations. This not only allows assessment of the bladder itself but also facilitates identification of dilated distal ureters, free peritoneal fluid, the pelvic genitalia, and a pelvic mass. A urine-filled bladder may also help localize gastrointestinal abnormalities, such as appendicitis and intussusception. In females, pelvic structures are examined with a full bladder and then emptied for the graded compression portion of the examination.

SONOGRAPHIC EVALUATION OF NEONATAL/PEDIATRIC ABDOMEN

The neonatal/pediatric sonographic examination should evaluate the abdomen and pelvis, with particular

BOX 26-1	General Pediatric Scanning Considerations

- Always use warm gel
- Keep infant warm and secure
  Wrap blankets around infant
  Use as little gel as possible
  Remove gel as soon as possible; it gets cold quickly
  - "Bottle, binky, and diaper"
    Glycogen and water bottles should be handy (dip binky into sugar solution; may repeat while scanning until able to give milk/formula)
    Examine gallbladder and pancreas quickly, then give infant bottle for remainder of examination
    Always keep dry diaper on infant
    Have plenty of distractions ready (e.g., noisy bright-colored toys, stickers, keys)
    Two sonographers to one child is preferred (one to scan, one to occupy child); if not possible, use the parent or nurse
  - Transducers
    Use highest frequency transducer for area image:
    0–1 yr: use 7.5 MHz linear
    1–2 yr: use 5–7.5 MHz linear, curved array, or sector
    >2± yr: use 5 MHz sector or linear
    Use sequential focusing and zoom instead of decreasing depth for better resolution
  - Take breaks
    If child becomes too stressed, give the child a rest
    Let mother hold child until calm
    Feasible to allow child to lie next to mother on stretcher to continue exam
  - Older child
    Explain procedure before child undresses
    Have mother and child touch the transducer and gel and be ready to "watch the movies"

BOX 26-2	Pediatric Ultrasound Examination Prep

Abdominal Ultrasound
0–2 yr: NPO × 4 hr
3–5 yr: NPO × 5 hr
6+ yr: NPO × 6 hr

Pelvic Ultrasound
0–9 yr: Plenty of juice or water 30 min before examination; no voiding 30 min before examination time
10+ yr: 32 oz water 1 hr before examination; no voiding

BOX 26-3	Normal Sonographic Measurements

Liver
- Infant: right lobe should not extend >1 cm below costal margin
- Older infants and children: right lobe should not extend below right costal margin

Biliary Ducts
- Neonates: CBD <1 mm
- Infants (up to 1 yr old): CBD <2 mm
- Older children: CBD <4 mm
- Adolescents: CBD <7 mm

Gallbladder Length
- Infants (under 1 yr old): 1.5–3 cm
- Older children: 3–7 cm

Pancreas (Size Increases with Age)
- Head: 1.0–2.2 cm
- Body: 0.4–1.0 cm
- Tail: 0.8–1.8 cm
- Duct: 1–2 mm

Spleen Length
- Infants (0–3 mo): 6.0 cm
- Children (>12 yr): 12.0 cm

Portal Vein Diameter
- Children <10 yr: 8.5 mm
- Children >10 yr: 10 mm

concentration on the right upper quadrant: liver, bile ducts and gallbladder, pancreas, spleen, and portal system.

The size and texture of the liver should be evaluated (Figure 26-1). The right hepatic lobe should not extend more than 1 cm below the costal margin in a young infant without pulmonary hyperaeration and should not extend below the right costal margin in older infants and children. The echogenicity is normally low to medium homogenicity with clear definition of the portal venous vasculature.

Careful evaluation of the biliary system should be made to exclude ductal dilatation (Figure 26-2). The common bile duct should measure less than 1 mm in neonates, less than 2 mm in infants up to 1 year old, less than 4 mm in older children, and less than 7 mm in adolescents and adults (Box 26-3). The gallbladder size and wall thickness should be assessed. In infants under 1 year of age, the gallbladder length is 1.5 to 3 cm, and in older children, it is 3 to 7 cm. The length of the gallbladder should not exceed the length of the kidney. Careful evaluation of the normal gallbladder should show a smooth-walled anechoic structure without internal echoes. Pericholecystic fluid should not be present.

The pancreas should be examined for size, echotexture, and evidence of dilatation of the pancreatic duct (Figure 26-3). The pancreatic head should measure 1.0 to 2.2 cm; the body, 0.4 to 1.0 cm; and the tail, 0.8 to 1.8 cm. The pancreatic duct should not exceed 1 to 2 mm. The size of the pancreas should increase with the child's age (Table 26-1). The normal texture is hypoechoic compared with the normal liver texture as little fatty tissue has invaded the islets of Langerhans.

The splenic size and texture should be evaluated (Figure 26-4). The upper limits of normal splenic length range from 6.0 cm in infants less than 3 months old to 12 cm in children over 12 years of age.

The diameter of the portal vein may be helpful in determining the presence of portal hypertension

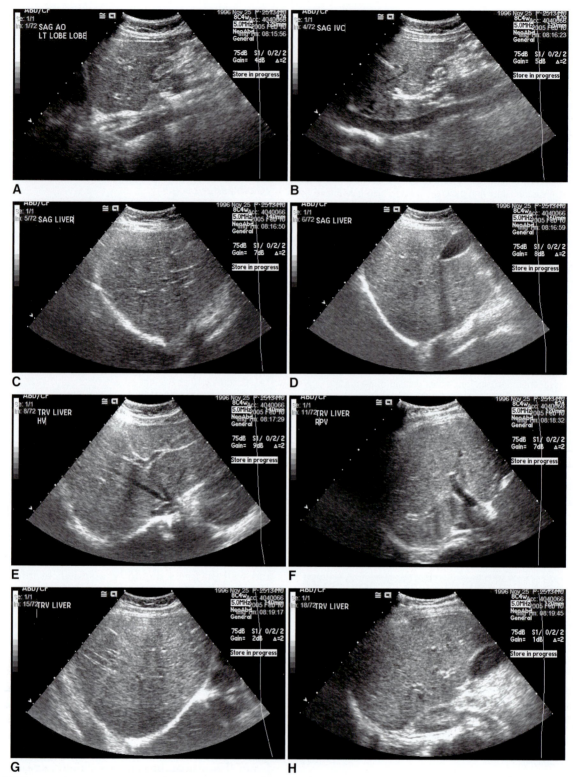

FIGURE 26-1 Normal pediatric liver. The liver is normal in size and contour without focal mass or marginal irregularity. **A,** Sagittal left lobe liver with aorta. **B,** Sagittal left lobe liver with inferior vena cava. **C,** Sagittal right lobe liver. **D,** Sagittal right lobe liver/gallbladder. **E,** Transverse liver with hepatic veins. **F,** Transverse liver with portal veins. **G,** Transverse liver with diaphragm. **H,** Transverse liver, gallbladder, and right kidney.

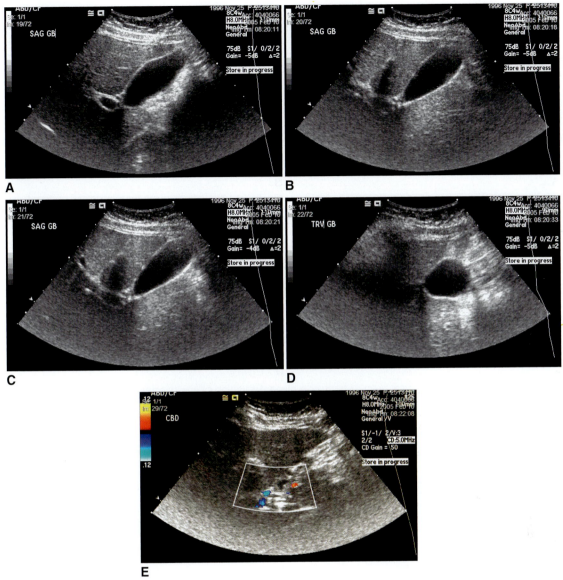

FIGURE 26-2 Normal pediatric gallbladder and common bile duct. Gallbladder is unremarkable without wall thickening, pericholecystic fluid, or cholelithiasis. No ductal dilatation is seen. **A-C,** Sagittal gallbladder. **D,** Transverse gallbladder. **E,** Transverse common bile duct, hepatic artery, and portal vein.

(Figure 26-5). The mean portal vein measurement is 8.5 mm in children less than 10 years of age and 10 mm in patients 10 to 20 years old. Color Doppler should be used to determine flow direction and patency.

PATHOLOGY

Neonatal Jaundice

During the first few weeks of life, many neonates experience transient jaundice. The cause of persistent jaundice in the neonate may be difficult to define because clinical and laboratory features may be similar in hepatocellular and obstructive jaundice. If bile obstruction, biliary atresia, or metabolic diseases are to be treated early before cirrhosis occurs, then diagnosis must be made

soon after delivery. Jaundice may be caused by either extrahepatic or intrahepatic obstruction to bile flow. The extrahepatic obstruction in the neonate includes conditions such as choledochal cyst, biliary atresia, or spontaneous perforation of the bile ducts. The intrahepatic causes of neonatal jaundice include hepatitis and metabolic disease. Systemic diseases that cause cholestasis include heart failure, shock, sepsis, neonatal lupus, histiocytosis, and severe hemolytic disease.

Obstructive and nonobstructive jaundice may be differentiated with sonographic evaluation. Unconjugated hyperbilirubinemia occurs in approximately 60% of normal term infants and in 80% of preterm infants. If the neonate has jaundice that persists beyond 2 weeks after delivery, sonography may be ordered to differentiate among the three most common causes for jaundice:

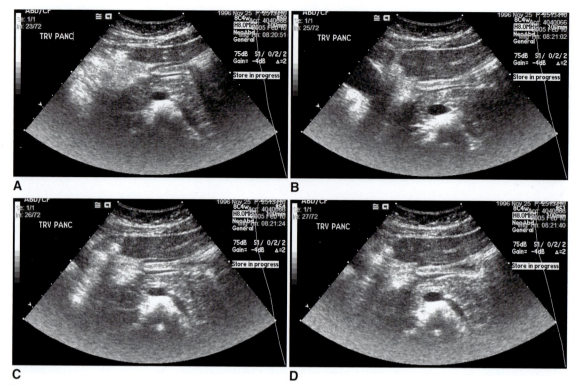

FIGURE 26-3 A-D, Normal pediatric pancreas seen in transverse plane. Evaluation of the pancreas is unremarkable without evidence of focal mass.

TABLE 26-1 | **Normal Dimensions of the Pancreas as a Function of Age**

Patient Age	Patients (N)	Maximum Anteroposterior Dimensions of Pancreas (cm ±1 Standard Deviation)		
		Head	Body	Tail
<1 mo	15	1.0 ± 0.4	0.6 ± 0.2	1.0 ± 0.4
1 mo–1 yr	23	1.5 ± 0.5	0.8 ± 0.3	1.2 ± 0.4
1–5 yr	49	1.7 ± 0.3	1.0 ± 0.2	1.8 ± 0.4
5–10 yr	69	1.6 ± 0.4	1.0 ± 0.3	1.8 ± 0.4
10–19 yr	117	2.0 ± 0.5	1.1 ± 0.3	2.0 ± 0.4

Data from Siegel MJ, Martin KW, Worthington JL: Normal and abnormal pancreas in children: US studies, *Radiology* 165:15-18, 1987.

hepatitis, biliary atresia, and choledochal cyst. With each of these conditions, the liver appears coarse and echogenic on ultrasound; various other conditions (e.g., hepatic inflammatory, obstructive, and metabolic processes) have a similar sonographic appearance. Other studies, such as hepatic **scintigraphy** or liver biopsy, may be necessary to narrow the differential considerations further. Ultrasound is useful in demonstrating the gallbladder with **inspissated** bile and biliary duct stones. Jaundice in infants and children may be due to cirrhosis, benign strictures, and neoplastic processes.

In an infant who has jaundice beyond the 2-week postdelivery date, a number of differentials are possible. In these patients, clinical and laboratory workup is necessary to identify the underlying infectious, metabolic, or structural causes of jaundice. Laboratory workup may include liver function tests, evaluation for hepatitis B

antigen, TORCH (to rule out maternal infections), workup for sepsis, metabolic screening, and sweat test. See Table 26-2 for clinical findings, sonographic findings, and differential considerations for the diseases and conditions discussed here.

Causes and Diagnosis of Neonatal Jaundice. The three most common causes of jaundice in the neonatal period are hepatitis, biliary atresia, and choledochal cyst.

Neonatal Hepatitis. Neonatal hepatitis is an infection of the liver that occurs within the first 3 months of birth. There are a number of causes of neonatal hepatitis, including infections, metabolic disorders, familial recurrent cholestasis, metabolism errors, or idiopathic causes. The infection reaches the liver through the placenta, via the vagina from infected maternal secretions, or through catheters or blood transfusions. Transplacental infection occurs most readily during the third

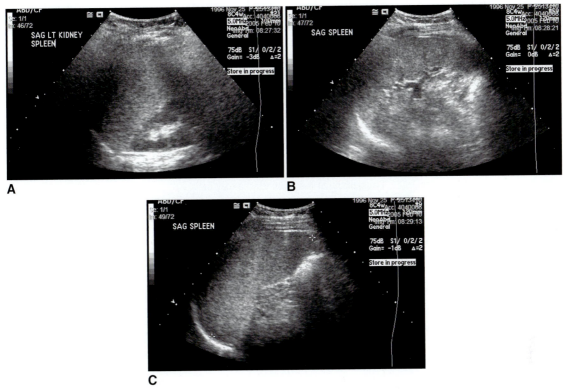

FIGURE 26-4 Normal pediatric spleen. The spleen is normal in size, contour with echogenicity measuring 10.9 cm in greatest pole-to-pole diameter. No focal masses are seen. **A,** Sagittal spleen and left kidney. **B,** Sagittal spleen with hilum. **C,** Sagittal spleen with measurement of the long axis.

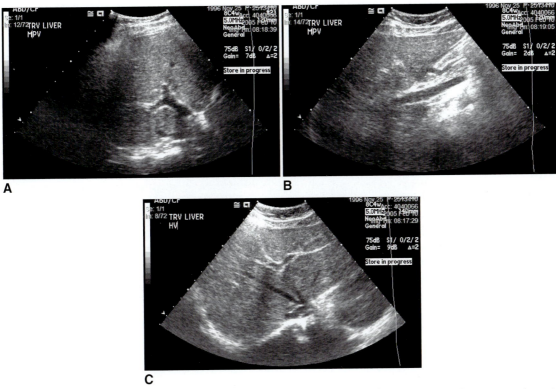

FIGURE 26-5 Normal pediatric portal vein. The portal vein is normal in size with normal flow patterns. **A,** Transverse main portal vein/right portal vein. **B,** Transverse main portal vein. **C,** Transverse left portal vein.

TABLE 26-2	Pediatric Abdominal Findings	
Clinical Findings	**Sonographic Findings**	**Differential Considerations**
Neonatal Hepatitis		
Hepatomegaly	Liver normal or enlarged	
Jaundice when obstruction is present	Liver parenchyma echogenic with decreased vascularization of peripheral portal venous structures	
	When severe, gallbladder may be small in size	
Biliary Atresia		
Persistent jaundice	Liver may be enlarged	
Acholic stools	Echogenicity of liver parenchyma may be normal or increased with slight decrease in visualization of portal structures	
Dark urine	Intrahepatic ducts not dilated	
Distended abdomen	Polysplenia may be present	
Choledochal Cyst		
Jaundice	Fusiform dilatation of the common bile duct with associated intrahepatic ductal dilatation	Duplicated gallbladder
Pain		Liver cyst
Palpable mass may be present	Multiple hypoechoic lesions in liver	Fluid in duodenum
Hemangioendothelioma	Hepatomegaly	Adenoma
First six months of life	Tumor is heterogeneous or isoechoic with cystic components	Focal nodular hyperplasia
Rapid growing benign tumor		Cirrhosis—regenerating nodules
Hepatomegaly	Calcification may be present	Hepatoblastoma
Congestive heart failure	Well circumscribed to poorly marginated	Biliary rhabdoma/sarcoma
Cutaneous hemangioma	Doppler may show AV shunt	Lymphoma
Serum alpha-fetoprotein level may be elevated		Metastasis
Hepatoblastoma		
Most common malignant tumor	Hepatomegaly	Adenoma
<5 years of age	Calcification may occur	Focal nodular hyperplasia
Palpable abdominal mass	Solitary heterogeneous mass	Cirrhosis—regenerating nodules
Elevated serum alpha-fetoprotein levels	Area around mass is hyperechoic	Hemangioendothelioma
Fever	Portal vein thrombosis	Biliary rhabdoma/sarcoma
Pain	Doppler shows high-velocity, low-resistance flow	Lymphoma
		Metastasis
Hypertrophic Pyloric Stenosis		
Male infants	Distended stomach	Pseudoechogenic muscle secondary to beam angulation
Projectile vomiting	Hypertrophied pyloric muscle with a canal >16 mm	Antropyloric canal posteriorly oriented
Dehydration and weight loss	Pyloric wall muscle >3.5 mm	Pylorospasm with minimal muscular hypertrophy
		Prostaglandin-induced HPS
Appendicitis		
RLQ pain	Noncompressible appendix	Meckel's diverticulum
Nausea, vomiting	Diameter >6 mm	Pelvic mass
Increased WBC	Rebound pain	Mesenteric adenitis
Fever		
Intussusception		
Colicky abdominal pain	Alternating hypoechoic and hyperechoic rings surrounding an echogenic center ("target sign")	Intestinal wall thickening
Vomiting		Inflammatory bowel
Bloody stools	Free peritoneal fluid	Colitis
Abdominal mass		Perforated appendix
		Viral disease
		Lymphoma
		Benign tumors

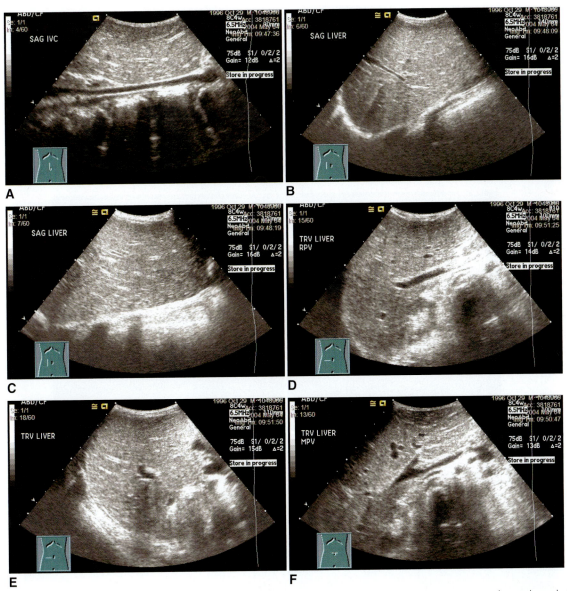

FIGURE 26-6 Liver size and texture should be evaluated in a patient with hepatitis. The liver may appear normal or enlarged. **A,** Sagittal liver/aorta. **B,** Sagittal liver/inferior vena cava. **C,** Sagittal liver. **D,** Transverse liver/right kidney. **E,** Transverse liver. **F,** Transverse liver.

trimester of pregnancy; the most common agents include syphilis, toxoplasma, rubella, and cytomegalovirus (CMV). Bacterial hepatitis is most commonly secondary to an upward spread of organisms from the vagina, infecting endometrium, placenta, and amniotic fluid. During delivery, direct contact with the viruses of herpes, CMV, human immunodeficiency virus (HIV), and *Listeria* may lead to hepatitis. Blood transfusions may contain the hepatitis virus, Epstein-Barr virus, or HIV. In addition, bacterial hepatitis or abscess formation may be obtained from an umbilical vein catheter after delivery.

▶ **Sonographic Findings.** Liver may be normal sized or enlarged (Figure 26-6). The parenchyma pattern is echogenic with decreased visualization of the peripheral portal venous structures. The biliary ducts and gallbladder are not enlarged. If the hepatocellular dysfunction is

severe, the gallbladder may be small in size because of the decreased volume of bile. The differential of neonatal hepatitis and biliary atresia may be difficult when the gallbladder is small; therefore, nuclear scintigraphy will allow visualization of the biliary function.

Biliary Atresia. Biliary atresia is the narrowing or underdevelopment of the biliary ductal system. This serious disease is seen more commonly in males and may result from inflammation of the hepatobiliary system. Biliary atresia may affect the intrahepatic or extrahepatic ducts and may or may not involve the gallbladder, although the latter is the most common form with absence of the gallbladder.

The clinical features of biliary atresia in the neonate include persistent jaundice, **acholic** stools, dark urine, and distended abdomen from hepatomegaly. Early

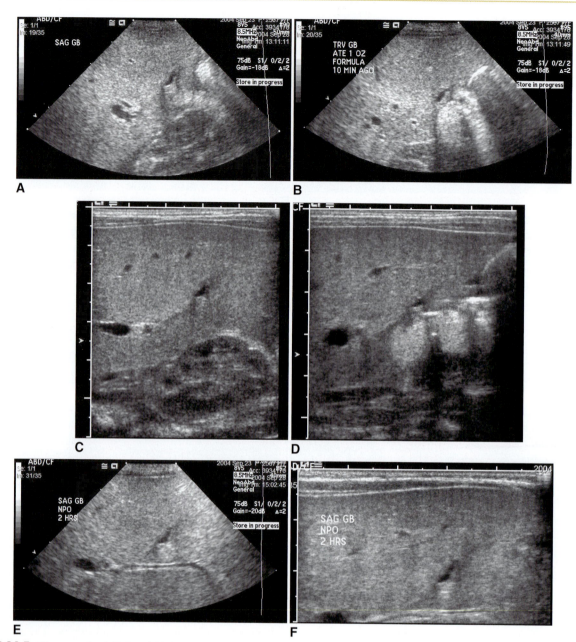

FIGURE 26-7 Biliary atresia. A 5-day-old infant with direct hyperbilirubinemia of unknown origin with liver congestion, inflammation, and ductal blockage. The liver is enlarged with a fairly homogeneous appearance. The neonate had eaten just before the study and the gallbladder was contracted and measured less than 1 cm. The patient was scanned after 2 hours and the gallbladder did not change in appearance. The common bile duct was not identified. **A,** Sagittal gallbladder. **B,** Transverse gallbladder after 1 oz formula. **C,** Sagittal gallbladder. **D,** Sagittal gallbladder. **E,** Sagittal gallbladder; NPO for 2 hours. **F,** Sagittal gallbladder; NPO for 2 hours.

surgical intervention may lead to the prevention of serious complications, which include cirrhosis, liver failure, and subsequent death.

Sonographic Findings. Sonographic findings in a neonate with biliary atresia may vary depending on the type and the severity of the disease (Figure 26-7). The liver size may be normal or enlarged. The echogenicity of the liver parenchyma may be normal or increased with slight decrease in visualization of the peripheral portal venous vasculature (indicative of fibrosis). The intrahepatic ducts are not dilated, although a remnant duct may

be identified with some types of atresia. A small triangular structure may be seen superior to the porta hepatis, which is a hypoplastic remnant of the biliary structure.

A normal sized gallbladder may be seen when the **atretic** common bile duct is distal to the insertion of the cystic duct. The finding of a small (less than 1.5 cm) gallbladder is nonspecific and may be seen with either hepatitis or biliary atresia. A change in the gallbladder size after a milk feeding suggests patency of the common hepatic and common bile ducts and is seen only with neonatal hepatitis.

The presence of polysplenia should also be made if the suspicion is biliary atresia because there is a high association of this abnormality. The abdomen should be examined for end-stage liver disease (i.e., ascites, hepatofugal flow, and collateral venous channels).

Choledochal Cyst. A **choledochal cyst** is an abnormal cystic dilation of the biliary tree, which most frequently affects the common bile duct. There are five types of choledochal cysts, fusiform dilation of the common bile duct (CBD) being the most common:

1. Fusiform dilation of the CBD
2. One or more diverticula of the CBD
3. Dilation of the intraduodenal portion of the CBD (choledochocele)
4. Dilation of the intrahepatic and extrahepatic ducts
5. Caroli's disease with dilation of intrahepatic ducts

The patient clinically presents with jaundice and pain. A palpable mass may be felt in the right upper quadrant. Sonography is used to differentiate the presence or absence of a gallbladder, dilation of the ductal system, and the presence or absence of a mass (Figure 26-8). When a choledochal cyst is present, there is usually fusiform dilation of the common bile duct with associated intrahepatic ductal dilation.

Causes and Diagnosis of Pediatric Jaundice. There are several causes of jaundice in the pediatric patient, including hepatocellular disease, hepatic neoplasms, cholelithiasis and choledocholithiasis, and cirrhosis. Only hepatitic neoplasms will be presented. The reader is referred to Chapters 10 and 11 for further discussion of the other abnormalities.

Liver Tumors

The two most common neoplasms in the pediatric population are the hemangioendothelioma and the hepatoblastoma.

Benign Liver Tumors. Approximately 40% of the liver tumors in children are benign, with hemangioma the most common. Mesenchymal hamartomas, adenomas, and focal nodular hyperplasia make up about half of benign liver tumors.

Hemangioma. This tumor is a vascular, mesenchymal mass characterized by active endothelial growth that may cause arteriovenous shunting, which, in turn, causes high-output heart failure in the infant (hemangioendothelioma). The vessel growth slows down as the tumor matures, but the existing vessels may form "lakes" within the lesion with little blood flow. The sonographic pattern is similar to that found in the adult.

Infantile Hemangioendothelioma. Infantile hepatic hemangioendothelioma is the most common benign vascular liver tumor of early childhood, occurring usually within the first six months of life (Figure 26-9). The mass is usually diagnosed in the first months of life as the mass grows rapidly, causing abdominal distention.

The clinical presentation for infants with hemangioendothelioma is hepatomegaly, which may be accompanied by congestive heart failure and cutaneous hemangioma. The serum alpha-fetoprotein level may be elevated. This benign tumor usually spontaneously regresses by 12 to 18 months of age.

🔖 **Sonographic Findings.** The most common sonographic appearance of hemangioendothelioma is that of multiple hypoechoic lesions and hepatomegaly. The tumor is usually heterogeneous or isoechoic and contains cystic components from the vascular-stroma structure (Figure 26-10). Speckled areas of calcification may be seen within the mass. The tumor may be well circumscribed or poorly marginated. The mass may be solitary or multicentric. Color Doppler shows high flow in the dilated vascular spaces and may be used to show the arteriovenous shunting that accompanies this lesion (Figure 26-11). The aortic caliper decreases in size inferior to the origin of the celiac artery. When arteriovenous shunting is severe, the celiac axis, hepatic artery, and veins are dilated and the infraceliac aorta is small.

Mesenchymal Hamartoma. This is a rare tumor in the asymptomatic infant under 2 years. The tumor has multiseptate cystic masses derived from periportal mesenchyma.

Adenoma. This tumor is not commonly seen in the infant unless liver disease is present (i.e., glycogen storage disease). Lab values will find the serum α-fetoprotein levels are normal. The sonographic appearance ranges from hyperechoic to hypoechoic and is nonspecific.

Malignant Liver Tumors. The distinction of the benign from malignant mass with sonography is not possible; only histologic diagnosis is definitive. However, the clinical history, laboratory results, and sonographic findings may provide a differential for the clinician. The two most common malignant tumors in childhood are the hepatoblastoma and hepatocellular carcinoma. The undifferentiated sarcoma and biliary rhabdomyosarcoma are rare. Metastases to the liver may arise from **neuroblastoma,** Wilms' tumor, leukemia, or lymphoma.

Hepatoblastoma. Hepatoblastoma is the most common primary malignant disease of the liver and occurs most frequently in children under 5 years of age, with the majority occurring in children under 2 years of age. The tumor is the third most common abdominal malignancy in children after **nephroblastoma (Wilms' tumor).** This tumor is sometimes considered the infantile form of hepatocellular carcinoma. The tumor may be familial. Hepatoblastoma has been associated with **Beckwith-Wiedemann syndrome, hemihypertrophy,** familial adenomatous polyposis, and precocious puberty.

Pathologically the tumor is single, solid, large, or mixed echogenicity, and poorly marginated, with small cysts and rounded or irregularly shaped deposits of calcium. The tumor may show areas of necrosis,

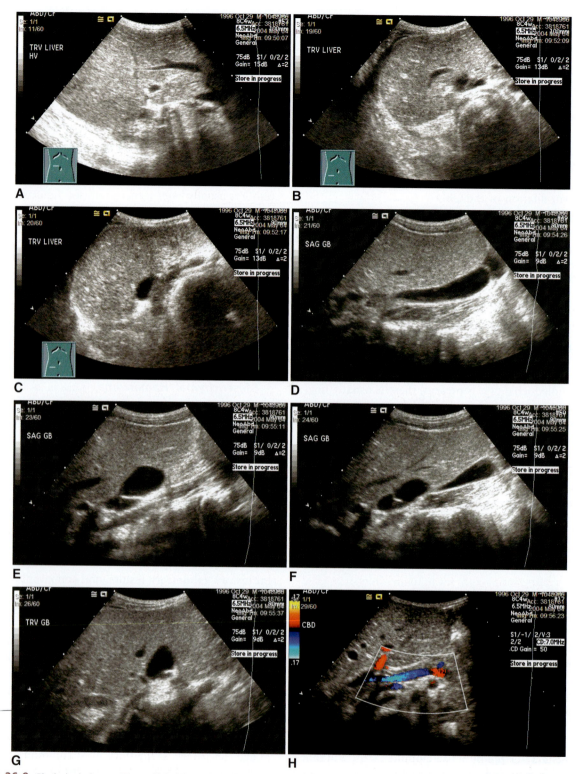

FIGURE 26-8 Choledochal cyst. The gallbladder is folded upon itself without evidence of gallstones or wall thickening. Adjacent to the gallbladder, to the right and extending posteriorly, is a thin-walled fluid collection, which measures 2 to 3 cm. The mass is separate from the gallbladder and does not demonstrate flow. It may represent choledochal cyst (type II) or less likely a duplicated gallbladder. **A,** Transverse liver/hepatic veins. **B,** Transverse liver with two cystic areas. **C,** Transverse liver. **D,** Sagittal gallbladder. **E,** Sagittal gallbladder with fold or separate cystic mass. **F,** Two cystic structures in area of gallbladder. **G,** Transverse gallbladder. **H,** Color shows common bile duct separate from vascular structures.

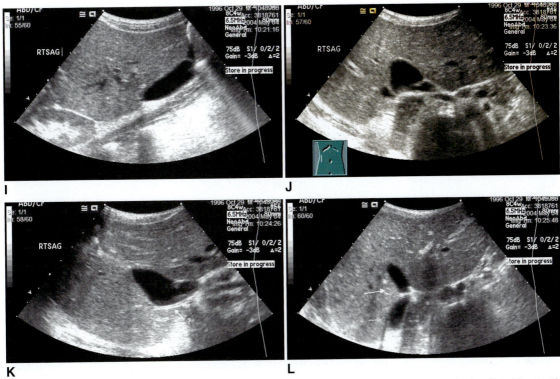

FIGURE 26-8, cont'd   **I,** Right sagittal gallbladder. **J,** Right sagittal gallbladder with fold. **K,** Right sagittal gallbladder. **L,** Right sagittal gallbladder shows two separate cystic structures *(arrows).*

hemorrhage, and calcification (Figure 26-12). It usually does not show diffuse infiltration; the remaining liver may be normal. The intrahepatic vessels are displaced or amputated by the mass. Color Doppler is useful to detect high-velocity flow in the malignant neovasculature.

Clinical findings include a palpable abdominal mass and an elevated serum alpha-fetoprotein level. Patients may be symptomatic with fever, pain, anorexia, and subsequent weight loss. The prognosis of the tumor is dependent on the resectability of the mass.

▶ **Sonographic Findings.** The sonographic appearance of the hepatoblastoma shows hepatomegaly with a solitary mass that may show some calcification (Figure 26-13). The heterogeneous mass is predominantly solid; however, there may be hypoechoic areas with necrosis or hemorrhage. The fleshy areas around the mass are often mildly hyperechoic. It becomes important to identify the hepatic vessels and hepatic veins. Portal vein thrombosis may be present. The Doppler flow pattern in the lesion shows a high-velocity, low-resistant flow pattern.

Hepatocellular Carcinoma. Hepatocellular carcinoma is the second most common malignant tumor in childhood. Half of the children have preexisting liver disease. The liver is a multicentric solid mass, usually without calcification and variable echogenicity on sonography. Color Doppler should be used to evaluate the portal venous structures to look for thrombus or tumor invasion.

Common Surgical Conditions

The pediatric patient may appear in the general ultrasound lab on an emergent basis for extreme abdominal pain with three common conditions: hypertrophic pyloric stenosis, appendicitis, and intussusception.

Hypertrophic Pyloric Stenosis. The **pyloric canal** is located between the stomach and duodenum. In some infants, the pyloric muscle can become hypertrophied, resulting in significantly delayed gastric emptying. Hypertrophy of the circular muscle of the pylorus is an acquired condition that narrows the pyloric canal (Figure 26-14). The pyloric canal itself is not intrinsically stenotic or narrowed, but it functions as if it were as a result of the abnormally thickened surrounding muscle.

Hypertrophic pyloric stenosis (HPS) appears most commonly in male infants between 2 and 6 weeks of age. Rarely, it becomes apparent at birth or as late as 5 months of age. The incidence of HPS is approximately 3 in 1000 neonates. Bile-free vomiting in an otherwise healthy infant is the most frequent clinical sign. As the pyloric muscle thickens and elongates, the stomach outlet obstruction increases and vomiting is more constant and projectile. Dehydration and weight loss may ensue. Peristaltic waves and reverse peristaltic waves crossing the upper abdomen may be observed during or after feeding as the stomach attempts to force its contents through the abnormal canal (**projectile vomiting**).

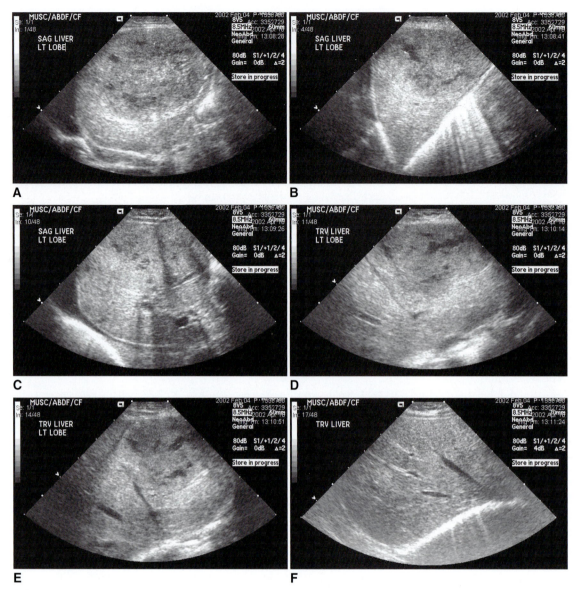

FIGURE 26-9 Infantile hemangioma. A 2-month-old infant with a liver hemangioma shows a well-circumscribed heterogeneous mass with focal areas of calcium in the left lobe of the liver. There is predominant flow around the mass. There were normal wave forms in both the main portal vein and the left hepatic artery. **A,** Sagittal left lobe liver with large heterogeneous mass. **B,** Sagittal left lobe liver with mass. **C,** Sagittal liver with mass; right pleural effusion superior to diaphragm. **D,** Transverse left lobe of liver with large mass. **E,** Transverse left lobe of liver with mass. **F,** Transverse liver inferior to the mass.

In these infants, palpation of an olive-shaped mass in the right upper quadrant is diagnostic and is treated by surgical pyloromyotomy. In infants with a suggestive history or an equivocal physical examination, diagnostic imaging is required to provide direct visualization of the pyloric muscle (Figure 26-15).

In pediatric imaging departments and in other ultrasound departments where there is appropriate expertise, sonography is the imaging method of choice to establish the diagnosis of HPS. If HPS is not a primary diagnostic consideration or if the sonogram is not diagnostic, conventional contrast radiography of the upper gastrointestinal tract is necessary to assess for other potential causes of vomiting (e.g., gastrointestinal reflux, antral web,

pylorospasm, hiatal hernia, and malrotation of the bowel) (Figure 26-16).

The neonate with projectile vomiting frequently is sent directly from the physician's office or the hospital emergency room. If the stomach is empty and HPS is not readily apparent, an oral feeding (i.e., glucose water or Pedialyte) is given to facilitate comprehensive visualization of the pyloric area (Figure 26-17). Conversely, an overly distended stomach can displace the pyloric muscle posteriorly, making sonographic delineation virtually impossible (Figure 26-18). In this instance, aspiration of gastric contents via a nasogastric tube may be required.

The infant is usually examined first in the supine and then in the right lateral decubitus position, which aids

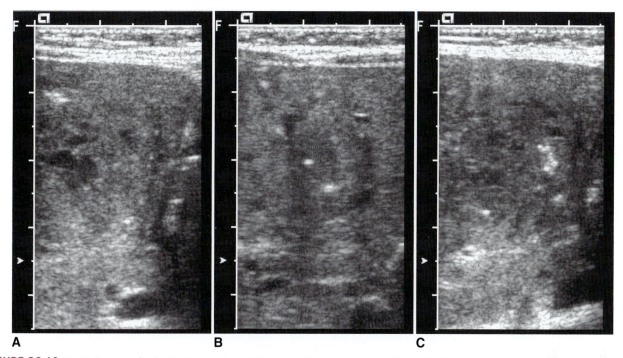

A   **B**   **C**

FIGURE 26-10 Sagittal views of infantile hemangioma. The mass often shows areas of calcification that appear echogenic on sonography. **A-C,** Mass with areas of calcification.

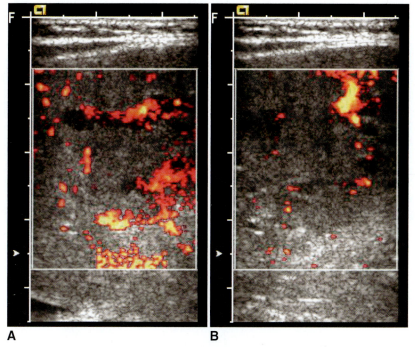

A   **B**

FIGURE 26-11 Infantile hemangioma. Color Doppler helps to define the vascularity of the mass and the relationship of the portal and hepatic veins to the mass lesion. **A,** Power Doppler shows increased vascularity within the mass. **B,** Power Doppler over the mass.

Continued

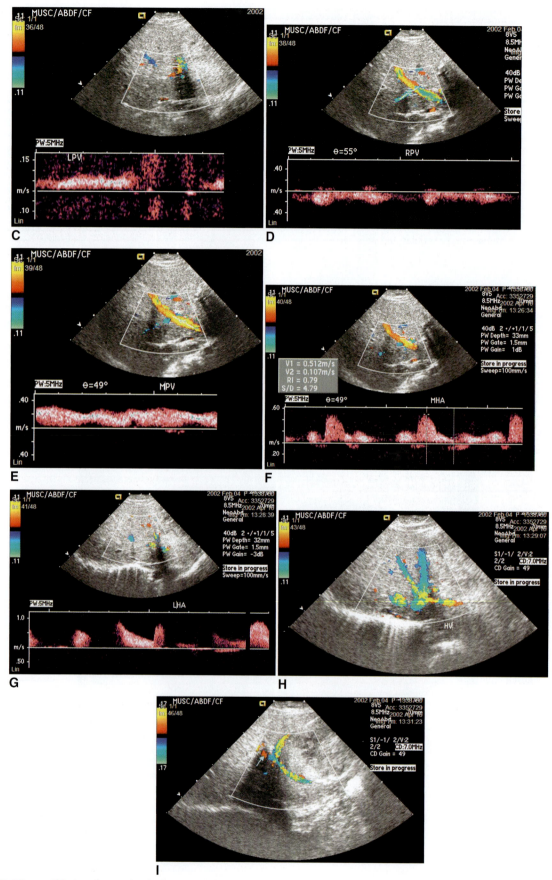

FIGURE 26-11, cont'd **C,** Left portal vein flow. **D,** Right portal vein flow. **E,** Main portal vein flow. **F,** Right hepatic artery flow. **G,** Left hepatic artery flow. **H,** Hepatic venous flow. **I,** Color flow in portal vein around the mass.

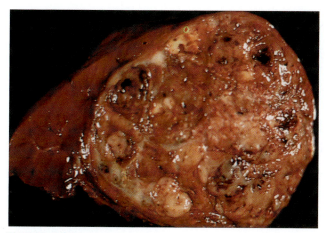

FIGURE 26-12 Hepatoblastoma. Lobular tumor with areas of necrosis.

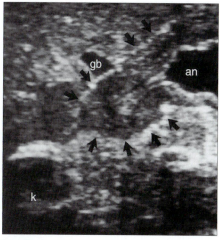

FIGURE 26-15 Transverse image of the right upper quadrant using the liver as an acoustic window in a 5-week-old boy with hypertrophic pyloric stenosis shows a longitudinal view of an elongated thickened pyloric muscle (arrows). The antrum (an) is filled with fluid. The gallbladder (gb) is anterior to the pyloric muscle, whereas the right kidney (k) is posterior and lateral.

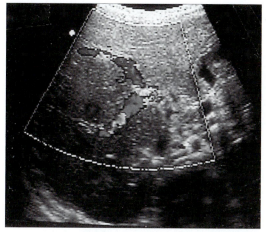

FIGURE 26-13 Hepatoblastoma. The portal veins are displaced by the large mass.

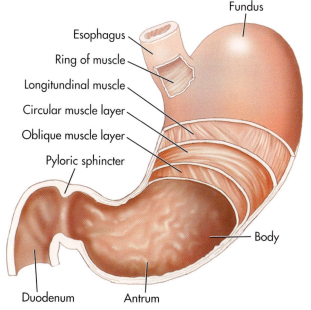

FIGURE 26-14 Diagram of hypertrophic pyloric stenosis. The pylorus muscle (sphincter) connects the antrum of the stomach with the duodenum of the small intestine.

in the visualization of the pylorus. A preliminary survey of the abdomen is performed to exclude abnormalities such as hydronephrosis or adrenal hemorrhage. Real-time imaging is then performed using a high-frequency linear array transducer (5 to 12 MHz). Longitudinal images of the pyloric muscle are obtained by placing the transducer transversely across the right upper quadrant, just below the level of the xiphoid process. The transducer is then rotated obliquely until the pyloric muscle is visualized in its long axis (Figure 26-19). The muscle is thickened and elongated and extends into the antrum; this appearance has been called the "cervix" sign. If fluid passes through the pyloric canal, it is often seen as a "double-track" in the crevices of the compressed mucosa. Other secondary signs include exaggerated gastric peristalsis and delayed gastric emptying.

Transverse short-axis images of the pyloric muscle are obtained from the right coronal plane. The gallbladder is initially identified, after which the transducer is angled medially until the "bull's eye" or "target" appearance of the hypertrophied pyloric muscle and echogenic central canal is noted (Figure 26-20). The pyloric muscle frequently has a nonuniform echo pattern, with the near and far fields appearing more echogenic.

If the diagnosis has not been established, the patient is then placed in a right lateral decubitus position and the transducer placed transversely in the right upper quadrant. This allows maximum visualization of the stomach and pyloric canal and is most advantageous for documenting the transit of gastric contents into the duodenum. The sonographer should determine the location of the superior mesenteric artery and vein to assess for malrotation, especially in the case of patients with negative findings of HPS.

FIGURE 26-16 A, Transverse image of the right upper quadrant using the liver as an acoustic window in a 4-week-old boy with projectile vomiting. There was to-and-fro peristalsis in the fluid-filled duodenal bulb *(db)* and descending duodenum *(dd)*. The descending duodenum tapered abruptly *(arrows)* and could not be traced distally. The right kidney *(k)* is posterior to the descending duodenum. A hypertrophied pyloric muscle was not identified. **B,** Right lateral view from a barium examination in the same patient shows the stomach, antrum *(an)*, duodenal bulb *(db)*, and descending duodenum *(dd)*. The descending duodenum tapers abruptly *(arrows)* and then spirals inferiorly. The barium examination delineates the surgically emergent malrotation, which could not be identified on the sonogram.

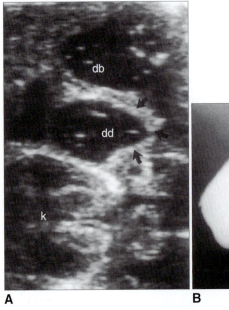

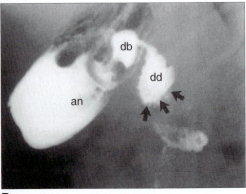

A   **B**

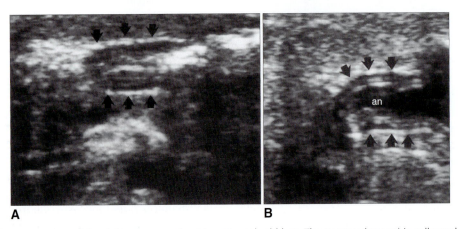

A   **B**

FIGURE 26-17 A, Transverse view of the right upper quadrant in a 5-week-old boy. The antrum *(arrows)* is collapsed and contains a linear echogenic centrum representing the interface between the lumen and mucosa. **B,** Transverse view of the right upper quadrant shows the antrum *(arrows)* in the same patient after administration of glucose water by bottle. The antrum *(an)* is now filled with fluid and is easy to differentiate from a hypertrophied pyloric muscle.

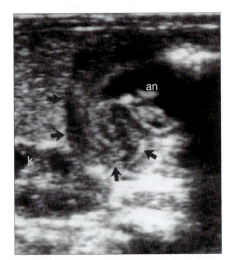

FIGURE 26-18 Transverse view of the right upper quadrant in a 5-week-old boy with hypertrophic pyloric stenosis. The fluid-distended antrum *(an)* has pushed the elongated pyloric muscle *(arrows)* posteriorly, precluding accurate measurement of the length of the pyloric canal. The kidney *(k)* is lateral and slightly posterior to the pyloric muscle.

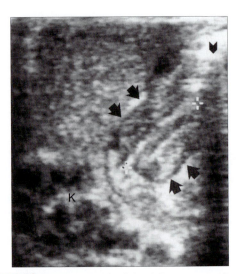

FIGURE 26-19 Transverse view of the right upper quadrant shows the longitudinal extent of the hypertrophied pyloric muscle *(arrows)*. The calipers measure the length of the pyloric muscle, which is 20 mm. The kidney *(K)* is posterior and lateral to the pyloric muscle. Gas *(arrowhead)* in the antrum is causing a reverberation artifact.

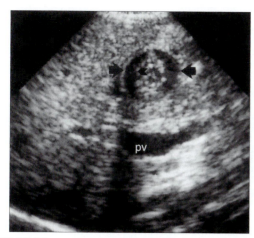

FIGURE 26-20 Coronal view of the right upper quadrant shows the hypertrophied pyloric muscle in transverse section. The diameter of the muscle *(arrows)* is measured from the outer borders. The muscle thickness *(left arrow to arrowhead)* is measured from the outer border to the mucosal-muscle interface. The portal vein *(pv)* is posterior to the pyloric muscle in this plane.

If there is not enough residual gastric fluid present, 60 to 120 ml of water may be administered either through a bottle or through a nasogastric tube. The stomach should not be overfilled because this displaces the pylorus posteriorly, making visualization more difficult.

Measurements. Sonographic measurement of pyloric muscle thickness enables the diagnosis of HPS. Pyloric muscle measurements can be made in both the short- and the long-axis planes. If the image is oblique, measurements will be overestimated. A muscle thickness of 3.5 mm or greater on the long-axis view, a channel length of 17 mm or greater, and a pyloric muscle length of 20 mm or greater are reliable indicators of HPS.

Individual muscle wall thickness, total diameter, and length of the pyloric canal are measured. The thickness is measured from the periphery of the hypoechoic muscle to its junction with the echogenic central canal. Diameter is measured between the peripheral margins of the hypoechoic muscle layer. Length is measured from the proximal to the distal extremes of the echogenic central canal.

Sonographic Findings. The sonographic diagnosis of HPS depends on the following findings: (1) visualization of a hypertrophied pyloric muscle with a canal measuring 17 mm or greater, (2) individual pyloric muscle wall thickness of 3.5 mm or greater, or (3) a pyloric muscle length of 20 mm or greater. An additional significant finding is the presence of active antegrade and reverse gastric peristalsis.

The differential considerations include pylorospasm, gastrointestinal reflux, and duodenal obstruction caused by stenosis or malrotation with bands or volvulus.

Appendicitis. After gastroenteritis, **appendicitis** is the most common acute abdominal inflammatory process in children. Appendicitis occurs when the appendiceal lumen becomes obstructed and subsequently infected. In infants and young children, the progression of acute appendicitis to perforation is more rapid than in older children and adults, sometimes occurring within 6 to 12 hours. Classic physical and laboratory findings may be absent or confusing, making the diagnosis difficult.

Right lower quadrant pain and vomiting are a common clinical presentation. In addition to appendicitis, diagnostic considerations include enteritis, inflammatory bowel disease, and lymphoma. In girls the differential broadens to include gynecologic processes, such as ovarian cysts and neoplasms and ovarian torsion.

Sonography has proven to be very accurate in confirming appendicitis. As in virtually all conditions, a survey examination of the abdomen is first performed to assess the upper abdomen and the kidneys and bladder. In girls the adnexal areas should be examined with the patient having a distended urinary bladder. The bladder should then be emptied to allow gradual graded compression over the area of the appendix with the linear or curved array transducer. The right flank and right lower quadrant are reexamined using a 5 to 12 MHz linear array transducer. The transducer is moved slowly over the abdomen using the graded compression technique. This technique allows the sonographer to carefully apply gentle pressure with the transducer over the region of the appendix. Be sure to explain to the patient what you are going to do before beginning the compression technique. This technique enables the sonographer to visualize the appendix by displacing adjacent bowel loops. The appendix is usually seen anterior and medial to the psoas muscle and lateral to the iliac vessels.

Nonvisualization of the appendix may occur for multiple reasons and is not a definite indication of a normal appendix. Appendiceal nonvisualization may result from any of the following: (1) being obscured by overlying bowel; (2) retrocecal position of the appendix; (3) overdistention or nondistention of the urinary bladder, which alters the position of the appendix and overlying bowel; or (4) lack of sonographer experience. Changing the patient's position and emptying or filling the urinary bladder may facilitate visualization of both the normal and abnormal appendix.

The normal appendix appears as a blind-ending, long, tubular structure in the longitudinal plane and as a bull's-eye in the transverse plane.

Sonographic Findings. Peristalsis is not seen in the appendix, allowing differentiation of normal appendix and small bowel. The appendix may be tortuous and therefore difficult to visualize in its entirety. The walls are not thickened, and the normal appendix compresses easily.

Sonographically the acutely inflamed appendix is noncompressible (Figure 26-21). The appendix is measured in the transverse plane, across the short axis, using the maximum diameter. An outer diameter greater than 6 mm with compression is consistent with appendicitis

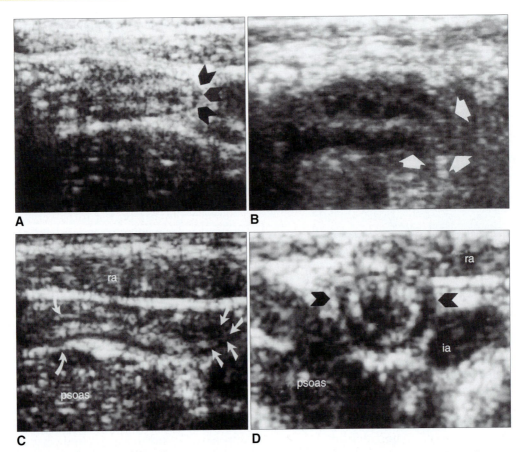

FIGURE 26-21 **A,** Longitudinal view of an inflamed appendix using the graded compression technique. The bulbous tip *(arrowheads)* is clearly defined. **B,** Longitudinal view of a fluid-filled inflamed appendix in a different child. The bulbous tip *(arrows)* is less easily seen. **C,** Longitudinal image of the right lower quadrant in a boy with appendicitis. The rectus abdominis muscle *(ra)* of the anterior abdominal wall is being compressed with the transducer to delineate the longitudinal extent of the appendix to its blind-ending tip *(arrows)*. The curved arrows demonstrate the alternating hyperechoic and hypoechoic bowel wall layers. The central echogenic band *(top curved arrow)* represents the interface between the lumen and mucosa. The most peripheral echogenic band *(bottom curved arrow)* represents the interface between the peripheral bowel wall muscle layer and the bowel wall covering. **D,** Transverse image of the right lower quadrant in the same patient demonstrates the inflamed appendix *(arrowheads)* in the transverse plane. The iliac artery *(ia)* and vein course parallel to the appendix. They can be differentiated from the bowel by using Doppler imaging or tracing their course in the longitudinal plane.

both in children and adults. An increase in echogenicity has been shown in the surrounding mesentery secondary to the inflammation. Localized pain produced by overlying transducer pressure is an additional finding consistent with appendicitis. Color Doppler is useful to document increased blood flow (hyperemia). Other findings in appendicitis may include free peritoneal fluid or a loculated fluid collection in the lower abdomen. Confirmation of an appendicolith in a symptomatic patient is virtually diagnostic (Figure 26-22). An **appendicolith** is hyperechoic, produces a classic acoustic shadow, may be single or multiple, and may be intraluminal or surrounded by a periappendiceal phlegmon or abscess. The right kidney may at times be hydronephrotic because of ureteral inflammation.

The perforated appendix may or may not be visualized. If decompressed, an abnormally thick bowel wall may be apparent. A localized, well-defined right lower quadrant phlegmon or abscess with or without an appendicolith may be present (Figure 26-23). Free peritoneal

fluid may be the lone abnormal sonographic finding. An abscess far removed from the right lower quadrant is another potential intraabdominal complication of an appendiceal perforation.

Enlarged lymph nodes may be a pitfall in diagnosing appendicitis. Patients with mesenteric lymphadenitis may present with prominent lymph nodes and symptoms of appendicitis with flulike symptoms previous to their illness. Color Doppler imaging may help the sonographer to determine the increased flow in the inflamed appendix from the enlarged node.

Intussusception. **Intussusception** is the most common acute abdominal disorder in early childhood. This condition occurs when the bowel prolapses into a more distal bowel and is propelled in an antegrade fashion. Telescoping of bowel in this manner causes obstruction. The ileum may invaginate into a more distal ileum, causing an ileoileal intussusception. If there is further progression through the ileocecal valve, an ileocecal intussusception results.

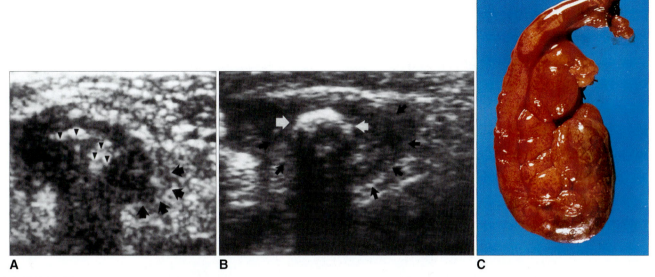

FIGURE 26-22 A, Longitudinal image of an inflamed appendix containing multiple echogenic foci *(arrowheads)* consistent with appendicoliths, which cast acoustic shadows. The blind-ending tip *(arrows)* confirms that the echogenic foci are within the appendix and are not gas moving through the small bowel. **B,** Transverse image of an inflamed appendix in a different patient. There is a solitary appendicolith *(white arrows)* located centrally within the lumen. The hypoechoic periphery *(black arrows)* results from edema. **C,** Gross pathology of acute appendicitis demonstrates inflammation extending to the serosa, which appears hyperemic.

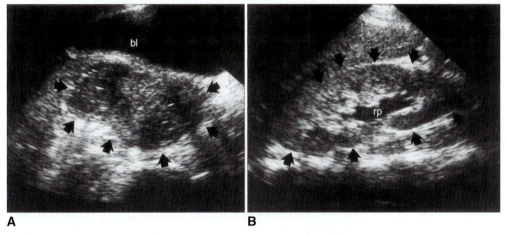

FIGURE 26-23 A, Midline sagittal image in a boy with an appendiceal abscess *(arrows)* posterior to the urinary bladder *(bl)*. The appendiceal abscess appears heterogeneous in echogenicity and is well demarcated from the surrounding bowel, which was actively peristaltic on real-time examination. **B,** Coronal image of the right kidney *(arrows)* in the same patient shows moderate hydronephrosis because of distal ureteral inflammation from the abscess. A fluid-filled right renal pelvis *(rp)* may be a secondary sign of a right lower quadrant or pelvic process.

Prolapse of the ileum into the cecum or beyond produces an ileocolic intussusception. Intussusception is usually seen in children between the ages of 6 months and 2 years. A higher incidence has been reported in males (2:1), along with a seasonal prevalence. Frequently, there is a history of an antecedent upper respiratory tract infection. Associated inflammation of lymphoid tissue in the ileocolic region may act as a lead point for the telescoping phenomenon.

Children may present with colicky abdominal pain, vomiting, and bloody (currant jelly) stools. Abdominal distention or a mass may also be palpable. In patients with

this classic clinical presentation, in whom there are no peritoneal symptoms or fever, preliminary abdominal radiographs followed by a barium or air enema are rapidly undertaken for both diagnostic confirmation and to attempt therapeutic reduction. Failure to reduce an intussusception mandates immediate surgical intervention.

Likewise, surgical intervention is indicated in patients with a classic clinical presentation of intussusception who have developed fever and peritoneal signs. In patients with a more vague clinical presentation, in whom intussusception remains suspect, an ultrasound examination is a helpful diagnostic undertaking.

▨ **Sonographic Findings.** The patient is examined in the supine position. A survey of the entire abdomen is performed, followed by an examination focusing on the bowel using a 5 to 12 MHz linear or curved array transducer.

The sonographic appearance of intussusception is of alternating hypoechoic and hyperechoic rings surrounding an echogenic center as seen in a short-axis view of the involved area. This is known as the **target sign** or **donut** (Figure 26-24). In the long axis view, hypoechoic layers on each side of the echogenic center result in a "pseudokidney" or "sandwich" sign appearance (Figure 26-25). The sonolucent ring is believed to represent the edematous infolded loop of the intussusceptum, whereas the echogenic central area represents its compressed mucosa. Other concentric rings are present resulting

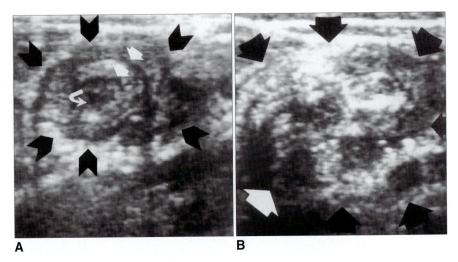

A   B

FIGURE 26-24 A, Transverse image of an intussusception *(arrowheads)* showing a target sign. There are several circumferential layers of increased and decreased echogenicity *(arrows)* because of the telescoping bowel. The lumen *(curved arrow)* contains fluid. **B,** In an image at a more superior level in the same patient, intussusception *(arrows)* is identified. The target sign is present, but instead of being round it is more C-shaped because the bowel loop is coiled on itself.

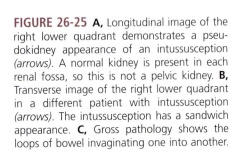

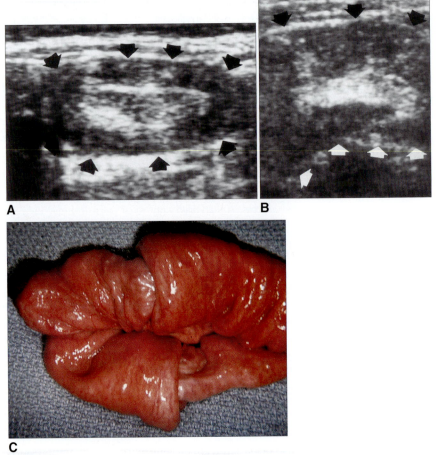

A   B

C

FIGURE 26-25 A, Longitudinal image of the right lower quadrant demonstrates a pseudokidney appearance of an intussusception *(arrows)*. A normal kidney is present in each renal fossa, so this is not a pelvic kidney. **B,** Transverse image of the right lower quadrant in a different patient with intussusception *(arrows)*. The intussusception has a sandwich appearance. **C,** Gross pathology shows the loops of bowel invaginating one into another.

from visualization of additional bowel wall layers within the intussusception. Free peritoneal fluid is not an uncommon finding with uncomplicated intussusception. Color Doppler may help to determine the success of an air reduction enema; if there is good color flow to all areas of the telescoping bowel, the chances are better for a reduction. Poor color Doppler may indicate ischemia to the area of affected bowel.

When an intussusception is documented sonographically, an associated cause, though relatively uncommon, should be sought. A double target sign has been reported as being diagnostic of intussuscepted Meckel's diverticulum. Other causes, such as a small bowel tumor or duplication cyst, may likewise be identified. Consideration of barium or air enema versus surgical intervention is as discussed earlier (Figure 26-26). Intussusception may be reduced with hydrostatic pressure or by air reduction. An edematous ileocecal valve may be seen on fluoroscopy that may mimic a residual intussusception. Sonography may be helpful in distinguishing between persistent intussusception and an edematous ileocecal valve. The edematous valve appears as a small sonolucent rim with an echogenic center. It is distinguishable from intussusception in that its cross-sectional diameter is smaller than that of an intussusception, and it lacks the concentric rings frequently seen in intussusception.

In addition to intussusception, conditions that can produce a target-like sonographic appearance include primary bowel tumors, such as lymphoma, and thickened bowel wall in post–stem cell transplant or bone

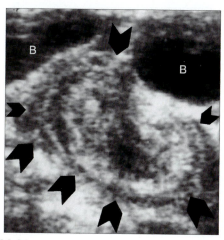

FIGURE 26-26 There are multiple, dilated fluid-filled bowel loops *(B)* located anterior to the intussusception *(arrowheads)*. The intussusception could not be reduced, a frequent occurrence when an ileocolic intussusception is encountered on contrast enema, mandating surgical intervention.

marrow transplant patients and in patients with inflammatory bowel disease.

Other Surgical Conditions. In addition to hyperpyloric stenosis, appendicitis, and intussusception, other conditions that may lead to surgical correction may be less frequently seen in the neonate. These conditions include mesenteric or omental cysts (often large in size), duplication cysts of the bowel, duodenal atresia, and meconium peritonitis. Older children may also present with duplication cysts of the bowel and hematomas of the bowel resulting from trauma.

The Neonatal and Pediatric Kidneys and Adrenal Glands

Sandra L. Hagen-Ansert

Sonography is the diagnostic imaging method of choice when a renal or an adrenal abnormality is suspected in the neonate or pediatric patient. There are numerous indications for renal imaging in the newborn period. One major indication is a renal abnormality detected during prenatal sonography. Some of the conditions or findings in the newborn associated with renal abnormalities are flank masses, abdominal distention, anuria, oliguria, hematuria, sepsis or urinary tract infection, meningomyelocele, **VATER** and **VACTER***L* anomalies, abnormal external genitalia, and prune belly syndrome. Still other indicators include skin tags (usually near the ear and associated with cardiac anomalies) or a two-vessel umbilical cord. These conditions usually indicate the renal study is for screening the kidneys with no particular renal symptoms present.

EXAMINATION PREPARATION

General aspects of the ultrasound examination of the neonate and pediatric patient are described in Chapter 26. Maintaining body temperature in the neonate is very important because small infants can lose a potentially dangerous amount of body heat quickly. Whenever possible, scanning through the portholes of an isolette provides an optimal environment for the premature or otherwise fragile neonate. When the examination is performed outside of the isolette, body heat loss can be minimized by the use of heat lamps and by exposing only the area of the body being interrogated.

Visualization of the urinary bladder, which includes assessment for distal ureteral dilation, is considered an important part of the renal sonographic examination (Figure 27-1). Because of the infant's tendency to urinate spontaneously, scanning is gently initiated over the suprapubic region. If the urinary bladder is not distended at this time or if voiding occurs before adequate detail can be obtained, this area can be examined after imaging of the kidneys and perirenal areas. Refilling of the urinary bladder is usually relatively rapid if the infant is fed or when parenteral fluids are being administered.

Long- and short-axis views of the kidneys and of the perirenal areas are initially obtained by scanning via the flanks to obtain coronal and axial images, via the anterior abdomen for longitudinal and transverse images, or both. When necessary, additional transverse and

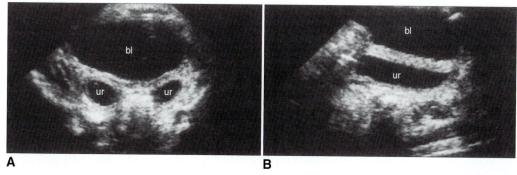

FIGURE 27-1 A, Transverse image of the pelvis in a 2-day-old infant with bilateral primary megaureter (nonobstructive dilation of the distal ureter). The urinary bladder *(bl)* is well distended. Bilateral dilation of the distal ureter *(ur)* is seen posterior to the bladder. **B,** Longitudinal view of the same patient shows the distal ureter *(ur)* entering the urinary bladder *(bl)*.

longitudinal views can be obtained with the infant in a prone position. Renal scanning before and after the infant voids may provide useful information. For example, development of, or increase in, **hydronephrosis** after voiding would suggest high-grade vesicoureteral reflux.

NORMAL ANATOMY AND SONOGRAPHIC FINDINGS

Kidneys

In the second trimester, the kidney develops from small renunculi that are composed of a central large pyramid with a thin peripheral rim of cortex. As the renunculi fuse progressively, their adjoining cortices form a column of Bertin. The former renunculi are at that point called "lobes." Remnants of these lobes with somewhat incomplete fusion, often termed "fetal lobulation," should not be confused with renal abnormalities or scars when imaging the kidney. These pyramids remain large even after birth in comparison with the thin rim of cortex that surrounds them. The glomerular filtration rate is low right after term birth but increases rapidly thereafter. The cortex continues to grow throughout childhood, whereas the pyramids become smaller. The larger amount of cortical fat is not present in the neonate and pediatric patient, thus allowing for clear distinction of the cortical-medullary junction.

The normal kidney in the neonate is characterized by a distinct demarcation of the cortex and medullary pyramids. The **medullary pyramids** are large and hypoechoic and should not be mistaken for dilated calyces or cysts. The surrounding **cortex** is quite thin, with echogenicity essentially similar to or slightly greater than that of normal liver parenchyma (Figure 27-2). Renal cortical echogenicity normally decreases to less than that of liver parenchyma, usually by 4 to 6 months of age.

The pediatric renal anatomy varies with the pediatric patient, depending on the age of the child. The adolescent and teenager have a sonographic renal anatomy similar to adult anatomy. The renal parenchyma consists of a peripheral cortex, the glomeruli, and several extensions to the edge of the renal sinus (column of Bertin). The medulla is more central and adjacent to the calyces. The normal cortex produces low-level, back-scattered echoes.

The medullary pyramids are relatively hypoechoic and arranged around the central, echo-producing renal sinus. The arcuate vessels are seen as intense specular echoes at the corticomedullary junction. The increased cortical echogenicity may result from glomeruli occupying a larger proportion of cortical volume and the location of 20% of the loops of Henle within the cortex as opposed to the medulla. In neonates and infants, the medullary pyramids are prominent and hypoechoic, and corticomedullary definition is accentuated (from a larger medullary volume).

The surrounding cortex is echogenic and thick, with the echogenicity essentially similar to or slightly greater than that of normal liver or splenic parenchyma (see Figure 27-2). Because of a paucity of fat in the renal sinus of the neonate, this area is generally hypoechoic and therefore indistinct. The **arcuate arteries,** which lie at the bases of the medullary pyramids, appear as punctate, intensely echogenic structures.

The contour of the neonatal kidney is usually lobulated from residual fetal lobulations. At the site of this fetal lobulation, a parenchymal triangular defect may be identified in the anterosuperior or inferoposterior aspect of the kidney as the *junctional parenchymal defect.* The normal renal length varies with the age of the infant (Figure 27-3).

Renal anomalies of number include renal agenesis and supernumerary kidney. Anomalies of position, form, and orientation include pelvic kidney, horseshoe kidney, crossed ectopy, and renal duplication. The reader is referred to Chapter 14 for further discussion of these anomalies.

Adrenal Glands

The normal adrenal glands are relatively larger and therefore more easily identified in the neonate than in

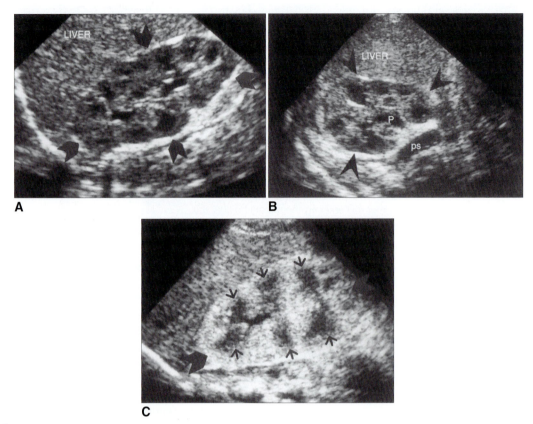

FIGURE 27-2 A, Coronal view of a normal right kidney *(arrowheads)* in a 3-day-old male with a left multicystic dysplastic kidney. The medullary pyramids appear as triangular hypoechoic areas. The cortex has the same echogenicity as the liver. **B,** Transverse view of the same kidney *(arrowheads)*. The hypoechoic psoas muscle *(ps)* is located posteromedial to the kidney. The nondilated renal pelvis *(P)* contains anechoic fluid. **C,** Normal kidney *(arrowheads)* in 13-day-old female. The increased echogenicity of the renal cortex compared with the normal liver parenchyma can be normal. The medullary pyramids appear large and hypoechoic *(arrows)*.

the older infant or young child. Each gland lies immediately superior to the upper pole of the kidney. The left adrenal gland extends slightly more medial than does the right. Sonographically the gland has an inverted "V" or "Y" shape in the longitudinal plane (Figure 27-4, *A*). In the transverse plane, the portion of the gland delineated has a linear or curvilinear outline (Figure 27-4, *B*). The adrenal medulla in the neonate is relatively thin, appearing as a distinctly echogenic stripe, surrounded by the more prominent and less echogenic adrenal cortex. When the kidney is absent or ectopic, the ipsilateral adrenal gland remains in the renal fossa, but as a result it may have an altered configuration (Figure 27-5).

Bladder

The normal urinary bladder is thin-walled in the distended state and should measure less than 3 mm. When empty, the wall thickness increases but remains less than 5 mm. The distal ureters may be seen at the bladder base if the child is well hydrated. The use of color Doppler may aid in the visualization of the distal ureter as it enters the posterior wall of the bladder.

PATHOLOGY OF RENAL AND ADRENAL ENLARGEMENT

The more common causes of renal and adrenal enlargement that can present as a palpable mass in the neonate are presented. Table 27-1 p. 715 lists the clinical and sonographic renal findings and differential considerations for the pathology discussed here.

Hydronephrosis

Hydronephrosis describes the dilation of the urinary collecting system and is a common finding in the younger patient. There are many causes of dilation of the collecting system, the most common being obstruction, reflux, or abnormal muscle development. Sonography is sensitive in detecting small amounts of fluid in the renal pelvis. The sonographer is able to determine the severity of the hydronephrosis, whether the condition is unilateral or bilateral, if the ureters and bladder are dilated, and the status of the renal parenchyma.

Sonographic features found in hydronephrosis include visible renal parenchyma surrounding a central cystic component, small peripheral cysts (dilated calyces) budding off a large central cyst (renal pelvis), and visualization of a dilated ureter. This must be distinguished from the noncommunicating cysts of multicystic dysplastic kidneys.

Ureteropelvic Junction Obstruction. The most common type of obstruction of the upper urinary tract is called **ureteropelvic junction obstruction.** It most often results from intrinsic narrowing or extrinsic vascular compression at the level of the ureteropelvic junction. Bilateral involvement may occur along with a contralateral multicystic dysplastic kidney or vesicoureteral reflux. The obstruction produces proximal dilation of the collecting system; however, the ureter is normal in caliber. There is an increased incidence of abnormalities of the contralateral kidney.

 Sonographic Findings. Sonographically, there is pelvocalyceal dilation without ureteral dilation (Figure 27-6, *A*). When the obstruction is pronounced, the dilated renal pelvis extends inferiorly and medially (Figure 27-6, *B*). If vesicoureteral reflux or primary megaureter is present, the ureter may be dilated. The best way to demonstrate the dilated ureters at the ureteropelvic junction is with a coronal scan plane.

Ureteral Obstruction. The ureter may be obstructed anywhere along its course or at the ureterovesical junction. An abscess or lymphoma may cause obstruction to the ureter, or the presence of a primary megaureter, atresia, or an ectopic ureter may be the cause of obstruction. With a primary megaureter, sonography shows hydronephrosis and hydroureter with a narrow segment of the distal ureter behind the bladder. The increased peristalsis in the ureter distal to the obstruction may be seen with sonography as the probe is held over the dilated ureter and the sonographer watches for the peristaltic movement. A diminished ureteral jet may be seen at the lower margin of the bladder with color Doppler on the side of the obstruction.

Bladder Outlet Obstruction. Bilateral hydronephrosis is frequently caused by obstruction at the level of the bladder or bladder outlet. The bladder may be obstructed by a neurogenic bladder, a pelvic mass, or a congenital

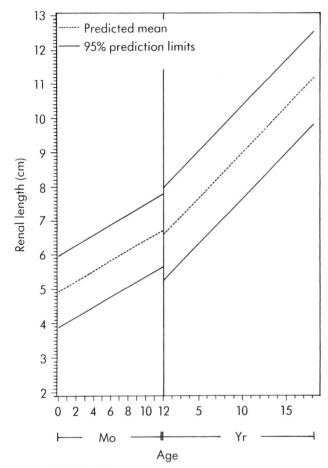

FIGURE 27-3 Normal renal length versus age.

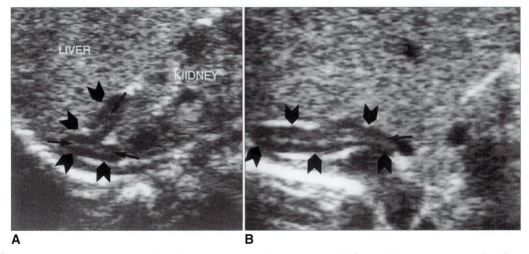

FIGURE 27-4 **A,** Coronal view of a normal adrenal gland *(arrowheads)* in a 1-day-old infant with ambiguous genitalia. The adrenal medulla *(arrows)* appears as a central echogenic stripe, surrounded by the less echogenic cortex. The adrenal gland has an inverted Y configuration. **B,** Transverse view through a portion of adrenal gland *(arrowheads)* demonstrating the curvilinear shape in this plane.

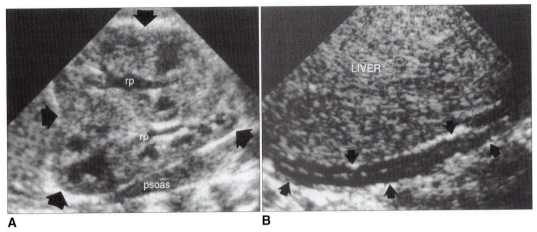

FIGURE 27-5 A, Crossed-fused renal ectopia *(arrows)* in a 1-day-old male with imperforate anus. Sonogram through the right flank demonstrates the renal pelvis *(rp)* of each kidney. **B,** Coronal image through the right flank demonstrates an elongated adrenal gland *(arrows)* resulting from the absence of a kidney in this renal fossa.

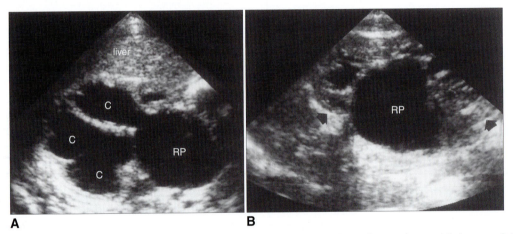

FIGURE 27-6 A, Ureteropelvic junction obstruction in a 2-week-old female infant with an abnormal prenatal ultrasound. Marked dilation of the renal pelvis *(RP)* and calyces *(C)* is present. Parenchymal loss is also noted. The distal ureter was not identified. Radionuclide imaging confirmed the diagnosis. **B,** Uteropelvic junction obstruction in a 1-day-old infant. Coronal image of the kidney *(arrows)* identifies marked dilation of the renal pelvis *(RP)*.

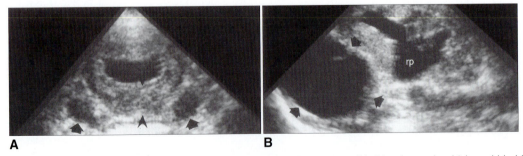

FIGURE 27-7 A, Posterior urethral valves in a male infant. Transverse view of the urinary bladder shows the thickened bladder wall *(arrowheads)*. Dilated distal ureters *(arrows)* are identified posterior to the bladder. **B,** Coronal view of the left kidney shows moderate pelvocaliectasis *(rp)*. A urinoma *(arrows)* is seen superior to the kidney.

anomaly, such as posterior urethral valves. **Posterior urethral valves** are the most common cause of bladder outlet obstruction in the male neonate. A pelvic mass or tumor may be the cause of the bladder obstruction, causing the bladder to be distended with a thickened wall. Vesicoureteral reflux may also be the cause of the dilated renal pelvis.

Sonographic Findings. The wall of the urinary bladder appears thickened and trabeculated (Figure 27-7, *A*). Midline sagittal imaging with caudal angulation through the bladder may allow visualization of the distended posterior urethra. Alternatively the posterior urethra can be imaged directly from a perineal approach. The resultant hydronephrosis and hydroureter are usually

TABLE 27-1 | Renal Findings

Clinical Findings	Sonographic Findings	Differential Considerations
Hydronephrosis		
Flank pain	Pelvocalyceal dilation Ureter is dilated when vesicoureteral reflux or primary megaureter is present	Parapelvic cyst Extrarenal sinus Congenital megacystis Multiple renal cysts Multicystic renal disease Functional dilation Duplicated collecting system
Posterior Urethral Valves		
Decreased urine output	Thickened bladder wall ("keyhole") Hydronephrosis Hydroureter	Megaureter
Multicystic Dysplastic Kidney		
	Unilateral multicystic mass in kidney Contralateral ureteropelvic junction	Hydronephrosis
Polycystic Renal Disease		
Pulmonary hypoplasia Potter's facies	Enlarged kidneys Echogenic kidneys	
Prune Belly Syndrome		
Absence of abdominal muscle Undescended testes Dilated bladder, ureter, prostatic urethra	Kidney is normal, hydronephrotic, or dysplastic Dysplastic enlarged kidneys Dilated ureters Dilated bladder	Posterior urethral valves
Congenital Mesoblastic Nephroma		
Found in children <1 yr	Hyperechoic or hypoechoic or mixed	Adrenal tumor Neuroblastoma Benign renal tumor Abscess
Neuroblastoma		
Nystagmus Unsteady gait	Mass usually in adrenal gland Echogenic Calcification Look for metastasis to liver	Adrenal tumor Benign renal tumor Abscess
Wilms' Tumor		
Hypertension Palpable abdominal or flank mass Weight loss, fever, anemia, pain	Complex mass in kidney Well-circumscribed mass Isoechoic to echogenic May have calcification Look for tumor extension into renal vein or inferior vena cava	Mesoblastic nephroma Renal cell carcinoma Retroperitoneal sarcoma Adrenal cortical carcinoma Multicystic renal hamartoma
Adrenal Hemorrhage		
Abdominal mass Jaundice Anemia	Ovoid enlargement of the gland Anechoic to hyperechoic	Adrenal neuroblastoma Adrenal cyst Adrenal neoplasm

bilateral. Urinary ascites or a perirenal urinoma can result from high-pressure vesicoureteral reflux, rupturing a calyceal fornix or tearing the renal parenchyma (Figure 27-7, *B*). The perirenal urinoma is usually anechoic, but septations may be noted. Other potential causes of perirenal urine extravasation include ureteropelvic junction obstruction, ureterovesical junction obstruction, and pelvic masses that obstruct the bladder or ureter (Figure 27-8).

Ectopic Ureterocele. Ectopic ureterocele occurs more commonly in females and more often on the left side. It results from an ectopic insertion and cystic dilation of the distal ureter of the upper moiety of a completely duplicated renal collecting system.

Sonographic Findings. The ectopic ureterocele, seen as a fluid mass within the urinary bladder, is located inferomedially to the ureteral insertion of the lower pole ureter (Figure 27-9, *A*, *B*). Postoperatively, following the

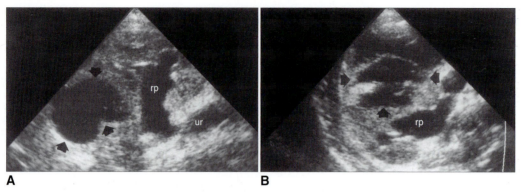

FIGURE 27-8 A, Sonogram of urinoma *(arrows)* in a 5-week-old with bilateral ureterovesical obstruction. Moderate pelvocaliectasis *(rp)* and dilation of the ureter *(ur)* are seen. **B,** Transverse image in the same patient identifies septations within the urinoma *(arrows)*.

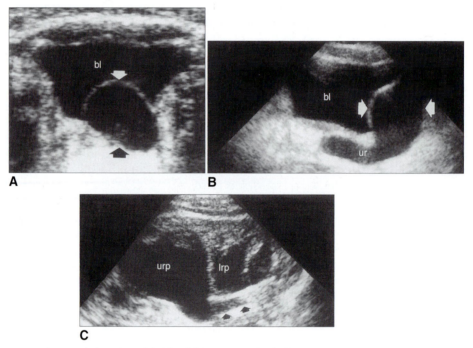

FIGURE 27-9 A, Transverse image of the urinary bladder *(bl)* in a 2-month-old female with pyelonephritis. A large, thin-walled ureterocele *(arrows)* is seen in the posterior aspect of the bladder. **B,** Longitudinal view of the bladder in the same patient shows the dilated ureter *(ur)* and ureterocele *(arrows)*. Low-level echoes seen in the ureter and ureterocele represent debris. **C,** Coronal view of the kidney in the same patient demonstrates a duplicated kidney with notable pelvocaliectasis of the upper pole segment *(urp)* and moderate pelvocaliectasis of the lower pole segment *(lrp)*. The ureter from the upper pole segment *(arrows)* is located medial to the lower pole renal pelvis.

incision of the ureterocele, the structure may be seen in a collapsed state. The sonographic delineation of an upper pole fluid mass, in continuity with a dilated ureter and the aforementioned ureterocele, is diagnostic of this entity (Figure 27-9, C). Distention and effacement or contraction of the ureterocele may be evident during the real-time study.

Prune Belly Syndrome

The **prune belly syndrome** (or abdominal muscle deficiency syndrome) is the triad of hypoplasia or deficiency of the abdominal musculature, cryptorchidism, and

urinary tract anomalies. This anomaly includes congenital absence or deficiency of the abdominal musculature, large hypotonic dilated tortuous ureters, a large bladder, a patent urachus, bilateral cryptorchidism, and a dilated prostatic urethra. Severely affected patients have urethral atresia and bilateral cystic renal dysplasia secondary to obstruction. Resultant pulmonary hypoplasia is fatal. The less severely affected neonates have a bladder with poor contractility without obstruction; however, the ureters may be ectatic and dilated. Reflux is a common problem with the prune belly syndrome.

Sonographic Findings. The sonographic findings vary depending on the severity of the syndrome. The most severely affected neonates show dysplastic echogenic kidneys. In the less severely affected, nonhydronephrotic kidneys with dilated ureters and a huge bladder are seen. This appearance may be similar to that of a neonate with posterior urethral valves. Physically the wrinkled "prune-like" abdomen aids in the clinical diagnosis.

Renal Cystic Disease

Multicystic Dysplastic Kidney. **Multicystic dysplastic kidney** (MCDK) is the most common cause of renal cystic disease in the neonate; when hydronephrosis is excluded, it is the most common cause of an abdominal mass in the newborn. The MCDK is a congenital, usually sporadic, renal dysplasia, which is thought to be secondary to severe, generalized interference with ureteral bud function during the first trimester. The malformation results from ureteral obstruction. High ureteral atresia and pyelocalyceal occlusion are almost always present.

In utero the obstruction interferes with ureteral bud division and inhibits the maturation of nephrons in the kidney. Thus, the collecting tubules enlarge, becoming cystic and grossly distorting the shape of the kidney. The remaining renal parenchyma becomes virtually nonfunctioning. Nearly half of the cases have contralateral abnormalities (i.e., ureteropelvic junction obstruction and vesicoureteral reflux).

Sonographic Findings. Sonographically the classic appearance of MCDK is of a unilateral mass resembling a "cluster of grapes," which represents multiple discrete noncommunicating cysts, the largest of which are peripheral. There is no identifiable renal pelvis (Figure 27-10). A less common hydronephrotic form of MCDK has been described in which a renal pelvis has been identified. The association with contralateral uteropelvic junction obstruction has been noted. Bilateral occurrence of MCDK is fatal.

At times, sonographic differentiation of MCDK from severe uteropelvic junction obstruction may be difficult. In such instances, radionuclide documentation of renal function usually indicates severe hydronephrosis. The use of ultrasound has led to conservative management of MCDK. These abnormal kidneys most often involute and disappear completely or result in a small dysplastic kidney. If there is evidence of growth, resection is usually undertaken.

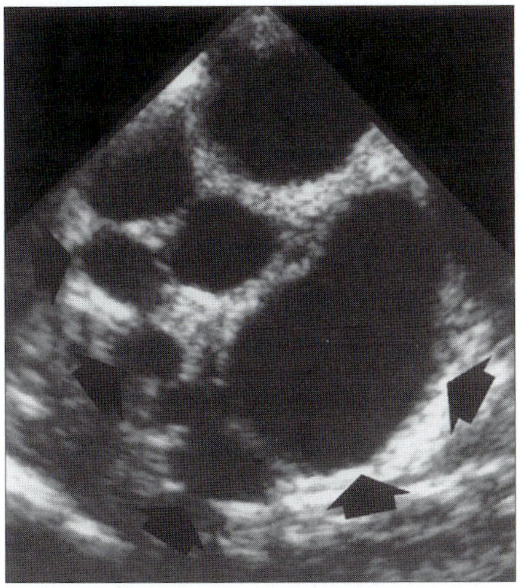

FIGURE 27-10 Multicystic dysplastic kidney *(arrows)* in a 3-week-old male. Axial view of the left flank demonstrates multiple, noncommunicating cysts of varying sizes. There was no apparent renal pelvis. Radionuclide imaging confirmed the diagnosis.

Medullary Cystic Disease. This disease is indistinguishable from juvenile nephronophthisis, as both cause renal failure in the child or adolescent. With sonography, the kidneys are small, echogenic, with cysts of variable sizes at the corticomedullary junction and elsewhere in the parenchyma.

Autosomal Recessive Polycystic Kidney Disease. **Polycystic renal disease** identified in the neonatal period is most often **autosomal recessive polycystic kidney disease** (**ARPKD**), also known as *infantile polycystic disease.* This disease is not common, occurring in 1 in 6000 to 14,000 births with a female predominance 2:1. It is transmitted by autosomal recessive inheritance. The typical pathologic presentation is diffuse enlargement, sacculations, and cystic diverticula of the medullary portions of the kidneys (Figure 27-11).

ARPKD is associated with biliary **ectasia** and hepatic fibrosis; the severity is proportional to the degree of renal involvement. The most severe form is seen in the neonatal stage, whereas the least severe form is seen in the infantile to juvenile stage. In the third trimester of pregnancy, the dilated kidneys occupy nearly the entire abdomen and cause the abdomen to protrude. The perinatal form is the most common and is characterized by varying degrees of renal tubular dilation and hepatic fibrosis. The kidneys are hyperechoic and enlarged with a hypoechogenic outer rim, which represents the cortex

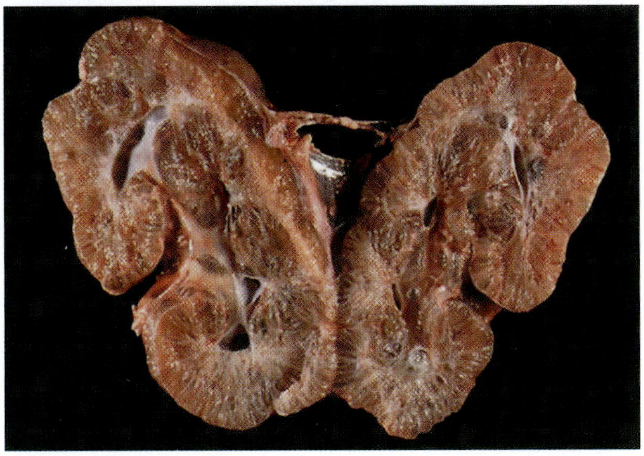

FIGURE 27-11 Gross pathology of autosomal-recessive polycystic kidney disease demonstrated bilateral renal enlargement with diffuse cyst replacing the tubules and collecting ducts.

compressed by the expanded pyramids. The degree of renal cystic disease determines the severity of renal dysplasia, which can lead to renal failure and eventual liver failure. **Pulmonary hypoplasia** with respiratory distress and **Potter facies** may also be associated findings.

In the juvenile form of ARPKD, symptoms can occur later in childhood. The renal tubular ectasia and the resultant renal symptomatology are overshadowed by hepatic fibrosis leading to portal hypertension and gastrointestinal bleeding. In this condition, the dilated renal collecting tubules produce an accentuated medullary echogenicity, and the renal cortex has an essentially normal appearance. Increased liver echogenicity reflects hepatic fibrosis.

Sonographic Findings. The most striking feature is bilateral renal enlargement with diffuse increased echogenicity and loss of definition of the renal sinus, medulla, and cortex. The less severe cases may show hepatosplenomegaly and portal hypertension, with the renal parenchyma normal to echogenic. In utero, oligohydramnios and nonvisualization of the bladder will also be apparent. (The lack of amniotic fluid volume in turn leads to the development of pulmonary hypoplasia.) This diagnosis may be made as early as 16 to 18 weeks of gestation in the presence of severe oligohydramnios and nonvisualization of the bladder.

The macroscopic cystlike appearance throughout both kidneys actually reflects dilated renal tubules that are generally less than 2 mm in diameter. The innumerable acoustic interfaces that present because of this morphologic abnormality result in notable echogenicity, obscuring corticomedullary demarcation. A thin, peripheral, hypoechoic renal rim may be demonstrated, representing either a compressed renal cortex or elongated thin-walled cystic spaces (Figure 27-12). Associated mild

hepatic fibrosis and ductal hyperplasia can produce a heterogeneous increase in echogenicity of liver parenchyma.

Autosomal Dominant Polycystic Kidney Disease. More than 90% of patients with **autosomal dominant polycystic kidney disease (ADPKD)** have a gene locus on the short arm of chromosome 16. There is wide variation in the severity of the disease. The adult dominant form of polycystic kidney disease usually appears during middle age. On rare occasions, however, it has been reported in a young infant. More typically the disease becomes manifest during the fourth decade of adulthood, with hypertension, hematuria, and enlarged kidneys. Cysts are macroscopic and of varying size and can also form in the liver, spleen, and pancreas. Cerebral berry aneurysms are also known to occur in 10% to 15% of patients with ADPKD. There is an increased incidence of renal cell carcinoma in patients with ADPKD. Sonography of parents and siblings of patients with ADPKD has proven helpful in identifying this abnormality in afflicted persons who are asymptomatic.

Sonographic Findings. On sonography the findings are similar to that of ARPKD. However, a lack of significant renal impairment, normal amniotic fluid volume (in utero), family history, or histologic sampling allows differentiation. The well-defined cysts affect both kidneys. The cysts are of varying sizes and can be identified in the kidneys in the adult as the tubular and ductal cells become engorged.

Renal Cysts

Just as in the adult patient, renal cysts may appear in the kidney and may be found associated with various

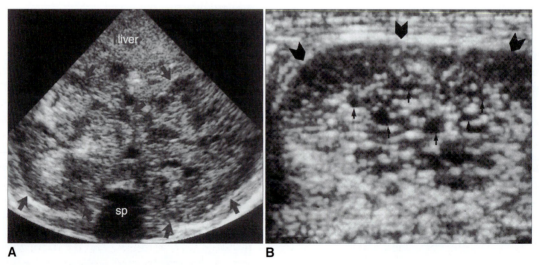

A   **B**

FIGURE 27-12 A, Autosomal-recessive polycystic kidney disease (ARPKD) in a 1-day-old male with abdominal distention. Transverse image of the upper abdomen using the liver as an acoustic window shows that the kidneys are enlarged and echogenic with a hypoechoic peripheral rim *(arrows); sp,* Spine. This appearance is typical for ARPKD. **B,** A 7-MHz linear image of the kidney *(arrowheads)* in the same patient reveals multiple small cysts *(arrows).* The high frequency allows resolution of the cysts.

syndromes like tuberous sclerosis and von Hippel-Lindau disease. Patients with the autosomal disease of tuberous sclerosis have a 40% incidence of having renal cysts, which may resemble polycystic renal disease. Angiomyolipomas may occur and be multiple; their echogenicity is determined by the amount of fatty tissue within the lesion. In patients with von Hippel-Lindau disease, there are multiple cysts with an increased incidence of renal cell carcinoma.

Infection of the Urinary Tract

Children are referred for sonography if there are suspicious of a urinary tract infection. Although infection of the urinary system is not as specific to image on sonography as a simple cyst, it is important for the clinician to order a sonogram to rule out the presence of other abnormalities of the kidney that may lead to the infection.

Acute Pyelonephritis. Clinical symptoms of acute pyelonephritis include sudden fever, flank pain, and tenderness. The infection usually begins in the bladder and ascends the ureter into the renal pelvis. On sonography, the renal size may be slightly enlarged with an altered renal parenchymal echogenicity secondary to the edema. As the infection spreads into the renal pyramids, there may be increased echogenicity in this triangular area. The renal pelvis and ureter may show some thickening secondary to the inflammation. The infection may be diffuse or localized. As the infection begins to wall itself into an abscess formation, a mixed echogenic pattern is demonstrated within the renal parenchyma. Sonography may be useful in following the patient after antibiotic therapy has been given to demonstrate the shrinkage of the lesion.

Chronic Pyelonephritis. This results when repeated episodes of acute pyelonephritis cause the kidney to become scarred and decreased in size. The outline of the kidney may be irregular as the parenchyma becomes scarred. The renal cortex becomes increasingly more echogenic than the liver parenchyma. The renal pyramids become difficult to separate from the renal parenchyma.

Renal Vein Thrombosis

Renal vein thrombosis is most likely to occur in the dehydrated or septic infant and is more prevalent in infants of diabetic mothers. One or both kidneys may be involved. There is renal enlargement, hematuria, proteinuria, and a low platelet count.

◤ Sonographic Findings. Thrombosis occurs initially in the small intrarenal venous branches, and at this stage the enlarged kidney has a nonspecific disordered heterogeneous internal echogenicity corresponding to the extent and severity of the process (Figure 27-13). If the thrombus reaches the renal vein or inferior vena cava, it

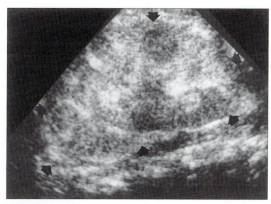

FIGURE 27-13 Renal vein thrombosis in a 5-day-old term newborn with hematuria. Coronal sonogram of the left flank demonstrates an enlarged kidney *(arrows)* with patchy areas of increased echogenicity.

may be directly visualized within these vascular structures. There may be coexistent adrenal hemorrhage, particularly on the left side where the adrenal vein drains directly into the renal vein. Calcification within the involved veins may eventually result. The use of color Doppler helps the sonographer to identify whether the flow is present, reversed, or obstructed.

Renal/Adrenal Tumors

The most common abdominal masses in the pediatric patient are renal in origin: hydronephrosis and multicystic renal dysplasia. Solid tumors of the kidney are far less common. When the child presents in the ultrasound department, it is the responsibility of the sonographer to determine the origin of the mass (whether it is part of the liver, kidney, biliary system, etc.), the internal pattern (cystic, solid, or mixed), and whether the mass has vascular flow. The most common renal tumors will be presented.

Congenital Mesoblastic Nephroma. The most common renal tumor of the neonate is **congenital mesoblastic nephroma** (also known as *fetal renal hamartoma* or *congenital Wilms' tumor*). This tumor is rare, occurring with a prevalence of 8 : 1,000,000 births. The mesoblastic nephroma consists of connective tissue elements that can completely replace renal tissue. This tumor is benign but is indistinguishable from a Wilms' tumor by any method of imaging. Because the tumor may invade adjacent structures, nephrectomy is indicated.

◤ Sonographic Findings. Sonographically, as with Wilms' tumor, this lesion is solid but may have a complex texture that includes hyperechoic, hypoechoic, or mixed echogenicity (Figure 27-14). The mass may extend through the renal capsule into the retroperitoneum. It is seen in children less than 1 year of age, whereas Wilms' tumor commonly occurs in children more than 1 year old.

Nephroblastoma (Wilms' Tumor). Wilms' tumor (**nephroblastoma**) is the most common intraabdominal

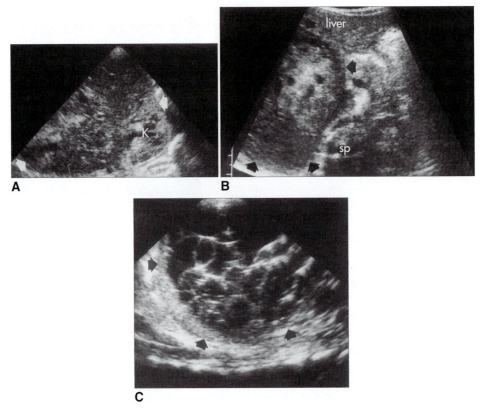

FIGURE 27-14 A, Mesoblastic nephroma in an 11-week-old infant with a renal mass *(arrows)*. Coronal image of the right flank identifies that the mass is predominantly solid, with some cystic areas, and arises from the right kidney *(K)*. **B,** Transverse view shows the mass *(arrows)* posterior to the liver and anterior and lateral to the spine *(sp)*. Nephrectomy and pathologic evaluation confirmed the diagnosis of mesoblastic nephroma. **C,** Wilms' tumor in a 7-month-old with an abdominal mass. Sonogram reveals a large mass with multiple cystic areas occupying the renal fossa *(arrows)*. This represents an unusual presentation of a Wilms' tumor; more frequently a large solid component is present in these masses.

malignant renal tumor in young children. The incidence of this tumor peaks between 2 and 5 years of age. This tumor is usually unilateral, although in a small percentage it may occur bilaterally. Wilms' tumor is bulky and expands within the renal parenchyma, resulting in distortion and displacement of the collecting system and capsule. Sonography is used for periodic renal monitoring in those at risk of developing Wilms' tumor, including patients with a previous Wilms' tumor or a family history of the disease. Periodic sonographic monitoring is also performed in patients with either proven or potential **nephroblastomatosis**. It is important to note that Wilms' tumor may occur spontaneously, and many pediatric laboratories will monitor both types of patients (those predisposed to the tumor and those with a history of Wilms' tumor) with sonography. In addition, sonography may be used to monitor the size of the tumor while the patient is treated with chemotherapy drugs to shrink the tumor. Therefore, the size of the tumor is documented and the appropriate time for surgery is chosen. Early surgical removal and treatment yield a favorable prognosis.

Sonographic Findings. The sonographic appearance of a Wilms' tumor is variable, extending from

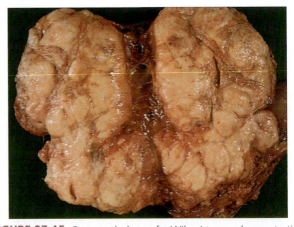

FIGURE 27-15 Gross pathology of a Wilms' tumor demonstrating the multinodular tumor replacing a large portion of the renal parenchyma.

homogeneous to complex texture (Figure 27-15). The mass usually has areas of echogenicity and may have calcifications within. The liquefaction may represent necrosis and hemorrhage. The borders are sharply marginated and well defined, but bulky, with a hypoechoic to hyperechoic rim surrounding the mass (Figure 27-16).

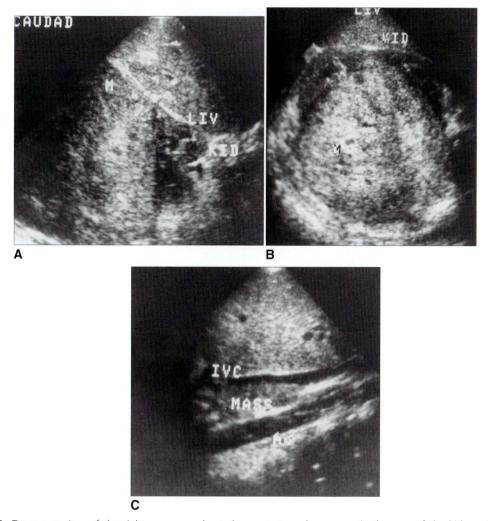

FIGURE 27-16 A, Transverse view of the right upper quadrant demonstrates a large mass in the area of the kidney displacing the liver anteriorly. **B,** The large mass representing a Wilms' tumor is heterogeneous and echogenic. **C,** Evaluation of the inferior vena cava shows extension of the tumor into the IVC.

The adjacent renal tissue becomes compressed with the growth of the mass. The large solid mass generally is seen to completely distort the renal sinus, pyramids, cortex, and contour of the kidney. The mass may be so large as to protrude into the hepatic capsule. Resultant hydronephrosis may be present.

Sonography is valuable in detecting extension of a Wilms' tumor into the renal vein, inferior vena cava, right atrium, and contralateral kidney. The tumor spreads through direct extension into the renal sinus and peripelvic soft tissues, the lymph nodes in the renal hilum, and the paraaortic areas. Careful evaluation of the renal vein, inferior vena cava, and right atrium of the heart are important to document the possible extension of the tumor. Documentation of tumor extension can have a significant bearing on the surgical approach to the patient. When the tumor extends into the right atrium, cardiopulmonary bypass may be necessary to resect the tumor completely.

Neuroblastoma. Neuroblastoma, a malignant tumor that arises in the sympathetic chain ganglia and adrenal medulla, may be detected on antenatal sonography or at birth. This is the second most common abdominal tumor of childhood, occurring between the ages of 2 months and 2 years. About half of these tumors arise in the medulla of the adrenal gland, although tumors have also been found in the neck, mediastinum, retroperitoneum, and pelvis. Clinical findings depend on the location of the tumor. Tumors that arise within the adrenal gland show an abdominal mass, hypertension, diarrhea, and bone pain if metastasis is involved.

Sonographic Findings. Neuroblastoma is usually highly echogenic. Intrinsic calcification may be identified (Figure 27-17). The smaller tumors may appear homogeneous and hyperechoic, whereas the large tumors are more complex in appearance. A cystic form of neuroblastoma has also been described. The adjacent kidney is displaced inferiorly and at times laterally. Doppler

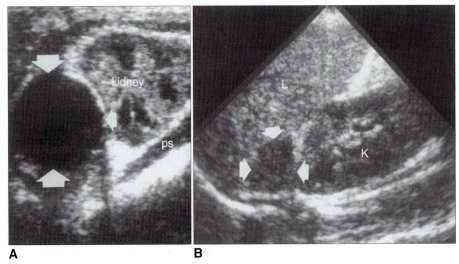

FIGURE 27-17 A, Adrenal hemorrhage in a 2-week-old male with a history of neonatal infections, increased bilirubin, and an abdominal mass. Coronal sonogram demonstrates a cystic mass *(arrows)* superior to the kidney. A normal adrenal gland was not identified. The psoas muscle *(ps)* is located posteriorly. **B,** Adrenal hemorrhage in a jaundiced 3-week-old female. Coronal view of the right upper quadrant reveals an echogenic mass *(arrows)* superior to the kidney *(K)* and posterior to the liver *(L)*.

evaluation may help to differentiate the tumor from an adrenal hemorrhage because there is increased vascularity within the neoplastic growth.

The disease spreads early and widely, so the majority of patients present with metastases. Careful sonographic evaluation of the liver should be made for evidence of metastatic disease. The mass also spreads around the aorta, celiac, and superior mesenteric arteries. This spread of tumor helps to distinguish a neuroblastoma from a Wilms' tumor because this tumor is well encapsulated, although it is somewhat homogeneous and heterogeneous. The neuroblastoma is poorly defined and heterogeneous with irregular hyperechoic areas caused by calcifications. Because intraspinal extension is reported to occur in as many as 15% of patients and because ultrasonography can successfully define the spinal canal in young infants, such examination should be considered in the initial assessment of the infant with suspected neuroblastoma.

Adrenal Hemorrhage

Difficult delivery, large size, infants of diabetic mothers, stress and hypoxia at delivery, septicemia, and shock all predispose the neonate to the development of an adrenal hemorrhage. The newborn with **adrenal hemorrhage,** however, may have none of these associated factors and still present with abdominal mass, jaundice, and anemia. Usually the hemorrhage is found secondary to other complications, such as uncontrolled bleeding, jaundice, intestinal obstruction, hypertension, adrenal abscess, or impaired renal function.

▸ **Sonographic Findings.** Sonographically, adrenal hemorrhage results in ovoid enlargement of the gland or a portion of the gland. The appearance of the hemorrhagic

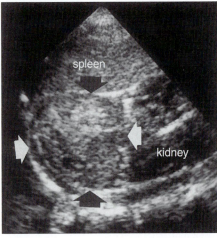

FIGURE 27-18 Adrenal neuroblastoma in a 1-week-old female with history of a left kidney mass on a fetal sonogram. Coronal image through the left flank reveals a large heterogeneous mass *(arrows)* displacing the left kidney inferiorly.

gland can range from anechoic to hyperechoic or may be a mixture of echogenicities, depending on the extent, age, and severity of the process (Figure 27-18). When enlargement is significant, a characteristic blunting of the superior pole of the underlying kidney is produced, along with inferior displacement of the kidney. The initial appearance of adrenal hemorrhage may render it indistinguishable from an adrenal neuroblastoma. Follow-up sonography can differentiate these two entities. Unlike a neoplasm, a hemorrhagic adrenal gland does not enlarge but rather decreases in size. Generally within 4 to 6 weeks, the lesion becomes appreciably smaller and subsequent calcification may be identified on the sonogram or radiographically.

The Neonatal and Pediatric Pelvis

Sandra L. Hagen-Ansert

OBJECTIVES

On completion of this chapter, you should be able to:
- Discuss the development of the ovaries and the male genital tract
- Describe normal sonographic appearance of the pediatric female pelvis and pediatric scrotum
- Describe when external genitalia may be seen by ultrasound
- Detail the sonographic findings and appearance of the congenital anomalies and pathologic conditions discussed in this chapter
- Describe the difference between true precocious puberty and precocious pseudopuberty
- Describe the complications and differential considerations for ovarian cysts

OUTLINE

The evaluation with high-resolution sonography of both the male and female pelvis is well documented. The development of the female genital system and the role embryology plays in congenital abnormalities of the female reproductive tract are presented in this chapter. Sonography has become an important imaging modality for the evaluation of the pelvis in the neonatal, pediatric, and adolescent patient. Frequently, uterine anomalies are associated with abnormalities of the urinary tract. The distended urinary bladder is used as a landmark to image the uterus, ovaries, and adnexal structures in the pelvis. In the male neonate or infant, the full bladder serves as an acoustic window to image the prostate gland, seminal vesicles, and pelvic musculature may be well seen. The most common abnormalities are presented in this chapter.

Multiple sonographic images are made in the transverse and sagittal planes with a 5- to 7.5-MHz phased array or curvilinear broad bandwidth or sector transducer. The neonatal images are obtained with a higher resolution transducer (7.5 to 12 MHz).

EMBRYOLOGY OF THE FEMALE GENITAL TRACT

Development of the Gonads

The first parts of the genital system to develop are the gonads. The gonads arise from the parts of the urogenital ridges called gonadal ridges. This ridge enlarges and frees itself from the mesonephros by developing a mesentery that becomes the mesovarium (Figure 28-1). At the same time, the coelomic epithelium covering the gonadal ridges grows and forms cords of cells, called primary sex cords, which grow into the mesenchyme of the developing gonads. The primordial germ cells originate in the wall of the yolk sac, migrate into the embryo, and enter the primary sex cords to give rise to the ova.

Development of the Ovaries

In embryos with a double "X" chromosome (female), differentiation of the gonads occurs later than in males. The primary sex cords converge to form a network of canals called the *rete ovarii*, which soon disappear with the primary sex cords. At the same time, the surface epithelium of the developing ovary gives rise to secondary sex cords, or cortical cords (Figure 28-2). As these cords grow in the ovary, primordial germ cells are incorporated into them. At about 16 weeks of gestation, the cortical cords break up into isolated cell clusters called primordial follicles, each of which contains an **oogonium** that is derived from the primordial germ cell. Each oogonium is surrounded by a layer of flattened follicular cells derived from the surface epithelial cells in the cortical cord. The oogonia multiply rapidly by mitosis, producing thousands of these primitive germ cells. Before birth, all oogonia enlarge to form primary **oocytes**. Most of them have entered the first meiotic prophase, but this process remains in an arrested state until puberty.

Development of the Genital Ducts

All embryos have identical pairs of genital ducts in the beginning. The female or **paramesonephric** ducts (see

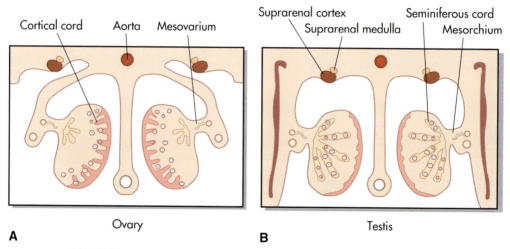

FIGURE 28-1 Development of the female (**A**) and male (**B**) gender at 7 weeks.

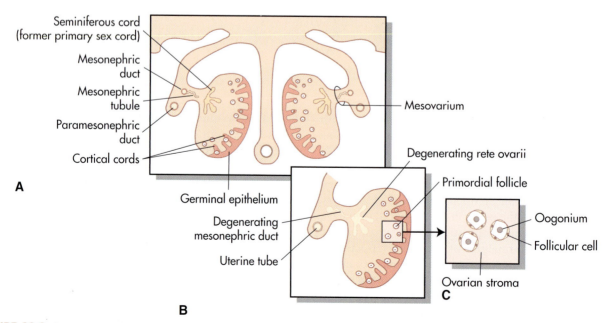

FIGURE 28-2 A, Fetus at 12 weeks of gestation shows the ovary beginning to develop. **B,** Ovary at 20 weeks, showing the primordial follicles formed from the cortical cords. **C,** Section from the ovarian cortex of a 20-week fetus showing three primordial follicles.

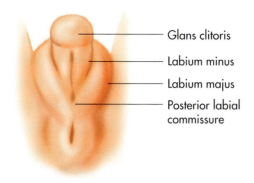

- Glans clitoris
- Labium minus
- Labium majus
- Posterior labial commissure

FIGURE 28-3 Development of the female external genitalia at 11 weeks.

Figure 28-2) develop into the female reproductive system. During the indifferent state of sexual development, both pairs of genital ducts are present. Even though the genetic sex of an embryo is determined at fertilization by the kind of sperm that fertilizes the ovum, there are no morphologic indications of maleness or femaleness until the 9th gestational week.

Development of the Female Genital Ducts

The paramesonephric ducts form most of the female genital tract. Their cranial parts form the uterine tubes and their caudal parts fuse to form the uterovaginal primordium, or canal, which develops into the uterus and part of the vagina. Contact of the uterovaginal primordium with the urogenital sinus induces paired endodermal outgrowths called sinovaginal bulbs to form. These bulbs fuse to form a solid vaginal plate. The central cells of this plate break down to form the vagina; the peripheral cells form the vaginal epithelium.

Development of the External Genitalia

Early in development, both sexes appear similar until the 9th week of gestation. External organs are fully developed by the 12th week. Both the urethra and vagina open into the urogenital sinus, which becomes the vestibule of the vagina. The urogenital folds become the labia minora, the labioscrotal swellings become the labia majora, and the phallus becomes the clitoris (Figure 28-3).

NORMAL SONOGRAPHIC APPEARANCE OF THE PEDIATRIC FEMALE PELVIS

The transabdominal sonographic evaluation of the neonatal and pediatric pelvic cavity requires a distended urinary bladder to act as an acoustic window to image the pelvic anatomy. It may be necessary to catheterize and fill the bladder with sterile water if there is difficulty in obtaining a distended urinary bladder. The use of sterile water as a contrast agent may be utilized to outline the vagina (hydrosonovaginography) in a pediatric patient with a pelvic mass or complex congenital abnormality of the genitourinary tract.

Bladder

The normal urinary bladder should have a smooth, thin wall. When the bladder is distended (the top of the bladder exceeds the fundus of the uterus), the bladder wall thickness should measure less than 3 mm, with a mean of 1.5 mm. When the bladder is empty or partially full, the wall will appear thicker but should not measure greater than 5 mm. The distal ureters are not routinely visualized unless they are dilated. Color Doppler allows adequate visualization of the ureters as they empty into the bladder. To image the ureteral jets, angle the probe caudally toward the base of the bladder and turn the color Doppler on with the gain slightly high, but not so high as to see extraneous color "ghost" echoes in the background. Hold the probe still for a several seconds and the jet flow should be noted, first on one side, then on the other.

The bladder neck and urethra may be demonstrated in either sex by angling the transducer inferiorly. The perineum or transrectal approach may also prove useful to image a urethral abnormality. Hydrosonourethrography is used with anterior urethral abnormalities, such as strictures, calculi, urethral valves, diverticula, and trauma.

The postvoid scan may be useful to provide information about the bladder emptying capability; sometimes it is necessary to demonstrate a change in bladder size to separate it from a pelvic cyst.

Uterus

In the newborn female, the uterus is prominent and thickened with a brightly echogenic endometrial lining caused by the hormonal stimulation received in utero. The uterus is pear shaped in configuration with the length, approximately 3.5 cm with a fundus-to-cervix ratio of 1:2. (The fundus is smaller than the cervix.)

The maternal hormones stimulate the initial size of the uterine cavity after birth; as these hormones decrease, so does the uterine size. The uterus assumes a teardrop shape, with the cervix consuming more area than the uterus (Figure 28-4). At 2 to 3 months of age, the uterus regresses to a prepubertal size and tubular configuration with the length measuring 2.5 to 3 cm, the fundus-to-cervix ratio 1:1, and the endometrial stripe echoes not visualized. Some endometrial fluid may be present.

The uterus increases in size after the age of 7 years, with the greatest increase in size occurring after the onset of puberty, when the fundus becomes much larger than the cervix (Table 28-1). It is not until puberty that the uterine shape and size dramatically change. The uterine

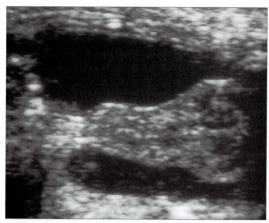

FIGURE 28-4 Neonatal uterus well seen within the pelvic cavity with ascitic fluid surrounding the teardrop-shaped uterine wall. The cervix consumes the majority of the total uterine length at this stage.

TABLE 28-1	Uterine Measurements	
Age	Uterine Length	Fundus-Cervix Ratio
Newborn	3.5 cm	1:2
Prepubertal (>2 months)	2.5–3 cm	1:1
Postpubertal	5–7 cm	3:1

Data from Comstock CH, Boal DK: Pelvic sonography of the pediatric patient, *Semin Ultrasound* 5:54-67, 1984.

length increases to 5 to 7 cm, and the fundus-to-cervix ratio becomes 3:1 (the fundus is now greater than the cervix). The echogenicity and thickness of the endometrial lining vary according to the phase of the menstrual cycle.

The uterus is supplied by the bilateral uterine arteries, which are branches of the internal iliac arteries. Color flow Doppler may demonstrate flow in the myometrial tissue with little or no flow in the endometrium.

Vagina

The physical examination of the uterus and vagina is difficult in the young patient and often is only performed under general anesthesia when an anomaly is suspected. The vagina is best imaged on the midline longitudinal image when the bladder is very distended. The vagina appears as a tubular structure posterior to the bladder and is in continuity with the uterine cervix. The mucosal walls cause a bright central echo within the tubular structure.

Ovary

Depending on the location, size, and age of the patient, evaluation of the ovary in the young patient may be a challenge. In the neonatal patient, the ovary may be

TABLE 28-2	Ovarian Volume Measurements
Premenarchal Age	Mean Ovarian Volume
0–5 yr	<1 cm³
6–8 yr	1.2 cm³
9–10 yr	2.1 cm³
11 yr	2.5 cm³ (±1.3)
12 yr	3.8 cm³ (±1.4)
13 yr	4.2 cm³ (±2.3)
Menstrual	9.8 cm³ (±5.8)

Data slightly modified from Cohen HL, Shapiro MA, Mandel FS, et al: Normal ovaries in neonates and infants: a sonographic study of 77 patients 1 day to 24 months old, AJR 160:583-586, 1993.

found anywhere between the lower pole of the kidneys and the true pelvis. The evaluation of ovarian size is most accurate when the volume is determined by using the prolate-ellipse formula:

$$\text{Volume in cubic centimeters} = \text{Length} \times \text{Height} \times \text{Width} \times 0.523$$

The mean ovarian volume is stable up to 5 years of age and ranges from 0.75 to 0.86 cm³ (Table 28-2). Ovarian volume gradually increases until puberty is reached. Usually the ovarian texture is homogeneous, but small follicles may be seen with ultrasound.

The appearance of the ovary in the neonatal period is heterogeneous secondary to tiny cysts. The larger cysts in the ovary are more commonly seen in female patients after their first year of life. The blood supply to the ovary is from the ovarian artery, which originates directly from the aorta and from the uterine artery, which supplies an adnexal branch to each ovary.

PATHOLOGY OF THE PEDIATRIC GENITAL SYSTEM

Congenital Anomalies of the Uterus and Vagina

The definitive diagnosis and classification of a congenital anomaly of the uterine cavity requires the visualization of the uterine cavity or cavities and the serosal margin(s). Before ultrasound, hysterosalpingography with laparoscopy was used to define the uterine cavity in the teenage and adult patient. With transabdominal and transvaginal ultrasound, the uterine cavities can now be defined. A newer technique in the older patient, sonohysterosalpingography, requires the injection of a small amount of contrast material into the cavity through a catheter threaded into the vagina and cervix to differentiate the uterine cavity and septa.

The uterus provides the endometrial canal for the site of implantation and growth for the intrauterine pregnancy. Developmental problems, interference with blood supply, or distortion of the uterine cavity may result in infertility or spontaneous abortion. Congenital uterine abnormalities occur in approximately 0.5% of females and are associated with an increased incidence of abortion and other obstetric complications later in life.

Congenital anomalies of the uterus and vagina in children are not common and usually present as an abdominal or pelvic mass secondary to obstruction. Also a high association of renal anomalies is found when abnormalities of the uterine cavity are discovered.

The uterus and upper third of the vagina are derived from the embryonic Müllerian (paramesonephric) ducts. These ducts must elongate, fuse, and form lumens between the 7th and 12th weeks of embryonic development. When this sequence fails to occur, one of the following types of Müllerian abnormalities results: improper fusion, incomplete development of one side, or incomplete vaginal canalization.

▧ **Sonographic Findings.** If Müllerian anomalies are encountered, the kidneys should be examined for ipsilateral renal agenesis or morphologic abnormalities (Figure 28-5) because these conditions are commonly associated with Müllerian anomalies. Uterine malformations may be suspected on the basis of abnormal configuration of the uterus on pelvic sonograms.

Müllerian Anomalies

The congenital abnormalities have been classified into six groups based on their prognosis for future fertility and their surgical correction (Figure 28-6):

Class I.   Segmental Müllerian agenesis or incomplete vaginal canalization is suspected when a young girl reaches puberty without menstruation. This condition produces a transverse vaginal septum or vaginal atresia. **Vaginal atresia** is diagnosed by the development of **hydrocolpos** (fluid-filled vagina), **hydrometrocolpos** (fluid-filled vagina and uterus), or **hematometrocolpos** (blood-filled vagina and uterus) (Figure 28-7). On sonographic examination, the cervix may be absent, with or without blood in the uterine or cervical cavities. This condition either presents in the neonatal period as a large cystic pelvic-abdominal mass because of stimulation from maternal hormones or is discovered at puberty. These findings also result from an imperforate hymen.

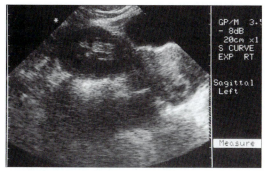

FIGURE 28-5 A pelvic kidney is seen adjacent to the bicornuate uterus on this sagittal transabdominal scan.

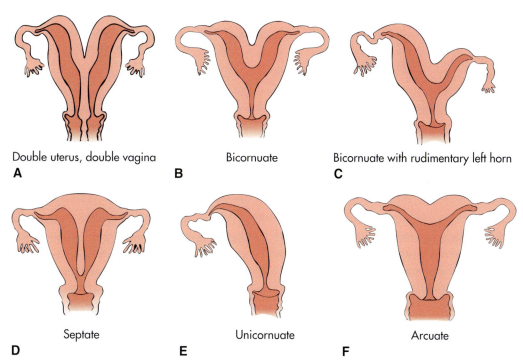

Double uterus, double vagina
A

Bicornuate
B

Bicornuate with rudimentary left horn
C

Septate
D

Unicornuate
E

Arcuate
F

FIGURE 28-6 Congenital uterine abnormalities. **A**, Uterus didelphys: double uterus and vagina. **B**, Bicornuate uterus. **C**, Bicornuate uterus with a rudimentary left horn. **D**, Septate uterus. **E**, Unicornuate uterus. **F**, Arcuate uterus.

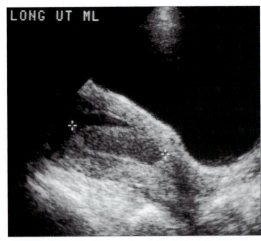

FIGURE 28-7 Transabdominal image along the midline of the pelvic cavity shows the distended urinary bladder anterior to the uterine cavity. A complex area within the endometrial canal represents both blood and fluid in the uterus and vagina (hematometrocolpos).

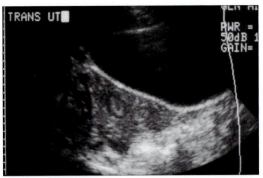

FIGURE 28-8 Transabdominal image of the bicornuate uterus showing two endometrial canals within the bilobed uterine horns.

Class II. **Unicornuate uterus** is related to infertility and pregnancy loss. Sonography demonstrates a uterus that is long and slender (cigar shaped) and deviated to one side. Usually, renal agenesis is apparent on the contralateral side. This is difficult to differentiate from the normal uterus by sonography, but the condition is suspected when the uterus appears small and laterally positioned.

Classes III through V. Classes III through V are more difficult to diagnose because they all have two uterine cavities, and their correct classification and treatment depend on the appearance of the external contour of the uterine fundus. In the nonpregnant state, a congenital malformation is often difficult to demonstrate and may mimic a fibroid.

Class III. **Uterus didelphys** is a complete duplication of the uterus, cervix, and vagina. This condition is not usually associated with fertility problems and does not generally require treatment. Sonography detects two endometrial echo complexes, which are best demonstrated during the secretory phase of the menstrual cycle when the endometrium is most prominent. Then the external contour of the uterus is helpful in distinguishing between the septate and the bicornuate uterus.

Class IV. **Bicornuate uterus** is a duplication of the uterus with a common cervix (Figure 28-8). This bilobed uterine cavity has wide-spaced cavities and a low incidence of fertility complications and is usually not treated. The exception is when one of the horns is rudimentary and noncommunicating. If an embryo implants in this rudimentary cavity, it may grow until about 12 to 16 weeks, when rupture of the uterine cavity occurs. In many cases the bicornuate uterus is diagnosed incidentally in early pregnancy, when a gestational sac is present in one horn and decidual

reaction in the other. The bicornuate uterus is best identified on the transverse sonogram through the superior portion of the two horns of the uterus. The image looks heart shaped on the transverse plane.

Class V. Class V involves a septate uterus in which two uterine cavities are closely spaced, with one fundus and sometimes two cervical canals or a vaginal septum. This condition has the highest incidence of fertility problems, and the septum may be hysteroscopically removed.

Class VI. Class VI is related to the exposure to the drug diethylstilbestrol (DES) in utero. DES is a synthetic preparation drug that possesses estrogenic properties. The drug is several times more potent than natural estrogens. This drug was used extensively in the 1970s during pregnancy to treat threatened and habitual abortion. An estimated 5 million to 10 million Americans received the drug during pregnancy. The drug was later found to cause vaginal malignancies in the daughters of mothers who were given the drug. The uterus is normal in size and shape externally; however, the cavity is "T"-shaped with an irregular contour. This condition may be difficult to diagnose with ultrasound.

Ambiguous Genitalia

The embryo has the potential to develop as a male or female. Errors in sexual development result in ambiguous genitalia or **hermaphroditism**. True hermaphrodites have both ovarian and testicular tissue. The internal and external genitalia are variable, although most true hermaphrodites have a 46,XX karyotype; however, some are mosaics (46,XX/46,XY).

Female pseudohermaphrodites have a 46,XX karyotype. The most common cause is congenital virilizing adrenal hyperplasia. An increased production of androgens leads to masculinization of the external genitalia (enlarged clitoris, abnormalities of the urogenital sinus, and partial fusion of the labia majora).

The external genitalia may also be masculinized by androgenic hormones, which reach it via the placenta from the maternal circulation. These hormones may be present in excessive amounts if the mother's suprarenal cortices are overactive or if she has received hormone therapy involving androgenic substances.

 Sonographic Findings. Sonography may be helpful in identifying the presence or absence of the uterus, vagina, and ovaries in utero or in neonates with ambiguous genitalia. However, the in utero cases can be difficult if a clear image cannot be made of the genital area. Sex assignment is based on results of karyotype analysis, gonadal biopsy, and knowledge of genital anatomy.

Precocious Puberty

Precocious pubertal development may be classified as true precocious puberty or precocious pseudopuberty. True precocious puberty is always **isosexual** (same sex) and involves the development of secondary sexual characteristics and an increase in the size and activity of the gonads. The uterus has an enlarged, postpubertal configuration (fundus to cervix ratio is 2:1 and 3:1), with an echogenic endometrial canal. The ovarian volume is enlarged (greater than 1 cubic cm), and functional cysts are often present.

Precocious pseudopuberty involves the maturation of secondary sexual characteristics, but not the gonad, as there is no activation of the hypothalamic-pituitary-gonadal axis. Excessive exogenous synthesis of gonadal steroids (by the adrenal gland, tumors, or cysts) is the most common cause of precocious pseudopuberty; prolonged exposure to exogenous gonadal hormones may mature the central nervous system and cause true precocious puberty in some children. Sonography is useful to detect the presence of a pelvic mass and a mature uterus.

 Sonographic Findings. Sonography is used to determine the volume and size of the ovaries, uterus, and cervix, and to exclude an ovarian neoplasm. The liver and the adrenal gland should also be assessed in these patients to rule out the presence of a lesion causing the precocious puberty.

PATHOLOGY OF THE PEDIATRIC OVARY

The development of the ovary begins in the fetal gestational period and continues during childhood. The growth process is dynamic. The neonatal ovaries are similar in function and anatomy to the pubertal and adult ovaries. Only the more common pathologies of the pelvis will be presented, including the ovarian cyst, ovarian torsion, and ovarian teratoma development (Table 28-3).

The typical neonatal and infant ovary is heterogeneous and cystic on ultrasound. Most cysts are less than 9 mm in diameter, with the mean diameter of the largest cyst measuring 7.5 mm. Ovarian cysts develop from ovarian follicles. The difference between a pathologic

TABLE 28-3	Common Neonatal Pathologic Conditions		
Female Pelvis			
	Clinical Findings	**Sonographic Findings**	**Differential Diagnosis**
Ovarian cyst	Asymptomatic palpable mass; complications include hemorrhage or torsion	Anechoic well-defined borders Internal echoes with hemorrhage	Mesenteric or duplication cyst Hydrometrocolpos Cystic meconium peritonitis Urachal cysts Anterior meningocele
Ovarian torsion	Severe abdominal pain	Enlarged ovary Fluid in cul-de-sac Fluid/debris secondary to hemorrhage	Appendicitis Gastroenteritis Pyelonephritis Pelvic inflammatory disease
Ovarian teratomas	Asymptomatic; increased size of tumor may cause abdominal pain or distention	Central complex/cystic cavity with debris Dermal plug Fat-fluid levels Calcifications	Appendicitis
Male Pelvis			
	Clinical Findings	**Sonographic Findings**	**Differential Diagnosis**
Epididymitis	Scrotal swelling, pain	Doppler shows increased flow	Torsion
Testicular torsion	Acute pain, swelling	Doppler shows absence of flow; compare to contralateral testis.	Epididymitis
		After 4 to 6 hours the testis becomes hypoechoic from swelling and edema.	
		If spermatic cord is torsed, the epididymis may become hypoechoic with a reactive hydrocele and skin thickening	

cyst and a physiologic mature follicle is primarily size; cysts larger than 2 cm are considered pathologic.

Factors that contribute to the follicular growth in utero include follicle-stimulating hormone (FSH), maternal estrogens, and human chorionic gonadotropin (hCG). The primary stimulus is FSH. This hormone is secreted by the pituitary gland and causes the increase in both the number and size of the small follicles. During the third trimester, the other hormones contribute to further follicular growth. At birth, the maternal estrogens and hCG levels fall with the separation of the placenta from the neonate. FSH levels decline secondary to the inhibitory mechanism of the hypothalamus pituitary ovary axis.

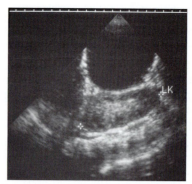

FIGURE 28-9 Sagittal image of the neonatal abdomen shows a large, well-defined anechoic structure anterior to the right kidney and inferior to the liver. This proved to be an ovarian cyst.

Neonatal Ovarian Cysts

The origin of the neonatal cyst may be the result of disordered folliculogenesis occurring in the fetal ovary. Most fetal cysts resolve spontaneously, but they may persist into the neonatal period. Small follicular cysts of 3 to 7 mm are a common and normal finding in neonatal ovaries. Pathologic evaluation of the cysts reveals follicular, corpus luteum, and theca lutein cysts. Their development may be the result of excessive stimulation of the fetal ovary by both placental and maternal hormones. There is a higher incidence of larger ovarian cysts in infants of mothers with toxemia, diabetes, and Rh isoimmunization, all of which are associated with a greater than normal release of placental chorionic gonadotropin.

Follicular cysts have been described in maternal and congenital hypothyroidism. Nonspecific pituitary glycoprotein hormone synthesis has been cited as the explanation for the follicular cysts seen in patients with juvenile hypothyroidism.

Complications. Most ovarian cysts regress spontaneously, but if they persist, complications may arise. The most common primary complications are hemorrhage and salpingotorsion. Torsion is more common in the larger cysts; clinically, patients present with pain, vomiting, fever, abdominal distention, leukocytosis, and peritonitis.

Hemorrhage may result from torsion or may occur spontaneously in a nontwisted cyst. If rupture occurs, hemorrhagic ascites, or peritonitis may be seen.

If the cyst is large, complications such as bowel obstruction, thorax compression with pulmonary hypoplasia, urinary tract obstruction, or incarceration with an inguinal hernia may occur.

Sonographic Findings. As discussed previously, the size of the ovarian cyst varies greatly with the larger cysts occupying nearly the entire abdomen, thus compressing the normal organs (Figure 28-9). The cyst may appear to be completely anechoic with well-defined borders or have internal echoes, if hemorrhage has occurred. The complicated cyst may contain fluid-debris level, a

retracting clot, or septa, or it may be completely filled with echoes producing a solid masslike appearance.

Differential Considerations. Sonography is able to characterize the mass, but the diagnosis must be confirmed histologically with a biopsy specimen. It may be difficult to separate an ovarian cyst from a mesenteric or enteric duplication cyst if the cyst is large and the normal ovary becomes displaced or distorted. Other abnormalities that should be considered include hydrometrocolpos, cystic meconium peritonitis, urachal cysts, and anterior meningocele. Neoplastic lesions, such as cystadenoma, cystic teratomas, and granulosa cell tumors, are rare in the neonate.

Ovarian Torsion

Torsion of the ovary may occur at any age, from the neonate to the adult. Most torsion problems, however, occur within the first two decades of life. The normal adnexa in young girls may be mobile, allowing torsion at the mesosalpinx with changes in intraabdominal pressure or body position. The ovary is extrapelvic in the neonate and infant, whereas in the older child the mass may be in the adnexal area. Torsion occurs more commonly when ovarian cysts or tumors are present. Torsion of the ovary and fallopian tube results from partial or complete rotation of the ovary on its vascular pedicle. This rotation compromises both arterial and venous flow, causing congestion of the ovarian parenchyma and, ultimately, hemorrhagic infarction.

Clinical symptoms include the severe onset of abdominal pain. In the infant this symptom may go unrecognized, which in turn may lead to necrosis of the ovary if surgical intervention is not performed quickly. Other causes of lower abdominal pain include appendicitis, gastroenteritis, pyelonephritis, or pelvic inflammatory disease.

Sonographic Findings. Sonographic findings may be nonspecific but may show enlargement of the affected ovary (Figure 28-10), fluid in the cul-de-sac, and other adnexal pathologic findings, such as cyst or tumor. A

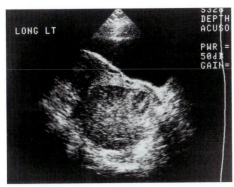

FIGURE 28-10 Sagittal image of an adolescent girl who presented with a severe onset of lower abdominal pain. The enlarged left ovary was shown just posterior to the distended urinary bladder. Color Doppler showed decreased flow around the ovary.

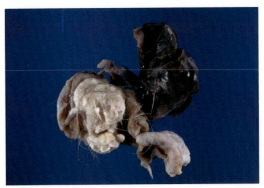

FIGURE 28-11 Gross pathology of a dermoid tumor filled with sebaceous debris representing teeth and fat.

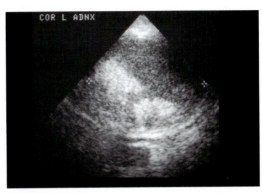

FIGURE 28-12 Transvaginal image of the dermoid tumor seen in a teenage girl. The tumor is filled with bright echogenic material representing the fat, bone, and teeth.

predominantly cystic or complex adnexal mass with a fluid-debris level or septa correlates with pathologic evidence of ovarian hemorrhage or infarction. The demonstration of multiple prominent follicles (greater than 8 to 12 mm) in the cortical (peripheral) portion of a unilaterally enlarged ovary has been reported as a specific sonographic sign of torsion. Color Doppler was not specific as the arterial blood flow was variable, depending on the extent of the torsion (complete or incomplete). Fluid in the cul-de-sac was found in the late manifestation of ovarian torsion.

If the ovary shows torsion and subsequent amputation, the ovary is seen to detach from the adnexa and migrate to the other sites in the abdomen. This mass is pedunculated with mesentery and omentum within the pedicle. Eventually these masses calcify and may be seen on a radiograph later in life.

Ovarian Teratomas

Ovarian tumors are uncommon in the neonate and adolescent. When found, germ cell tumors account for 60% of ovarian neoplasms in patients younger than 20 years of age. The spectrum of germ cell tumors ranges from benign mature teratomas to the malignant varieties, which include the dysgerminomas, embryonal carcinomas, endodermal sinus tumors, immature teratomas, choriocarcinomas, and mixed tumors. The most common pediatric germ cell tumor is the benign mature teratoma or dermoid cyst.

Benign teratomas have a wide spectrum of sonographic characteristics. They can have a central cystic cavity filled with sebaceous debris that is surrounded by a variety of skin appendages, a squamous epithelial layer, and a thick capsule (Figure 28-11). A nubbin of tissue, called the dermal plug or mural nodule, is frequently found in the wall of a teratoma. Other findings may include a solid or complex mass with fat-fluid levels, hair-fluid levels, and calcification. Most dermoid tumors range between 5 and 15 cm in size.

Clinically, most patients with a dermoid tumor are asymptomatic. When the tumor becomes large, abdominal pain or distention may occur. The most frequent complication of a teratoma is torsion, which may occur in 16% to 40% of cases. The pain may mimic appendicitis if located on the right side of the abdomen.

Sonographic Findings. Sonography recognizes the dermoid tumor as a complex mass with a heterogeneous appearance (Figure 28-12). Mural nodules and echogenic foci with acoustic shadowing are typical findings on ultrasound. In the neonatal period, less shadowing is seen in the lesion than is evident when a lesion is observed in adolescent girls.

THE SCROTUM

The examination of the neonatal scrotum should be made with a high-frequency linear array transducer to obtain the best resolution and widest field of view. The pediatric scrotum may be evaluated with the high-frequency curvilinear array transducer. The scrotum should be carefully palpated to detect any abnormalities in the scrotal parenchyma. As in the adult, a small towel may be placed vertically between the legs, under the scrotal sac to elevate and immobilize the testes. If the scrotum is red and painful, the stand-off pad may be used to avoid touching the sensitive area. The sonographer should examine both testes with sonography to compare the volume and echogenicity to one another. Routine color Doppler should be performed to detect the low-velocity and low-volume blood flow that is usually seen in the scrotum. Careful adjustment of Doppler controls should be made to eliminate background noise and look for the low-velocity flow patterns that can be confirmed by pulsed Doppler spectral evaluation.

The Prostate

The prostate in the young boy is more ellipsoid in shape than the conical shape seen in the adult male. The echogenicity of the gland is hypoechoic and homogeneous. The same formula may be used to calculate the volume as is used for the ovary:

$$\text{Volume in cubic centimeters} = \text{Length} \times \text{Height} \times \text{Width} \times 0.523$$

The normal volume of the prostate for boys 7 months to 13 years ranges between 0.4 mL and 5.2 mL. The seminal vesicles may be identified on the transverse plane

as small, hypoechoic structures giving the appearance similar to wings of a seagull.

EMBRYOLOGY OF THE MALE GENITAL TRACT

The fetal testes produce androgens that cause the masculinization of the external genitalia. The phallus elongates to form the penis (Figure 28-13). This sonographic finding is known as the "**turtle**" **sign** in obstetric sonography. The urogenital folds fuse on the ventral surface of the penis to form the spongy urethra. The labioscrotal swellings grow toward the median plane and fuse to form the scrotum. The line of fusion of the labioscrotal folds is called the scrotal raphe.

NORMAL SONOGRAPHIC APPEARANCE OF THE SCROTUM

The normal scrotal sac contains two testes that appear homogeneous with low- to medium-level echogenicity (Figure 28-14). They are usually spherical or oval in shape with a diameter of 7 to 10 mm. The echogenic line

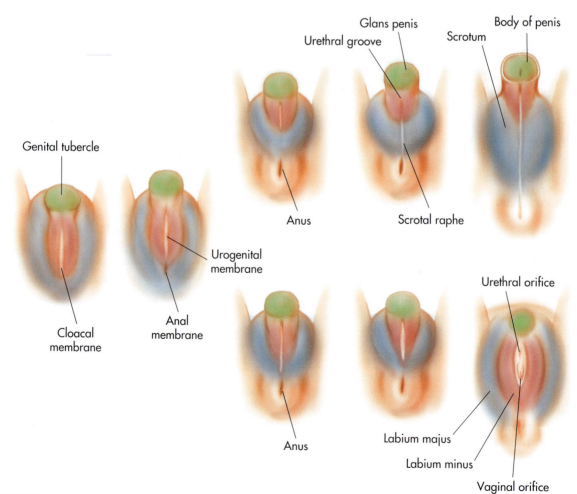

FIGURE 28-13 Sexual characteristics begin to develop during the 9th week and are fully differentiated by the 12th week.

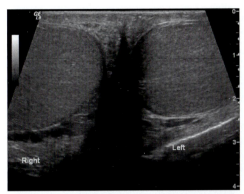

FIGURE 28-14 Transverse sonographic imaged in a normal patient demonstrating both testes to compare the size, echogenicity, and texture.

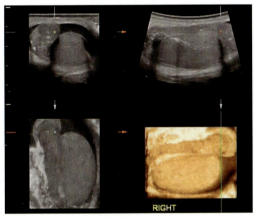

FIGURE 28-15 Three-dimensional rendering of the testis and epididymis. A small hydrocele is surrounding the testis.

of the mediastinum testis and the epididymis are usually not seen in the neonate but will be seen after puberty. After puberty the testis measures 3 to 5 cm in length and 2 to 3 cm in depth and width. The normal volume of the neonate and infant is approximately 1 cm³. The tunica albuginea is imaged as a thin echogenic line surrounding the testis. The intratesticular vessels may occasionally be seen as a hypoechoic linear band that fills in with color Doppler. In the very small neonate and infant, the flow velocity may be so small and so low that it may be difficult to record with color Doppler. The most reliable patency of the testicular artery is made when the Doppler sample volume is placed in the center of the testis. When seen, the flow should be symmetrical in both testes. Care should be made to have proper Doppler controls set to record the low flow by making sure the wall filter is not too high, that the gains are not set too low, that the pulse repetition frequency (PRF) is set correctly, and that the proper transducer frequency is used. Power Doppler may eliminate some of these pitfalls.

The epididymis is seen along the posterior lateral aspect of the testis. The epididymal head is triangular in shape and is isoechoic to slightly hyperechoic when compared with the testis (Figure 28-15). The body of the epididymis is isoechoic or slightly hypoechoic to the testis. It is more difficult to image the tail of the epididymis unless it is surrounded by fluid such as a hydrocele. There is no visible flow in the epididymis until after puberty.

CONGENITAL ABNORMALITIES OF THE SCROTUM

Cryptorchidism

Between the 25th and 32nd gestational weeks, the testis descends via the inguinal canal into the scrotum. The testes should be located within the scrotal sac at birth or by 6 weeks after birth. A small percentage of male infants have undescended testes. The testicular descent continues during the first year of life, so that by the end of the first year, only less than 0.8% of infants have true **cryptorchidism**, and in 10% to 25% it is bilateral. The malpositioned testis may lie anywhere in the pelvis, although most are found at or below the inguinal canal (Figure 28-16). The localization of the undescended testis is important because cryptorchidism is associated with increased risks of malignancy, infertility, and torsion. The bilateral absence of testes is **anorchidism**, whereas **monorchidism** is the absence of one testis (usually the left testis).

SCROTAL PATHOLOGY

Acute Scrotal Pain

The most common causes of acute pain and swelling in the pediatric male patient include testicular torsion, epididymitis (with or without orchitis), torsion of the testicular appendages, testicular traumas, acute hydrocele, and incarcerated hernia.

Testicular Torsion and Epididymitis. Testicular torsion and epididymitis are the two most common causes of the acute scrotum in the male neonate, infant, and adolescent patient. It is important to distinguish the two abnormalities, as torsion is a surgical emergency and epididymitis is medically treated. Doppler is the key factor in determining the presence or absence of flow within the testicle. Torsion will show an absence of flow in the affected testes, whereas epididymitis will have increased flow. Intermittent or incomplete torsion may present a varying flow pattern, but one that is diminished as compared to the normal contralateral testicular flow pattern.

The sonographic findings in testicular torsion may show the testis to be normal in echogenicity early, but after 4 to 6 hours the testis becomes hypoechoic from swelling and edema. After 24 hours the testis becomes heterogeneous secondary to hemorrhage and infarction. If the spermatic cord is torsed, the epididymis may become hypoechoic with a reactive hydrocele and skin

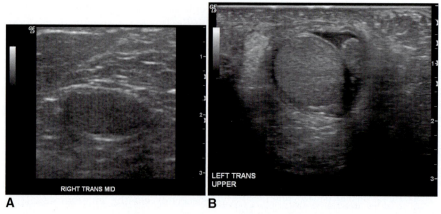

FIGURE 28-16 Undescended right testicle **(A)** with normal left testicle **(B)**. The undescended testis is smaller and hypoechoic compared with the normal left testis. The right testicle was located within the right inguinal canal.

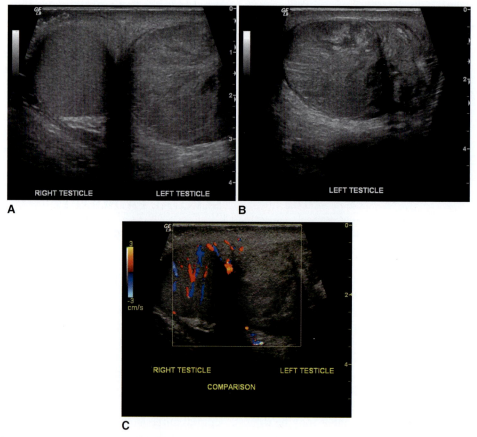

FIGURE 28-17 Left spermatic cord torsion in adolescent with a history of scrotal pain of a duration greater than 24 hours. **A**, Transverse image showing both testes. The left testis is enlarged and heterogeneous. **B**, Sagittal image of the left testis. The infracted testis has a mixed echo pattern caused by the hemorrhage, necrosis, and vascular congestion associated with spermatic cord torsion exceeding 24 hours. **C**, Transverse color Doppler image showing normal perfusion to the right testis with absence of detectable signal on the left side. Paratesticular blood flow is increased around the abnormal testis.

thickening. The spermatic cord may be seen as twisted and enlarged (Figure 28-17).

Color Doppler usually shows decreased or absent flow in the affected testes. If the torsion is incomplete, the flow is normal or slightly decreased. In epididymitis, there is increased flow in the epididymis with extension into the testes if the infection has spread to this area. Ischemia may cause decreased flow in the area.

Scrotal Masses

Sonography has become an important imaging modality in the detection of scrotal masses in the young male patient. Sonography is able to distinguish between an intratesticular and extratesticular mass, which is significant because intratesticular masses are malignant and extratesticular masses are benign (Figure 28-18). It is

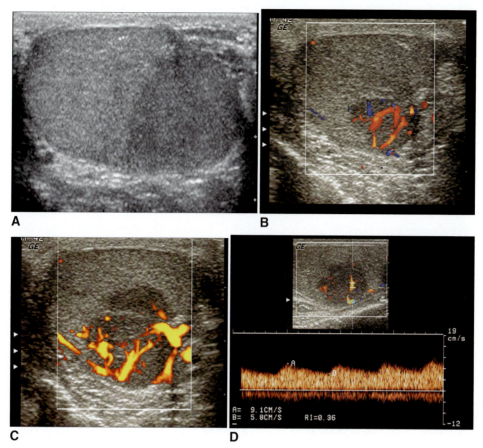

FIGURE 28-18 Germ cell tumor. **A,** Transverse image shows heterogeneous echo texture throughout the testis. The tumor is primarily hypoechoic. **B,** Color Doppler shows distortion of the normal vessel architecture within the testis. Increased flow is seen within the mass. **C,** Power Doppler clearly shows the distorted vasculature of the testis within the mass. **D,** Spectral Doppler waveforms obtained within the mass show low resistance with prominent end diastolic velocities characteristic of tumor flow.

important to note that 80% of the testicular tumors are malignant. In the pediatric age group, there are two peak incidences of testicular tumors: in children under 3 years of age, the incidence of malignancy in a cryptorchid testis is increased (seminomas [malignant] and gonadoblastomas [benign] may be found). In childhood, testicular tumors are rare (less than 1% of all childhood neoplasms and 2% for solid malignant tumors). The reader is referred to Chapter 23 for further discussion of such lesions.

The Neonatal Hip

Sandra L. Hagen-Ansert

OBJECTIVES

On completion of this chapter, you should be able to:
- Discuss anatomy of the neonatal hip
- Describe normal movements of the hip
- Describe sonographic evaluation of the neonatal hip, including technique and protocol
- Describe the normal sonographic appearance of the neonatal hip

- Describe the sonographic evaluation of the neonatal hip for developmental displacement of the hip
- Define the Barlow and Ortolani maneuvers
- Differentiate between subluxation of the hip and dislocation of the hip

OUTLINE

Sonographic evaluation of the neonatal hip has received wide clinical acceptance in the diagnosis and management of developmental dysplasia of the hip. There are two conditions for which sonography offers advantages over other imaging modalities: (1) developmental dislocation or dysplasia of the hip, which is seen in the first year of life, and (2) hip pain, which may be caused by inflammatory or traumatic conditions.

To determine if sonography of the neonatal hip is indicated, do the following:

- Rule out developmental displacement of the hip.
- Check for septic arthritis or joint effusion.
- Check for proximal focal femoral deficiency.

ANATOMY OF THE HIP

The anatomy of the upper leg consists of many parts, including bones and joints, nerves, arteries, superficial veins, and muscles (Figure 29-1). The thigh is the upper part of the lower extremity. The anterior surface of the thigh is continuous with the inguinal region of the abdomen. The posterior surface of the thigh is inferior to the gluteal region, which is at the back of the pelvis and hip joint.

Bones and Joints

The sacroiliac joints unite the two hip bones with the sacral part of the vertebral column. The pubic symphysis is where the two hip bones unite with each other anteriorly.

The hip bones are the fusion of three separate bones: the ilium, ischium, and pubis. Together they form the **pelvic girdle**. The bone of the upper thigh is the femur. The femur is surrounded by muscles, ligaments, and tendons. The upper part of the femur, the head, articulates with the hip bone to make the hip joint.

Femoral Artery

The femoral artery is the principal artery of the upper thigh. This artery is a continuation of the external iliac

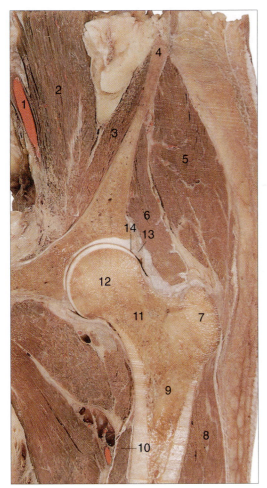

FIGURE 29-1 Coronal section, looking from the front toward the back.
1. External iliac artery
2. Psoas major
3. Iliacus
4. Iliac crest
5. Gluteus medius
6. Gluteus minimus
7. Greater trochanter
8. Vastus lateralis
9. Shaft of femur
10. Vastus medialis
11. Neck of femur
12. Head of femur
13. Acetabular labrum
14. Rim of acetabulum

artery and enters the thigh beneath the inguinal ligament. The femoral artery branches into the profunda femoris artery, which is the main artery supply for the thigh muscles.

Sciatic Nerve

The sciatic nerve is the largest nerve in the upper thigh. This nerve enters the gluteal region from the pelvis to run caudally down the back of the thigh.

Fascia Lata

The deep fascia of the thigh, the **fascia lata**, forms a tough connective tissue surrounding the muscles. The part of the fascia on the lateral part of the thigh is the iliotibial tract as it extends from the iliac crest to the lateral condyle of the tibia. The **saphenous opening** is a gap in the fascia lata that is found about 4 cm inferior and lateral to the pubic tubercle. The great saphenous vein passes through the saphenous opening to enter the femoral vein.

Muscles

The muscles of the thigh fall into three categories: anterior or extensor, medial or adductor, and posterior or hamstring (Table 29-1).

Femoral Triangle

The **femoral triangle** describes a region at the front of the upper thigh, just below the inguinal ligament. The inguinal ligament forms one side of the triangle, whereas the other two sides are formed by adductor longus (medially) and sartorius (laterally) (see Figure 29-1). The contents of the femoral triangle include the femoral canal, femoral vein and artery, and femoral nerve. The femoral vein and artery and the femoral canal are enclosed in a connective tissue sleeve called the femoral sheath.

The contents of the femoral triangle are separated from the more deeply lying hip joint by muscles; the pectineus is medial and the iliacus is lateral. In the middle is the psoas major muscle (found at the middle of the head of the femur). The psoas major becomes tendinous and separates the femoral artery from the capsule of the joint at this point.

Gluteal Region

The gluteal region (buttock) extends from the iliac crest to the gluteal fold and from the midline over the sacrum to the greater trochanter of the femur (Figure 29-2). It includes the area at the back of the hip joint. The large gluteus maximus muscle overlies other muscles superior and posterior to the hip joint. The gluteus maximus is a powerful extensor of the hip.

The gluteus medius and gluteus minimus pass from the outer surface of the hip bone to the greater trochanter. Together they act as abductors of the hip joint. Their most important function is to prevent adduction and keep the pelvis level during walking.

The tensor fasciae latae is a smaller muscle arising from the outer, front part of the iliac crest. The tensor fasciae latae is inserted into the iliotibial tract of the fascia lata. With this attachment, it assists the gluteus maximus with extension of the knee.

Below the lower borders of the gluteus medius and minimus the following muscles are found: piriformis, obturator externus with the gemelli at its upper and lower borders, and quadratus femoris (see Figure 29-2). The **sciatic nerve** and most other structures that leave the pelvis to enter the gluteal region do so by passing under the border of the piriformis. Together, these muscles act as a lateral rotator of the femur.

Hip Joint

The articulation of the head of the femur with the acetabulum of the hip bone forms the **hip joint** (Figure 29-3). The joint is not directly palpable because it is surrounded and protected by muscles of the upper thigh. The greater trochanter of the femur forms a palpable knob at the side of the region. The psoas tendon crosses the center of the hip joint just inferior to the inguinal ligament at the top of the femoral triangle. The pectineus muscle is medial to the tendon. The femoral vein and canal are anterior to the pectineus muscle. Lateral to the tendon is the iliacus muscle, with the femoral nerve anterior. The gluteus minimus muscle is the immediate cover for the upper part of the hip joint, whereas the obturator externus is found winding below it from front to back. The piriformis muscle is immediately posterior

TABLE 29-1	Muscles	
Muscle Group	**Supplied By**	**Muscles**
Anterior compartment/extensor muscles (front of thigh)	Femoral nerve	**Quadriceps femoris** (rectus femoris plus three vastus muscles)—insert into patella, which is attached to patellar ligament • The vastus muscles arise from the femur • The rectus femoris arises from the hip bone above the acetabulum—acts as a flexor of the hip and extensor of the knee **Sartorius** muscle with longest fibers in the body, crosses the front of the thigh obliquely from the anterior superior iliac spine laterally to the upper medial side of the tibia
Medial compartment/adductor muscles (inner thigh)	Obturator nerve	**Adductor longus** muscle **Adductor magnus** muscle
Posterior compartment/hamstring muscles	Sciatic nerve	**Biceps femoris**—outer hamstring **Vastus lateralis**—part of quadriceps

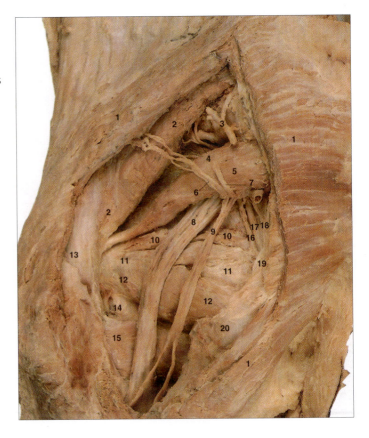

FIGURE 29-2 Left gluteal region (after most of the gluteus muscle and all veins have been removed).
1. Gluteus maximus
2. Gluteus medius
3. Superior gluteal artery
4. Superior gluteal nerve
5. Piriformis
6. Inferior gluteal nerve
7. Inferior gluteal artery
8. Sciatic nerve
9. Posterior femoral cutaneous nerve
10. Superior gemellus
11. Obturator internus
12. Inferior gemellus
13. Greater trochanter
14. Obturator externus
15. Quadratus femoris
16. Nerve to obturator internus (11)
17. Internal pudendal artery
18. Pudendal nerve
19. Sacrotuberous ligament
20. Ischial tuberosity

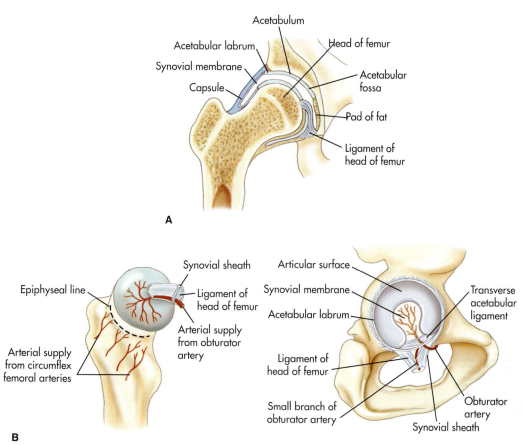

FIGURE 29-3 Coronal section of the right hip joint **(A)** and articular surfaces of the right hip joint and arterial supply of the head of the femur **(B)**.

to the joint, whereas the obturator internus and the gemelli and quadratus femoris are lower down (see Figure 29-2).

Bones of the Hip Joint. The rounded shape of the femur and the cup shape of the acetabulum form the "ball and socket" hip joint (see Figure 29-3). The acetabulum is made deeper by a rim of fibrocartilage called the *acetabular labrum*. The bony deficiency at the lower part of the acetabulum (acetabular notch) is covered by a band of fibrous tissue called the *transverse ligament*. From this point, a rounded ligament (ligament teres) passes upward inside the joint to be attached to the pit or fovea in the head. In the younger child, this ligament contains an artery to supply the femoral head. The artery usually disintegrates by 7 years of age.

Ligaments of the Hip Joint. The hip joint is surrounded by a tough capsule. Anteriorly to the femur, it is attached to the intertrochanteric line (Figure 29-4). Posteriorly, it does extend as far as the intertrochanteric crest but only to halfway along the neck of the femur (Figure 29-5). Therefore, the posterior part of the neck is inside the capsule (intracapsular), and part of the neck is outside it (extracapsular).

The outside of the capsule is reinforced by ligaments. The most important is the iliofemoral ligament, which blends with the front of the capsule (see Figure 29-1).

This ligament is the shape of an inverted "Y" or "V" passing from the anterior inferior iliac spine to each end of the intertrochanteric line. It is one of the strongest ligaments in the body and is very important for standing and maintaining correct upright balance.

Movements of the Hip

The movements of the hip are somewhat limited in range because of the tight fit between the femur and acetabulum and because the hip bone is immobile (Figure 29-6). Following are the hip movements and their actions:

1. Flexion—bending forward
2. Extension—bending backward
3. **Abduction**—moving sideways outward
4. **Adduction**—moving sideways inward
5. Medial rotation
6. Lateral rotation

The primary flexors of the hip are the psoas major, iliacus, and rectus femoris. Extension is limited to 20 degrees by tension in the iliofemoral ligament and the flexor muscles, and it is brought about by the hamstrings and gluteus maximus.

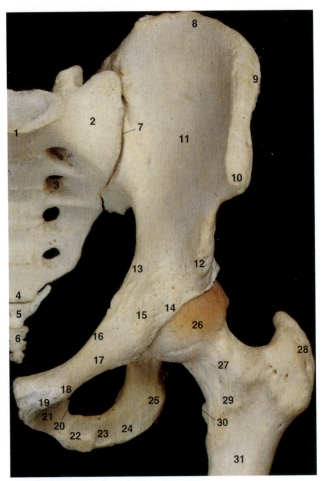

FIGURE 29-4 Anterior view of left hip bone and femur, with sacrum and coccyx.

1. Sacral promontory
2. Ala of sacrum
3. Second anterior sacral foramen
4. Apex of sacrum
5. First coccygeal vertebra, with transverse process
6. Fused coccygeal vertebrae
7. Sacroiliac joint
8. Iliac crest
9. Tubercle of iliac crest
10. Anterior superior iliac spine
11. Iliac fossa
12. Anterior inferior iliac spine
13. Arcuate line of ilium
14. Rim of acetabulum
15. Iliopubic eminence
16. Pectineal line (pectin) of pubis
17. Superior ramus of pubis
18. Pubic tubercle
19. Pubic crest
20. Obturator foramen
21. Body of pubis
22. Inferior ramus of pubis
23. Site of union of pubic and ischial rami (22 and 24)
24. Ramus of ischium
25. Ischial tuberosity
26. Head of femur
27. Neck
28. Greater trochanter
29. Intertrochanteric line
30. Tip of lesser trochanter
31. Shaft of femur

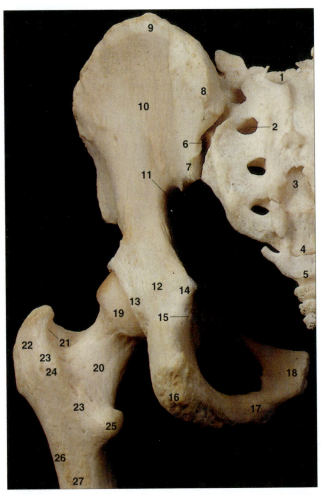

FIGURE 29-5 Posterior view of left hip bone and femur with sacrum and coccyx.

An example of hip adduction is crossing your legs when in a seated position, an action performed by the adductor group of muscles. In abduction, the limbs are opened by the gluteus medius and minimus muscles. The more important function of these muscles, however, is to prevent adduction, which is the function they perform during walking.

Recall that the head and shaft of the femur lie at an angle to one another (about 120 degrees), and the axis about which rotation movements take place is not along the line of the shaft of the femur but along a line drawn from the head of the femur to the lower end of the bone between the condyles. Medial and lateral rotation is related to this principle. When the trochanter moves forward, the femur rotates medially, and when the trochanter moves backward, the femur rotates laterally. Thus, the medial rotators are the anterior fibers of gluteus medius and minimus. The lateral rotators are the small muscles at the back of the joint—piriformis, obturator internus, and quadratus femoris, with assistance of the gluteus maximus.

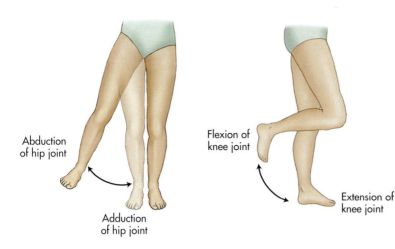

Abduction
of hip joint

Adduction
of hip joint

Flexion of
knee joint

Extension of
knee joint

FIGURE 29-6 Anatomic terms used in relation to movement of the hip.

SONOGRAPHIC EVALUATION OF THE HIP

Sonography has the advantage over conventional radiography in imaging the fine detail of the neonatal hip. The cartilaginous femoral head, the cartilaginous acetabular rim, and labrum are clearly visible with sonography. The size, shape, and position of the femoral head can be assessed sonographically well before the bones are ossified enough to be seen on radiography. The motion of the femoral head in the acetabulum under stress can also be tested. The shape of the acetabulum can be evaluated. With sonography, the morphologic development of the cartilaginous and bony acetabulum, labrum, and femoral head; the degree to which the femoral head is covered by the labrum; and the position of the femoral head in the acetabulum at rest are assessed during motion and stress.

Indications for neonatal hip sonography include the presence of risk factors for **developmental displacement of the hip (DDH)**, an abnormal hip examination, and the need to evaluate the response to treatment.

Sonography can be performed until the femoral head ossifies. Ossification of the femoral head begins between 2 and 8 months of age, occurs earlier in girls than boys, and is often complete by 1 year of age. Once the femoral head is completely ossified, it is difficult to obtain adequate sonographic images because of beam artifact interference.

Sonographic Technique

Sonography of the neonatal hip is performed with a high-frequency linear-array transducer. For average-weight neonates up to 3 months of age, a high-frequency transducer of at least 7.5 MHz is used. Infants 3 to 7 months may be imaged with a 5.0-MHz transducer; and after 7 months, a 3-MHz transducer can be used. The premature infant may be imaged with a 12-MHz transducer.

To achieve a satisfactory examination, the infant should be relaxed and as comfortable as possible. Feeding before or during the examination helps to soothe the infant. Make sure the room is warm and keep blankets close for warmth. Toys and other distractions help to quiet the infant so the examination may be performed. Parental assistance is often helpful, with the mother or father sitting on the bed or next to the infant to help keep the infant calm.

The primary sonographic imaging is performed from the lateral or posterolateral aspect of the hip while moving the hip from the neutral position at rest into one in which the hip is flexed. The infant is lying in the supine position with the feet toward the sonographer. The transducer is shifted from the right to the left hand when examining each hip; the right hip is examined with the transducer in the sonographer's left hand and the left hip is examined with the transducer in the right hand.

Sonographically the femoral head is hypoechoic because it is cartilaginous and contains a focal echogenic ossification nucleus (Figure 29-7). The femoral head sits within the acetabulum, which is echogenic and has a deep concave configuration. Two thirds of the head should be covered by the labrum. The labrum is narrow and has a triangular shape. The labrum is composed of hyaline cartilage and is hypoechoic, except at its tip, which is echogenic due to its fibrous content. The femoral head should be stable within the acetabulum with stress after 4 weeks of age. During the neonatal period (the first 4 weeks of life), there is physiologic laxity of the ligaments about the hip that makes the hip unstable.

Throughout the examination, the sonographer is able to assess the position and stability of the femoral head in addition to assessing the development of the acetabulum. In the normal infant, the femoral head is congruently positioned within the acetabulum. Mild displacement, **subluxation**, is when the head is either in contact with part of the acetabulum or is displaced, but partly covered. On the other hand, a *dislocated* hip has

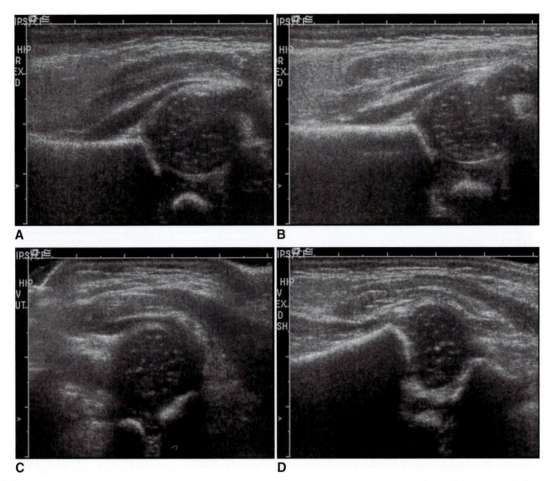

FIGURE 29-7 Normal ultrasound images of the neonatal hip. **A,** Right hip coronal: flexion/abduction. **B,** Left hip coronal: flexion/abduction. **C,** Right hip transverse: neutral. **D,** Right hip transverse: flexion/adduction/push.

TABLE 29-2	Dynamic Sonography Classification of the Hip			
View and Maneuver	**Normal**	**Laxity with Stress (Subluxable)**	**Subluxed**	**Dislocatable/Dislocated**
Coronal/neutral	N	N	A	A
Coronal/flexion	N	N	A	A
Coronal/flexion (posterior lip) No stress-piston stress	N	N-A	A	A
Transverse/flexion Abduction-adduction	N	N-A	N-A	A
Transverse/neural	N	N	A	A

A, Abnormal; *N,* normal.

no contact with or coverage by the acetabulum. The principle of treatment is that a subluxed hip in the neutral or rest position will seat itself with flexion and abduction.

The stability of the hip is determined through guided motion and the application of gentle stress. The stress maneuvers are the imaging counterparts of the clinical Barlow and Ortolani maneuvers. The Barlow test determines whether the hip can be dislocated. The Ortolani test determines the opposite if the dislocated hip can be reduced.

Sonographic Protocol

The basic hip anatomy is imaged in four different views: (1) coronal/neutral, (2) coronal/flexion, (3) transverse/flexion, and (4) transverse/neutral. A two-word combination is used to label the views according to the plane of the body (coronal or transverse) and the position of the hips (neutral or flexed). The primary objective of the dynamic hip assessment is to determine the position and stability of the femoral head and the development of the acetabulum (Table 29-2).

Coronal/Neutral View. This view is performed with the infant in the supine position from the lateral aspect of the hip joint, with the plane of the transducer oriented coronally with respect to the hip joint (Figure 29-8). The femur is stabilized with a physiologic amount of flexion. The plane must demonstrate the midportion of the acetabulum with the straight iliac line superiorly and the inferior tip of the os ilium medially within the acetabulum (Figure 29-9). The echogenic tip of the labrum should also be visualized. The alpha and beta angles may be measured from this view. A stability test can be performed in this view by gently pushing and pulling the infant's leg. This helps to verify deformity of the acetabulum and to identify craniodorsal movement of the femoral head under pressure (Table 29-3).

In the normal coronal/neutral view, the femoral head is resting against the bony acetabulum. The acetabular roof should have a concave configuration and cover at least half of the femoral head. The hypoechoic cartilage of the acetabular roof extends lateral to the acetabular lip, terminating in the echogenic labrum. When a hip

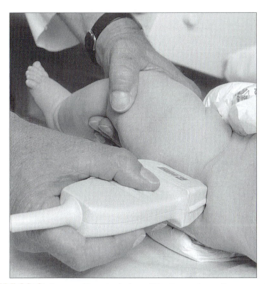

FIGURE 29-8 Coronal/neutral view. The transducer is coronal with respect to the hip. The femur is in physiologic neutral for the infant (slight hip flexion).

TABLE 29-3	Neonatal Hip Technique: Coronal/Neutral View
View: Coronal/Neutral	**Sonographic Findings**
Normal	• Femoral head rests against the bony acetabulum • Acetabular roof has concave configuration, covers half of femoral head • Hypoechoic cartilage acetabular roof extends lateral to the acetabular lip, terminates in echogenic labrum
Subluxed/dislocated	• Femoral head gradually migrates laterally and superiorly with decreased coverage of femoral head
Hip dysplasia	• Acetabular roof is irregular and angled • Labrum is defected superiorly; becomes echogenic and thickened
Frankly dislocated	• Labrum may be deformed

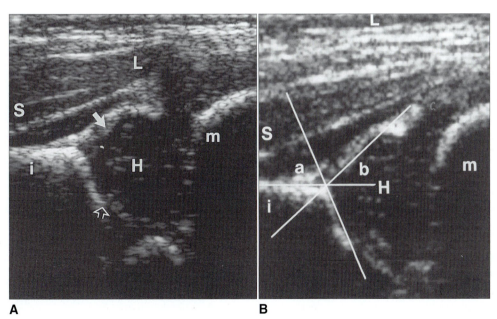

A   **B**

FIGURE 29-9 A, Normal hip sonogram shows sonolucent femoral head resting against the bony acetabulum. Note: Fibrocartilaginous tip of labrum *(solid arrow)* and junction of bony ilium and triradiate cartilage *(open arrow).* **B,** Normal hip sonograph with alpha, *a,* and beta, *b,* angles used in measurement. *H,* Femoral head; *L,* lateral; *S,* superior; *i,* iliac; *m,* femoral metaphysis.

becomes subluxed, or dislocated, the femoral head gradually migrates laterally and superiorly with progressively decreased coverage of the femoral head (Figure 29-10).

In hip dysplasia, the acetabular roof is irregular and angled, and the labrum is defected superiorly and becomes echogenic and thickened. When the hip is frankly dislocated, the labrum may be deformed. Echogenic soft tissue is interposed between the femoral head and the bony acetabulum. A combination of deformed labrum and fibrofatty tissue prevents the hip from being reduced.

The acetabulum may be assessed visually or with the alpha and beta angles, noting the depth and angulation of the acetabular roof, as well as the appearance of the labrum. This can be seen in both coronal/neutral and coronal/flexion views and described verbally. The classification of hip joints may also be based on the measurement of the alpha and beta angles. The alpha angle measures the inclination of the posterior and superior osseous acetabular rim with respect to the lateral margin of the iliac bone. The beta angle is formed by the baseline iliac bone and the inclination of the anterior cartilaginous acetabular roof, with the labrum the key landmark. The software available on ultrasound systems makes it possible to evaluate these angles.

Coronal/Flexion View. The transducer is maintained in the lateral position while the hip is moved into a 90-degree angle of flexion. The transducer is then moved in an anteroposterior direction with respect to the body to visualize the entire hip (Figure 29-11). The curvilinear

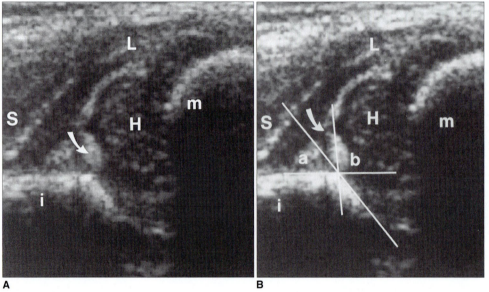

FIGURE 29-10 A, Dislocated hip sonogram shows displacement of femoral head laterally with deformity of labrum *(curved arrow)*. **B,** Dislocated hip sonogram with abnormal alpha *(a)* and beta *(b)* angles. *H,* Femoral head; *L,* lateral; *S,* superior, *i,* iliac line; *m,* femoral metaphysis.

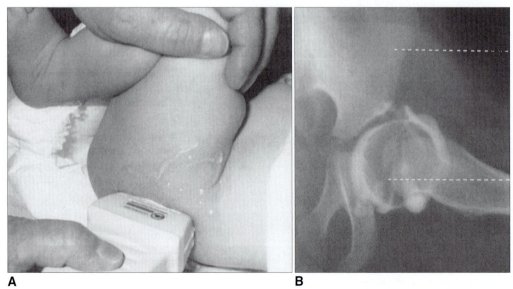

FIGURE 29-11 Coronal/flexion view. Transducer is coronal to flexed femur (A).

margin of the body femoral shaft is identified anterior to the femoral head. In the midportion of the acetabulum, the femoral head is surrounded by echoes from the bony acetabular components (Figure 29-12). Superiorly the lateral margin of the iliac bone is seen, and the transducer position should be adjusted so that it becomes a straight horizontal line. A normal hip gives the appearance of a "ball on a spoon" in the midacetabulum. The femoral head is the ball, the acetabulum forms the spoon, and the iliac line is the handle (Table 29-4). As the transducer is moved posteriorly, the scan plane is over the posterior margin of the acetabulum showing the posterior lip of the triradiate cartilage.

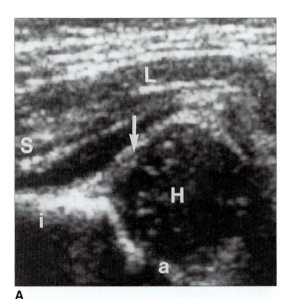

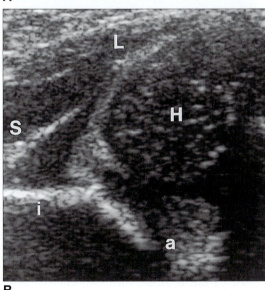

FIGURE 29-12 A, Normal coronal/flexion view is identified with femoral head resting against acetabulum. **B,** Dislocated hip shows soft tissue echoes in acetabulum that may prevent hip from being reduced without surgical intervention. *a,* Acetabulum; *H,* femoral head; *i,* iliac line; *L,* lateral; *S,* superior; *arrow,* labrum.

In subluxation, the femoral head is displaced laterally, posteriorly, or both, with respect to the acetabulum. Between the femoral head and the bony reflections soft tissue echoes from the medial acetabulum are seen. In dislocation, the femoral head is completely out of the acetabulum. With superior dislocations, the femoral head may rest against the iliac bone. In posterior dislocations, the femoral head is seen lateral to the posterior lip of the triradiate cartilage. The acetabulum is usually not visualized in a dislocation because the bony shaft of the femur blocks the view.

There are two components to this view. The first involves a "push and pull" maneuver. In many clinical sites, the pediatric orthopedist, the radiologist, or the experienced pediatric sonographer performs this examination. In the normal hip, the femoral head is never seen over the posterior lip of the acetabulum (Figure 29-13). When instability is present, a portion of the femoral head appears over the posterior lip of the triradiate cartilage as the femur is pushed. With a pull, the head disappears from the plane. In a dislocated hip, the femoral head may be located over the posterior lip and may or may not move out of the plane with traction.

The second component of the dynamic examination is performed over the midacetabulum. The **Barlow maneuver** is performed with adduction and gentle pushing against the knee (Figure 29-14). In the normal hip, the femoral head will remain in place against the acetabulum. With subluxation or dislocation, the head will migrate laterally and posteriorly, and there will be echogenic soft tissue between the femoral head and the acetabulum.

Transverse/Flexion View. In the transverse view, the transducer is rotated 90 degrees and moved posteriorly into a posterolateral position over the hip joint (Figure 29-15). The bony shaft of the femur gives off bright reflected echoes anteriorly, adjacent to the femoral head. The echoes from the bony acetabulum appear posteriorly to the femoral head, and in the normal hip, a "U" configuration is produced (Figure 29-16). The relationship of the femoral head to the acetabulum is observed during flexion of the hip from adduction to abduction. The deep "U" configuration is produced with maximum abduction; in adduction the "V" appearance is seen. Be careful that the transducer is posterior enough to image the medial acetabulum, or the hip may appear falsely displaced (Table 29-5).

The hip is then stressed with a gentle posterior push (Barlow maneuver). In the normal hip, the femoral head will remain deeply in the acetabulum in contact with the ischium with stress. In subluxation, the hip will be normally positioned or mildly displaced at rest and there will be further lateral displacement from the medial acetabulum with stress, but the femoral head will remain in contact with a portion of the ischium.

With **frank dislocation,** the hip will be laterally and posteriorly displaced to the extent that the femoral head has no contact with the acetabulum, and the normal "U"

TABLE 29-4	Neonatal Hip Technique: Coronal/Flexion View	
View: Coronal/Flexion	**Sonographic Findings**	**Maneuver Changes**
Normal	• Curvilinear margin of the body femoral shaft anterior to the femoral head • In midacetabulum, the femoral head is surrounded by echoes from the bony acetabular components • Superiorly seen is lateral margin of the iliac bone; transducer position adjusted to become straight horizontal line • A normal hip gives the appearance of a "ball on a spoon" in the midacetabulum	"Push and pull": The femoral head is never seen over the posterior lip of the acetabulum Barlow: Femoral head remains in place in acetabulum
Subluxed/dislocated	Subluxation: • Femoral head displaced laterally, posteriorly, or both, with respect to acetabulum • Soft-tissue echoes seen between femoral head and bony reflections from medial acetabulum Dislocation: • Femoral head completely out of acetabulum • With superior dislocations, femoral head may rest against iliac bone • In posterior dislocations, femoral head seen lateral to posterior lip of triradiate cartilage • Acetabulum not visualized in a dislocation	"Push and pull": Portion of femoral head appears over the posterior lip of the triradiate cartilage as femur is pushed; with pull, femur may or may not disappear from the plane Barlow: Head migrates laterally and posteriorly; echogenic soft tissue between femoral head and acetabulum

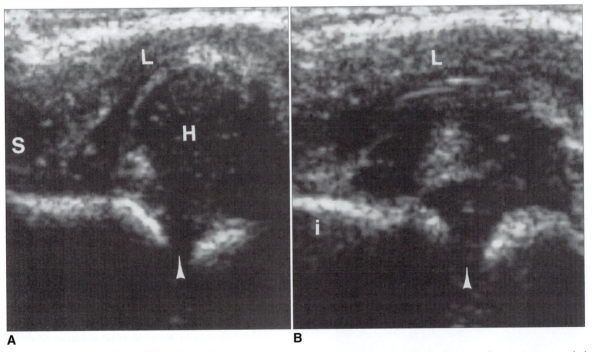

FIGURE 29-13 A, Push maneuver shows displacement of femoral head over posterior acetabular lip. **B,** Pull maneuver reveals head no longer positioned over triradiate cartilage *(arrowhead)* of posterior lip of acetabulum. *H,* Femoral head; *L,* lateral, *S,* superior line; *i,* iliac line.

configuration cannot be obtained (Figure 29-17). The process of dislocation and reduction can be visualized in unstable hips in the transverse/flexion view. With abduction, the dislocated hip may be reduced, and this represents the sonographic counterpart of the **Ortolani maneuver.**

Transverse/Neutral View. From the transverse/flexion view, the leg is brought down into a neutral position. The transducer is now horizontal to the acetabulum from the lateral aspect of the hip (Figure 29-18). The plane passes through the femoral head into the acetabulum at the center of the triradiate cartilage. The exam is

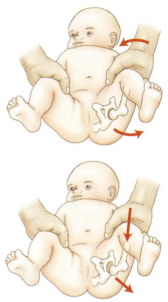

FIGURE 29-14 Barlow maneuver.

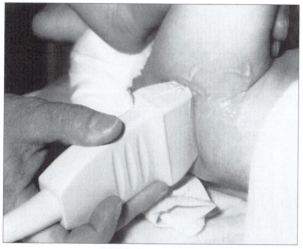

FIGURE 29-15 Transverse/flexion view. The transducer is in the axial plane posterolaterally over the hip joint with the hip flexed.

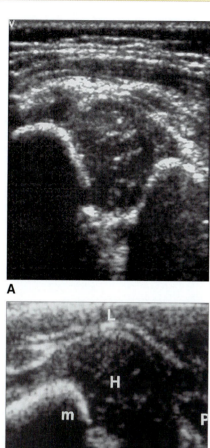

FIGURE 29-16 A, Normal transverse/flexion view shows "U"-shaped configuration that is not present in **(B)** dislocated hip. *H,* Femoral head; *i,* ischium; *m,* femoral metaphysic; *L,* lateral; *P,* posterior.

begun caudally over the bony shaft of the femur. Moving cephalad, the transition from bone to cartilage in the proximal femur becomes apparent, and the circular cross section of the spherical femoral head is identified (Table 29-6).

In the normal hip, the sonolucent femoral head is positioned against the bony acetabulum over the triradiate cartilage (see Figure 29-18, *B*). The images of the sonogram represent the parts of a flower. The femoral head is the flower; the echoes from the ischium posteriorly and pubis anteriorly represent the leaves at its base. The stem is formed by echoes that pass through the triradiate cartilage into the area of acoustic shadowing created by the osseous structures.

In this view, malpositioned hips show soft tissue echoes between the femoral head and acetabulum (see

Figure 29-18, *C*). The width and configuration of the gap depend on the nature of the displacement. With subluxation, the femoral head usually moves posteriorly and remains in contact with the posterior aspect of the acetabulum. With more severe cases, the lateral displacement accompanies posterior migration. Most dislocations are lateral, posterior, and superior.

PATHOLOGY OF THE NEONATAL HIP

Dislocation of the Hip

Neonatal hip dislocation can be acquired, teratogenic, or developmental. Acquired causes of hip dislocation can be traumatic or nontraumatic (i.e., neuromuscular diseases). Teratogenic dislocations occur in utero and are

TABLE 29-5	Neonatal Hip Technique: Transverse/Flexion View	
View: Transverse/Flexion	**Sonographic Findings**	**Maneuver Changes**
Normal	• Bony shaft of femur gives bright reflected echoes anteriorly, adjacent to the femoral head • Echoes from the bony acetabulum appear posteriorly to the femoral head, and in the normal hip, a "U" configuration is produced • Relationship of the femoral head to the acetabulum observed during flexion of hip from adduction to abduction • Deep "U" configuration produced with maximum abduction; in adduction the "V" appearance is seen	Barlow: Femoral head will remain deeply in the acetabulum in contact with the ischium with stress
Subluxed/dislocated	• Femoral head is displaced • "U" configuration of normal metaphysis and ischium is not seen	Subluxation: Hip normally positioned or mildly displaced at rest; further lateral displacement from medial acetabulum with stress, but femoral head will remain in contact with portion of ischium
Frankly dislocated	Hip will be laterally and posteriorly displaced to the extent that the femoral head has no contact with the acetabulum, and the normal "U" configuration cannot be obtained	

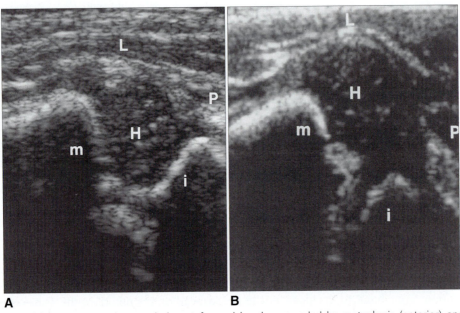

FIGURE 29-17 A, Normal hip sonogram shows echolucent femoral head surrounded by metaphysis (anterior) and ischium (posterior), forming a "U" around femoral head. **B,** Dislocated hip sonogram shows sonolucent femoral head displaced posterolaterally. The "U" configuration of normal metaphysis and ischium is not seen. *H,* Femoral head; *L,* lateral; *P,* posterior; *i,* ischium; *m,* metaphysis.

associated with neuromuscular disorders. Developmental dislocation of the hip was formerly known as *congenital hip dysplasia.* The term *congenital hip dysplasia* covered a wide spectrum of pathology that usually occurs after birth. Therefore, the term has been replaced by *developmental displacement of the hip (DDH).* This new term includes dysplastic, subluxated, dislocatable, and dislocated hips.

The sonographic appearance of the femoral head is described as normal, subluxed, or dislocated. Stability testing is reported as normal, lax, subluxable, dislocatable, and reducible or irreducible. Sonographic description of the acetabulum is assessed visually and is described as normal, immature, or dysplastic.

Developmental Displacement of the Hip

A displacement of the hip is a relatively common congenital abnormality and can be diagnosed in the early neonatal period. Before sonography, plain film

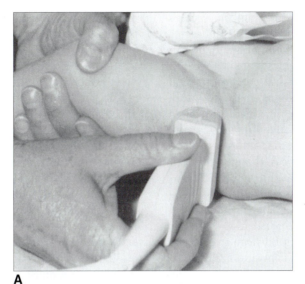

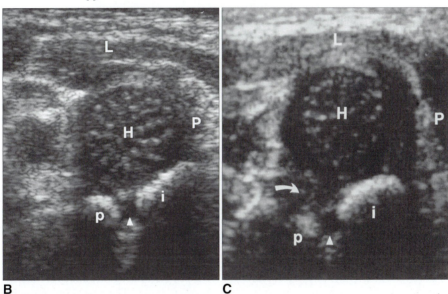

FIGURE 29-18 Transverse/neutral view. **A,** Transducer is perpendicular to neutral femoral head in the plane of acetabulum. **B,** Normal hip sonogram shows sonolucent femoral head centered over triradiate cartilage with pubis (anterior) and ischium (posterior). **C,** Subluxed hip sonogram shows sonolucent femoral head displaced posterolaterally with gap between pubis and femoral head *(arrow)*. *H,* Femoral head; *L,* lateral; *P,* posterior; *i,* ischium; *arrowhead,* triradiate cartilage; *p,* pubis.

TABLE 29-6	Neonatal Hip Technique: Transverse/Neutral View
View Transverse/ Neutral	**Sonographic Findings**
Normal	Sonolucent femoral head is positioned against the bony acetabulum over the triradiate cartilage
Subluxed/dislocated	Femoral head usually moves posteriorly, and remains in contact with the posterior aspect of the acetabulum

radiographs were used to confirm the diagnosis of a dysplastic hip. Today, sonography has replaced radiography because it does not require the neonate to be sedated, no ionizing radiation is used, and the soft tissues are well defined with high-frequency ultrasound. Moreover, the ultrasound examination may be repeated as often as necessary to follow the progression of treatment.

Incidence of Developmental Displacement of the Hip. The incidence of DDH is small, ranging between 1.5 and 1.7 per 1000 live births. When lesser degrees of abnormality such as subluxation are included, as many as 10 infants per 1000 live births may show some features of the disorder.

Multiple risk factors may contribute to the condition. It usually affects the firstborn child, with females affected more frequently than males. The left hip is most commonly affected with only a small number of cases affecting both hips. The condition affects Caucasians more than the African-American population. A breech birth is also a risk factor in DDH, as is low birth weight. Other risk factors include maternal hypertension, fetal growth restriction, oligohydramnios, premature rupture of membranes, prolonged gestation, increased birth weight, Potter's syndrome, and neonatal intensive care.

Causes of Developmental Displacement of the Hip. The primary cause of DDH is thought to be a gradual migration of the femoral head from the acetabulum because of the loose, elastic joint capsule. In addition, other factors—such as genetic, mechanical, and physiologic—are thought to play a role.

In the newborn period, the femoral head may dislocate in a lateral and posterosuperior position relative to the acetabulum (Figure 29-19). When this occurs, the femoral head can usually be reduced without deformity to the joint. However, when the dislocation is not recognized early, the muscles tighten and limit movement, which causes the acetabulum to become dysplastic because it lacks the stimulus of the femoral head. In turn, the ligamentous structures stretch and fibrofatty tissue occupies the acetabulum, making it impossible to return the femoral head into the acetabulum.

Genetic factors show that there is a 6% chance that a child will be affected if a sibling has DDH and a 36%

chance if one sibling and one parent are affected. There is a 12% chance that an affected individual will have a child with DDH.

As for the mechanical causes of DDH, oligohydramnios, breech presentation, and the primigravid uterus are considered risk factors because each limits the mobility of the hip in its own way. Oligohydramnios limits mobility because there is less than a normal amount of amniotic fluid present for the fetus to move freely within the amniotic sac. In breech presentation, the fetus's hip rests against the maternal sacrum and is usually flexed, which limits movement. This usually affects the left hip. The frank breech presentation of the fetus is the highest risk because the hips are maximally flexed and the knees are extended. The primigravid uterus is smaller than the multigravida uterus and is therefore more confining and thus limits mobility.

Physical Examination for Developmental Displacement of the Hip

A careful physical examination is critical for the diagnosis of developmental displacement of the hip (Figure 29-20). By visual inspection, the dislocated hip shows asymmetric skin folds and shortening of the affected thigh. The knee is lower in position on the affected side when the patient is supine and the knees are flexed (**Galeazzi sign**).

If the physical examination is abnormal at birth, sonography of the hip should be done within 1 to 2 weeks of age. Hip instability may resolve on its own. Newborns with a risk factor for DDH can be examined at 4 to 6 weeks.

Two basic maneuvers are helpful in the diagnosis of DDH. The Barlow maneuver determines if the hip can be dislocated. The Ortolani maneuver determines if the dislocated femoral head can be reduced back into the acetabulum.

The Barlow Maneuver. For this maneuver, the patient lies in the supine position with the hip flexed 90 degrees and adducted (see Figure 29-16). Downward and outward pressure is then applied. If the hip can be

Dislocation of the hip

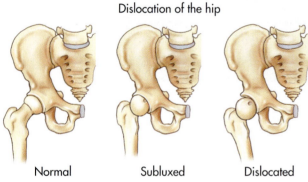

Normal   Subluxed   Dislocated

FIGURE 29-19 Dislocation of the hip.

Early signs (dislocation of right hip)

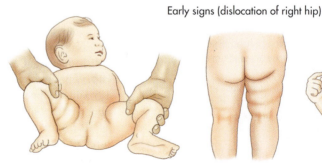
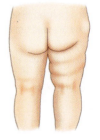
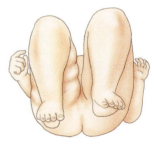

FIGURE 29-20 Physical signs of developmental displacement of the hip.

Limitation of abduction   Asymmetry of skin folds
                                 Prominence of trochanter   Shortening of femur

dislocated, the examiner will feel the femoral head move out of the acetabulum with his fingers.

The Ortolani Maneuver (Figure 29-21). The patient lies in the supine position. The examiner's hand is placed around the hip to be examined, with the fingers over the femoral head. The examiner's middle finger lies over the greater trochanter and the thumb is over the lesser trochanter. The hip is flexed 90 degrees and the thigh is abducted. Movement in the normal hip should feel smooth. In cases of DDH, a "clunk" is appreciated as the femoral head returns into the acetabulum. A "click" does not imply DDH. Each hip should be examined individually.

Sonographic Technique for Developmental Displacement of the Hip

Two sonographic techniques are used in the diagnosis of DDH: static (morphologic) and dynamic. Although the dynamic approach is more commonly used and preferred, the techniques are not mutually exclusive. Results of these procedures are presented next.

Static Technique. Professor Reinhard Graf, an Austrian orthopedic surgeon, introduced this technique in the United States in 1980. The standard sonographic image is acquired in the coronal plane at the midacetabular level. This image includes the femoral head, acetabulum, labrum, and the iliac bone as it meets the triradiate cartilage. This produces a coronal image of the hip, which has a configuration of a lazy "Y."

Graf's Classification of Neonatal Hips. According to Graf, there are four types of neonatal hip displacements (Box 29-1). The neonatal hip is classified according to its alpha and beta angles (Box 29-2). Type I hips are normal and require no further evaluation. Type II

hips must be monitored and follow-up studies are required. Types III and IV hips must be treated.

Sonographic signs of developmental displacement of the hip include a shallow dysplastic acetabulum, delayed ossification of the femoral head (in either a lateral or posterior direction), increased thickness of the acetabular cartilage, an alpha angle greater than 60 degrees, and a beta angle of less than 55 degrees. A "normal" sonogram does not absolutely exclude DDH, although the sensitivity and specificity of sonography approach 100%.

Dynamic Technique. Harcke and Graf formulated basic standards for dynamic hip sonography, which is currently used in most clinical situations today. All scanning is performed from the lateral or posterolateral aspect of the hip. The hip is imaged in orthogonal planes: coronal (longitudinal) and transverse (axial). Images of the hip are obtained in the coronal-extension/flexion and transverse-extension/flexion positions.

With the hip flexed, the femur is moved through a range of abduction and adduction, with stress views performed in the flexed position.

The infant is lying in a supine position with the feet toward the sonographer. It is wise to leave the diaper on

---

BOX 29-1 | Graf's Classification of Neonatal Hips

- A normal hip has an alpha angle of less than 60 degrees and is classified as a type I hip.
- A type II hip has an alpha angle between 43 and 60 degrees.
- A type III hip has an alpha angle of less than 43 degrees and a beta angle greater than 77 degrees.
- A type IV hip has an alpha angle less than 43 degrees and the beta angle is immeasurable.

BOX 29-2 | Graf's Alpha and Beta Angles

Graf used a series of lines and angle measurements to evaluate the morphology of the acetabulum:
1. The baseline connects the osseous acetabular convexity to the point where the joint capsule and perichondrium unite.
2. The inclination line connects the osseous acetabular convexity to the labrum.
3. The acetabular roofline connects the lower edge of the medially acetabular roof to the osseous acetabular convexity.

The alpha and beta angles are measured based on the above lines. The alpha angle is the angle between the baseline and the acetabular roofline and represents the osseous acetabulum (Figure 29-22). The alpha angle is normally greater than 60 degrees. The beta angle is the angle between the baseline and the inclination line. This angle evaluates the formation and size of the cartilaginous acetabulum and is normally less than 55 degrees. The alpha angle reflects changes in the osseous portion of the acetabulum, which occur gradually. The beta angle reflects changes in the cartilaginous acetabulum, which occur more quickly than do changes in the osseous acetabulum and may therefore be more sensitive than the alpha angle (Figure 29-23).

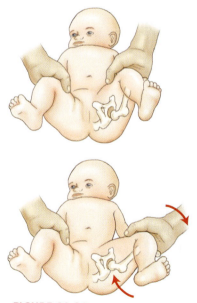

FIGURE 29-21 Ortolani maneuver.

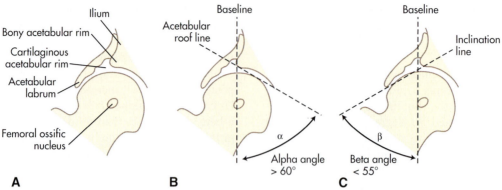

FIGURE 29-22 A, Anatomy of the lateral view of the hip. **B,** Alpha angle of the hip by Graf. **C,** Beta angle of the hip by Graf.

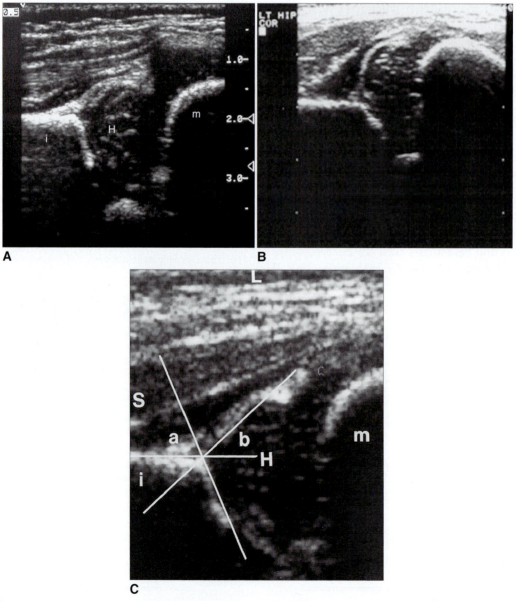

FIGURE 29-23 A, Normal hip in the coronal/neutral view. The femoral head *(H)* sits deep within the bony acetabulum. **B,** In comparison, an abnormal hip shows the femoral head positioned laterally and superiorly. **C,** Beta angle of the hip by Graf.

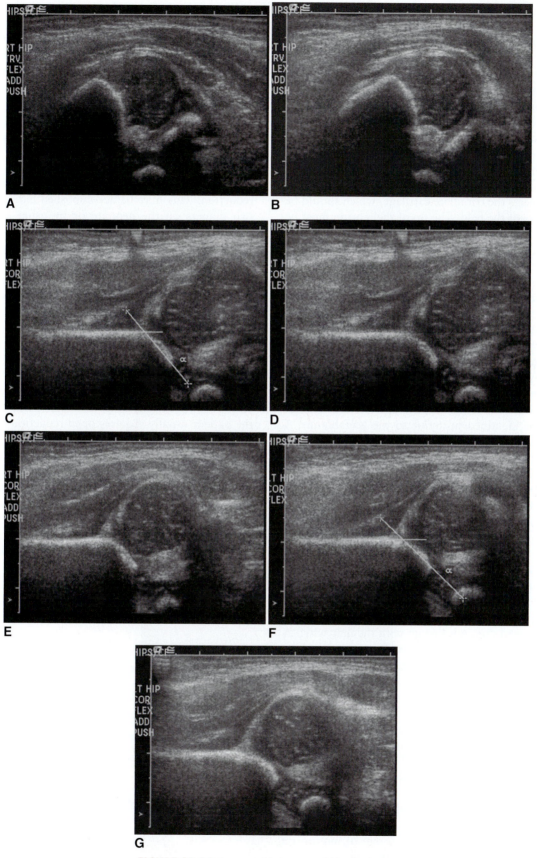

FIGURE 29-24 Sonographic images of hip dysplasia.

through the examination and expose only the side of the hip being examined. The sonographer should hold the left leg with the left hand and hold the transducer in the right hand. When the right hip is examined, the sonographer should hold the transducer in the left hand and use the right hand to manipulate the leg.

The examination begins with a coronal-neutral or coronal-flexion image. For the coronal-neutral image, the hip is held in 15 to 20 degrees of flexion. This is considered physiologic. For the coronal-flexion image, the hip is held in 90 degrees of flexion. The images in the standard or midacetabular plane include the iliac bone as it meets the triradiate cartilage, which should be in the middle of the field. The tip of the labrum must be included in this image.

The sonographic images differ in that the echogenic femoral metaphysis is seen in the coronal-neutral position, but not in the coronal-flexion position. Both images are obtained with the transducer held in the coronal axis of the hip. In both cases, the femoral head should rest against the osseous acetabulum. Approximately two thirds of the femoral head should be covered by the labrum. Stress can be applied in the coronal-flexion position through piston action of the hip. This is accomplished by pushing and pulling the hip in an anterior and posterior direction. If the hip is unstable, the femoral head will be identified posterior to the acetabulum. A coronal-extension image may also be obtained.

The transverse-flexion position is made with the transducer held in the axial plane while the hip is held in 90 degrees of flexion. The hip is pushed posteriorly and adducted in an attempt to dislocate the hip. This is analogous to the Barlow maneuver. If the hip dislocates, the examiner should be able to feel the femoral head dislocate. The hip is then pulled and abducted to attempt to reduce a dislocatable hip. This is analogous to the Ortolani maneuver. The transverse extension can also be obtained (Figure 29-24).

If the femoral head dislocates laterally, the center of the femoral head does not line up with the iliac wing. A line drawn through the iliac wing will pass through the medial aspect of the femoral head. If the femoral head dislocates posteriorly, only an echogenic arc (which represents one side of the head) is seen.

A stress view can be obtained with a "piston maneuver." The hip is placed in 90 degrees of flexion and pressure is applied in the anterior and posterior direction. The transducer is held in the axial plane along the posterior and lateral aspect of the hip.

Hips are classified according to their behavior under stress as normal, unstable, or dislocated. The normal neonatal femoral head cannot be displaced out of the acetabulum, but it can have up to 6 mm of motion on the left and 4 mm of motion on the right during abduction and adduction because of physiologic laxity.

Unstable hips are further divided into subluxable and dislocatable. A subluxable hip is one in which the proxi-

mal femur moves (more than 6 mm on the left and 4 mm on the right) within the acetabulum, but it cannot be displaced out of it. A dislocatable hip is one in which the proximal femur can be displaced out of the acetabulum, but it can be reduced. A dislocated hip is one in which the femoral head is displaced out of the acetabulum and cannot be reduced.

Treatment of Developmental Displacement of the Hip

The initial treatment of uncomplicated DDH is closed reduction. This may be accomplished either by placing two diapers on the neonate or by using a spica cast, Pavlik harness (Figure 29-25), or brace. The hip should be positioned in flexion, with abduction and external rotation. The position of the femoral head relative to the acetabulum can be determined with sonography. If the patient has a cast, a "window" must be cut into the cast so that the transducer can be placed directly on the skin.

Causes of failure of closed reduction include inversion of the labrum or capsule and invagination of the iliopsoas muscle, which can be imaged most efficiently by sonography and magnetic resonance imaging (MRI). If closed reduction fails or if the dislocation is teratogenic, the patient usually requires open reduction.

Screening

Development of both sides of the neonatal hip (the acetabulum and femoral head) requires the femoral head to be seated normally within the acetabulum. If the femoral head and acetabulum are not in their normal position, both sides of the hip will develop abnormally. This will

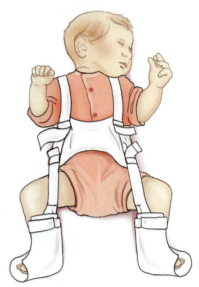

FIGURE 29-25 Pavlik harness may be used in the treatment of hip dysplasia.

cause abnormal morphology and function. If the diagnosis is made early and treatment is instituted promptly, a potentially abnormal hip may develop normally.

The most important factor influencing outcome is the age at which the diagnosis is made and treatment initiated. Treatment should begin before the patient walks. Sonography has been found to be more sensitive than physical examination in the detection of DDH. The goal of screening sonography of the neonatal hip is to establish an early diagnosis so that treatment can be instituted as early as possible. Currently, sonography is used in the neonatal period if the physical examination is abnormal, or if risk factors or associated congenital anomalies are present.

The Neonatal Spine

Sandra L. Hagen-Ansert

OBJECTIVES

On completion of this chapter, you should be able to:
- Describe the sonographic technique to image the neonatal spinal column
- Describe the sonographic appearance of normal anatomy of the spinal cord, the dura, the nerve roots, and the cauda equina
- Describe how to determine the level of the lumbar vertebrae in the sonographic examination
- List the common pathologic conditions of the spinal cord and their sonographic appearances

OUTLINE

The spinal canal and its contents can be demonstrated sonographically with great clarity in the neonatal period. Among the indications for spine sonography are conditions, such as occult **tethered spinal cord** and various **dysraphic** conditions, and to determine the relationship of back masses and midline cutaneous deformities to the spinal canal. High-resolution imaging of the spinal canal has been a clinically accepted tool for examining the neonate. Clinically the infant may present with a dimple on the posterior surface of the body along the spinal canal. Although it is not uncommon for the buttocks to contain a shallow dimple near the anus, at times the dimple appears unusually deep or asymmetric. Other indications that an abnormality may be present include a hemangioma or a raised midline area, a hairy patch, or even a tail-like projection from the lower spine. The dimple may also be suspicious if it is more than 1 inch from the anus. These findings may suggest the possibility of an underlying maldevelopment of the spinal cord or the adjacent elements, known as *occult dysraphic lesions*. Spinal dysraphism includes disorders of the spine involving absent or incomplete closure of the neural tube. The severity of the defect ranges from mild **spina bifida** **occulta** to severe **spina bifida aperta.** If these abnormalities are not recognized early, the patient may have difficulty walking or experience other neurologic problems in infancy or childhood.

Advantages of sonography include the ability to perform the procedure easily and at the bedside without ionizing radiation. The availability of high-frequency transducers now leaves operator inexperience as the main reason for unsuccessful neonatal spinal sonography. The sonographer may observe the spinal cord as it pulsates normally within the spinal canal. The vascular supply to the spinal canal may be evaluated with color Doppler ultrasound. The development of fluid collections, cysts, or fatty tumors (lipomas) is easily seen. Malformations of the spinal cord may be imaged and will be presented in this chapter.

EMBRYOGENESIS

The defects of the spinal canal occur in the first 8.5 weeks of life as the fetal nervous system develops. The neural tube and the subsequent spinal cord arise from ectodermal cells. The surface ectoderm separates from the neural tube, with the mesoderm coming to lie between the neural tube and the ectoderm. The mesoderm forms the bony spine, meninges, and muscle. Incomplete separation of the neural tube from the ectoderm may result in cord tethering, **diastematomyelia,** or a dermal sinus. Premature separation of the cutaneous ectoderm from the neural tube can result in abnormal mesenchymal elements, such as lipomas forming between the neural tube and skin. If the neural tube fails to fold and fuse in the midline, defects such as **myelomeningocele** occur. Disorders of the distal cord may lead to fibrolipomas of the **filum terminale.**

ANATOMY OF THE VERTEBRAL COLUMN AND SPINAL CORD

The vertebral column extends from the base of the skull to the tip of the coccyx along the posterior surface of the body. The vertebral column is the central bony stabilizer of the body. Within the vertebral cavity lie the spinal cord, the roots of the spinal nerves, and the covering meninges, which provide protection for the vertebral column.

The vertebral column consists of 33 vertebrae: 7 cervical, 12 thoracic, 5 lumbar, 5 sacral (fused to form the sacrum), and 4 coccygeal fused bones (Figure 30-1). The

pads of fibrocartilage, called intervertebral disks, are found between each vertebra and allow flexibility in the spine.

Vertebrae

Each vertebra consists of a rounded body anteriorly and a vertebral arch posteriorly (Figure 30-2). These enclose a space called the *vertebral foramen*, through which run the spinal cord and its coverings. The *vertebral arch* consists of a pair of cylindrical pedicles, which form the sides of the arch, and a pair of flattened laminae, which complete the arch posteriorly. The vertebral arch gives rise to seven processes: one spinous, two transverse, and four articular. The two superior articular processes of one vertebral arch articulate with the two inferior articular processes of the arch above, forming two synovial joints.

The pedicles are notched on their upper and lower borders, forming the superior and inferior vertebral notches. On each side, the superior notch of one vertebra and the inferior notch of an adjacent vertebra together form the intervertebral foramen. These foramina transmit the spinal nerves and blood vessels.

In the neonate, problems typically occur in the lower back near the area of the lumbar vertebrae and the

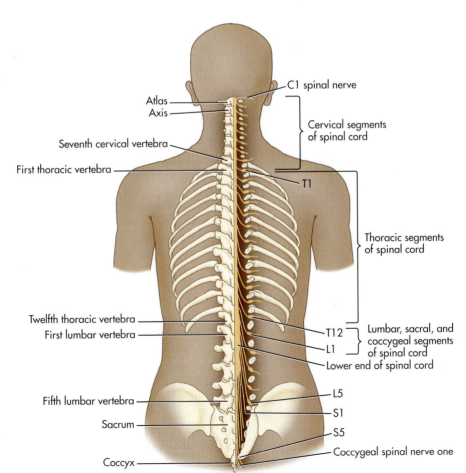

Atlas
Axis
Seventh cervical vertebra
First thoracic vertebra
Twelfth thoracic vertebra
First lumbar vertebra
Fifth lumbar vertebra
Sacrum
Coccyx

C1 spinal nerve
Cervical segments of spinal cord
T1
Thoracic segments of spinal cord
T12
L1
Lumbar, sacral, and coccygeal segments of spinal cord
Lower end of spinal cord
L5
S1
S5
Coccygeal spinal nerve one

FIGURE 30-1 Spinal cord. Posterior view of the spinal cord showing the origins of the roots of the spinal nerves. On the right, the laminae have been removed to expose the right half of the spinal cord and the nerve roots.

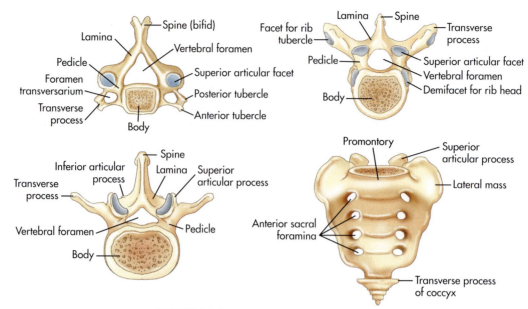

FIGURE 30-2 Basic features of the vertebrae.

sacrum. Characteristics of the lumbar vertebrae may be described as follows:

- The body is large and oval.
- The pedicles are strong and directed posterior.
- The laminae are thick.
- The vertebral foramina are triangular.
- The transverse processes are short, flat, and quadrangular and project backward.
- The articular surfaces of the superior articular processes face medially, and those of the inferior articular processes face laterally.

Sacrum

The sacrum consists of five bones fused together. The upper border articulates with the fifth lumbar vertebra. The narrow inferior border articulates with the coccyx. Laterally the sacrum articulates with the two iliac bones to form the sacroiliac joints. The anterior and upper margin of the first sacral vertebra bulges forward as the posterior margin of the pelvic inlet and is known as the sacral promontory.

The vertebral foramina are present and form the sacral canal. The laminae of the fifth sacral vertebra, and sometimes those of the fourth also, fail to meet in the midline and form the sacral hiatus (Figure 30-3). The sacral canal contains the anterior and posterior roots of the sacral and coccygeal spinal nerves, the filum terminale, and fibrofatty material. It also contains the lower part of the subarachnoid space down as far as the lower border of the second sacral vertebra.

The anterior and posterior surfaces of the sacrum each have four foramina on each side for the passage of the anterior and posterior rami of the upper four sacral nerves.

Intervertebral Disks

The intervertebral disks are responsible for one fourth of the length of the vertebral column. They are thickest in the cervical and lumbar regions where the movements of the vertebral column are greatest. Each disk consists of a peripheral part, the annulus fibrosus, and a central part, the nucleus pulposus (Figure 30-4). The annulus fibrosus consists of fibrocartilage. The nucleus pulposus is an ovoid mass of gelatinous material containing a large amount of water, a small number of collagen fibers, and a few cartilage cells. It is normally under pressure and situated slightly nearer to the posterior than to the anterior margin of the disk.

Ligaments and Nerves

The anterior and posterior longitudinal ligaments run as continuous bands down the anterior and posterior surfaces of the vertebral column from the skull to the sacrum. The small meningeal branches of each spinal nerve innervate the joints between the vertebral bodies.

Spinal Cord

The spinal cord is a cylindrical, grayish white structure that begins above at the foramen magnum, where it is continuous with the medulla oblongata of the brain. It terminates below in the adult at the level of the lower border of the first lumbar vertebra. In the younger child, it is relatively longer and ends at the upper border of the third lumbar vertebra (Figure 30-5).

Inferiorly the cord tapers off into the **conus medullaris**, from the apex of which a prolongation of the pia mater, the filum terminale, descends to be attached to the back of the coccyx. The cord has a deep longitudinal

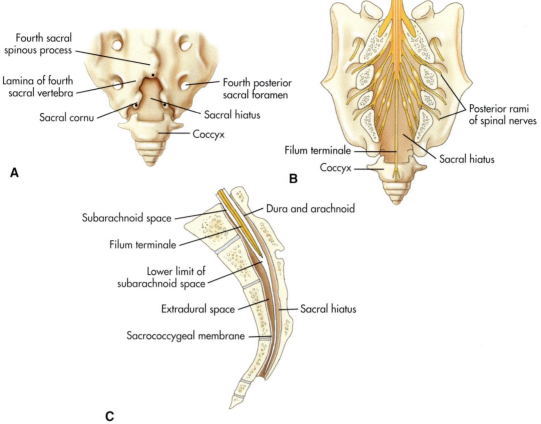

FIGURE 30-3 A, The sacral hiatus. The black dots indicate the position of the important bony landmarks. **B,** The dural sheath (thecal sac) around the lower end of the spinal cord and spinal nerves in the sacral canal; the laminae have been removed. **C,** Longitudinal section through the sacrum.

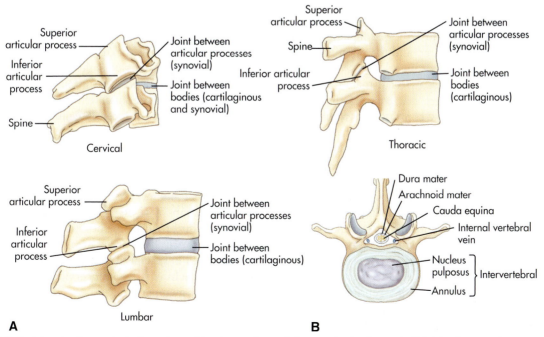

FIGURE 30-4 A, Joints in the cervical, thoracic, and lumbar regions of the vertebral column. **B,** Third lumbar vertebra seen from above showing the relationship between intervertebral disk and cauda equina.

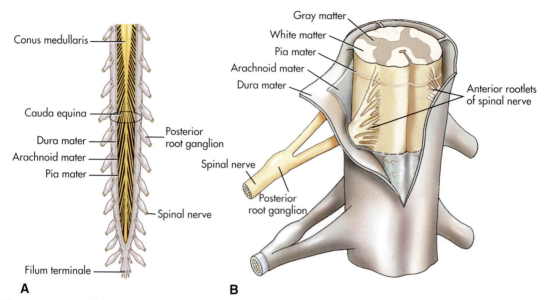

FIGURE 30-5 A, Lower end of the spinal cord and the cauda equina. **B,** Section through the thoracic part of the spinal cord showing the anterior and posterior roots of the spinal nerves and meninges.

fissure in the midline anteriorly, the anterior median fissure, and on the posterior surface a shallow furrow, the posterior median sulcus.

Roots of the Spinal Nerves

Along the length of the spinal cord are attached 31 pairs of spinal nerves. The spinal nerve roots unite to form a spinal nerve. The lower nerve roots together are called the **cauda equina.**

Meninges of the Spinal Cord

The spinal cord is surrounded by three meninges: the dura mater, the arachnoid mater, and the pia mater (see Figure 30-5).

The dura mater is the most external membrane and is a dense strong, fibrous sheet that encloses the spinal cord and cauda equina. It is continuous through the foramen magnum with the meningeal layer of dura covering the brain. Inferiorly, it ends on the filum terminale at the level of the lower border of the second sacral vertebra.

The arachnoid mater is a delicate impermeable membrane covering the spinal cord, and it lies between the pia mater internally and the dura mater externally. It is separated from the dura by the subdural space, which contains a thin film of tissue fluid. The arachnoid is separated from the pia mater by a wide space, the subarachnoid space, which is filled with cerebrospinal fluid.

The pia mater is a vascular membrane that closely covers the spinal cord. It is continuous above the neck through the foramen magnum with the pia covering the brain; below it fuses with the filum terminale.

SONOGRAPHIC EVALUATION OF THE NEONATAL SPINAL COLUMN

The incomplete ossification of the posterior spinal elements allows sonography to provide a broad panoramic view of the neonatal spinal canal and its contents. A posterior approach is used with the patient prone or lateral decubitus, but the examination could be performed with the baby in an upright (against the mother's abdomen) or sitting position. It is crucial that the spine be flexed enough to separate the posterior spinal elements. When prone, this is accomplished by having the baby lie over a small pillow or a rolled towel. Slight elevation of the upper part of the body will better distend the caudal aspect of the thecal sac. Care must be taken that flexion is not so extreme as to compromise the infant's breathing. This consideration is amplified if the baby has been sedated. The infant usually falls asleep during the procedure once the warm coupling gel is applied and the transducer is gently rubbed along the spine canal.

The sonographer should use the highest frequency transducer available to obtain the greatest soft tissue detail. Small neonates will require a higher frequency (7.5 MHz or higher) than a chunky baby, who would require perhaps a 5- to 7-MHz transducer. The linear array transducer works the best to completely scan along the spinal canal. The curved array or sector transducers are best used in special situations where the body surface is curved, such as the craniocervical junction or at the margin of a **meningocele.**

Scanning is performed in the midline sagittal (longitudinal) and axial (transverse) planes, the latter mainly between the spinous processes. Sagittal images are oriented with the baby's head toward the left on the viewing screen, similar to conventional abdominal images. On transverse scans, the patient's right side is to the left of the monitor.

Because most examinations are performed to exclude an occult tethered spinal cord, determining the vertebral level of the tip of the conus medullaris is most important, and accordingly, the lumbar spinal canal receives the most attention. The entire spinal canal is examined, however, at multiple levels.

The depth of field is adjusted so the vertebral bodies are at the bottom of the image. The spinal canal is usually easily identified, and the depth of the image is adjusted accordingly. It is helpful to scan the sacral region first, where the canal is easily identified by the stepwise ascent of the sacral vertebral elements, and then follow the spinal canal in a cranial direction. A stand-off pad may be used between the transducer and the skin surface to examine the soft tissue dorsal to the spine, such as looking for a sinus tract. Oscillations of the spinal cord and roots of the cauda equina are observed best when the image persistence or frame averaging is minimized.

Sonographic Anatomy of the Spinal Canal

With sonography, the spinal canal is defined anteriorly by the echogenic posterior vertebral body surfaces and posteriorly by the posterior dorsal spinal elements, some of which might be incompletely ossified (Figure 30-6). The dura is visible as an echogenic line just internal to these osseous borders. The spinous processes appear as inverted "U"s. Laminae are seen when scanning slightly off midline and appear similar to overlapping roof tiles. The coccyx is mostly or completely unossified and therefore hypoechoic.

The spinal cord is hypoechoic with slightly echogenic borders and an echogenic line extending longitudinally along its midline. This central echo complex represents or is close to the cord's central canal (Figure 30-7).

The size and shape of the spinal cord vary along its length. Its diameter is narrowest in the midthoracic and thoracolumbar junctions (Figure 30-8). Transverse dentate ligaments of the cord are sometimes visible. The cord tapers caudally at the conus medullaris.

The nerve roots that surround the spinal cord are echogenic. They are especially noticeable at and below the conus forming the cauda equina. Dorsal and ventral nerve roots can have a spider-like configuration at the tip of the conus in the transverse view. Clusters of normal nerve roots might be mistaken for an echogenic intra-canalicular mass. Nerves, however, will be observed to move and change configuration as one scans along the canal in real time. In transverse views, nerve roots might appear as an echogenic clump in the middle of the spinal canal or as bilateral clusters, sometimes in an upside down "V" configuration. Another potential false-positive finding is the bilateral dorsal and ventral roots at the tip of the conus that can superficially mimic a split cord (diastematomyelia). Although they appear similar on the sonographic image, they are readily distinguished during real-time scanning in both projections, above and below the area of concern.

The spinal cord and roots of the cauda equina are normally observed to move. This is best seen with minimal frame persistence. Dorsoventral oscillations occur at the frequency of the heartbeat, and there is also a superimposed motion, which occurs with respirations. These movements are variably present in neonates but are almost always seen after 1 or 2 months of age.

Level of the Conus Medullaris. The single most important determination is usually the level of the tip of the tapered conus medullaris (Figure 30-9). The normal level is in the upper lumbar canal, above the superior endplate of L3, with most cords ending above L2.

The lumbar vertebral level may be determined by looking at the baby's back during the scanning examination. A transverse projection across the midline from the lowest palpable rib end is often L2. A similar projection

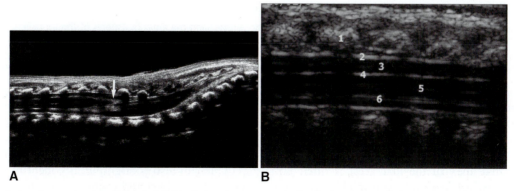

FIGURE 30-6 A, Lumbosacral spine. Extended field of view image reveals detailed anatomy of the course and contour of the neonatal lumbosacral spine. The tip of the conus medullaris is clearly visible. **B,** Normal ultrasound of the neonatal spinal canal defined anteriorly by the echogenic posterior body surfaces and posteriorly by the posterior dorsal spinal elements. *1,* Posterior elements or spinous processes; *2,* posterior arachnoid-dural layer bordering spinal canal; *3,* subarachnoid space filled with cerebrospinal fluid; *4,* posterior margin of the spinal cord; *5,* spinal cord with central echo complex; *6,* anterior margin of the spinal cord.

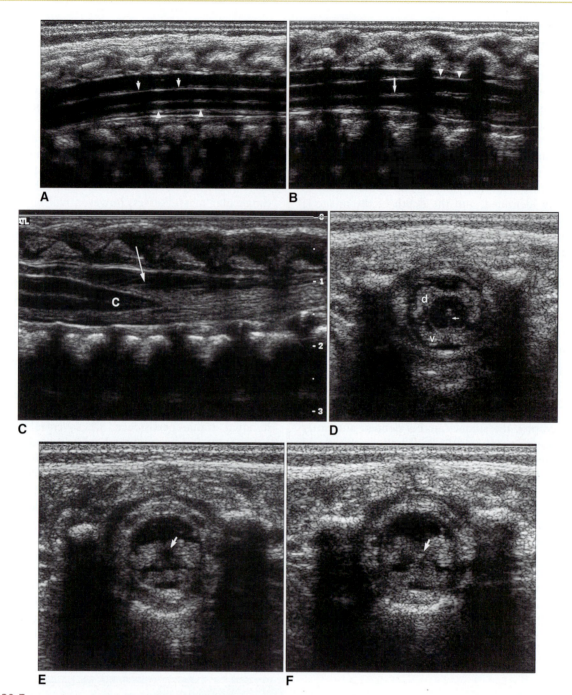

FIGURE 30-7 Normal spinal cord. **A,** Sagittal view shows the posterior *(arrows)* and the anterior aspects of the thoracic spinal cord *(arrowheads)*. Normal thoracic spinal cord is more anteriorly positioned within the vertebral canal than the more distal spinal cord. **B,** Normal widening of the lumbar spinal cord *(arrowheads)*. The central spinal canal is visible as an echogenic line *(arrow)*. **C,** Tip of the conus medullaris *(c)* should taper gradually. Individual nerve rootlets are visible *(arrow)*. **D,** On transverse view of the lumbar spinal cord, dorsal *(d)* and ventral *(v)* nerve rootlets, as well as the anterior median fiffusre, are visible *(arrow)*. **E,** Transverse view near the tip of the conus medullaris demonstrates the relatively hypoechoic substance of the cord *(arrow)* in the center of the more echogenic nerve rootlets. **F,** The beginning of the filum terminale is seen as a central, slightly echogenic focus *(arrow)* in the transverse plane.

from the palpated apex of the iliac crest is often L5. One can count vertebral levels on ultrasound by counting caudad from the lowest rib-bearing vertebra or by counting cranial from the caudal end of the thecal sac (usually S2), from the coccyx, or from the lumbosacral junction.

One can also sonographically identify the lowest rib over each kidney and follow it medially to its vertebral body. That level can be assigned as T12, although it could be off by a level if the patient has 11 or 13 pairs of ribs. If the conus tip is midlumbar, its exact level might need to be determined by a correlative radiograph. The

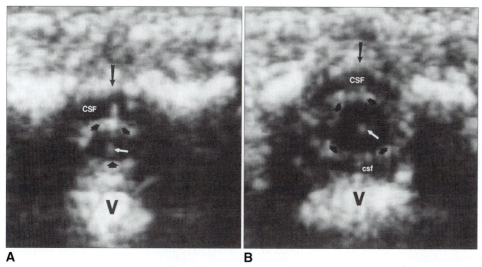

FIGURE 30-8 A, Thoracic **(A)** and lumbar **(B)** spine of a normal 5-day-old cord. The spinal cord is hypoechoic with slightly echogenic borders and an echogenic line extending longitudinally along its midline (central echo complex). *V,* Vertebrae; *CSF,* cerebrospinal fluid.

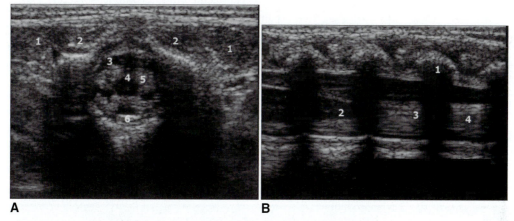

FIGURE 30-9 A, Level of conus—transverse view. The nerve roots are echogenic as they surround the spinal cord. *1,* Paravertebral muscles; *2,* laminae of vertebral arches; *3,* subarachnoid space filled with cerebrospinal fluid; *4,* spinal cord with central echo complex; *5,* paired dorsal and ventral nerve roots; *6,* vertebral body. **B,** Normal conus medullaris—sagittal view. The tapered conus medullaris shows the end of the spinal cord. *1,* Posterior elements or spinous processes; *2,* cauda medullaris; *3,* filum terminale; *4,* cauda equina and nerve roots.

conus tip is carefully noted in both longitudinal and transverse sonographic projections, and this position is marked on the skin by a radiopaque marker, such as a nipple "B-B" marker.

Most tethered cords are unquestionably low and correlative radiographs are not usually necessary. Sometimes the conus tip is obscured by an overlying posterior spinal element, but this is more often a problem in older infants and children. In those cases the conus level is inferred to be lying between the lowest level showing cord and the adjacent caudal level, which contains only the cauda equina.

PATHOLOGY OF THE NEONATAL SPINAL COLUMN

Spinal sonography is performed primarily to study the contents of the spinal canal. The most common request is to search for the occult tethered cord. Other problems, such as lipoma, hydromyelia and diastematomyelia, cysts of the spinal cord, and myelomeningocele, are presented (Figure 30-10). For a more extensive discussion of spinal anomalies, the reader is referred to Chapter 59. Table 30-1 lists the clinical findings, sonographic findings, and differential considerations for spinal anomalies.

Tethered Spinal Cord

The tethered spinal cord is a pathologic fixation of the spinal cord in an abnormal caudal location, so that the cord suffers mechanical stretching, distortion, and ischemia with daily activities, growth, and development. The tethered spinal cord, in addition to being in a more caudal location, is often fixed eccentrically within the canal (Figure 30-11). Spinal cord oscillations might be diminished in the tethered cord. If cord oscillations are present distant from the site of tethering, they are often dampened or absent closer to the point of fixation. This normal brisk oscillation of the cord is not as apparent in normal neonates as it is in older infants; therefore, looking for dampened or absent oscillations in neonates with tethered cords has limited usefulness (false positives). Most nonoscillating cords in neonates are normal and are not due to tethering. These oscillations usually diminish as the child grows, presumably because the cord is anchored and is being stretched (Figure 30-12).

Lipoma

A **lipoma** is a benign tumor composed of fat cells. Spinal lipomas are fatty masses that have a connection with the spinal cord. These lipomas may be further divided into four categories of intradural lipomas, lipomyelocele, lipomyelomeningocele, and fibrolipomas of the filum terminale. Intradural lipomas are situated in a subpial position in a dorsal cleft of the open spinal cord. The lipomyelocele is analogous to the myelocele, whereas there is a covering of attached lipoma and intact skin. In patients with lipomyelomeningocele, there is expansion of the subarachnoid space ventral to the placode.

Fibrolipomas of the filum terminale are a unique form of lipoma that may represent a variant of normal development. On sonography, this is seen as a thickened, echogenic filum terminale, sometimes with an undulating contour. However, when associated with a tethered cord, it is usually accompanied with a mass of the lower cord or filum terminale. This anomaly comprises 20% to 50% of the spinal dysplasias. This mass often has lipomatous elements and can be continuous with the subcutaneous tissues and present as a fatty lump on the lower back. Lipomas can be isolated to the filum terminale or extend to and infiltrate the spinal cord and conus medullaris to varying degrees. Lipomas are usually echogenic and may present as a small or large mass (Figure 30-13).

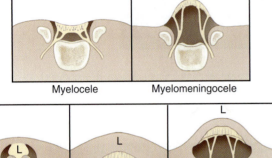

FIGURE 30-10 Open neural tube defects and examples of occult dysraphisms. Each diagram is positioned with the dorsal side up, the position one would use when scanning the spine of an infant (*L*, lipoma).

TABLE 30-1	Spinal Anomalies	
Abnormality	**Definition/Clinical Findings**	**Sonographic Findings**
Tethered spinal cord	Tethered cord is a group of complicated developmental malformations of the spinal cord Benign; terrible consequences if not treated As children grow, the spinal cord is not able to grow because of the abnormal structures holding onto the cord Children may have pain or lose function of legs, bowel, or bladder Fatty mass may be present on mid to lower back Increased areas of pigmentation Dimples on back Large collections of hair on back	Cord fixed centrally within spinal canal Decreased cord oscillations
Lipoma	Fatty lump on lower back	Echogenic small to large mass
Hydromyelia	Increased fluid in the central canal of the spinal cord	Prominence of central canal at caudal end of cord Focal hydromyelia present cephalad to site of tethered cord
Diastematomyelia	A congenital fissure of the spinal cord, frequently associated with spina bifida cystica	Cord split at one or more sites by osseous cartilaginous or fibrous septum Vertebral column is always abnormal
Cysts of spinal cord	Well-marginated mass	Anechoic mass in cauda equina region
Myelomeningocele	Spina bifida with a portion of the spinal cord and membranes protruding	Flat nontubulated cord with nerve roots extending into the defect
Meningocele	Congenital hernia in which the meninges protrude through a defect in the skull or spinal column	Shows only fluid within the sac May have fine, lacelike strands into the sac Cord may be eccentric or tethered

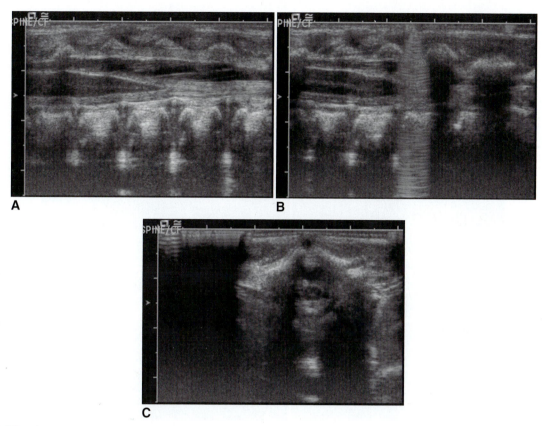

FIGURE 30-11 Tethered spinal cord. **A** and **B,** Longitudinal scans of the lumbosacral spine show how the spinal cord extends below the L3 vertebra before tapering into a conus. **C,** Transverse lumbar spine. The tethered spinal cord shows the cord is fixed eccentrically within the canal.

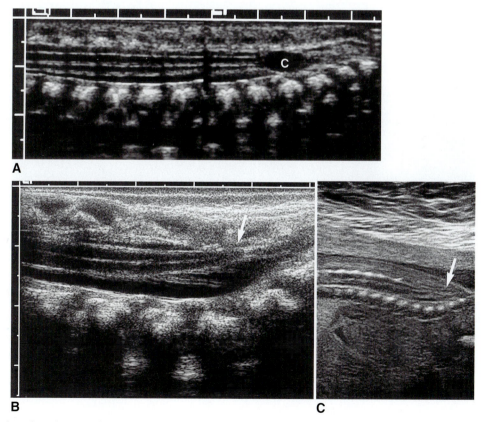

FIGURE 30-12 Tethered cord. **A,** Newborn with an interposed filar cyst (C). **B,** Newborn. **C,** Fetus at 30 weeks with a tethered cord in the setting of the VATER association. The *arrow* indicates the point of tethering. The term *VATER* is an acronym describing an association that may include vertebral defects, imperforate anus, tracheoesophageal fistula, and radial and renal anomalies.

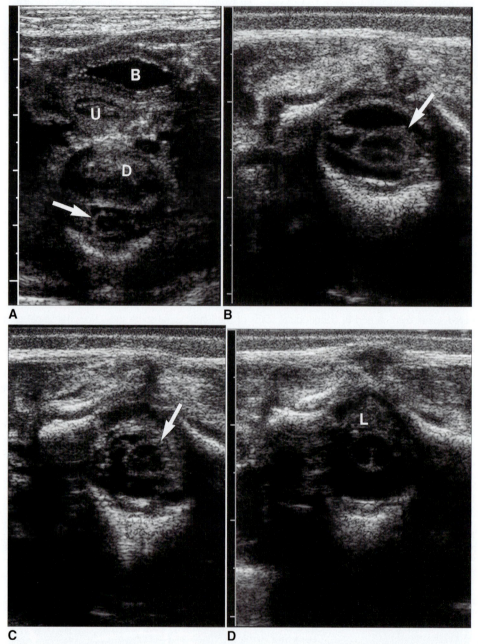

FIGURE 30-13 Intradural juxtamedullary lipoma in a 2-week-old girl. **A,** Transverse view of the pelvis shows the partially full urinary bladder (*B*), the newborn uterus (*U*), and an intervertebral disk space of the sacrum (*D*). The spinal cord is too low and is visible from an anterior approach *(arrow)*. Traditional views of the spine scanning the neonatal back (**B, C,** and **D**) are progressively inferior transverse views revealing the rightward skew of the abnormally low spinal cord *(arrow)* that is also pulled into an abnormally dorsal position by the lipoma *(L)*.

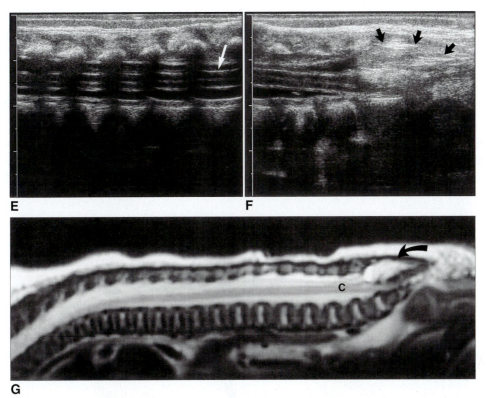

FIGURE 30-13, cont'd E and **F**, Sagittal views of the low cord *(white arrow)* with the clearly visible tethering lipoma *(black arrows).* **G,** The correlative sagittal T2-weighted MRI, oriented to match the sonogram, reveals the abnormally low cord *(C)* and the lipoma *(curved black arrow).*

Hydromyelia and Diastematomyelia

Hydromyelia is another sonographically observable abnormality of the spinal cord that can be seen in variable degrees. One should be aware that slight prominence of the central canal at the caudal end of the cord is a common finding in neonates. Focal hydromyelia is often present just cephalad to the site of tethering in dysraphic conditions such as myelomeningocele or lipomyelomeningocele. Hydromyelia might also accompany diastematomyelia (Figure 30-14), a condition in which there is sagittal division of the cord into two hemicords, each containing a central canal, a single dorsal horn, and a single ventral horn. The cord is split at one or more sites by an osseous, cartilaginous, or fibrous septum. The two segments of the cord can be seen most clearly on transverse views. They might rejoin caudal to the cleft. The vertebral column is virtually always abnormal on plain radiography in patients with diastematomyelia.

Cysts of the Spinal Cord

Small cysts in the filum terminale might be remnants of a terminal ventricle or an arachnoid pseudocyst and have no significance. A cyst in the cauda equina region may be seen with a thick filum terminale.

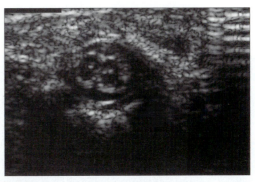

FIGURE 30-14 Diastematomyelia. Transverse scan of the lumbar spinal canal shows left and right hemicords. Each hemicord has an eccentric central canal.

Myelomeningocele or Myeloschisis

The primary reason for studying the cord in cases of clinically obvious myelomeningocele or **myeloschisis** is to exclude additional cord pathology, such as diastematomyelia. Intraoperative sonography has been successfully used to detect the margin of the skin defect. The anatomy of the cord, adhesion of the cord to the dorsal aspect of the spinal canal cephalad to the defect, and the appearance of the neural placode and nerve roots in the defect can all be seen on a sonogram.

Sonography is used to distinguish a meningocele from a myelomeningocele or if the dysraphic defect is skin covered (Figure 30-15). Myelomeningocele shows a flat nontabulated cord (neural placode) with nerve roots extending into the defect. The nerve roots rise from the neural placode with dorsal roots lateral and ventral roots medial. In contrast, a meningocele shows nothing but fluid within the sac. However, a meningocele can also contain fine lacelike strands extending into the sac. These fibers are finer than nerve roots and are strands of lining tissue, such as arachnoid. Although the spinal cord is tabulated and does not enter the sac in a meningocele, the cord might be focally eccentric in the canal and even be tethered by a focal adhesion (Figure 30-16).

Other Indications and Associations

Midline cutaneous abnormalities over the lower back have been the most common reason for requesting neonatal spinal sonography. Midline dimples over the lower back occur in approximately 2% to 4.3% of newborns.

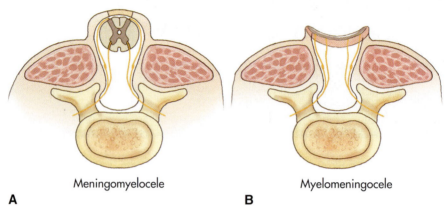

Meningomyelocele Myelomeningocele

A B

FIGURE 30-15 A, Meningomyelocele is a hernia of the spinal cord and membranes through a defect in the vertebral column. **B,** Myelomeningocele is seen in patients with spina bifida with a portion of the spinal cord and membranes protruding through the defect.

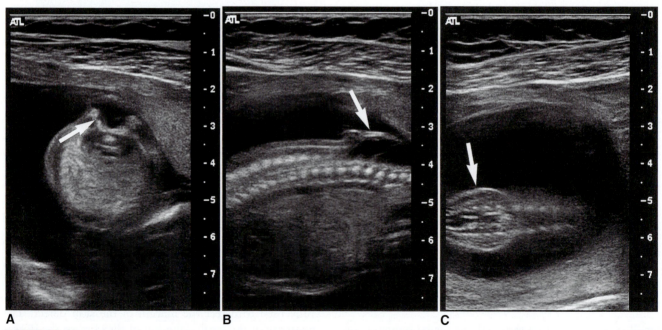

A B C

FIGURE 30-16 Lumbosacral myelomeningocele. Transverse **(A)**, sagittal **(B)**, and coronal **(C)** views of an 18-week fetus with a lumbosacral myelomeningocele. The transverse view shows the open nature of the posterior elements of the affected vertebral ring *(arrow)*. The sagittal view shows the protuberance of the covering membrane and neural placode *(arrow)*. The coronal view shows the thin nature of the covering membrane *(arrow)*.

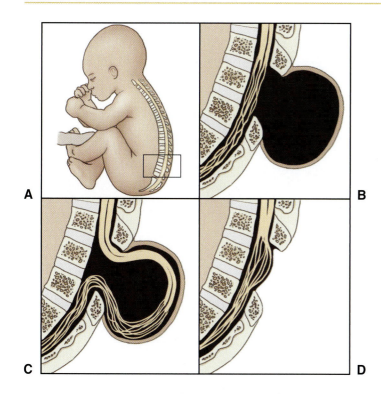

FIGURE 30-17 Spina bifida classifications. Meningoceles **(B)** contain only fluid, while myelomeningoceles **(C)** also contain neural elements. The defect is uncovered in myeloschisis **(D)**.

Most are low sacral or coccygeal pits without an associated tethered cord. A tract can sometimes be seen and followed, especially if it is fluid filled or if it disrupts normal soft tissue planes (Figure 30-17). The soft tissue interfaces are continuous echogenic lines between skin, subcutaneous fat, muscle, and fascia. A sinus tract will disrupt the echogenic line with possible extension to the dura. However, dural penetration is difficult to ascertain or exclude on sonography. The neonatal coccyx is usually of very low echogenicity and should not be mistaken for a cyst or fluid collection.

During the first month of gestation, the neural tube is closing, whereas neural and epithelial tissues are differentiating from the overlying ectoderm. The concurrence of these events might explain the coincidence of midline cutaneous and spinal defects. Midline hair patches, fatty lumps, skin tags, pigmented nevi, lumbar dimples, aplasia cutis, and hemangiomas over the back should prompt a search for an occult tethered spinal cord. Hemangiomas seem to have a high association with tethered spinal cord. Tethered cord has an association with neonates with imperforate anus.

abduction to move away from the body

abscess localized collection of pus

absorption process of nutrient molecules passing through wall of intestine into blood or lymph system

accessory spleen results from the failure of fusion of separate splenic masses forming on the dorsal mesogastrium; most commonly found in the splenic hilum or along the splenic vessels or associated ligaments

acholic describes absence or deficiency of bile secretion or failure of bile to enter the alimentary tract (secondary to obstruction); the stool is claylike and colorless

acidic a type of solution that contains more hydrogen ions than hydroxyl ions

acidosis an actual increase in the acidity of blood due to an accumulation of acids (as in diabetic acidosis or renal disease) or an excessive loss of bicarbonate (as in renal disease)

acini cells cells that perform exocrine function

acinus (acini) glandular (milk-producing) component of the breast lobule; each breast has hundreds of lobules, each of which contains one or several acini

acoustic emission occurs when an appropriate level of acoustic energy is applied to the tissue, the microbubbles first oscillate and then rupture; the rupture of the microbubbles results in random Doppler shifts appearing as a transient mosaic of colors on a color Doppler display

acoustic impedance measure of a material's resistance to the propagation of sound; expressed as the product of acoustic velocity of the medium and the density of the medium ($Z = pc$)

acromioclavicular joint (AC) the joint found in the shoulder that connects the clavicle to the acromion process of the scapula

acute tubular necrosis acute damage to the renal tubules; usually resulting from ischemia associated with shock

Addison disease condition caused by hyposecretion of hormones from the adrenal cortex

adduction to move toward the body

adenoma tumor of glandular tissue; smooth, round homogeneous benign tumor of the adrenal cortex; benign thyroid neoplasm characterized by complete encapsulation

adenomyomatosis small polypoid projections

adenosis in the breast, overgrowth of the stromal and epithelial elements of the acini within the terminal ductal lobular unit (TDLU) of the breast; a component of a fibrocystic condition

adrenal hemorrhage hemorrhage that occurs when the fetus is stressed during a difficult delivery or a hypoxic insult

adrenocorticotropic hormone (ACTH) a hormone secreted by the pituitary gland

afferent arteriole small artery that carries blood into the glomerulus of the nephron

aliasing improper Doppler-shift information from a pulsed wave Doppler or color Doppler instrument when the true Doppler shift exceeds one half the pulse repetition frequency

alimentary canal also known as the gastrointestinal tract; includes the mouth, pharynx, esophagus, stomach, duodenum, and small and large intestines

alkaline a type of solution that contains more hydroxyl ions than hydrogen ions

alkalosis an actual increase in blood alkalinity due to an accumulation of alkalies or reduction of acids

amplitude strength of an ultrasound wave measured in decibels

ampulla of Vater small opening in the duodenum in which the pancreatic and common bile duct enter to release secretions

amylase enzyme secreted by the pancreas to aid in the digestion of carbohydrates

amyloidosis metabolic disorder marked by amyloid deposits in organs and tissue

anaplastic carcinoma rare, undifferentiated carcinoma occurring in middle age

anastomosis a communication between two blood vessels without any intervening capillary network

anechoic without echoes; simple cyst on ultrasound should be anechoic

anembryonic pregnancy (blighted ovum) ovum without an embryo

anemia abnormal condition in which blood lacks either a normal number of red blood cells or a normal concentration of hemoglobin

aneurysm permanent localized dilation of an artery, with an increase in diameter of 1.5 times its normal diameter

angle of incidence angle at which the ultrasound beam strikes the interface between two types of tissue

angle of reflection angle at which the ultrasound beam is reflected from an interface; the angle of reflection equals the angle of incidence

anisotropy the quality of comprising varying values of a given property when measured in different directions

anorchidism bilateral absence of testes

anterior pararenal space space located between the anterior surface of the renal fascia and the posterior area of the peritoneum

antiradial plane of imaging on ultrasound of the breast that is perpendicular to the radial plane of imaging. The radial plane of imaging uses the nipple as the center point of an imaginary clock face imposed on the breast, such that the radial 12 o'clock plane is a line extending upward toward the top of the breast; similarly, the radial 9 o'clock plane extends straight out to the right aspect of the breast, and so on; three-dimensional measurements of a breast mass can be recorded using sagittal transverse or radial/antiradial planes

aorta (AO) largest arterial structure in the body; arises from the left ventricle of the heart to supply blood to the head, upper and lower extremities, and abdominopelvic cavity by descending into the abdominal cavity to branch into iliac vessels at the level of the umbilicus

apnea spontaneous breathing that stops for any reason

apocrine metaplasia from of fibrocystic change in the breast in which the epithelial cells of the acini undergo alteration (metaplasia); the epithelial cells assume a columnar shape similar to sweat (apocrine) glands; this process can lead to cyst formation, hyperplasia, and other fibrocystic changes

aponeurosis bandlike flat tendons connecting muscle to the bone

appendicitis inflammation of the appendix

appendicolith a fecalith or calcification located in the appendix

aqueductal stenosis blockage of the duct connecting the third and fourth ventricles, which causes their dilation

arcuate arteries small arteries that lie at the bases of the renal pyramids and appear as echogenic structures

areola the pigmented skin surrounding the breast nipple

arrhythmia any irregular heartbeat; also called dysrhythmia

arteries vascular structures that carry blood away from the heart

arteriosclerosis thickening and hardening of arterial walls

arteriovenous fistula communication between an artery and vein

ascites accumulation of serous fluid in the peritoneal cavity

asphyxia severe hypoxia, or inadequate oxygenation

asymptomatic without symptoms; in the case of breast cancer screening, only asymptomatic women are eligible for a screening mammogram, a fast, low-cost mammogram; a screening mammogram is different from a diagnostic mammogram, which is a more extensive examination for evaluation of a specific symptom or an abnormal finding

atherosclerosis condition in which the aortic wall becomes irregular from plaque formation

atretic describes congenital absence or closure of a normal body opening or tubular structure

atrium (trigone) of the lateral ventricles the ventricle is measured at this site (junction of the anterior, occipital, and temporal horn) on the axial view

attenuation reduction in the amplitude and intensity of a sound wave as it propagates through a medium; attenuation of ultrasound waves in tissue is caused by absorption and by scattering and reflection

atypical ductal hyperplasia (ADH) see **atypical hyperplasia**

atypical hyperplasia abnormal proliferation of cells with atypical features involving the terminal ductal-lobular unit (TDLU), with an increased likelihood of evolving into breast cancer; in atypical ductal hyperplasia (ADH), the pathologist recognizes some, but not all, of the features of ductal carcinoma in situ (DCIS); atypical lobular hyperplasia (ALH) shows some, but not all, of the features of lobular carcinoma in situ (LCIS); ALH and LCIS are now grouped by some authors under the term *lobular neoplasia*

atypical lobular hyperplasia (ALH) see **atypical hyperplasia** and **lobular neoplasia**

auscultation method of listening to the heart sounds with a stethoscope

autoimmune hemolytic anemia anemia caused by antibodies produced by the patient's own immune system

autosomal dominant polycystic kidney disease (ADPKD) congenital polycystic kidney disease that usually presents during middle age

autosomal recessive polycystic kidney disease (ARPKD) rare, congenital polycystic renal disease (infantile polycystic disease)

axial plane placement of the transducer above the ear (above the canthomeatal line)

axial resolution refers to the minimum distance between two structures positioned along the axis of the beam where both structures can be visualized as separate objects

axilla armpit; the axilla contains the lymph nodes that drain the majority of the breast tissue; in cases of invasive breast cancer, the lymph nodes are sampled to stage the cancer and direct further treatment

Baker's cyst synovial fluid collection in the posterior fossa

bare area area superior to the liver that is not covered by peritoneum so that the inferior vena cava may enter the chest

Barlow maneuver the patient lies in the supine position with the hip flexed 90 degrees and adducted; downward and outward pressure is applied; if the hip is dislocated, the examiner will feel the femoral head move out of the acetabulum

baseline shift movement of the zero Doppler-shift frequency or zero flow speed line up or down on a spectral display

Beckwith-Wiedemann syndrome hereditary disorder transmitted as an autosomal recessive trait; clinical manifestations include umbilical hernia (exomphalos), macroglossia, and gigantism, often accompanied by visceromegaly and dysplasia of the renal medulla; also called exophthalmos-macroglossia-gigantism (EMG) syndrome

bicornuate uterus duplication of the uterus (two horns and one vagina)

bile bile pigment, old blood cells, and the by-products of phagocytosis are known together as *bile*

biliary atresia closure or absence of some or all of the major bile ducts

bilirubin yellow pigment in bile formed by the breakdown of red blood cells

blood urea nitrogen (BUN) laboratory measurement of the amount of nitrogenous waste and creatinine in the blood; waste products accumulate in the blood when kidneys malfunction

body mechanic theory and practice of using the correct muscles to complete a task safely, efficiently, and without undue strain on any joints or muscles

body of the pancreas located in the midepigastrium anterior to the superior mesenteric artery and vein, aorta, and inferior vena cava

Bowman's capsule the cup-shaped end of a renal tubule enclosing a glomerulus; site of filtration of the kidney; contains water, salts, glucose, urea, and amino acids

bradycardia a heart rate of less than 60 bpm

brainstem part of the brain connecting the forebrain and the spinal cord; consists of the midbrain, pons, and medulla oblongata

branchial cleft cyst remnant of embryonic development that appears as a cyst in the neck

breast differentiated apocrine sweat gland with the functional purpose of secreting milk during lactation

breast cancer (breast carcinoma) breast cancer involves two main types of cells: ductal and lobular; ductal cancer, accounting for approximately 85% of breast cancer cases, includes many subtypes, such as medullary, mucinous, tubular, apocrine, or papillary types; in addition, very early or preinvasive breast cancer is generally ductal in type; this preinvasive breast cancer is also called *in situ*, *noninvasive*, or *intraductal* breast cancer; another commonly used term for this early type of cancer is *ductal carcinoma in situ (DCIS)*

breast cancer screening screening for breast cancer involves annual screening mammography (starting at age 40), monthly breast self-examination (BSE), and regular clinical breast examination (CBE)

Breast Imaging Reporting and Data System (BI-RADS) trademark system created by the American College of Radiology (ACR) to standardize mammographic reporting terminology, to categorize breast abnormalities according to the level of suspicion for malignancy, and to facilitate outcome monitoring; BI-RADS was made a mandatory part of mammogram reports by federal legislation (Mammography Quality Standards Act of 1994)

breast self-examination (BSE) part of breast cancer screening; every woman is encouraged to perform breast self-examination monthly starting at age 20; BSE is usually best performed at the end of menses

Budd-Chiari syndrome thrombosis of the hepatic veins

buffer chemical compound that can act as a weak acid or a base to combine with excess hydrogen or hydroxyl ions to neutralize the pH in blood

bull's eye (target) lesion hypoechoic mass with echogenic central core (abscess, metastasis)

bursa a saclike structure containing thick fluid that surrounds areas subject to friction, such as the interface between bone and tendon

bursitis (shoulder) inflammation of the shoulder bursa from repeated motion

calcitonin a thyroid hormone that is important for maintaining a dense, strong bone matrix and regulating the blood calcium level

calyx part of the renal collecting system adjacent to the pyramid that collects urine and is connected to the major calyx

capillaries minute vessels that connect the arterial and venous systems

cardiac orifice entrance of the esophagus into the stomach

cardiomyopathy disease of the myocardial muscle layer of the heart that causes the heart to dilate secondary to regurgitation and also affects cardiac function

carpal tunnel entrapment of the median nerve as it runs through the carpal bones of the wrist; results from repeated flexion and extension of the wrist and also from mechanical pressure against the wrist

cartilage interface sign echogenic line on the anterior surface of the cartilage surrounding the humeral head

cauda equina bundle of nerve roots from the lumbar, sacral, and coccygeal spinal nerves that descend nearly vertically from the spinal cord until they reach their respective openings in the vertebral column

caudal pancreatic artery branch of the splenic artery that supplies the tail of the pancreas

caudate lobe smallest lobe of the liver; lies posterior to the left lobe and anterior to the inferior vena cava; superior border is the ligamentum venosum

caudate nucleus area of the brain that forms the lateral borders of the anterior horns, anterior to the thalamus

cavernous transformation of the portal vein periportal collateral channels in patients with chronic portal vein obstruction

cavum septum pellucidum prominent structure best seen in the midline filled with cerebrospinal fluid in the premature infant

celiac axis first major anterior artery to arise from the abdominal aorta inferior to the diaphragm; it branches into the hepatic, splenic, and left gastric arteries

centripetal artery terminal intratesticular arteries arising from the capsular arteries

cerebellum area of the brain that lies posterior to the brainstem below the tentorium

cerebrum largest part of the brain consisting of two equal hemispheres

Chiari malformation congenital defect in which the cerebellum and brainstem are pulled toward the spinal cord (banana sign); frontal bossing or *lemon head* is also evident on ultrasound

cholangitis inflammation of the bile duct

cholecystectomy removal of the gallbladder

cholecystitis acute or chronic inflammation of the gallbladder

cholecystokinin hormone secreted into the blood by the mucosa of the upper small intestine; stimulates contraction of the gallbladder and pancreatic secretion of enzymes

choledochal cyst cystic growth on the common bile duct that may cause obstruction

choledocholithiasis stones in the bile duct

cholelithiasis gallstones in the gallbladder

cholesterolosis variant of adenomyomatosis; cholesterol polyps; also called *cholesterosis*

choroid plexus echogenic cluster of cells important in the production of cerebrospinal fluid that lie along the atrium of the lateral ventricles

cistern reservoir for cerebrospinal fluid

clapper-in-the-bell sign hypoechoic hematoma found at the end of a completely retracted muscle fragment

clinical breast examination (CBE) examination of the breast by a health care provider as part of breast cancer screening; every woman is encouraged to have a thorough CBE in conjunction with her routine health care assessment; between ages 20 and 40, CBE is advised every 3 years; from age 40 on, CBE should be performed by the woman's regular health care provider annually

C-loop of the duodenum forms the lateral border of the head of the pancreas

collateral circulation circulation that develops when normal venous channels become obstructed

collateral vessels ancillary vessels that develop when portal hypertension occurs

color flow velocity in each direction is quantified by allocating a pixel to each area; each velocity frequency is allocated a color; flow toward the transducer may be red; flow away from the transducer may be blue

column of Bertin   band of cortical tissue that separates the renal pyramids; a prominent column of Bertin may mimic a renal mass on sonography

comet tail artifact   a series of closely spaced reverberation echoes

common bile duct   duct that extends from the point where the common hepatic duct meets the cystic duct; drains into the duodenum after it joins with the main pancreatic duct

common duct   refers to common bile or hepatic ducts when cystic duct is not seen

common femoral arteries   arteries originating from the iliac arteries and seen in the inguinal region into the upper thigh

common hepatic artery   artery arising from the celiac trunk to supply the liver

common hepatic duct   bile duct system that drains the liver into the common bile duct

common iliac arteries   a division of the abdominal aorta at the level of the umbilicus to supply blood to the lower extremities

compression   region of increased particle density

confluence of the splenic and portal veins   junction of the splenic and portal veins that occurs in the midabdomen and serves as the posterior border of the pancreas

congenital mesoblastic nephroma   most common benign renal tumor of the neonate and infant

continuous wave (CW) Doppler   one transducer continuously transmits sound, and one continuously receives sound; used in higher-velocity flow patterns

contrast   the feature of a radiographic image that affects the ability to visualize detail and detect lesions

contrast-enhanced sonography   diagnostic medical sonography performed after administration of an ultrasound contrast agent

conus medullaris   the caudal end of the spinal cord

Cooper's ligaments   connective tissue septae that connect perpendicularly to the breast lobules and extend out to the skin; considered the fibrous "skeleton" supporting the breast glandular tissue

coronal plane   transducer is perpendicular to the anterior fontanelle in the coronal axis of the head

corpus callosum   prominent group of nerve fibers that connect the right and left sides of the brain; found superior to the third ventricle

corpus luteum cyst   small endocrine structure that develops within a ruptured ovarian follicle and secretes progesterone and estrogen; it may persist until the 20th to 24th week of pregnancy

cortex   outer parenchyma of an organ; in the kidney, it is the outer parenchyma that contains the renal corpuscle and proximal and distal convoluted tubules of the nephron; outer parenchyma of the adrenal gland that secretes steroid hormones; liver cortex is thin in the neonate, with echogenicity similar to or slightly greater than that of the normal liver parenchyma

Courvoisier's sign   enlargement of the gallbladder caused by a slow, progressive obstruction of the distal common bile duct from an external mass such as adenocarcinoma of the pancreatic head

creatinine (Cr)   a product of metabolism; laboratory test measures the ability of the kidney to get rid of waste; waste products accumulate in the blood when the kidneys are malfunctioning

cremasteric artery   small artery arising from the inferior epigastric artery (a branch of the external iliac artery), which supplies the peritesticular tissue, including the cremasteric muscle

cremasteric muscle   an extension of the internal oblique muscle that descends to the testis with the spermatic cord; contraction of the cremasteric muscle shortens the spermatic cord and elevates the testis

Crohn's disease   inflammation of the bowel, accompanied by abscess and bowel wall thickening

cross-talk   leakage of strong signals in one direction channel of a Doppler receiver into the other channel; can produce the Doppler mirror-image artifact

crus of the diaphragm   muscular structure in the upper abdomen at the level of the celiac axis

cryptorchidism   failure of the testes to descend into the scrotum; testicles remain within the abdomen or groin and fail to descend into the scrotal sac

crystal   special material in the ultrasound transducer that has the ability to convert electrical impulses into sound waves

cubital tunnel   entrapment of the ulnar nerve as it runs through the elbow; can result from repeated twisting of the forearm and mechanical pressure against the elbow when sonographers rest it on the exam table while scanning

culling   process by which the spleen removes nuclei from the red blood cells as they pass through

Cushing's syndrome   condition caused by hypersecretion of hormones from the adrenal cortex

cyanosis   bluish discoloration of the skin and mucous membranes caused by lack of oxygen in the blood

cycle   a sequence of events occurring at regular intervals; sound waves are generated over a period of time; the time required to produce each cycle depends on the frequency of the transducer

cyst   fluid-filled sac of variable size; cysts in the breast usually result either from obstruction of the terminal duct draining the normal fluid secretions from the acinar units of the lobule or from overproduction of fluid from the acini; cysts are typically simple (anechoic, sharply marginated) or complex (thick, irregular wall, internal debris, internal echoes, intracystic mass)

cyst aspiration   common diagnostic and interventional breast procedure that involves placing a needle through the skin of the breast into a cystic mass and pulling fluid out of the cyst through the needle; in the case of a palpable cyst, this procedure can be performed in a physician's office; in the case of a small, complex, or nonpalpable cyst, image guidance (usually with ultrasound) can be used to facilitate the aspiration

cystic duct   duct that connects the gallbladder to the common hepatic duct

cystic fibrosis   inherited disorder of the exocrine glands; symptoms include mucus buildup within the lungs and other areas of the body

cystic medial necrosis   weakening of the arterial wall

Dandy-Walker malformation abnormal development of the fourth ventricle, often accompanied by hydrocephalus

decibel (dB) unit used to quantitatively express the ratio of two amplitudes or intensities; decibels are not absolute units, but express one sound level or intensity in terms of another or in terms of a reference (e.g., the amplitude 10 cm from the transducer is 10 dB lower than the amplitude 5 cm from the transducer)

deferential artery arises from the vesicle artery (a branch of the internal iliac artery) and supplies the vas deferens and epididymis

deQuervain's disease specific type of tendonitis involving the thumb that can result from gripping the transducer

developmental displacement of the hip abnormal condition of the hip that results in congenital hip dysplasia; includes dysplastic, subluxated, dislocatable, and dislocated hips

diagnostic breast imaging also called *consultative*, *workup*, or *problem-solving mammography* or *breast imaging*; this type of breast imaging examination is more intensive than routine screening mammography; diagnostic breast imaging is usually directed either toward a specific clinical symptom of possible breast cancer or toward an abnormal finding on a screening mammogram; the goal of diagnostic breast imaging is to categorize the abnormality according to the level of suspicion for cancer (see Breast Imaging and Reporting System [BI-RADS])

diaphragm broad muscle that separates the thoracic and abdominopelvic cavities and forms the floor of the thoracic cavity

diastematomyelia a congenital fissure of the spinal cord, frequently associated with spina bifida cystica

diffuse hepatocellular disease disease that affects hepatocytes and interferes with liver function

dissecting aneurysm tear in the intima or media of the abdominal aorta

diverticulum a pouchlike herniation through the muscular wall of a tubular organ that occurs in the stomach, the small intestine, or most commonly, the colon

dome of the liver most superior aspect of the liver at the level of the diaphragm

Doppler angle the angle that the reflector path makes with the ultrasound beam; the most accurate velocity is recorded when the beam is parallel to flow

Doppler sample volume the sonographer selects the exact site to record Doppler signals and sets the sample volume (gate) at this site

Doppler shift the difference between the receiving echo frequency and the frequency of the transmitted beam

dorsal pancreatic artery branch of the splenic artery that supplies the body of the pancreas

dorsiflexion upward movement of the hand or foot

dromedary hump normal variant that occurs on the left kidney as a bulge of the lateral border

duct of Santorini small accessory duct of the pancreas found in the head of the gland

duct of Wirsung largest duct of the pancreas that drains the tail, body, and head of the gland; it joins the common bile duct to enter the duodenum through the ampulla of Vater

duodenal bulb first part of the duodenum

dynamic range ratio of the largest to smallest signals that an instrument or component of an instrument can respond to without distortion

dyspnea a shortness of breath or the feeling of not getting enough air, which may leave a person gasping

dysraphic describes anomalies associated with incomplete embryologic development

dysuria painful or difficult urination

ectasia dilation of any tubular vessel

ectopic kidney kidney located outside of the normal position, most often in the pelvic cavity

ectopic ureterocele ectopic insertion and cystic dilation of distal ureter of duplicated renal collecting system; occurs more commonly in females and on left side

efferent arteriole small artery that carries blood from the glomerulus of the nephron and conducts blood to the peritubular capillaries that surround the renal tubule

ejaculatory ducts ducts that connect the seminal vesicle and the vas deferens to the urethra at the verumontanum

endocrine process of secreting into the blood or lymph circulation to have a specific effect on tissues in another part of the body

enhancement increase in echo amplitude from reflectors that lie behind a weakly attenuating structure

epicondylitis (lateral and medial) inflammation of the periosteum in the area of the insertion of the biceps tendon into the distal humerus; can result from repeated twisting of the forearm

epididymal cyst cyst filled with clear, serous fluid located in the epididymis

epididymis anatomic structure that lies posterior and lateral to the testes in which the spermatozoa accumulate

epididymitis infection and inflammation of the epididymis

epigastric above the umbilicus and between the costal margins

epigastrium area between the right and left hypochondrium that contains part of the liver, duodenum, and pancreas

epineurium the covering of a nerve that consists of connective tissue

epiploic foramen opening to the lesser sac

ergonomics the science of designing a job to fit the individual worker

erythrocyte red blood cell

erythropoiesis production of red blood cells

euthyroid refers to a normal functioning thyroid gland

exocrine process of secreting outwardly through a duct to the surface of an organ or tissue or into a vessel

extracorporeal membrane oxygenation (ECMO) treatment for infants with severe respiratory failure who have not responded to maximal conventional ventilator support

extrahepatic outside the liver

falciform ligament ligament that attaches the liver to the anterior abdominal wall and undersurface of the diaphragm

false pelvis portion of the pelvic cavity that is above the pelvic brim, bounded posteriorly by the lumbar vertebrae, laterally by the iliac fossae and iliacus muscles, and anteriorly by the lower anterior abdominal wall

falx cerebri (interhemispheric fissure) echogenic fibrous structure (portion of the dura mater) that separates the cerebral hemispheres

fascia lata deep fascia of the thigh

fasciculi term describing a small bundle of muscles, nerves, and tendons

fecalith calcified deposit within the appendix; appendicitis develops when the appendix becomes blocked by hard fecal matter; also called fecolith

femoral triangle description of a region at the front of the upper thigh, just below the inguinal ligament

femoral veins upper part of the venous drainage system of the lower extremity found in the upper thigh and groin that empties into the inferior vena cava at the level of the diaphragm

fibroadenoma most common benign solid tumor of the breast, consisting predominantly of fibrous and epithelial (adenomatous) tissue elements; these masses tend to develop in young women (even teenagers), to run in families, and can be multiple; a fibroadenoma is usually a benign-appearing mammographic mass (round, oval, or gently lobular and well circumscribed) with a correlating sonographic mass that is well defined and demonstrates homogeneous echogenicity

fibrocystic condition (FCC) also called *fibrocystic change* or *fibrocystic breast*, this condition represents many different tissue processes within the breast that are all basically normal processes that over time can get exaggerated to the point of causing symptoms or mammographic changes that raise concern for breast cancer; the main fibrocystic tissue processes are adenosis, epitheliosis, and fibrosis; these processes can cause symptoms such as breast lumps and pain as well as mammographic changes such as cysts, microcalcifications, distortion, and masslike densities; common pathologic changes of FCC include apocrine metaplasia, microcystic adenosis, sclerosing adenosis, and many others; only a few fibrocystic tissue processes are associated with an increased risk of subsequent development of breast cancer; see **atypical hyperplasia**

film/detector contrast contrast that is inherent in the film type and the processing techniques that is not changeable by the operator

filum terminale slender tapering terminal section of the spinal cord

fine needle aspiration the use of a fine-gauge needle to obtain cells from a mass

first generation agents contrast agents containing room air (i.e., Albunex)

focal nodular hyperplasia (FNH) liver tumors with an abundance of Kupffer cells; sonographically, they are isoechoic to the surrounding normal liver tissue

focal zone the region over which the effective width of the sound beam is within some measure of its width at the focal distance

focused assessment with sonography for trauma (FAST) limited examination of the abdomen or pelvis to evaluate free fluid or pericardial fluid

follicular carcinoma occurs as a solitary mass within the thyroid gland

fontanelle soft space between the bones; the space is usually large enough to accommodate the ultrasound transducer until the age of 12 months

frame rate rate at which images are updated on the display; dependent on frequency of the transducer and depth selection

frank dislocation the hip is laterally and posteriorly displaced to the extent that the femoral head has no contact with the acetabulum and the normal "U" configuration cannot be obtained on ultrasound

Fraunhofer zone the field farthest from the transducer during the formation of the sound beam

free hand technique method of performing an ultrasound-guided procedure without the use of a needle guide on the transducer

fremitus refers to vibrations produced by phonation and felt through the chest wall during palpation; a technique used in conjunction with power Doppler to identify the margins of a lesion

frequency number of cycles per second that a periodic event or function undergoes; number of cycles completed per unit of time; the frequency of a sound wave is determined by the number of oscillations per second of the vibrating source

frequency shift amount of change in the returning frequency compared with the transmitting frequency when the sound wave hits a moving target, such as blood in an artery

Fresnel zone the field closest to the transducer during the formation of the sound beam

fusiform aneurysm circumferential enlargement of a vessel with tapering at both ends

gain measure of the strength of the ultrasound signal; can be expressed as a simple ratio or in decibels; overall gain amplifies all signals by a constant factor regardless of the depth

Galeazzi sign on physical examination, the knee is lower in position on the affected side of the neonate with developmental displacement of the hip (DDH) when the patient is supine and the knees are flexed

gallbladder (GB) storage pouch for bile

gamma rays physically similar to x-rays but generated spontaneously from the decay of radioactive isotopes

gantry the "hole" in the center of a computed tomography scanner

gastrin endocrine hormone released from the stomach (stimulates secretion of gastric acid)

gastroduodenal artery branch of the common hepatic artery that supplies the stomach and duodenum

gastrohepatic ligament helps support the lesser curvature of the stomach

gastrophrenic ligament ligament that helps support the greater curvature of the stomach

gastrosplenic ligament ligament between the stomach and the spleen; helps support stomach and spleen

gate the sample site from which the signal is obtained with pulsed Doppler

Gaucher's disease one of the storage diseases in which fat and proteins are deposited abnormally in the body

germinal matrix fragile periventricular tissue (includes the caudate nucleus) that easily bleeds in the premature infant

Gerota's fascia another term for the renal fascia; the kidney is covered by the renal capsule, perirenal fat, Gerota's fascia, and pararenal fat

glomerulus network of capillaries that are part of the filtration process in the kidney

glucagon hormone that stimulates the liver to convert glycogen to glucose; produced by alpha cells

goiter any enlargement of the thyroid, focal or diffuse, regardless of cause

Graves' disease autoimmune disorder characterized by a diffuse toxic goiter, exophthalmos, and cutaneous manifestations

gray scale B-mode scanning technique that permits the brightness of the B-mode dots to be displayed in various shades of gray to represent different echo amplitudes

gray-scale harmonic imaging (GSHI) allows detection of contrast-enhanced blood flow and organs with gray-scale ultrasound; in the harmonic-imaging mode, the echoes from the oscillating microbubbles have a higher signal-to-noise ratio than found in conventional ultrasound; regions with microbubbles (e.g., blood vessels and organ parenchyma) are better visualized

greater omentum double fold of the peritoneum attached to the duodenum, stomach, and large intestine; helps support the greater curve of the stomach; known as the "fatty apron"

greater sac primary compartment of the peritoneal cavity; extends across the anterior abdomen from the diaphragm to the pelvis

gutters most dependent areas in the flanks of the abdomen and pelvis where fluid collections may accumulate

Guyon's canal or tunnel a fibrous tunnel that contains the ulnar artery and vein, ulnar nerve, and some fatty tissue

gynecomastia hypertrophy of residual ductal elements that persist behind the nipple in the male, causing a palpable, tender lump; there is generally no lobular (glandular) tissue in the male; a breast mass resulting from gynecomastia must be distinguished from male breast cancer

harmonic imaging in the HI mode, the ultrasound system is configured to receive only echoes at the second harmonic frequency, which is twice the transmit frequency

Hartmann's pouch small part of the gallbladder that lies near the cystic duct where stones may collect

Hashimoto's thyroiditis chronic inflammation of the thyroid gland caused by the formation of antibodies against normal thyroid tissue

haustra normal segmentation of the wall of the colon

head of the pancreas portion of the pancreas that lies in the C-loop of the duodenum; the gastroduodenal artery is the anterolateral border and the common bile duct is the posterolateral border

Heimlich maneuver emergency treatment to clear an upper airway obstruction that is preventing normal breathing

Heister's valves tiny valves found within the cystic duct

hematocele blood within the sac surrounding the testes

hematochezia passage of bloody stools

hematocrit the percentage of the total blood volume containing the red blood cells, white blood cells, and platelets

hematometrocolpos blood-filled vagina and uterus

hematopoiesis blood cell production

hemihypertrophy excessive development of one side or one half of the body or an organ

hemoglobin protein found in red blood cells that binds with oxygen and releases it in the capillaries of tissue

hemolytic anemia anemia resulting from hemolysis of red blood cells

hemoperitoneum collection of bloody fluid in the abdomen or pelvis secondary to trauma or surgical procedure

hemorrhage collection of blood

hemosiderin pigment released from hemoglobin process

hepatic artery (HA) common hepatic artery arises from the celiac trunk and courses to the right of the abdomen and branches into the gastroduodenal artery and proper HA

hepatic flexure point at which the ascending colon arises from the right lower quadrant to bend to form the transverse colon

hepatic veins largest tributaries that drain the liver and empty into the inferior vena cava at the level of the diaphragm

hepatocellular carcinoma (HCC) a common liver malignancy related to cirrhosis; the carcinoma may present as a solitary massive tumor, multiple nodules throughout the liver, or diffuse infiltrative masses in the liver; HCC can be very invasive

hepatocellular disease classification of liver disease where hepatocytes (liver cells) are the primary problem, as opposed to obstruction of bile secretion

hepatocyte a parenchymal liver cell that performs all functions ascribed to the liver

hepatofugal flow away from the liver

hepatopetal flow toward the liver

hepatorenal syndrome condition affecting both the liver and the renal system

hermaphroditism condition in which both ovarian and testicular tissues are present

hertz (Hz) unit for frequency, equal to 1 cycle per second

hilum area of kidney where vessels, ureter, and lymphatics enter and exit

hip joint formed by the articulation of the head of the femur with the acetabulum of the hip bone

Hodgkin disease malignant disease that involves lymphoid tissue

holoprosencephaly congenital defect characterized by abnormal single ventricular cavity with some form of thalami fusion; caused by an extra chromosome, the prosencephalon fails to divide into hemispheres during embryonic development

homeostasis maintenance of normal body physiology

horseshoe kidney congenital malformation in which both kidneys are joined together by an isthmus, most commonly at the lower poles

Hounsfield unit the numeric scan for representing the different tissue characteristics by their x-ray (or "electron") density

hydrocele fluid within the sac surrounding the testes

hydrocephalus   ventriculomegaly in the neonate; abnormal accumulation of cerebrospinal fluid within the cerebral ventricles, resulting in compression and frequently destruction of brain tissue

hydrocolpos   fluid-filled vagina

hydrometrocolpos   collection of fluid in the vagina and uterus

hydromyelia   dilation of the central canal of the spinal cord

hydronephrosis   dilation of the renal collecting system

hydrops   massive enlargement of the gallbladder

hypercalcemia   elevated levels of calcium in the blood

hyperechoic   echo texture that is more echogenic than the surrounding tissue; hyperechoic masses in the breast are nearly always benign

hyperglycemia   uncontrolled increase in glucose levels in the blood

hyperlipidemia   congenital condition in which there are elevated fat levels that may cause pancreatitis

hyperparathyroidism   disorder associated with elevated serum calcium level, usually caused by a benign parathyroid adenoma

hyperplasia   an increase in the number of cells of a body part that results from an increased rate of cellular division

hypertension   high blood pressure, >130/90 mm Hg

hyperthyroidism   overactive thyroid gland

hypertrophic pyloric stenosis (HPS)   thickened muscle in the pylorus that prevents food from entering the duodenum; occurs more frequently in males

hypoechoic   having relatively weak echoes; opposite of hyperechoic (having relatively strong echoes)

hypoglycemia   deficiency of glucose in the blood

hypophosphatasia   congenital condition characterized by decreased mineralization of the bones resulting in "ribbonlike" and bowed limbs, underossified cranium, and compression of the chest; early death often occurs; Chapter 22 defines as "low phosphate level, which can be seen with hyperparathyroidism"

hypotension   low blood pressure, <115/75 mm Hg; decreased systolic and diastolic blood pressure below normal; may occur with shock, hemorrhaging, infection, fever, cancer, anemia, neurasthenia, and Addison's disease

hypothyroidism   underactive thyroid gland

hypovolemia   diminished blood volume

hypoxia   decreased oxygen in the body

ileus   dilated loops of bowel without peristalsis; associated with various abdominal problems, including pancreatitis, sickle cell crisis, and bowel obstruction

iliac arteries   arteries that originate from the bifurcation of the aorta at the level of the umbilicus

iliac veins   receive tributaries from the lower extremities and drain into the inferior vena cava

incarcerated hernia   confinement of a part of the bowel; the visceral contents cannot be reduced

induced acoustic emission   see **acoustic emission**

infarction   an interruption in the blood supply to an area that may lead to necrosis of the area

inferior mesenteric artery (IMA)   artery that arises from the anterior aortic wall at the level of the third or fourth lumbar vertebra to supply the left transverse colon, descending colon, sigmoid colon, and part of the rectum

inferior mesenteric vein (IMV)   vein that drains the left third of the colon and upper colon and joins the splenic vein

inferior vena cava (IVC)   largest abdominal vessel formed by the union of the common iliac veins; flows posterior to the liver to enter the right atrium of the heart

infiltrating (invasive) ductal carcinoma   cancer of the ductal epithelium; most common general category of breast cancer, accounting for approximately 85% of all breast cancers; this cancer usually arises in the terminal duct in the terminal ductal-lobular unit (TDLU); if the cancerous cells remain within the duct without invading the breast tissue beyond the duct wall, this is ductal carcinoma in situ (DCIS); if the cancerous cells invade breast tissue (invasive ductal carcinoma or IDC), the cancer may spread into the regional lymph nodes and beyond; of the many subtypes of IDC, the most common is infiltrating ductal carcinoma, not otherwise specified (IDC-NOS)

infiltrating (invasive) lobular carcinoma (ILC)   cancer of the lobular epithelium of the breast, arises at the level of the terminal ductal-lobular unit (TDLU); accounts for 12% to 15% of all breast cancers

inguinal ligament   ligament between the anterior superior iliac spine and the pubic tubercle

inspissated   thickened by absorption, evaporation, or dehydration

insulin   hormone that causes glycogen formation from glucose in the liver that allows circulating glucose to enter tissue cells; failure to produce insulin results in diabetes mellitus

intensity   power per unit area

interface   surface forming the boundary between media having different properties

internal os   inner surface of the cervical os

international normalized ratio (INR)   a method developed to standardize prothrombin time (PT) results among laboratories by accounting for the different thromboplastin reagents used to determine PT

interstitial pregnancy   pregnancy occurring in the cornu of the uterus

intertubercular plane   lowest horizontal imaginary line that joins the tubercles on the iliac crests to help divide the abdominopelvic cavity into nine regions

intrahepatic   within the liver

intraperitoneal   within the peritoneal cavity

intravenous (IV) injection   administration of a drug or contrast agent via a needle or catheter placed in a vein

intravenous (IV) therapy   the practice of giving liquid substances directly into a vein

intravenous urography (IVU)   procedure used in radiography wherein contrast is administered intravenously to help visualize the urinary system

intussusception   bowel prolapses into distal bowel (telescoping) and is then propelled in an antegrade fashion

islets of Langerhans   portion of the pancreas that has an endocrine function and produces insulin, glucagon, and somatostatin

isoechoic echo texture that resembles the surrounding tissue; in the breast, isoechoic masses can be difficult to identify

isolated systolic hypertension condition that occurs when systolic pressure is above 140 mm Hg but diastolic pressure remains below 90 mm Hg

isosexual concerning or characteristic of the same sex

isthmus small piece of thyroid tissue that connects the lower lobes of the gland

IUP intrauterine pregnancy

jaundice excessive bilirubin accumulation causes yellow pigmentation of the skin; first seen in the whites of the eyes

junctional fold small septum within the gallbladder, usually arising from the posterior wall

juxtathoracic near the chest wall (thorax)

kilohertz (kHz) 1000 Hz

Klatskin's tumor cancer at the bifurcation of the hepatic ducts; may cause asymmetric obstruction of the biliary tree

Kupffer cells special hepatic cells that remove bile pigment, old blood cells, and the by-products of phagocytosis from the blood and deposit them into the bile ducts

laminar normal pattern of vessel flow; flow in the center of the vessel is faster than it is at the edges

lateral arcuate ligament thickened upper margin of the fascia covering the anterior surface of the quadratus lumborum muscle

lateral resolution the minimum distance between two objects where they still can be displayed as separate objects

left crus of the diaphragm arises from the sides of the bodies of the first two lumbar vertebrae

left gastric artery artery that arises from the celiac axis to supply the stomach and lower third of the esophagus

left hepatic artery small branch supplying the caudate and left lobes of the liver

left hypochondrium left upper quadrant of the abdomen that contains the left lobe of the liver, spleen, and stomach

left lobe of the liver lobe that lies in the epigastrium and left hypochondrium

left portal vein the main portal vein branches into the left and right portal veins to supply the liver

left renal artery artery that arises from the posterolateral wall of the aorta directly into the hilum of the kidney

left renal vein leaves the renal hilum, travels anterior to the aorta and posterior to the superior mesenteric artery to enter the lateral wall of the inferior vena cava

lesser omentum membranous extension of the peritoneum that suspends the stomach and duodenum from the liver; helps to support the lesser curvature of the stomach

lesser sac peritoneal pouch located behind the lesser omentum and stomach

leucopoiesis white blood cell formation stimulated by presence of bacteria

leukocyte white blood cell

leukocytosis increase in the number of leukocytes

leukopenia abnormal decrease of white blood corpuscles; may be drug induced

lienorenal ligament ligament between the spleen and kidney that helps support the greater curvature of the stomach

ligament fibrous band of tissue connecting bone or cartilage to bone that aids in stabilizing a joint

ligamentum teres termination of the falciform ligament; seen in the left lobe of the liver

ligamentum venosum transformation of the ductus venosus in fetal life to closure in neonatal life; it separates left lobe from caudate lobe; shown as echogenic line on the transverse and sagittal images

linea alba fibrous band of tissue that stretches from the xiphoid to the symphysis pubis

linea semilunaris Slightly curved line on the ventral abdominal wall that marks the lateral border of the rectus abdominis; visible as a shallow groove when that muscle is tensed

lipase pancreatic enzyme that acts on fats; enzyme is elevated in pancreatitis and remains increased longer than amylase

lipoma common benign tumor composed of fat cells

liver function tests specific laboratory tests that look at liver function (aspartate or alanine aminotransferase, lactic acid dehydrogenase, alkaline phosphatase, and bilirubin)

lobular carcinoma in situ (LCIS) see **lobular neoplasia**

lobular neoplasia term preferred by many authors to replace *atypical hyperplasia* and *lobular carcinoma in situ (LCIS)*, neither considered a true cancer nor treated as such

longus colli muscle wedge-shaped muscle posterior to the thyroid lobes

loop of Henle portion of a renal tubule lying between the proximal and distal convoluted portions; reabsorption of fluid, sodium, and chloride occurs in the proximal convoluted tubule and the loop of Henle

lymph alkaline fluid found in the lymphatic vessels

lymphadenopathy any disorder characterized by enlargement of the lymph nodes or lymph vessels

lymphoma malignancy that arises from lymphoid tissue and primarily affects the lymph nodes, spleen, or liver

main lobar fissure boundary between the right and left lobes of the liver; seen as hyperechoic line on the sagittal image extending from the portal vein to the neck of the gallbladder

main portal vein vein formed by union of the splenic vein and superior mesenteric vein; serves as the posterior border of the pancreas; enters the liver at the porta hepatis

major calyces (infundibula) areas of the kidney that receive urine from the minor calyces to convey to the renal pelvis

malpighian corpuscles small masses found in the white pulp; lymph node in the spleen

mammary layer the middle of three layers of breast tissue recognized on breast ultrasound between the skin and the chest wall that contains the ductal, glandular, and stromal portions of the breast

Marfan's syndrome hereditary disorder of connective tissue, bones, muscles, ligaments, and skeletal structures

McBurney's point located by drawing a line from the right anterosuperior iliac spine to the umbilicus; at approximately midpoint of this line lies the root of the appendix

McBurney's sign   site of maximum tenderness in the right lower quadrant; usually with appendicitis

mechanical index (MI)   MI is equal to the peak negative pressure of the ultrasound wave divided by the square root of the frequency of the ultrasound wave. It provides an estimate of the degree of bioeffects a given set of ultrasound parameters will induce. Low MI values are typically used during CES to reduce microbubble destruction

Meckel's diverticulum   congenital sac or blind pouch found in the lower portion of the ileum; a remnant of the proximal part of the yolk stalk

medial arcuate ligament   thickened upper margin of the fascia covering the anterior surface of the psoas muscle

mediastinum testis   linear structure within the midline of the testes

medulla of the adrenal gland   central tissue of the adrenal gland that secretes epinephrine and norepinephrine

medulla of the kidney (also known as the pyramid)   inner portion of the renal parenchyma that contains the loop of Henle

medullary carcinoma   neoplastic growth that accounts for 10% of thyroid malignancies

medullary pyramids   large and hypoechoic in the neonate

megahertz (MHz)   1,000,000 Hz

meninges   three membranes enclosing the brain and spinal cord

meningocele   open spinal defect characterized by protrusion of the spinal meninges

mesentery   a fold from the parietal peritoneum that attaches to the small intestine, anchoring it to the posterior abdominal wall

mesothelium   single layer of cells that forms the peritoneum's fifth layer of the bowel

metabolism   physical and chemical changes that occur within the body

metastatic disease   tumor that develops away from the site of the organ; most common form of neoplasm of the liver; most common primary sites are colon, breast, and lung

microcalcifications   tiny echogenic foci with a nodule that may or may not shadow

minor calyces   area of the kidneys that receives urine from the renal pyramids; form the border of the renal sinus

mirror image   artifactual gray-scale, color-flow, or Doppler signal appearing on the opposite side (from the real structure or flow) of a strong reflector

molecular imaging agents   contrast agents that exhibit affinity towards a specific tissue (e.g., tumor cells, thrombus) or a biologic process

mononucleosis   acute infection caused by the Epstein-Barr virus; can cause hepatomegaly

monorchidism   absence of one testis, usually the left one

Morison's pouch   right posterior subhepatic space located anterior to the kidney and inferior to the liver where fluid may accumulate

mucosa   mucous membrane; thin sheet of tissue that lines cavities of the body that open to the outside; it is the first layer of bowel

multicentric breast cancer   breast cancer occurring in different quadrants of the breast at least 5 cm apart; multicentric cancers are more likely to be of different histologic types than a multifocal cancer is

multicystic dysplastic kidney disease (MCDK)   multiple cysts replace normal renal tissue throughout the kidney; usually causes renal obstruction; most common cause of renal cystic disease in the neonate; may have contralateral ureteral pelvic junction obstruction

multifocal breast cancer   breast cancer occurring in more than one site within the same quadrant or the same ductal system of the breast

multinodular goiter   nodular enlargement of the thyroid associated with hyperthyroidism

multiple reflection   several reflections produced by a pulse encountering a pair of reflectors; reverberation

Murphy's sign   positive sign implies exquisite tenderness over the area of the gallbladder upon palpation

muscle   a type of tissue consisting of contractile cells or fibers that affects movement of an organ or part of the body

muscularis   third layer of bowel

myelin   substance forming the sheath of Schwann cells

myelomeningocele   defect in which the spinal cord and nerve roots are exposed, often adhering to the fine membrane that overlies them

myeloschisis   cleft spinal cord resulting from failure of the neural tube to close

naked tuberosity sign   the deltoid muscle is on the humeral head; seen with a full-thickness tear of the rotator cuff

nasal cannula   device for delivering oxygen by way of two small tubes inserted into the nostrils

nasal catheter   a piece of tubing longer than a cannula that is inserted through the nostril and into the back of the patient's mouth to provide continual oxygen

neck of the pancreas   small area of the pancreas between the head and the body; anterior to the superior mesenteric vein

neonate   infant during the first 28 days of life

neoplasm   any new growth (benign or malignant)

nephron   functional unit of the kidney; includes a renal corpuscle and a renal tubule

nerve   conduit for impulses sent to and from the muscles and central nervous system (CNS)

neuroblastoma   malignant adrenal mass that is seen in pediatric patients; hemorrhagic tumor principally consisting of cells resembling neuroblasts

neuroectodermal tissue   early embryonic tissue that will eventually develop into the brain and spinal cord

nodular hyperplasia   degenerative nodules within the thyroid

non-Hodgkin lymphoma   malignant disease of lymphoid tissue seen in increased frequency in individuals over 50 years of age

nonpalpable   cannot be felt on clinical examination; nonpalpable breast mass is one that is usually identified on screening mammogram and is too small to be felt as a breast lump on breast self-examination (BSE) or clinical breast examination (CBE)

nonresistive vessels that have high diastolic component and supply organs that need constant perfusion (internal carotid artery, hepatic artery, and renal artery)

nosocomal infection a hospital-acquired infection

Nyquist limit the Doppler-shift frequency above which aliasing occurs; one half the pulse repetition frequency

Nyquist sampling limit in pulsed Doppler, the Doppler signal must be sampled at least twice for each cycle in the wave if the Doppler frequencies are to be detected accurately

obstructive disease classification of liver disease where main problem is blocked bile excretion within the liver or biliary system

obstructive jaundice excessive bilirubin in the bloodstream caused by an obstruction of bile from the liver

Occupational Safety and Health Act (OSHA) federal law passed in 1970 to ensure that every working man and woman in the nation has safe and healthful working conditions

omentum pouchlike extension of the visceral peritoneum from the lower edge of the stomach, part of the duodenum, and the transverse colon

oocyte the early or primitive ovum before it has developed completely

oogonium cell produced at an early stage in the formation of an ovum

Ortolani maneuver patient lies in the supine position; the examiner's hand is placed around the hip to be examined with the fingers over the femoral head; the hip is flexed 90 degrees and the thigh is abducted

ostomy surgical procedure in which an opening is made to allow the passage of urine from the bladder or intestinal contents from the bowel to a surgically created opening, or stoma, in the wall of the abdomen

oximetry noninvasive method of monitoring blood oxygen levels

Paget's disease surface erosion of the nipple (reddened area with flaking and crusting) that results from direct invasion of the skin of the nipple from underlying breast cancer

palpable can be felt on clinical examination; palpable breast lump is one that is identified on clinical breast examination (CBE) or breast self-examination (BSE)

pampiniform plexus multiple veins that drain the testicles; when a varicocele is present, dilation and tortuosity may develop

pancreatic ascites fluid accumulation caused by a rupture of a pancreatic pseudocyst into the abdomen; free-floating pancreatic enzymes are dangerous to surrounding structures

pancreatic duct duct that travels horizontally through the pancreas to join the common bile duct at the ampulla of Vater

pancreatic pseudocyst "sterile abscess" collection of pancreatic enzymes that accumulate in the available space in the abdomen (usually in or near the pancreas)

pancreaticoduodenal arteries arteries that help supply blood to the pancreas along with the splenic artery

pancreatitis inflammation of the pancreas; may be acute or chronic

papillary carcinoma most common form of thyroid malignancy

paralytic ileus dilated, fluid-filled loops of bowel without peristalsis secondary to obstruction, decreased vascularity, or abnormal metabolic state

paramesonephric ducts (müllerian ducts) either of the paired ducts that form adjacent to the mesonephric ducts in the embryo

parathyroid hormone (PTH) hormone that is secreted by parathyroid glands, which regulates serum calcium levels

parathyroid hyperplasia enlargement of multiple parathyroid glands

parietal peritoneum layer of the peritoneum that lines the abdominal wall

patient focused care (PFC) national movement to recapture the respect and goodwill of the American public and to ensure that every patient receives the best possible medical care

peau d'orange French term that means *skin of the orange*; descriptive term for skin thickening of one breast that, on clinical breast examination, resembles the skin of an orange; such an appearance can result from an inflammatory breast condition (mastitis), simple edema, or skin involvement from underlying breast cancer; the thickening is caused by the pores of the skin opening to allow edema to directly evaporate through the skin, as inflammatory disease has blocked the lymphatic drainage of fluids building up in those tissues

pelvic cavity lower portion of the abdominopelvic cavity that contains part of the large intestine, the rectum, urinary bladder, and reproductive organs

pelvic girdle formation of the hip bones by the ilium, ischium, and pubis

pennate featherlike pattern of muscle growth

perineurium the connective tissue that surrounds muscle

perirenal space located directly around the kidney; completely enclosed by renal fascia

peristalsis rhythmic dilation and contraction of the gastrointestinal tract as food is propelled through it

peritoneal cavity potential space between the parietal and visceral peritoneal layers

peritoneal lavage invasive procedure that is used to sample the intraperitoneal space for evidence of damage to viscera and blood vessels

peritoneal recess slitlike spaces near the liver; potential space for fluid to accumulate

peritonitis inflammation of the peritoneum

periventricular leukomalacia (PVL) echogenic white matter necrosis (WMN) best seen in the posterior aspect of the brain or adjacent to the ventricular structures

phagocytosis process by which cells engulf and destroy microorganisms and cellular debris; "cell-eating"; for example, the red pulp destroys the degenerating red blood cells

Phalen's sign (Phalen's test, Phalen's maneuver, or Phalen's position) an increase in wrist compression due to hyperflexion of the wrist for 60 seconds; this test is done with the patient holding the forearms upright and pressing the ventral side of the hands together

pheochromocytoma   benign adrenal tumor that secretes hormones that produce hypertension

phrenocolic ligament   one of the ligaments between the spleen and splenic flexure of the colon

Phrygian cap   gallbladder variant in which part of the fundus is bent back on itself

piezoelectric effect   generation of electric signals as a result of an incident sound beam on a material that has piezoelectric properties; in a reverse piezoelectric effect, an element exposed to an electric shock will begin to vibrate and transmit a sound wave

pitting   process by which the spleen removes abnormal red blood cells

plantar flexion   pointing of the toes toward the plantar surface of the foot

polycystic renal disease   poorly functioning enlarged kidneys

polycythemia   overproduction of red blood cells

polycythemia vera   chronic, life-shortening condition of unknown etiology involving bone marrow elements; characterized by an increase in red blood cell mass and hemoglobin concentration

polyp   small, tumorlike growth that projects from the surfaces of mucous membranes

polysplenia   condition in which there is more than one spleen; associated with cardiac malformations

porcelain gallbladder   calcification of the gallbladder wall

porta hepatis   central area of the liver where the portal vein, common duct, and hepatic artery enter

portal confluence   see *confluence of the splenic and portal veins;* this triad makes the area appear slightly more echogenic

portal vein   vein formed by the union of the superior mesenteric vein and splenic vein near the porta hepatis of the liver

portal venous hypertension   caused by increased resistance to venous flow through the liver; sonographic findings include dilation of the portal, splenic and mesenteric veins; reversal of portal venous blood flow; and the development of collateral vessels

portal venous system   comprises the splenic, inferior mesenteric, superior mesenteric, and portal veins

positive contrast agent   radiopaque medium used in imaging; iodine and barium are positive contrast agents

posterior pararenal space   space found between the posterior renal fascia and the muscles of the posterior abdominal wall

posterior urethral valve   the presence of a valve in the posterior urethra; occurs only in male fetuses; most common cause of bladder outlet obstruction in the male neonate

power   rate of energy flow over the entire beam of sound; in general terms it is the rate at which energy is transmitted and is often measured in watts (W) or milliwatts (mW)

prehypertension   blood pressure readings associated with prehypertension are 120 mm Hg to 139 mm Hg systolic pressure, and 80 mm Hg to 89 mm Hg diastolic pressure

primary hyperparathyroidism   oversecretion of parathyroid hormone, usually from a parathyroid adenoma

projectile vomiting   condition found in pyloric stenosis in the neonatal period; after drinking, the infant experiences projectile vomiting secondary to the obstruction

prune-belly syndrome   dilation of the fetal abdomen secondary to severe bilateral hydronephrosis and fetal ascites; fetus also has oligohydramnios and pulmonary hypoplasia

pseudoaneurysm   pulsatile hematoma that results from leakage of blood into soft tissues abutting the punctured artery with fibrous encapsulation and failure of the vessel wall to heal

pseudocyst   a space or cavity that contains fluid but has no true endothelial lining membrane

pseudo-dissection   condition seen in a patient with aortic dissection; no intimal flap is seen, only hypoechoic thrombus near the outer margin of the aorta with echogenic laminated clot

psoas major muscle   begins at the level of hilum of the kidneys and extends inferiorly along both sides of the spine into the pelvis

pudendal artery   the internal and external pudendal arteries partially supply the scrotal wall and epididymis and occasionally the lower pole of the testis

pulmonary hypoplasia   small, underdeveloped lungs with resultant reduction in lung volume; secondary to prolonged oligohydramnios or as a consequence of a small thoracic cavity

pulse   a way to measure heart rate; recorded as beats per minute (bpm)

pulse duration   the time interval required for generating the transmitted pulse; it is calculated by multiplying the number of cycles in the pulse by the period

pulse pressure   the difference between the systolic and diastolic blood pressures

pulse repetition frequency (PRF)   in pulse-echo instruments, it is the number of pulses launched per second by the transducer

pulsed wave (PW) Doppler   sound is transmitted and received intermittently with one transducer

pyloric canal   canal located between the stomach and duodenum

pyocele   pus located between the visceral and parietal layers of the tunica vaginalis

pyogenic   pus producing

pyogenic abscess   pus-forming collection of fluid

pyramidal lobe   lobe of the thyroid gland that is present in a small percentage of patients; extends superiorly from the isthmus

radial   plane of imaging on ultrasound of the breast; see **antiradial**

range ambiguity   artifact produced when echoes are placed too close to the transducer because a second pulse was emitted before they were received

rarefaction   region of decreased particle density

real-time   ultrasound instrumentation that allows the image to be displayed many times per second to achieve a "real-time" image of anatomic structures and their motion patterns

rectouterine pouch   area in the pelvic cavity between the rectum and the uterus where free fluid may accumulate

rectus abdominis muscle   muscle of the anterior abdominal wall

recurrent rami   terminal ends of the centripetal (intratesticular) arteries that curve backward toward the capsule

red pulp   tissue composed of reticular cells and fibers (cords of Billroth); surrounds the splenic sinuses

reducible hernia   capable of being replaced in a normal position; the visceral contents can be returned to normal intra-abdominal location

refractile shadowing (edge artifact)   the bending of the sound beam at the edge of a circular structure, resulting in the absence of posterior echoes

refraction   change in the direction of propagation of a sound wave transmitted across an interface where the speed of sound varies

renal agenesis   interruption in the normal development of the kidney resulting in absence of the kidney; may be unilateral or bilateral

renal artery stenosis   narrowing of the renal artery; historically, this has been difficult to evaluate sonographically

renal capsule   first layer adjacent to the kidney that forms a tough, fibrous covering

renal corpuscle   the initial filtering component of nephrons in the kidneys; consists of the Bowman's capsule and the glomerulus

renal ectopia (ectopic kidney)   a kidney that is not located in its usual position, usually found in the pelvic cavity

renal hilum   area in the midportion of the kidney where the renal vessels and ureter enter and exit

renal hypoplasia   incomplete development of the kidney, usually with fewer than five calyces

renal pelvis   area in the midportion of the kidney that collects urine before entering the ureter

renal pyramid   one of several conical masses of tissue that form the kidney medulla; the base of each pyramid adjoins the kidney's cortex; the apex terminates at a renal calyx; the pyramids consist of the loops of Henle and the collecting tubules of the nephrons

renal sinus   central area of the kidney that includes the calyces, renal pelvis, renal vessels, fat, nerves, and lymphatics

renal vein thrombosis   obstruction of the renal vein resulting in an enlarged and edematous kidney

resistance   passive force in opposition to another active force; occurs when tissue exerts pressure against the vascular flow

resistive   vessels that have little or reversed flow in diastole and supply organs that do not need a constant blood supply (e.g., external carotid artery and brachial arteries)

resistive index   peak systole minus peak diastole divided by peak systole (S-D/S = 5 RI); an RI of 0.7 or less indicates good perfusion; an RI of 0.7 or higher indicates decreased perfusion

resolution   ability of the transducer to distinguish between two structures adjacent to one another

resonance   condition where a driven mechanical vibration is of a frequency similar to a natural vibration frequency of the structure

respiration   the process of inhaling and exhaling air

rete testis   network of the channels formed by the convergence of the straight seminiferous tubules in the mediastinum testis; these channels drain into the head of the epididymis

reticuloendothelial cells   certain phagocytic cells (found mainly in the liver and spleen) make up the reticuloendothelial system (RES), which plays a role in the defense against infection and synthesis of blood proteins and hematopoiesis

retromammary layer   deepest of the three layers of the breast noted on breast ultrasound; the retromammary layer is predominantly fatty and can be thin; the retromammary layer separates the active breast glandular tissue from the pectoralis fascia overlying the chest wall muscles

retroperitoneum   space behind the peritoneal lining of the abdominal cavity

reverberation   multiple reflections

right crus of the diaphragm   arises from the sides of the bodies of the first three lumbar vertebrae

right gastric artery   artery that supplies the stomach

right hepatic artery   artery that supplies the gallbladder via the cystic artery

right hypochondrium   right upper quadrant of the abdomen that contains the liver and gallbladder

right lobe of the liver   largest lobe of the liver

right portal vein   the main portal vein branches into the right and left portal veins to supply the lobes of the liver

right renal artery   artery that arises from the posterolateral wall of the aorta and travels posterior to the inferior vena cava to enter the hilum of the kidney

right renal vein   vein that leaves the renal hilum to enter the lateral wall of the inferior vena cava

ring-down   artifact resulting from a continuous stream of sound emanating from an anatomic site

rotator cuff injury   repeated motion results in fraying of the rotator cuff muscle tendons; this injury increases with age and is even more prevalent when work-related stresses are added; repeated arm abduction contributes to this injury by restricting blood flow to the soft tissues of the shoulder

rugae   inner folds of the stomach wall

saccular aneurysm   localized dilatation of the vessel

sagittal plane   vertical plane through the longitudinal axis of the body that divides it into two portions; in neonatal imaging, perpendicular to the coronal plane with the transducer in the anterior fontanelle

sandwich sign   occurs when a vessel or organ is surrounded by a tumor on either side

saphenous opening   gap in the fascia lata, which is found 4 cm inferior and lateral to the pubic tubercle

sciatic nerve   largest nerve in the upper thigh

scintigraphy   photographing the scintillations emitted by radioactive substances injected into the body to determine the outline and function of structures in which the radioactive substance collects or is secreted

scrotal cavity   in the male, a small outpocket of the pelvic cavity containing the testes

scrotum   sac containing the testes and epididymis

secondary hyperparathyroidism   enlargement of the parathyroid glands in patients with renal failure or vitamin D deficiency

second generation agents agents containing heavy gases (i.e., Optison)

secretin hormone released from small bowel as antacid; stimulates secretion of bicarbonate

section thickness thickness of the scanned tissue volume perpendicular to the scan plane; also called slice thickness

seminal vesicles reservoirs for sperm located posterior to the bladder

sentinel node represents the first lymph node along the axillary node chain; this is the node chain the surgeon examines for evidence of metastasis

sepsis spread of an infection from its initial site to the bloodstream

septa testis multiple septa formed from the tunica albuginea that course toward the mediastinum testis and separate the testicle into lobules

septicemia infection in the blood

seroma accumulation of serous fluid within tissue

serosa fourth layer of bowel; thin, loose layer of connective tissue, surrounded by mesothelium covering the intraperitoneal bowel loops

serum amylase pancreatic enzyme that is elevated during pancreatitis

serum calcium laboratory value that is elevated with hyperparathyroidism

shadowing reduction in echo amplitude from reflectors that lie behind a strongly reflecting or attenuating structure

sickle cell anemia inherited disorder transmitted as an autosomal recessive trait that causes an abnormality of the globin genes in hemoglobin

sickle cell crisis condition in sickle cell anemia in which the malformed red cells interfere with oxygen transport, obstruct capillary blood flow, and cause fever and severe pain in the joints and abdomen

slice thickness thickness of a section in the patient that contributes to echo signals on any one image

sludge low-level echoes found along the posterior margin of the gallbladder; move with change in position

specific gravity laboratory test that measures how much dissolved material is present in the urine

speckle the granular appearance of images and spectral displays that is caused by the interference of echoes from the distribution of scatterers in tissue

spectral analysis analysis of the entire frequency spectrum

spectral broadening change in the spectral width that increases with flow disturbance

speed error propagation speed that is different from the assumed value (1.54 mm/μs)

spermatic cord structure made up of vas deferens, testicular artery, cremasteric artery, and pampiniform plexus that suspends the testis in the scrotum

spermatocele cyst within the vas deferens containing sperm

spherocytosis condition in which erythrocytes assume a spheroid shape; hereditary

sphincter of Oddi small muscle that guards the ampulla of Vater

sphygmomanometer device used to measure blood pressure

spiculation finger-like extension of a malignant tumor; usually appears as a small line that radiates outward from the margin of a mass

spina bifida aperta open (non–skin-covered lesions) neural tube defects, such as myelomeningocele and meningocele

spina bifida occulta closed (skin-covered lesions) neural tube defects, such as spinal lipoma and tethered cord

spinal degeneration intervertebral disk degeneration results from bending and twisting and improper sitting

splenic agenesis complete absence of the spleen

splenic artery one of the three vessels that arise from the celiac axis to supply the spleen, pancreas, stomach, and greater omentum; forms the superior border of the pancreas

splenic flexure the transverse colon travels horizontally across the abdomen and bends at this point to form the descending colon

splenic hilum site where vessels and lymph nodes enter and exit the spleen; located in the middle of the spleen

splenic sinuses long, irregular channels lined by endothelial cells or flattened reticular cells

splenic vein vein that drains the spleen; travels horizontally across the abdomen (posterior to the pancreas) to join the superior mesenteric vein to form the portal vein; serves as the posterior medial border of the pancreas

splenomegaly enlargement of the spleen

standard precautions the basic infection control guidelines used to reduce the risks of infection spread through the following three transmission modes: airborne infections, droplet infection, and contact infection

sternocleidomastoid muscles large muscles anterolateral to the thyroid

strangulated hernia an incarcerated hernia with vascular compromise

strap muscles groups of three muscles (sternothyroid, sternohyoid, and omohyoid) that lie anterior to the thyroid

subacute (deQuervain's) thyroiditis inflammatory condition of the thyroid, sometimes occurring after a viral respiratory infection

subcostal plane the upper horizontal imaginary line that joins the lowest point of the costal margin on each side of the body to help divide the abdominopelvic cavity into nine regions

subcutaneous layer most superficial of the three layers of the breast identified on breast ultrasound, the subcutaneous layer is mainly fatty; it is located immediately beneath the skin and superficial to the mammary layer; the subcutaneous layer can be very thin and difficult to recognize

subependyma fragile area beneath the ependyma that is subject to bleeding in the premature neonate; site of hemorrhage for the germinal matrix

subependymal cyst cyst that occurs at the site of a previous bleed in the germinal matrix

subhepatic inferior to the liver

subject contrast affected by the absorption characteristics of the tissue being imaged and the imaging parameters

subluxation   occurs when the femoral head moves posteriorly and remains in contact with the posterior aspect of the acetabulum

submucosa   one of the layers of the bowel, under the mucosal layer; contains blood vessels and lymph channels

subphrenic   below the diaphragm

sulcus   groove on the surface of the brain that separates the gyri

superficial inguinal ring   triangular opening in the external oblique aponeurosis

superior mesenteric artery   artery that arises inferior to the celiac axis to supply the proximal half of the colon and the small intestine; serves as the posterior border to the body of the pancreas

superior mesenteric vein   drains the small bowel and cecum, transverse and sigmoid colon; travels vertically to join the splenic and portal veins; serves as a posterior landmark to the body of the pancreas and anterior border to the uncinate process of the head

suprapubic   above the symphysis pubis

synovial sheath   membrane surrounding a joint, tendon, or bursa that secretes a viscous fluid called synovia

tachycardia   heart rate more than 100 beats per minute

tail of Spence   a normal extension of breast tissue into the axillary or arm pit region

tail of the pancreas   tapered end of the pancreas that lies in the left hypochondrium near the hilum of the spleen and upper pole of the left kidney

target (donut) sign   characteristic of gastrointestinal wall thickening consisting of an echogenic center and a hypoechoic rim; frequently associated with sectional areas of the gastrointestinal tract; the muscle is hyperechoic, and the inner core is hypoechoic

temporal resolution   ability of the system to accurately depict motion

tendinitis/tendonitis (tendinopathy, tendinosis, or tenosynovitis)   inflammation of a tendon

tendon   fibrous tissue connecting muscle to bone

tentorium cerebelli   echogenic V-shaped "tent" structure in the posterior fossa that separates the cerebellum from the cerebrum

terminal ductal-lobular unit (TDLU)   smallest functional portion of the breast involving the terminal duct and its associated lobule containing at least one acinus (tiny milk-producing gland); the TDLU undergoes significant monthly hormone-induced changes and radical changes during pregnancy and lactation; it is the site of origin of nearly all significant pathologic processes involving the breast, including all elements of fibrocystic condition, fibroadenomas, and in situ and invasive breast cancer, both lobular and ductal

testicle   male gonad that produces hormones that induce masculine features and production of spermatozoa

testicular artery   artery arising from the aorta just distal to each renal artery; it divides into two major branches supplying the testis medially and laterally

testicular vein   the pampiniform plexus forms each testicular vein; the right testicular vein drains directly into the inferior vena cava, whereas the left testicular vein drains into the left renal vein

tethered spinal cord   fixed spinal cord that is positioned in an abnormal position

thalamic-caudate groove or notch   the region at which the thalamus and caudate nucleus join; the most common location of germinal matrix hemorrhage

thalamus   two ovoid brain structures located midbrain, situated on either side of the third ventricle superior to the brain stem

thalassemia   group of hereditary anemias occurring in Asian and Mediterranean populations

Thompson's test   a test used to evaluate the integrity of the Achilles tendon that involves plantar flexion with squeezing of the calf

thoracic outlet syndrome   nerve entrapment can occur at different levels, resulting in a variety of symptoms

thrombocyte   blood platelet

thyroglossal duct cyst   congenital anomaly that presents in the midline of the neck anterior to the trachea

thyroiditis   inflammation of the thyroid

thyroid-stimulating hormone (TSH)   hormone secreted by the pituitary gland that stimulates the thyroid gland to secrete thyroxine and triiodothyronine

time gain compensation (TGC)   also referred to as *depth gain compensation (DGC)*; ability to compensate for attenuation of the transmitted beam as the sound wave travels through tissues in the body; usually, individual pod controls allow the operator to manually change the amount of compensation necessary for each patient to produce a quality image

Tinel's sign (Hoffmann-Tinel sign, Tinel's symptom, or Tinel-Hoffmann sign)   pins-and-needles type tingling felt distally to a percussion site; sensation can be either an abnormal or a normal occurrence (i.e., hitting the elbow creates a tingling in the distal arm)

TIPS   transjugular intrahepatic portosystemic shunt

tissue-specific ultrasound contrast agent   a type of contrast agent whose microbubbles are removed from the blood and taken up by specific tissues in the body; one example is the contrast agent Sonazoid

transducer   any device that converts energy from one form to another

transpyloric plane   horizontal plane that passes through the pylorus, the duodenal junction, the neck of the pancreas, and the hilum of the kidneys

trigger finger   inflammation and swelling of the tendon sheath in a finger entraps the tendon and restricts motion of the finger

trigone   see **atrium (trigone) of the lateral ventricles**

true aneurysm   permanent dilation of an artery that forms when tensile strength of the arterial wall decreases

tunica adventitia   outer layer of the vascular system

tunica albuginea   inner fibrous membrane surrounding the testicle

tunica intima   inner layer of the vascular system

tunica media   middle layer of the vascular system; veins have thinner tunica media than arteries

tunica vaginalis   membrane consisting of a visceral layer (adherent to the testis) and a parietal layer (adherent to the scrotum) lining the inner wall of the scrotum; a potential space between these layers is where hydroceles may develop

turtle sign   sonographic finding when the phallus elongates to form the penis

tympany   predominant sound heard over hollow organs (stomach, intestines, bladder, aorta, gallbladder)

ultrasound contrast agent   a substance that alters the amplitude of reflected ultrasound signals (echoes). Commercially available UCAs used for human applications are composed of encapsulated microbubbles that are less than 10 microns in diameter

umbilical   around the navel

uncinate process   small, curved tip of the pancreatic head that lies posterior to the superior mesenteric vein

unicornuate uterus   anomaly of the uterus in which only one horn and tube develop

ureteropelvic junction obstruction   most common neonatal obstruction of the urinary tract; results from intrinsic narrowing or extrinsic vascular compression

ureters   retroperitoneal structures that exit the kidney to carry urine to the urinary bladder

urethra   small, membranous canal that excretes urine from the urinary bladder

urinary bladder   muscular retroperitoneal organ that serves as a reservoir for urine

urinary incontinence   the uncontrollable passage of urine

urinoma   cyst containing urine

urolithiasis   stone within the urinary system

uterus didelphys   complete duplication of the uterus, cervix, and vagina

VACTERL   *v*ertebral abnormalities, *a*nal atresia, *c*ardiac abnormalities, *t*racheoesophageal fistula, and *r*enal and *l*imb abnormalities; VATER excludes cardiac and limb anomalies

vagina atresia   failure of the vagina to develop

valvulae conniventes   normal segmentation of the small bowel

varicocele   dilated veins caused by obstruction of the venous return from the testicle

vas deferens   tube that connects the epididymis to the seminal vesicle

vasa previa   condition that occurs when the umbilical cord vessels cross the internal os of the cervix

vasa vasorum   tiny arteries that supply the walls of blood vessels

veins   collapsible vascular structures that carry blood back to the heart

velocity   speed of the ultrasound wave; determined by tissue density

ventriculitis   inflammation or infection of the ventricles that appears as echogenic linear structures along the gyri; may also appear as focal echogenic structures within the white matter

ventriculoperitoneal (VP) shunt   a tube that is placed by a neurosurgeon to relieve intracranial pressure due to increased cerebrospinal fluid (hydrocephalus)

verumontanum   junction of the ejaculatory ducts with the urethra

vesicouterine pouch   pouch formed by the deflection of the peritoneum from the bladder to the uterus

villi   inner folds of the small intestine

viscera   the internal organs (*sing.* viscus)

visceral peritoneum   layer of peritoneum that covers the abdominal organs

vital signs   medical measurements used to ascertain how the body is functioning

volar   the anterior portion of the body when in anatomic position

wall echo shadow (WES) sign   sonographic pattern found when the gallbladder is packed with stones

wandering spleen   spleen that has migrated from its normal location in the left upper quadrant

wave   propagation of energy that moves back and forth or vibrates at a steady rate

wavelength   distance over which a wave repeats itself during one period of oscillation

white pulp   tissue composed of lymphatic tissue and lymphatic follicles

Wilms' tumor   nephroblastoma; most common malignant tumor in the neonate and infant

work-related musculoskeletal disorders (WRMSD)   current term to describe occupational injury; defined as injuries that result in restricted work, days away from work, MSD symptoms that remain for seven or more days, and MSD requiring medical treatment beyond first aid

Aehlert B: *Mosby's comprehensive pediatric emergency care*, St. Louis, 2007, Mosby
Figure 3-25, *A*

Chapleau W, Pons PT: *Emergency medical technician: making the difference*, St. Louis, 2007, Mosby/JEMS
Figure 3-25, *B*

Chervenak FA and others: Fetal cystic hygroma: cause and natural history, *N Eng J Med* 309:822, 1985
Figure 58-39, *A*

Damjanov I, Linder J: *Pathology: a color atlas*, St. Louis, 2000, Mosby
Figures 9-6; 9-13; 10-29; 10-33; 10-35; 10-46; 10-53; 10-56; 10-61; 10-64; 10-66; 11-18; 11-22; 11-33; 11-40; 11-48; 12-7; 12-23; 12-24; 12-29; 12-32; 12-33; 12-36; 12-37; 12-39; 12-40; 12-44; 15-14; 15-16; 20-18; 22-7; 22-13; 22-15; 22-17; 22-18; 22-20; 22-22; 22-24; 22-25; 25-26; 25-31; 25-34; 25-40; 25-46; 26-12; 26-22, *C*; 26-25, *C*; 27-11; 27-15, 42-21, *A*; 42-24; 42-29, *A*; 42-30; 42-31; 42-34

England MA: *Color atlas of life before birth*, St Louis, 1983, Mosby
Figure 47-14, *A*

Hadlock FP, Shah YP, Kanon DJ, Lindsey JV: Fetal crown-rump length: reevaluation of relation to menstrual age (5–18 weeks) with high resolution real time US, *Radiology* 182:501, 1992
Figures 47-26, 47-28

Henningsen C: *Clinical guide to ultrasonography*, St. Louis, 2004, Mosby
Figures 14-52, *A*, *B*; 14-53, *A*, *B*; 21-29, *A-F* (modified); 25-27; 25-29, *A-C*; 25-32, *A-D*; 25-35, *A*, *B*; 26-13; 29-12, *A*, *B*; 29-16, *A*, *B*; 29-23, *A-C*; 53-13; 53-20; 53-25, *A*, *B*; 53-28; 59-13; 59-32, *A*, *B*; 59-38, *A*, *B*; 59-45, *A*, *B*; 64-4, *A-C*; 64-8, *A*, *B*; 64-22, *A*

Kremkau FW: Principles and instrumentation. In Merritt CRB, editor: Doppler color imaging, New York, 1992, Churchill Livingstone
Figure 6-31

Kremkau FW: *Principles and pitfalls of real-time color-flow imaging.* In Bernstein EF, editor: *Vascular diagnosis*, ed 4, St Louis, 1993, Mosby
Figures 6-28, *A-C*; 6-29, *A-E*; 6-33

Kremkau FW: *Semin Roentgenol* 27:6–16, 1992
Figures 6-25, 6-27, *B*

Kremkau FW, Taylor KJW: *J Ultrasound Med* 5:227, 1986
Figure 6-6

Kremkau FW: J *Vasc Technol* 15:265–266, 1991. Reprinted with permission by the Society for Vascular Ultrasound (SVU).
Figure 6-27, *C*

Maternal Fetal Medicine Foundation, Washington, D. C.
Figure 47-30 (redrawn)

Mayden KL and others: Cystic adenomatoid malformation in the fetus: Ultrasound evaluation, *Am J Obstet Gynecol* 148:349, 1984.
Figure 60-8, *A*, *B*

McMinn RMH: *Functional and clinical anatomy*, St. Louis, 1999, Mosby
Figures 13-1, *A-D*; 13-24; 16-17; 17-1, *A-D*; 17-24; 20-25, *A*; 25-1; 25-2; 25-4; 25-5; 29-1; 29-2; 29-4; 29-5

Nyberg DA et al, editors: *Transvaginal ultrasound*, Mosby, 1992, St. Louis
Figure 41-33

Nyberg DA, Mahony BS, Pretorius DH, editors: *Diagnostic ultrasound of fetal anomalies: text and atlas*, St Louis, 1990, Mosby
Figure 53-23

Potter PA, Perry AG, *Fundamentals of nursing*, ed 7, St. Louis, 2009, Mosby
Figures 3-3, *A*; 3-6, *A*, *B*; 3-9, *B*; 3-12, *A-C*; 3-13; 3-14; 3-18, *B*; 3-20, *A-E*

Queenan JT: *Modern management of the Rh problem*, ed 2, Hagerstown, PA, 1977, Harper & Row Medical. http://lwww.com
Figure 52-8

Rumack C, Wilson S, Charboneau W: *Diagnostic ultrasound*, ed 4, St Louis, 2011, Mosby
Figures 21-30; 21-41, *A*, *B*; 21-43, *A*, *B*; 21-44, *A*, *B*; 25-36, *A*, *B*; 25-38, *A*, *B*; 25-39, *A-C*; 27-3; 29-8; 29-9, *A*, *B*; 29-10, *A*, *B*; 29-11; 29-13, *A*, *B*; 29-15; 29-18, *A-C*; 30-6, *A*; 30-7, *A-F*; 30-8, *A*, *B*; 30-12, *A-C*; 30-13, *A-G*; 30-16, *A-C*; 41-20; 41-25; 42-9; 42-13; 42-15; 42-20; 48-14; 59-22; 63-18

Taylor KJW, Holland S: *Radiology* 174:297–307, 1990.
Figure 6-23, *A-E*

Thibodeau GA, Patton KT: *The human body in health and disease*, ed 5, St Louis, 2010, Mosby
Figure 7-4

Young AP: *Kinn's the administrative medical assistant: an applied learning approach*, ed 7, Philadelphia, 2011, Saunders
Figures 3-1; 3-2; 3-3, *B*; 3-5, *A*; 3-21; 3-22; 3-24